Critical Care Exami
and Board Review

Critical Care Examination and Board Review

Ronaldo Collo Go, MD
Faculty
Division of Pulmonary, Critical Care, and Sleep Medicine
Mount Sinai Beth Israel
New York, New York
Division of Pulmonary, Critical Care, and Sleep Medicine
Crystal Run Health Care
Middletown, New York

New York   Chicago   San Francisco   Athens   London   Madrid   Mexico City
Milan   New Delhi   Singapore   Sydney   Toronto

Critical Care Examination and Board Review

1 2 3 4 5 6 7 8 9   DSS   23 22 21 20 19 18

ISBN 978-1-259-83435-6
MHID 1-259-83435-2

This book was set in minion pro by Cenveo® Publisher Services.
The editors were Andrew Moyer and Regina Y. Brown.
The production supervisor was Catherine Saggese.
Project Management was provided by Kritika Kaushik, Cenveo Publisher Services.

This book is printed on acid-free paper.

Library of Congress Cataloging-in-Publication Data

Names: Go, Ronaldo Collo, editor.
Title: Critical care examination and board review / editor, Ronaldo Collo Go.
Description: New York : McGraw-Hill Education, [2018] | Includes
    bibliographical references.
Identifiers: LCCN 2018015423 | ISBN 9781259834356 (adhesive - soft : alk.
    paper)
Subjects: | MESH: Critical Care | Examination Questions
Classification: LCC RC86.9 | NLM WX 18.2 | DDC 616.02/8076—dc23
LC record available at https://na01.safelinks.protection.outlook.com/?

McGraw-Hill Education books are available at special quantity discounts to use as premiums and sales promotions or for use in corporate training programs. To contact a representative, please visit the Contact Us pages at www.mhprofessional.com

Contents

Contributors

Samuel Acquah, MD
Director
Medical Intensive Care Unit
Division of Pulmonary, Critical Care, and Sleep Medicine
Mount Sinai Hospital
New York, New York

Mais N. Al-Kawaz, MD
Resident
Department of Neurology
Weill Cornell Medicine
New York, New York

Uschi Auguste, MD
Fellow
Division of Cardiology
Mount Sinai Beth Israel
New York, New York

Edward W. Bahou, MD
Clinical Neurophysiology Fellow
Mount Sinai Hospital
New York, New York

Christian Becker, MD, Ph.D
Associate Medical Director, eHealth Center
Director, Research & Quality
Westchester Medical Center Health Network
Associate Professor
New York Medical College
Department of Medicine
Division of Pulmonary, Critical Care, and Sleep Medicine
Valhalla, New York

Saad A. Bhatti, MD
Surgical Trauma ICU
Elmhurst Hospital
Queens, New York

Eric Bondarsky, MD
Assistant Director of Critical Care
NYU Langone Orthopedic Hospital
Division of Pulmonary, Critical Care, and Sleep Medicine
New York, New York

Karen Braich, MD
Fellow
Division of Nephrology
Icahn School of Medicine at Mount Sinai
Mount Sinai Hospital
New York, New York

Sidney Braman, MD
Professor of Medicine
Director of Pulmonary Disease Management
Icahn School of Medicine at Mount Sinai
Mount Sinai Hospital
New York, New York

Jennifer Cabot, MD
Fellow
Department of Anesthesiology and Critical Care Medicine
Memorial Sloan Kettering Cancer Center
New York, New York

Joseph Cerminara, MD
Resident
Department of Anesthesiology
Roswell Park Cancer Institute
Buffalo, New York

Hala El Chami, MD
Fellow
Division of Pulmonary, Critical Care, and Sleep Medicine
Tufts Medical Center
Boston, Massachusetts

James F. Crismale, MD
Transplant Hepatology/Gastroenterology Fellow
Icahn School of Medicine at Mount Sinai
New York, New York

Melissa Dakkak, DO
Cardiology Fellow
University of Arizona School of Medicine
Division of Cardiology
Banner University Medical Center Tucson
Tucson, Arizona

Ananda Dharshan, MD
Clinical Assistant Professor
Assistant Professor of Oncology
Department of Anesthesiology
Jacobs School of Medicine and Biomedical Sciences
State University of New York at Buffalo
Buffalo, New York
and
Associate Director of Intensive Care Unit
Roswell Park Cancer Institute
Buffalo, New York

Sakshi Dua, MD
Pulmonary and Critical Care Medicine Fellowship Program
   Director
Division of Pulmonary, Critical Care, and Sleep Medicine
Assistant Professor of Medicine
Icahn School of Medicine at Mount Sinai
Mount Sinai Hospital
New York, New York

Maureen Dziura, MD
Fellow
Division of Pulmonary, Critical Care, and Sleep Medicine
Tufts Medical Center
Boston, Massachusetts

Oleg Epelbaum, MD
Division of Pulmonary, Critical Care, and Sleep Medicine
Westchester Medical Center
Assistant Professor
New York Medical College
Valhalla, New York

Rania Esteitie, MD
Assistant Professor of Medicine
Tufts University School of Medicine
Division of Pulmonary, Critical Care, and Sleep Medicine
Boston, Massachusetts

Marianna Fedorenko, PharmD, BCPS
Clinical Pharmacy Specialist, Infectious Diseases
Department of Pharmacy
Mount Sinai Beth Israel
New York, New York

Steven H. Feinsilver, MD
Director, Center for Sleep Medicine
Division of Pulmonary Medicine
Lenox Hill Hospital
Professor of Medicine
Hofstra Northwell School of Medicine
New York, New York

Jason Filopei, MD
Assistant Professor of Medicine
Pulmonary, Critical Care, and Sleep Medicine, Icahn School
   of Medicine
Assistant Director
Medical Intensive Care Unit
Mount Sinai Beth Israel
New York, New York

Brandon Foreman, MD
Assistant Clinical Professor of Neurology & Rehabilitation
   Medicine
Associate Director for Neurocritical Care Research
Division of Neurocritical Care
University of Cincinnati
231 Albert Sabin Way
Cincinnati, Ohio

Matthew Frank, MD
Resident
Department of Internal Medicine
Mount Sinai Beth Israel
New York, New York

Allison Ann Froehlich, MD
Department of Endocrinology
Lehigh Valley Hospital
Stroudsburg, Pennsylvania

Blesit George, DO
Department of Emergency Medicine
Orange Regional Medical Center
Middletown, New York

Anousheh Ghezel-Ayagh, MD
Department of Infectious Disease
Crystal Run Health Care
Middletown, New York

Aamir Gilani, MD
Division of Pulmonary, Critical Care, and Sleep Medicine
Orange Regional Medical Center
Middletown, New York

Anna Collo Go, MD
Gullas Medical School
Cebu, Philippines

Evangeline Collo Go, MD
Obstetrics and Gynecology (retired)

Ronaldo Collo Go, MD, FCCP
Faculty
Division of Pulmonary, Critical Care, and Sleep Medicine
Mount Sinai Beth Israel
New York, New York
Division of Pulmonary, Critical Care, and Sleep Medicine
Crystal Run Health Care
Middletown, New York

Diana Gritsenko, PharmD
Multispecialty Clinical Pharmacist
Department of Pharmacy
Yale-New Haven
New Haven, Connecticut

Steven Grundfast, MD
Division of Pulmonary, Critical Care, and Sleep Medicine
Crystal Run Healthcare
Middletown, New York

Raghad Hussein, MD
Associate
Critical Care Medicine
Geisinger Medical Center
Danville, Pennsylvania

Margaret Huynh, DO
Department of Neurology & Rehabilitation Medicine
University of Cincinnati Gardner Neuroscience Institute
University of Cincinnati
Cincinnati Ohio

Yumiko Kanei, MD
Program Director
Interventional Cardiology
Division of Cardiology
Mount Sinai Beth Israel
New York, New York

Candice Kim, MD
Cardiology Fellow
University of Arizona School of Medicine
Division of Cardiology
Banner University Medical Center Tucson
Tucson, Arizona

Murali G. Krishna, MD
Division of Pulmonary, Critical Care, and Sleep Medicine
Orange Regional Medical Center
Middletown, New York

Michael H. Kroll, MD
Professor of Medicine
Chief of the Section of Benign Hematology
UT MD Anderson Cancer Center
Houston, Texas

Gregg M. Lanier, MD
Director of Pulmonary Hypertension, Associate Director
   of Heart Failure
Assistant Professor of Medicine, New York Medical College
Westchester Medical Center
Valhalla, New York

Vijay Lapsia, MD
Assistant Professor of Medicine
Medical Director, Mount Sinai Kidney Center
Icahn School of Medicine at Mount Sinai
Mount Sinai Hospital
New York, New York

Mikyung Lee, MD
Director of Infectious Disease Fellowship Program
Associate Professor of Medicine
Icahn School of Medicine at Mount Sinai
Mount Sinai Hospital
New York, New York

Young Im Lee, MD
Assistant Professor of Medicine
Pulmonary, Critical Care, and Sleep Medicine, Icahn School
   of Medicine
Director
Medical Intensive Care Unit
Mount Sinai Beth Israel
New York, New York

Ronni Levy, MD
Division of Pulmonary, Critical Care, and Sleep Medicine
Crystal Run Healthcare
Middletown, New York

Riffat Mannan, MD
Assistant Professor of Pathology
University of Pennsylvania
Philadelphia

Michael McBrine, MD
Assistant Professor of Medicine
Tufts Medical School
Division of Pulmonary, Critical Care, and Sleep Medicine
Boston, Massachusetts

Alexander E. Merkler, MD
Assistant Professor of Neurology
Department of Neurology/Neurocritical Care
Weill Cornell Medicine
New York, New York

Osmaan Minhas, DO
Resident
Department of Family Medicine
Orange Regional Medical Center
Middletown, New York

Sajid A. Mir, MD
Program Director
Department of Internal Medicine
Adjunct Clinical Professor
Touro Medical College
Orange Regional Medical Center
Middletown, New York

Lina Miyakawa, MD
Assistant Professor
Icahn School of Medicine
Division of Pulmonary, Critical Care, and Sleep Medicine
Mount Sinai Beth Israel
New York, New York

Chika Nwulu, MD
Division of Internal Medicine
Crystal Run Healthcare
Middletown, New York

Sergio Obligado, MD
Adjunct Clinical Professor
Touro Medical College
Department of Nephrology
Orange Regional Medical Center
Middletown, New York

Maria Osundele, PharmD, CGP, BCPS
Clinical Pharmacy Manager
Orange Regional Medical Center
Middletown, New York

Stephen M. Pastores, MD
Professor of Medicine and Anesthesiology, Weill Cornell
    Medical College of Cornell University
Program Director, Critical Care Medicine
Vice-Chair of Education
Department of Anesthesiology and Critical Care Medicine
Memorial Sloan Kettering Cancer Center
New York, New York

Shanna K. Patterson, MD
Assistant Professor of Neurology
Director, Electromyography Laboratory
Mount Sinai West and St. Luke's Hospitals
Associate Director, Neurology Residency
Mount Sinai Hospital
New York, New York

Eduardo Pinto, MD
Department of Internal Medicine
Crystal Run Healthcare
Middletown, New York

Imrana Qawi, MD
Assistant Professor of Medicine
Tufts School of Medicine
Division of Pulmonary, Critical Care,
    and Sleep Medicine
Tufts Medical Center
Boston, Massachusetts

Romeo Quilitan, MD
Department of Internal Medicine
Crystal Run Healthcare
Middletown, New York

Timothy Quinn, MD
Clinical Assistant Professor
Assistant Professor of Oncology
Department of Anesthesiology, Critical Care, and
    Pain Medicine
Jacobs School of Medicine and Biomedical Sciences
State University of New York at Buffalo
and
Roswell Park Cancer Institute
Buffalo, New York

Kartik Ramakrishna, MD
Assistant Professor
Division of Pulmonary, Critical Care, and Sleep Medicine
Drexel University College of Medicine
Philadelphia

Navitha Ramesh, MD
Division of Pulmonary, Critical Care, and Sleep Medicine
Geisinger Wyoming Valley Medical Center
Wilkes-Barre, Pennsylvania

Dulya Santikul, DO
Program Director
Department of Internal Medicine
Adjunct Clinical Professor
Touro Medical College
Orange Regional Medical Center
Middletown, New York

Thomas Schiano, MD
Medical Director, Adult Liver Transplantation
Director of Clinical Hepatology
Director, Intestinal Transplantation
Recanati/Miller Transplantation Institute
Division of Liver Diseases
Professor of Medicine
Icahn School of Medicine
Mount Sinai Medical Center
New York, New York

Khalid Sherani, MD
Fellow
Department of Anesthesiology and Critical Care Medicine
Memorial Sloan Kettering Cancer Center
New York, New York

Jason A. Stamm, MD
Clinical Associate Professor of Medicine
Lewis Katz School of Medicine at Temple University
and
Associate
Division of Pulmonary and Critical Care and Sleep Medicine
    Geisinger Medical Center
Danville, Pennsylvania

Arvind Sundaram, MD
Associate
Critical Care Medicine
Geisinger Medical Center
Danville, Pennsylvania

Prakash Goutham Suryanarayana, MD
Assistant Professor of Medicine
University of Arizona School of Medicine
Division of Cardiology
Banner University Medical Center Tucson
Tucson, Arizona

Maher Tabba, MD
Fellowship Director
Assistant Professor of Medicine
Tufts University School of Medicine
Division of Pulmonary, Critical Care, and Sleep Medicine
Boston, Massachusetts

Faisal Tamimi, MD
Fellow
Division of Pulmonary, Critical Care, and Sleep Medicine
Tufts Medical Center
Boston, Massachusetts

Sohaib Tariq, MD
Fellow
Division of Cardiology
Westchester Medical Center
Valhalla, New York

Mayanka Tickoo, MD
Fellow
Division of Pulmonary, Critical Care, and Sleep Medicine
Tufts Medical Center
Boston, Massachusetts

Yaojie Wu, MD
Clinical Neurophysiology Fellow
Mount Sinai Hospital
New York, New York

Srikanth Yandrapalli, MD
Chief Resident
Department of Internal Medicine
Westchester Medical Center
Valhalla, New York

Han Yu MD
Resident
Department of Internal Medicine
New York Presbyterian – Queens
New York, New York

Songyang Yuan, MD
Assistant Professor of Medicine
Icahn School of Medicine at Mount Sinai
Department of Pathology
Mount Sinai Hospital
New York, New York

Nicole K. Zagelbaum, DO, MPH
Resident
Department of Internal Medicine
Westchester Medical Center
Valhalla, New York

Samer El Zarif, MD
Division of Pulmonary, Critical Care, and
    Sleep Medicine
Orange Regional Medical Center
Middletown, New York

Preface

Discernment of critical care medicine is derived from multiple factors: an understanding of the basics of medicine, access to the most current evidence, clinical experience, and openness to palliative care. Based on these factors, I wanted to create a one stop reference for critical care.

McGraw-Hill's Critical Care Examination and Board Review is an evidence-based multidisciplinary perspective to critical care medicine. The format of each chapter is text material followed by questions and answers. Authors are from major academic centers discussing not only the basic principles in their field but also the most current studies.

Current guidelines from various specialties are incorporated including their levels and/or grades of recommendation. Nomenclature on the stratification of quality of evidence and categories of recommendation vary per country and guideline but generally are similar. This book is ideal for the critical care fellow or intensivist studying for the critical care boards, medical student, resident, or any other healthcare provider interested in critical care.

It was an amazing journey working on this book and I hope it will strengthen your fund of knowledge to help you pass your critical care boards.

Acid–Base Disorders

Nicole K. Zagelbaum, DO, MPH, Osmaan Minhas, DO, Sajid A. Mir, MD, and Sergio Obligado, MD

INTRODUCTION

The human body needs to regulate free hydrogen ions (H⁺) within a narrow window in order to maintain proper protein structure and function. In the process of metabolizing carbohydrates, proteins, and fats, 15,000 mmol of volatile acid, carbon dioxide (CO_2), is generated and another 50 to 100 mEq of nonvolatile acid is also produced.[1] Despite this, free hydrogen ion concentration is maintained at level of 40 nmol/L (10^{-6} mmol/L).[2] When describing hydrogen concentration of physiologic solutions, we refer to the pH of the solution rather than the actual concentration. The pH of a solution is defined by the following equation:

$$pH = -\log[H^+]$$

The pH compatible with human life is in the range of 6.8 to 7.8.[3] In order to maintain serum pH in this range, the human body requires the following:[2]

- an effective buffer system to prevent wide fluctuations of pH in response to small additions or subtractions of acid,
- the ability to excrete volatile acids (CO_2) via the lungs, and
- the ability to excrete nonvolatile acids (sulfuric acid, phosphoric acid, and ammonium) via the kidneys.

The bicarbonate/carbon dioxide buffer system is how clinicians usually analyze acid–base balance at the bedside. Carbon dioxide and bicarbonate are easily measured; bicarbonate is important simply because of its high concentration in the blood.

Carbon dioxide effectively becomes an acid when dissolved in solution as described in the following reaction:

$$CO_2 \leftrightarrow CO_2 + H_2O \leftrightarrow H_2CO_3 \leftrightarrow H^+ + HCO_3^-$$
$$\text{Gas Phase} \qquad \text{Aqueous Phase}$$

The relationship of these reactants can be described by the Henderson-Hasselbalch equation:[4]

$$pH = \frac{6.1 + \log[HCO_3^-]}{0.03 \times Paco_2}$$

where $Paco_2$ is the partial pressure of CO_2 in arterial blood. The amount of CO_2 dissolved in solution is proportional to the partial pressure of CO_2 (Pco_2), which is in equilibrium with $Paco_2$ of alveolar air. The solubility constant of CO_2 is 0.03.[2]

The effectiveness of the buffering system can be appreciated when studying this equation. One measure used to quantify strength of acid in solution is the dissociation constant, or pKa. In general, a weak acid will be the most effective buffer when pH is within 1 log of its pKa. Bicarbonate is not an excellent buffer at physiological pH (its pKa is only 6.1). However, because CO_2 and bicarbonate can be independently regulated (by the lungs and kidneys, respectively), bicarbonate can be an effective buffer.[2] Of course, other extracellular buffers such as phosphates and plasma proteins do contribute to preserving pH; however, they are not considered to be as important. Intracellular buffers, such as hemoglobin, are very important to the initial buffering of respiratory acidosis and alkalosis, and will be discussed later in the chapter.

Although the values change depending on the laboratory or reference, generally, acidemia refers to serum pH less than 7.35 and alkalemia refers to serum pH more than 7.45. We refer to acidosis as the physiologic process that leads to an acidemia, which can be either a fall in bicarbonate or a rise in $Paco_2$. Conversely, alkalosis is due to processes that increase bicarbonate or decrease $Paco_2$. Additionally, an acid–base disturbance is defined as *metabolic* if the primary process driving it is due to a change in serum bicarbonate, and as *respiratory* if it's driven by a change in $Paco_2$. Table 1-1 summarizes these processes.

Renal Role in Acid–Base Homeostasis

Although the lungs can assist in excreting carbonic acid, the 50 to 100 mEq of nonvolatile acid (eg, sulfuric acid and phosphoric acid) that is generated by the body each day must be excreted in the urine. There are 2 steps to excretion of nonvolatile acid:

1. Reabsorption of the entire filtered bicarbonate load (mostly by the proximal tubule)
2. Secretion of hydrogen by the distal tubule

TABLE 1-1 Acid–Base Disturbances With Appropriate Responses. Adapted from Berend et al[4]

Acid–Base Disturbance	Appropriate Response
Metabolic acidosis	$pH < 7.35$ and $[HCO_3^-] < 22$ mEq/L
Respiratory compensation	$Paco_2 = 1.5 \times [HCO_3^-] + 8 \pm 2$ mmHg
Metabolic alkalosis	$pH > 7.45$ and $[HCO_3^-] > 26$ mEq/L
Respiratory compensation	$Paco_2 = [HCO_3^-] + 15$ mmHg
Respiratory acidosis	$pH < 7.35$ and $Paco_2 > 45$ mmHg
Acute metabolic compensation (< 24 h)	$[HCO_3^-]$ increases by 1 mEq/L for every 10-mmHg rise in $Paco_2$ *or* change in $pH = 0.008 \times (40 - Paco_2)$
Chronic metabolic compensation (> 48 h)	$[HCO_3^-]$ increases by 4 mEq/L for every 10-mmHg rise in $Paco_2$ *or* change in $pH = 0.003 \times (40 - Paco_2)$
Respiratory alkalosis	$pH > 7.45$ and $Pco_2 < 35$ mmHg
Acute metabolic compensation (< 24 h)	$[HCO_3^-]$ decreases by 2 mEq/L for every 10-mmHg fall in $Paco_2$ *or* change in $pH = 0.008 \times (40 - Paco_2)$
Chronic metabolic compensation (> 48 h)	$[HCO_3^-]$ decreases by 4 mEq/L for every 10-mmHg fall in $Paco_2$ *or* change in $pH = 0.003 \times (40 - Paco_2)$

HCO_3^- = bicarbonate; $Paco_2$ = partial pressure of carbon dioxide in arterial blood; Pco_2 = partial pressure of carbon dioxide.

Although the nephron can pump protons against an electrochemical gradient, the minimum urine pH that it can generate is about 4.5 to 5. This pH only corresponds to a proton load of about 0.04 mEq/L, which is far less than the 50 to 100 mEq of hydrogen that needs to be excreted each day.[2] Hence, most of the free hydrogen that is secreted into the lumen is bound to titratable acids (primarily hydrogen phosphate [HPO_4^{2-}] or ammonia [NH_3]). On a typical diet, 10 to 40 mEq of H^+ is excreted bound to titratable acid, and another 30 to 60 mEq is bound to NH_3. If more acid needs to be excreted (as in the case of underlying acidosis), then the kidney can generate more NH_3 by metabolizing glutamine in the proximal tubule in order to buffer that excess H^+ in the urine.

METABOLIC ACIDOSIS

As mentioned above, a pH below 7.35 is considered acidemia. Metabolic acidosis is defined as a pathological process that results in decreased bicarbonate ion concentration. If serum bicarbonate is less than 22 mEq/L, and the serum pH is less than 7.35, then a metabolic acidosis is present.[4] In general, there are 3 physiologic mechanisms for metabolic acidosis:

1. increased generation of acid (eg, diabetic ketoacidosis),
2. increased bicarbonate loss (eg, diarrhea), and
3. inability to excrete acid (eg, renal tubular acidosis).[1]

When there is an increase in serum hydrogen ion concentration due to generation of acid or inability to excrete acid, the following reaction is driven to the right:[2]

$$H^+ + HCO_3^- \leftrightarrow H_2CO_3 \leftrightarrow CO_2 + H_2O$$

This ultimately leads to consumption of the major extracellular buffer, bicarbonate. If the etiology of acidosis is due to increased bicarbonate loss (as in diarrhea) the reaction is driven to the left, and H^+ is ultimately generated in the reaction.

The normal physiologic response to an acid load is to minimize the change in pH via several mechanisms:

- extracellular buffering (by serum bicarbonate),
- intracellular and bone buffering (by hemoglobin and phosphate from bone), and
- respiratory compensation (increase in ventilation to excrete $Paco_2$).

These intracellular and extracellular buffer mechanisms are particularly important to prevent excessive drops in serum pH. Up to 60% of acid loads will be taken up by intracellular and bone buffers. For example, if 12 mEq of hydrogen ions is added to serum, the serum bicarbonate will only fall by a total of 5 mEq because of intracellular and bone buffering.[5]

The fall in serum pH leads to stimulation of peripheral and central chemoreceptors, which are located on the ventrolateral medullary surface and carotid and aortic bodies, respectively. This stimulation results in a rise of alveolar ventilation by increasing tidal volume and respiratory rate. The increased respiratory response typically begins within 1 to 2 hours and results in a fall in $Paco_2$. The fall in $Paco_2$ in response to metabolic acidosis will approximately follow the Winter equation:

$$Paco_2 = 1.5 \times [HCO_3^-] + 8 \pm 2 \text{ mmHg}$$

If the $Paco_2$ is higher than what is predicted by the above equation, then it suggests an additional respiratory acidosis. Conversely, a $Paco_2$ that is lower than predicted suggests a simultaneous respiratory alkalosis.

Anion Gap

Once a metabolic acidosis has been identified and the respiratory compensation is calculated, the next step in acid–base analysis involves calculating the anion gap (AG). The serum anion gap is defined as

$$\text{Serum Anion Gap} = [Na^+] - ([Cl^-] + [HCO_3^-])$$

Of course, there is no true electrolyte gap, as the law of electroneutrality dictates that all cations must be equal to all anions. It is inconvenient to measure all the anions in every patient, particularly given how small in concentration some electrolytes are. Since sodium, chloride, and bicarbonate are present in very large concentrations in the serum and can display the largest variability, we can monitor them and identify

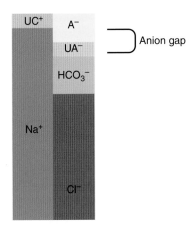

FIGURE 1-1 Schematic of the anion gap.

the presence of unmeasured anions (UA^-) if the anion gap rises. The typical unmeasured ions include lactate, phosphate, citrate, sulfate, and, most importantly, albumin. Accumulation of 1 of these UA^- causes an increase in the anion gap because of the buffering by bicarbonate of hydrogen produced by these anions:[2]

$$H^+UA^- + NaHCO_3 \leftrightarrow H_2CO_3 + Na^+ + UA^-$$
$$\leftrightarrow H_2O + CO_2 + Na^+ + UA^-$$

Hence, bicarbonate is consumed when buffering the excess hydrogen, leaving only the sodium and UA^-. Chloride concentration remains unchanged in this equation, and therefore, the calculated anion gap will rise.

Albumin accounts for about 75% of the anion gap, so falls in albumin must be accounted for when the calculation is made.[4] The "normal" anion gap in most labs runs in the range of 3 to 12 mEq/L; the typical correction for low albumin is to add 2.5 mEq/L to the calculated anion gap for every drop of albumin of 1 g/dL (Fig. 1-1).

It should be noted that an abnormally low anion gap can occur in scenarios where there is an excess of unmeasured cation (UC^+), which is commonly seen in multiple myeloma (the monoclonal protein is positively charged), lithium toxicity, or hypercalcemia. A negative anion gap occurs in bromide or iodide toxicity because they cause a pseudohyperchloremia.[4]

Delta/Delta

When an anion gap acidosis is identified, the next step is to ensure that there is not a mixed metabolic acid–base disturbance. Because there is a predictable relationship between the fall in bicarbonate and the increase in the anion gap, the clinician can identify a concurrent non-gap acidosis or metabolic alkalosis by analyzing the ratio of the increase in the anion gap compared to the fall in serum bicarbonate. This is referred to as the *delta-delta*.[4] For example, in diabetic ketoacidosis, the increase in the anion gap compared to the fall in bicarbonate should be close to 1 to 1. In diabetic ketoacidosis, if the change in the anion gap is significantly greater (5 mEq is the typical error range) than the fall in bicarbonate, we expect a

concomitant metabolic alkalosis to be present. Similarly, if the change in bicarbonate is more than 5 mEq greater than the change in the anion gap, then we would predict a mixed non-gap acidosis to be present as well. So, the equation for diabetic ketoacidosis is the following:

$$\Delta AG - \Delta HCO_3 = 0 \pm 5$$

In lactic acidosis, the ratio is 0.6 (ie, for every 1 mEq/L rise in the anion gap, the serum bicarbonate falls by 0.6 mEq/L). This difference is probably due to the lower renal clearance of lactate as compared to ketoacids. Hence, the formula for lactic acidosis would be adjusted slightly:[5]

$$0.6 \times \Delta AG - \Delta HCO_3 = 0 \pm 5$$

Causes of High Anion Gap Acidosis

There is a wide differential diagnosis that has to be considered when an elevated anion gap is diagnosed. The most common categories are lactic acidosis, ketoacidosis (eg, diabetic, alcoholic, starvation induced), uremic acidosis, and drug or toxin ingestion. A helpful mnemonic to remember the different etiologies is GOLD MARRK (Table 1-2).[4]

Lactic Acidosis

Lactic acid is produced from the metabolism of pyruvic acid during the process of anaerobic glycolysis. The digestive tract is responsible for over 50% of the body's lactic acid production.[4,5] Skeletal muscle, brain tissue, skin, and red blood cells (RBCs) also produce lactate, which is metabolized by both the liver and the kidneys. Causes of lactic acidosis can be categorized by subtype (A or B), depending on the mechanism.[6] Type A lactic acidosis is the result of decreased tissue perfusion or decreased oxygen delivery that occurs in shock or carbon monoxide toxicity. Anaerobic glycolysis is increased in these conditions, resulting in higher levels of lactic acid. In the setting of shock, reduced perfusion of the liver results in a simultaneous decrease in lactate metabolism. Type B lactic acidosis occurs when mitochondrial or liver function is impaired. The conversion of lactate to pyruvate requires adequate liver and mitochondrial function. If either of these is impaired, lactic acid may accumulate. Metformin and certain antiviral medications (such as zidovudine or stavudine) also can inhibit mitochondrial function. Cyanide toxicity results in

TABLE 1-2 Gold Marrk

Glycols: propylene and ethylene
5-**o**xoproline (pyroglutamic acid)
L-lactate (standard)
D-lactate (short bowel syndrome)
Methanol
Aspirin
Renal failure
Rhabdomyolysis
Ketoacidosis

type B lactic acidosis because cyanide binds the final enzyme of the mitochondrial cytochrome complex (ie, the electron transfer chain), interrupting normal mitochondrial oxidative phosphorylation.[6]

Ketoacidosis

Ketoacidosis occurs when glucose is not available to cells due to a lack of insulin, glucose depletion, or cellular dysfunction. The 2 major types of ketoacidosis that are seen in clinical practice are diabetic ketoacidosis and alcoholic/starvation ketosis. In these conditions, there are 2 mechanisms that result in the development of ketoacidosis:

1. increase in free fatty acid delivery due to increased lipolysis, and
2. change in hepatocyte function so that free fatty acids are converted to ketoacids and not triglycerides.[2,5]

During insulin deficiency (which occurs in type 1 diabetes or in starvation states), fatty acids undergo lipolysis. High serum glucagon causes fatty acyl coenzyme A (CoA) molecules within hepatocytes to be converted to ketones (acetoacetate and β-hydroxybutyrate).[2,5] These ketones are preferentially taken up and oxidized by the brain and kidneys. In patients with starvation or alcoholic ketosis, the rate of uptake of ketones by these organs approximates the rate of generation, and hence, acidosis tends not to be as severe.[7] The presence of low levels of insulin in starvation limits ketosis to some degree. A more detailed discussion of diabetic ketoacidosis can be seen in Chapter 22.

It should be noted that the major type of ketone synthesized is dependent on etiology of the patient's ketoacidosis. The concentrations of each ketone are based on cellular reduction-oxidation (redox) levels, or in other words, the ratio of nicotinamide adenine dinucleotide phosphate (NADP) to NADPH (the reduced form) in the body. In diabetic ketoacidosis, the average β-hydroxybutyrate–acetoacetate ratio is 5 to 2. In alcoholic ketoacidosis, the ratio is 20 to 1.[5] Notably, urine dipstick testing measures acetoacetate and β-hydroxybutyrate, whereas blood serum ketone levels register only β-hydroxybutyrate (Fig. 1-2).

Toxins and Drug Ingestions

There are several toxins and drugs that increase levels of endogenous acids upon ingestion. In the case of aspirin (acetylsalicylic acid), the therapeutic range in the serum is usually 20 to 35 mg/dL. When levels exceed 40 to 50 mg/dL, patients will present with signs of intoxication.[5] Early clinical symptoms include tinnitus, vertigo, nausea, vomiting, and diarrhea. Severe overdose can cause hyperthermia, altered mental status, coma, and death.[8] The major anions that accumulate in salicylate poisoning are ketoacids and lactic acid, as salicylate concentrations in serum are very small and do not significantly contribute to the anion gap.[5] Salicylate toxicity stimulates respiratory centers in the brainstem, leading to a respiratory alkalosis in addition to the anion gap acidosis.

The mainstay of management of salicylate toxicity includes administration of intravenous sodium bicarbonate to alkalinize the serum to a pH of 7.5 to 7.55. Salicylic acid diffuses easily into central nervous system (CNS) tissue, whereas salicylate ions can be trapped in alkaline serum and urine, and excreted.[8,9] In a patient who presents with severe neurologic symptoms, renal failure, or fluid overload, hemodialysis should be initiated. Because salicylate is a small molecule with a small volume of distribution, hemodialysis is very effective to enhance elimination of the drug and should be continued until serum levels are below 20 mg/dL.[9]

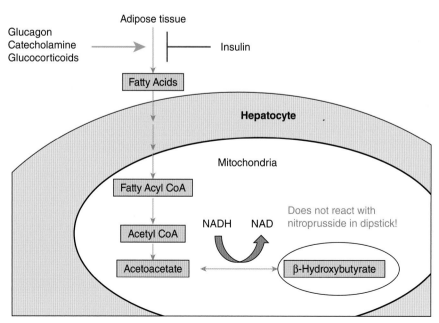

FIGURE 1-2 Ketoacid generation in alcoholic and diabetic ketoacidosis.

Acetaminophen is another common over-the-counter medication that can cause an elevated gap acidosis in patients who are chronic users and simultaneously malnourished. The metabolic acidosis is secondary to the build-up of pyroglutamic acid.[4]

Methanol and ethylene glycol are toxic alcohols available in automotive antifreeze and commercial solvents that, when ingested, are metabolized by alcohol dehydrogenase and aldehyde dehydrogenase (the enzymes that metabolize alcohol) into toxic metabolites. Methanol, which is available in a number of commercial preparations and in illicit distillations of alcohol (moonshine), is metabolized to formaldehyde and then to formic acid.[9] Formic acid is extremely toxic to the retina and leads to blindness, coma, and death. Ethylene glycol, common in antifreeze, gets metabolized to glycolate and oxalate, which precipitate in the kidney to cause tubular injury and obstruction.[2] Treatment of these toxic ingestions involves aggressive hydration to maximize renal clearance and use of fomepizole, a competitive inhibitor of alcohol dehydrogenase. It is recommended that fomepizole be administered if any of the below criteria are met:[10,11]

1. Documented recent history of ingesting methanol or ethylene glycol and serum osmolal gap more than 10
2. Strong clinical suspicion of methanol or ethylene glycol poisoning with 2 of the following:
   a. Arterial pH less than 7.3
   b. Serum bicarbonate less than 20 mEq/L
   c. Osmol gap more than 10
   d. Urinary oxalate crystals present

Hemodialysis may be required in cases of severe ingestions, acidemia, or renal failure.[10,11] It should also be noted that patients with methanol ingestion should be treated with folic acid (50 mg every 6 hours), as it assists with metabolism of formic acid to CO_2 and water.[12]

Use of the *osmolal gap* can aid early diagnosis of toxic alcohol ingestions. If a patient with metabolic acidosis and an unexplained anion gap presents to the emergency room, the osmolal gap calculation should be performed to rule out a toxic alcohol ingestion. The measured serum osmolality is compared to the calculated osmolality to determine if a foreign substance with a low molecular weight and high osmolal activity is present. Examples of such substances are methanol, ethylene glycol, isopropyl alcohol, or propylene glycol. The osmolal gap calculation is as follows:

$$\text{Calculated P}_{osm} = 2[Na^+] + \frac{glucose}{18} + \frac{BUN}{2.8} + \frac{[ethanol]}{3.7} \text{ (if Present)}$$

A normal osmolal gap is less than 10 mOsm/L; however, there is a wide range in the general population. This variance leads to potential problems with using the osmolal gap in a clinical setting. In addition, other clinical situations may involve elevated osmolal gaps, specifically, lactic acidosis, alcoholic ketoacidosis, and diabetic ketoacidosis.[4] It should be noted that the osmolal gap in methanol and ethylene glycol ingestion may only be elevated for several hours after ingestion before the alcohols are metabolized into their anion forms. Nevertheless, an osmolal gap greater than 20 has a specificity of 85% for ingestion of a toxic alcohol.[13]

Uremic Acidosis

Uremic acidosis is a complication of advanced renal failure that occurs when the kidney is unable to excrete daily dietary acids. When glomerular filtration rate (GFR) begins to fall, the kidney will increase ammonium (NH_4^+) excretion to maintain acid balance. However, once the GFR falls to more significant levels (15–20 cc/min), daily nonvolatile acid generation cannot be excreted completely and serum bicarbonate falls to levels between 12 and 20 mEq/L.[2] Severe acidosis usually does not occur due to buffering by release of calcium salts from the bone. This can produce a calcium loss over time that results in osteopenia in patients with advanced (stage 4 and 5) chronic kidney disease. There are also several unmeasured anions that accumulate in this process that increase the anion gap. Sulfates accumulate from sulfuric acid, which is generated from the metabolism of amino acids containing sulfur (methionine, cysteine, homocysteine, and taurine). Other unmeasured anions that accumulate due to decreased GFR are phosphate, urate, and hippurate.

Normal Anion Gap Metabolic Acidosis

Normal anion gap metabolic acidosis is due to loss of bicarbonate in the gastrointestinal (GI) tract, failure to reabsorb bicarbonate in the proximal tubule, or inability to secrete hydrogen in the distal tubule (Table 1-3). The renal causes are collectively termed renal tubular acidosis (RTA). In a normal anion gap metabolic acidosis, bicarbonate decreases relative to chloride in a roughly 1-to-1 ratio. As a result, a commonly used synonym of normal anion gap acidosis is hyperchloremic metabolic acidosis.[4,5]

The urinary anion gap (UAG) is a useful tool to help distinguish GI losses of bicarbonate from impaired urinary hydrogen excretion. In patients with acidosis, compensatory increased ammonium excretion is expected. Although urinary ammonium is not typically measured, we can make inferences about its excretion based on the difference between the major cations and anions in the urine: sodium, potassium, and chloride.[4,5] Hence, the UAG is defined as

$$UAG = (Na^+ + K^+) - Cl^-$$

In metabolic acidosis due to diarrhea, normal renal compensation leads to an increase in NH_4^+ excretion, which would generate a negative UAG, since chloride excretion would have to increase to maintain electroneutrality. In most cases of RTA or advanced renal failure where ammonium excretion cannot be increased, the UAG will be 0 or positive. It should be noted that proximal RTA may cause a positive UAG due the excretion of another anion other than chloride, namely bicarbonate.[5]

TABLE 1-3 Etiologies for Normal Anion Gap Metabolic Acidosis

Gastrointestinal loss of bicarbonate
- Diarrhea
- Laxative abuse
- Enterocutaneous fistulas
- Ureterosigmoidostomy or other urinary diversions

Renal bicarbonate loss
- Type 2 (proximal) renal tubular acidosis
  - Fanconi syndrome
  - Wilson disease
  - Multiple myeloma, amyloid
  - Sjögren syndrome
  - Toxins: lead, cadmium, mercury
- Medication induced (carbonic anhydrase inhibitors)
  - Acetazolamide
  - Topiramate

Impaired renal excretion of hydrogen
- Advanced renal disease
- Type 1 (distal) renal tubular acidosis
  - Wilson disease
  - Primary hyperparathyroidism
  - Medullary sponge kidney
  - Sjögren syndrome and other autoimmune diseases
  - Drugs: amphotericin, ifosfamide, lithium
  - Multiple myeloma
- Type 4 (hyperkalemic) renal tubular acidosis
  - Diabetic kidney disease
  - Hypoaldosteronism
  - Angiotensin-converting enzyme inhibitors, angiotensin receptor binders, cyclosporine, nonsteroidal anti-inflammatory drugs, spironolactone, heparin

Ingestions or toxins
- Ammonium chloride
- Toluene
- Cholestyramine

Dilutional acidosis with normal saline

Gastrointestinal Loss of Bicarbonate

Intestinal fluids tend to be alkaline, and as a result, increased loss of these fluids in the form of diarrhea, enterocutaneous fistula, or villous adenoma lead to a hyperchloremic acidosis. Laxative abuse causes a non-gap acidosis for the same reason. If a patient had a ureterosigmoidostomy after a cystectomy in the treatment of bladder cancer, there is frequently a postrenal loss of bicarbonate in the urine due to exchange of chloride for bicarbonate by the intestinal epithelial cells.[5]

Renal Tubular Acidosis

Acid handling in the kidney is facilitated by 3 mechanisms:

1. secretion of hydrogen ions at the distal tubule,
2. reabsorption of bicarbonate at the proximal tubule, or
3. generation of NH_3, which buffers the urine by binding hydrogen ions in the filtrate.

Disruption of these mechanisms corresponds with the respective type of RTA.[5]

A type 1 (distal) RTA is due to impairment of hydrogen ion secretion in the distal collecting tubule. This prevents lowering of urine pH to less than 5.3, which is necessary to excrete excess hydrogen in the form of titratable acid (phosphate and sulfate) and NH_4^+.[5] Impaired proton secretion can be seen in autoimmune disorders such as Sjögren syndrome, systemic lupus erythematosus, or rheumatoid arthritis (RA). Amphotericin B can cause increased membrane permeability and a subsequent leak of H^+ ions back in the serum. Type 1 RTA is associated with urine pH more than 5.5, plasma HCO_3 less than 15, and renal stones.

Type 2 (proximal) RTA is due to the impairment of bicarbonate reabsorption at the proximal tubule. This can be caused by genetic disorders such as Wilson disease, multiple myeloma, autoimmune conditions, or carbonic anhydrase inhibitors (acetazolamide or topiramate). The acidosis in this condition tends to be milder than type 1 RTA and frequently concurrent Fanconi syndrome can be observed, as other elements of proximal tubule function are affected.

Type 4 (distal or hyperkalemic) RTA is usually due to aldosterone deficiency or resistance. The hyperkalemia causes impaired NH_3 generation, and prevents proper buffering of urinary hydrogen ions. Nonsteroidal anti-inflammatory drugs (NSAIDs), angiotensin-converting enzyme (ACE) inhibitors, beta-blockers, and cyclosporine can also produce this effect. Type 4 RTA is common in diabetic kidney disease as a result of hyporeninemic hypoaldosteronism.

Dilutional Acidosis

A common cause of iatrogenic hyperchloremic acidosis is large administration of unbuffered crystalloid solutions (eg, normal saline).[4] This most commonly is seen in surgical and trauma patients, where large amounts of saline solution are given to resuscitate unstable patients. In these cases, the normal bicarbonate of the serum is diluted down before appropriate renal compensation can take place to excrete supplemental ammonium and chloride.

Treatment

In general, treatment of metabolic acidosis is aimed at treating the underlying disorder. For example, in lactic acidosis due to hypotension or sepsis, appropriate volume resuscitation, pressors, inotropes, and antibiotics should be administered to improve tissue perfusion. Similarly, for diabetic ketoacidosis, intravenous insulin will stop lipolysis and ketogenesis. The benefits of supplemental bicarbonate therapy to replete the bicarbonate deficit and increase pH remains controversial. Severe acidosis decreases myocardial contractility and impairs responsiveness to catecholamines.[7,14] Hence, treatment of severe acidosis is recommended by some experts when pH falls under 7.2.[15] It must be noted that the benefit of this practice remains unproven.[6] There are 2 potential problems that can occur with aggressive bicarbonate replacement:

1. intracellular acidification due to increase in CO_2 generation, and
2. a fall in ionized calcium with a rise in pH, resulting in decreased myocardial contractility.

In patients with renal failure, volume overload may become an issue when sizeable amounts of sodium bicarbonate crystalloid solutions are administered. Hemodialysis could theoretically be a safer modality to correct acidosis as it can prevent hypocalcemia, hypervolemia, and intracellular acidification while removing lactate ions.[6] However, a hemodynamically unstable patient may be challenging to dialyze safely. Controlled prospective studies are needed to evaluate the potential benefits of dialysis for treatment of lactic acidosis. Even the choice of resuscitation fluids remains controversial with patients in shock; use of chloride-rich isotonic solutions has been shown to be associated with worsening acute kidney injury (AKI). However, randomized, prospective trials have not verified a benefit to buffered (bicarbonate-added) solutions, as far as improved outcomes.[6,16,17]

In diabetic ketoacidosis (DKA), it has been proposed that severe acidosis can affect insulin binding to the insulin receptor.[18] However, small randomized controlled trials have not shown a clear benefit of alkali administration to patients with diabetic ketoacidosis.[19] There are theoretical risks of bicarbonate therapy, such as worsening hypokalemia, slower resolution of ketonemia, cerebral edema, and paradoxically worsening cerebral spinal fluid (CSF) acidosis, although none of these adverse effects was conclusively demonstrated. At this time, nonbuffered solutions are recommended as the initial resuscitation solutions.

As discussed in prior sections, urinary alkalinization is a useful treatment to improve toxic alcohol and salicylate clearance. Isotonic buffered crystalloid solution should be used in these situations (eg, addition of 3 amps or 150 mEq sodium bicarbonate to a D5 water solution). Other electrolytes need to be monitored closely, as alkalization can lead to hypokalemia and hypocalcemia. Chronic metabolic acidosis should be treated with oral bicarbonate therapy, as it may relieve dyspnea (due to pulmonary compensation), reduce bone buffering, and potentially reduce progression of chronic kidney disease.[20,21]

METABOLIC ALKALOSIS

Metabolic alkalosis is defined as pH more than 7.42 and bicarbonate more than 26 mmol/L. The typical respiratory response to metabolic alkalosis is an increase in $Paco_2$ by 0.75 mmHg per 1 mEq/L increase in HCO_3^-.[4,22] Complete respiratory adjustment occurs in 24 to 36 hours.

Metabolic alkalosis is a result of either GI losses of hydrogen and chloride, renal losses of hydrogen and chloride, intracellular shifts of hydrogen ions, or contraction alkalosis (Fig. 1-3). Whatever the cause for generation of the metabolic alkalosis, a mechanism for maintenance of the alkalosis has to be present as well, since the kidneys should be able to filter excess bicarbonate into the urine relatively easily.[4,22] Usually, the mechanism for maintenance of a high serum bicarbonate is a reduction in GFR with concomitant increased tubular sodium bicarbonate reabsorption and increased distal proton excretion at the distal tubule. Other possible etiologies for maintenance of metabolic alkalosis are hyperaldosteronism (primary or secondary), hypokalemia, or chloride depletion.[2] In cases of volume depletion and secondary hyperaldosteronism, the fall in GFR leads to decreased proximal tubule sodium delivery to the juxtaglomerular apparatus, which stimulates renin release, which in turn causes aldosterone production by the adrenal gland. Hyperaldosteronism causes increased cortical and medullary hydrogen ion secretion by activating type A intercalated cells (Fig. 1-4).[4]

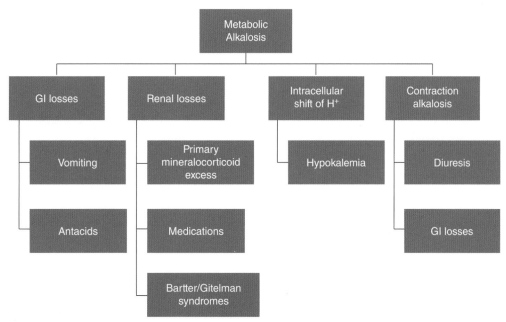

FIGURE 1-3 Multiple causes of metabolic alkalosis. GI = gastrointestinal.

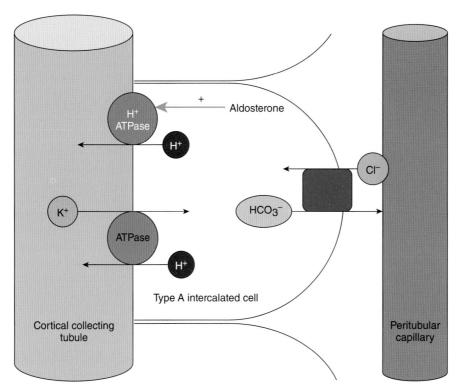

FIGURE 1-4 Hydrogen adenosine triphosphatase (ATPase) activity in the type A intercalated cell in distal tubule is enhanced by aldosterone.

Gastrointestinal Losses

Gastrointestinal fluid and electrolyte losses can significantly impact ion concentration and lead to volume depletion. Decreased effective circulating volume leads to proximal tubule retention of water (H_2O), sodium (Na^+), and HCO_3^-. Common clinical scenarios resulting in metabolic alkalosis as a result of GI losses are the following:

- **Vomiting.** Excessive vomiting or nasogastric suction of upper gastric secretions have several effects. Gastric secretions have high concentrations of hydrogen chloride, which, when lost, directly leads to alkalosis and hypochloremia. Per the mechanism described above, simultaneous volume depletion maintains the alkalosis due to proximal tubule reabsorption of sodium with bicarbonate and activation of the renin-angiotensin system.
- **Antacids.** Antacids are commonly comprised of calcium carbonate or magnesium hydroxide. When antacid medications are ingested in a large quantity, alkali (CO_3^- or OH^-) is absorbed and can lead to a mild alkalosis. This alkali typically can be excreted, unless a fall in GFR occurs. If hypercalcemia develops from ingestion of these calcium carbonate salts, the increased calcium levels decrease action at both the antidiuretic hormone (ADH) receptors and thick ascending limb Na-K-2Cl cotransporter, leading to inappropriate diuresis and subsequent volume depletion. In addition, the associated malabsorption can lead to osmotic diarrhea, further worsening volume depletion and ability to excrete excess alkali loads.[23]

Renal Losses

Metabolic alkalosis can also occur from urinary loss of hydrogen due to mineralocorticoid excess, sodium and chloride wasting syndromes such as Bartter and Gitelman syndromes, hypokalemia, diuretic use, and iatrogenic administration. Renal processes that cause hypokalemia can perpetuate alkalosis due to action of the type A intercalated cell (see Fig. 1-4) and the principal cell (Fig. 1-5),[23] both of which are in the cortical collecting duct of the nephron.

- **Mineralocorticoid excess.** Mineralocorticoids act to open sodium channels for increased sodium reabsorption at the principal cells in the collecting tubule; in order to maintain electroneutrality, potassium is passively secreted into the tubule (see Fig. 1-5). The most common cause of mineralocorticoid excess is primary hyperaldosteronism (including Conn syndrome and bilateral adrenal hyperplasia), Cushing syndrome, congenital adrenal hyperplasia, and Liddle syndrome.
- **Bartter/Gitelman syndromes.** Bartter and Gitelman syndromes are autosomal recessive disorders characterized by mutations in nephron transporters that lead to sodium and chloride wasting states. The ensuing volume depletion leads to activation of the renin-angiotensin aldosterone system (RAAS), which ultimately results in hypokalemia and metabolic alkalosis via similar mechanisms outlined above. There are several classifications of Bartter syndrome, all resulting in dysfunction in the thick ascending limb (mimics use of a loop diuretic). Gitelman syndrome is caused by a

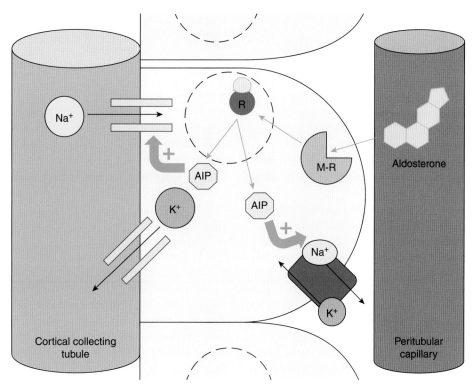

FIGURE 1-5 Mechanism of aldosterone on principal cells. AIP = aldosterone induced protein; K^+ = potassium ion; M-R = mineralocorticoid receptor; Na^+ = sodium ion; R = ribosome.

defect in the thiazide-sensitive Na-Cl cotransporter and is also characterized by hypomagnesemia.[23]

- **Intracellular H^+ Shift.** In chronic potassium deficiency, the body adjusts to create metabolic alkalosis in several ways. There is an intracellular exchange of hydrogen for potassium in order to maintain electroneutrality. In addition, the kidneys compensate by upregulating potassium hydrogen ATPase (see Fig. 1-4). This leads to an increase in potassium at the expense of hydrogen loss, exacerbating metabolic alkalosis.
- **Contraction Alkalosis.** Contraction alkalosis occurs in clinical scenarios in which the amount of fluid that is lost is high in chloride and relatively low in bicarbonate. The extracellular volume contracts around a constant bicarbonate concentration (due to decreased GFR and impaired bicarbonate excretion).[2] The most common causes of contraction alkalosis are diuretic use, sweat, and gastric losses, as outlined above.
- **Alkali Administration.** In certain iatrogenic situations, patients may develop metabolic alkalosis if large amounts of bicarbonate or other alkalis are administered. This may be seen in the setting of a cardiac arrest, when sodium bicarbonate is administered rapidly. In addition, in cases of hemorrhagic shock in which large amounts of blood products are administered ($\geq$ 10 units), metabolic alkalosis can be seen, due to metabolism of sodium citrate (used as an anticoagulant in the packed cells) to sodium bicarbonate.[24]

Diagnosis

Use of a spot urine chloride can be useful to distinguish among the potential etiologies of alkalosis. Metabolic alkalosis can be considered chloride "responsive" if urine chloride is less than 25 mEq/, or "resistant" if urine chloride is more than 40 mEq/L. Chloride-responsive metabolic alkalosis is due to vomiting, volume depletion, the subsiding of a diuretic medication's effect, villous adenoma, and congenital chloridorrhea.[4] These conditions respond well to sodium chloride and potassium chloride administration. If diuresis is needed, acetazolamide, spironolactone, amiloride, or triamterene can be used. In chloride-resistant states, which can be due to primary hyperaldosteronism, Bartter and Gitelman syndromes, or severe hypokalemia, administration of sodium chloride and/or potassium chloride will not correct the alkalosis. Primary aldosteronism, Liddle syndrome, chronic licorice ingestion, and mineralocorticoid excess will have metabolic alkalosis with hypertension. Bartter and Gitelman syndromes are associated with hypotension or normotension.

RESPIRATORY ACIDOSIS

During the metabolism of carbohydrates and fats, the body generates 15,000 mmol of CO_2 that has to be excreted via the lungs.[2,25] As discussed earlier in the chapter, dissolved CO_2 combines with water to form carbonic acid (H_2CO_3):

$$CO_2 + H_2O \leftrightarrow H_2CO_3$$

The carbonic acid generated is buffered by intracellular proteins (primarily hemoglobin [Hgb]) and delivered to the lungs as seen in the equation below.

$$H_2CO_3 + Hgb^- \leftrightarrow HHgb + HCO_3^-$$

In the alveoli, the process is reversed: Hgb binds O_2 and releases H^+, and CO_2 is excreted.

The main stimulus for ventilation is the reduction of arterial oxygen (Pao_2) and an elevation in arterial CO_2 ($Paco_2$). The chemosensitive areas of the respiratory center in the medulla sense cerebral interstitial changes in pH. $Paco_2$ is the major stimulus to respiration, as very minute changes in $Paco_2$ can induce changes in minute ventilation; a rise in $Paco_2$ of 1 mmHg can increase minute ventilation by 1 to 4 L.[25] This contrasts with the response to hypoxemia in that minute ventilation may not increase significantly until Pao_2 is less than 60 mmHg.[25]

Respiratory acidosis, defined as pH less than 7.35 and $Paco_2$ more than 45, can be acute (< 24 hours) or chronic (> 24 hours). There are 2 phases of metabolic compensation with any drop in arterial pH due to an elevation in $Paco_2$. The initial buffering that occurs is due to intracellular protein buffering (mostly due to hemoglobin, as discussed above). This immediate buffering causes a rise of bicarbonate by 1 mEq for every 10 mmHg increase in $Paco_2$. Interestingly, although the extracellular buffers assist in buffering an acute increase in extracellular hydrogen due to metabolic acidosis, the response to acute rise in Pco_2 is not as efficient. This is because serum bicarbonate cannot buffer proton that is released from Pco_2:

$$H_2CO_3 + HCO_3^- \leftrightarrow H_2CO_3 + HCO_3^-$$

Hence, the intracellular buffers (eg, hemoglobin) are the only available buffer to proton released from dissolved Pco_2.[25]

After 48 hours or so, renal compensation results in a 4 mEq increase in bicarbonate for every 10 mmHg increase in $Paco_2$.[1,2] Low serum pH leads to an increase in hydrogen excretion in the distal tubule to accompany bicarbonate reabsorption in the proximal tubule. It should be noted that due to frequent and aggressive use of diuretics in patients with respiratory acidosis (to treat volume overload), an inappropriate metabolic alkalosis may be evident. This causes a higher CSF pH, which is sensed by the central medullary chemoreceptors, and in turn, decreases ventilatory drive and worsens chronic respiratory acidosis.

Causes

Respiratory acidosis has several systemic physiologic consequences and as a result may present with variable and nonspecific findings. Psychological symptoms include somnolence, psychosis, agitation, and delirium (from hypercarbia to brain tissue). Respiratory consequences include dyspnea (from CO_2 delivery to metabolic chemoreceptors in brainstem and carotid body) and respiratory failure (hypercapnia resulting from decreased respiratory drive). Neurologic manifestations include lethargy and coma.

The etiology of respiratory acidosis also can be characterized as central/CNS, airway, parenchymal, neuromuscular, and miscellaneous (Fig. 1-6). Central causes result in a depression of the respiratory center through pharmacologic effects or direct injury. Airway obstruction commonly leads to an increase in physiologic dead space and may also present with hypoxemia. Neuromuscular disease may lead to limited ventilation capacity as a result of physiologic limitation (scoliosis/obesity) and/or extreme fatigue of central and accessory respiratory musculature. In patients requiring mechanical ventilation for acute respiratory failure due to pneumonia or ARDS, a permissive hypercapnia strategy may be utilized. In these patients, tidal volume is kept low in order to prevent lung injury from barotrauma, which may cause significant hypoventilation and hypercapnia.

Acute Respiratory Acidosis

Causes of acute respiratory acidosis are numerous, as discussed above. Pneumonia, severe asthma, suppression of the respiratory center after cardiac arrest, and drug overdose are common causes in patients without underlying lung disease.

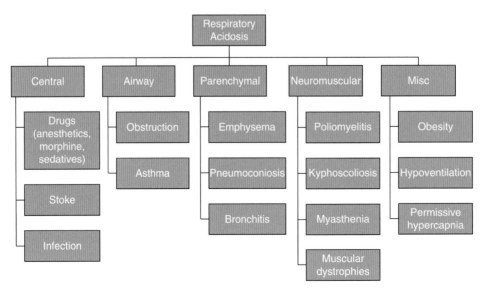

FIGURE 1-6 Causes of respiratory acidosis.

Obstructive sleep apnea can be considered an acute cause of respiratory acidosis since the rise in CO_2 occurs primarily at night, and once in the awake state, improves, hence renal compensation does not have time to occur completely.

Chronic Respiratory Acidosis

Chronic respiratory acidosis with concurrent hypercapnia is associated with chronic lung disease, including chronic obstructive pulmonary disorder (COPD) and cystic fibrosis. In extremely obese patients with the obesity hypoventilation (Pickwickian) syndrome, the increased weight of the chest wall leads to increased work of breathing and inspiratory weakness, leading to hypoventilation. In addition, decreased respiratory responsiveness to increased $Paco_2$ and hypoxemia has been suggested as playing a role.[26,27]

It is believed that the respiratory centers become less sensitive to CO_2 during states of chronic hypercapnia, and hypoxia becomes the main stimulus to respiration. In addition, aggressive use of diuretics to treat edema in cor pulmonale increases serum bicarbonate levels (contraction alkalosis), which further increase the serum pH and blunt the expected increase in ventilation stimulated by hypercapnia. In normal states, hypoxia does not stimulate severe hyperventilation because the fall in $Paco_2$ causes a rise in pH, which suppresses medullary-induced ventilation. In chronic CO_2-retaining states, ventilation will be enhanced once Po_2 falls below 80 because a respiratory alkalosis never develops despite high CO_2 levels in the CSF, and medullary centers will not be suppressed.[28]

Diagnosis

As previously outlined, acute respiratory acidosis is a result of an acute decrease in ventilation or a worsening of alveolar ventilation in patients who have decreased pulmonary reserve. In contrast, chronic respiratory acidosis is the result of an ongoing disease process. In patients who present with hypercapnic respiratory failure, immediate labs and arterial blood gas (ABG) should be taken. Also of note is that while ABGs are preferred, venous blood gas (VBG) analysis may also be used but will result in a higher $Paco_2$ and lower Pao_2.[29] As discussed above, if the pH is significantly below normal, acute respiratory acidosis is likely present (due to limited intracellular buffering). If arterial pH is near normal, then chronic respiratory acidosis is likely, as the patient has had time for renal compensation to take effect. In acute or chronic respiratory acidosis, $Paco_2$ is elevated, yet pH remains markedly low despite a high serum bicarbonate generated by renal compensatory mechanisms.

Alveolar–Arterial Gradient

In the event of hypercapnia and hypoxemia leading to respiratory failure, the alveolar–arterial gradient (A-a gradient) is useful to distinguish extrapulmonary versus interstitial disease. It compares arterial oxygen with alveolar oxygen pressure in ambient air; a large difference, or gradient, suggests diffusion defect, ventilation/perfusion (V/Q) mismatch, right-to-left shunt, or increased O_2 extraction. A normal or low A-a gradient suggests hypoventilation or low partial pressure of inspired oxygen (Pio_2).[30] The normal value (5–10 mmHg) will change depending on age and fraction of inspired oxygen (Fio_2). The A-a gradient is seen below. Pao_2 is alveolar O_2, Pao_2 is arterial O_2, $Paco_2$ is arterial CO_2, Fio_2 is fraction of inspired oxygen (21% on room air), and atmospheric pressure is 760 pascals (Pa) in conventional units, 101.33 kPa in SI units.

$$\text{A-a gradient} = Pao_2 - Pao_2 = [(Fio_2) \times (\text{Atmospheric Pressure} - H_2O \text{ Pressure}) - (Paco_2/0.8)] - Pao_2$$

Normal Gradient Estimate = (Age/4) + 4 *or* 2.5 + 0.21 × Age

Treatment

Treatment of acute respiratory acidosis usually is aimed at treatment of underlying disease. If these methods are ineffective alone, efforts to increase ventilation using noninvasive or invasive mechanical ventilation frequently are necessary.

Bicarbonate administration for acute respiratory acidosis can be useful in severe acidemia (pH < 7.15), particularly in the setting of a patient on a ventilator when tidal volumes need to be minimized to decrease barotrauma associated with high peak and plateau pressures. This permissive hypercapnia strategy may improve outcomes in patients with acute respiratory distress syndrome (ARDS) who are difficult to oxygenate, and prevent ventilator lung injury.[31] Some experts suggest use of sodium bicarbonate (100 mEq) in a D5W solution, to be infused for a goal pH of 7.3.[32] Potential risks of sodium bicarbonate administration include worsening intracellular acidemia (because of increased generation of CO_2, which can pass across cell membranes), worsening volume overload (due to volume of intravenous bicarbonate), and CNS effects (increased intracranial pressure and decrease in seizure threshold).[25,33]

Sodium bicarbonate therapy is not required for patients with chronic respiratory acidosis since renal compensation will usually be adequate to maintain a reasonable (> 7.2) systemic pH. Treatment is aimed at therapy for the underlying disease. Excessive oxygen should be avoided given that these patients' drive for respiration is frequently dependent on hypoxia. Feeding patients lower carbohydrate diets may be useful to decrease the respiratory quotient and reduce CO_2 production.[34] Weight loss should be encouraged in obese patients to assist alveolar ventilation. Nocturnal positive pressure ventilation can be considered in some COPD patients as well as in patients with obstructive sleep apnea.

Of note, it is important to be cautious with potassium wasting diuretics in hypercapnic patients because they could cause a secondary metabolic alkalosis, which would suppress respiratory drive further. Theoretically, acetazolamide may be used to correct this metabolic alkalosis; however, it needs to be used cautiously, as correction of bicarbonate to a normal level (24–28 mEq) would lead to a severe acidemia for which a patient with intrinsic lung disease may not be able to compensate.[25,35,36]

RESPIRATORY ALKALOSIS

Respiratory alkalosis can be identified by a decreased $Paco_2$ (primary hypocapnia), decreased HCO_3^-, and a subsequent increase in systemic pH. There are several simultaneous metabolic consequences. Acute alkalosis affects renal clearance of electrolytes as well as intracellular shifts of Na^+, K^+, and PO_4^-, causing transient ion imbalances, although these mechanisms are incompletely understood.[35] The fall in CO_2 leads to a shift of H^+ from intracellular buffers that causes the early compensation for alkalosis. The equation below is driven to the right to make up for loss of $Paco_2$ due to hyperventilation:

$$H^+ + HCO_3^- \leftrightarrow H_2CO_3 \leftrightarrow H_2O + Pco_2$$

This leads to release of hydrogen from intracellular buffers (hemoglobin and lactic acid):

$$HBuff \rightarrow H^+ + Buff^-$$

This additional hydrogen will be buffered by extracellular bicarbonate and will reduce bicarbonate by approximately 2 mEq for every 10-mmHg decrease in Pco_2.[2] Over several days, the change in $Paco_2$ stimulates renal compensation and prevents the excretion of H^+. Typically in respiratory alkalosis, blood $Paco_2$ ranges from 15 to 40 mmHg.[36] In chronic respiratory alkalosis, the renal compensation leads to a 4- to 5-mEq decrease in HCO_3^- levels for every 10-mmHg decrease in $Paco_2$.[22,23]

There are also several systemic changes that are exacerbated based on the patient's underlying chronic disease pathology. Decreased bicarbonate levels lead to cerebral vasoconstriction, reduced oxygenation of CNS, and subsequent somnolence, mental confusion, dizziness, and lethargy. Hypoxia leads to a "left" shift to the oxygen dissociation curve, decreasing oxygen unloading and increasing risk of arrhythmias and cardiovascular events. In addition, respiratory alkalosis leads to increased anionic charge of albumin, which promotes calcium binding and results in a fall in ionized calcium, which can cause paresthesia symptoms.[22]

Causes

Respiratory alkalosis has been noted to be common in patients admitted to the intensive care unit (ICU), and therefore, understanding the etiology is critical in order to treat the underlying disease process. Respiratory hyperventilation can be caused by acute events, including drug ingestion, pain, CNS stimulants, respiratory stimulants, and environmental conditions. Chronic alkalosis may reflect an underlying disease process, including heart failure, anemia, and hepatic failure. It is interesting to note that acute hypoxia needs to be severe to trigger respiratory alkalosis because alkalemic pH tends to inhibit the respiratory center, which dampens the initial hyperventilation. However, in chronic hypoxemic states, because the kidney will compensate for alkalosis by decreasing proton secretion, a greater degree of hyperventilation can occur, leading to a greater fall in Pco_2 (Fig. 1-7).[2]

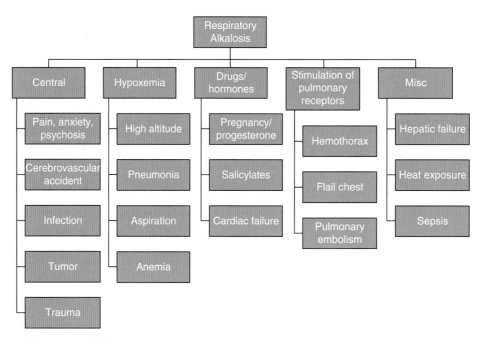

FIGURE 1-7 Causes of respiratory alkalosis.

QUESTIONS

1. A 45-year-old male painter with past medical history of drug abuse presents to the emergency department with slurred speech and difficulty walking. His symptoms came on when he was on the job painting in the basement of a house.

   Vital signs: BP 88/43 mmHg, RR 26 breaths/min, HR 100 beats/min, Temp 99°F
   Lethargic but arousable with diffuse muscle weakness
   Dry mucous membranes
   Lungs clear
   Regular rate and rhythm, no murmurs
   Abdomen soft and nontender

   Labs:

WBC	$15 \times 10^3/\mu L$
Hgb	14.2 g/dL
Plt	$312 \times 10^3 \ \mu L$
Sodium	136 mEq/L
Potassium	2 mEq/L
Chloride	118 mEq/L
CO_2	12 mEq/L
BUN	52 mg/dL
Creatinine	1.5 mg/dL
Phosphorus	3 mg/dL
Plasma osmolality	280 mOsm/kg H_2O

   Urine:

pH	6
EtOH	Negative

   Toxicity Screen:
   Marijuana +
   Benzodiazepine +

   Arterial Blood Gas:

pH	7.29
Pco_2	26 mmHg

   What is the most likely cause of the patient's clinical condition?

   A. Methanol ingestion
   B. Toluene inhalation
   C. Aspirin overdose
   D. Alprazolam overdose

2. A 37-year-old woman with history of diabetes and alcohol abuse presents in unresponsive state to the emergency department. According to her son, she complained of blurred vision before losing consciousness.

   Home medications: metformin

   Vital signs: BP 99/43 mmHg, RR 26 breaths/min, HR 107 beats/min, Temp 98.4°F
   Somnolent
   Dry mucous membranes
   Lungs clear
   Tachycardic, no murmurs
   Abdomen soft and nontender
   No edema, cyanosis, or clubbing

   Arterial Blood Gas:

pH	6.724
Pco_2	20 mmHg

   Labs:

BUN	56 mg/dL
Creatinine	2.4 mg/dL
Sodium	134 mEq/L
Potassium	5.2 mEq/L
Chloride	100 mEq/L
CO_2	5 mEq/L
Calcium	8.3 mg/dL

   UA:

pH	5.5
Specific gravity	1.020
Blood	Negative
Ketones	trace ketones
Ethanol	12 mg/dL
Glucose	122 mg/dL
Lactate	3 mg/dL
Plasma osmolality	321 mOsm/kg H_2O
Phosphorous	3.7 mg/dL

   Blood work for ethanol, salicylates, and acetaminophen is negative. What is the most appropriate treatment strategy for this patient?

   A. Aggressive resuscitation with a buffered crystalloid solution
   B. IV fomepizole and emergent hemodialysis
   C. Intravenous bicarbonate solution to induce urinary alkalinization
   D. IV fomepizole alone

3. A 64-year-old man is hospitalized with confusion, nausea, and dizziness.

   PMHx: hypertension, atrial fibrillation, hyperlipidemia, chronic diarrhea

   PSHx: superior mesenteric artery embolus 2 years ago, s/p resection of large section of small bowel

   Home medications: rosuvastatin, metoprolol, warfarin, and enalapril; no over-the-counter drugs or supplements

Vital signs: BP 108/60 mmHg, RR 19 breaths/min, HR 96 beats/min, Temp 99°F
AAO × 1, confused to place and time
Mucous membranes moist
Lungs clear to auscultation
Heart regular rate and rhythm
Abdomen soft and nontender, normoactive bowel sounds
No edema

Labs:

BUN	14 mg/dL
Sodium	140 mEq/L
Potassium	3.8 mEq/L
Chloride	106 mEq/L
CO_2	17 mEq/L
Glucose	90 mg/dL
Lactate	Normal
Plasma osmol	296 mOsm/kg H_2O

Arterial blood gas:

pH	7.37
Pco_2	36 mmHg

Which of the following is the most likely diagnosis?

A. D-lactic acidosis
B. Ethylene glycol or methanol poisoning
C. Propylene glycol toxicity
D. Pyroglutamic acidosis

4. A 37-year-old man with a history of depression was found by his son unresponsive in his garage with a suicide note lying nearby. On arrival to hospital, patient demonstrated rapid and shallow Kussmaul breathing with a Glasgow coma score of 4.

Vital signs: BP 110/85 mmHg, RR 26 breaths/min, HR 100 beats/min, Temp 98.7°F
Pupils reactive to light
Lungs clear to auscultation
Heart tachycardic and without murmurs
Abdomen is soft and nontender
No edema

Arterial blood gas:

pH	6.79
Pco_2	37 mmHg
Po_2	115 mmHg

Drug toxicity screen and testing of salicylic acid and acetaminophen were negative.

Labs:

BUN	45 mg/dL
Creatinine	2.1 mg/dL
Sodium	135 mEq/L
Potassium	3.8 mEq/L
Chloride	106 mEq/L
CO_2	8.4 mEq/L
Calcium	6.8 mEq/L
Glucose	180 mg/dL
Lactate	2.5 mmol/L
Ethanol	undetectable
Plasma osmol	320 mOsm/kg H_2O

Which of the following statements about this patient is FALSE?

A. A normal osmol gap would be expected to be less than 10 mOsm/kg.
B. Fomepizole followed by hemodialysis is appropriate treatment for this patient.
C. Urine alkalinization via administration of sodium bicarbonate to increase urinary excretion of the toxin is sufficient treatment for this patient.
D. Antifreeze is a common source of the alcohol causing this patient's poisoning.

5. A 24-year-old woman with depression presents to the emergency department with lethargy, confusion, and vomiting 18 hours after ingesting 100 unknown pills from a bottle in her parents' medicine cabinet.

Vital signs: BP 100/55 mmHg, RR 28 breaths/min, HR 122 beats/min, Temp 100°F
Lungs clear to auscultation
Tachycardic but regular
Abdomen soft
No edema in lower and upper extremities

Labs:

pH	7.56
Pco_2	22 mmHg
Sodium	144 mEq/L
Potassium	3.2 mEq/L
Chloride	100 mEq/L
HCO_3^-	19 mEq/L
Creatinine	1.4 mg/dL
Albumin	5 mg/dL
LFTs	within normal limit (WNL)

What is the most accurate characterization of the patient's acid–base abnormality?

A. Respiratory alkalosis with concomitant metabolic alkalosis
B. Respiratory alkalosis with concomitant anion gap acidosis
C. Metabolic alkalosis with combined metabolic anion gap acidosis
D. Respiratory alkalosis with anion gap acidosis and metabolic alkalosis

6. An 84-year-old woman who resides at a nursing home is sent to the emergency department with 2 to 3 days of abdominal pain, nausea, vomiting, and low-grade fever. The patient is severely demented and can provide no history. Abdominal x-ray (Fig. 1-8) is seen below.

Home medications: diphenhydramine 25 mg, calcium carbonate 600 mg bid, amlodipine 5 mg, Colace 100 mg, and a multivitamin

Vital signs: BP 105/80 mmHg, RR 18 breaths/min, HR 100 beats/min, O₂ sat 99% room air
Cachexic elderly woman
Clear to auscultation
Regular rate and rhythm, no murmurs
Abdomen is distended, diffuse tenderness to palpation, hypoactive bowel sounds
Awake and alert × 1, no focal neurological deficits

Labs:

Sodium	136 mEq/L
Potassium	3 mEq/L
Chloride	90 mEq/L
CO₂	36 mEq/L
BUN	56 mg/dL
Glucose	116 mg/dL
Calcium	10.6 mg/dL
Creatinine	2 mg/dL
Albumin	4.7 mg/dL
Urine chloride	10 mEq/L
pH	7.47
Pco₂	51 mmHg

What is the mechanism of her acid–base abnormality?

A. Upper GI losses of hydrogen and chloride
B. Diuretic-induced metabolic alkalosis
C. Milk-alkali syndrome
D. Dilutional acidosis

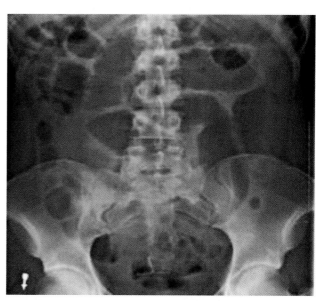

FIGURE 1-8 Abdominal x-ray on admission.

7. A 31-year-old woman with chronic pain syndrome is hospitalized with dyspnea and general failure to thrive.

Vital signs: BP 105/65 mmHg, RR 14 breaths/min, HR 110 beats/min, Temp 98°F, Weight 42 kilograms (kgs)
Appears anxious and uncomfortable
Temporal muscle wasting
Lungs clear to auscultation
Heart tachycardic, but regular rate and rhythm, no murmurs
Abdomen soft, nontender

Labs:

Sodium	130 mEq/L
Potassium	2.0 mEq/L
Chloride	80 mEq/L
CO₂	46 mEq/L
BUN	56 mg/dL
Calcium	8.5 mg/dL
Creatinine	1.6 mg/dL
Albumin	1.9 g/dL

Urine:

Chloride	46 mEq/L
Potassium	57 mEq/L
Sodium	46 mEq/L

What is the likely cause of this patient's metabolic alkalosis?

A. Diuretic use
B. Laxative use
C. Intractable vomiting
D. Gitelman syndrome

8. A 32-year-old man with myotonic dystrophy presents for follow-up from a recent hospitalization for the treatment of pneumonia. He reports worsening dyspnea over the last 6 months.

Vital signs: BP 129/77 mmHg, RR 18 breaths/min, HR 90 beats/min, Temp 99 °F
Appears anxious and uncomfortable
Mild crackles heard over the right lower lung field
Regular rate and rhythm, no murmurs

Arterial Blood Gas:

pH	7.36
Pco_2	57 mmHg
Po_2	85 mmHg (room air)
HCO_3^-	31 mEq/L

Chest radiograph shows hypoinflation and an improving infiltrate in the upper portion of the right lower lobe. Which of the following most accurately describes the acid–base status and A-a gradient expected in this patient?

A. Chronic respiratory acidosis, appropriate metabolic compensation, widened A-a gradient
B. Chronic respiratory acidosis, appropriate metabolic compensation, normal A-a gradient
C. Acute respiratory acidosis, metabolic acidosis, widened A-a gradient
D. Chronic respiratory acidosis, concurrent metabolic acidosis, normal A-a gradient

9. A 67-year-old man with COPD and CHF (normal EF) presents to the emergency department with shortness of breath and intermittent associated cough with white sputum. He reported chronic lower extremity edema. His exam was consistent with rhonchi and wheezes as well as 2+ lower extremity edema. His chest x-ray on admission reveals hyperinflation, but no infiltrates or pulmonary edema.

His Admission ABG:

pH	7.36
Pco_2	55 mmHg
HCO_3^-	31 mEq/L
Po_2	55 mmHg

He was started on intravenous steroids, furosemide, bronchodilators via nebulizer, and empiric antibiotics. He initially improved but on hospital day 3, he appeared more lethargic and confused. Repeat lab work and ABG was as follows:

pH	7.41
Pco_2	70 mmHg
HCO_3^-	43 mEq/L
Sodium	142 mEq/L
Potassium	3.5 mEq/L
Chloride	98 mEq/L
Creatinine	1.5 mg/dL

Which of the following most accurately describes this patient's current acid–base status?

A. Primary respiratory acidosis with appropriate metabolic compensation
B. Primary metabolic alkalosis with appropriate respiratory compensation
C. Mixed metabolic alkalosis and respiratory alkalosis
D. Mixed metabolic alkalosis and respiratory acidosis

10. A 40-year-old woman with past medical history of diabetes and acute lymphoblastic leukemia is admitted with respiratory failure due to pneumonia. Labs on admission reveal relatively normal renal function but neutropenia and anemia. Her ICU stay is significant for persistent fevers despite appropriate broad-spectrum antibiotic therapy. By hospital day 4, she is started on amphotericin B to cover for invasive aspergillosis. On day 8, the following labs were obtained:

Labs:

Sodium	144 mEq/L
Potassium	2.6 mEq/L
Chloride	125 mEq/L
CO_2	10 mEq/L
BUN	35 mg/dL
Calcium	8.2 mg/dL
Creatinine	1.6 mg/dL
Albumin	3 g/dL

Urine:

pH	6
Sodium	35 mEq/L
Chloride	60 mEq/L
Potassium	46 mEq/L

Which of the following is the most likely cause of this patient's metabolic findings?

A. Type 1 renal tubular acidosis
B. Type 2 renal tubular acidosis
C. Type 4 renal tubular acidosis
D. Diarrhea

11. A 60-year-old woman with type 2 diabetes mellitus (DM) and hypertension presents to the emergency department with nausea, vomiting, and abdominal pain for 3 days. She reports an acute diarrhea illness 1 week prior to admission.

Home medications: lisinopril, metformin, metoprolol

Vital signs: BP 95/55 mmHg, RR 30 breaths/min, HR 112 beats/min, O_2 sat 97% room air
Lethargic, but arousable
No jugular venous distension
Lungs clear to auscultation
Tachycardic but regular rhythm, no murmurs
Abdomen soft, nontender
No edema

Labs:

Sodium	124 mEq/L
Potassium	5.5 mEq/L
Chloride	85 mEq/L
CO_2	5 mEq/L
BUN	94 mg/dL
Glucose	232 mg/dL
Calcium	7.6 mg/dL
Creatinine	9.2 mg/dL
Phosphorus	9 mg/dL
Albumin	3 mg/dL
Lactic acid	10.7 mmol/L
pH	7.15
Pco_2	15 mmHg

A CT of the abdomen and pelvis with contrast revealed no evidence of mesenteric ischemia, colitis, or other intra-abdominal process. Which of the following statements about the treatment of this patient with sodium bicarbonate is FALSE?

A. Sodium bicarbonate therapy can result in hypernatremia and fluid overload.

B. Sodium bicarbonate therapy can result in hypocalcemia and worsen myocardial contractility.

C. Sodium bicarbonate therapy can increase generation of carbon dioxide.

D. Sodium bicarbonate can aid in renal excretion of metformin via ion-trapping in tubules.

12. A 50-year-old man presents to the emergency department with trauma to the abdomen following a motorized vehicle accident.

Vital signs: BP 80/55 mmHg, RR 30 breaths/min, HR 124 beats/min, O_2 sat 97% room air
Lethargic, but arousable
No jugular venous distension
Lungs clear to auscultation
Tachycardic but regular rhythm, no murmurs
Abdomen distended, tender

Labs: Pending

On abdominal CT, spleen demonstrates branching hyperdensities, consistent with rupture. A splenic subcapsular hematoma is also noted. He is transfused 2 units of packed red blood cells and taken to the operating room where he undergoes splenectomy with no complications. During his procedure, an additional 3 units of packed red blood cells are dispensed.

Overnight, the patient is given broad-spectrum antibiotics, morphine, norepinephrine, and normal saline. He requires another 5 units of packed RBC overnight. The following morning, the patient is found to be anxious and has vomited twice.

Upon re-evaluation:

Vital signs: BP 100/70 mmHg, RR 20 breaths/min, HR 95 beats/min
Appears anxious
No jugular venous distension
Lungs clear to auscultation
Tachycardic but regular rhythm, no murmurs
Abdomen distended, tender

Labs:

Sodium	132 mEq/L
Potassium	2.5 mEq/L
Chloride	80 mEq/L
CO_2	41 mEq/L
BUN	35 mg/dL
Calcium	6.0 mg/dL
Creatinine	1.6 mg/dL
Albumin	2.3 g/dL

Arterial Blood Gas:

pH	7.49
Pco_2	50 mmHg
Po_2	60 mmHg

What is the most likely pathogenesis of the patient's current condition?

A. Metabolic alkalosis due to vomiting

B. Metabolic alkalosis due to conversion of excess citrate to bicarbonate via the tricarboxylic acid (TCA) cycle

C. Respiratory alkalosis secondary to hyperventilation due to uncontrolled pain

D. Underlying pulmonary embolism as a complication of recent abdominal surgery

ANSWERS

1. B. Toluene inhalation

Toluene is widely used in many industrial solvents, acrylic paints, and paint thinners. Toxicity may be a result of environmental, accidental, or intentional exposure. It is the most widely abused inhaled volatile drug; it causes a euphoric effect when sniffed. Toluene is metabolized to benzoic acid and then to hippuric acid. These anions are very readily excreted into the urine as sodium and potassium salts. Most patients with toluene ingestion present with hypovolemia, hypokalemia, and a normal anion gap acidosis.[37]

Methanol ingestion (and frequently ethanol) would cause a high anion gap acidosis (choice A). Aspirin overdose causes a mixed respiratory alkalosis with high anion gap acidosis (choice C). Benzodiazepine overdose typically presents with a respiratory acidosis due to suppression of respiratory drive (choice D).

2. B. IV fomepizole and emergent hemodialysis

Methanol, also known as *wood alcohol*, is sometimes consumed as a substitute for ethanol, and initial presentation after ingestion resembles ethanol intoxication. Patients may present with drowsiness, seizures, or vision changes or loss. A report from the American Association of Poison Control Centers stated that 44 out of 979 methanol poisoning victims had major complications.[38]

Methanol is metabolized by the body first to formaldehyde by alcohol dehydrogenase and then formic acid (Fig. 1-9). Formate is the unmeasured anion that causes the elevated anion gap and is toxic to the retina, causing the visual changes classically associated with methanol toxicity.

Fomepizole (Antizol) is the antidote for both methanol and ethylene glycol poisoning. It works by competitively inhibiting alcohol dehydrogenase and thereby preventing the conversion of methanol to its toxic metabolites. This slower rate of production allows the liver to process the metabolites at a manageable rate and prevents organ damage.

In severe methanol poisoning, hemodialysis should be used to rapidly remove methanol from the body. The combination of hemodialysis and medical treatment (fomepizole) has been shown to decrease mortality and permanent neurological damage in severe cases.[14,38,39] Hemodialysis is recommended in any patient with metabolic acidosis or manifesting evidence of end organ damage (renal failure or blindness). Another option that is not listed is that intravenous ethanol is an effective alcohol dehydrogenase inhibitor. However, observational studies suggest that ethanol has a much higher incidence of adverse reactions compared to fomepizole. The main adverse effect associated with ethanol is central nervous system depression.[40]

Choice A is incorrect, as simple volume resuscitation, although indicated, is insufficient treatment for toxic alcohol ingestion. Intravenous bicarbonate (choice C) is useful for short-term treatment of acidosis, but in the setting of such severe renal failure, it will not treat methanol ingestion adequately.

3. A. D-lactic acidosis

D-lactic acid is produced by fermentation of carbohydrates by colonic bacteria. The body typically produces L-lactic acid, and our endogenous lactate dehydrogenase cannot metabolize the D-lactate variant. Increased absorption of D-lactic acid typically occurs in patients with short bowel syndrome; it can also occur in cases of high carbohydrate load or decreased colonic motility. D-lactic acidosis causes mental status changes and patients present with encephalopathy.[2] This condition can also present with a normal anion gap acidosis due to renal excretion of lactate with a cation such as sodium.

Choices B and C are incorrect, as they should have an elevated osmolal gap (> 10 mOsm/kg H_2O). Pyroglutamic acidosis (choice D) causes a gap acidosis in the setting of chronic acetaminophen use, which this patient denies.

4. C. Urine alkalinization via administration of sodium bicarbonate to increase urinary excretion of the toxin is sufficient treatment for this patient.

Ethylene glycol is an alcohol found in antifreeze, de-icing solutions, and windshield wiper fluid. Due to its sweet taste, it is often ingested by children, alcohol abusers seeking an alternative to alcohol, and by persons attempting suicide. Its primary metabolites, glycolic acid and oxalate, are the unmeasured anions responsible for the high anion gap metabolic acidosis. In cases where ingestion is suspected, laboratory testing for ethylene glycol specifically may not be available, so clinicians should use other laboratory findings to make a diagnosis; this is where measuring an osmolal gap is useful (choice A).

As in the treatment for methanol ingestion, fomepizole can be given to block the conversation of ethylene glycol to its toxic metabolites (choice B). Sodium bicarbonate may increase urinary excretion and decrease tissue toxicity; however, it should not be used without fomepizole or hemodialysis (in this patient with end organ damage). It should also be noted that sodium bicarbonate administration may paradoxically further nephrotoxicity by raising urine pH and increasing the precipitation of oxalate crystals in the kidney (choice C).[41-43]

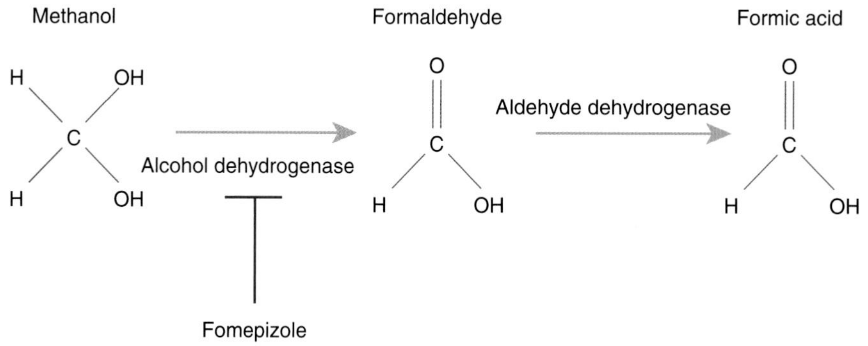

FIGURE 1-9 Conversion of methanol to formic acid.

5. D. Respiratory alkalosis with anion gap acidosis and metabolic alkalosis

Aspirin overdose classically presents with hyperventilation, gastric irritation, and tinnitus. Supratherapeutic doses of salicylate directly stimulate the respiratory center in the medulla. Therefore, aspirin toxicity produces a primary respiratory alkalosis along with an anion gap acidosis. As a result of this mixed picture, blood pH may be within normal limits in the setting of increased anion gap.

The acidosis produced by aspirin overdose is multifactorial. In addition to being an endogenous acid itself, aspirin causes uncoupling of oxidative phosphorylation and inhibition of the Krebs cycle. This inhibition results in an accumulation of organic acids and an increased production of lactic acid. Aspirin can also impair renal function, which results in further accumulations of organic acids, such as phosphoric and sulfuric acids.

There is no antidote for aspirin, so the goal of therapy is to limit absorption and enhance elimination. Patients are treated with gastric lavage, activated charcoal, and supportive measures, such as hydration and correct acid–base disturbances. The airway should be stabilized and mechanical ventilations provided, if required. Hemodialysis may be indicated in severe cases.[44-46]

Analysis of this patient's acid–base status is complex. Analysis of the arterial blood gas reveals a respiratory alkalosis with acidosis slightly greater than expected; analysis of the serum chemistry shows an anion gap of 25, which suggests an elevated anion gap acidosis. Calculation of the delta anion gap/delta bicarbonate ratio suggests that the fall in bicarbonate was much less than the increase in the anion gap (ratio > 3), which suggests a concomitant metabolic alkalosis (probably from vomiting). Answer choices A, B, and C are incorrect.

6. A. Upper GI losses of hydrogen and chloride

This patient's x-ray showed peristaltic ileus. Due to her nausea and vomiting, it is likely that she has metabolic alkalosis due to gastric losses of H^+ and Cl^-. Her volume-depleted state causes high aldosterone levels and activation of the type A intercalated cell, which stimulates hydrogen secretion (see Fig. 1-4). The high level of aldosterone in combination with gastric losses leads to a hypokalemic metabolic alkalosis.

In evaluation of metabolic alkalosis, urine chloride is helpful. Urine chloride less than 25 mEq/L can suggest gastrointestinal loss, contraction alkalosis, and late diuretic use. Urine chloride more than 40 mEq/L can suggest primary hyperaldosteronism, hypokalemia, Gitelman syndrome, and Bartter syndrome. Diuretic-induced metabolic alkalosis (choice B) is incorrect due to the low urine chloride. Diuretics could cause a low urine chloride if the diuretic has not been given in 24 hours, but there is no reason to suspect surreptitious diuretic use in this nursing home patient. Although the patient has a slightly high calcium, which might suggest milk-alkali syndrome (choice C), her calcium is not high enough to cause AKI, and in fact, her high calcium level is likely due to hemoconcentration (high albumin level). The patient does not have a dilutional acidosis; in fact, she has a contraction alkalosis (choice D).

7. A. Diuretic use

For patients presenting with nonspecific symptoms, a careful history and physical examination (with key portions, including vital signs, body mass index (BMI), and parotid gland swelling) are important to assess. In this case, this patient's BMI and physical exam are consistent with an eating disorder with associated dehydration/electrolyte abnormalities. Her urine chemistries, however, suggest that her alkalosis is due to diuretic abuse rather than vomiting. Her urine chloride is greater than 40, which suggests a chloride-resistant metabolic alkalosis. In this patient, who likely suffers from an eating disorder, diuretic use has to be suspected. Diuretics (both thiazide and loop diuretics) block the kidneys' ability to appropriately resorb sodium chloride, which results in an increased urine chloride concentration. In addition, the increased delivery of sodium to the distal tubule leads to sodium reabsorption at the convoluted tubule (activated by aldosterone) and excretion of potassium in exchange, which partially explains this patient's profound hypokalemia.

Vomiting often presents with a concurrent hypovolemia and stimulates renin and aldosterone activity. As a result, the kidneys actively resorb Na, HCO_3^-, and Cl, thus reducing the amount of urine Cl to less than 25 mEq/L (choice C).

In contrast, laxative use depends on the mechanism of the drug of choice, but usually causes loss of bicarbonate in the diarrhea, and causes a non-gap metabolic acidosis with hypokalemia (choice B). Although Gitelman syndrome would present with a chloride-resistant metabolic alkalosis, it is usually diagnosed in children and would not explain the physical exam findings in this patient (choice D).

8. B. Chronic respiratory acidosis, appropriate metabolic compensation, normal A-a gradient

Mechanisms that affect A-a gradient include ventilation/perfusion (V/Q) mismatch, right-to-left shunting, diffusion limitation, hypoventilation (drugs, obesity, etc), and reduced inspired oxygen tension. In this example, muscular weakness results in a pure hypoventilation syndrome, which results in a chronic respiratory acidosis. There would be metabolic compensation, as this patient does not have renal failure or metabolic insufficiency. There is a simultaneous acute respiratory acidosis as a result of infection and pulmonary effusions as described by radiography and physical exam. The A-a gradient would be normal.

9. D. Mixed metabolic alkalosis and respiratory acidosis

This patient is experiencing clinical manifestations of acute on chronic CHF/COPD exacerbation, as evidenced by his medical history and physical exam of dyspnea and lower extremity edema. His initial arterial blood gas (ABG) reflects expected findings in a COPD patient with chronic respiratory acidosis and appropriate renal compensation. Although it may initially appear that the repeat ABG reflects an improvement in this patient's overall status because pH is normalized, this represents an inappropriate alkalosis (contraction alkalosis from diuretic use). This rise in pH has suppressed his ventilatory drive further, causing worsening hypercarbia and mental status.

10. A. Type 1 renal tubular acidosis

Amphotericin B is a broad-spectrum antifungal agent used in the treatment of systemic and life-threatening fungal infections. Amphotericin B exerts its antifungal effect by binding cholesterol in fungal membranes and causing the formation of pores; this same effect can occur in human renal tubular membranes. This process affects the distal renal tubular membrane permeability, resulting in tubular dysfunction. Nephrotoxicity can manifest with normal anion gap metabolic acidosis due to distal tubular dysfunction. Urine pH is typically low, and hypokalemia is also prominent. In addition, patients will typically have polyuria and hypomagnesemia. Modern formulations of Amphotericin B are lipid based, although an improvement in nephrotoxic side effects compared to older formulations is unclear.[47]

Type 2 (proximal) RTA (choice B), more common in infiltrative diseases such as Sjögren syndrome and multiple myeloma, usually will have a lower urine pH and a less severe metabolic acidosis (serum bicarbonate > 12 mEq/L). Type 4 RTA (choice C) typically is associated with hyperkalemia. Urine studies with diarrhea should have a negative urine anion gap (choice D).

11. D. Sodium bicarbonate can aid in renal excretion of metformin via ion-trapping in tubules.

This patient presents with lactic acidosis due to metformin toxicity. The patient presumably developed acute renal failure from her GI illness, which inhibited normal metformin urinary excretion and, as a result, caused accumulation of metformin in the plasma. Metformin toxicity causes a type B lactic acidosis due to formation of lactate in the splanchnic bed of the small intestine and impairs oxidative phosphorylation in mitochondria.

The use of sodium bicarbonate in all patients with lactic acidosis is controversial, but in general, it is appropriate to use it in any patient with a pH less than 7.2. Potential complications of bicarbonate therapy are fluid overload, hypernatremia (if isotonic solutions are not used), hypokalemia (due to intracellular shift), and, most worrisome, potential worsening of intracellular pH (from generation of CO_2) and fall in ionized serum calcium (choices A, B, and C). In cases of lactic acidosis due to metformin toxicity, it is recommended that dialysis is used in severe acidosis (pH < 7 or lactate > 20) or with renal failure. Intravenous bicarbonate is not useful to increase clearance of the metformin via ion-trapping, as in the case of aspirin overdose (choice D).[14,48]

12. B. Metabolic alkalosis due to conversion of excess citrate to bicarbonate via the tricarboxylic acid (TCA) cycle

Although RBC transfusion has been considered a safe procedure, recent evidence demonstrates increased complications from massive blood transfusions (> 10 units of RBC) in patients, as a result of citrate toxicity. Citrate, a common anticoagulant added to blood products, is normally converted to bicarbonate by the liver via the TCA cycle.[22] Hence, citrate is usually metabolized to bicarbonate and filtered by nephrons.[49] If renal perfusion is suboptimal, as frequently occurs in patients with hypovolemic shock, bicarbonate will not be excreted appropriately. In addition, the excess citrate in the serum leads to chelation of magnesium and calcium, and subsequent hypocalcemia, which can result in nausea, vomiting, anxiety, and even cardiac dysfunction. Infusion rates of greater than 1 unit of PRBC in 5 minutes can result in citrate toxicity. Complications of citrate toxicity have also been shown in cases of recurrent nonmassive transfusions. Patients with liver disease are also at higher risk.[24,50]

Choice A is incorrect, as the patient's volume depletion, although possibly partially responsible for impairing some of the bicarbonate excretion, is not the main etiology of the patient's alkalosis. Choice C is incorrect because the patient has an appropriate respiratory acidosis as compensation for metabolic alkalosis. Choice D is incorrect since a pulmonary embolism should cause a respiratory alkalosis, not a metabolic alkalosis.

REFERENCES

1. Emmett M, Szerlip H. Approach to the adult with metabolic acidosis. In: Post TW, ed. UpToDate. Waltham, MA: UpToDate Inc. http://www.uptodate.com. Accessed July 15, 2017.
2. Rose BD, Post T. Chapter 10: Acid-base phsiology. In: Rose BD, Post TW. *Clinical Physiology of Acid-Base and Electrolyte Disorders*. New York, NY: McGraw-Hill; 2001:300-324.
3. Rennke HG, Denker BM. *Renal Pathophysiology, the Essentials*. 3rd ed. Philadelphia, PA: Lippincott Williams and Wilkins; 2010.
4. Berend K, de Vries AP, Gans RO. Physiological approach to assessment of acid-base disturbances. *N Engl J Med*. 2014; 371(15):1434-1445.
5. Rose BD, Post T. Chapter 19: Metabolic acidosis. In: Rose BD, Post TW. *Clinical Physiology of Acid-Base and Electrolyte Disorders*. New York, NY: McGraw-Hill; 2001:578-646.
6. Kraut JA, Madias NE. Lactic acidosis. *N Engl J Med*. 2014; 371(24):2309-2319.

7. Kamel KS, Halperin ML. Acid-base problems in diabetic keto-acidosis. *N Engl J Med*. 2015;372(6):546-554.

8. Klig JE, Sharma A, Skolnik AB. Case records of the Massachusetts General Hospital. Case 26-2014. A 21-month-old boy with lethargy, respiratory distress, and abdominal distention. *N Engl J Med*. 2014;371(8):767-773.

9. Marc Ghannoum M, Mardini K. Chapter 69: Elimination enhancement of poisons. In: Skorecki K, Chertow G, Marsden P, Taal M, Yu A. *Brenner and Rector's: The Kidney*. 10th ed. Philadelphia, PA: Elsevier; 2015; 2180.

10. Barceloux DG, Bond GR, Krenzelok EP, Cooper H, Vale JA; American Academy of Clinical Toxicology Ad Hoc Committee on the Treatment Guidelines for Methanol Poisoning. American Academy of Clinical Toxicology practice guidelines on the treatment of methanol poisoning. *J Toxicol Clin Toxicol*. 2002; 40(4):415-446.

11. Barceloux DG, Krenzelok EP, Olson K, Watson W. American Academy of Clinical Toxicology practice guidelines on the treatment of ethylene glycol poisoning. Ad hoc committee. *J Toxicol Clin Toxicol*. 1999;37(5):537-560.

12. Nazir S, Melnick S, Ansari S, Kanneh HT. Mind the gap: a case of severe methanol intoxication. *BMJ Case Rep*. 2016;2016.

13. Krasowski MD, Wilcoxon RM, Miron J. A retrospective analysis of glycol and toxic alcohol ingestion: utility of anion and osmolal gaps. *BMC Clin Pathol*. 2012;12:1.

14. Kraut JA, Madias NE. Treatment of acute metabolic acidosis: a pathophysiologic approach. *Nat Rev Nephrol*. 2012;8(10): 589-601.

15. Adrogue HJ, Madias NE. Management of life-threatening acid-base disorders. First of two parts. *N Engl J Med*. 1998; 338(1):26-34.

16. Yunos NM, Bellomo R, Hegarty C, Story D, Ho L, Bailey M. Association between a chloride-liberal vs chloride-restrictive intravenous fluid administration strategy and kidney injury in critically ill adults. *JAMA*. 2012;308(15):1566-1572.

17. Young P, Bailey M, Beasley R, et al; SPLIT Investigators; ANZICS CTG. Effect of a buffered crystalloid solution vs saline on acute kidney injury among patients in the intensive care unit: the SPLIT randomized clinical trial. *JAMA*. 2015;314(16): 1701-1710.

18. Sonne O, Gliemann J, Linde S. Effect of pH on binding kinetics and biological effect of insulin in rat adipocytes. *J Biol Chem*. 1981;256(12):6250-6254.

19. Chua HR, Schneider A, Bellomo R. Bicarbonate in diabetic keto-acidosis—a systematic review. *Ann Intensive Care*. 2011;1(1)23.

20. Chapter 3: Management of progression and complications of CKD. *Kidney Int Suppl (2011)*. 2013;3(1):73-90.

21. de Brito-Ashurst I, Varagunam M, Raftery MJ, Yaqoob MM. Bicarbonate supplementation slows progression of CKD and improves nutritional status. *J Am Soc Nephrol*. 2009;20(9): 2075-2084.

22. Naureckas ET, Solway J. Chapter 306e: Disturbances of respiratory function. In: Kasper D, Fauci A, Hauser S, Longo D, Jameson J, Loscalzo J, eds. *Harrison's Principles of Internal Medicine*. 19th ed. New York, NY: McGraw-Hill; 2014. http://accessmedicine.mhmedical.com/content.aspx?bookid=1130&sectionid=63652933. Accessed February 16, 2018.

23. Rose BD, Post T. Chapter 18: Metabolic alkalosis. In: Rose BD, Post TW. *Clinical Physiology of Acid-Base and Electrolyte Disorders*. New York, NY: McGraw-Hill; 2001:551-577.

24. Bicakci Z, Olcay L. Citrate metabolism and its complications in non-massive blood transfusions: association with decompensated metabolic alkalosis+respiratory acidosis and serum electrolyte levels. *Transfus Apher Sci*. 2014;50(3):418-426.

25. Rose BD, Post T. Chapter 20: Respiratory acidosis. In: Rose BD, Post TW. *Clinical Physiology of Acid-Base and Electrolyte Disorders*. New York, NY: McGraw-Hill; 2001:647-672.

26. Rochester DF, Enson Y. Current concepts in the pathogenesis of the obesity-hypoventilation syndrome. Mechanical and circulatory factors. *Am J Med*. 1974;57(3):402-420.

27. Zwillich CW, Sutton FD, Pierson DJ, Greagh EM, Weil JV. Decreased hypoxic ventilatory drive in the obesity-hypoventilation syndrome. *Am J Med*. 1975;59(3):343-348.

28. Murray J, Nadel J. *Textbook of Respiratory Medicine*. Philadelphia, PA: Saunders; 1994.

29. Walkey AJ, Farber HW, O'Donnell C, Cabral H, Eagan JS, Philippides GJ. The accuracy of the central venous blood gas for acid-base monitoring. *J Intensive Care Med*. 2010;25(2):104-110.

30. Helmholz HF Jr. The abbreviated alveolar air equation. *Chest*. 1979;75(6):748.

31. Kregenow DA, Rubenfeld GD, Hudson LD, Swenson ER. Hypercapnic acidosis and mortality in acute lung injury. *Crit Care Med*. 2006;34(1):1-7.

32. Hyzy RC, Hidalgo J. Permissive hypercapnia. In: Post TW, ed. *UpToDate*. Waltham, MA: UpToDate Inc. http://www.uptodate.com. Accessed May 7, 2017.

33. Tuxen DV. Permissive hypercapnic ventilation. *Am J Respir Crit Care Med*. 1994;150(3):870-874.

34. Donahoe M. Nutritional support in advanced lung disease. The pulmonary cachexia syndrome. *Clin Chest Med*. 1997; 18(3):547-561.

35. Krapf R, Jaeger P, Hulter HN. Chronic respiratory alkalosis induces renal PTH-resistance, hyperphosphatemia and hypocalcemia in humans. *Kidney Int*. 1992;42(3):727-734.

36. Krapf R, Beeler I, Hertner D, Hulter HN. Chronic respiratory alkalosis. The effect of sustained hyperventilation on renal regulation of acid-base equilibrium. *N Engl J Med*. 1991; 324(20):1394-1401.

37. Camara-Lemarroy CR, Rodríguez-Gutiérrez R, Monreal-Robles R, González-González JG. Acute toluene intoxication—clinical presentation, management and prognosis: a prospective observational study. *BMC Emerg Med*. 2015;15:19.

38. Spalding CT, Briones F, Tzamaloukas AH. Outcomes of severe methanol intoxication treated with hemodialysis: report of seven cases and review of literature. *Hemodial Int*. 2002;6(1):20-25.

39. Manuchehri AA, Alijanpour E, Daghmechi M, et al. A case of methanol poisoning leading to prolonged respirator dependency with consequent blindness and irreversible brain damage. *Caspian J Intern Med*. 2015;6(3):180-183.

40. Lepik KJ, Levy AR, Sobolev BG, et al. Adverse drug events associated with the antidotes for methanol and ethylene glycol poisoning: a comparison of ethanol and fomepizole. *Ann Emerg Med*. 2009;53(4):439-450.e10.

41. Singh R, Arain E, Buth A, Kado J, Soubani A, Imran N. Ethylene glycol poisoning: an unusual cause of altered mental status and the lessons learned from management of the disease in the acute setting. *Case Rep Crit Care*. 2016;2016:9157393.

42. Erickson HL. Case report of a fatal antifreeze ingestion with a record high level and impressive renal crystal deposition. *Case Rep Crit Care*. 2016;2016:3101476.

43. Schoen JC, Cain MR, Robinson JA, Schiltz BM, Mannenbach MS. Adolescent presents with altered mental status and elevated anion gap after suicide attempt by ethylene glycol ingestion. *Pediatr Emerg Care.* 2016;32(10):688-690.

44. Quintero Parra N, Wurgaft Kirberg A, Orellana Araya Y, Arellano Lorca J, Rojas Wettig L, Pefaur Penna J. Haemodialysis management for salicylate intoxication. *Nefrologia.* 2009;29(2):182-183.

45. Farid H, Wojcik MH, Christopher KB. A 19-year-old at 37 weeks gestation with an acute acetylsalicylic acid overdose. *NDT Plus.* 2011;4(6):394-396.

46. Musumba CO, Pamba AO, Sasi PA, English M, Maitland K. Salicylate poisoning in children: report of three cases. *East Afr Med J.* 2004;81(3):159-163.

47. Sawaya BP, Briggs JP, Schnermann J. Amphotericin B nephrotoxicity: the adverse consequences of altered membrane properties. *J Am Soc Nephrol.* 1995;6(2):154-164.

48. Kalantar-Zadeh K, Uppot RN, Lewandrowski KB. Case records of the Massachusetts General Hospital. Case 23-2013. A 54-year-old woman with abdominal pain, vomiting, and confusion. *N Engl J Med.* 2013;369(4):374-382.

49. Neal MD, McDaniel LM, Forsythe RM. Chapter 7: Massive transfusions and coagulopathy. In: Tisherman SA, Forsythe RM, eds. *Trauma Intensive Care (Pittsburgh Critical Care Medicine).* New York, NY: Oxford University Press; 2013;73-84.

50. Li K, Xu Y. Citrate metabolism in blood transfusions and its relationship due to metabolic alkalosis and respiratory acidosis. *Int J Clin Exp Med.* 2015;8(4):6578-6584.

Electrolyte Disorders

*Sergio Obligado, MD, Romeo Quilitan, MD, Eduardo Pinto, MD,
Dulya Santikul, DO, Blesit George, DO, and Steven Grundfast, MD*

INTRODUCTION

Critically ill patients have disturbances in multiple organ systems and hence are at risk for serious imbalances in electrolyte and water handling. Electrolyte disorders are extremely prevalent in the ICU: Hyponatremia can be found in 18% of ICU patients,[1] hypokalemia in 21%,[2] hypomagnesemia in more than 50%,[3] hypocalcemia in 20%,[4] and hypophosphatemia in 28%.[5] This chapter will outline these disturbances with an emphasis on pathophysiology and treatment of electrolyte problems more commonly seen in the intensive care unit.

SODIUM DISORDERS

Plasma sodium (Na) concentration is the principal determinant of the relative volume of extracellular fluid.[6] It is the major extracellular solute, whereas potassium is the major intracellular solute. Total solute activity, also called osmotic activity and expressed in osmoles (osm), is the sum of the individual osmotic activities of all the solute particles in the solution. For monovalent ions, the osmotic activity in milliosmoles (mOsm) per unit volume is equivalent to the concentration of the ions in milliequivalents (mEq) per unit volume.

Example: Osmotic activity in isotonic saline (0.9% NaCl)

0.9% NaCl = 154 mEq Na/L + 154 mEq Cl/L = 308 mOsm/L

Osmolarity is the osmotic activity per volume of solution, whereas osmolality is the osmotic activity per kilogram of water (mOsm/kg H_2O). Osmolality is used to describe the osmotic activity of body fluids. Since the weight of body fluids is basically equal to the weight of water, there is little difference between osmolality and osmolarity of body fluids. The effective osmolality or osmotic activity in 2 solutions is called tonicity. Water passes from the solution of lower osmotic activity to the solution of higher osmotic activity. The tendency for water to move into and out of cells is determined by the relative tonicity of intracellular and extracellular fluids. Because of the ability of water to pass freely across membranes, the intracellular and extracellular space have equivalent osmolality, normally about 280 mOsm/kg (Fig. 2-1). However, the intracellular space comprises a larger percentage of total body water (about 60%).

Urea is freely permeable across cell membranes. An increase in the urea concentration in extracellular fluid increases the osmolality of the extracellular fluid but does not increase the tonicity of the extracellular fluid or cause a net movement of water out of cells. Azotemia (increase in blood urea nitrogen [BUN]) is a hyperosmotic condition but not a hypertonic condition.

Major solutes in extracellular fluid include sodium, chloride, glucose, and urea. Plasma osmolality is estimated by the following equation:

$$\text{Plasma Osmolality} = (2 \times Na) + Glucose/18 + BUN/2.8$$
$$= (2 \times 140) + 90/18 + 14/2.8$$
$$= 290 \text{ mOsm/kg } H_2O$$

Solutes other than sodium, chloride, glucose, and urea are present in extracellular fluid, so measured plasma osmolality will be greater than calculated plasma osmolality; this osmolar gap is normally as much as 10 mOsm/kg H_2O. An increase in the osmolar gap occurs when certain toxins (ethanol, methanol, ethylene glycol, or unidentified toxins that accumulate in renal failure) are in the extracellular fluid.

Hyponatremia

Most hyponatremic states, defined as Na less than 135 mEq/L, are secondary to hypotonic, low osmolality conditions and are classified based on extracellular fluid volume status. Intravascular volume is not easily measured, which necessitates clinical determination by history, physical exam, and laboratory results.[7] Three laboratory tests necessary in the workup of hyponatremia are serum osmolality, urine osmolality, and urine sodium.

Isotonic hyponatremia is defined as a serum osmolarity of 280 to 295 mOsm. The differential includes distinguishing pseudohyponatremia from hypertriglyceridemia, hyperglobulinemia, and hyperproteinemia (> 10 g/dL). Hypertonic hyponatremia is defined as serum osmolarity of greater than 295 mOsm. The differential includes hyperglycemia,

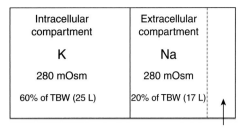

FIGURE 2-1 The relative volumes of intracellular and extracellular compartments of a 70-kg man. TBW = total body water.

mannitol, sorbitol, glycine, and intravenous immunoglobulin (IVIG). Hypotonic hyponatremia is defined as serum osmolarity of less than 280 mOsm.

Further characterization of hypotonic hyponatremia is dependent on evaluation of urine osmolality and urine sodium. Hypovolemic hypotonic hyponatremia is suggested by urine osmolality greater than 450 mOsm/kg. Urine sodium of less than 20 mEq/L suggests vomiting, diarrhea, third space loss, trauma, or sweating. Urine sodium greater than 20 mEq/L suggest diuretics, mineralocorticoid deficiency, salt wasting nephropathy, renal tubular acidosis, metabolic alkalosis, cerebral salt wasting syndrome, and osmotic diuresis. Hypervolemic hypotonic hyponatremia is suggested by urine osmolality of greater than 100 mOsm/kg. Urine sodium of less than 20 mEq/L or greater than 20 mEq/L if recently diuresed would suggest congestive heart failure (CHF), cirrhosis, nephrotic syndrome, low arterial volume, and low aldosterone. A urine osmolality greater than 100 mOsm/kg indicates impaired ability of the kidneys to dilute urine, usually secondary to elevated levels of antidiuretic hormone (ADH). Urine sodium is usually low due to secondary renal sodium conservation resulting from activation of the renin-angiotensin-aldosterone system despite total body volume overload. A urine sodium level greater than 20 mEq/L suggests renal failure.

Euvolemic hypotonic hyponatremia has a serum osmolarity of less than 280 mOsm and no edema. A urine osmolarity of greater than 100 mOsm/kg with a urine sodium level greater than 20 mEq/L suggests hypothyroidism, glucocorticoid deficiency, syndrome of inappropriate antidiuretic hormone secretion (SIADH), stress, or drug use. A urine osmolarity of less than 100 mOsm/kg with a urine sodium level less than 20 mEq/L suggests primary polydipsia and low solute intake like beer potomania.

Treatment of Hyponatremia

Treatment of hyponatremia is dependent on duration (acute [≤ 48 hours] versus chronic [> 48 hours]), symptoms, and severity. Hyponatremia is presumed chronic (unless there is clear evidence to the contrary), hence, cerebral symptoms ultimately determine the treatment of hyponatremia. Symptoms include headache, nausea, vomiting, fatigue, gait disturbance, confusion, seizures, obtundation, coma, and respiratory arrest. Mild hyponatremia (Na 130–134 mEq/L) generally requires a less aggressive therapeutic approach than severe hyponatremia (Na ≤ 120 mEq/L).[8-12] In most cases, the rate of rise of serum sodium should not exceed 0.5 mEq/L/h and should not exceed 8 mEq/L in any given 24-hour period, or 18 mEq/L in 48 hours.

Emergent treatment is warranted with neurologic symptoms, and the goal is to increase serum sodium rapidly by 4 to 6 mEq/L over a period of 3 to 4 hours. To raise the serum sodium by 1.5 mEq/L in men and 2 mEq/L in women, give a 100-cc bolus of 3% saline over 10 minutes. If neurologic symptoms persist or worsen, boluses can be repeated twice.[10-12] Plasma sodium should be checked in 2 to 3 hours initially and then every 3 to 4 hours until the patient is stable.

Correction begins with calculation of sodium deficit, as determined by the formula:

$$\text{Sodium Deficit (mEq)} = \text{Normal TBW} \times (\text{Goal P}_{Na} - \text{Current P}_{Na})$$

Normal total body water (TBW) is approximately 60% lean body weight of men and 50% lean body weight of women. A 3% sodium chloride solution contains 513 mEq of sodium per liter and a 0.9% sodium chloride solution contains 154 mEq of sodium per liter.

The rationale for the goals of treatment begins with osmolytes. Osmolytes are small molecules, such as glutamate and taurine, that can be synthesized or transported out of the cell to help prevent osmotic damage to neurons. Under osmotic stress (increases or decreases in serum sodium), neurons are capable of altering their solute concentrations by changing osmolyte concentration. Normally, during hyponatremia, osmolytes will be transported out of the cell to prevent water from diffusing into the neuron, thereby preventing an increase in cell volume. These protective mechanisms take time to occur. Astrocytes will take 24 to 48 hours to release sufficient osmolytes to restore cell volume to normal. However, loss of these osmolytes will leave the astrocyte susceptible to hypertonic injury. The rapid correction of hyponatremia will lead to apoptosis of astrocytes, causing osmotic demyelination.[8] This syndrome is associated with progressive quadriplegia, dysphagia, dysarthria, and alterations in consciousness that occur days after treatment. This underscores the need to correct chronic (occurring over > 48 hours) hyponatremia more slowly, whereas acute hyponatremia may be corrected more quickly since astrocytes have not had sufficient time to release osmolytes. Disease states that increase the risk of osmotic demyelination include alcoholism, liver failure, malignant disease, hypokalemia, serum sodium less than 120 mEq/L, and malnutrition.

There are no controlled trials validating overcorrection treatment strategies, although experimental studies in animals support that lowering serum sodium prevents osmotic demyelination.[13] In addition, a small series of patients with hyponatremia who have overcorrected has demonstrated that lowering serum sodium is well tolerated.[14] Expert panels recommend lowering serum sodium to goal levels for patients who are at high risk for osmotic demyelination and who have overcorrected at the 24-hour mark. They recommend that sodium should be lowered by replacing free water urinary losses with 5% dextrose in water (D5W) or by giving 2 to 4 μg of desmopressin intravenously (IV) every 8 hours with boluses of 3 mL/kg D5W over 1 hour and rechecking serum sodium after each bolus.[7] For patients with chronic hyponatremia in clinically euvolemic and hypervolemic states, vasopressin receptor antagonists can be utilized but must be initiated in the hospital setting. Conivaptan is a combined vasopressin 1a receptor (V1aR) and V2R receptor antagonist available only as IV formulation and initiated with a 20-mg bolus over 20 minutes and then 20 to 40 mg/day. Adverse effects include headache, thirst, and hypokalemia. It should not be used for more than 4 days because of drug-interaction effects with other medications metabolized by the hepatic CYP3A4 enzymes.[7] Tolvaptan, an oral V2R antagonist, is initiated at 15 mg and then titrated to a maximum of 60 mg/day if the sodium level remains less than 135 mEq/L. Side effects include dry mouth, increased urinary frequency, thirst, dizziness, and orthostatic hypotension.

Vaptans are not indicated for hypovolemic hyponatremia because simple volume expansion would be expected to increase sodium levels secondary to decreased vasopressin release and resultant aquaresis. In addition, these agents will likely not be effective in patients with a creatinine level greater than 2.5 mg/dL. They should be avoided in patients with underlying liver disease or cirrhosis due to the potential of inducing further liver injury. In 1 trial of polycystic kidney disease patients treated with tolvaptan, a significant number of patients developed elevations of the liver enzyme alanine aminotransferase (ALT) of 3 times normal levels.[7]

Hypernatremia

Hypernatremia, defined as a sodium concentration greater than 145 mEq/L, commonly occurs secondary to free water loss in excess of sodium loss. This can be seen in diabetes insipidus, from hypotonic fluid losses such as those that occur in gastrointestinal loss secondary to osmotic diarrhea, or in osmotic diuresis.[15] Rarely, it can occur because of excessive sodium intake in relation to free water intake (usually iatrogenic). The state of intravascular volume can be used as a reflection of the state of extracellular volume.

Patients with acute hypernatremia can exhibit symptoms that include lethargy, weakness, irritability, seizures, and coma. In those with chronic hypernatremia, lasting more than 48 hours, fewer symptoms occur because of osmotic adaptation.

Signs of hypernatremia are usually exhibited as volume depletion and include dry mucous membranes, decreased skin turgor, postural hypotension, and jugular venous pressure less than 5 cm H_2O. In patients with heart failure taking loop diuretics, signs of volume expansion can be seen, including peripheral edema and pulmonary edema.

Treatment of Hypernatremia

It is important to remember that all patients with hypovolemia, regardless of serum sodium concentration, should be administered isotonic crystalloid solutions first to improve tissue perfusion. After hypovolemia is corrected with isotonic fluids (normal saline or lactated Ringer solution), the next step is to calculate and replace the free water deficit using the following formula:

$$\text{Current TBW} \times \text{Current } P_{Na} = \text{Normal TBW} \times \text{Normal } P_{Na}$$
$$\text{Current TBW} = \text{Normal TBW} \times (140/\text{Current } P_{Na})$$

Normal TBW is usually 60% of lean body weight in men and 50% of lean body weight in women. However, in hypernatremia associated with free water deficits, normal TBW should be approximately 10% less than usual:

$$\text{TBW Deficit (L)} = \text{Normal TBW} - \text{Current TBW}$$

In patients with hypovolemic hypernatremia, free water deficits should be replaced slowly, over 48 to 72 hours, to prevent cerebral edema. Generally, one-half of TBW deficit is replaced in the first 24 hours and the rest over the next 48 hours. Replacement should include insensible water losses, and frequent monitoring of sodium and other electrolytes should be performed over the first 24 hours.

POTASSIUM DISORDERS

Ninety-eight percent of potassium is located intracellularly, with 2% found extracellularly. This large gradient is a major determinant for setting the thresholds of cellular action potentials, mainly in the cardiac and neuromuscular cells.[16] Maintaining a distribution of potassium in the extracellular fluid within the narrow margin of 3.5 to 5.5 mEq/L is critical for normal cell function.[17] This homeostasis is maintained by the sodium-potassium—adenosine triphosphatase (Na-K-ATPase) pump in the cell membrane,[18] and the total body potassium content is primarily preserved by the kidneys (Fig. 2-2). Disruption of renal function or the action of the Na-K-ATPase pump can lead to hyperkalemia or hypokalemia.

Hyperkalemia

The approach to evaluating a patient with hyperkalemia requires evaluation of each of the following possibilities:

- laboratory error and pseudohyperkalemia
- potassium shift from intracellular to extracellular
- decreased renal excretion of potassium

An electrocardiogram (ECG) is recommended as soon as a hyperkalemia is suspected.[16] As hyperkalemia worsens, impulse generation is suppressed, resulting in bradycardia, conduction blocks, and ultimately cardiac arrest.[19]

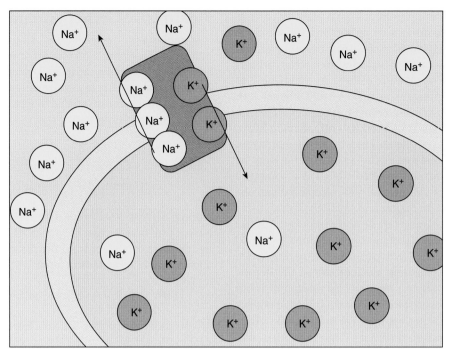

FIGURE 2-2 The sodium-potassium–adenosine triphosphatase (Na-K-ATPase) pump. Three sodium ions are moved out of the cell while 2 potassium ions are moved intracellularly. Adenosine triphosphate hydrolysis is required for each action of the pump. The result is a slightly negative intracellular charge and slightly positive extracellular charge.

Pseudohyperkalemia is an elevation in the measured serum potassium concentration due to potassium movement out of the cells (in vitro) without the true effect on cells.[20] This should be suspected when there is no obvious cause for hyperkalemia in an asymptomatic patient who has no electrocardiographic manifestations of hyperkalemia. Examples of pseudohyperkalemia include prolonged specimen storage, hemolysis during venipuncture, repeated fist clenching and a tight tourniquet, thrombocytosis, and leukemoid reaction with white blood cell (WBC) count greater than 50×10^3/mL.[18]

Potassium shift from the intracellular to extracellular compartment can be seen in insulin deficiency, metabolic acidosis, β-adrenergic antagonists, drugs that inhibit Na-K-ATPase, and hyperkalemic periodic paralysis. Acute cell tissue breakdown (eg, tumor lysis syndrome, rhabdomyolysis, or massive transfusion) causes potassium to be released into the extracellular space.[21,22]

Decreased renal excretion of potassium can be due simply to fall in glomerular filtration rate (GFR), which leads to decreased glomerular filtration of potassium, and hence reduced excretion. Even if GFR remains normal, potassium excretion may be reduced considerably if potassium secretion is impaired at the cortical collecting duct. At this section of the tubule, sodium diffuses through the electroneutral sodium channel (ENaC) and down its concentration gradient. Potassium will then diffuse out of the cell, down its concentration gradient, and into the tubule lumen, in order to maintain electroneutrality (Fig. 2-3). Processes that interfere with this sodium-potassium transport cause hyperkalemia as well; examples of this are an impaired renin-aldosterone axis

(eg, caused by angiotensin-converting enzyme [ACE] inhibitors and spironolactone), inhibition of ENaC function (caused by amiloride), and decreased distal tubular sodium delivery and urine flow (in acute kidney injury [AKI] and CHF).[22] Table 2-1 outlines common medications that cause hyperkalemia.

Clinical Manifestations of Hyperkalemia

Clinical effects of mild to moderate hyperkalemia are usually nonspecific and may include generalized weakness, fatigue, paresthesia, nausea, vomiting, intestinal colic, and diarrhea. Severe hyperkalemia may lead to life-threatening conditions such as cardiac blocks/arrhythmias and muscle weakness/paralysis.[21]

The ECG changes that occur with hyperkalemia are relatively characteristic and can sometimes point to hyperkalemia as etiology of symptoms before laboratory results are available. However, studies have shown that the ECG may not be sensitive to the severity of hyperkalemia in chronic cases.[23] In general, the progression of ECG follows a pattern:[24]

1. Shortened QT and peaked T waves
2. Progressive lengthening of PR and QRS
3. Disappearance of P wave and development of a sine-wave pattern

In general, alterations in T-wave morphology and QT shortening occur when the serum potassium is above 6, whereas progressive lengthening of PR and QRS occur at higher serum potassium levels (> 7 mEq/L). However, one cannot predict ECG changes based on a given serum potassium level[23,25] (and vice versa), as other factors affect cardiac conduction, such as

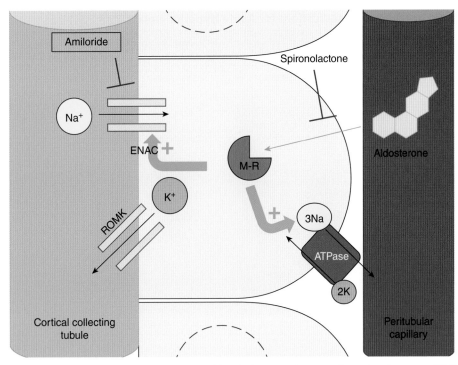

FIGURE 2-3 Aldosterone diffuses across the cell membrane and binds the cytosolic mineralocorticoid receptor (M-R). Aldosterone binding to M-R leads to an increase in the number of open electroneutral sodium channels (ENaC) and increased activity of the sodium-potassium–adenosine triphosphatase (Na-K-ATPase) pump. Potassium diffuses into the tubule via a renal outer membrane potassium (ROMK) channel.

associated hypocalcemia and hypomagnesemia. Patients with end-stage renal disease (ESRD) and chronic kidney disease (CKD) are less likely to manifest ECG changes with hyperkalemia, as it is thought that they manifest tolerance to hyperkalemia.[26] In any event, the sign-wave pattern is an ominous sign and it will progress to asystole if not treated.

TABLE 2-1 Medications That Commonly Cause Hyperkalemia

Mechanism	Medication
Potassium release from cells	• Beta-blockers • Digitalis (overdose) • Succinylcholine • Aminocaproic acid • Isoflurane
Inhibition of aldosterone production	• ACE inhibitors • Angiotensin receptor blockers • NSAIDs • Aliskiren (renin inhibitor) • Heparin • Calcineurin inhibitors
Inhibition or antagonism of effects of aldosterone	• Spironolactone • Eplerenone • Amiloride • Triamterene • Trimethoprim • Pentamidine

ACE = angiotensin-converting enzyme; NSAIDs = nonsteroidal anti-inflammatory drugs.

Treatment of Hyperkalemia

Hyperkalemia can be classified into the following 3 categories:[16]

- mild: K^+ = 5.5–6.5 mEq/L;
- moderate: K^+ more than 6.5–7.5 mEq/L; and
- severe: K^+ more than 7.5 mEq/L.

Treatment of hyperkalemia consists of 3 main steps (summarized in Table 2-2):[18]

1. Stabilizing the cardiac membrane
2. Shifting potassium from extra- to intracellular space
3. Removing potassium from the body

First, intravenous calcium is given if there are ECG changes, in order to stabilize the myocardial cell membrane by antagonizing excitation.[16,21] Intravenous calcium is recommended in any patient with ECG changes or symptoms of hyperkalemia (muscle weakness or paralysis), or if potassium is 6.5 mEq/L or higher.[26] Second, therapy should be given to shift potassium from extracellular to intracellular space in any patient with moderate to severe hyperkalemia (or ECG changes). Insulin with or without glucose and β_2-adrenergic agonists (eg, salbutamol/albuterol) decrease serum potassium by stimulating the Na-K-ATPase pump, shifting potassium intracellularly in exchange for sodium.[22] β_2-Adrenergic stimulants combined with insulin have been shown to have an additive effect and also have been shown to reduce the incidence of insulin-induced hypoglycemia.[27,18] Sodium bicarbonate, which causes a mild shift of potassium into cells due

TABLE 2-2 Summary of Treatment Medications for Acute Hyperkalemia[26,31]

Agent	Effect	Dose	Onset of Action	Duration of Treatment	Adverse Effect
Calcium gluconate (10% solution)	Stabilizes cell membrane	1 g IV over 10 min	Immediate	60 min, can be repeated	Arrhythmia
Regular insulin	Intracellular shift	10 units IV push (with 25 g of dextrose unless glucose ≥ 250)	20 min	Lasts 4–6 h	Hypoglycemia within 1 h is very common (up to 75% of patients)
Albuterol	Intracellular shift	10 to 20 mg in 4 mL of saline by nebulization over 10 min	30 min	60 min	Tachycardia, arrhythmia
Sodium bicarbonate	Intracellular shift	150 mEq in 1 L of 5% dextrose in water over 2–4 h	Hours		Volume overload
Furosemide	Renal excretion	40 mg every 12 h (may need to add saline if patient is not in heart failure)	15 min	6 h	Volume depletion, worsening azotemia
Sodium polystyrene sulfonate	GI excretion	15–30 g PO every 4–6 h	Unpredictable	Hours	Intestinal necrosis

GI = gastrointestinal; IV = intravenous; PO = orally.

to a rise in systemic pH, is preferably given to patients who are acidotic. In hemodialysis patients with hyperkalemia, it has only a moderate effect if given as prolonged infusion.[22] Overall, the efficacy of sodium bicarbonate for treatment of acute hyperkalemia is of modest benefit at most.

Third, total body potassium is reduced by other methods. In patients with normal to moderately impaired renal function, loop or thiazide diuretics can be used to increase renal excretion of potassium.[18] Gastrointestinal cation exchange resins, such as sodium polystyrene sulfonate (SPS), bind potassium in the gastrointestinal tract in exchange for other cations, such as sodium or calcium. The efficacy of SPS in the treatment of hyperkalemia has been debated. A recent retrospective study suggests that SPS is effective in reducing potassium by 1 mEq/L but is associated with intestinal necrosis.[22,28] Earlier studies have suggested that sorbitol or sorbitol mixed with SPS causes intestinal necrosis.[23-27] Recent animal study have suggested SPS can cause intestinal necrosis alone.[28] Despite this, SPS is still used in persistent hyperkalemia if a newer cation exchange resin such as patiromer is unavailable, other methods have failed to improve, and renal function is not restored. Patients in the postoperative setting and/or those who have gastrointestinal ileus or underlying bowel disease (eg, infection with *Clostridium difficile*) are at higher risk for intestinal necrosis and should not receive SPS. Patiromer is a newer cation exchange resin that has been studied for use in CKD patients with chronic hyperkalemia; it has not yet been studied for acute therapy of hyperkalemia, so it cannot be recommended for treatment of acute hyperkalemia.[29] Renal replacement therapy (RRT) is the definitive treatment in severe hyperkalemia. Any patient with persistent hyperkalemia despite appropriate interventions described above should be initiated on hemodialysis. In addition, patients with severe AKI (creatinine 2–3 times baseline or oliguria) should be considered for urgent hemodialysis.[26] Intermittent hemodialysis provides a substantially higher potassium clearance than continuous forms of RRT.[22] Rebound hyperkalemia, due to extracellular shift of potassium from the intracellular compartment, can occur in 30% of patients an hour after intermittent hemodialysis, so repeat potassium should be checked a couple hours after completion of treatment.[30]

Hypokalemia

Hypokalemia is defined as a decreased level of potassium in the bloodstream (< 3.5 mEq/L). Hypokalemia generally occurs because of 1 of the following mechanisms:

- poor oral intake,
- intracellular potassium shift,
- gastrointestinal losses, or
- urinary losses.

Increased entry of potassium into the cell can lead to hypokalemia, although these effects are usually temporary and are most prominent in patients who are already deficient in total body potassium. As discussed above, insulin, albuterol, and dobutamine all increase the activity of the Na-K-ATPase pump and hence stimulate intracellular shift.[32] A rise in the extracellular pH will also lead to a fall in serum potassium levels; in general, this fall is typically mild and the serum potassium concentration falls by less than 0.4 mEq/L for every 0.1 unit rise in pH.[31]

Severe hypokalemia due to intracellular shift can occur in patients with hypokalemic periodic paralysis, which is a rare disorder characterized by recurrent muscle paralysis due to hypokalemia. Hypokalemic periodic paralysis typically is inherited in families, passed down in an autosomal dominant pattern. It can also be acquired in association with thyrotoxicosis. The paralysis occurs when potassium moves intracellularly after a stimulus such as carbohydrate load or exercise. The patient manifests with weakness of extremities, more commonly of the proximal lower extremity muscles (although upper extremities may be affected as well) and hyporeflexia. In between attacks, the neurologic exam is typically normal. The hypokalemia during these attacks can be severe; serum potassium levels may drop as low as 1.5 to 2 mEq/L.[33] The exact pathogenesis of the disease is not clear, but in most cases of familial disease (70%), the mutation is in the gene that encodes the dihydropyridine-sensitive calcium channel in skeletal muscle. When the etiology is thyrotoxicosis, the mechanism of intracellular shift is increased sensitivity of Na-K-ATPase to catecholamine. Untreated, potassium tends to return to normal in 6 to 24 hours and paralysis resolves.[33]

Other etiologies of hypokalemia are a poor oral intake of potassium, or gastrointestinal and urinary losses. Poor oral intake of potassium alone rarely causes hypokalemia, mainly because the kidney has the ability to reduce urinary potassium excretion to 5 to 25 mEq/day if necessary. Usually, another cause of hypokalemia (such as volume depletion) will compound poor oral intake, which will exacerbate hypokalemia.[33]

Gastrointestinal losses as seen in diarrhea (either infectious, secretory, or osmotic) or vomiting will lead to hypokalemia. Under normal physiologic conditions, only 5 to 10 mEq of potassium are lost in stool. However, acute or chronic diarrhea can cause significant potassium losses in the stool; in severe diarrhea, such as villous adenoma or cholera states, a patient can lose over 100 mEq of potassium per day from the stool. In contrast, vomitus doesn't contain a lot of potassium (only 5–10 mEq/L). The high hydrogen and chloride losses in the gastric fluid lead to an increased filtered bicarbonate load at the glomerulus. Hence, bicarbonate reabsorption is overwhelmed in the proximal tubule; the result is increased sodium and bicarbonate delivery to the cortical collecting tubule. The volume depletion associated with vomiting activates the renin-angiotensin-aldosterone system and causes aggressive sodium reabsorption at the cortical collecting duct and associated potassium excretion, accompanied by bicarbonate as the nonabsorbable anion.

Urinary losses of potassium are seen in increased mineralocorticoid activity (either from primary or secondary hyperaldosteronism), and from urinary potassium secretion at the cortical collecting duct. The hypokalemia that accompanies diuretic therapy is again primarily due to increased delivery of sodium to the distal nephron where aldosterone activates the electroneutral sodium channel (and resultant potassium secretion by the renal outer medullary potassium [ROMK] channel). See Figure 2-4 and Figure 2-5 for summaries of diuretic effects on the nephron. Please note that although loop diuretics do indeed inhibit the Na-K-2Cl channel of the thick ascending limb, the major mechanism of hypokalemia is the increased delivery of sodium to that aldosterone-sensitive portion of the nephron. The mechanism for

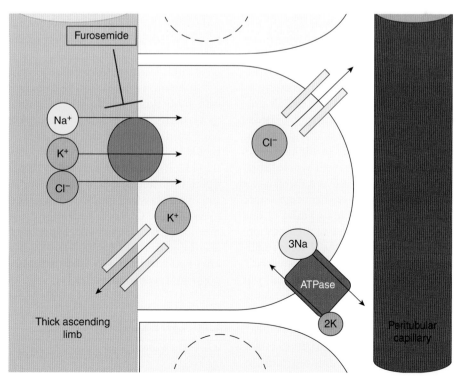

FIGURE 2-4 Thick ascending limb and loop sensitive Na-K-2Cl cotransporter. Bartter syndrome is due to mutation of this cotransporter and inhibited by furosemide.

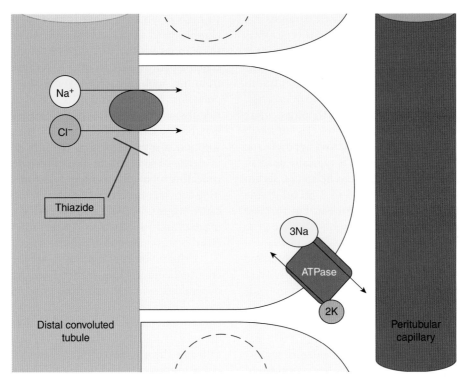

FIGURE 2-5 Distal convoluted tubule and thiazide-sensitive Na-Cl cotransporter. The same cotransporter that is inhibited by thiazides is also the channel that is mutated in Gitelman syndrome.

hypokalemia for the genetic disorders of Bartter and Gitelman syndromes is identical to the mechanism for diuretic use.[33]

Clinical Manifestations

Clinical manifestations occur with hypokalemia usually at a level less than 3 mEq/L. Weakness usually begins in the lower extremities and spreads to the trunk and upper extremities.[32] Severe potassium depletion can lead to muscle cramps, rhabdomyolysis, and myoglobinuria.[34,35] A variety of arrhythmias may be seen in patients with hypokalemia. These include premature atrial and ventricular beats, sinus bradycardia, paroxysmal atrial or junctional tachycardia, atrioventricular block, and ventricular tachycardia or fibrillation.[33] In addition, electrocardiogram abnormalities often are seen with hypokalemia. The earliest ECG changes associated with hypokalemia are a decrease in the T wave amplitude and ST-segment depression. With more profound hypokalemia (potassium < 3 mEq/L), one can expect T-wave inversions, with PR interval prolongation, widening QRS complex, and an increase in the U-wave amplitude (a U wave is described as a positive deflection after the T wave, best seen in V_2 and V_3).[36] There is certainly variability in the relationship between ECG changes and serum potassium levels; however, 90% of patients with a potassium less than 2.7 mEq/L will manifest some ECG evidence of hypokalemia.[33]

Treatment of Hypokalemia

The initial treatment is to replace the potassium deficit and to correct the underlying cause. The correlation between total body potassium deficit and serum potassium varies significantly between patients and is in part due to alteration in distribution of potassium across the membrane. As discussed above, acidemia, hyperglycemia, catecholamine surges, and periodic paralysis can alter potassium movement across the cell membrane. In chronic hypokalemia, one can assume that for every 1 mEq/L fall in serum potassium, there is a potassium deficit of at least 200 mEq.[33] It is important to monitor potassium closely while correcting to prevent overcorrection.

Potassium chloride can be given intravenously in patients who have symptomatic and/or more severe hypokalemia (potassium < 3 mEq/L). In addition, patients who have underlying cardiac disease and have higher risk for arrhythmia should be treated more aggressively, even if the hypokalemia is mild.[37] It can be administered as 10 mEq IV if given through a peripheral line, and 20 mEq IV doses if given through a central line. Potassium should be replaced orally in cases of mild hypokalemia. Of note, patients with gastrointestinal losses may also have concomitant hypomagnesemia which should also be corrected aggressively. Potassium-sparing diuretics are usually restricted to those patients who are refractory to potassium supplementation.

CALCIUM DISORDERS

In adults, 99% of the total body calcium (Ca) is sequestered in the skeleton, in the form of hydroxyapatite ($Ca_{10}[PO4]_6[OH]_2$). The remaining 1% of total body calcium can be found in plasma, extracellular fluid, and intracellular space. About 40% of serum

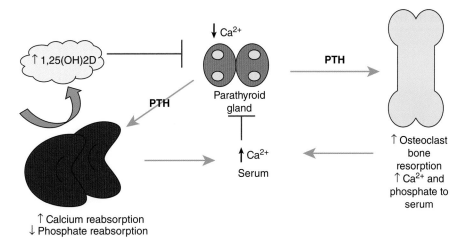

FIGURE 2-6 Effect of parathyroid hormone (PTH) on calcium and phosphorous handling by bone and kidney. Low serum calcium stimulates PTH secretion from the parathyroid gland. PTH has stimulatory effects on calcium resorption in bone and calcium reabsorption by kidney. PTH also stimulates production of 1,25-dihydroxyvitamin D (1,25[OH]2D), which in turn inhibits PTH release.

calcium is bound to albumin (varies depending on pH), 50% is ionized and biologically active, and the remaining 10% is complexed to other anions like citrate and phosphate.[38,39] Free ionized calcium is necessary for bodily function such as muscle contraction, nerve conduction, and blood coagulation. Because calcium is highly protein bound, serum albumin levels need to be considered when interpreting serum calcium measurements. A measured serum calcium that is low may not accurately represent a low ionized calcium. At the bedside, an estimate of "adjusted serum calcium" can be done with the following formula:

$$\text{Adjusted Total Ca}^{2+} = \text{Measured Total Ca}^{2+} + [0.8 \times (4 - \text{Measured Serum Albumin})]$$

If any question remains regarding actual ionized Ca^{2+}, then ionized calcium should be measured. It should be noted that disturbances in pH, and other circulating chemicals such as citrate, phosphate, and paraprotein can influence total serum calcium and are not factors in the above equation. The extracellular fluid maintains ionized calcium concentration within a tight range via an interplay of 3 hormones that act on specific cells in the bone, gut, and kidney (Fig. 2-6).

The parathyroid gland detects ionized plasma calcium via the calcium-sensing receptor (CaSR), which is stimulated by low calcium concentrations, and leads to release of parathyroid hormone (PTH).[38] Parathyroid hormone mobilizes calcium (and phosphate) by stimulating bone resorption from osteoclast cells. It also enhances calcium reabsorption from the thick ascending limb and distal convoluted tubules in the kidney. The other effect of PTH in the kidney is to stimulate conversion of 25-hydroxyvitamin D_3 (25[OH]D) to the active form, 1,25-dihydroxyvitamin D_3 (1,25[OH]2D) (Fig. 2-7). This activated form of vitamin D acts to increase calcium absorption by the transient receptor potential channel TRPV6 expressed in the small and large intestines. 1,25-vit D also appears to act on bone to mobilize calcium and

phosphate by increasing the number of mature osteoclasts. Calcitonin is also important in calcium regulation and is secreted by the thyroid gland to prevent bone resorption.

Hypocalcemia

The differential diagnosis of hypocalcemia is broad and can be categorized by deficiency of parathyroid hormone, deficiencies of vitamin D, medication use, or miscellaneous etiologies (Table 2-3). Both low and high serum magnesium states can cause hypocalcemia by functional hypoparathyroidism. The hypocalcemia induced by these states tends to be relatively mild and reversible.[38] Hypomagnesemia interferes with PTH receptor activation of intracellular secondary messenger systems that lead to target organ action when PTH binds. Severe hypomagnesemia also causes decreased PTH secretion. The major effect of hypomagnesemia leads to functional PTH resistance and prevents the normal physiologic response to hypocalcemia.

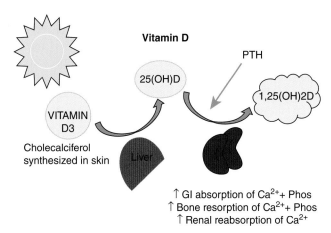

FIGURE 2-7 Metabolism of vitamin D. Activation of vitamin D_3 (vit D_3) requires adequate liver and kidney function in addition to parathyroid hormone (PTH) stimulation. 1,25(OH)2D = 1,25-dihydroxyvitamin D_3; 25(OH)D = 25-hydroxyvitamin D_3.

TABLE 2-3 Etiologies for Hypocalcemia

Disorders of inadequate parathyroid hormone (PTH) production
- Primary hypoparathyroidism (encompasses congenital and autoimmune etiologies)
  - PTH gene mutations
  - Constitutively active mutations of calcium-sensing receptor
  - Parathyroid gland mutations
- Postsurgical (following thyroidectomy) and postradiation
- Secondary to infiltrative diseases such as hemochromatosis and thalassemia, Wilson disease, and infiltrating tumor
- Hypermagnesemia
- Hypomagnesemia

Inadequate vitamin D production
- Nutritional deficiency, malabsorption
- Lack of sunlight exposure
- Cirrhosis
- Chronic kidney disease

PTH resistance
- Hypomagnesemia
- Pseudohypoparathyroidism

Vitamin D resistance (rickets)

Pseudohypocalcemia substances interfering with laboratory assay for total calcium
- Gadolinium

Hyperphosphatemia
- Hyperphosphatemia due to advanced chronic kidney disease
- Massive phosphate intake due to oral supplements and enemas
- Tumor lysis syndrome
- Rhabdomyolysis

Drug induced
- Intravenous bisphosphonate
- Foscarnet
- Imatinib

Acute pancreatitis

Rapid transfusion of blood products containing citrate

Saline-induced calciuresis

Hungry bone syndrome
- Post-thyroidectomy
- Postparathyroidectomy

On the other hand, hypermagnesemia mimics hypercalcemia and inhibits the CaSR, which in effect inhibits PTH release from parathyroid cells. Patients with pancreatitis can be extremely ill, and low serum calcium is commonly seen due to the precipitation of Ca^{2+}-containing salts in the inflamed pancreatic tissue. The severity of hypocalcemia in pancreatitis frequently correlates with severity of illness. Any situation in which acute hyperphosphatemia develops, such as acute or chronic kidney disease, tumor lysis syndrome, rhabdomyolysis, or ingestion of phosphate-containing laxatives, has the potential to cause hypocalcemia. In chronic kidney disease, there is an additional mechanism in that the kidney is unable to adequately convert 25(OH)D to 1,25(OH)2D. It is also important to consider the pseudohypocalcemia that occurs after administration of gadolinium-based contrast media. Gadolinium complexes with the calorimetric assays and interferes with measurement of serum calcium.[40] This effect will

usually be seen immediately after contrast administration and should resolve rapidly. In patients with CKD, where gadolinium excretion is prolonged, this spurious hypocalcemia may take longer to resolve. Measurement of ionized calcium will differentiate true from pseudohypocalcemia.

Clinical Manifestations of Hypocalcemia

Hypocalcemia presents with neuromuscular irritability and tetany. The spectrum of symptoms can be as mild as paresthesias of the hands and feet, muscle cramps, or perioral numbness. However, severe hypocalcemia can cause more dramatic symptoms such as laryngospasm, seizures (focal and generalized), or carpopedal spasm. It may also present with nonspecific symptoms such as irritability, fatigue, anxiety, confusion, hallucinations, and psychosis. Tetany usually occurs when serum ionized calcium falls below 4.3 mg/dL (total serum calcium of 7.0 mg/dL). Myocardial dysfunction also may occur due to prolongation of phase 2 of the action potential, which manifests as prolongation of the QTc interval. This increases risk of serious arrhythmias such as torsade de pointes (albeit at a lower rate than in hypomagnesemia and hypokalemia). Severity of clinical manifestations also depends on whether the hypocalcemia occurs acutely or gradually. Since calcium is mostly protein bound, the variation and severity of symptoms are also affected by conditions that increase or decrease protein binding. On physical examination, findings of neuromuscular irritability are manifested as Trousseau sign, which is the induction of carpopedal spasm brought about by inflation of a sphygmomanometer. Chvostek sign is elicited by tapping on the facial nerve, which causes contraction of the ipsilateral facial muscle. These physical findings may not always be sensitive enough to be elucidated in all patients with hypocalcemia.

Treatment of Hypocalcemia

Treatment of hypocalcemia is aimed at alleviating symptoms and maintaining an acceptable ionized calcium, without inducing calcium-phosphate precipitation or causing significant hypercalciuria[40] (Table 2-4). In patients with moderate to severe symptoms, intravenous calcium gluconate should be administered (1 g = 1 amp = 10 mL of 10% solution). Two grams of IV calcium gluconate can be infused slowly over 10 minutes, followed by a continuous infusion (usually 11 g of calcium in a 1-L D5W solution). Goals of therapy are to control symptoms, improve the QT interval, and keep the ionized calcium in the lower end of normal range. Ionized calcium should be monitored closely during infusion (every 4 hours).

For asymptomatic or mild hypocalcemia, oral therapy is more appropriate. Oral calcium supplements, in conjunction with vitamin D metabolites (ergocalciferol, calcitriol) are mainstays of therapy. In addition, given its hypocalciuric effect, thiazide diuretics can be used as well to maintain serum calcium. Calcium carbonate and calcium citrate are both appropriate oral supplements and should be administered in multiple doses, with meals, for maximum absorption. If hypoparathyroidism is an etiology of hypocalcemia, then

TABLE 2-4 Indications and Treatment of Hypocalcemia

Indications	Treatment
• Seizures, tetany, spasms • Prolonged QTc • Acute serum corrected calcium ≤ 7.5 mg/dL	• Calcium gluconate 1–2 g IV in 10–20 min to prevent cardiac arrest • Calcium chloride 1–2 g IV • Continuous calcium gluconate infusion in D5W and avoid concomitant bicarbonate or phosphate drips to prevent precipitation
• Paresthesias • Serum corrected calcium 7.5–8 mg/dL or ionized calcium 3–3.2 mg/dL	• Calcium carbonate or calcium citrate 1500–2000 mg PO daily in divided doses • If no improvement with symptoms or levels, can switch to IV
• Hypocalcemia and hypoparathyroidism	• Calcium with activated vitamin D (1,25[OH]2D) + recombinant PTH
• Hypocalcemia and hypomagnesemia	• Supplementation with magnesium in addition to calcium

1,25(OH)2D = 1,25-dihydroxyvitamin D$_3$; D5W = 5% dextrose in water; IV = intravenous; PO = orally; PTH = parathyroid hormone.

activated vitamin-D therapy (1,25[OH]2D) is important to use to improve oral absorption. Although vitamin D$_2$ (ergocalciferol) or vitamin D$_3$ (cholecalciferol) can also be used, it is important to note that in the presence of renal insufficiency or low PTH levels, these forms of vitamin D may not be converted to their more active metabolites. Magnesium deficiency needs to be treated with magnesium supplements as well if magnesium deficiency is contributing to hypocalcemia.

Hypercalcemia

In general, hypercalcemia occurs because of abnormal movement of calcium to the extracellular fluid from the GI tract, skeleton, or kidney. Factitious or artifactual hypercalcemia can occur when calcium is bound to serum proteins, increasing the total serum calcium, but the ionized calcium is normal. An example of this is seen in severe volume depletion and subsequent increase in serum albumin, which causes an increase in total serum calcium. An analogous situation has been described in Waldenstrom macroglobulinemia as well.[41]

When considering the etiology of hypercalcemia, it is important to differentiate between parathyroid-mediated hypercalcemia and nonparathyroid causes (Fig. 2-8). A PTH level above normal (> 70 pg/mL) makes parathyroid-mediated hypercalcemia the likely diagnosis. However, it should be noted that even a normal PTH level (> 35 pg/mL) in the setting of hypercalcemia represents loss of feedback suppression of PTH, and hence also suggests primary hyperparathyroidism as the likely etiology.[42] A PTH level that is suppressed (< 20 pg/mL) suggests a nonparathyroid-mediated hypercalcemia.

Hypercalcemia from parathyroid disease is common, although it typically does not cause severe hypercalcemia that leads to admission to an intensive care unit (ICU). Typically, symptoms are mild or completely asymptomatic. It is caused

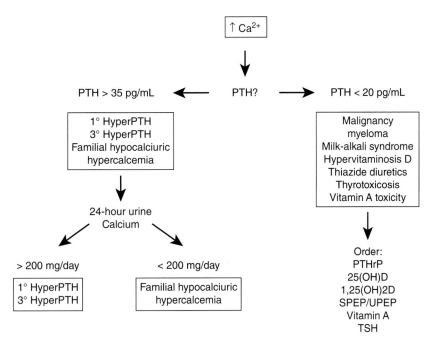

FIGURE 2-8 Initial workup of hypercalcemia. PTH = parathyroid hormone; PTHrP = parathyroid hormone–related protein; SPEP = serum protein electrophoresis; TSH = thyroid-stimulating hormone; UPEP = urine protein electrophoresis. (Reprinted with permission from Horwitz MJ, Hodak SP, Stewart AF. Non-parathyroid hypercalcemia. In: Rosen CJ, ed. *Primer on the Metabolic Bone Disease and Disorders of Mineral Metabolism.* 8th ed. Oxford, UK: Wiley-Blackwell; 2013: 562-571.).

TABLE 2-5 Nonparathyroid Causes of Hypercalcemia

Cancer
- Osteolytic hypercalcemia
- Humoral hypercalcemia of malignancy (parathyroid hormone–related protein)
- 1,25-vit D producing tumors (lymphoma)

Granulomatous disorders (also 1,25-vit D mediated)

Endocrine disorders
- Hyperthyroidism
- Pheochromocytoma
- Adrenal insufficiency

Milk-alkali syndrome

Medication induced
- Thiazide diuretics
- Vitamin D toxicity
- Vitamin A toxicity
- Lithium
- Foscarnet
- Teriparatide (recombinant human parathyroid hormone)
- Theophylline

End-stage liver disease

Chronic kidney disease (could be iatrogenic or due to parathyroid disease)

Immobility

by a benign solitary adenoma in 80% of cases (malignancy is the etiology in < 1% of cases).[43] Rarely, a patient with "acute parathyroid crisis" can cause severe symptoms, leading to hospitalization.

Nonparathyroid causes of hypercalcemia are diverse and are listed in Table 2-5. Malignancy causes hypercalcemia via various methods, namely via production of PTH-related protein (PTHrP; squamous carcinomas of any origin but most commonly breast and renal carcinomas), via local osteolytic metastases (breast cancer and myeloma), and via activation of 1,25(OH)2D (lymphoma). Of note, ectopic production of actual parathyroid hormone also has been described but is exceedingly rare.[41]

Iatrogenic hypercalcemia due to medications are an important cause of hypercalcemia. Hypercalcemia due to total parenteral nutrition administration has also been described, usually due to excessive administration of calcium in the solution. Thiazide diuretics increase distal convoluted tubule calcium reabsorption and commonly cause mild hypercalcemia. Lithium has also been shown to cause hypercalcemia in up to 5% of patients via multiple mechanisms. Chronic kidney disease patients are prone to hypercalcemia due to frequent use of activated vitamin D (calcitriol) as well as calcium-based phosphate binders.[41]

Clinical Manifestations of Hypercalcemia

Mild hypercalcemia is defined as serum calcium level of less than 12 mg/dL. Patients with this level of hypercalcemia may be asymptomatic, or they may have nonspecific symptoms

such as constipation and fatigue. Patients with moderate hypercalcemia, defined as serum calcium of 12 to 14 mg/dL, will manifest symptoms depending on how quickly the condition occurred. Patients may be asymptomatic or may experience polyuria, polydipsia, muscle weakness, or altered mental status. Severe hypercalcemia (serum calcium > 14 mg/dL) will usually have severe manifestations of the above symptoms.

Neuropsychiatric manifestations of hypercalcemia can be similar to symptoms of hypocalcemia: anxiety, depression, cognitive dysfunction, confusion, lethargy, stupor, and coma. Gastrointestinal symptoms such as constipation, anorexia, and nausea may occur.

Serum calcium persistently above 11 mg/dL induces nephrogenic diabetes insipidus due to decreased concentrating ability of the kidneys.[44] Chronic hypercalcemia also leads to nephrolithiasis formation due to prolonged hypercalciuria. Moderate hypercalcemia can lead to acute kidney injury from a fall in GFR mediated by renal vasoconstriction, as well as volume depletion from the above-mentioned diabetes insipidus.[45]

Elevated calcium can cause cardiovascular disease by shortening the myocardial action potential, which predisposes patients to dysrhythmias such as supraventricular tachycardia and ventricular tachycardia. Prolonged hypercalcemia predisposes patients to calcium deposition in the coronary arteries, heart valves, and myocardium.

Treatment of Hypercalcemia

Treatment of hypercalcemia is aimed at restoring optimal renal function to allow for renal clearance of calcium and treatment of the underlying disorder. In general, patients with moderate to severe hypercalcemia (> 12 mg/dL) tend to be volume depleted because of nephrogenic diabetes insipidus and require adequate volume expansion.[46,47] Normal saline should be administered liberally initially, with the addition of loop diuretics only when volume overload is evident. Saline-induced natriuresis causes increased calcium excretion (calciuresis); the addition of loop diuretics to further the calciuresis is of controversial benefit. Calcitonin can be effective initially to decrease serum calcium concentrations in patients with moderate to severe hypercalcemia. It increases urinary calcium excretion and inhibits bone resorption by interfering with osteoclasts. However, its effect tends to be short lived (48–72 hours) due to the development of tachyphylaxis.[48]

Treating the underlying condition is critical. If the mechanism of hypercalcemia is bone resorption due to humoral hypercalcemia or local bone metastases, then use of a bisphosphonate is important to interfere with osteoclast recruitment and function. Intravenous bisphosphonate therapy is highly effective for treatment of severe hypercalcemia.[48] The medications used most frequently are zoledronate and pamidronate. It is important to take into account 2 points when considering bisphosphonate therapy: First, bisphosphonates are cleared by the kidney and could potentially exacerbate renal failure in patients with significant kidney injury, and second, the onset of action is delayed for about 48 hours, so treatment with calcitonin and volume expansion is important initially. Of note, there are studies for the use of the RANKL inhibitor, denosumab, for hypercalcemia of malignancy, and it may be useful in patients with significant renal failure, as it is not known to worsen renal failure.[48]

If the etiology of the hypercalcemia is believed to be an activation of 1,25(OH)2D, as in granulomatous disease, then bisphosphonate therapy may not be as effective. Rather, steroids are more useful, as they decrease calcitriol production by mononuclear cells.

If the patient has severe hypercalcemia with life-threatening symptoms and renal failure refractory to therapy with saline and diuretics, then hemodialysis with a low calcium dialysate bath should be considered to treat hypercalcemia and azotemia.

PHOSPHATE DISORDERS

The majority of total body phosphorus (85%) is sequestered as bone in the form of hydroxyapatite crystals. Another 14% of phosphorus is stored within intracellular soft tissue, and the final 1% of remaining body phosphorus is found in serum. The intracellular and serum forms of phosphorus exist as a negatively charged phosphate ion, which is composed of a central phosphorus molecule and 4 oxygen molecules.[49,50] This form of phosphorus is what is measured in serum on standard laboratory tests. In serum, it exists in the forms of HPO_4^{2-}, $H_2PO_4^-$, and PO_4^{3-}; the ratio of these ions depends on serum pH, proteins, and other cations.[49] Although normal serum phosphate levels are only 2.5 to 4.5 mg/dL, it is also the major intracellular anion and has concentrations of 100 times that level within cells.

The primary determinants of serum phosphate levels are dietary phosphorus intake and renal phosphate excretion. An average diet consists of approximately 800 to 1200 g of phosphorus per day. This phosphorus is absorbed primarily in the jejunum by active $Na-PO_4$ transporters, which are stimulated by 1,25-vit D.[51] Ingested phosphorus is either sequestered by bone, moved into the intracellular compartment (stimulated by insulin), or excreted by the kidneys.[52] Under normal physiologic conditions, most of the phosphate filtered at the glomerulus is reabsorbed by the proximal tubule, and the remaining 5% to 20% is excreted. Parathyroid hormone stimulates internalization of the $Na-PO_4$ cotransporter from the tubular membrane, allowing more phosphate to be excreted.[53]

In general, PTH regulates serum calcium levels, with effects on phosphorus as a secondary effect (see Fig. 2-7). On the other hand, fibroblast growth factor (FGF) 23 primarily responds to serum phosphate levels and dietary phosphorus intake. Produced by osteoblasts and osteoclasts, it decreases expression of the $Na-PO_4$ cotransporter in the proximal tubule (allowing for more phosphorous excretion), inhibits 1,25-vit D production, and decreases PTH expression in the parathyroid glands. All the effects of FGF promote a decrease in serum phosphorous.[54]

Hyperphosphatemia

Hyperphosphatemia occurs due to acute phosphate load, impaired excretion, or movement of intracellular phosphate into the extracellular space. In general, hyperphosphatemia is accompanied by hypocalcemia due to calcium and phosphate precipitation in tissue.

Large extracellular shifts of phosphate occur after tissue injury, as in the case of rhabdomyolysis. Muscle injury causes release of phosphate, potassium, and myoglobin into the extracellular space. As myoglobin is filtered by the glomerulus, it causes tubular injury (heme pigment–induced nephropathy) and decreased GFR. Hence, phosphorous excretion becomes impaired, exacerbating hyperphosphatemia. Treatment of rhabdomyolysis centers around adequate volume resuscitation and attempts to induce polyuria to decrease intratubular myoglobin cast formation.[55] Saline should be administered aggressively (1–2 L/h initially to try to induce a diuresis); prospective studies with mannitol and bicarbonate have not been conclusively beneficial. Use of diuretics in pigment-induced nephropathy remains controversial as well.[56]

Tumor lysis syndrome is another example of massive extracellular movement of phosphate leading to hyperphosphatemia. Cytotoxic therapy leads to massive tumor cell death in cancer populations suffering from acute leukemia and high-grade lymphoma.[57] Subsequent cellular release of phosphorus and nucleic acids, which are subsequently metabolized to uric acid, deposit in the nephron and cause tubular injury. Since hypouricemic therapy is used prophylactically in high-risk patients, calcium phosphate deposition in the renal tubules (nephrocalcinosis) has become the major etiology for acute kidney injury in tumor lysis syndrome.[58]

It has been documented that extracellular shift of phosphate can also occur in severe lactic acidosis (primarily due to tissue cell death and subsequent release of phosphate).[59] Diabetic ketoacidosis (DKA) can occasionally cause hyperphosphatemia due to insulin deficiency and decreased cellular phosphate uptake. However, most patients with DKA are in a true state of total body phosphate depletion due to the prominent phosphaturia associated with osmotic diuresis.[60]

Oral intake of large amounts of phosphate-based laxative solutions (Fleet phospho soda) have been associated with hyperphosphatemia and associated nephrocalcinosis. These colonoscopy preparation solutions provide 11 g of phosphate (compared to 1 g associated with a normal diet). In the setting of volume depletion or CKD, acute phosphate nephropathy can develop.[61]

Either acute or chronic renal failure is associated with hyperphosphatemia due to a reduction in the filtered phosphate load (because of a reduced number of functioning nephrons). Once GFR falls to less than 20 cc/min, phosphate reabsorption is maximally suppressed (due to increase in PTH and FGF levels). At this point, serum phosphorus will rise, leading to a higher filtered phosphate by remaining nephrons.[54] Other less common causes of hyperphosphatemia include vitamin D toxicity, bisphosphonate use, and familial tumoral calcinosis.

Treatment of Hyperphosphatemia

The approach to treatment depends on whether hyperphosphatemia is acute or chronic. In acute hyperphosphatemia, initial treatment includes isotonic saline administration to increase phosphaturia, and limiting phosphate administration in parenteral and enteral feeds. Monitoring of the calcium phosphate product is important, as levels exceeding 60 mg^2/dL^2 is associated with calcium phosphate precipitation in the renal tubules and acute kidney injury.[62] This is particularly important in diseases such as tumor lysis syndrome, where hemodialysis can actually prevent further kidney injury. It has been recommended that dialysis is initiated when the calcium phosphorus product reaches 70 mg^2/dL^2.

For chronic hyperphosphatemia, as occurs in chronic kidney disease, treatment involves limiting dietary phosphate intake and decreasing GI absorption with oral phosphate binders. Calcium-based phosphate binders (calcium acetate and calcium carbonate) are effective for controlling phosphorus absorption, with the main side effect being hypercalcemia. Aluminum hydroxide, although extremely effective for short-term use, is avoided for chronic use due to the potential for aluminum toxicity.[63] Newer phosphate binders such as sevelamer and lanthanum can be used if hypercalcemia becomes problematic.

Hypophosphatemia

Hypophosphatemia has been estimated to occur in 2% of all hospitalized patients, but in up to 28% of ICU patients.[5] Usually, the etiology is decreased phosphorus ingestion due to disrupted dietary intake. This contrasts to the outpatient population, in which low serum phosphorus usually is a result of increased renal phosphate excretion (due to primary hyperparathyroidism and vitamin D deficiency).[54]

Hypophosphatemia is the key electrolyte abnormality in refeeding syndrome, which occurs due to increased cellular phosphate uptake when feeding is initiated in malnourished patients, alcoholics, and postoperative patients. Refeeding syndrome usually occurs within 2 to 5 days of introducing carbohydrates to a malnourished patient and is marked by severe hypophosphatemia and hypokalemia, as both of these electrolytes will move intracellularly in response to insulin secretion. Insulin stimulates intracellular glucose movement and synthesis of ATP and 2,3-diphosphoglycerate (2,3-DPG), which depletes the inorganic phosphate pools.[64,65] Inability to sufficiently provide these phosphorylated intermediates leads to tissue hypoxia, myocardial dysfunction, and respiratory failure. Most fatalities from refeeding syndrome are due to cardiac complications[53]; hypophosphatemia leads to reversible cardiac dysfunction, congestive heart failure, and even ventricular arrhythmia.[66] Several studies have shown that repletion of phosphorus in hypophosphatemic patients improves cardiac index and stroke volume.[67,68] Respiratory muscle dysfunction due to hypophosphatemia is a major concern as well, and failure to wean from a ventilator has been demonstrated in hypophosphatemic patients.[69,70] Other complications, such as

neurologic symptoms (tremors, paresthesias, delirium, and seizures) and rhabdomyolysis have been described.[70,71]

Drugs that cause intracellular shift of phosphate, such as catecholamines, epinephrine, and β-adrenergic receptor agonists, have all been implicated in reducing serum phosphate levels.[49] In addition, acetazolamide and theophylline can promote phosphaturia due to inhibition of renal phosphate reabsorption in the proximal tubule.[72,73]

Increased phosphate excretion in urine is well described in DKA as well. In addition, the obligatory treatment with insulin leads to intracellular movement of phosphate, which worsens hypophosphatemia, in a manner similar to the refeeding syndrome.[49]

Lastly, spurious hypophosphatemia and hyperphosphatemia have been described due to very high serum protein concentrations in patients with multiple myeloma. The high monoclonal protein concentration can interfere with the laboratory phosphate assay. Before intravenous phosphorous replacement is ordered in a patient with myeloma and asymptomatic hypophosphatemia, pseudo-hypophosphatemia has to be considered and serum deproteinization should be performed.[74,75]

Treatment of Hypophosphatemia

Given that moderate hypophosphatemia (serum phosphate 1–2.5 mg/dL) can theoretically affect respiratory function, ventilated patients should be treated aggressively with intravenous phosphate. In addition, for severe hypophosphatemia (serum phosphate < 1 mg/dL), intravenous therapy is always indicated. The recommended dose is 0.08 mmol/kg of body weight for acute hypophosphatemia and 0.16 mmol/kg for more chronic malnutrition states. Intravenous phosphorus can be safely administered over 2 to 6 hours.[76,77] However, given that intravenous phosphate therapy can cause acute hypocalcemia, patients with mild or moderate hypophosphatemia who are not in respiratory failure should be treated with oral phosphorus.[53]

MAGNESIUM DISORDERS

Serum magnesium represents 0.3% of the total amount of magnesium in the body. Magnesium is found in bone (53%), muscle (27%), and soft tissues (19%).[78] Most is ionized (62%), and the rest is either bound to protein, particularly albumin (33%), or forms complexes with citrate and phosphate (12%).[79] Most of the body's magnesium in the different compartments does not equilibrate easily, unlike other electrolytes.[80]

Absorption of magnesium through the gut varies according to the amount of magnesium in the diet. For example, a diet that has a magnesium content of 20 mEq/day is found to have a 42% rate of absorption. A low magnesium diet of 3 mEq/day shows a 79% absorption, while absorption decreased to 27% in the setting of a high magnesium diet of 53 mEq/day.[81] Magnesium is absorbed mainly through the ileum and jejunum.

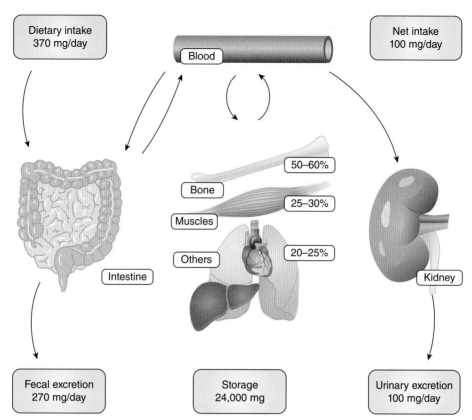

FIGURE 2-9 Magnesium homeostasis. (Reprinted with permission from Baaij JH, Hoenderop JG, Bindels, RJ. Magnesium in man: implications for health and disease. *Physiol Rev.* 2015;95:1-46.)

Mostly, the kidneys achieve magnesium homeostasis. Assuming that daily intake of magnesium is 370 mg, the intestines have a net absorption of 100 mg. The kidneys then filter 2400 mg, of which 2300 mg is reabsorbed by the renal tubules with, a net excretion of 100 mg, thereby matching the intestinal absorption. Figure 2-9 summarizes this graphically.

Magnesium plays a crucial role in many physiologic processes. It is a cofactor in more than 300 enzymatic reactions in energy metabolism and ATP synthesis. It is involved in hormone-receptor binding, calcium-channel function, muscle contraction, neuronal activity, cardiac excitability, vasomotor tone, and neurotransmitter release.[82] Derangements in body magnesium concentrations usually coexist with a secondary electrolyte disorder, and have clinical implications as well.

Most cases of hypomagnesemia are asymptomatic.[83] As mentioned above, the serum magnesium level represents less than 1% of the total body serum. This makes the diagnosis of hypomagnesemia difficult, as the level does not correlate well with body stores, and most cases are asymptomatic. Many have tried different ways of measuring magnesium that better reflect total body stores, including 24-hour urinary excretion of magnesium. This is inconvenient clinically as the specimen needs to be collected over 24 hours to account for circadian variations in excretion.

Hence, a normal serum level should not necessarily rule out the presence of total body magnesium deficits. Suspicion of magnesium deficiency should exist in cases where it is to be expected, particularly in cases of malnutrition, alcoholism, hypokalemia, and hypocalcemia.

Hypermagnesemia

Hypermagnesemia is an uncommon laboratory finding, especially in the absence of renal failure or magnesium ingestion. Symptomatic hypermagnesemia is even less common. This disorder has a low incidence of occurrence because the kidney is able to eliminate excess magnesium by rapidly reducing its tubular reabsorption to almost negligible amounts.

Hypermagnesemia is defined as serum levels greater than 2.2 mg/dL. Symptoms are uncommon until levels are above 4 to 6 mg/dL and may include nausea, vomiting, lethargy, headaches, flushing, and diminished deep tendon reflexes. Bradycardia, hypotension, absent deep tendon reflexes, fixed and dilated pupils, and prolongation of QRS, PR, and QT intervals may result from levels above 6.0 mg/dL. Severe cases (usually > 10 mg/L) may cause coma, asystole, muscle paralysis leading to flaccid quadriplegia, and respiratory failure and cardiac arrest in extreme cases.[84]

Most commonly, hypermagnesemia is induced by administration or use of magnesium-containing agents such as ingestion of Epsom salts, use of magnesium-based laxatives or enemas, or administration of magnesium agents in the setting of renal failure. Parenteral administration of magnesium in pre-eclampsia patients with normal renal function has been reported to cause symptomatic hypermagnesemia, particularly when serum levels reach 4 to 8 mg/dL.[85] However, these patients recover easily with discontinuation of magnesium, particularly if renal function is intact.

Treatment is cessation of the offending magnesium-containing agent, administration of intravenous fluids together with a loop diuretic, and calcium salts to antagonize the cardiac effects of magnesium. Hemodialysis is used for severe acute hypermagnesemia.[86]

Hypomagnesemia

Hypomagnesemia (defined as serum levels below 1.7 mg/dL) has been found in about 7% to 11% of hospitalized patients[87] and approximately 65% of critically ill patients.[3] Disturbance in magnesium in critically ill patients may lead to significant clinical consequences (eg, cardiac arrhythmias, neuropsychiatric problems, and other electrolyte abnormalities such as hypokalemia and hypocalcemia) that may affect prognosis, morbidity, and mortality of patients.[88] Critically ill patients who are hypomagnesemic have been shown to have a higher mortality (as high as 74%) compared to that of normomagnesemic patients.[89]

Aside from poor dietary intake, the 2 major mechanisms causing hypomagnesemia are GI losses and renal losses. Diarrhea causes inadequate water reabsorption along the GI tract. Since water reabsorption is a prerequisite for magnesium resorption, magnesium deficiency ensues. Laxative use predisposes patients to hypomagnesemia via essentially the same mechanism. Renal losses can be from tubular defects, diabetes mellitus, alcoholism, and drugs. Alcoholism causes magnesium deficiency through several mechanisms: renal magnesium wasting, impaired magnesium resorption due to diarrhea and vomiting associated with alcohol intake, and withdrawal. Neuromuscular manifestations include a positive Chvostek and Trousseau sign, generalized seizures, migraines, vertigo, ataxia, nystagmus, and athetoid and choreiform movements.[90] Plausible mechanisms include lowering of the threshold for neural stimulation associated with hypomagnesemia, increased glutamate release in the neuromuscular junction, and allowing calcium influx into the presynaptic nerves with subsequent release of neurotransmitters.[88]

Cardiovascular effects of hypomagnesemia include prolonged PR and QT intervals, supraventricular dysrhythmias (eg, atrial fibrillation, atrial tachycardia, and premature atrial complexes), ventricular tachycardia, and ventricular fibrillation. It must be emphasized that a normal serum magnesium concentration does not preclude intracellular magnesium depletion so magnesium deficiency should always be considered when dealing with these arrhythmias. Although there is a higher incidence of cardiac dysrhythmias among hypomagnesemic patients following acute myocardial infarction or coronary artery bypass grafting (CABG), the data is still insufficient to warrant routine administration of magnesium in these scenarios.[91,92]

The presence of hypomagnesemia, particularly at levels less than 1.2 mg/dL, almost always is associated with hypocalcemia, given the close relationship between magnesium and calcium, as mentioned above. In particular, a form of PTH resistance occurs when the magnesium level is below 1 mg/dL. In severe cases of magnesium deficiency, there is direct inhibition of PTH secretion.[93-95]

More than 50% of clinically significant hypokalemia has concomitant magnesium deficiency, particularly in patients receiving diuretics.[95,96] Hypokalemia accompanied by hypomagnesemia is often refractory to treatment with potassium administration, unless the hypomagnesemia is corrected first. The mechanism is not completely clear but could be due to inhibition of Na-K-ATPase, which promotes renal potassium wasting and secretion.[97] Distal potassium secretion could also be stimulated by hypomagnesemia because the ROMK channel in the cortical collecting duct is inhibited by intracellular magnesium.[94] Finally, it has been shown that in normal individuals, magnesium infusion decreases renal potassium excretion.[96]

Of note, drugs that are associated with hypomagnesemia include diuretics, proton-pump inhibitors, cisplatin/carboplatin, and antimicrobials (particularly aminoglycosides, pentamidine, rapamycin, amphotericin B, and foscarnet).

In general, patients who present with signs and symptoms of hypomagnesemia, and those who are at risk for it, should be promptly treated. There is no clear consensus of how magnesium deficiency should be replaced. Most recommendations agree that moderate to severe symptomatic hypomagnesemia should be treated with intravenous supplementation, while cases with no symptoms to minimal symptoms are treated through the oral route. Advanced cardiac life support guidelines do have clear guidelines for magnesium therapy for torsade de pointes and pre-eclampsia; they recommend giving a loading dose of 1 to 2 g intravenously over 15 minutes followed by 0.5 to 1 g/h infusion.

In the hospital settings, the oral route may not be well tolerated for various reasons, particularly for its GI side effects. The following regimen has been recommended:[97,98]

- If the plasma magnesium is less than 1 mg/dL, give 4 to 8 g over 12 to 24 hours, and repeat as needed.
- If the plasma magnesium is 1 to 1.5 mg/dL, give 2 to 4 g over 4 to 12 hours.
- If the plasma magnesium is 1.6 to 1.9 mg/dL, give 1 to 2 g over 1 to 2 hours.

It is important to remember that magnesium does not equilibrate easily between all tissue compartments, and it may take a few days to several weeks. Hence, the correction of the serum magnesium does not necessarily mean total body magnesium has been corrected. Therefore, even after the serum level is normalized, therapy needs to be continued for a few more days orally or parenterally in patients with normal renal function. In patients with renal failure, caution needs to be exercised and close monitoring of levels is important. More often than not, unless hypomagnesemia is severe, removing or treating the cause of the hypomagnesemia would be sufficient.

QUESTIONS

1. A 52-year-old man with history of chronic alcohol (ETOH) abuse, chronic obstructive pulmonary disease (COPD), hypertension (HTN), and previous gastrointestinal (GI) bleed presented to the emergency department (ED) with 3 to 4 days of altered mental status. He was lethargic and drowsy but communicating appropriately when aroused. His girlfriend reported decreased food intake but excessive beer consumption of approximately 30 cans in the past 3 days.

   On physical exam, he was afebrile. His blood pressure was 120/80 mmHg, his pulse was 80 beats/min, his respiratory rate was 20 breaths/min, and his oxygen saturation was 93% on room air. He appeared disheveled but not dehydrated. He had no pupillary abnormalities, and deep tendon reflexes were normal with no focal neurologic deficits. In addition, he had palmar erythema and a few spider angiomas on the chest.

   Labs:

Hematocrit	44%
White blood cells	6.9×10^3 µL
Platelets	142×10^3 µ/L
Blood urea nitrogen	3 mg/dL
Serum osm	98 mOsm/kg
Urine Na	6 mmol/L
Thyroid-stimulating hormone	0.5 mIµ/L
International normalized ratio	1.0
Sodium	107 mEq/L
Chloride	69 mEq/L
Potassium	4.0 mEq/L
Creatinine	0.4 mg/dL
Urine osm	97 mOsm/kg
Alcohol level	268 mg/dL
Albumin	2.4 g/dL

   What is the most likely cause?

   A. Hypovolemia
   B. Syndrome of inappropriate antidiuretic hormone secretion
   C. Pseudohyponatremia
   D. Poor solute intake

2. For the patient in question 1, what is the next step?

   A. No IV fluids, institution of proper nutrition with increased content of electrolytes and protein
   B. 3% saline at 75 mL/h
   C. 0.9% saline at 150 mL/h
   D. Desmopressin

3. A 55-year-old woman is brought to the ED after a week of binge drinking. On physical exam, her blood pressure is 130/76 mmHg, her heart rate is 102 beats/min, and her weight is 70 kg. She is lethargic and mumbling incoherently. In the ED, the patient has a generalized tonic-clonic seizure, which resolves with IV lorazepam.

   Labs:

Sodium	110 mEq/L
Potassium	3.8 mEq/L
Alcohol	250 mg/dL
Serum osm	230 mOsm/kg
Glucose	92 mg/dL
Urine osm	312 mOsm/kg
Creatinine	0.4 mg/dL

   How should this patient be managed at this time?

   A. IV hypertonic saline (3%) at 70 mL/h for 4 hours
   B. IV hypertonic saline (3%) at 200 mL/h for 4 hours
   C. IV normal saline (0.9%) at 100 mL/h
   D. IV normal saline (0.9%) at 1000 mL/h

4. For the patient in question 3, after 8 hours of therapy, a serum chemistry profile reveals a sodium level of 118 mEq/L. The patient is now euvolemic and more responsive. What is the next step in this patient's management?

   A. Continue current therapy, recheck sodium every 6 hours
   B. Start IV ceftriaxone
   C. Stop IV fluids and administer a 1-time dose of IV furosemide 80 mg
   D. Stop IV fluids, restrict free water intake, and monitor serum sodium closely

5. A 72-year-old man with a history of asthma-COPD overlap syndrome, diabetes mellitus type 2, hypertension, and recent diagnosis of lung cancer presents for routine follow-up to his primary care physician. He has mild dyspnea on exertion. His appetite has been good and he denies weight loss, nausea, vomiting, or diarrhea. He has had a recent normal colonoscopy and he is up to date with his eye exams. His only medications are fluticasone-propionate, albuterol, lisinopril, and metformin. Physical exam reveals blood pressure of 120/70 mmHg without orthostasis, heart rate of 72 beats/min, respiratory rate of 22 breaths/min, and pulse oximetry of 97% on room air.

   Labs:

Complete blood count	normal
Glucose	100 mg/dL
Sodium	122 mEq/L
Serum osm	250 mOsm/L
Urine osm	450 mOsm/L
Potassium	3.5 mEq/L
Blood urea nitrogen	7 mg/dL
Creatinine	0.9 mg/dL
Urine Na	64 mEq/L

What is the most likely cause of hyponatremia?

A. Pseudohyponatremia
B. SIADH
C. Diuretic use
D. Adrenal insufficiency

6. For the patient in question 5, which of the following is the best treatment at this time?

A. 3% saline infusion
B. 0.9% saline infusion
C. Furosemide
D. Fluid restriction or tolvaptan

7. A 40-year-old woman complains of unabated thirst that began 3 weeks ago. She is constantly drinking and goes to the bathroom approximately 6 times per night. She has lost 6 pounds over the last few weeks and has started on lithium for bipolar disorder. She is hemodynamically stable.

Labs:
Sodium	149 mEq/L
Urine osm	120 mOsm/kg

What is the mostly likely diagnosis?

A. Diuretic-induced dehydration
B. Central diabetes insipidus
C. Nephrogenic diabetes insipidus
D. None of the above

8. With an initial urine osmolarity of 120 mOsm/kg, which of the following findings on a desmopressin test would be most consistent with a diagnosis of central diabetes insipidus?

A. Reduction in urine osmolarity to 60 mOsm/L following vasopressin administration
B. Reduction in urine osmolarity to 110 mOsm/L following vasopressin administration
C. Increase in urine osmolarity to 130 mOsm/L following vasopressin administration
D. Increase in urine osmolarity to 400 mOsm/L following vasopressin administration

9. A 43-year-old man was admitted to the hospital 6 days earlier for an intracranial hemorrhage requiring emergency evacuation. His medical history includes poorly controlled hypertension and rheumatoid arthritis. On hospital day 6, his serum sodium level is noted to be 121 mEq/L. He has been receiving 0.9% normal saline since admission, and his sodium level has been gradually decreasing from 141 mEq/L, the level at admission.

Labs:
Sodium	121 mEq/L
Serum osm	520 mOsm/kg
Creatinine	0.6 mg/dL
Urine Na	89 mmol/L
Urine osm	588 mOsm/kg
Urinalysis	specific gravity of 1.030 with no blood or protein fractional excretion of uric acid is elevated at 83.8% TSH and random cortisol are normal

On exam, the patient has a blood pressure of 105/50 mmHg and pulse of 98/min. His mucous membranes are dry, and he has poor skin turgor and no detectable edema. His urine output has been 2 to 4 L/day despite fluid restriction of less than 1.5 L/day initiated 2 days earlier. His sodium level has continued to decline after fluid restriction. What is the most likely cause of this patient's hyponatremia?

A. Hypothyroidism
B. SIADH
C. Adrenal insufficiency
D. Cerebral salt wasting syndrome

10. For the patient in question 9, what is the next step?

A. Fluid restrict to 1200 mL/d
B. Furosemide 80 mg IV daily
C. Continue 0.9% normal saline plus Na tablets 2 g qid
D. Both A and B

11. A 74-year-old man presents with 2 days of dizziness. Today, the patient states he felt like he was going to pass out. Patient states he was prescribed sulfamethoxazole/trimethoprim for acute sinusitis by his primary care doctor 5 days ago.

Past medical history: congestive heart failure, diabetes, hypertension, chronic kidney disease stage 3

Medications: carvedilol 6.25 mg PO BID, aspirin 81 mg, lisinopril 5 mg PO once daily, metformin 1000 mg PO BID, simvastatin 20 mg PO once daily

ECG in ED (Fig. 2-10):

Labs:
White blood cells	$8 \times 10^3/\mu L$
Hemoglobin	14 g/dL
Platelets	$194 \times 10^3/\mu L$
Sodium	132 mEq/L
Potassium	6.9 mEq/L
Chloride	112 mEq/L
Calcium	8.3 mEq/L
Phosphorous	6.5 mg/dL
CO_2	13 mEq/L
BUN	38 mg/dL
Creatinine	2.7 mg/dL (baseline 1.8 mg/dL)

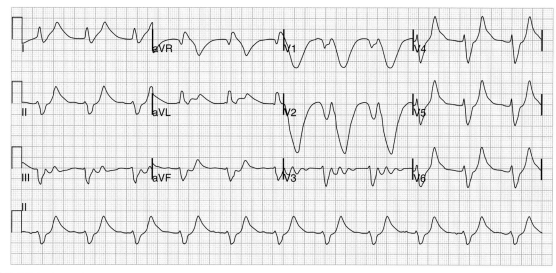

FIGURE 2-10 ECG on admission.

What would be the immediate initial treatment for this patient?

A. Calcium gluconate
B. Emergent dialysis
C. Sodium bicarbonate 50 mEq IV push
D. Sodium polystyrene sulfonate (Kayexalate) 15 g orally

12. For the patient in question 11, what would be the next step?

A. Albuterol 10 to 20 mg in 4 mL of saline by nebulization over 10 min
B. 25 g of dextrose and 10 units of regular insulin
C. Sodium polystyrene sulfonate (Kayexalate) 15 g orally
D. A and B

13. A 56-year-old woman presents to the ED with complaints of fatigue, muscle aches, and generalized weakness. She reports that she was recently started on a new antihypertensive medication a few weeks ago and attributes her symptoms to this medication. ECG is shown below (Fig. 2-11).

What was the new medication that this patient was recently prescribed?

A. Spironolactone
B. Hydrochlorothiazide
C. Metoprolol
D. Diltiazem

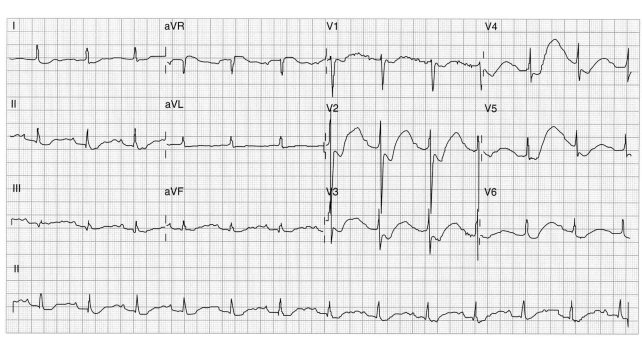

FIGURE 2-11 ECG on admission.

14. A 55-year-old man with known cardiomyopathy and coronary artery disease presents with carpopedal spasm. He denies any other symptoms on admission. ECG shows normal sinus rhythm (NSR), left ventricular hypertrophy (LVH), and QTc of 550 ms. His blood pressure is 80/50 mmHg. Physical exam reveals dry mucous membranes, clear lungs, and no significant edema. In ED it is difficult to obtain intravenous access, but after several tries, a 22-gauge IV is successfully placed on his right hand.

Labs:

Sodium	146 mEq/L
Potassium	3.9 mEq/L
Calcium	6.0 mg/dL
CO_2	27 mEq/L
BUN	19 mg/dL
Creatinine	1.2 mg/dL
Albumin	4.8 g/dL
Magnesium	2.1 mg/dL

In addition to obtaining more reliable access, what should be the next step in management?

A. Calcium carbonate 650 mg PO BID
B. Calcitriol 0.25 mg PO daily
C. Give 1 g calcium chloride IV over 10–20 minutes
D. Give 1 g calcium gluconate IV in 10–20 minutes

15. In a patient with hypocalcemia, which of the following is needed to determine if vitamin D supplementation is needed?

A. 25(OH)D level
B. 1,25(OH)2D level
C. Magnesium level
D. PTH level

16. A 75-year-old man presents with weakness and decreased urine output. His medical history is significant for atrial fibrillation and hypertension. In the ED, his blood pressure (BP) is 138/60 mmHg, his pulse is 100 beats/min, and his respiratory rate is 16 breaths/min. Physical exam is significant for a lethargic man, in no acute distress. His heart rate is irregularly irregular, lungs are clear to auscultation, and he has no significant edema.

Labs:

Hemoglobin	8.2 g/dL
Total protein	12.2 g/dL
Creatinine	15 mg/dL
Potassium	5.9 mEq/L
Calcium	13.5 mg/dL
Albumin	2.5 g/dL
BUN	119 mg/dL
Sodium	135 mEq/L
CO_2	13.3 mEq/L
Phosphorus	< 1 mg/dL

What is the etiology of hypophosphatemia?

A. Increased renal phosphate excretion due to inhibition of phosphate reabsorption due to hyperparathyroidism
B. Severe malnutrition leading to decrease phosphorus intake
C. Spurious hypophosphatemia due to interference of laboratory measurement of phosphorus by elevated concentrations of monoclonal immunoglobulins
D. Fanconi syndrome due to multiple myeloma

17. For the patient in question 16, what is the appropriate management?

A. Aggressive intravenous fluid resuscitation, followed by intravenous furosemide to improve calciuresis
B. Intravenous fluids with isotonic fluids followed by intravenous bisphosphonate therapy
C. Intravenous fluids with an isotonic bicarbonate solution and subcutaneous calcitonin twice daily
D. Initiation of renal replacement therapy

18. A 51-year-old man with history of alcoholism presents with altered mental status. In the ED, he is found to be confused and lethargic. His neighbor reports that he had been on a drinking binge for the past week.

On examination, he is cachexic with poor hygiene and very lethargic. His blood pressure is 105/67 mmHg, his pulse is 112 beats/min and regular, his respiratory rate is 22 breaths/min, his temperature is 96°F, and his weight is 72 kg. His dentition is poor, and his lungs reveal bilateral rhonchi. His abdomen is soft, and he has hepatomegaly appreciated. He has trace lower extremity edema. Skin reveals abrasions and bruises.

Labs:

Sodium	121 mEq/L
CO_2	18 mEq/L
Creatinine	0.8 mg/dL
Albumin	2.1 g/dL
Potassium	3.6 mEq/L
BUN	10 mg/dL
Calcium	7.8 mg/dL
Phosphorus	2.2 mg/dL

The patient is started on a 0.9% saline solution supplemented with dextrose initially; his sodium improves over the next 48 hours. He is treated with thiamine, potassium, and antibiotics for presumed aspiration pneumonia. Initially he improves; however, on day 3, he develops worsening shortness of breath and hypoxia. Chest x-ray reveals pulmonary edema.

Repeat Labs:

Sodium	129 mEq/L
Potassium	3.3 mEq/L
Phosphorus	1.0 mg/dL

What is the etiology of this patient's hypophosphatemia?

A. Secondary hyperparathyroidism
B. Refeeding syndrome
C. Hyperphosphaturia due to saline administration
D. Rhabdomyolysis

19. What is the appropriate management of the patient above?

   A. Intravenous furosemide and intravenous potassium phosphate 15 mmol over 4 hours
   B. Intravenous furosemide and oral phosphorus replacement of 1000 mg/day
   C. Hypertonic saline at 50 mL/h and intravenous potassium phosphate 15 mmol over 4 hours
   D. Intravenous potassium phosphate 30 mmol over 1 hour

20. An 18-year-old man with recently diagnosed acute lymphoblastic leukemia is admitted for initiation of chemotherapy. Physical exam is significant for bulky cervical lymphadenopathy, enlarged tonsils, and mild hepatosplenomegaly. Laboratory data on admission reveals WBC of $92 \times 10^3/\mu L$, Hgb of 8.8 g/dL, and platelets of $50 \times 10^3/\mu L$. Comprehensive metabolic panel at that time is within normal limits, although LDH was 5100 IU. He is initiated on intravenous fluids and allopurinol 300 mg twice daily. On day 2, he is started on vincristine, daunorubicin, and prednisolone. On day 3, he starts complaining of weakness and shortness of breath. His heart rate is 120 beats/min, his BP is 100/55 mmHg, and his temperature is 100.4°F.

Labs:

Creatinine	3.2 mg/dL
Calcium	5.4 mg/dL
Uric acid	6.2 mg/dL
CO$_2$	15 mEq/L
Phosphorus	12.8 mg/dL
Potassium	6.2 mEq/L

Urine output in the past 24 hours is 320 mL.

Which of the following is true about tumor lysis syndrome?

A. Bicarbonate-based solution and urinary alkalinization can prevent calcium phosphorus precipitation in tissue.
B. Rasburicase can be used to prevent calcium phosphorous precipitation during tumor lysis.
C. Hemodialysis should be started once the calcium phosphorus product is greater than 60 mg^2/dL^2.
D. Aggressive IV fluids should be used for prophylaxis in high-risk patients to try to obtain a urine output of 2 cc/kg/h.

21. A 70-year-old man presented to the ED with delirium and severe respiratory distress. He was found with atrial fibrillation at a rapid ventricular rate. He was admitted to the intensive care unit and promptly intubated. He has a history of hypertension and takes hydrochlorothiazide 25 mg daily. He also has been on pantoprazole 40 mg daily for recurrent gastroesophageal reflux disease (GERD). He does not smoke nor drink alcohol. Chest radiograph showed no pneumonia but mild pulmonary congestion. On physical exam, he had a positive Chvostek sign.

Labs:

Sodium	132 mg/dL
CO$_2$	23 mEq/L
Creatinine	1.1 mg/dL
Calcium	6.1 mg/dL
Magnesium	0.9 mg/dL
Potassium	3.1 mEq/L
BUN	18 mg/dL
Chloride	100 mEq/L
Albumin	2.1 mg/dL

PTH and 25-vit D were both low.

What is/are the possible risk factor(s) for this patient's hypomagnesemia?

A. Chronic hydrochlorothiazide use
B. Chronic proton-pump inhibitor use
C. Age more than 65 years
D. Only A and B

22. Which of the following is true about hypomagnesemia?

   A. Hypomagnesemia can cause secondary hypoparathyroidism and increase resistance of tissues to PTH and vitamin D.
   B. Hypomagnesemia causes 25-vit D deficiency.
   C. Refractory hypomagnesemia should be corrected only after the correction of underlying hypocalcemia.
   D. All of the above

23. A 69-year-old woman with history of hypertension and diabetes presents with severe back pain, weakness, and confusion. Symptoms have been progressively worsening for 3 weeks. In the ED, she is confused and unable to get out of bed. Her BP is 80/40 mmHg, her pulse is 100 beats/min, her respiratory rate is 22 breaths/min, and she was afebrile. Her mucous membranes are dry, her lungs are clear to auscultation, and she displays no edema. She has 4/5 muscle weakness in all extremities. She has a 3-cm palpable mass of right breast.

Radiology of lumbar spine reveals lytic lesions.

Labs:

Sodium	147 mEq/L
BUN	75 mg/dL
Albumin	2.3 g/dL
Potassium	4.7 mEq/L
Creatinine	3.4 mg/dL
Phosphorus	6.2 mg/dL
CO_2	18 mEq/L
Calcium	14.2 mg/dL
Parathyroid hormone	16 pg/mL

What is the next appropriate treatment?

A. Normal saline at 200 cc/h
B. Normal saline at 200 cc/h and furosemide 40 mg IV
C. Normal saline at 200 cc/h and zoledronic acid 4 mg IV over 15 minutes
D. Normal saline at 200 cc/h and calcitonin 4 IU subcutaneously

24. What is the likely mechanism of hypercalcemia in the patient in question 23?

A. Humoral hypercalcemia of malignancy (release of systemic PTHrP)
B. Conversion of 25-vit D to 1,25-vit D
C. Local activation of osteoclasts by tumor cells
D. Ectopic secretion of PTH by tumor cells

25. A 31-year-old woman with history of hypertension and lupus nephritis, currently gravid at 32 weeks develops severe hypertension (BP 180/110 mmHg) and worsening proteinuria (> 3 g of proteinuria). She is admitted to the labor and delivery unit and started on labetalol and IV magnesium 2 g/h as a continuous infusion. Admission labs are also significant for a creatinine of 1.8 mg/dL. Which of the following is FALSE about the use of IV magnesium in this patient?

A. The therapeutic range for IV magnesium for seizure prophylaxis is 4.8 to 8.4 mg/dL.
B. She is at higher risk for magnesium toxicity due to her renal insufficiency.
C. Monitoring for loss of deep tendon reflexes should be done every 6 hours in this patient.
D. Cardiac symptoms of magnesium toxicity should be treated with IV calcium gluconate.

ANSWERS

1. D. Poor solute intake

   Hyponatremia from poor solute intake (beer potomania) is secondary to water intoxication with relatively low solute intake. ADH secretion will be (appropriately) negligible and urine osmolality will be maximally dilute. In a patient whose diet is comprised of mostly beer, there will be a very low solute intake (< 250 mOsm/day). Hence, despite a maximally dilute urine (50 mOsm/L), the maximum urine volume will be 5 Liters before the patient will be unable to excrete additional free water (250 mOsm ÷ 50 mOsm/L = 5 Liters).[99,101] Introduction of more solute will lead to a brisk aquaresis, which causes rapid correction of sodium and places the patient at risk for osmotic demyelination syndrome. Patients typically have a low serum osmolarity (although it can be high if there is an acute alcohol load), low urine sodium, and low urine osmolarity. In some patients with beer potomania, loss of the urea concentration gradient can impair some of the dilution capacity, but urine osmolality should still be relatively low.[102] Hyponatremia in alcoholics also can be caused by hypovolemia, pseudohyponatremia from hypertriglyceridemia, SIADH, cerebral salt wasting syndrome, and CHF. Clues for diagnosis are history of ETOH abuse, binge drinking, and poor dietary intake.

   Choice A is incorrect since he shows no evidence of hypovolemia by vital signs, physical exam, or renal indices. Choice B is incorrect, since urine osmolality is less than 100. Pseudohyponatremia (choice C) is incorrect, as his serum osmolality is truly low, which suggests hypotonic hyponatremia.

2. A. No IV fluids, institution of proper nutrition with increased content of electrolytes and protein

   The patient will have brisk diuresis with the introduction of a solute, which may cause serum sodium to correct too quickly, as sufficient urine osmoles will be excreted to allow for free water excretion. Management recommendations include institution of proper meds and proper nutrition[7]; no IVF should be started unless the patient is symptomatic. Given the chronicity of the hyponatremia, the malnourished state, and the history of alcoholism, this patient is at high risk for osmotic demyelination syndrome. Hence, serum sodium should be checked every 2 hours, and the goal is a sodium increase less than 8 mEq/L in 24 hours and less than 18 mEq/L in 48 hours. Hypotonic solution (D5W) can be given if necessary to decrease correction rate, and desmopressin (choice D) should only be administered if serum sodium corrects by more than 10 mEq/L per 24 hours.

Giving normal saline (choice C) or 3% saline (choice B) might overcorrect the sodium in the 24-hour time period.

3. A. IV hypertonic saline (3%) at 70 mL/h for 4 hours

This patient is exhibiting severe neurologic manifestations of hyponatremia, so the appropriate treatment is to raise serum tonicity by 4 to 6 mEq in the first 3 to 4 hours or until symptoms have resolved. Usually increasing the sodium by 4 to 6 mEq will improve the most severe neurologic manifestations of hyponatremia. In order to raise the serum sodium 4 mEq/L in a 70-kg woman (35 Liters TBW) over 4 hours, one needs to first calculate the sodium deficit:

$$\text{Sodium Deficit} = \text{Normal TBW} \times (\text{Goal } P_{Na} - \text{Current } P_{Na})$$
$$\text{Sodium Deficit} = (70 \text{ kg} \times 0.5) \times (114 - 110) = 140 \text{ mEq}$$

This 140 mEq of sodium is equal to about 300 mL of 3% saline (140/500). This needs to be given in 4 hours or approximately 70 mL/h.

Choice B would correct a sodium deficit of about 300 mEq in 4 hours, which would theoretically correct her by more than 8 mEq in 4 hours. Choices C and D would be unlikely to rapidly correct her serum sodium by 4 mEq in a short time period given that her urine osmolality is relatively high and she is not clearly volume depleted by exam.

4. D. Stop IV fluids, restrict free water intake, and monitor serum sodium closely

Therapy for hyponatremia must be closely monitored because overly rapid correction can cause fluid shifts in the brain and result in often fatal osmotic demyelination. A safe rate of correction in the first 24 hours is less than 9 mEq/L. As treatment has already corrected the patient's sodium level from 110 to 118 mEq/L over 8 hours and her neurologic condition has improved, therapy should be targeted to slow the rise of serum sodium. At this point, stopping hypertonic saline and restricting free water should slow the rise of sodium. If the sodium level continues to rise despite these measures, hypotonic solution (D5W) must be administered, and administration of desmopressin should be considered. This will ensure that the target level of correction is not exceeded. Continuing current therapy (choice A) would certainly cause an overcorrection. Furosemide (choice C) will not slow the rate of correction. Intravenous ceftriaxone (choice B) does not play a role in this case.

5. B. SIADH

The patient has a low serum sodium level with a low serum osmolarity and clinically does not appear to be either volume overloaded or depleted. Therefore, he has hypotonic, euvolemic hyponatremia, which can result from ectopic production of ADH from his lung cancer. His normal glucose level makes pseudohyponatremia secondary to hyperglycemia unlikely (choice A). He is not on diuretics, making choice C incorrect. Adrenal insufficiency (choice D) will typically present with orthostasis or relatively low blood pressure, and labs will frequently show at least mild hyperkalemia.

6. D. Fluid restriction or tolvaptan

Fluid restriction to 500 to 1500 mL/day is the initial treatment for hyponatremia secondary to SIADH. The serum osmolarity subsequently rises and causes increased water excretion to maintain a steady urinary pH. Fluid is also removed from insensible water loss. Tolvaptan is an ADH-receptor antagonist and reduces water permeability in the collecting ducts. Tolvaptan is second-line treatment in patients who are euvolemic or hypervolemic and should not be used concurrently with fluid restriction during the dosing phase.

A 3% saline infusion (choice A) could be considered if the patient had more severe hyponatremia with mental status changes consistent with cerebral edema. A 0.9% saline infusion (choice B) would be used if the patient were volume depleted. He has many signs that he is not volume depleted, including normal renal function, normal blood pressure without orthostatic decline, and no history of vomiting or diarrhea. Furosemide (choice C) is incorrect because there are no signs of volume overload.

7. C. Nephrogenic diabetes insipidus

Lithium causes nephrogenic diabetes insipidus by inhibiting the tubules' ability to insert aquaporins into the tubular membrane in response to ADH. Hence, these patients will excrete a relatively dilute urine (urine osmolality less than serum osmolality) despite a high serum sodium and the presence of ADH in serum. Central diabetes insipidus (choice B), although a possibility, is less likely, given that patient is on lithium for bipolar disorder and lithium is well known to cause ADH resistance. The distinction between nephrogenic diabetes insipidus and central diabetes insipidus can be made via desmopressin administration. Choice A is incorrect as patient is not taking diuretics. See Table 2-6.

TABLE 2-6 Sodium Disorders and How They are Diagnosed

Sodium Disorders	Diagnosis	Water Restriction Interpreted When Urine Osmolarity Stabilized or Plasma Osmolarity > 295 mOsm/kg and/or Desmopressin	Plasma and Urine ADH
Primary polydipsia	Sodium < 137 mEq/L and urine osmolarity < ½ serum osmolarity	• Water restriction causes urine osmolarity > 500 mOsm/kg • No effect with desmopressin	
Nephrogenic diabetes insipidus	Sodium > 142 mEq/L and urine osmolarity < serum osmolarity	• Water restriction causes submaximal response with urine osmolarity • Desmopressin causes up to 45% increase in urine osmolarity in partial nephrogenic DI • Desmopressin causes no increase in urine osmolarity in complete nephrogenic DI	• Nephrogenic DI excluded if urine osmolarity increases with increasing levels of ADH
Central diabetes insipidus	Sodium > 142 mEq/L and urine osmolarity < serum osmolarity	• Water restriction causes submaximal response with urine osmolarity • Desmopressin causes 15–50% increase of urine osmolarity in partial central DI • Desmopressin causes urine osmolarity > 300 mOsm/kg in complete central DI	• Central DI excluded if appropriate increase in serum and urine ADH with increasing plasma osmolarity

ADH = antidiuretic hormone; DI = diabetes insipidus.

8. **D. Increase in urine osmolarity to 400 mOsm/L following vasopressin administration**

Choices A and B are incorrect because administration of vasopressin would not cause a reduction in urine osmolarity in either central or nephrogenic diabetes insipidus. Choice C is incorrect because in nephrogenic diabetes insipidus, urine osmolarity rises less than 50% over the preadministration osmolarity. Choice D is correct because urine osmolarity increased more than 50% over preadministration osmolarity, which is consistent with central diabetes insipidus.

9. **D. Cerebral salt wasting syndrome**

Cerebral salt wasting (CSW) syndrome is an uncommon cause of hyponatremia in patients suffering from subarachnoid hemorrhage or following neurosurgical procedures. In 1 study of 189 hyponatremic patients following neurosurgery, 7 were thought to have CSW.[103] The mechanism of cerebral salt wasting is believed to be secondary to (1) decreased sympathetic input, which impairs sodium and urate reabsorption in the proximal tubule and also impairs aldosterone and renin release, and (2) increased secretion of brain natriuretic peptide (BNP) causes further reduction in sodium reabsorption and renin release. Because of impaired proximal sodium handling, patients with CSW tend to have high urine volume and sodium output, which causes volume depletion and an appropriate increase in ADH secretion in response, causing hyponatremia. These patients may demonstrate signs of volume depletion with fluid restriction as a result. Differentiation from SIADH can be difficult, as CSW will also have low serum BUN and uric acid, yet a high urine sodium excretion. Some authors have suggested a higher BNP or fractional excretion of uric acid is more consistent with CSW.[99] Differentiation of the 2 diseases ultimately requires close observation of response to fluid restriction; CSW should manifest clinical signs of volume depletion with a fluid restriction.[7]

Choices A and C are incorrect, as normal thyroid-stimulating hormone and random cortisol levels were reported. Choice B is incorrect because of the evidence of volume depletion by exam during fluid restriction.

10. **C. Continue 0.9% normal saline plus Na tablets 2 g QID**

Cerebral salt wasting syndrome is a volume-depleted state treated with intravenous administration of isotonic or hypertonic fluids. Therefore, choices A, B and D are incorrect because they add to the volume depleted state rather than correcting it, as in choice C.

11. **A. Calcium gluconate**

The patient has the sine wave on ECG. Hyperkalemia causes decreased membrane excitability of the cardiac muscles; via unclear mechanisms, calcium antagonizes this effect of potassium. Hence, calcium gluconate should be administered first in a hyperkalemic patient with any ECG changes consistent with hyperkalemia or a potassium greater than 6.5 mEq/L to stabilize the cardiac membrane.[26] The effect of intravenous calcium is rapid but is short lived. Therefore, calcium should not be administered as monotherapy for hyperkalemia but should rather be combined with therapies that drive extracellular potassium into cells. The dose of calcium gluconate can be repeated after 5 minutes if the ECG changes persist or recur.[32]

Emergent dialysis (choice B) is incorrect as it would not be the next *immediate* treatment. It may be indicated if medical therapy is unsuccessful in treating hyperkalemia, or if this patient's renal function continues to deteriorate. Sodium bicarbonate (choice C) can be used to try to shift potassium intracellularly (after membrane stabilization with calcium gluconate); however, it is frequently not particularly effective.[104,105] Kayexalate (choice D) should be administered only after calcium is given, and also following treatment with modalities that shift potassium intracellularly (eg, insulin, albuterol, bicarbonate).

12. D. A and B (Albuterol 10 to 20 mg in 4 mL of saline by nebulization over 10 min, and 25 g of dextrose and 10 units of regular insulin)

Following treatment with IV calcium to stabilize the membrane, the next appropriate step is to give agents that shift potassium intracellularly. Treatment with dextrose and insulin is effective to drive potassium intracellularly, and will decrease serum potassium concentration by 0.5 to 1.2 mEq/L.[104] Insulin can be given without dextrose if the serum glucose is more than or equal to 250 mg/dL.[106] Monitoring for hypoglycemia is important, as hypoglycemia is common following treatment with intravenous insulin (particularly in patients with renal insufficiency).[107] Albuterol via nebulizer is also quite effective in shifting potassium intracellularly and should be administered with dextrose and insulin in hyperkalemic patients. Albuterol can have the effect of transiently lowering serum potassium by 0.5 to 1.5 mEq/L[104] and has an effect that lasts about 2 hours.[26] Although sodium polystyrene (choice C) is useful for decreasing total body potassium, it tends to take a long time to be effective and frequently requires multiple doses.

13. B. Hydrochlorothiazide

Hydrochlorothiazide is a thiazide diuretic used for the treatment of hypertension. One of the common side effects of this drug is hypokalemia, as well as hypomagnesemia, hypercalcemia, and hyponatremia. The mechanism of renal potassium wasting is increased delivery of sodium to the cortical collecting duct where sodium is exchanged for potassium). The characteristic ECG finding of hypokalemia is the U wave (positive deflection following inverted T wave) seen on this ECG, most pronounced in leads V_1 through V_5.

Spironolactone (choice A) is a potassium-sparing diuretic and therefore would not cause hypokalemia. Diltiazem (choice D) is a calcium-channel blocker with no effect on potassium handling. Metoprolol (choice C) is a beta-blocker, which causes PR prolongation and bradycardia on ECG. It can cause mild hyperkalemia due to inhibition of potassium entry into cells.

14. D. Give 1 g calcium gluconate IV in 10–20 minutes

Intravenous calcium gluconate is indicated due to symptomatic hypocalcemia and prolonged QTc. Calcium gluconate,

however, should not be administered faster than 10 to 20 minutes, since it can precipitate dysrhythmias. Calcium chloride (choice C) is an alternative to calcium gluconate; however, given the patient's poor peripheral access, calcium gluconate would be a safer treatment due to risks of tissue necrosis with calcium chloride in the event of extravasation.

Choice A, oral calcium, is given for patients with mild or chronic hypocalcemia and mild symptoms such as oral paresthesia. Choice B, calcitriol, will be helpful to improve oral calcium absorption, but is not the next appropriate step in such a symptomatic patient.

15. A. 25(OH)D level

25-hydroxyvitamin D, which is hydroxylated by the liver, has a relatively long half-life (several weeks), making it the best indicator of vitamin D stores in the body. On the other hand, 1,25(OH)2D levels (choice B) reflect PTH activity to stimulate renal conversion of 25(OH)D to activated 1,25(OH)2D. Serum magnesium (choice C) is involved in calcium metabolism and levels should be checked to prevent tissue resistance to the effects of PTH. However, magnesium levels would not affect vitamin D stores. Parathyroid hormone (choice D) increases renal tubule calcium reabsorption and calcium resorption of bones during states of hypocalcemia. However, this would not reflect the body's overall vitamin D stores.

16. C. Spurious hypophosphatemia due to interference of laboratory measurement of phosphorus by elevated concentrations of monoclonal immunoglobulins

Hypercalcemia due to multiple myeloma that is associated with renal failure should also be accompanied by significant hyperphosphatemia due to increased phosphorous release from bone coupled with impaired phosphorus excretion. Hypophosphatemia in such a patient should be viewed with skepticism.

Choice A would be incorrect, as the patient does not have hyperparathyroidism as the cause of hypercalcemia. Hyperparathyroidism rarely causes such severe hypercalcemia and renal failure. In addition, the hypophosphatemia associated with hyperparathyroidism tends to be mild (not < 1 mg/dL, even if it was a true lab value). Although patients with myeloma can have associated malnutrition (choice B) and Fanconi syndrome (choice D), both are also incorrect since the hypophosphatemia is not a true value.

17. D. Initiation of renal replacement therapy

The appropriate treatment for a patient with so many severe electrolyte derangements (hyperkalemia, hypercalcemia, acidosis) and significant azotemia is initiation of hemodialysis. Although intravenous fluids can be attempted initially, aggressive intravenous fluids could potentially lead to volume overload in a patient with such severe renal disease. Hence, dialysis is really a better option than trying to induce calciuresis (choice A). In addition, renal failure of this magnitude would be a relative contraindication to intravenous bisphosphonate therapy (choice B). Intravenous bicarbonate could potentially increase calcium phosphorus precipitation and worsen tissue injury and renal calcinosis. Hence, choice C is also incorrect.

18. B. Refeeding syndrome

The patient developed refeeding syndrome due to dextrose administration in a chronically malnourished state. The introduction of dextrose causes secretion of insulin, which stimulates movement of potassium and phosphorus into cells and synthesis of ATP and 2,3-DPG. Phosphate stores become depleted, leading to cellular dysfunction, and in this patient, myocardial dysfunction causes acute congestive heart failure.

Choice A, secondary hyperparathyroidism, is incorrect since it typically manifests with hyperphosphatemia. Although saline administration does increase phosphaturia (choice C), the severity of hypophosphatemia is typically mild. Choice D, rhabdomyolysis, is incorrect because it typically also causes hyperphosphatemia (and hyperkalemia).

19. A. Intravenous furosemide and intravenous potassium phosphate 15 mmol over 4 hours

In a patient with respiratory failure who has moderate hypophosphatemia (1–2.5 mg/dL), appropriate treatment is intravenous potassium phosphate (0.08–0.16 mmol/L) over 4 hours. Lasix is also indicated to treat congestive heart failure from acute myocardial dysfunction associated with refeeding syndrome. Choice B (oral phosphorus replacement) is inappropriate, since respiratory failure is an indication for aggressive phosphate administration. Hypertonic saline (choice C) is not appropriate in mild hyponatremia and congestive heart failure. Choice D is incorrect due to the potential dangers of rapid infusion of intravenous phosphate therapy (arrhythmia and acute hypocalcemia).

20. D. Aggressive IV fluids should be used for prophylaxis in high-risk patients to try to obtain a urine output of 2 cc/kg/h

Tumor lysis syndrome is an oncological emergency caused by massive tumor cell death and release of uric acid, phosphorus, and potassium. Clinical features include hypocalcemia and hyperphosphatemia due to calcium phosphorus precipitation. Renal failure can occur through 2 methods: acute urate nephropathy or nephrocalcinosis. Urate nephropathy can be prevented with allopurinol (a xanthine oxidase inhibitor, which inhibits breakdown of xanthine to uric acid), and if patients have a uric acid greater than 8 mg/dL, rasburicase. Rasburicase is a recombinant urate oxidase that catalyzes the breakdown of uric acid to a much more soluble product, allantoin.[108] It is recommended that aggressive IV fluid administration be utilized to induce a polyuria, so choice D is correct.

Although urinary alkalinization (choice A) could theoretically increase uric acid solubility and excretion, it can also increase calcium phosphorus precipitation in tissue and the nephron, and hence should be avoided. Hemodialysis should be initiated in any patient whose calcium-phosphate product is greater than or equal to 70 mg^2/dL^2 (not 60 mg^2/dL^2, as in choice C). Rasburicase is used to prevent urate nephropathy, not calcium phosphorus precipitation, so choice B is incorrect.

21. D. Only A and B (Chronic hydrochlorothiazide use and chronic proton-pump inhibitor use)

Loop and thiazide diuretics can cause hypomagnesemia. There have been a number of reported cases of hypomagnesemia correlated to the chronic use of proton-pump inhibitors (PPI), with an average use of 5.5 years.[109] One of the largest studies to date showed association between hypomagnesemia and PPI use, but only in those patients who are on diuretics.[109] Advanced age (choice C) has no association to hypomagnesemia by itself.

22. A. Hypomagnesemia can cause secondary hypoparathyroidism and increase resistance of tissues to PTH and vitamin D.

Hypomagnesemia impairs hypocalcemia-induced PTH release and decreases the sensitivity of the tissues to PTH and vitamin D metabolites (in effect, causing secondary hyperparathyroidism). By itself, hypomagnesemia does not cause low 25(OH)D levels (choice B), as 25(OH)D levels are a better indicator of total body stores. Hypocalcemia due to secondary hyperparathyroidism induced by hypomagnesemia is rapidly corrected by administration of magnesium. Of note, PTH and calcitonin have a profound effect on magnesium homeostasis since higher PTH levels can increase magnesium reabsorption in the kidney and gut, and increase magnesium release from bone. Choice C is incorrect, as hypocalcemia does not need to be corrected to improve serum magnesium levels.

23. D. Normal saline at 200 cc/h and calcitonin 4 IU subcutaneously

The initial treatment of severe hypercalcemia, regardless of underlying origin, is to expand plasma volume in order to improve renal function and increase calciuresis. Saline should be used aggressively in this patient because she is clearly volume depleted by exam. In addition, because of its efficacy in the first 48 hours of therapy (before tachyphylaxis develops), calcitonin is useful to improve calcium until more definitive treatment is started. Of note, intranasal calcitonin is not effective for treatment of hypercalcemia, so it should be administered by subcutaneous or intramuscular route.[110]

Choice A (normal saline at 200 cc/h) is incorrect since calcitonin should be added to increase bone resorption by interfering with osteoclasts. Furosemide (choice B) should not be used in a volume-depleted patient, as it will worsen her prerenal azotemia and renal function.

Although zoledronic acid (choice C) has been shown to improve calcium in patients with hypercalcemia due to malignancy, her acute kidney injury is a relative contraindication to treatment at this time. If the patient's renal function improves with aggressive hydration to a more reasonable GFR, bisphosphonate therapy can be administered with less risk. Risks of bisphosphonates depend on indication, duration of therapy, and dose. Acute kidney injury can occur, particularly at higher dose of zoledronic acid and if administered in less than 15 minutes. In addition, patients with elevated creatinine (creatinine > 1.4 mg/dL or GFR < 60 ml/min/1.732 m^2) have a higher risk of AKI than patients with normal renal function.[111] Risk of AKI can be reduced by adjusting dose of bisphosphonate for creatinine clearance. The other rare but feared complication of bisphosphonates (and denosumab) is osteonecrosis of the jaw, which is a type of avascular necrosis.[111]

24. **C. Local activation of osteoclasts by tumor cells**

The patient in the case likely has breast cancer and her complaints of back pain suggest bone metastases. Although breast cancer cells can in some cases secrete systemic PTHrP, the typical mechanism of hypercalcemia is via local stimulation of osteoclasts (osteolytic lesions), so choice A is incorrect. Breast cancer does not stimulate synthesis of 1,25-vit D, which can happen in lymphoma or sarcoidosis, so choice B is incorrect. Ectopic secretion of PTH by tumor cells (choice D) is a very rare cause of hypercalcemia in malignancy.

25. **C. Monitoring for loss of deep tendon reflexes should be done every 6 hours in this patient.**

Magnesium infusion is recommended by most guidelines as therapy for seizure prophylaxis for patients with preeclampsia and has been shown by randomized controlled trials to be effective in preventing eclampsia.[112] The goal of therapy is to maintain a serum magnesium level between 4.8 and 8.4 mg/dL (hence, choice A is true).[113] In general, magnesium infusion is safe and toxicity is uncommon in patients with normal renal function. However, patients with abnormal renal function are at higher risk for toxicity (choice B), and should be monitored closely.[114] Symptoms of magnesium toxicity are related to the level of magnesium, and loss of deep tendon reflexes (DTR) tend to occur at levels greater than 7 mEq/L. All patients on IV magnesium should have DTR monitored at least every 2 hours (hence, choice C is false); patients with renal insufficiency should have serum magnesium levels checked frequently.[115] Respiratory depression and cardiac toxicity occur after loss of DTR and should be treated with IV calcium gluconate (15 to 30 mL of a 10 % solution [1500 to 3000 mg]) over 5 minutes (hence, choice D is true).

REFERENCES

1. Funk GC, Lindner G, Druml W, et al. Incidence and prognosis of dysnatremias present on ICU admission. *Intensive Care Med.* 2010;36(2):304-311.
2. Hessels L, Hoekstra M, Mijzen LJ, et al. The relationship between serum potassium, potassium variability and in-hospital mortality in critcally ill patients and a before-after analysis on the impact of computer-assisted potassium control. *Crit Care.* 2015;19(4):1-11.
3. Ryzen E, Wagers PW, Singer FR, Rude RK. Magnesium deficiency in a medical ICU population *Crit Care Med.* 1985;13(1):19-21.
4. Zaloga GP. Hypocalcemia in critically ill patients. *Crit Care Med.* 1992;20(2):251-262.
5. Kruse JA, Al-Douahji M, Carlson RW. Hypophosphatemia in critically ill patients: incidence and associations. *Crit Care Med.* 1992;20(40):S104.
6. Overgaard-Steensen C, Ring T. Clinical review: practical approach to hyponatraemia and hypernatraemia in critically ill patients. *Crit Care Med.* 2016;17(1):206.
7. Verbalis JG, Goldsmith SR, Greenberg A, Korzelius C, Schrier RW, Sterns RH. Diagnosis, evaluation, and treatment of hyponatremia: expert panel recommendations. *Am J Med.* 2013;126(10 Suppl 1):S1-42.
8. Sterns RH. Disorders of plasma sodium—causes, consequences, and correction. *New Eng J Med.* 2015;372(1):55-65.
9. Marino PL. Chapter 32: Hypertonic and hypotonic conditions. In: Marino, ed. *The ICU Book.* 3rd ed. Philadelphia, PA: Lippincott, Williams and Wilkins; 2007: 595-610.
10. Sterns RH, Nigwekar SU, Hix JK. The treatment of hyponatremia. *Semin Nephrol.* 2009;29(3):282-299.
11. Karp BL, Laureno R. Pontine and extrapontine myelinolysis: a neurologic disorder following rapid correction of hyponatremia. *Medicine (Baltimore).* 1993;72(6):359-373.
12. Schrier BL, Gross P, Gheorghiade M, et al; SALT Investigators. Tolvaptan, a selective oral vasopressin V2-receptor antagonist, for hyponatremia. *New Engl J Med.* 2006;355(20):2099-2112.
13. Gankham Kengne F, Soupart A, Pochet R, Brion JP, Decaux G. Re-induction of hyponatremia after rapid overcorrection of hyponatremia reduces mortality in rats. *Kidney Int.* 2009;76(6):614-621.
14. Perianayagam A, Sterns RH, Silver SM, Mayo R, Hix J, Kouides R. DDAVP is effective in preventing and reversing inadvertent overcorrection in hyponatremia. *Clin J Am Soc Nephrol.* 208;3(2):331-336.
15. Liamis G, Filippatos TD, Elisaf MS. Evaluation and treatment of hypernatremia: a practical guide for physicians". *Postgrad Med.* 2016;128(3):299-306.
16. Pepin J, Shields C. Advances in diagnosis and management of hypokalemia and hyperkalemic emergencies. *Emerg Med Pract.* 2012;14(2):1-17.
17. Palmer BF. Regulation of potassium homeostasis. *Clin J Am Soc Nephrol.* 2015;10(6):1050-1060.
18. Mount DB. Causes and evaluation of hyperkalemia. In: Post TW, ed. UpToDate, Waltham, MA: UpToDate, Inc. http://www.uptodate.com. Accessed November 29, 2016.
19. Freeman K, Feldman JA, Mitchell P, et al. Effects of presentation and electrocardiogram on time to treatment of hyperkalemia. *Acad Emerg Med.* 2008;15(3):239-249.
20. Smellie WS. Spurious hyperkalaemia. *BMJ.* 2007;334(7595):693-695.

21. Mushiyakh Y, Dangaria H, Qavi S, Ali N, Pannone J, Tompkins D. Treatment and pathogenesis of acute hyperkalemia. *J Community Hosp Intern Med Perspect.* 2012;1(4).

22. Lehnhardt A, Kemper MJ. Pathogenesis, diagnosis and management of hyperkalemia. *Pediatric Nephrol.* 2011;26(3): 377-384.

23. Montague BT, Ouellette JR, Buller GK. Retrospective review of the frequency of ECG changes in hyperkalemia. *Clin J Am Nephrol.* 2008;3(2):324-330.

24. Petrov DB. Images in clinical medicine. An electrocardiographic sine wave in hyperkalemia. *N Engl J Med.* 2012;366(19):1824.

25. Acker CG, Johnson JP, Palevsky PM, Greenberg A. Hyperkalemia in hospitalized patients: causes, adequacy of treatment, and results of an attempt to improve physician compliance with published therapy guidelines. *Arch Intern Med.* 1998;158(8):917-924.

26. Rossignol P, Legrand M, Kosiborod M, et al. Emergency management of severe hyperkalemia: guideline for best practice and opportunities for the future. *Pharmacol Res.* 2016;113(Pt A): 585-591.

27. Cohen R, Ramos R, Garcia CA, et al. Electrocardiogram manifestations in hyperkalemia. *World J Cardiovasc Dis.* 2012;2(2): 57-63.

28. Sterns RH, Rojas M, Berstein P, Chennupati S. Ion-exchange resins for the treatment of hyperkalemia: are they safe and effective? *J Am Soc Nephrol.* 2010;21(5):733-735.

29. Bakris GL, Pitt B, Weir MR, et al. Effect of patiromer on serum potassium level in patients with hyperkalemia and diabetic kidney disease: the AMETHYST-DN randomized clinical trial. *JAMA.* 2015;314(2):151-161.

30. Weisberg LS. Management of severe hyperkalemia. *Crit Car Med.* 2008;36(12):3246-3251.

31. Mount D. Clinical manifestations and treatment of hypokalemia in adults. In: Post TW, ed. UpToDate, Waltham, MA: UpToDate, Inc. http://www.uptodate.com. Accessed November 20, 2016.

32. Mount DB, Zandi-Nejad K. Disorders of potassium balance. In: Brenner BM, ed. *Brenner and Rector's: The Kidney.* 8th ed. Philadelphia, PA: WB Saunders Co; 2008: 547.

33. Rose BD, Post TW. Hypokalemia. In: Rose BD, ed. *Clinical Physiology of Acid-Base and Electrolyte Disorders.* 5th ed. New York, NY: McGraw-Hill; 2001: 836-887.

34. Comi G, Testa D, Cornelio F, et al. Potassium depletion myopathy: a clinical and morphological study of six cases. *Muscle Nerve.* 1985;8(1):17-21.

35. Shintani S, Shiigai T, Tsukagoshi H. Marked hypokalemic rhabdomyolysis with myoglobinuria due to diuretic treatment. *Eur Neurol.* 1991;31(6):396-398.

36. Yelamanchi VP, Molnar J, Ranade V, Somberg JC. Influence of electrolyte abnormalities on interlead variability of ventricular repolarization times in 12-lead electrocardiography. *Am J Ther.* 2001;8(2):117-122.

37. Wahr JA, Parks R, Boisvert D, et al. Preoperative serum potassium levels and perioperative outcomes in cardiac surgery patients. Multicenter Study of Perioperative Ischemia Research Group. *JAMA.* 1999;281(23):2203-2210.

38. Favus MI, Goltzman D. Regulation of calcium and magnesium. In: Rosen CJ, Boillon R, eds. *Primer on the Metabolic Bone Disease and Disorders of Mineral Metabolism.* 8th ed. Oxford, UK: Wiley-Blackwell; 2013: 173-179.

39. Hogan J. Goldfarb S. Regulation of calcium and phosphate balance. In: Post TW, ed. UpToDate, Waltham, MA: UpToDate, Inc. http://www.uptodate.com. Accessed November 25, 2016.

40. Schafer AL, Shoback D, Hypocalcemia: definition, etiology, pathogenesis, diagnosis and management. In: Rosen CJ, ed. *Primer on the Metabolic Bone Disease and Disorders of Mineral Metabolism.* 8th ed. Oxford, UK: Wiley-Blackwell; 2013: 572-577.

41. Horwitz MJ, Hodak SP, Stewart AF. Non-parathyroid hypercalcemia. In: Rosen CJ, ed. *Primer on the Metabolic Bone Disease and Disorders of Mineral Metabolism.* 8th ed. Oxford, UK: Wiley-Blackwell; 2013: 562-571.

42. Shane E. Diagnostic approach to hypercalcemia. In: Post TW, ed. UpToDate, Waltham, MA: UpToDate, Inc. http://www.uptodate.com. Accessed January 29, 2017.

43. Silverberg SJ. Primary hyperparathyroidism. In: Rosen CJ, ed. *Primer on the Metabolic Bone Disease and Disorders of Mineral Metabolism.* 8th ed. Oxford, UK: Wiley-Blackwell; 2013: 543-552.

44. Rose BD, Post TW. Hyperosmolal states—hypernatremia. In: Rose BD. *Physiologic Approach to Acid-Base and Electrolyte Disorders.* 5th ed. New York, NY: McGraw-Hill; 2001:756.

45. Lins LE. Reversible renal failure caused by hypercalcemia: a retrospective study. *Acta Med Scand.* 1978;203(4):309-314.

46. Bilezikian JP. Clinical review 51: management of hypercalcemia. *J Clin Endocrinol Metab.* 1993;77(6):1445-1449.

47. Stewart. Hypercalcemia associated with cancer. *N Eng J Med.* 2005;352(4):373-379.

48. Dietzek A, Connolly K, Cotugno M, Bartel S, McDonnell AM. Denosumab in hypercalcemia of malignancy: a case series. *J Oncol Pharm Pract.* 2015;21(2):143-147.

49. Bugg NC, Jones JA. Hypophoshatemia: pathophysiology, effects and management on the intensive care unit. *Anaesthesia.* 1998;53(9):895-902.

50. Stubbs Y. Overview of the causes and treatment of hyperphosphatemia, In: Post TW, ed. UpToDate, Waltham, MA: UpToDate, Inc. http://www.uptodate.com. Accessed June 15, 2017.

51. Juan D, Liptak P, Gray TK. Absorption of inorganic phosphate in the human jejunum and its inhibition by salmon calcitonin. *J Clin Endocrinol Metab.* 1976;43(3):517-522.

52. Murer H. Homer Smith Award. Cellular mechanisms in proximal tubular Pi reabsorption: some answers and more questions. *J Am Soc Nephrol.* 1992;2(12):1649-1665.

53. Amanzadeh J, Reilly RF Jr. Hypophosphatemia: an evidenced-based approach to its clinical consequences and management. *Nat Clin Pract Nephrol.* 2006;2(3):136-148.

54. Lederer E. Regulation of serum phosphate. *J Physiol.* 2014; 592(18):3985-3995.

55. Brown CV, Rhee P, Chan L, et al. Preventing renal failure in patients with rhabdomyolysis: do bicarbonate and mannitol make a difference? *J Trauma.* 2004;56(6):1191-1196.

56. Slater MS, Mullins RJ. Rhabdomyolysis and myoglobinuric renal failure in trauma and surgical patients: a review. *J Am Coll Surg.* 1998;186(6):693-716.

57. Hande KR, Garrow GC. Acute tumor lysis syndrome in patients with high-grade non-Hodgkins lymphoma. *Am J Med.* 1993;94(2):133-139.

58. Boles JM, Dutel JL, Briere J. Acute renal failure caused by extreme hyperphosphatemia after chemotherapy of acute lymphoblastic leukemia. *Cancer.* 1984;53(11):2425-2429.

59. O'Connor LR, Klein KL, Bethune JE. Hyperphospatemia in lactic acidosis. *N Engl J Med*. 1977;297(13):707-709.

60. Kebler R, McDonald FD, Cadnapaphornchai P. Dynamic changes in serum phsophorous levels in diabetic ketoacidosis. *Am J Med*. 1985;79(5):571-576.

61. Lieberman DA, Ghormley J, Flora K. Effect of oral sodium phosphate colon preparation on serum electrolytes in patients with normal serum creatinine. *Gastrointest Endosc*. 1996;43(5):467-469.

62. Howard SC, Jones DP, Pui CH. The tumor lysis syndrome. *New Engl J Med*. 2011;364(19):1844-1854.

63. Pierides AM, Edwards WG Jr, Cullum UX Jr, McCall JT, Ellis HA. Hemodialysis encephalopathy with osteomalacic fractures and muscle weakness. *Kidney Int*. 1980;18(1):115-124.

64. Skipper A. Refeeding syndrome or refeeding hypophosphatemia: a systematic review of cases. *Nutr Clin Pract*. 2012;27(1):34-40.

65. Crook MA, Hally V, Panteli JV. The importance of the refeeding sydrome. *Nutrition*. 2001;17(7-8):632-637.

66. Ognibene A, Ciniglio R, Greifenstein A, et al. Ventricular tachycardia in acute myocardial infarction: the role of hypophosphatemia. *South Med J*. 1994;87(1):65-69.

67. O'Connor LR, Wheeler WS, Bethune JE. Effect of hypophosphatemia on myocardial performance in man. *New Engl J Med*. 1977;297(17):901-903.

68. Zazzo JF, Troché G, Ruel P, Maintenant J. High incidence of hypophosphatemia in surgical intensive care patients. *Intensive Care Med*. 1995;21(10):826-831.

69. Aubier M, Murciano D, Lecocguic Y, et al. Effects of hypophosphatemia on diaphragmatic contractility in patients with acute respiratory failure. *New Engl J Med*. 1985;313(7):420-424.

70. Knochel JP, Barcenas C, Cotton JR, Fuller TJ, Haller R, Carter NW. Hypophosphatemia and rhabdomyolysis. *J Clin Invest*. 1978;62(6):1240-1246.

71. Mehller PS, Winkelman AB, Andersen DM, Gaudiani JL. Nutritional rehabilitation: practical guidelines for refeeding the anorectic patient. *J Nutr Metab*. 2010; 2010.

72. Collin AA, Hochberg Z, Kraiem Z. Maintenance theophylline therapy in children: effect on urinary calcium, phosphate and cyclic AMP excretion. *Acta Paediatr Scand*. 1987;76(2):367-368.

73. Kelepouris E, Agus ZS. Effects of diuretics on calcium and phosphate transport. *Semin Nephrol*. 1988;8(3):273-281.

74. Weisbord SD, Chaudhuri A, Blauth K, Derubertis FR. Monoclonal gammopathy and spurious hypophosphatemia. *Am J Med Sci*. 2003;325(2):98-100.

75. Mandry JM, Posner MR, Tucci JR, Eil C. Hyperphosphatemia in multiple myeloma due to a phosphate binding immunoglobulin. *Cancer*. 1991;68(5):1092-1094.

76. Lentz RD, Brown DM, Kjellstrand CM. Treatment of severe hypophosphatemia. *Ann Intern Med*. 1978;89(6):941-944.

77. Rosen GH, Boullata JI, O'Rangers EA, Enow NB, Shin B. Intravenous phosphate repletion regimen for critically ill patients with moderate hypophosphatemia. *Crit Care Med*. 1995;23(7):1204-1210.

78. Elin RJ. Magnesium: the fifth but forgotten electrolyte. *Am J Clin Pathol*. 1994;102(5):616-622.

79. Elin RJ. Assessment of magnesium status. *Clin Chem*. 1987;33(11):1965-1970.

80. McLean RM. Magnesium and its therapeutic uses: a review. *Am J Med*. 1994;96(1):63-76.

81. Graham LA, Caesar JJ, Burgen A. Gastrointestinal absorption and excretion of magnesium 28 in man. *Metab Clin Exp*. 1960;9:646-659.

82. Fawcett WJ, Haxby EJ, Male DA. Magnesium: physiology and pharmacology. *Br J Anaesth*. 1999;83(2):302-320.

83. Zaloga GP. Interpretation of serum magnesium level. *Chest*. 1989;95(2):257-258.

84. de Baaij JH, Hoenderop JG, Bindels RJ. Magnesium in man: implications for health and disease. *Physiol Rev*. 2015;95(1):1-46.

85. Moriasaki H, Yamamoto S, Morita Y, Kotake Y, Ochiai R, Takeda J. Hypermagnesemia-induced cardiopulmonary arrest before induction of anesthesia for emergency cesarean section. *J Clin Anesthes*. 2000;12(3):224-226.

86. Rude RK. Chapter 70: Magnesium depletion and hypermagnesemia. In: Rosen CJ, Compston JE, Lian JB, eds. *Primer on the Metabolic Bone Diseases and Disorders of Mineral Metabolism*. 7th ed. Washington DC: JW Wiley; 2008; 325-328.

87. Whang R, Oei TO, Aikawa J. Predictors of clinical hypomagnesemia, hypokalemia, hypophophatemia, hyponatremia, and hypocalcemia. *Arch Intern Med*. 1984;144(9):1794-1796.

88. Tong GM, Rude RK. Magnesium deficiency in critical illness. *J Intensive Care Med*. 2005;20(1):3-17.

89. Zafar MH, Wani JI, Karim R, Mir MM, Koul PA. Significance of serum magnesium levels in critically ill patients. *Int J App Basic Med Res*. 2014;4(1):34-37.

90. Ramadan NM, Halvorson H. Low brain magnesium in migraine. *Headache*. 1989;29(9):590-593.

91. Ramee SR, White CJ, Svinarich JT, Watson TD, Fox RF. Torsade de pointes and magnesium deficiency. *Am Heart J*. 1985;109(1):164-167.

92. Satur CM. Magnesium and cardiac surgery. *Ann R Coll Surg Engl*. 1997;79(5):349-354.

93. Rude RK, Oldham SB, Singer FR. Functional hypoparathyroidism and parathyroid hormone end-organ resistance in human magnesium deficiency. *Clin Endocrinol*. 1976;5(3):209-224.

94. Huang CL, Kuo E. Mechanism of hypokalemia in magnesium deficiency. *J Am Soc Nephrol*. 2007;18(10):2649-2652.

95. Wong N, Sutton RA, Navichak V, Quame GA, Dirks JH. Enhanced distal absorption of potassium by magnesium-deficient rats. *Clin Sci (Lond)*. 1985;69(5):626-639.

96. Heller BI, Hammarsten JF, Stutzman FL. Concerning the effects of magnesium sulfate on renal function, electrolyte excretion, and clearance of magnesium. *J Clin Invest*. 1953;32(9):858-861.

97. Yu A, Lam AQ. Evaluation and treatment of hypomagnesemia. In: Post TW, ed. UpToDate, Waltham, MA:UpToDate, Inc. http://www.uptodate.com. Accessed December 18, 2016.

98. Kraft MD, Btaiche IF, Sacks GS, Kudsk KA. Treatment of electrolyte disorders in adult patients in the intensive care unit. *Am J Health Syst Pharm*. 2005;62(16):1663-1682.

99. Momi J, Tang CM, Abcar AC, Kujubu DA, Simm JJ. Hyponatremia-What is cerebral salt wasting? *Perm J*. 2010;14(2):62-65.

100. Nijer S, Ghosh AK, Dubrey SW. Hypocalcaemia, long QT interval and atrial arrhythmias. *BMJ Case Rep*. 2010;2010: bcr0820092216.

101. Rose BD, Post TW. Hypoosmolal states—hyponatremia. *Clinical Physiology of Acid-Base and Electrolyte Disorders*. New York, NY: McGraw-Hill; 2001.

102. Nimesh B, Kafle P, Panda M. Beer potomania: a case report. *BMJ Case Rep*. 2010;2010.

103. Hannon MJ, Finucane FM, Sherlock M. Clinical review: disorders of water homeostasis in neurosurgical patients. *J Clin Endocrinol Metab.* 2012;97(5):1423-1433.

104. Rose BD, Post TW. Hyperkalemia. *Clinical Physiology of Acid-Base and Electrolyte Disorders.* 5th ed. New York, NY: McGraw-Hill; 2001: 888-930.

105. Blumberg A, Weidmann P, Shaw S, Gnadinger M. Effect of various therapeutic approaches on plasma potassium and major regulating factors in terminal renal failure. *Am J Med.* 1988;85(4):507-512.

106. Mount. DB. Treatment and prevention of hyperkalemia in adults. In: Post TW, ed. UpToDate, Waltham, MA: UpToDate, Inc. http://www.uptodate.com. Accessed November 26, 2016.

107. Allon M, Copkney C. Albuterol and insulin for treatment of hyperkalemia in hemodialysis patients. *Kidney Int.* 1995;38(5):869-872.

108. Goldman S, Holcenberg JS, Finklestein JZ, et al. A randomized comparison between rasburicase and allopurinol in children with lymphoma or leukemia at high risk for tumor lysis. *Blood.* 2001;97(10):2998-3003.

109. Danziger J, William JH, Scott DJ, et al. Proton-pump inhibitor use is associated with low serum magnesium concentrations. *Kidney Int.* 2013;83(4):692-699.

110. Dumon JC, Magritte A, Body JJ. Nasal human calcitonin for tumor-induced hypercalcemia. *Calcif Tissue Int.* 1992;52(1):18-19.

111. Berenson JR, Yellin O, Crowley JEA. Prognostic factors and jaw and renal complications among multiple myeloma patients treated with zoledronic acid. *Am J Hematol.* 2011;86(1):25-30.

112. Magee LA, Pels A, Rey E, von Dadelszen P; SOGC Hypertension Guideline Committee. Diagnosis, evaluation and management of hypertensive disorders of pregnancy: executive summary. *J Obstet Gynaecol Can.* 2014;36(7):575-576.

113. Sibai BM, Lipshitz J, Anderson GD, Dilts PV. Reassessment of intravenous MgSO$_4$ therapy in preeclampsia-eclampsia. *Obstet Gynecol.* 1981;57(2):199-202.

114. Smith JM, Lowe RF, Fullerton J, Currie SM, Harris L, Felker-Kantor E. An integrative review of the side effects related to the use of magnesium sulfate for pre-eclampsia and eclampsia management. *BMC Pregnancy Childbirth.* 2013;13(1):34.

115. Lu JF, Nightingale CH. Magnesium sulfate in eclampsia and pre-eclampsia: pharmacokinetic principles. *Clin Pharmacokinet.* 2000;38(4):305-314.

Hemodynamic Monitoring

Mayanka Tickoo, MD, Ronaldo Collo Go, MD, and Michael McBrine, MD

INTRODUCTION

Patients are usually transferred to the intensive care unit (ICU) due to their hemodynamic instability. Interpretation of hemodynamic monitoring is crucial to delivery of prompt and appropriate intervention.

PHYSIOLOGY

One of the goals of the cardiovascular system is to ensure optimum oxygen delivery to peripheral tissues. Oxygen delivery to the tissues (Do_2, mL O_2/min) is defined as the arterial oxygen content (Cao_2, mL O_2/dL) times the cardiac output (CO, L/min), described as

$$Do_2 \text{ (mL } O_2/\text{min)} = CO \text{ (L/min)} \times Cao_2 \text{ (mL } O_2/\text{dL)} \times 10$$

Where CO (L/min) = Heart Rate (HR, beats/min) × Stroke Volume (SV, L/beat), and Cao_2 (mL O_2/dL) = (1.34 × [Hgb (g/dL)] × Sao_2) + (0.0031 × Pao_2 [mmHg]), where Hgb is hemoglobin, Sao_2 the arterial saturation of oxygen, and Pao_2 is arterial pressure of oxygen.[1,2]

Oxygen consumption (Vo_2) is the amount of oxygen utilized by the tissues and is defined by the following equation:

$$VO_2 = \text{Transported Arterial Oxygen } (Dao_2)$$
$$- \text{Transported Venous Oxygen } (Dvo_2)$$

Given its negligible contribution, the dissolved oxygen in plasma can be omitted and the equation simplified, using the arterial concentration of carbon dioxide ($Caco_2$), the venous concentration of carbon dioxide ($Cvco_2$), and the venous saturation of oxygen (Svo_2):

$$VO_2 = (CO \times Caco_2 \times 10) - (CO \times Cvco_2 \times 10)$$
$$VO_2 = CO \times Hgb \times 13.4 \times (Sao_2 - Svo_2)$$

Normal oxygen consumption is 250 mL of oxygen per minute. When there is a stress or imbalance, the body compensates by increasing cardiac output or by increasing oxygen extraction at the tissue level. Increased oxygen extraction can be seen when there is a larger arterial-venous oxygen saturation difference and when the mixed venous oxyhemoglobin saturation (Svo_2) is lower than normal. The body also tries to compensate during these times of stress by redistributing blood to these areas of greatest extraction and with selective vasoconstriction of other capillary beds.[1,2]

Several of these parameters can be measured using various techniques that are static, intermittent, or continuous. In an acute critical illness, it is preferable to perform hemodynamic monitoring at least intermittently, if not continuously. Not only does this type of monitoring help determine progression of the disease process, but it also can evaluate the success or failure of the interventions performed.[3-5]

As mentioned above, cardiac output is the heart rate times stroke volume. Stroke volume is the amount of blood ejected per beat and depends on preload (end-diastolic tension), contractility, and afterload (end-systolic tension).[3] Preload is determined by the pressure gradient between capacitance veins and the right atrium. Pressure in capacitance veins is determined by mean systemic pressure (MSP), right atrial pressure (RAP), and systemic vascular resistance (SVR) via the following equation:

$$\text{Venous Return} = (MSP - RAP)/SVR^{3,5}$$

This is regulated by the sympathetic nervous system on the splanchnic circulation and will adapt to maintain adequate venous return.[6]

According the Frank-Starling law, the increase in myocyte stretching increases the strength of contraction, stroke volume, and afterload. This forms the concept of fluid responsiveness.[3] However, there is a point at which further stretching does not further increase the contraction, thus forms the concept of fluid unresponsiveness[3] (Fig. 3-1).

BLOOD PRESSURE MONITORING

Blood pressure (BP) is CO × SVR. Blood pressure has two components: systolic blood pressure (SBP) and diastolic blood pressure (DBP). Mean arterial pressure (MAP), or average pressure in one cardiac cycle, can be calculated as: [(2 × Diastolic) + Systolic] divided by 3 or MAP = 1/3 (SBP − DBP) + DBP. Generally, the MAP goal is more than or equal to 65 mmHg.

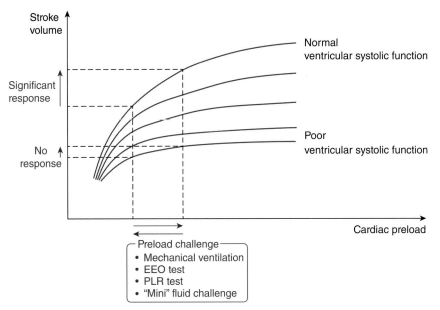

FIGURE 3-1 Frank-Starling relationship. The slope of the Frank-Starling curve depends on the ventricular systolic function. Then, one given level of cardiac preload does not help in predicting fluid responsiveness. By contrast, dynamic tests include a preload challenge (either spontaneous, induced by mechanical ventilation, or provoked, by passive leg raising, end-expiratory occlusion, or fluid infusion). Observing the resulting effects on stroke volume allows for the detection of preload responsiveness. EEO = end expiratory occlusion; PLR = passive leg raising.[7] (Source: Monnet X, Marik PE, Teboul JL. Prediction of fluid responsiveness: an update. *Ann Intensive Care.* 2016;6(111):1-11.)

Noninvasive monitoring is often the initial modality, given its ease of use and ubiquitous availability.[8] However, hemodynamic instability or vasopressor dependence demand continuous or more frequent assessment of BP than a noninvasive system can provide.

Arterial Catheter

Invasive arterial monitoring is performed by placing a hollow catheter in a peripheral (radial or brachial) or central (axillary or femoral) artery. Arterial pressure changes are continuously transmitted to a noncompressible fluid column that is connected via noncompliant tubing to an electromanometric transducer at the end. The transducer converts mechanical displacement into an electrical signal that generates a waveform. The systolic arterial pulse pressure increases and the diastolic arterial pulse pressure decreases the further away the vessel is from the thoracic aorta. This phenomenon leads to different waveform morphologies,[9,10] depending on where the arterial catheter is placed (Fig. 3-2).

Overdamping (Fig. 3-3) of the system with high resistance or an inefficient transmission of pressure leads to an underestimation of pressure. Conversely, underdamping with either low resistance or excessive oscillation

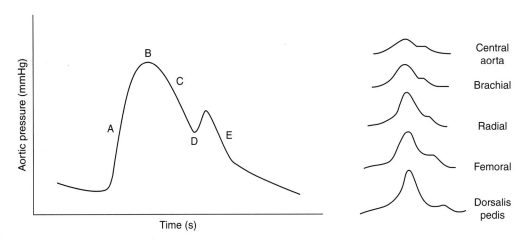

FIGURE 3-2 (A) Systolic upstroke or anacrotic limb reflects the left ventricle contraction. (B) Peak systole. (C) Decreasing systole. (D) Incisura or aortic valve closure. (E) Diastole. (Right panel from: Gorny DA. Arterial blood pressure measurement technique. Figure 2. AACN Clin Issues *Crit Care Nurs.* 1993;4(1):66-80. All rights reserved. Used with permission.).

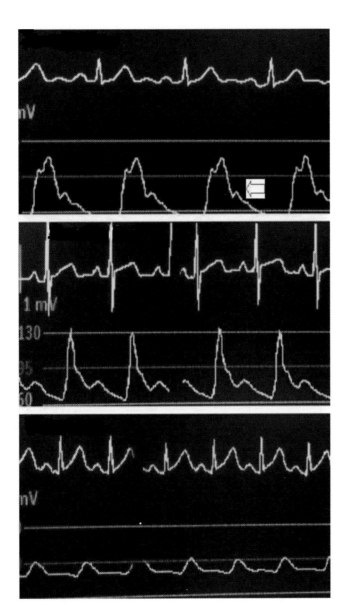

FIGURE 3-3 Invasive arterial waveform in red (A) showing systolic upstroke and a dicrotic notch (arrow), followed by downstroke. (B) An underdamped waveform (can overestimate systolic and underestimate diastolic pressure). (C) An overdamped waveform (can underestimate systolic and overestimate diastolic waveform). Note the mean arterial pressure is less prone to errors related to under- or overdamping.

overestimates the actual pressure of the system. The air-fluid interface of the catheter system must be leveled at the phlebostatic axis. This axis is the junction of a vertical line drawn from the fourth intercostal space at the sternum and a horizontal line drawn from the midpoint of a line from the anterior to the posterior of the chest. The phlebostatic axis is a reflection of the level of the atrium in either an upright or supine patient.[1] It also must be zeroed to establish hydrostatic zero, a reference point for accuracy. If the air-fluid interface is below this point, the pressure will be falsely high, and if the air-fluid interface is above this point, pressure will be falsely low.

In addition to the influences of the mean arterial pressure, the arterial waveform is influenced by stroke volume, vascular capacitance, peripheral vascular resistance, and heart rate. A reduction in vascular compliance will result in elevated systolic pressures, while reduced volume diminishes vascular recoil, leading to low diastolic pressures.[11,12]In patients who are hypovolemic, the incisura or dicrotic notch may appear later in the waveform.

Mechanical ventilation has a profound influence on both right- and left-sided heart pressures when compared to spontaneously breathing patients. While on the ventilator, intrathoracic pressure increases during inspiration. Subsequently, the right ventricular (RV) preload decreases and afterload increases, causing a reduction in the RV stroke volume. This decrease in RV stroke volume causes a decrease in left ventricular (LV) filling after a 2- to 3-beat phase lag and, therefore, decreases the LV stroke volume. This beat-to-beat variation in stroke volume and pulse pressure is more pronounced in hypovolemic patients, and is also influenced by tidal volume, inspiratory pressure, and positive end-expiratory pressure (PEEP). In patients with low tidal volumes and decreased lung compliance, this variation in stroke volume is often masked.[11,12]

Risks of invasive arterial monitoring include vascular injury, such as a hematoma, or wall dissection. Infection, embolization, or thrombosis of the distal vasculature can also occur and can lead to limb-threatening ischemia.[13]

FLUID RESPONSIVENESS

The decision to give fluids is based on the increase in stroke volume, but all fluid responders are not necessarily hypovolemic and do not necessarily require volume expansion.[14] The iatrogenic phenomenon called *volume overload* gives credence to this idea. Analysis of the Frank-Starling curve and extravascular lung water (EVLW) shows that as the patient becomes less fluid responsive, the EVLW and edema increase.[14-16] (Fig. 3-4) This is worse in patients with prior endothelial damage such as sepsis, acute respiratory distress syndrome (ARDS), and burns.[14-16] In addition, natriuretic peptides cleave membrane-bound proteoglycans and glycoproteins off the membrane permeability–regulating endothelial glycocalax and, consequently, increase fluid into the interstitial spaces.[14-21]

Fluid response challenges can be given with a trial of fluid bolus or a passive leg raise (PLR). A PLR is a reversible preload challenge involving a 250- to 500-mL bolus of blood and can be measured in patients with arrhythmias, spontaneous breathing, low tidal volumes, and low lung compliance.[7,22] The best sensitivity and specificity is an increase in CO greater than 10%, with a sensitivity of 85% and specificity of 91%.[23] Cardiac output effects of PLR reach their maximum within 1 minute. Therefore, continuous monitoring is advocated. PLR can induce changes in: (1) peak velocities of carotids or femoral arteries; (2).bioreactance; (3) cardiac output via pulse contour analysis of arterial wave via photoplethysmography; and (4) in end-tidal CO_2.[7]

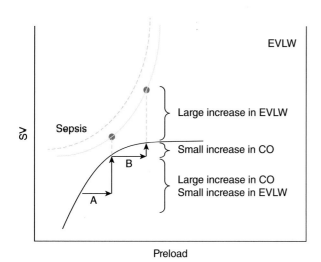

FIGURE 3-4 Superimposition of the Frank-Starling and Marik-Phillips curves demonstrating the effects of increasing preload on SV and lung water in a patient who is preload responsive (A) and nonresponsive (B). With sepsis, the EVLW curve is shifted to the left. EVLW = extravascular lung water; CO = cardiac output; SV = stroke volume. (Source: Marik PE Lemson J. Fluid responsiveness: an evolution of our understanding. *Brit J Anaesth*. 2014;112(4):617-620.)

Central venous pressure was thought to monitor volume status and fluid responsiveness, but recent literature suggests it is a poor indicator of either.[14,24] Static measurements such as pulmonary artery occlusive pressure (PAOP), global end-diastolic volume via transpulmonary thermodilution, and flow time of aortic flow via transesophageal Doppler are poor indicators due to the variability of Frank-Starling mechanics from person to person and from time to time.[25-27] Certain authors still found the utility of measuring the central venous pressure (CVP) in shock, since it can be marker of organ perfusion (MAP – CVP), and elevated CVP is associated with acute kidney injury (AKI).[27-29]

There has been a focus toward dynamic interactions between the heart and lung during positive-pressure ventilation. Dynamic preload indices such as pulse-pressure variation (PPV) and stroke volume variation (SVV) are based on physiologic changes occurring in the preload and afterload conditions of the ventricles with positive-pressure ventilation, as described earlier in the chapter. A stroke volume (and pulse pressure) variation of more than 13% indicates fluid responsiveness in a patient.[30]

Several devices in common clinical use (pulse index continuous cardiac output [PiCCO], lithium dilutional cardiac output [LiDCO], pressure recording analytical method [PRAM]) are based on arterial pulse waveform or contour analysis. These devices may also include indicator dilution cardiac output for calibration of the pulse contour. The principle of pulse contour analysis is that the area under the curve of the systolic portion of the arterial waveform is proportional to the stroke volume.[12] These systems also allow for calculation of pulse-pressure variation (direct, waveform analysis) or stroke-volume variation (indirect, pulse contour analysis).

Both pulse-pressure variation and stroke-volume variation are useful indicators of volume responsiveness in a patient in shock.[31,32] The accuracy of pulse waveform–based devices is limited in patients with arrhythmias, decreased arterial compliance, and aortic diseases like aortic insufficiency and severe atherosclerosis.

Limitations of pulse pressure variation and stroke volume variation include needing tidal volumes greater than 8 mL/kg and a sinus rhythm, and having a patient not spontaneously breathing. They are also limited in the following clinical scenarios: ARDS, intra-abdominal hypertension, and right-heart failure. In ARDS, tidal volumes are advocated to be 6 mL/kg but can be transiently increased to 8 mL/kg, and fluid responsiveness would be defined as PPV of 3.5% or greater, or SVV of 2.5% or greater.[33] However, the low compliance prevents transmission of alveolar pressures to intravascular and cardiac pressures, therefore limiting its use.[34] In intra-abdominal hypertension, the respiratory variations of stroke volume are not necessarily related to volume status.[35-37] Right ventricular failure can cause increased afterload that might suggest false positive PPV and SVV.[27]

BIOIMPEDENCE

Bioimpedance cardiography is based on the principle that the thorax is a fluid-filled cylinder (filled with tissue fluid, pulmonary and venous blood volume, and aortic blood volume) that has an intrinsic resistance to the flow of current, or impedance. With systolic and diastolic changes in the fluid content of the thorax, the impedance of the thorax changes. This change in current or impedance is measured by applying low-voltage electrodes on the chest and detecting the difference between systole and diastole. Cardiac output is subsequently calculated with the assumption that the change in voltage correlates with the change in stroke volume.[38] In the clinical setting, however, several reports describing a poor correlation between cardiac output using pulmonary artery catheters (PAC) and bioimpedance monitors in cardiac surgery,[39] as well as in critically ill patients.[30,40] Given its low fidelity, newer monitoring devices have since been developed.

BIOREACTANCE

Noninvasive cardiac output monitoring (NICOM; eg, CHEE-TAH NICOM)[41] is a device based on the principle of bioreactance. While bioimpedance depends on the fluid content of the entire thorax, bioreactance measures changes in current during pulsatile blood flow in the large thoracic arteries like the aorta. By measuring the phase shift in applied current caused by the pulsatile flow, SV can be calculated.[42] The system detects the heart rate and generates a display of cardiac output using HR and SV (CO = SV × HR). Manual or automated entry of mean arterial pressure (MAP) allows for calculation of systemic vascular resistance. Stroke volume variation can be calculated before and after a fluid bolus (or passive leg raise) to assess fluid responsiveness. NICOM is a completely non-invasive system, utilizing special sensor pads with transmitting and receiving sensors applied to the thorax. Several studies have shown correlation between CO determined by bioreactance systems and PACs.[43] Use of electrocautery and external pacemakers, as well as severe aortic insufficiency or aortic pathology, might limit the accuracy of this system. Weight, hemoglobin, MAP, and oxygen saturation are the initial parameters needed. Passive leg raise or 250% mL normal saline bolus is needed to calculate stroke volume index (SVI). An SVI of greater than 10% suggests fluid responsive hypotension.

END-EXPIRATORY OCCLUSION TEST

Insufflation from mechanical ventilation can decrease cardiac preload and impede venous return. Interruption of mechanical ventilation will stop this impedence.[7] Therefore, cardiac preload increases, which can cause an increase in cardiac output. The end-expiratory occlusion (EEO) should be greater than 15 seconds due to transit through the pulmonary circulation, and it appears to have utility in ARDS.[44,45] Analysis is via pulse contour and echocardiography, with a 4% increase of the velocity-time integral (VTI) of the left ventricular outflow tract defining fluid responsiveness.[46]

RESPIRATORY SYSTOLIC VARIATION TEST

In the respiratory systolic variation test (RSVT), fluid responsiveness is determined by a decrease in systolic blood pressure after 3 standardized mechanical ventilator breaths with increased airway pressure.[47] Its accuracy appears to be equivalent to PPV and SVV.[48]

END-TIDAL CO_2

Along with diastolic blood pressure, end-tidal CO_2 ($ETCO_2$) has been considered a surrogate marker of coronary perfusion pressure and myocardial blood flow.[47] Therefore, an $ETCO_2$ of greater than 10 mmHg has been suggested with improved survival compared to an $ETCO_2$ of 10 mmHg or less.[49-51] It also has been suggested that changes in $ETCO_2$ can correlate to changes in CO when metabolic conditions and minute ventilation are constant.[52] Garcia and colleagues showed that changes in $ETCO_2$ during PLR in mechanically ventilated patients with acute circulatory failure under fixed minute ventilation and constant CO_2 production correlate with changes in CO to predict fluid responsiveness, with 5% or greater $ETCO_2$ or 12% or greater CO during PLR-predicted fluid responsiveness with sensitivity 90.5% (confidence interval [CI], 69.9–98.8%) and 95.2% (5% CI, 76.2–99.9%) and specificity 93.7% (95% CI, 69.9–99.8%).[52]

ECHOCARDIOGRAPHIC INDICES TO DETERMINE FLUID RESPONSIVENESS AND ULTRASOUND TO DETERMINE ETIOLOGY OF HYPOTENSION

Echocardiogram has been used to determine fluid-responsive hypotension and the etiology of the hypotension. It measures dynamic changes induced by heart-lung interactions or postural changes.[3] Two changes may occur with positive-pressure ventilation: increased intrathoracic pressure may decrease venous return and therefore may decrease stroke volume, and increased transpulmonary pressure compresses pulmonary arteries and therefore increases right ventricular afterload.[3] Postural changes often are elicited via the passive leg raise. Stroke volume, VTI, or BP is measured before and after the maneuver. A supine patient's legs are raised to 30% to 45%, causing 250 to 300 mL of blood to return to the heart. An increase of 10% to 15% or greater suggests fluid responsiveness.[3]

In the appropriate clinical setting, fluid-responsive hypotension may be suggested by echocardiographic visualization of a small left ventricle; the "kissing," or touching, papillary muscles during systole via M-mode on parasternal short-axis (PSAX) view; and/or hyperdynamic left ventricle with end-diastolic area in PSAX less than 10 cm^2.[3,53]

The same principle applies for a hyperdynamic and small right ventricle. However, a dilated right ventricle might preclude the use of fluid to improve the hypotension.

Another way to determine fluid-responsive hypotension is to evaluate the inferior vena cava (IVC). In a spontaneously breathing patient, an IVC diameter of less than 20 mm correlates with CVP or an RAP of less than 10 mm, and an IVC diameter of greater than 20 to 25 mm with no respiratory variation correlated with a CVP or RAP of greater than 10 mm.[53,54] In addition to the diameter, respiratory variation of greater than 25%, or 40% in mechanically ventilated patients, has suggested fluid responsiveness, but its utility in spontaneously breathing patients is less likely.[7,53,55,56] Other literature suggests that respiratory variation as low as 12% to 18% can still suggest fluid responsiveness, and this phenomenon is abolished when RAP or CVP is more than 10 mm.[3] This method is still controversial and other authors have proposed correlating IVC findings with the development of B-lines on thoracic ultrasound as a guide to stop fluid resuscitation (Fig. 3-5).[57]

The superior vena cava (SVC) can also be used to determine fluid responsiveness. A collapsibility index of 36% is used via the equation $100 \times ([D_{max} - D_{min}]/D_{min})$.[3] The need for a transesophageal echocardiogram to assess this variation may limit its use in the acute setting.

Another approach is to determine stroke volume variation via measurements of respiratory variation in VTI in the left ventricular outflow tract or respiratory variations in peak aortic flow. Respiratory variations of 20% or more predict fluid responsiveness in a patient who is mechanically

Point of Care Ultrasound *Fluid Resuscitation Guide*

- using IVC and lung ultrasound -

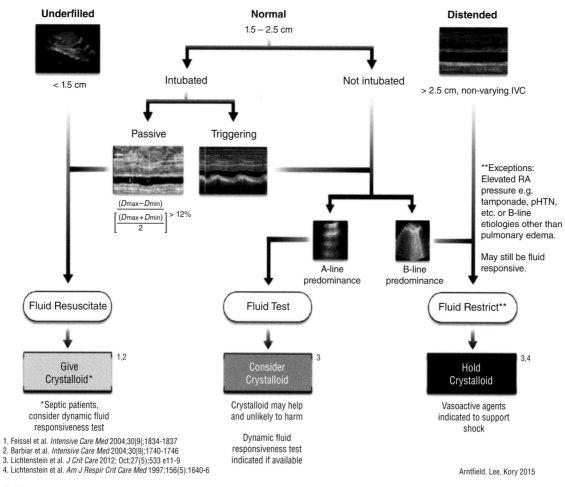

FIGURE 3-5 Point-of-care ultrasound fluid resuscitation guide. (Reprinted with permission from Lee C, Kory P, Arntfield R. Development of a fluid resuscitation protocol using inferior vena cava and lung ultrasound. *J Critical Care.* 2016;31(1):96-100.)

ventilated, and has a tidal volume of 8 mL/kg, a sinus rhythm, and normal abdominal pressure.[53]

A multicenter prospective study comparing several echographic indices such as respiratory variations of pulse pressure, SVC, IVC, and the maximal Doppler velocity in left ventricular outflow tract ($Vmax_{Ao}$) found that changes in respiratory variations of $\Delta Vmax_{Ao}$ had the best sensitivity and respiratory variations of the SVC had the best specificity in predicting fluid responsiveness after passive leg raise.[58] Another study found that passive leg raise may be the most useful parameter to determine fluid responsiveness in an unstable patient, and respiratory variation in the vena cava still needs confirmation studies.[59]

Point-of-care ultrasound might also suggest the etiology of hemodynamic compromise. McConnell sign of RV dysfunction with akinesis of the mid free wall but normal motion of the apex can suggest acute pulmonary embolism. Cardiac tamponade can be suggested by early diastole RV collapse,

late diastole right atrial (RA) collapse, exaggerated tricuspid and decreased mitral diastolic inflow on inspiration, dilated IVC with no respiratory variation, and the presence of pericardial effusion. Focal wall motion abnormality on echocardiogram could suggest acute coronary syndrome. Presence of lung point sign or bar code sign on thoracic ultrasound can suggest pneumothorax. Presence of fluid in abdominal ultrasound can suggest hemoperitoneum.

In a recent systematic review, Thiele and colleagues compared the available systems (thermodilution, bioreactance, bioimpedance, Doppler, and pulse contour analysis) with the Fick method in multiple clinical scenarios.[60] Based on the available data, this study found that Doppler-based techniques have comparable accuracy to thermodilution, while bioimpedance devices were less reliable. There is not much data regarding pulse contour analysis, but these devices are probably less accurate in the setting of hemodynamic instability. See Table 3-1 for a complete listing of all these devices.

TABLE 3-1 **Hemodynamic Monitoring Devices**

Device	Principle	Type	Advantages	Disadvantages	Additional Parameters
Swan	Fick or thermodilution	Invasive	Considered gold standard	Infection, thrombosis, dependent on observer interpretation, poorly correlates with mortality/morbidity outcomes	
CCO Swan	Thermodilution	Invasive	Provides continuous instead of intermittent measure of CO		
NICOM	Bioreactance	External sensor pads	Noninvasive	Electric interference, lower accuracy in AI	SVI
PiCCO	PCA with thermodilution to calibrate pulse contour	Subclavian/ IJ CVC and central arterial catheter	Good correlation with invasive CO in hemodynamic instability	CVC dependent	SVV
LiDCO	PCA with lithium dilution to calibrate pulse contour initially, then root mean square for subsequent measurements	Central or peripheral vein and central or peripheral arterial catheter	Good correlation with invasive CO in hemodynamic instability	Needs recalibration after any major hemodynamic or arterial impedance change	SVV, PPV
FloTrac	PCA with standardized demographic variables (age, sex, height, weight) for arterial impedance estimation	Central or peripheral arterial catheter	Easy to use, no external calibration	Poor correlation with CO in hemodynamic instability or arrhythmias	SVV, SVI
PRAM	PCA; real-time analysis of pressure-wave morphology throughout cardiac cycle	Central or peripheral arterial catheter	No external calibration	Not enough data for validation	SVV, PPV
Doppler	Velocity-time integral in RV and LVOT		Noninvasive (transthoracic) or minimally invasive (transesophageal)	Highly operator dependent (accurate positioning of probe along direction of blood flow)	

AI = aortic insufficiency; CCO = continuous cardiac output; CO = cardiac output; CVC = central venous catheter; IJ = internal jugular; LVOT = left ventricular outflow tract; PCA = pulse contour analysis; PPV = pulse pressure variation; RV = right ventricle; SVI = stroke volume index; SVV = stroke volume variation.

RIGHT HEART CATHETERIZATION

Overall, the use of pulmonary artery catheter (PAC) has been on the decline in the past several years. Randomized control trials in several ICU patient populations have not shown a significant difference in mortality rates or length of stay with the use of PACs.[61-66] The SUPPORT group investigators showed that PAC use is associated with higher mortality, longer ICU stays, and increased costs in critically ill patients.[67] Despite this recent literature, PAC is still used to determine different types of shock, diagnosis of pulmonary hypertension, valvular heart disease, and shunts.

The typical PAC has 4 lumens: (1) the proximal lumen (right atrial port) for venous sampling and intravenous infusion of cardiac output injectate; (2) the distal lumen (pulmonary artery port) for pulmonary artery sampling and SVo_2; (3) balloon lumen; and (4) thermistor lumen.[68] The pulmonary catheter is typically 110 cm long and can be inserted in the internal jugular vein, subclavian vein, brachial artery, or femoral vein (Table 3-2). The balloon is inflated in the right atrium, and both the distance from insertion and the cardiac chamber waveforms aide in determining the catheter's location (Table 3-3). While the patient is supine, the transducer should be set to 0 at the midthoracic level, halfway between the anterior sternum and bed surface.

The pulmonary artery wedge pressure (PAWP), also called pulmonary capillary wedge pressure (PCWP) or pulmonary artery occlusion pressure (PAOP), is measured by inflating the balloon with 1 to 1.5 mL of air when the distal tip is in the pulmonary artery in lung zone 3 at end expiration, and at end diastole (P waves on echocardiogram [ECG]).[66,68] Measuring both the PA and PAWP in lung zone 3 is important because the vessels are all patent during respiration (arterial pressure > venous pressure > alveolar pressure)[68]

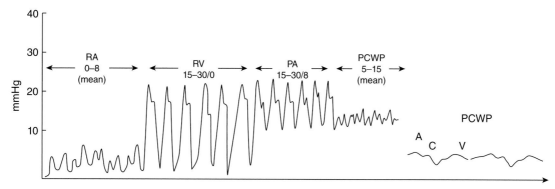

FIGURE 3-6 Pulmonary artery catheter waveforms as a Swan-Ganz catheter is floated through the right heart chambers. A = left atrial contraction; C = mitral valve closure; V = left ventricular contraction. (Left panel: Reproduced with permission from Bashore TM, et al. Heart Disease. In: Papadakis MA, McPhee SJ, Rabow MW. eds. *Current Medical Diagnosis & Treatment* 2018. New York, NY: McGraw-Hill; 2018.)

enabling an estimation of the highest pressure in the system. The following scenarios suggest that the catheter is in zone 3: PAWP is less than pulmonary artery diastolic pressure (PADP) by at least 1 to 5 mmHg, and a change of less than 50% in the PAWP with increases in PEEP in mechanically ventilated patients, with the catheter tip below the left atrium on chest x-ray.

Cardiac output is obtained via the Fick method or thermodilution. According to the Fick method, total oxygen consumption (Vo_2) by the lungs, or other peripheral tissues, is the product of blood flow through the lungs (CO) and the arteriovenous oxygen content difference ($Cao_2 - Cvo_2$) (Table 3-4). In steady state, the Vo_2 is commonly estimated, and cardiac output can be calculated using the difference in the pulmonary artery O_2 saturation and the O_2 saturation in the right atrium, thereby yielding CO as follows:[2]

$$CO = \frac{\text{Oxygen Consumption } (Vo_2)}{\text{Arteriovenous } O_2 \text{ Content Difference } (Cao_2 - Cvo_2)}$$

In the intermittent thermodilution technique for cardiac output estimation, a known volume of an injectate (usually normal saline) at known temperature (usually room temperature) is injected into the right atrium. The cooled blood traverses to the pulmonary artery, and the thermistor in the PAC measures the change in blood temperature. The cardiac output is inversely proportional to the mean decrease in blood temperature over the time of transit of cooled blood (area under the curve). This is usually measured 3 times, and an average is accepted as the CO to increase accuracy. Cardiac index, which is CO per unit of body surface area, can also be derived from this measurement. Continuous cardiac output PACs (Swan-Ganz CCO PACs) utilize the principle of thermodilution to calculate and display CO. These devices use a thermal filament located at the catheter tip with a continuous inflow of indicator temperature infusate (Fig. 3-6).

In addition, measurement of arterial pressure and CVP at the time of the procedure also allows for estimation of systemic vascular resistance (SVR = 80 × [MAP − CVP]/CO) as well as pulmonary vascular resistance (PVR = 80 × [mPAP − PCWP]/CO)], where mPAP is mean pulmonary artery pressure, and PCWP is pulmonary capillary wedge pressure.

The Svo_2 can be measured from the pulmonary artery, as there is an adequate mixing of blood from the coronary sinus, inferior vena cava, and superior vena cava. This measurement can be performed intermittently or continuously via reflection spectrophotometry. High Svo_2 is seen in hyperoxia, hypothermia, anesthesia, therapeutic paralysis, or sepsis. Low Svo_2 is seen with anemia or hemorrhage, hypoxia,

TABLE 3-2   Relative Distance of Cardiac Chambers From the Site of Insertion of Pulmonary Artery Catheter

Site	Distance to the:		
	RA	**RV**	**PA**
Internal jugular	15–20 cm	30 cm	40 cm
Subclavian	15–20 cm	30 cm	40 cm
Femoral	30 cm	40 cm	50 cm
Brachial			
Right	40 cm	50 cm	60 cm
Left	50 cm	60 cm	70 cm

PA = pulmonary artery; RA = right atrium; RV = right ventricle.

TABLE 3-3   Range of Normal Pressures in Various Cardiac Chambers Using Pulmonary Artery Catheterization

Cardiac Chamber Pressure	Normal Values
Right atrial pressure/central venous pressure	0–8 mmHg
Right ventricular pressure	15–30 mmHg/2–8 mmHg
Pulmonary artery pressure	15–30 mmHg/8–15 mmHg
Pulmonary artery wedge pressure	5–15 mmHg

TABLE 3-4 Normal Range of Hemodynamic Variables Derived Using Pulmonary Artery Catheterization

Variable	Formula	Normal Values
Cardiac output	$\dfrac{\text{Oxygen Consumption (Vo}_2)}{\text{A-V O}_2 \text{ Content Difference } (\text{Cao}_2 - \text{Cvo}_2)}$	4.0–8.0 L/min
Cardiac index	$\dfrac{\text{Cardiac Output (L/min)}}{\text{Body Surface Area (m}^2)}$	2.2–4.2 L/min/m²
Systemic vascular resistance (SVR)	$\dfrac{(\text{MAP} - \text{CVP}) \times 80}{\text{Cardiac Output (L/min)}}$	800–1200 dynes/s/cm⁵
Pulmonary vascular resistance (PVR)	$\dfrac{(\text{mPAP} - \text{PAOP}) \times 80}{\text{Cardiac Output (L/min)}}$	125–250 dynes/s/cm⁵
Stroke volume	$\dfrac{\text{Cardiac Output (L/min)}}{\text{Heart Rate (beats/min)}}$	60–120 mL/beat

A-V = atrioventricular; CVP = central venous pressure; MAP = mean arterial pressure; mPAP = mean pulmonary artery pressure; PAOP = pulmonary artery occlusive pressure.

shock, arrhythmias, shivering, hyperthermia, poor pain control, or seizures. The central venous oxyhemoglobin saturation (Scvo₂) is often used as a surrogate for Svo₂, as it can be drawn from the distal port of a central catheter terminating in the SVC. It does not require a PAC. The Svo₂ typically is greater than the Scvo₂, as the Scvo₂ is primarily drawing on blood from the SVC alone. Exceptions include anesthesia, when cerebral metabolism is depressed, and shock, in which circulation is diverted from the splanchnic circulation with subsequent increased oxygen extraction.

Shunt assessment is considered in patients with pulmonary artery saturation greater than 75%. Oxygen saturation measurements are obtained from the superior vena cava, inferior vena cava, right atrium high, right atrium middle, right atrium low, right ventricle, and pulmonary artery.[69] An oxygen saturation step-up greater than 7% suggests a left-to-right shunt in the atrium, such as in an atrial septal defect. An oxygen saturation step-up greater than 5% suggests a left-to-right shunt in ventricles, such as in a ventricular septal defect, or in the great vessels such as in patent ductus arteriosus.

QUESTIONS

1. A 62-year-old man with a history of paraplegia and a chronic indwelling suprapubic catheter is admitted into the ICU due to hemodynamic instability. He is fluid resuscitated, cultures are obtained, and he is started on empiric antimicrobial therapy. Norepinephrine is initiated for his persistently low blood pressure and an arterial line is placed for blood pressure monitoring. The nurse calls you over after she notices that the automated systolic cuff pressures are significantly higher than the arterial line pressures. Which of the following statements could explain the discrepancy?

   A. With lower blood pressure (systolic below 95), automated blood pressure measurements are often falsely higher than intra-arterial systolic pressure measurements.
   B. The resistance in the arterial line system set up is too high (overdamped), leading to an underestimation of systemic arterial pressure.
   C. The automated cuff is currently placed on the leg and is usually 10% to 20% percent higher than that in the brachial artery.
   D. All of the above.

2. For the patient in question 1, you examine the arterial line tracing and note a good waveform. What would your next best step be?

   A. Compare the mean arterial pressure obtained from both the noninvasive measurement and the invasive measurement.
   B. Ask the nurse to use the systolic measurement obtained from the noninvasive measurement and not from the arterial line.
   C. Ask the nurse to draw an arterial blood gas from the arterial line to ensure that it is an arterial line and not a venous line.
   D. Ask the nurse to decrease the resistance in the arterial line, as it is overdamped.

3. An elderly patient with septic shock from a urinary source is admitted into the ICU. The physical exam findings are suggestive of a fluid depleted state. Microbiologic cultures are obtained and antibiotics are initiated. A central line is placed, and CVP is measured at 6 mmHg. What is the optimal next best step?

   A. Fluid resuscitate until the CVP is greater than 12 mmHg.
   B. Fluid resuscitate until the CVP is between 8 and 12 mmHg.
   C. Hold fluids, as her CVP is within the normal range.
   D. Start fluid resuscitation, and use the CVP in conjunction with physical exam findings, lab values, and other noninvasive techniques to decide when to stop fluid resuscitation.

4. For the patient in question 3, after 2 Liters of normal saline, a subsequent CVP is obtained and reported as 3 mmHg. Her urine output has increased, and a lactate is downtrending. What is the next best step?

   A. Continue fluid resuscitation.
   B. Change antibiotics, as the decreased CVP suggests inadequate microbial coverage.

C. Clarify with nursing staff the location of the transducer placement and whether the level changed between measurements.

D. Obtain a computed tomography scan (CT) of the abdomen to look for a perinephric abscess.

5. An elderly patient presented to the hospital with chest discomfort for the past several days. Her ECG was without evidence of acute ST elevations but did show Q waves inferiorly. She is medically managed with heparin drip, nitrates, and Lasix but gradually develops worsening shortness of breath and is intubated. She has persistently high oxygen requirements despite attempts at diuresis, and her PEEP is gradually increased to a level of 14. A Swan-Ganz catheter is placed to help guide inotrope titration. An end-expiration PCWP is measured and found to be 34 mmHg. Subsequently, the thermodilution method is used to calculate CO. What factors may affect the validity of the PCWP reported?

A. Measurement at end inspiration
B. The high level of PEEP
C. The PAC placed in zones 1 or 2
D. All of the above

6. What factors may contribute to an underestimation of the CO?

A. Aortic regurgitation
B. Tricuspid regurgitation
C. Right-to-left intracardiac shunt
D. Pulmonary hypertension

7. An elderly gentleman is brought to the hospital after a neighbor found him to be obtunded on a wellness check. There is no further history available from the patient, family, or medical record. He is markedly hypotensive with no fever, leukocytosis, or obvious nidus of infection. He is empirically fluid challenged with no hemodynamic improvement. A Swan-Ganz catheter is being considered to help differentiate the etiology of his shock state. The use of routine Swan-Ganz catheter placement in shock is associated with which of the following?

A. Shorter ICU stays
B. Improved 30-day mortality
C. Less vasopressor use
D. None of the above

8. Which hemodynamic profile is most consistent with cardiogenic shock?

A. Low CO, low PCWP, high SVR
B. Low CO, high PCWP, high SVR
C. High CO, normal PCWP, low SVR
D. None of the above

9. A young man is admitted into the hospital with severe abdominal pain and shortness of breath. He admits to daily alcohol use and is markedly tender in the epigastric area. His lipase is markedly elevated and his chest x-ray shows bilateral infiltrates. His respiratory status worsens and he is electively intubated. Given the bilateral infiltrates and concern for ARDS, lung protective ventilator strategies are utilized with targeted tidal volumes around 6 mL/kg. He is aggressively fluid resuscitated but develops profound hypotension requiring vasopressors. An arterial line is placed and his SVV is measured. What factors limit the effectiveness of SVV?

A. Spontaneous breathing
B. Targeted tidal volume of 6 mL/kg
C. Atrial fibrillation
D. All of the above

10. For the patient in question 9, the tidal volume is temporarily increased, and his SVV is measured at 6%. What is the next best step?

A. Continue fluid resuscitation with normal saline
B. Continue fluid resuscitation with albumin
C. Stop fluid resuscitation
D. Stop fluid resuscitation and recheck SVV later

11. A 42-year-old patient with lupus and pulmonary hypertension is admitted into the ICU with fever, hypotension, and a lobar pulmonary infiltrate. Despite 30 mL/kg of bolus fluid resuscitation, the patient remains hypotensive with a blood pressure of 90/50 mmHg (mean arterial pressure of ~63 mmHg). A PAC is inserted that shows a CVP of 10 mmHg. Cardiac output is measured at 6 L/min. What is the systemic vascular resistance in this patient?

A. 10 dynes/cm^2
B. 200 dynes/cm^2
C. 700 dynes/cm^2
D. 1400 dynes/cm^2

12. For the patient in question 11, what is the etiology of shock?

A. Cardiogenic
B. Neurogenic
C. Septic
D. Hypovolemic

13. Which of the following choices correctly matches the waveform with an etiology (Fig. 3-7)?

A.   I = overwedging
B.   II = mitral regurgitation
C.   III = complete heart block
D.   IV = ventricular septal defect

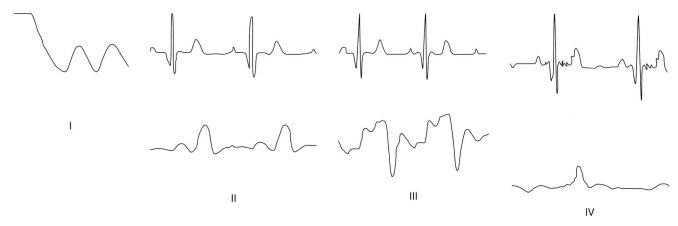

I

II

III

IV

FIGURE 3-7 Pulmonary artery catheter waveforms from I to IV.

ANSWERS

1. D. All of the above

   There are numerous reasons for a discrepancy in systolic blood pressure measurements between automated noninvasive measurements and intra-arterial measurements. Recent data has suggested that at lower blood pressures, a noninvasively measured systolic blood pressure will usually be higher than intra-arterial sampling without significant deviation in the mean arterial pressures (choice A). If the resistance in the arterial line is too high, there will be less mechanical displacement and subsequent lowering of the electrical signal, ultimately leading to a diminished blood pressure reading (choice B). Finally, studies suggest that in normal adults, systolic blood pressure readings are often higher in the legs than in the arms (choice C).

2. A. Compare the mean arterial pressure obtained from both the noninvasive measurement and the invasive measurement.

   In the setting of a good arterial waveform, there is little reason to doubt if the line is truly arterial or if the line is overdamped (choices C and D). Likewise, there is no reason to use the systolic measurement from the noninvasive measurement over the arterial line (choice B). One would expect that the mean arterial pressure obtained both invasively and noninvasively would roughly correlate. If the measurements do not correlate, given the good arterial waveform, that measurement should be used preferentially.

3. D. Start fluid resuscitation, and use the CVP in conjunction with physical exam findings, lab values, and other noninvasive techniques to decide when to stop fluid resuscitation.

   Historically, the management of sepsis involved targeting a CVP between 8 and 12 mmHg, based on early goal directed therapies as described by Rivers et al.[70] However, more recent data has suggested that CVP is not an entirely accurate marker of fluid responsiveness by itself.

Consequently, basing fluid resuscitation strategies on this number alone is not advisable (choices A, B, and C). Using CVP in conjunction with other modalities is more appropriate.

4. C. Clarify with nursing staff the location of the transducer placement and whether the level changed between measurements.

   In the setting of improving laboratory and physical exam findings, one should question the validity of a decreasing CVP (choice C). It is possible that there has been operator error in setting or changing the level at which the transducer was zeroed. Usually, the transducer is zeroed at the level of the right atrium. This level is usually taken to be at the fourth intercostal space in the midaxillary line while the patient is lying supine. Changing antibiotics, pursuing a CT, or increasing IV fluids (choices A, B, and D) based on 1 possibly spurious reading is not indicated yet.

5. D. All of the above

   Numerous factors can affect PCWP readings. Inspiration on positive-pressure ventilation causes increases in pleural and alveolar pressures. Therefore, PCWP should be interpreted at end expiration so thoracic and atmospheric pressures have equalized and PCWP is not influenced by changing thoracic pressures (choice A). Positive end expiratory pressure (PEEP) may influence PCWP but its clinical significance maybe negligible. True value of PCWP can be estimated by subtracting 1/2 of the PEEP if lung compliance normal or 1/4 if lung compliance reduced (choice B). The tip of the PAC should be in zone 3, where alveolar pressure (Palv) is less than pulmonary artery pressure (Ppa) and pulmonary venous pressure (Ppv) and there is a direct connection to left atrium. In Zone 1, Palv is greater than Ppa and Ppv. In Zone 2, Palv Ppa is greater than Palv which is greater than Ppv. There is no direct column of blood with left atrium in Zone 1 and 2. Verification of the location can be performed with the tip below left atrium on chest radiograph. Placement of the tip of PAC in Zone 1 or 2 will have variable PCWP due to respiratory swings or overestimated PCWP readings (choice C).

6. **B. Tricuspid regurgitation**

The thermodilution technique involves injecting an indicator substance that is cooler than blood through the proximal port of the PAC. As the blood flows past the distal port of the PAC, the thermistor records the temperature change over time. The area under this curve is inversely proportional to the pulmonary artery flow rate, which is reflective of the CO. Consequently, any intervention that lowers the change in temperature measured will suggest a higher CO. Any intervention that minimizes the time under the curve will also suggest a higher CO. A right-to-left shunt (choice C) leads to the cooler injectate leaking over to the left side of the heart, and thus the thermistor does not detect as much temperature change. A left-to-right shunt will lead to a diluted injectate and a lower temperature change as well. Tricuspid regurgitation (choice B) will cause the injectate to reflux back into the vena cava and delay the appearance of the injectate at the thermistor. This "prolonged washout" leads to an underestimation of the CO. Neither aortic regurgitation (choice A) nor pulmonary hypertension (choice D) has an effect on thermodilution.

7. **D. None of the above**

The routine use of a Swan-Ganz catheter in patients with shock has not been associated with improved outcomes. In fact, some studies suggest an increase in 30-day mortality. Overall, there remain a few widely accepted indications for a Swan-Ganz catheter, including pulmonary hypertension, cardiogenic shock, and unexplained or unknown volume status in shock, and it is also used for the evaluation of intrinsic cardiac disease such as shunts, valvular disease, or congenital heart disease.

8. **B. Low CO, high PCWP, high SVR**

Cardiogenic shock is characterized by low CO, high PCWP, and high SVR. Hypovolemic shock (choice A) is differentiated from cardiogenic shock by a low PCWP. Distributive shock (choice C) is characterized by a low SVR.

9. **D. All of the above**

Stroke volume variation is a useful tool to help assess fluid responsiveness. An SVV greater than 13% suggests that a patient may still be on the steep part of the Frank-Starling curve and would benefit from further fluid resuscitation if he or she is hypotensive. However, this technique has only been validated in nonspontaneously breathing patients who are mechanically ventilated at larger tidal volumes (> 8 mL/kg), and who are in a sinus rhythm.

10. **D. Stop fluid resuscitation and recheck SVV later**

An SVV greater than 13% is suggestive of fluid responsiveness. With an SVV of 6%, administering more fluids

(choices A and B) is not indicated. While it is prudent to stop IV fluids (choice C), it is important to remember that fluid responsiveness is not a static endpoint. Frequent reassessment of a patient's fluid needs is prudent. Thus, choice D is the best answer.

11. **C. 700 dynes/cm²**

Systemic vascular resistance is calculated as the difference in mean arterial pressure and central venous pressure divided by the cardiac output and multiplied by 80: $80 \times ([MAP - CVP]/CO)$. In this case, the MAP is 63 mmHg (1/3 Systolic Blood Pressure + 2/3 Diastolic Blood Pressure) and the CVP is 10. The SVR is then calculated to be ~700 dynes/cm².

12. **C. Septic**

Classically, a low SVR helps to differentiate septic shock from hypovolemic and cardiogenic shock. The hemodynamic profile described in this vignette is most consistent with distributive shock with hypotension (MAP < 65 despite adequate fluid resuscitation) and a low SVR. Given the clinical scenario with fever and a lobar infiltrate, it is most likely septic shock related to a pulmonary source.

13. **D. IV = ventricular septal defect**

Figure 3-8 shows an overdamped pulmonary artery waveform detected by a rapid flush test and not overwedging (choice A is wrong). Overdamping occurs secondary to an air bubble in the lumen or a kinked/occluded catheter. A characteristic gradual decline in pressure as compared to the sharp decline post flush is visualized.

An overwedged PAWP tracing (choice A) is secondary to the balloon obstructing the distal tip of the vessel or if the tip is pressed against a vessel wall. A normal PAWP waveform consists of 3 positive deflections and 2 negative deflections. The A wave represents atrial contraction and is usually seen after the P wave on ECG. The X descent represents atrial relaxation. Following is the C wave, which reflects movement of the tricuspid/mitral valve toward the atrium during ventricular systole. The V wave is attributable to the filling of the atria during systole and may occur simultaneously with the T wave on ECG. Finally, the Y descent occurs after the opening of the tricuspid/mitral valve and as the atria empty. Pulmonary arterial catheter waveforms and their etiologies are seen in Table 3-5.

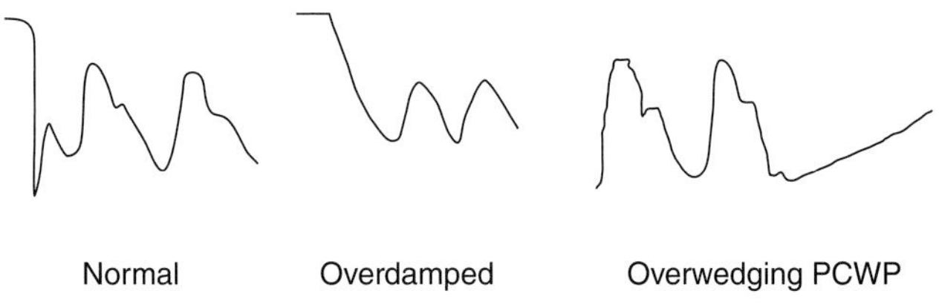

Normal   Overdamped   Overwedging PCWP

FIGURE 3-8 Comparison between the rapid flush test normal wave form and overdamped wave form to overwedging waveform.

TABLE 3-5 Types of Pulmonary Arterial Catheter Waveforms and Their Etiologies

Pulmonary Arterial Waveforms	Etiologies
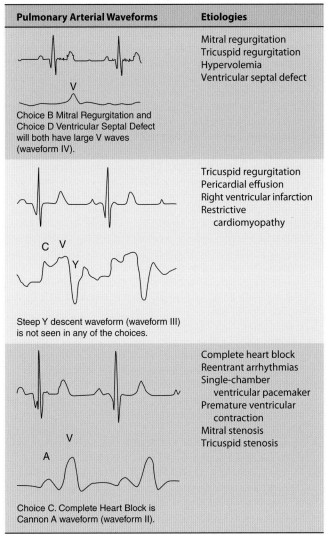 Choice B Mitral Regurgitation and Choice D Ventricular Septal Defect will both have large V waves (waveform IV).	Mitral regurgitation Tricuspid regurgitation Hypervolemia Ventricular septal defect
Steep Y descent waveform (waveform III) is not seen in any of the choices.	Tricuspid regurgitation Pericardial effusion Right ventricular infarction Restrictive cardiomyopathy

Choice C. Complete Heart Block is Cannon A waveform (waveform II).	Complete heart block
	Reentrant arrhythmias
	Single-chamber
	    ventricular pacemaker
	Premature ventricular
	    contraction
	Mitral stenosis
	Tricuspid stenosis

Choices A, B, and C do not match with their corresponding images.

REFERENCES

1. Marino PL. Chapter 1: Circulatory blood flow. In: Marino, ed. *The ICU Book*. Philadelphia, PA: Lippincott, Williams, & Wilkins; 2007: 3-19.
2. Marino PL. Chapter 2: Oxygen and carbon dioxide transport. In: Marino, ed. *The ICU Book*. Philadelphia, PA: Lippincott, Williams, & Wilkins; 2007: 21-38.
3. Miller A, Mandeville J. Predicting and measuring fluid responsiveness with echocardiography. *Echo Res Pract*. 2016;3(2):G1-G12.
4. Vignon P, Repessé X, Bégot E, et al. Comparison of echocardiographic indices used to predict fluid responsiveness in ventilated patients. *Am J Respir Crit Care Med*. 2017;195(8):1022-1032.
5. Bentzer P, Griesdale D, Boyd J, et al. Will this hemodynamically unstable patient respond to a bolus of intravenous fluids? *JAMA*. 2016;316(12):1298-1309.
6. Gelman S. Venous function and central venous pressure: a physiologic story. *Anesthesiology*. 2008;108(4):735-748.
7. Monnet X, Marik PE, Teboul JL. Prediction of fluid responsiveness: an update. *Ann Intensive Care*. 2016;6(111):1-11.
8. Lehman LW, Saeed M, Talmor D, Mark R, Malhotra A. Methods of blood pressure measurement in the ICU. *Crit Care Med*. 2013;41(1):34-40.
9. Esper SA, Pinsky MR. Arterial waveform analysis. *Best Pract Res Clin Anaesthesiol*. 2014;28(4):363-380.
10. Gorny DA. Arterial blood pressure measurement technique. *AACN Clin Issues Crit Care Nurs*. 1993;4(2):66-80.
11. Nirmalan M, Dark PM. Broader applications of arterial pressure wave form analysis. *Continuing Educ Anesth Crit Care Pain*. 2014;14(6):284-290.
12. Hofer CK, Cecconi M, Marx G, della Rocca G. Minimally invasive haemodynamic monitoring. *Eur J Anaesthesiol*. 2009;26(12):996-1002.
13. O'Horo JC, Maki DG, Krupp AK, Safdar N. Arterial catheters as a source of bloodstream infection: a systematic review and meta-analysis. *Crit Care Med*. 2014;42(6):1334-1339.
14. Marik PE, Lemson J. Fluid responsiveness: an evolution of our understanding. *Br J Anaesth*. 2014;112(4):617-620.
15. Marik PE, Desai H. Goal directed fluid therapy. *Curr Pharm Des*. 2012;18(38):6215-6224.
16. Lee WL, Slutsky AS. Sepsis and endothelial permeability. *N Engl J Med*. 2010;363(7):689-691.
17. Bruegger D, Jacob M, Rehm M, et al. Atrial natriuretic peptide induces shedding of endothelial glycocalyx in coronary vascular bed of guinea pig hearts. *Am J Physiol Heart Circ Physiol*. 2005;289(5):H1993-H1999.
18. Bruegger D, Schwartz L, Chappell D, et al. Release of atrial natriuretic peptide precedes shedding of the endothelial glycocalyx equally in patients undergoing on- and off-pump coronary artery bypass surgery. *Basic Res Cardiol*. 2011;106(6):1111-1121.
19. Jacob M, Chappell D. Reappraising Starling: the physiology of the microcirculation. *Curr Opin Crit Care*. 2013;19(4):282-289.
20. Sakka SG, Klein M, Reinhart K, Meier-Hellmann A. Prognostic value of extravascular lung water in critically ill patients. *Chest*. 2002;122(6):2080-2086.
21. Chung FT, Lin SM, Lin SY, Lin HC. Impact of extravascular lung water index on outcomes of severe sepsis patients in a medical intensive care unit. *Respir Med*. 2008;102(7):956-961.
22. Monnet X, Bleibtreu A, Ferré A, et al. Passive leg raising and end-expiratory occlusion tests perform better than pulse pressure variation in patients with low respiratory system compliance. *Crit Care Med*. 2012;40(1):152-157.
23. Monnet X, Marik P, Teboul JL. Passive leg raising for predicting fluid responsiveness: a systematic review and meta-analysis. *Intensive Care Med*. 2016;42(12):1935-1947.
24. Marik PE, Cavallazzi R. Does the central venous pressure (CVP) predict fluid responsiveness? An update meta-analysis and a plea for some common sense. *Crit Care Med*. 2013;41(7):1774-1781.
25. Michard F, Teboul JL. Predicting fluid responsiveness in ICU patients: a critical analysis of the evidence. *Chest*. 2002;121(6):2000-2008.
26. Osman D, Ridel C, Ray P, et al. Cardiac filling pressures are not appropriate to predict hemodynamic response to volume challenge. *Crit Care Med*. 2007;35(1):64-68.
27. Monnet X, Marik PE, Teboul JL. Prediction of fluid responsiveness: an update. *Ann Intensive Care*. 2016;6(111):1-11.
28. Legrand M, Dupuis C, Simon C, et al. Association between systemic hemodynamics and septic acute kidney injury in critically ill patients: a retrospective observational study. *Crit Care*. 2013;17(6):R278.

29. Marik PE. Iatrogenic salt water drowning and the hazards of a high central venous pressure. *Ann Intensive Care.* 2014;4:21.

30. Fagnoul D, Vincent JL, Backer de D. Cardiac output measurements using the bioreactance technique in critically ill patients. *Crit Care.* 2012;16(6):460.

31. Yang X, Du B. Does pulse pressure variation predict fluid responsiveness in critically ill patients? A systematic review and meta-analysis. Crit Care. 2014;18(6):650.

32. Zhang Z, Lu B, Sheng X, Jin N. Accuracy of stroke volume variation in predicting fluid responsiveness: a systematic review and meta-analysis. *J Anesth.* 2011;25(6):904-916.

33. Myatra SN, Prabu SR, Divatia JV, Monnet X, Kulkarni AP, Teboul JL. The changes in pulse pressure variation or stroke volume variation after a "tidal volume challenge" reliably predict fluid responsiveness during low tidal volume ventilation. *Crit Care Med.* 2017;45(3):415-421.

34. Monnet X, Bleibtreu A, Ferré A, et al. Passive leg raising and end-expiratory occlusion tests perform better than pulse pressure variation in patients with low respiratory system compliance. *Crit Care Med.* 2012;40(1):152-157.

35. Diaz F, Erranz B, Donoso A, Salomon T, Cruces P. Influence of tidal volume on pulse pressure variation and stroke volume variation during experimental intra-abdominal hypertension. *BMC Anesthesiol.* 2015;15:127.

36. Duperret S, Lhuillier F, Piriou V, et al. Increased intra-abdominal pressure affects respiratory variations in arterial pressure in normovolaemic and hypovolaemic mechanically ventilated healthy pigs. *Intensive Care Med.* 2007;33(1):163-171.

37. Jacques D, Bendjelid K, Duperret S, Colling J, Piriou V, Viale JP. Pulse pressure variation and stroke volume variation during increased intra-abdominal pressure: an experimental study. *Crit Care.* 2011;15(1):R33.

38. Saugel B, Cecconi M, Wagner JY, Reuter DA. Noninvasive continuous cardiac output monitoring in perioperative and intensive care medicine. *Br J Anaesth.* 2015;114(4):562-575.

39. Spiess BD, Patel MA, Soltow LO, Wright IH. Comparison of bioimpedance versus thermodilution cardiac output during cardiac surgery: evaluation of a second-generation bioimpedance device. *J Cardiothorac Vasc Anesth.* 2001;15(5):567-573.

40. Squara P, Rotcajg D, Denjean D, Estagnasie P, Brusset A. Comparison of monitoring performance of bioreactance vs. pulse contour during lung recruitment maneuvers. *Crit Care.* 2009;13(4):R125.

41. Squara P, Denjean D, Estagnasie P, Brusset A, Dib JC, Dubois C. Noninvasive cardiac output monitoring (NICOM): a clinical validation. *Intensive Care Med.* 2007;33(7):1191-1194.

42. Cheetah Medical Technology: How does it work? Cheetah Medical Web site. http://www.cheetah-medical.com/bioreactance. Accessed July 10, 2017.

43. Marik PE. Noninvasive cardiac output monitors: a state of the art review. *J Cardiothorac Vasc Anesth.* 2013;27(1):121-134.

44. Monnet X, Osman D, Ridel C, Lamia B, Richard C, Teboul JL. Predicting volume responsiveness by using the end-expiratory occlusion in mechanically ventilated intensive care unit patients. *Crit Care Med.* 2009;37(3):951-956.

45. Silva S, Jozwiak M, Teboul JL, Persichini R, Richard C, Monnet X. End-expiratory occlusion test predicts preload responsiveness independently of positive end-expiratory pressure during acute respiratory distress syndrome. *Crit Care Med.* 2013;41(7):1692-1701.

46. Jozwiak M, Teboul JL, Richard C, Monnet X. Predicting fluid responsiveness with echocardiography by combining end-expiratory and inspiratory occlusions. *Ann Intensive Care.* 2017;45(11):e1131-e1138.

47. Preisman S, Kogan S, Berkenstadt H, Perel A. Predicting fluid responsiveness in patients undergoing cardiac surgery: functional haemodynamic parameters including the respiratory systolic variation test and static preload indicators. *Br J Anaesth.* 2005;95(6):746-755.

48. Trepte CJ, Eichhorn V, Haas SA, et al. Comparison of an automated respiratory systolic variation test with dynamic preload indicators to predict fluid responsiveness after major surgery. *Br J Anaesth.* 2013;111(5):736-742.

49. Sutton RM, French B, Meaney PA, et al; American Heart Association's Get With The Guidelines–Resuscitation Investigators. Physiologic monitoring of CPR quality during adult cardiac arrest: a propensity-matched cohort study. *Resuscitation.* 2016;106:76-82.

50. Sanders AB, Kern KB, Otto CW, Milander MM, Ewy GA. End-tidal carbon dioxide monitoring during cardiopulmonary resuscitation. A prognostic indicator for survival. *JAMA.* 1989;262(10):1347–1351.

51. Levine RL, Wayne MA, Miller CC. End-tidal carbon dioxide and outcome of out-of-hospital cardiac arrest. *N Engl J Med.* 1997;337(5):301-306.

52. Garcia MIM, Cano AG, Romero MG, Pintado RM, Madueno VP, Morove JCD. Non-invasive assessment of fluid responsiveness by changes in partial end-tidal CO_2 pressure during a passive leg raising maneuver. *Ann Intensive Care.* 2012;2:9.

53. Prekker ME, Scott NL, Hart D, Sprenkle MD, Leatherman JW. Point-of-care ultrasound to estimate central venous pressure: a comparison of three techniques. *Crit Care Med.* 2013;41(3):833–841.

54. Jardin F, Vieillard-Baron A. Ultrasonographic examination of the venae cavae. *Intensive Care Med.* 2006;32(2):203-206.

55. Muller L, Bobbia X, Toumi M, et al. Respiratory variations of inferior vena cava diameter to predict fluid responsiveness in spontaneously breathing patients with acute circulatory failure: need for a cautious use. *Crit Care.* 2012;16(5):R188.

56. Wallace DJ, Allison M, Stone MB. Inferior vena cava percentage collapse during respiration is affected by the sampling location: an ultrasound study in healthy volunteers. *Acad Emerg Med.* 2010;17(1):96-99.

57. Lee C, Kory P, Arntfield R. Development of a fluid resuscitation protocol using inferior vena cava and lung ultrasound. *J Critical Care.* 2016;31(1):96-100.

58. Vignon P, Repessé X, Bégot E, et al. Comparison of echocardiographic indices used to predict fluid responsiveness in ventilated patients. *Am J Respir Crit Care Med.* 2017;195(8):1022-1032.

59. Bentzer P, Griesdale D, Boyd J, et al. Will this hemodynamically unstable patient respond to a bolus of intravenous fluids? *JAMA.* 2016;316(12):1298-1309.

60. Thiele R, Bartels K, Gan T. Cardiac output monitoring: a contemporary assessment and review. *Crit Care Med.* 2015;43(1):177-185.

61. Wiener R, Welch H. Trends in the use of the pulmonary artery catheter in the United States, 1993–2004. *JAMA.* 2007;298(4):423-429.

62. Gershengorn HB, Wunsch H. Understanding changes in established practice: pulmonary artery catheter use in critically ill patients. *Crit Care Med.* 2013;41(12):2667-2676.

63. Harvey S, Harrison DA, Singer M, et al. Assessment of the clinical effectiveness of pulmonary artery catheters in management of patients in intensive care (PAC-Man): a randomised controlled trial. Lancet. 2005;366(9484):472–477.

64. Yu DT, Platt R, Lanken PN, et al. Relationship of pulmonary artery catheter use to mortality and resource utilization in patients with severe sepsis. *Crit Care Med*. 2003;31(12):2734-2741.

65. Afessa B, Spencer S, Khan W, LaGatta M, Bridges L, Freire AX. Association of pulmonary artery catheter use with in-hospital mortality. *Crit Care Med*. 2001;29(6):1145-1148.

66. Rajaram SS, Desai NK, Kalra A, et al. Pulmonary artery catheters for the adult patients in intensive care. *Cochrane Database Syst Rev*. 2013;(2):CD003408.

67. Connors AFJ, Speroff T, Dawson NV, et al. The effectiveness of right heart catheterization in the initial care of critically ill patients. SUPPORT Investigators. *JAMA*. 1996;276:889-897.

68. Brierre SP, Summer W, Happel KI, Taylor DW. Interpretation of pulmonary artery catheter tracings. *Clin Pulm Med*. 2002;9(6):335-341.

69. Rosenkraz S, Preston IR. Right heart catheterization: best practice and pitfalls in pulmonary hypertension. *Eur Respir Rev*. 2015;24(138):642-652.

70. Rivers E, Nguyen B, Havstad S, et al. Early goal-directed therapy in the treatment of severe sepsis and septic shock. *NEJM*. 2001;345(19):1368-1377.

Shock

Mayanka Tickoo, MD, Ronaldo Collo Go, MD, and Michael McBrine, MD

INTRODUCTION

Shock is a profound state of circulatory failure that leads to a reduction in delivery and impaired utilization of oxygen and other nutrients at the end-organ level. At first, these changes cause reversible injury and, if prolonged, lead to irreversible cellular damage.[1,2] Shock is a common syndrome encountered in the intensive care unit (ICU) and is associated with a high mortality rate.[1-3] Consequently, early recognition, prompt exploration of its etiology, and effective management of shock can greatly influence clinical outcomes.

Fundamentally, shock is a state of circulatory collapse relating to an aberration in preload (hypovolemic shock), pump function (cardiogenic and obstructive shock), or afterload (distributive shock). Early signs of shock include alterations in vital signs (tachycardia, tachypnea, and hypotension) and clinical evidence of end-organ hypoperfusion. Specifically, end-organ hypoperfusion can manifest as an acute alteration in mental status, a decrease in capillary refill, and a decrease in urine output (< 0.5 mL per kg of body weight per hour). Laboratory abnormalities may include alterations in lactate levels and mixed venous oxygen saturations.

INITIAL APPROACH TO A PATIENT IN SHOCK

The initial approach to a patient in shock involves an assessment of the cause as well as simultaneous management of the shock (Tables 4-1 and 4-2). As resuscitative efforts are initiated, a close examination of the available history, clinical examination, laboratory findings, and radiographs is warranted. As noted above, shock is characterized by a hypoperfused state, manifested by low blood pressure (BP). Both cardiac output (CO) and systemic vascular resistance (SVR) contribute to BP, as demonstrated by the equation BP = CO × SVR. The various types of shock are characterized by distinct alterations in either or both parameters. A thorough understanding of this relationship is advantageous when managing a patient in shock.

Patients with decreased cardiac output and increased systemic vascular resistance will often have cool extremities, delayed capillary refill, and a narrow pulse pressure,

often referred to as *cold shock*. The underlying etiology in this situation is either hypovolemic, cardiogenic, or obstructive. Hypovolemic shock is characterized by a low intravascular volume, which can be seen via low or flat jugular venous pressure (JVP), and low cardiac filling pressures. Also, an etiology for volume loss usually is apparent. Cardiogenic shock, on the other hand, is often associated with elevated intravascular volume, manifesting as an elevated JVP, elevated cardiac filling pressures, extremity edema, or crackles on lung exam. Myocardial ischemia on an electrocardiogram (ECG), elevated cardiac biomarkers, or evidence of structural impairment on echocardiography also may be seen. Obstructive shock is often more difficult to recognize and requires a high index of suspicion. Adjunct investigations such as an echocardiogram, computed tomography (CT) scan, or a chest x-ray are often needed to diagnose obstructive shock. Conversely, distributive shock (septic or otherwise) is characterized by a normal to high cardiac output state with a low SVR, or impaired oxygen extraction in the periphery. However, it is important to recognize that these classical descriptors of shock are not mutually exclusive and, can in fact, coexist.

Hypovolemic Shock

Hypovolemic shock is characterized by a low preload. The decreased pressure in the capacitance system creates a weaker gradient to the right atrium, clinically characterized by low venous pressures. The initial compensatory mechanism activates a sympathetic response that causes peripheral vasoconstriction in order to maintain adequate systemic arterial pressures and thereby perfuse distal tissues. A shift in the left ventricular end systolic pressure-volume relationship also occurs as a part of this response. The left ventricle (LV) tries to generate a higher pressure for a lower left ventricular end diastolic volume (positive inotropy) and there is also an increase in heart rate (positive chronotropy). These changes augment the cardiac output. Initially, the body is able to compensate and maintain perfusion to vital organs such as the brain and the heart. However, if the initial insult is not reversed and there is continued volume loss beyond 40% of the total body volume,[3] there is a left shift in the diastolic pressure-volume relationship with increased diastolic stiffening of the LV.

TABLE 4-1 Common Causes of Shock and Their Prevalence

Type of Shock	Description	Prevalence
Hypovolemic shock	Hemorrhage (trauma, variceal bleed, coagulopathy, post-partum hemorrhage), severe diarrhea or vomiting	16%
Cardiogenic shock	Myocardial ischemia, acute decompensated heart failure, acute valve rupture	16%
Obstructive shock	Cardiac tamponade, tension pneumothorax, massive pulmonary embolism	2%
Distributive shock	Sepsis, anaphylaxis, acute spinal cord transection, acute adrenal insufficiency	66%

(Data from Vincent JL, De Backer D. Circulatory shock. *N Engl J Med.* 2013; 369(18):1726–1734).

Poor filling of the LV ensues, resulting in a lower stroke volume, which further decreases preload. Ultimately, diminished end organ tissue perfusion activates the release of systemic inflammatory mediators that can directly suppress the myocardium and perpetuate refractory shock.

Treatment of hypovolemic shock relies on early identification of and control of the underlying source with adequate fluid resuscitation to maintain cardiac output. There have been numerous studies that have examined what the optimal fluid is for resuscitation in hypovolemic shock. The Saline versus Albumin Fluid Evaluation (SAFE) investigators[4] reported no significant difference in outcomes, including 28-day mortality, in patients receiving 4% albumin versus normal saline in medical and surgical ICU patients. The higher cost of albumin and lack of clear benefit have made colloids a second-line agent. Other investigators[5,6] have also found no significant difference in outcomes such as 28-day mortality, as well as ICU and hospital length of stay when comparing patients treated with colloids versus crystalloids. Use of hydroxyethyl starch for resuscitation also has been discredited due to increased risk of acute kidney injury, renal replacement therapy, and mortality.[7]

Resuscitative strategies for hemorrhagic shock are somewhat different from those strategies described above. The underlying premise of resuscitation in this setting is to utilize blood products over crystalloids. In the recently published progmatic, randomized optimal platelet and plasma ratios (PROPRR) study, a 1:1:1 (plasma to platelets to packed red blood cells) transfusion strategy did not show a significant difference in mortality at 24 hours or 30 days when compared to a 1:1:2 ratio. However, the 1:1:1 group achieved better hemostasis and had fewer deaths attributed to exsanguination. In addition, there were no significant differences in safety with respect to the development of acute respiratory distress, venous thromboembolic events, coagulation abnormalities, or transfusion-associated complications.[8] The literature also suggests that the use of tranexamic acid leads to favorable outcomes in both civilian[9] and military trauma settings[10] in the management of hemorrhagic shock. The end point of resuscitation, again, has not been clearly defined but essentially entails achieving hemostasis while maintaining tissue perfusion.

TABLE 4-2 Hemodynamic Profiles in Shock

Shock type	CO/CI	PCWP	SVR	Svo$_2$	Comments
Hypovolemic	Low	Low	Normal/high	Low	
Cardiogenic	Low	High	High	Low	
Acute MR	Low forward CO				Giant V waves on PAOP tracing
Acute VSD	Low forward CO			Step up in oxygen saturation between RA and RV	
RV failure		Normal/low			Elevated RA and RV pressures with normal PAOP
Obstructive	Low	High	High	Low	
Massive PE					PAD > PCWP by > 5 mmHg, increase in PVR
Tamponade					Equalization of pressures (RA, PA diastolic, and wedge) within 5 mmHg
Distributive	Normal/ high	Low/normal	Low	High	Decreased oxygen extraction by peripheral tissues
Late Septic	Normal/low		Can be high		

CI = cardiac index; CO = cardiac output; MR = mitral regurgitation; PA = pulmonary artery; PAD = pulmonary arterial diastolic pressure; PCWP = pulmonary capillary wedge pressure; PVR = pulmonary vascular resistance; RA = right atrium; RV = right ventricle; Svo$_2$ = venous oxygen saturation; SVR = systemic vascular resistance; VSD = ventricular septal defect.

Cardiogenic Shock

Cardiogenic shock is characterized by inadequate tissue and/or end-organ perfusion due to cardiac dysfunction. It is defined via persistent hypotension (systolic blood pressure < 80 to 90) with a severe reduction in the cardiac index (< 1.8 L/min per m^2 without support or < 2 to 2.2 L/min per m^2 with support) in the setting of adequate filling pressures (left ventricle end-diastolic pressure > 18 mmHg or right ventricle end-diastolic pressure of 10–15 mmHg). The incidence is estimated at 5% to 8% of ST elevation myocardial infarcts and 2.5% of non–ST elevation myocardial infarcts.[11] The most common underlying etiology remains acute myocardial dysfunction with associated left ventricular failure but can also be caused by right ventricular dysfunction, wall rupture, tamponade, or valvular pathology.

Based on data collected from several national registries, both the incidence and mortality from cardiogenic shock seem to be decreasing. Presumably, this decrease is a result of early reperfusion strategies now employed for ischemic heart disease.[11] Despite these improvements, increasing age, prior myocardial infarction (MI), oliguria, and physical exam findings suggestive of poor perfusion have been identified as independent predictors of increased mortality.[12]

From a pathophysiologic perspective, cardiogenic shock as a result of myocardial ischemia has been described as a "downward spiral." Myocardial perfusion depends on the pressure gradient between the coronary arterial system and the left ventricle, and on the duration of diastole. When stroke volume and cardiac output decrease after an initial ischemic insult, hypotension leads to a further decrease in myocardial perfusion. This decrease in perfusion leads to worsening ischemia and progressive myocardial dysfunction. Ultimately, without intervention, this downward spiral leads to death.[13]

As noted above, most patients with cardiogenic shock have evidence of significant coronary artery disease, particularly either left main disease or triple vessel disease. This fact is important because compensatory hyperkinesis normally develops in unaffected segments to help maintain cardiac output. The inability to augment CO, because of previous infarction or high-grade coronary stenosis, is an important risk factor for cardiogenic shock and death.[14] Consequently, early revascularization strategies have been shown to improve long-term outcomes, as evidenced in the SHOCK trial. More specifically, primary percutaneous coronary intervention (PCI), when available, is preferred as compared to fibrinolytic therapy.[15]

Although the data supporting early PCI is convincing, the data in support of routine intra-aortic balloon pump (IABP) insertion is less robust. No clear-cut mortality benefit has been seen to date.[16] Consequently, the American College of Cardiology/American Heart Association (ACC/AHA) guidelines on ST-elevation myocardial infarction (STEMI) recommended an IABP as a stabilizing measure in patients with acute MI and cardiogenic shock that is not quickly reversed with pharmacologic therapy.[17]

Percutaneous mechanical circulatory devices are continuous flow pumps designed to augment end-organ perfusion, reduce intracardiac filling pressures, reduce myocardial oxygen consumption, and augment coronary perfusion. As of yet, they have not been shown to improve clinical outcomes but are being used in a variety of situations, including cardiogenic shock, as recommended by the ACC.[18]

Extracorporeal membrane oxygenation (ECMO) is a cardiopulmonary support device that can be used for respiratory failure and/or shock. With venovenous bypass, ECMO primarily helps in respiratory failure by bypassing the pulmonary circulation and uses an artificial membrane to remove carbon dioxide and provide oxygen. With venoarterial bypass, an extracorporeal pump is used to support systemic circulation. There is a growing amount of data, albeit from observational and case control studies, that ECMO may improve outcomes for those in cardiogenic shock.[19,20]

Mechanical Causes of Cardiogenic Shock

Both ventricular septal defects and acute mitral regurgitation can be seen in the days following acute myocardial infarction. Classically, these complications occur in the range of 2 to 7 days after a myocardial infarction. An increased risk is seen in patients with disease involving the left anterior descending artery for ventricular septal defects and the posterior descending artery for acute mitral regurgitation. However, diffuse disease with poor collateral circulation can also be the underlying cause. Prompt action is necessary as clinical deterioration can be sudden. Both of these diagnoses need to be differentiated from rupture of the left ventricular free wall. In fact, ventricular septal rupture can be difficult to distinguish from acute mitral regurgitation on a pulmonary arterial catheter because both can produce dramatic V waves. However, the classic finding is a left-to-right intracardiac shunt, which manifests as an increase in oxygen saturation from the right atrium to the right ventricle (step-up; see Chapter 3, "Hemodynamic Monitoring"). Bedside echocardiography again helps to distinguish between the 2, and surgical repair usually is necessary.[15]

Obstructive Shock

Obstructive shock can often be classified as either mechanical or secondary to pulmonary vascular diseases. The mechanical etiologies often present with hypotension due to a decreased preload rather than right ventricle (RV) or left ventricle (LV) failure. In contrast, the physiology seen in the pulmonary vascular etiologies is consistent with RV failure. Three important types of obstructive shock are pericardial tamponade, tension pneumothorax, and massive pulmonary embolism.

Pericardial Tamponade

Cardiac tamponade is a clinical syndrome that is caused by the rapid accumulation of fluid, pus, blood, clots, or gas within the pericardial space. This process results in impaired diastolic filling and reduced cardiac output. Classically, the clinical picture includes distended jugular veins, an exaggerated inspiratory decrease in arterial systolic pressure (pulsus paradoxus), arterial hypotension, and diminished heart sounds on cardiac auscultation.[21] Bedside ECG plays a major role in the identification of cardiac tamponade and in the assessment of its hemodynamic significance.[22] Hemodynamic significance is present when intrapericardial pressure exceeds intracardiac pressure. On echocardiography, this can be visualized either by the diastolic collapse of the right atrium or the right ventricle. In general, the right-sided structures are more prone to collapse than the left-sided structures due to their thinner walls. Other echocardiographic findings include inferior vena cava (IVC) dilatation associated with less than a 50% reduction in its diameter during inspiration due to impaired filling of the right-sided structures. Finally, from a Doppler perspective, augmented variation in the flow across both the mitral and tricuspid valves during respiration can be measured. Specifically, a 30% inspiratory decrease in flow across the mitral valve is considered diagnostic.[23] This change in flow is reflective of the right ventricle's inability to outwardly expand during inspiration with subsequent underfilling of left-sided structures and bulging of the septum into the LV. These respiratory changes ultimately can lead to a decrease in stroke volume and form the basis of the pathophysiology behind pulsus paradox. However, these changes in flow should not be used in isolation to diagnose tamponade. When a diagnosis of pericardial tamponade is confirmed, either percutaneous or surgical drainage is necessary.

Tension Pneumothorax

A pneumothorax can occur if there is a breach through the visceral or parietal pleura. This breach creates a 1-way valve where air enters but cannot escape[24-37] (Table 4-3). In a healthy, spontaneously breathing patient, the normal intrapleural pressure (IPP) is approximately –5 to –8 cm H_2O, with the potential to reach –80 cm H_2O at forced maximal inspiratory effort. In a ventilated patient, the IPP is often greater than +20 cm H_2O due to the application of positive pressure. The literature has used several different definitions for tension pneumothorax, which have included mediastinal shift, the hiss of air on

thoracic needle decompression, and hemodynamic compromise. Ultimately, the diagnosis of a tension pneumothorax is mostly clinical and a delay in treatment can be catastrophic.

Chest radiographs may be used to confirm the presence of a pneumothorax in stable patients. However, waiting for a radiograph should not precede emergent decompression in patients with a high suspicion of tension pneumothorax and the following scenarios: hypoxia less than 92%; hypotension (systolic blood pressure [SBP] < 90%); respiratory rate (RR) less than 10; altered mental status; or cardiac arrest.[24]

Decompression can be initially achieved via needle thoracostomy, followed by tube thoracostomy. Needle decompression involves insertion of a 14-gauge (4.5-cm) needle in the second/third intercostal space (ICS) at the midclavicular line (MCL). Failure to decompress the pleural space has been attributed to increases in chest wall thickness up to 5 cm in that location, needle obstruction, loculated pneumothoraces, or large air leaks.[24,38] The fourth/fifth ICS at the midaxillary line has less muscle tissue and fat and is another potential location.[24,39] After needle thoracostomy has been inserted, tube thoracostomy is placed and usually suction is applied.

Massive Pulmonary Embolism

The distinction between submassive pulmonary embolism (PE) and massive PE is predominantly dependent on hypotension, either an SBP less than 90 mmHg or a 40-mmHg drop in BP for at least 15 minutes.[40] Fibrinolysis has been advocated as the initial mode of treatment for those in shock, as it has been shown to reduce mortality by up to 55% in some studies.[40-45] While alteplase 100 mg intravenously (IV) for 2 hours is the drug of choice, there have been reports that use 50 mg IV for those patients at higher perceived risk of bleeding.[40-45] In general, a partial thromboplastin time (PTT) should be obtained after the infusion finishes and systemic heparin initiated when the PTT is less than 80 seconds or twice the upper limit of normal. If the PTT is greater than 80 seconds, a repeat PTT should be obtained after 4 hours. The presence of the McConnell sign on a transthoracic echo (TTE), hypokinesis of the RV free wall and base, with sparing of the apex, may help to differentiate RV failure secondary to PE from chronic RV failure.

There are controversies regarding fluid management in obstructive shock. Based on the pathophysiology of an overloaded right ventricle, with septal bowing and LV dysfunction, volume loading may further increase right ventricular overload.[46] In contrast, for some patients, diuresis may be more beneficial than volume loading.[47] Ultimately, the etiology of the obstructive shock state needs to be corrected and either fluids or diuretics should be used judiciously on a patient-by-patient basis.

Distributive Shock

Low peripheral vascular resistance and a normal to increased cardiac output characterize distributive shock. It is often described as *warm shock* because of the characteristic flushed skin, warm extremities, high respiratory rates, and bounding

TABLE 4-3 Clinical Signs of a Pneumothorax[24]

Clinical Signs of Pneumothorax in Spontaneously Breathing Patients	Clinical Signs of Pneumothorax in Ventilated Patients
• Chest pain and/or respiratory distress (100%) • Tachycardia and decreased air entry (50–75%) • Hypoxia, tracheal deviation, hypotension (< 25%) • Cyanosis, hyper-resonance, altered mental status, hypomobile ipsilateral chest, epigastric pain (< 10%)	• Subcutaneous emphysema (100%) • Tachycardia (95%) • Decreased breath sounds (87%) • Hyper-resonance (85%) • Hypotension (81%) • Cyanosis (75%) • Hypoxia (70%) • Tracheal deviation (60%)

pulses with a normal capillary refill. If the shock state persists over the subsequent 72 hours, patients will often enter cold shock, which is characterized by cold and mottled extremities and associated with weak pulses, hypothermia, and vasoconstriction. This transition from a warm shock state to a cold shock state generally has been associated with a poorer prognosis and is considered a separate entity from sepsis-induced cardiomyopathy. The most common etiology of distributive shock is septic shock, which is discussed in Chapter 18, "Sepsis." Other etiologies include anaphylaxis, neurogenic shock, some forms of endocrinologic conditions such as hypothyroidism (myxedema coma), and adrenal insufficiency (AI).

Neurogenic Shock

Neurogenic shock can consist of 3 different subtypes, which are not mutually exclusive. Distributive neurogenic shock secondary to a disruption of the sympathetic pathway with unopposed parasympathetic excitation leads to hypotension and bradycardia. This phenomenon is seen in spinal cord injuries and neuromuscular diseases such as Guillain-Barré syndrome.

Patients are bradycardic and hypotensive but have warm limbs and good capillary refill. Central venous pressure (CVP), stroke volume (SV), SVR, and CO are low due to unopposed vagal stimulation. With a spinal cord injury, limbs above the level of the injury will have normal perfusion, while limbs below the level of the injury will have warm and dry characteristics. Treatment involves the early use of vasopressors to avoid fluid overload with a mean arterial pressure (MAP) goal of 85 to 90 mmHg.[48,49] Norepinephrine is the pressor of choice, and phenylephrine is generally avoided because of bradycardia; however, caution is warranted due to some patients being hypersensitive to vasopressors with subsequent uncontrolled hypertension (HTN).[48]

The second subtype is cardiogenic neurogenic shock, which is seen secondary to catecholamine stunning of the myocardium after subarachnoid hemorrhages or ischemic strokes, particularly from a right insula insult. Finally, hypopituitarism, as seen in traumatic brain injury, also occurs.[48]

Patients are "cold and wet" from peripheral vasoconstriction and generally are hypotensive and tachycardic. Systemic vascular resistance, CVP, pulmonary capillary wedge pressure (PCWP), and end-diastolic volume index (EDVI) can be high, with a low SV and CO.[48]

The third subtype, neuroendocrine neurogenic shock, is associated with hypotension that is not responsive to vasopressors. In this situation, the administration of hydrocortisone is both diagnostic and therapeutic. Cosyntropin tests are not helpful, as they are reflective of adrenal gland function and not the effected organ. Consequently, they would be falsely normal.[48]

Anaphylactic Shock

Anaphylaxis is defined as an allergic or hypersensitivity reaction that is rapid in onset. The diagnosis requires satisfying 1 of 3 criteria,[50] as seen in Table 4-4.

Risk factors for poor outcomes and/or severe reactions include peanut and tree nut allergies, underlying pulmonary and cardiac disease, asthma, delayed epinephrine administration, previous anaphylactic reactions, advanced age, and mast cell disease.[50] Serum tryptase is a marker of mast cell degranulation and can help confirm the diagnosis. However, it may not be readily available and may actually be low in food allergies.[50-52] A value of 2 µg/L or more has a sensitivity of 73% and specificity of 98% and usually increases within 30 minutes of the exposure and can remain elevated for 6 to 8 hours.[53,54]

Initial treatment begins with epinephrine 0.01 mg/kg (max, 0.5 mg) administration intramuscularly (IM) in the anterolateral thigh, and it can be repeated every 5 to 15 minutes. This is a strong recommendation based on an excellent quality of evidence. If the patient is not responding to IM therapy, an IV infusion with 1:1,000,000 at 1 µg/min can be started. This recommendation is weaker and based on a lesser quality of evidence. Epinephrine can also be given IM, via inhalation, sublingually, and endotracheally, if necessary.[50] Epinephrine causes vasoconstriction, bronchodilation, and suppression of histamine, mast cell, and basophil release. While epinephrine is the most important therapy, there are adjunctive therapies available as well. Both H1 and H2 antihistamines as well as corticosteroids can be administered. Although they relieve itching and urticaria and theoretically

TABLE 4-4 Diagnostic Criteria for Anaphylactic Shock

Criteria 1	Criteria 2	Criteria 3
Acute onset of illness within minutes, with pruritus, flushing, hives, stridor, and/or angioedema, and either:	Exposure to a likely allergen with > 2 of the following:	Exposure to a known allergen with subsequent hypotension
A) Respiratory symptoms, such as wheezing, stridor, dyspnea, or hypoxemia; or	A) Skin involvement (pruritus, flushing, hives, angioedema) B) Respiratory involvement (wheezing, stridor, hypoxia, dyspnea)	
B) Hypotension or end-organ damage, such as collapse, syncope, or incontinence	C) End-organ damage (hypotension, collapse, syncope, or incontinence) D) Gastrointestinal involvement (vomiting, pain, diarrhea)	

prevent a biphasic reaction, there is no data to suggest either intervention improves outcomes. Given the prevalence of angioedema and stridor, airway compromise is common, and intubation is often necessary. Crystalloid boluses for hypotension along with glucagon for refractory hypotension can also be used. Glucagon is given as a 1- to 5-mg IV bolus over 5 minutes followed by a 5- to 15-μg/min infusion that is titrated to effect.[55-61]

Shock Secondary to Adrenal Insufficiency

Adrenal insufficiency is the deficiency of glucocorticoids with or without an associated deficiency of mineralocorticoids and/or androgens. The adrenal cortex has 3 zones, which secrete specific hormones. The zona glomerulosa produces and secretes aldosterone, which regulates the renin-angiotensin system and extracellular potassium.[62] The zona fasciculata secretes cortisol in response to corticotropin and vasopressin.[62] The zona reticularis creates and secretes the androgens androstenedione, dehydroepiandrosterone, and the sulfate ester of dehydroepiandrosterone.[62] The clinical manifestations of adrenal insufficiency are dependent on which hormone is deficient, and many of these signs and symptoms are not specific. These symptoms may include fatigue, gastrointestinal (GI) upset, anorexia, dry and itchy skin, skin hyperpigmentation, fever, loss of hair, postural hypotension, hyponatremia, hypokalemia, anemia, lymphocytosis, eosinophilia, hypercalcemia, and hypoglycemia.[62] From a diagnostic perspective, the goal is to confirm low cortisol levels; determine if adrenal insufficiency is primary, secondary, or tertiary; and find the underlying cause.[62-65] Treatment depends on the type of adrenal insufficiency and its acuity or chronicity. In acute AI, glucocorticoid replacement via 100 mg IV hydrocortisone followed by 100 to 200 mg in 5% dextrose in water (D5W) is given. Fluids and electrolytes may need to be repleted.

Pheochromocytoma

Pheochromocytomas are epinephrine-secreting tumors, and 80% arise from the adrenal medulla.[66-68] Intermittent or continuous HTN associated with headaches, palpitations, and diaphoresis are common associated symptoms. However, this tumor also can present as shock. Epinephrine has a greater affinity for α-adrenergic receptors than β-adrenergic receptors. At low doses, epinephrine causes tachycardia via cardiac β_1 receptors and hypotension via β_2 receptors in skeletal muscle blood vessels.[66] Higher doses lead to hypertension via the α receptors in the peripheral vascular system.[66] Because there may be an increased release of epinephrine into the vascular system during a biopsy, aspiration of this tumor caries a risk of hypertensive crisis. The diagnostic process begins with an initial screening via plasma-free metanephrines or urine-deconjugated differential metanephrines. When compared to urine or plasma catecholamines, the metanephrines have a higher sensitivity, 98% to 99%, likely due to their longer half-life and continuous production.[68] An anatomic survey via

CT or magnetic resonance imaging (MRI) is performed after the biochemical screening. If the CT and/or MRI is negative and there still remains a strong clinical suspicion, iodine-123 metaiodobenzylguanidine (MIBG) scintigraphy can be performed. This nuclear medicine exam can identify areas of functional uptake of the norepinephrine-like compound. If negative, other tracers can be used such as somatostatin receptors (SSTRs) and indium-11–DTPA–octreotide. Ultimately, treatment is surgical after α blockade and fluid administration.

Vasoplegic Shock

Vasoplegic syndrome has been defined as hypotension in the setting of a cardiac index greater than 2.5 L/min/m, right atrial pressure less than 5 mmHg, left atrial pressure less than 10 mmHg, and an SVR less than 800 dynes/s/cm[5] while on a norepinephrine infusion.[69,70] The incidence of this phenomenon post-cardiac surgery has been reported to be as high as 8% to 10%. Risk factors include diabetes mellitus and drugs such as the preoperative use of heparin, angiotensin-converting enzyme (ACE) inhibitors, calcium channel blockers, and protamine.[69-77] Chronic use of ACE inhibitors leads to tissue accumulation, which decreases angiotensin II and increases bradykinin levels.[69] Bradykinins are vasodilators and are catabolized in the lungs, which are excluded in cardiopulmonary bypass.[69] Vasopressin deficiency has also been implicated as a cause of vasoplegic shock. This deficiency may be secondary to hyponatremia, atrial receptor activation, atrial natriuretic peptide, and autonomic dysfunction.[69,78,79] Norepinephrine may sometimes be sufficient, but the use of either vasopressin or methylene blue as a 2-mg/kg 20-min infusion has been suggested as treatment. Methylene blue competes with nitric oxide, binding to the iron heme moiety of soluble guanylate cyclase, decreasing levels of cyclic guanosine monophosphate (cGMP) and causing vasodilation.[69,80] Angiotensin II supplementation has been suggested to improve this type of shock.

RESUSCITATION

Resuscitation begins with adequate IV or intraosseous (IO) access to administer fluids and medications. Poiseuille law states that the flow (Q) of a liquid is related to its inherent viscosity (n), the pressure gradient (p) across the tubing, and the length (L) and diameter (r) of the tubing. To maximize flow, the system should consist of the shortest length of IV access, the largest diameter of IV, the maximal pressure, and the lowest viscosity. In other words, a large-bore IV is preferred to a small-bore IV; a short cannula is preferred to a long cannula; large proximal vascular access is preferred to small distal access; and upper extremities are preferred over lower extremities. In practical terms, an 18-gauge (G) peripheral IV will allow for the faster infusion of fluids than a central triple lumen catheter[81] (Table 4-5). Intraosseous access (14G to 15G, with 15 mm, 25 mm, or 45 mm length) has a 60 to 100 mL/min flow rate and is a reasonable alternative to central venous access in the initial resuscitation effort due to

TABLE 4-5 Flow Rates of Intravenous Catheters

Intravenous Catheter	Rate of Flow With Gravity (mL/min)	Rate of Flow With Pressure (mL/min)	Rate of Flow With Bionector (mL/min)	Percentage Increase With Pressure	Percentage Decrease With Bionector
14G 50-mm cannula	236.1	384.2	138.3	62.7%	−41.4%
14G 14-cm Abbocath	197	366	131.3	85.8%	−33.4%
16G 50-mm cannula	154.7	334.4	109.6	116.2%	−29.2%
14G 15-cm Leadercath	117.3	211.1	101.1	80%	−13.8%
18G 45-mm cannula	98.1	153.1	80.3	56%	−18.1%
16G distal port triple lumen central line	69.4	116.1	67.4	67.3%	−2.88%
20G 33-mm cannula	64.4	105.1	58.5	63.2%	−9.17%
22G 25-mm cannula	35.7	71.4	34.7	100%	−2.80%
18G proximal port triple lumen central line	29.7	79.3	28.7	167%	−3.37%

Reprinted with permission from Reddick AD, Ronald J, Morrison WG. Intravenous fluid resuscitation: was Poiseuille right? *E Merg Med J.* 2011;28(3):201-202.

the higher success rates and shorter procedure times in some studies.[82] However, some of this data comes from the time pre-dating ultrasound-assisted procedures. In adults, they can be placed on the proximal humerus, proximal tibia, distal tibia, femur, iliac crest, or sternum. Blood work can be obtained via IO once 2 mL of the initial draw is discarded, though certain values (white blood cells, platelets, sodium, potassium, and calcium) do not seem to correlate well with plasma levels.[83]

Resuscitative efforts in shock are focused on restoring perfusion and ensuring oxygen delivery to end-organ tissues. Oxygen delivery is the product of CO, the oxygen carrying capacity of the blood, and arterial oxygen saturation. Each of these components needs to be addressed and the underlying etiology of the shock state identified so that the appropriate fluid choice is made. While the choice of initial fluid for resuscitation is discussed in other sections, a discussion of the end points of fluid resuscitation will follow here.

While it is universally agreed that patients in shock need to be fluid resuscitated, what is less clear is how much fluid they need. There is no single best answer, as each clinical situation is different and individual patient needs differ accordingly. What is clear is that each patient's ongoing fluid requirement needs to be readdressed frequently. Physical exam findings are an integral part of this decision process, as noted earlier in this chapter, but other data is often required.

For the past 15 years, MAPs, CVPs, lactates, and the saturation of oxygen in the venous capillaries ($Scvo_2$) have been used to help determine adequate end points of fluid resuscitation. More recent data has suggested that these static endpoints may not be reflective of true fluid responsiveness. Furthermore, there is a growing body of literature that suggests that over-resuscitation may be harmful as well.[84] Consequently, more dynamic assessments of fluid responsiveness have been studied and these invasive and noninvasive devices have been discussed in depth earlier (See Chapter 3).

In addition to the previously mentioned devices and maneuvers, point-of-care ultrasound is increasingly being used in ICUs, and there has been an increasing amount of data supporting its use. Specifically, ultrasound imaging of the IVC to assess volume status has been studied. There is data suggesting that IVC diameter is reflective of central venous pressure.[85] Perhaps more importantly, changes in IVC diameter of 12% to 18% during respiration have been associated with fluid responsiveness.[86]

In addition, using lung ultrasonography to stop fluid resuscitation once B-lines are visualized has been examined. Some research has suggested that when A-lines convert to B-lines during fluid resuscitation, there is a correlation to a pulmonary artery occlusion pressure of 18.[87] Thus B-lines, which correlate with interstitial pulmonary edema, may also correlate with adequate filling pressures in the heart for some patients. The FALLS-protocol (fluid administration limited by lung sonography) was created to help guide in both the diagnostic workup and fluid management of the shock state.[88]

Ultimately, the decision to stop fluid resuscitation is based on multiple modalities, including physical exam findings, laboratory values, and measurements obtained from invasive and noninvasive devices.

The goal of resuscitation is to establish perfusion and minimize end-organ injury while dealing with the primary cause of the shock state. To this end, management of the airway using invasive mechanical ventilation, if needed, as well as appropriately timed renal replacement therapy for volume, electrolyte, and acid–base management is equally important.

Vasoactive Agents

Norepinephrine acts on both α_1 and β_1 receptors causing vasoconstriction and a mild increase in cardiac output.

Norepinephrine has become the preferred drug in septic and other types of shock due its ability to raise SVR without causing significant renal or mesenteric side effects.[89,90]

Phenylephrine works on α_1 receptors causing vasoconstriction and a reflex bradycardia. Classically, it has been used when profound tachycardia exists and as an alternative to other front-line agents. However, the side effects of decreased stroke volume, reduced splanchnic blood flow, and reduced oxygen delivery have made this a less desirable agent.[91]

Epinephrine is a strong β_1 agonist with moderate β_2 and α_1 effects as well. Clinically, at low doses of epinephrine, the β_1 receptor effects predominate. However, at higher doses, the α_1 receptor effect predominates, producing increased SVR in addition to an increased CO. Epinephrine is most often used for the treatment of anaphylaxis, as a second-line agent in septic shock, and for management of hypotension following coronary artery bypass grafting. The deleterious side effects include tachycardia and splanchnic vasoconstriction, the latter of which appears to be greater than either norepinephrine or dopamine in equivalent doses.[92]

Vasopressin levels in septic shock have been reported to be lower than anticipated for a shock state.[93] The repletion of this relative deficiency has been the ideology behind its use as a vasopressor in septic shock. However, more recent data have suggested that it offers no significant improvement in short-term mortality but may reduce the requirement of other vasopressors.[94] Vasopressin doses above 0.03 units/min have been associated with coronary and mesenteric ischemia and skin necrosis.

Dopamine has a variety of dose-dependent effects, although this has recently been questioned. At low doses, it primarily affects dopamine receptors in the renal, mesenteric, cerebral, and coronary beds, resulting in selective vasodilation. At moderate doses, it increases cardiac output by stimulating β_1 receptors. At higher doses, it causes vasoconstriction by acting on α_1 receptors. Recent data has suggested that dopamine is more arrhythmogenic than norepinephrine and is associated with a higher mortality rate in patients with septic shock.[95,96]

Midodrine is a prodrug that, upon deglycination, forms an active metabolite desglymidodrine. Desglymidodrine stimulates α_1-adrenergic receptors of the arteriolar and venous vasculature, leading to vasoconstriction and elevation of BP. Recent data suggests that it may reduce the duration of IV vasopressors during the recovery phase from septic shock and may be associated with a reduction in length of stay in the ICU.[97]

Dobutamine is an inotrope with predominant β_1 receptor activity with mild α and β_2 activity. Primarily, it causes an increased CO with decreased SVR that be manifested by slightly lower blood pressure. Primarily, its use is in cardiogenic shock.

Milrinone is a phosphodiesterase inhibitor that has both inotropic and vasodilatory effects. Its use is primarily in heart failure but has been limited by its vasodilatory effects.

Angiotensin II is considered a vasopressor adjunct for refractory septic shock on norepinephrine or epinephrine and other types of vasodilatory shock. ATHOS 3, a multinational, double blinded randomized trial, showed that the addition of angiotensin II to patients already on high dose vasopressors had an improvement in blood pressure at hour 3 after start of angiotensin II infusion compared to placebo (odds ratio 7.96 (95% confidence interval [CI] 4.76–13.3; $P < 0.001$) and at 48 hours, Sequential Organ Failure Assessment (SOFA) improvement was greater with angiotensin II group compared to placebo (-1.75 vs -1.28 P 0 = 0.01).[98]

QUESTIONS

1. A 73-year-old man with history of chronic kidney disease and hypertension presented to the hospital with weakness, confusion, and a productive cough. His initial chest x-ray is consistent with a left upper lobe pneumonia, and he is hypotensive on initial examination. Based on his weight of 68 kg, he is fluid resuscitated with 3 Liters of normal saline, and a central line is placed. His white blood cell count is elevated; he has a mild increase in his serum creatinine. His blood pressure subsequently improves and he is started on ceftriaxone and azithromycin after blood and sputum cultures are obtained. He is admitted into the ICU, and on arrival, the nursing staff notes his blood pressure to be 75/58 mmHg with a heart rate of 100 beats/min. A vasopressor is ordered. What is the next best step?

   A. Order an echocardiogram to see if he has any evidence of underlying congestive heart failure or wall motion abnormalities suggestive of acute myocardial ischemia.
   B. Switch to albumin for further fluid resuscitation as he has already received 3 Liters of normal saline and is hypotensive.
   C. Re-examine the patient, assess urine output, and order a bedside ultrasound of the lungs and IVC to assess for fluid responsiveness.
   D. Order a CT of the chest, abdomen, and pelvis to ensure adequate source control.

2. For the patient in question 1, which vasopressor would you order?

   A. Neo-Synephrine
   B. Norepinephrine
   C. Epinephrine
   D. Dopamine

3. A 55-year-old obese man who is an active smoker and has a history of chronic diastolic heart failure and diabetes mellitus presented to the hospital with progressive shortness of breath. His symptoms initially started with a "cold"

and he put himself on "bedrest" in order to recuperate. He is markedly tachypnic on initial examination with an oxygen requirement of 6 Liters via nasal cannula to keep his oxygen saturation above 90%. His blood pressure is within normal limits and his initial chest x-ray is without evidence of heart failure or pneumonia. His initial troponin is mildly elevated but his echocardiogram is without any ischemic changes. His D-dimer is markedly elevated, so he is sent for a computed tomography angiography (CTA) scan of his chest to rule out pulmonary embolism. On his way back from his CT, he abruptly becomes hypotensive and more hypoxemic. You prepare for an emergent intubation, and a nurse informs you that the radiologist called and said there is evidence of a saddle embolus on the CTA. What is the next best step?

A. Ensure that there are no contraindications for thrombolytic therapy, and if not, administer tissue plasminogen activator (tPA).
B. Order a stat echocardiogram to see if there is any evidence of right ventricular strain, and assess his need for thrombolytic therapy.
C. Bolus 1 Liter of normal saline to try to improve his blood pressure.
D. Call interventional radiology to discuss emergent catheter-guided thrombolysis.

4. Which of the following would be an absolute contraindication for the administration of tPA?

A. Uncontrolled hypertension
B. Age more than 75
C. History of ischemic stroke more than 3 months prior
D. None of the above

5. You arrive to work in the ICU in the morning and are given verbal sign-out regarding a patient admitted overnight. The admitting physician tells you that emergency medical services (EMS) were called to the patient's home by a neighbor who thought the patient looked unwell. On their arrival, EMS noted she was confused, short of breath, and hypotensive. She was intubated in the field for worsening respiratory distress, and eventually started on norepinephrine due to persistent hypotension. A review of available hospital medical records showed a history of chronic obstructive pulmonary disease (COPD), breast cancer, and frequent urinary tract infections with multidrug-resistant organisms. Urine and blood cultures were obtained, she was started on cefepime and vancomycin for a presumed urinary tract infection. She was also given 3 Liters IV fluids. On your exam, you note a thin woman, weighing 40 kg, with cool skin and an elevated JVP, whose vasopressor requirement has not decreased at all. Her urine culture returns without growth, and her family arrives. They mention that the patient has been feeling more short of breath over the past month. What is your next best step?

A. Order a CT of her abdomen and pelvis to look for a perinephric abscess, as the persistent hypotension suggests inadequate source control.
B. Continue fluid resuscitation, as the patient is still hypotensive.
C. Discontinue cefepime and start meropenem, as the patient likely has a multi-drug–resistant bacteria that is not being covered by cefepime.
D. Order an echocardiogram to assess for a possible pericardial effusion.

6. Which answer is most suggestive of tamponade physiology on right heart catheterization?

A. Elevated RA pressure, elevated RV pressure, elevated PA pressure, decreased LA pressure, decreased LV pressure
B. Normal RA pressure, normal RV pressure, elevated PA pressure, increased LA pressure, increased LV pressure
C. Equalization of diastolic pressures in all chambers
D. Normal RA pressure, normal RV pressure, normal PA pressure, normal LA pressure, normal LV pressure

7. A 65-year-old man presents to the hospital with pneumonia and septic shock. Which of the below follows best practice?

A. Daily assessment of antibiotics with consideration of de-escalation or discontinuation
B. Administration of systemic glucocorticoids if a vasopressor requirement develops
C. Central line placement for monitoring of CVP and $Scvo_2$ per ICU protocols
D. Tight glycemic control with blood glucose measurements less than 110 mg/dL

8. Which of the following is an example of adequate source control?

A. Drainage of the pleural space in a patient with empyema
B. Removal of a central line in a patient with persistently positive blood cultures and erythematous skin around the device
C. Removal of an infected artificial prosthesis
D. All of the above

9. You have admitted a 55-year-old man with a history of cirrhosis to the ICU. He has been diagnosed with pneumonia, has no risk factors for hospital-acquired pathogens, and is in shock on vasopressors. His initial lactate was measured at 5.4 mmol/L. You initiate antibiotics directed at community-acquired pneumonia and start aggressive fluid resuscitation based on his weight of 70 kg. Five hours later, he is hemodynamically improved and making

adequate amounts of urine. You re-measure a lactate and find that it has not decreased. What is your next best step?

A. Obtain a CT of the chest and abdomen/pelvis to ensure adequate source control.
B. Continue with aggressive fluid resuscitation for the next 4 hours and repeat a lactate.
C. Consider alternative reasons why the lactate may not have decreased.
D. Broaden antibiotics to cover healthcare-associated pneumonia.

10. An 82-year-old woman with history of diabetes mellitus, hypertension, and mild dementia is admitted into the ICU at a small community hospital with an acute large inferior wall infarct. The hospital does not have PCI capability. Her respiratory rate is 26 breaths/min, her pulse is 106 beats/min, and her blood pressure is 108/55 mmHg. Best practice would include which of the following?

A. Placement of an intra-aortic balloon pump and transfer to another facility for PCI
B. Administration of thrombolytics at the local hospital
C. Transfer to another facility for PCI
D. Start medical management with aspirin, nitrates, and heparin

11. An 82-year-old woman is admitted for STEMI. Her family is offered PCI but decides against an interventional approach. She is medically managed with aspirin, nitrates, and heparin. On hospital day 4, she develops hypotension and worsening tachycardia. Right heart catheterization (RHC) is discussed with the family and performed, and shows a step-up in oxygenation from the right atrium to the right ventricle of 7%. Which of the following is the most likely diagnosis?

A. Acute mitral valve regurgitation
B. Ventricular septal wall rupture
C. Worsening left ventricular failure
D. Tamponade

12. What are the consequences of continued volume loss beyond 40% of total body volume?

A. Stiffening of the LV in diastole, worsening systolic filling, and decreased stroke volume
B. Hyperdynamic LV function that compensates for a decreased SVR
C. Elevated end-diastolic pressure and diminished cardiac output
D. Increased SVR

13. A 35-year-old man has been admitted in the intensive care unit for acute respiratory distress syndrome secondary to influenza. He has been intubated for 1 week. The nurse calls you to tell you that his oxygen saturation dropped to 70% and his systolic blood pressure also dropped into the 70s. He is afebrile. She has already started to give him a

1-Liter bolus of normal saline. On physical examination he was noted to be diaphoretic and tachypnic. Crepitus was noted on palpation of the right side of his neck and anterior chest wall. On the ventilator, the peak airway pressure is markedly elevated at 60 cm H_2O. A chest radiograph is ordered (Fig. 4-1).

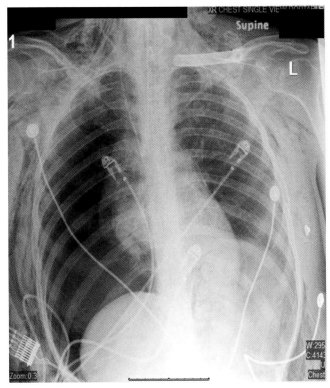

FIGURE 4-1 Chest radiograph after the hypotension has occurred.

What is the next best step?

A. Large-bore tube thoracostomy
B. Chest radiograph STAT
C. Needle decompression
D. Bag-valve-mask ventilation

14. A 40-year-old woman with spontaneous pneumothorax had a chest tube placed yesterday. She is noted to have an air leak today. What is the next step?

A. Observe
B. Change chest tube
C. Place on suction and increase pressure to −30 cm H_2O
D. Open thoracotomy and pleurectomy

15. A 42-year-old woman with a history of anxiety disorder and migraines complains of headache. In the emergency department, she reveals she also has midsternal chest pain. Electrocardiogram showed ST elevations in the anterior leads. Troponin was 2. She had a cardiac catheterization, and the left ventriculogram shows apical ballooning with

basal hyperkinesis. She had anterior motion of the mitral valve, touching the left ventricular septum. Her blood pressure started to drop. Crystalloid resuscitation was started but did not improve the blood pressure. What is the next step?

A. Phenylephrine
B. Dobutamine
C. Dopamine
D. Norepinephrine

ANSWERS

1. C. Re-examine the patient, assess urine output, and order a bedside ultrasound of the lungs and IVC to assess for fluid responsiveness.

   This scenario describes a patient in septic shock who has been appropriately managed with early fluid and antibiotic administration after cultures were obtained. The reoccurrence of hypotension after the initial improvement warrants further attention. The primary question is whether this patient needs more fluid or needs a pressor to be started. While there is no perfect single test to answer this question, using a combination of physical exam findings, ultrasound examination, and invasive or noninvasive assessments of fluid responsiveness is appropriate. While ordering an echocardiogram (choice A) may be appropriate, it will not answer the question of fluid responsiveness by itself. Albumin (choice B) is likely a noninferior choice for fluid resuscitation, but again, we do not know if more fluid administration is appropriate at this time. Finally, obtaining a CT (choice D) may help with source control, but his initial improvement argues against the need for further diagnostics until he is stabilized again.

2. B. Norepinephrine

   To date, there have been numerous studies looking at vasopressors. Norepinephrine is the currently recommended first-line agent for septic shock by the Surviving Sepsis Campaign based on its ability to increase SVR without significant renal or mesenteric side effects. The lack of significant tachycardia argues against using Neo-Synephrine (choice A). Dopamine (choice D) has been associated with a greater number of arrhythmogenic events and is not a recommended first-line agent. Epinephrine (choice C) is a reasonable alternative to norepinephrine but is not currently a first-line recommendation.

3. A. Ensure that there are no contraindications for thrombolytic therapy, and if not, administer tissue plasminogen activator (tPA).

   There is much debate about the management of patients with submassive pulmonary embolism. However, this scenario describes a patient with massive PE and hypotension.

Current guidelines are in support of thrombolysis in this patient population. An echocardiogram (choice B) is unlikely to add useful information in this hypotensive patient, but may be of benefit in patients with submassive PE. Intravenous fluids (choice C) may be of some benefit if the patient is thought to be fluid depleted, but not as the primary intervention. At some institutions, catheter-guided thrombolysis (choice D) may be an option but, in this acutely hypotensive patient, is not the best first choice.

4. D. None of the above

   The absolute contraindications to fibrinolytic therapy include prior intracranial hemorrhage, known intracranial neoplasms or vascular abnormalities, recent ischemic stroke (within 3 months), suspected dissection, active bleeding, and recent trauma. Uncontrolled hypertension (choice A), age more than 75 (choice B), and history of ischemic stroke more than 3 months prior (choice C) are all relative contraindications.

5. D. Order an echocardiogram to assess for a possible pericardial effusion.

   The patient described above was initially thought to be in septic shock from a urinary source. She has been adequately fluid resuscitated and started on broad-spectrum antibiotics, and has not improved. In addition, the suspected urinary source is now without evidence of infection. Alternative etiologies of shock should be investigated. Her history of breast cancer along with her cool skin and elevated JVP are suggestive of possible obstructive shock. In the setting of a negative urine culture and these physical exam findings, a perinephric abscess seems less likely (choice A). Based on her weight of 40 kg, she has already received adequate initial fluid resuscitation (choice B). The negative culture data argues against the benefit of adjusting her antibiotic regimen at this time (choice C).

6. C. Equalization of diastolic pressures in all chambers

   Classically, in tamponade, a right heart catheterization will show equalization of the average diastolic pressure in all chambers. Choices A, B, and D are incorrect.

7. A. Daily assessment of antibiotics with consideration of de-escalation or discontinuation

   Systemic glucocorticoids (choice B) are recommended for refractory septic shock despite vasopressors, but not initially. At present, there is no compelling data that suggests that measuring CVP and $Scvo_2$s in a protocolized manner leads to better outcomes for patients in septic shock (choice C). Furthermore, the NICE-SUGAR investigators showed an increase in mortality with tight glycemic control (choice D).[99] Daily consideration of antibiotic necessity (choice A) is an integral part of the management of a patient in septic shock.

8. **D. All of the above**

   All of the options (A, B, and C) describe good source control practices.

9. **C. Consider alternative reasons why the lactate may not have decreased.**

   The improving hemodynamics and adequate urine production after antibiotics and fluid administration are suggestive of a patient who is improving while being treated for septic shock. Lactate clearance is a helpful indication of perfusion, but its production and clearance are complicated by numerous factors, including liver function. In a patient with cirrhosis, who is otherwise improving, there is no acute need to perform a CT chest and abdomen to evaluate for adequate source control (choice A). There may be benefit of repeating a lactate (choice B), but an elevated level by itself in a cirrhotic would not be reason enough to continue aggressive fluid resuscitation in an otherwise improving patient. Other assessments of fluid responsiveness should be obtained. Broadening antibiotics is not indicated at this time (choice D).

10. **C. Transfer to another facility for PCI**

    Current guidelines prefer PCI (choice C) over thrombolytics (choice B), even if this requires transfer to another facility. While intra-aortic balloon pump insertion (choice A) is advocated as a stabilizing measure in hypotensive patients, this patient is hemodynamically stable. Finally, medical management (choice D) is indicated, but transfer for PCI is the optimal choice.

11. **B. Ventricular septal wall rupture**

    In the days following an inferior wall infarct, both acute mitral valve regurgitation (choice A) and ventricular septal wall rupture (choice B) can occur. However, the presence of a step-up in oxygenation on right heart catheterization is more indicative of a ventricular septal wall rupture. Both worsening left ventricular failure (choice C) and tamponade (choice D) could cause hypotension, but these diagnoses are not consistent with a step-up in oxygenation. Patent ductus arteriosus has a step-up of greater than 5%. Ventricular septal defect (VSD) is associated with a step-up of greater than 5%. Atrial septal defect has a step-up of greater than 7%.

12. **A. Stiffening of the LV in diastole, worsening systolic filling, and decreased stroke volume**

    With continued volume loss, there is a left shift in the diastolic pressure-volume relationship, which leads to worsening filling and decreased stroke volume (choice A). Initially, the LV is hyperdynamic (choice B) to try to compensate, but as volume loss persists, the diastolic pressure-volume relationship shifts. Elevated end-diastolic pressures and diminished cardiac output (choice C) are more consistent with cardiogenic shock and not hypovolemic shock. Increased SVR (choice D) is not consistent with hypovolemic shock.

13. **C. Needle decompression**

    A pneumothorax can be primary if there is no underlying pulmonary disease, or secondary if there is an underlying pulmonary disease. Pneumothoraces can also be differentiated by size although there is general consensus regarding how this is measured.[100] The Collins method suggest that the size of the pneumothorax is a function of interpleural distance (ID) where %Collins = 4.2 + 4.7 (A+B+C).[101,102] A means the maximal apical interpleural distance; B is the interpleural distance in the midpoint of upper half of the lung, and C is the interpleural distance at the midpoint of lower half of the lung.[101,102] The Rhea method uses the following equation: %Rhea = 5+1(35/12)(A+B+C).[103] The Light Index uses the following equation: %Light = 100 – 100 $(b/a)^3$ where a is average diameter of hemithorax and b is average diameter of lung.[104]

    According to the British Thoracic Society (BTS), large pneumothorax is defined as the distance between the chest wall and lung rim at the hilum larger than 2 cm, and small pneumothorax is considered if that distance is less than 2 cm whereas the American guidelines suggest measurement should take place between the apex and the cupola.[100,105] 2 cm is not just an arbitrary number but this is believed to represent 50% pneumothorax.[100,105] However, symptoms are classically more dependent on the location of the pneumothorax rather than its size.[100,105]

    The patient in this scenario has developed a tension pneumothorax, as suggested by the hemodynamic compromise and the developing mediastinal shift on chest radiograph. The best initial treatment is to evacuate the air in the pleural space via needle decompression. The definitive treatment would be to prevent its reoccurrence. Confirmation of a pneumothorax via chest radiography is often not a prerequisite of treatment since these patients can further deteriorate rapidly.

    Needle thoracostomy is preferred over tube thoracostomy for the initial management of a tension pneumothorax.[105,106] (Level of Evidence [LOE] A) It is performed by first sterilizing the anterior chest and subsequently inserting a 14G to 16G, 3- to 5-cm needle in the second intercostal space. Ideally, the insertion site should be at the MCL, superior to the third rib, and at least 1 to 2 cm from the sternal edge to avoid hitting the internal thoracic artery. It has been argued that this location might not be effective due to the thickness of the chest wall. The literature suggests a mean chest wall thickness of 42.79 mm (95% confidence interval [CI], 38.78–46.81) at the second ICS MCL with a failure rate of 38% (95% CI, 24–54). In contrast, the fourth to fifth ICS at the midaxillary line has been associated with a thickness of 39.85 mm (95% CI, 28.70–51.00) and a failure rate of 31% (95% CI, 10–64).[105,106]

Finally, the fourth to fifth ICS at the anterior axillary line has been reported to have a thickness of 34.33 mm (95% CI, 28.20–40.47) and a failure rate of 13% (95% CI, 8–22).[105,106] In addition to increased depth, failure to decompress can also be a result of kinking or clots. This might prompt finding a different location. Needle aspiration can drain up to 2.5 Liters of air. In a primary spontaneous pneumothorax, needle aspiration might be sufficient for treatment. In a secondary spontaneous pneumothorax, tube thoracostomy should be performed within 24 hours of needle thoracostomy (LOE A). There is no benefit from using a large-bore chest tube over a small-bore chest tube (LOE D).[105]

Obtaining a chest radiograph (choice B) might be helpful but is likely to delay the necessary treatment. Starting bag-valve-mask ventilation (choice D) might worsen the pneumothorax. A chest tube (choice C) may ultimately be warranted, but needle thoracostomy is easier and faster to perform.

14. **A. Observe**

Conservative management of a pneumothorax via a chest tube can still be successful up to 14 days after the initial event.[105] Consequently, continued observation is the best strategy at present. In a patient with a persistent air leak for more than 48 hours, thoracic surgery consultation may be warranted to evaluate for a possible bronchopleural fistula (choice D). However, given that only 24 hours have elapsed, this is likely premature. Pleurodesis might be contemplated for inoperable cases. Surgical options include video-assisted thoracoscopy and open thoracotomy with pleurectomy.

Increasing the suction might further allow the apposition of the visceral and parietal pleural layers.[105,107] However, the administration of suction early in the course can lead to re-expansion pulmonary edema and higher levels of suction (choice C) can lead to hypoxemia, air steal, and perpetuation of air leaks.[107-109] There is no role for changing the chest tube at this time (choice B).

15. **A. Phenylephrine**

Left ventricular outflow tract obstruction is caused by systolic anterior motion of the mitral valve, usually the anterior leaflet, contacting the septum. This is a mechanical obstruction of the blood flow. This can be caused in the setting of hypertrophic cardiomyopathy or Takotsubo cardiomyopathy or stress cardiomyopathy. In addition to the systolic apical ballooning of the left ventricle and hyperkinesis of the basal walls, atypical echographic variants of stress cardiomyopathy include mid-ventricular hypokinesis with sparing of the apex, basal hypokinesis with sparing of the mid-ventricle and apex, focal type usually anterolateral segment of the left ventricle, and global hypokinesis. Differential includes acute coronary syndrome, pheochromocytoma and myocarditis. Coronary angiography is necessary to rule out obstructive coronary artery disease. However, its presence does not eliminate the presence of concommittant stress cardiomyopathy if the location of the obstruction does not correlate with abnormal echographic findings. Therefore, diagnosis is based on the presence of new transient LV dysfunction, ECG changes and/or elevated cardiac enzymes, and exclusion of the differential diagnosis.[110-117] In the setting of hypotension, treatment consists of fluid resuscitation and β-adrenergics to improve heart rate and "atrial kick." Phenylephrine is the preferred pressor due to lack of inotropic or chronotropic effects; therefore, it decreases heart rate and increases afterload. Dobutamine (choice B), dopamine (choice C), and norepinephrine (choice D) increase heart rate and contractility and can worsen symptoms.[110-112]

REFERENCES

1. Todd RS, Turner KL, Moore FA. Chapter 35: Shock: General. In: Gabrielli, Layon, Yu, eds. *Civetta, Taylor, and Kirby's Critical Care*. Philadelphia, PA: Lippincott, Williams, & Wilkins; 2009:813-834.

2. Vincent JL, De Backer D. Circulatory shock. *N Engl J Med*. 2013;369(18):1726-1734.

3. ATLS Subcommittee, et al. Advanced Trauma Life Support (ATLS): The Ninth Edition. *J Trauma Acute Care Surg*. 2013;74(5):1363-1366.

4. Finfer S, Bellomo R, Boyce N, French J, Myburgh J, Norton R. A comparison of albumin and saline for fluid resuscitation in the intensive care unit. *N Engl J Med*. 2004;350(22):2247-2256.

5. Perel P, Roberts I, Ker K. Colloids versus crystalloids for fluid resuscitation in critically ill patients. *Cochrane Database Syst Rev*. 2013;(2):CD000567.

6. Annane D, Siami S, Jaber S, et al. Effects of fluid resuscitation with colloids vs crystalloids on mortality in critically ill patients presenting with hypovolemic shock: the CRISTAL randomized trial. *JAMA*. 2013;310(17):1809-1817.

7. Zarychanski R, Abou-Setta AM, Turgeon AF, et al. Association of hydroxyethyl starch administration with mortality and acute kidney injury in critically ill patients requiring volume resuscitation: a systematic review and meta-analysis. *JAMA*. 2013;309(7):678-688.

8. Holcomb JB, Tilley BC, Baraniuk S, et al. Transfusion of plasma, platelets, and red blood cells in a 1:1:1 vs a 1:1:2 ratio and mortality in patients with severe trauma: the PROPPR randomized clinical trial. *JAMA*. 2015;313(5):471-482.

9. CRASH-2 trial collaborators; Shakur H, Roberts I, Bautista R, et al. Effects of tranexamic acid on death, vascular occlusive events, and blood transfusion in trauma patients with significant haemorrhage (CRASH-2): a randomized, placebo-controlled trial. *Lancet*. 2010;376(9734):23-32.

10. Morrison JJ, Dubose JJ, Rasmussen TE, Midwinter MM. Military application of tranexamic acid in trauma emergency resuscitation (MATTERs) study. *Arch Surg*. 2012;147(2):113-119.

11. Reynolds HR, Hochman JS. Cardiogenic shock: current concepts and improving outcomes. *Circulation*. 2008;117(5):686-697.

11. Jeger RV, Radovanovic D, Hunziker PR, et al; AMIS Plus Registry Investigators. Ten-year trends in the incidence and treatment of cardiogenic shock. *Ann Intern Med*. 2008;149(9):618-626.

12. Hasdai D, Holmes DR Jr, Califf RM, et al. Cardiogenic shock complicating acute myocardial infarction: predictors of death. GUSTO Investigators. Global Utilization of Streptokinase and Tissue-Plasminogen Activator for Occluded Coronary Arteries. *Am Heart J.* 1999;138(1 Pt 1):21-31.

13. Hollenberg SM, Kavinsky CJ, Parrillo JE. Cardiogenic shock. *Ann Intern Med.* 1999;131(1):47-59.

14. Califf RM, Bengtson JR. Cardiogenic shock. *N Engl J Med.* 1994;330(24):1724-1730.

15. Hochman JS, Sleeper LA, Webb JG, et al. Early revascularization in acute myocardial infarction complicated by cardiogenic shock. SHOCK Investigators. Should we emergently revascularize occluded coronaries for cardiogenic shock. *N Engl J Med.* 1999;341(9):625-634.

16. Thiele H, Zeymer U, Neumann FJ, et al; IABP-SHOCK II Trial Investigators. Intraaortic balloon support for myocardial infarction with cardiogenic shock. *N Engl J Med.* 2012;367(14):1287-1296.

17. O'Gara PT, Kushner FG, Ascheim DD, et al. 2013 ACCF/AHA guideline for the management of ST-elevation myocardial infarction: executive summary: a report of the American College of Cardiology Foundation/American Heart Association Task Force on Practice Guidelines. *Circulation.* 2013;127(4):529-555.

18. Rihal CS, Naidu SS, Givertz MM, et al.; Society for Cardiovascular Angiography and Interventions (SCAI), Heart Failure Society of America (HFSA), Society of Thoracic Surgeons (STS), American Heart Association (AHA), and American College of Cardiology (ACC). 2015 SCAI/ACC/HFSA/STS clinical expert consensus statement on the use of percutaneous mechanical circulatory support devices in cardiovascular care: endorsed by the American Heart Association, the Cardiological Society of India, and Sociedad Latino Americana de Cardiologia Intervencion; affirmation of value by the Canadian Association of Interventional Cardiology-Association Canadienne de Cardiologie d'intervention. *J Am Coll Cardiol.* 2015;65(19):2140-2141.

19. Combes A, Leprince P, Luyt CE, et al. Outcomes and long-term quality-of-life of patients supported by extracorporeal membrane oxygenation for refractory cardiogenic shock. *Crit Care Med.* 2008;36(5):1404-1411.

20. Chang CH, Chen HC, Caffrey JL, et al. Survival analysis after extracorporeal membrane oxygenation in critically ill adults: a nationwide cohort study. *Circulation.* 2016;133(24):2423-2433.

21. Ristic AD, Imazio M, Adler Y, et al. Triage strategy for urgent management of cardiac tamponade: a position statement of the European Society of Cardiology Working Group on Myocardial and Pericardial Diseases. *Eur Heart J.* 2014;35(34):2279-2284.

22. Cheitlin MD, Armstrong WF, Aurigemma GP, et al. ACC/AHA/ASE 2003 guideline for the clinical application of echocardiography. *Circulation.* 2003;108(9):1146-1162.

23. Klein AL, Abbara S, Agler DA, et al. American Society of Echocardiography clinical recommendations for multimodality cardiovascular imaging of patients with pericardial disease: endorsed by the Society for Cardiovascular Magnetic Resonance and Society of Cardiovascular Computed Tomography. *J Am Soc Echocardiogr.* 2013;26(9):965-1012.

24. Leigh-Smith S, Harris T. Tension pneumothorax—time for a rethink? *Emerg Med J.* 2005;22(1):8-16.

25. Steier M, Ching N, Roberts EB, et al. Pneumothorax complicating continuous ventilatory support. *J Thorac Cardiovasc Surg.* 1974;67(1):17-23.

26. Barton ED. Tension pneumothorax. *Curr Opin Pulm Med.* 1999;5(4):269-274.

27. Holloway VJ, Harris JK. Spontaneous pneumothorax: is it under tension? *J Accid Emerg Med.* 2000;17(3):222-223.

28. Hollins GW, Beattie T, Harper I, Little K. Tension pneumothorax: report of two cases presenting with acute abdominal symptoms. *J Accid Emerg Med.* 1994;11(1):43-44.

29. Jones R, Hollingsworth J. Tension pneumothoraces not responding to needle thoracocentesis. *Emerg Med J.* 2002;19(2):176-177.

30. Leigh-Smith S, Davies G. Tension pneumothorax—eyes may be more diagnostic than ears. *Emerg Med J.* 2003;20(5):495-496.

31. Askins DC. Spontaneous tension pneumothorax during sexual intercourse. *Ann Emerg Med.* 1984;13(4):303-306.

32. Boon D, Llewellyn T, Rushton P. A strange case of a tension pneumothorax. *Emerg Med J.* 2002;19(5):470-471.

33. Friend KD. Prehospital recognition of tension pneumothorax. *Prehosp Emerg Care.* 2000;4(1):75-77.

34. Slay RD, Slay LE, Luehrs JG. Transient ST elevation associated with tension pneumothorax. *JACEP.* 1979;8(1):16-18.

35. Vermeulen EG, Teng HT, Boxma H. Ventral tension pneumothorax. *J Trauma.* 1997;43(6):975-976.

36. Wilkinson D, Moore E, Wither P, et al. ATLS on the ski slopes—a steamboat experience. *J Trauma.* 1992;32(4):448-451.

37. Werne CS, Sands MJ. Left tension pneumothorax masquerading as anterior myocardial infarction. *Ann Emerg Med.* 1985;14(2):164-166.

38. Pattison GT. Needle thoracocentesis in tension pneumothorax: insufficient cannula length and potential failure. *Injury.* 1996;27(10):758.

39. Rawlins R, Brown KM, Carr CS, Cameron CR. Life threatening haemorrhage after anterior needle aspiration of pneumothoraces. A role for lateral needle aspiration in emergency decompression of spontaneous pneumothorax. *Emerg Med J.* 2003;20(4):383-384.

40. Kucher N, Goldhaber SZ. Management of massive pulmonary embolism. *Circulation.* 2005;112(2):e28-e32.

41. The Urokinase Pulmonary Embolism Trial: a national cooperative study. *Circulation.* 1973;47(suppl II):II-1-II-108.

42. Tibbutt DA, Davies JA, Anderson JA,. Comparison by controlled clinical trial of streptokinase and heparin in treatment of life-threatening pulmonary embolism. *Br Med J.* 1974;1(5904):343-347.

43. Ly B, Arnesen H, Eie H, Hol R. A controlled clinical trial of streptokinase and heparin in the treatment of major pulmonary embolism. *Acta Med Scand.* 1978;203(6):465-470.

44. Dotter CT, Seaman AJ, Rosch J. Streptokinase and heparin in the treatment of pulmonary embolism: a randomized comparison. *Vasc Surg.* 1979;13(1):42-52.

45. Jerjes-Sanchez C, Ramirez-Rivera A, de Lourdes Garcia M. Streptokinase and heparin versus heparin alone in massive pulmonary embolism: a randomized controlled trial. *J Thromb Thrombolysis.* 1995;2(3):227-229.

46. Mercat A, Diehl JL, Meyer G, Teboul JL, Sors H. Hemodynamic effects of fluid loading in acute massive pulmonary embolism. *Crit Care Med.* 1999;27(3):540-544.

47. Ternacle J, Gallet R, Mekontso-Dessap A, et al. Diuretics in normotensive patients with acute pulmonary embolism with right ventricular dilatation. *Circ J.* 2013;77(10):2612-2618.

48. Muehlschlegel S, Greer DM. *Neurogenic Shock.* 2008: 925-933.

49. Stratman RC, Wiesner AM, Smith KM, et al. Hemodynamic management after spinal cord injury. *Orthopedics.* 2008;31(3):252-255.

50. Campbell RL, Li JTC, Nicklas RA, Sadosky AT; Members of the Joint Task Force; Practice Parameter Workgroup. Emergency department diagnosis and treatment of anaphylaxis: a practice parameter. *Ann Allergy Asthma Immunol.* 2014;113(6):599-608.

51. Lin RY, Schwartz LB, Corry A, et al. Histamine and tryptase levels in patients with acute allergic reactions: an emergency department-based study. *J Allergy Clin Immunol.* 2000;106(1 Pt 1):65-71.

52. Wang J, Sampson HA. Food anaphylaxis. *Clin Exp Allergy.* 2007;37(5):651-660.

53. Brown SG, Blackman KE, Heddie RJ. Can serum mast cell tryptase help diagnose anaphylaxis? *Emerg Med Australas.* 2004;16(2):120-124.

54. Schwartz LB. Diagnostic value of tryptase in anaphylaxis and mastocytosis. *Immunol Allergy Clin North Am.* 2006;26(3):451-463.

55. Schummer W, Schummer C, Wippermann J, Fuchs J. Anaphylactic shock: is vasopressin the drug of choice? *Anesthesiology.* 2004;101(4):1025-1027.

56. Schummer C, Wirsing M, Schummer W. The pivotal role of vasopressin in refractory anaphylactic shock. *Anesth Analg.* 2008;107(2):620-624.

57. Thomas M, Crawford I. Best evidence topic report. Glucagon infusion in refractory anaphylactic shock in patients on beta-blockers. *Emerg Med J.* 2005;22(4):272-273.

58. Lang D, Alpern MB, Visintainer PF, Smith ST. Elevated risk of anaphylactoid reaction from radiographic contrast media is associated with both beta-blocker exposure and cardiovascular disorders. *Arch Intern Med.* 1993;153(17):2033-2040.

59. Toogood JH. Beta blocker therapy and the risk of anaphylaxis. *CMAJ.* 1987;137(7):587-588.

60. Sherman MS, Lazar EJ, Eichacker P. A bronchodilator action of glucagon. *J Allergy Clin Immunol.* 1988;81(5 Pt 1):908-911.

61. Pollack CV. Utility of glucagon in the emergency department. *J Emerg Med.* 1993;11(2):195-205.

62. Charmandari E, Nicolaides NC, Chrousos GP. Adrenal insufficiency. *Lancet.* 2014;383(9935):2152-2167.

63. Arlt W, Allolio B. Adrenal insufficiency. *Lancet.* 2003; 361(9372): 1881-1893.

64. Bornstein SR. Predisposing factors for adrenal insufficiency. *N Engl J Med.* 2009;360(22):2328-2339.

65. Neary N, Nieman L. Adrenal insufficiency: etiology, diagnosis, and treatment. *Curr Opin Endocrinol Diabetes Obes.* 2010;17(3):217-223.

66. Ford J, Rosenberg F, Chan N. Pheochromocytoma manifesting with shock presents a clinical paradox: a case report. *CMAJ.* 1997;157(7):923-935.

67. Steppan J, Shields J, Lebron R. Pheochromocytoma presenting as acute heart failure leading to cardiogenic shock and multiorgan failure. *Case Rep Med.* 2011;2011:596354.

68. Parenti G, Zampetti B, Rapizzi E, Ercolino T, Giache V, Mannelli M. Updated and new perspectives on diagnosis, prognosis, and therapy of malignant pheochromocytoma/paraganglioma. *J Oncol.* 2012;2012:872713.

69. Shanugam G. Vasoplegic syndrome—the role of methylene blue. *Eur J of Cardiothorac Surg.* 2005;28(5):705-710.

70. Ozal E, Kuralay E, Yildirim V, et al. Preoperative methylene blue administration in patients at high risk for vasoplegic syndrome during cardiac surgery. *Ann Thorac Surg.* 2005;79(5):1615-1619.

71. Cremer J, Martin M, Redl H. Systemic inflammatory response syndrome after cardiac operations. *Ann Thorac Surg.* 1996;61(6):1714-1720.

72. Levin RL, Degrange MA, Bruno GF, et al. Methylene blue reduces mortality and morbidity in vasoplegic patients after cardiac surgery. *Ann Thorac Surg.* 2004;77(2):496-499.

73. Argenziano M, Chen JM, Choudhri AF, et al. Management of vasodilatory shock after cardiac surgery: identification of predisposing factors and use of a novel pressor agent. *J Thorac Cardiovasc Surg.* 1998;116(6):973-980.

74. Taylor K. SIRS—the systemic inflammatory response syndrome after cardiac operations. *Ann Thorac Surg.* 1996;61(6):1607-1608.

75. Mekontso-Dessap A, Houël R, Soustelle C, Kirsch M, Thébert D, Loisance DY. Risk factors for post-cardiopulmonary bypass vasoplegia in patients with preserved left ventricular function. *Ann Thorac Surg.* 2001;71(5):1428-1432.

76. Leyh RG, Kofidis T, Strüber M, et al. Methylene blue: the drug of choice for catecholamine-refractory vasoplegia after cardiopulmonary bypass. *J Thorac Cardiovasc Surg.* 2003;125(6):1426-1431.

77. Jones CW, Pickering BT. Comparison of the effects of water deprivation and sodium chloride imbibition on the hormone content of the neurohypophysis of the rat. *J Physiol.* 1969;203(2):449-458.

78. Zucker IH, Gorman AJ, Cornish KG, Huffman LJ, Gilmore JP. Influence of left ventricular receptor stimulation on plasma vasopressin in conscious dogs. *Am J Physiol.* 1983;245(6):R792-R799.

79. Sehested J, Wacker B, Forssmann WG. Natriuresis after cardiopulmonary bypass: relationship to urodilatin, atrial natriuretic factor, antidiuretic hormone, and aldosterone. *J Thorac Cardiovasc Surg.* 1997;114(4):666-671.

80. Haijjar LA, Vincent JL, Barbosa Gomes Galas FR, et al. Vasopressin versus norepinephrine in patients with vasoplegic shock after cardiac surgery: the VANCS randomized trial. *Anesthesiology.* 2017;126(1):85-93.

81. Reddick AD, Ronald J, Morrison WG. Intravenous fluid resuscitation: was Poiseuille right? *Emerg Med J.* 2011;28(3):201-202.

82. Leidel BA, Kirchhoff C, Bogner V, Braunstein V, Biberthaler P, Kanz KG. Comparison of intraosseous versus central venous vascular access in adults under resuscitation in the emergency department with inaccessible peripheral veins. *Resuscitation.* 2012;83(1):40-45.

83. Miller LJ, Philbeck TE, Montez D, Spadaccini CJ. A new study of intraosseous blood for laboratory analysis. *Arch Pathol Lab Med.* 2010;134(9):1253-1260.

84. Boyd JH, Forbes J, Nakada TA, Walley KR, Russell JA. Fluid resuscitation in septic shock: a positive fluid balance and elevated central venous pressure are associated with increased mortality. *Crit Care Med.* 2011;39(2):259-265.

85. Prekker ME, Scott NL, Hart D, Sprenkle MD, Leatherman JW. Point-of-care ultrasound to estimate central venous pressure: a comparison of three techniques. *Crit Care Med.* 2013;41(3):833-841.

86. Barbier C, Loubières Y, Schmit C, et al. Respiratory changes in inferior vena cava diameter are helpful in predicting fluid responsiveness in ventilated septic patients. *Intensive Care Med.* 2004;30(9):1740-1746.

87. Lichtenstein D, Mezière G, Lagoueyte JF, et al. A-lines and B-lines: Lung ultrasound as a bedside tool for predicting pulmonary artery occlusion pressure in the critically ill. *Chest.* 2009;136(4):1014-1020.

88. Lichtenstein DA. BLUE-protocol and FALLS-protocol: two applications of lung ultrasound in the critically ill. *Chest.* 2015;147(6):1659-1670.

89. LeDoux D, Astiz ME, Carpati CM, Rackow EC. Effects of perfusion pressure on tissue perfusion in septic shock. *Crit Care Med.* 2000;28(8):2729-2732.

90. Desjars P, Pinaud M, Bugnon D, Tasseau F. Norepinephrine therapy has no deleterious renal effects in human septic shock. *Crit Care Med.* 1989;17(5):426-429.

91. Reinelt H, Radermacher P, Kiefer P, et al. Impact of exogenous beta-adrenergic receptor stimulation on hepatosplanchnic oxygen kinetics and metabolic activity in septic shock. *Crit Care Med.* 1999;27(2):325-331.

92. De Backer D, Creteur J, Silva E, Vincent JL. Effects of dopamine, norepinephrine, and epinephrine on the splanchnic circulation in septic shock: which is best? *Crit Care Med.* 2003;31(6):1659-1667.

93. Landry DW, Levin HR, Gallant EM, et al. Vasopressin deficiency contributes to the vasodilation of septic shock. *Circulation.* 1997;95(5):1122-1125.

94. Polito A, Parisini E, Ricci Z, Picardo S, Annane D. Vasopressin for treatment of vasodilatory shock: an ESICM systematic review and meta-analysis. *Intensive Care Med.* 2012;38(1):9-19.

95. De Backer D, Aldecoa C, Njimi H, Vincent JL. Dopamine versus norepinephrine in the treatment of septic shock: a meta-analysis. *Crit Care Med.* 2012;40(3):725-730.

96. Vasu TS, Cavallazzi R, Hirani A, Kaplan G, Leiby B, Marik PE. Norepinephrine or dopamine for septic shock: systematic review of randomized clinical trials. *J Intensive Care Med.* 2012;27(3):172-178.

97. Whitson MR, Mo E, Nabi T, et al. Feasibility, utility, and safety of midodrine during recovery phase from septic shock. *Chest.* 2016;149(6):1380-1383.

98. Khanna A, English SW, Wang XS, et al; ATHOS-3 Investigators. Angiotensin II for treatment of vasodilatory shock. *N Engl J Med.* 2017;377(5):419-430.

99. NICE-SUGAR Study Investigators. Intensive versus conventional glucose control in critically ill patients. *NEJM.* 2009;360:1283-1297.

100. Baumann MH, Strange C, Heffner JE, et al. Management of spontaneous pneumothorax. An American College of Chest Physicians Delphi Consensus Statement. *Chest.* 2001;119:590-602.

101. Salazar AJ, Aguirre DA, Ocampo J, Camacho JC, Diaz XA. Evaluation of three pneumothorax size quantification methods on digitized chest X-ray films using medical-grade grayscale and consumer-grade color displays. *J Digit Imaging.* 2014;27(2):280-286.

102. Collins C, Lopez A, Mathie A, Wood V, Jackson J, Roddie M. Quantification of pneumothorax size on chest radiographs using interpleural distances: regression analysis based on volume measurements from helical CT. *AJS.* 1995;165:1127-1130.

103. Rhea JT, DeLuca SA, Greene RE. Determining the size of pneumothorax in the upright patient. *Radiology.* 1982;144:733-736.

104. Light RW. Management of spontaneous pneumothorax. *Am J Respir Crit Care Med.* 1993;148:245-248.

105. McDuff A, Arnold A, Harvey J; BTS Pleural Disease Guideline Group. Management of spontaneous pneumothorax: British Thoracic Society pleural disease guideline 2010. *Thorax.* 2010;65 (Suppl 2):ii18-ii31.

106. Laan DV, Thiels CA, Pandian TK, Schiller HJ, Murad MH, Aho JM. Chest wall thickness and decompression failure: a systematic review and meta-analysis comparing anatomic locations in needle thoracostomy. *Injury.* 2016;47(4):797-804.

107. Pavlin J, Cheney FW Jr. Unilateral pulmonary edema in rabbits after reexpansion of collapsed lung. *J Appl Physiol Respir Environ Exerc Physiol.* 1979;46(1):31-35.

108. Munnell ER. Thoracic drainage. *Ann Thorac Surg.* 1997;63(5): 1497-1502.

109. Pierson DJ. Persistent bronchopleural air-leak during mechanical ventilation: a review. *Respir Care.* 1982;27(4):408-415.

110. De Backer O, Debonnaire P, Geaert S, Missault L, Gheeraert P, Muyldermans L. Prevalence, associated factors and management implications of left ventricular outflow tract obstruction in Takotsubo cardiomyopathy: a two-year, two-center experience. *BMC Cardiovasc Dis.* 2014;14:147.

111. Chockalingam A, Tejwani L, Aggarwal K, Dellsperger KC. Dynamic left ventricular outflow tract obstruction in acute myocardial infarction with shock: cause, effect, and coincidence. *Circulation.* 2007;116(5):e110-e113.

112. Reynolds H, Hochman JS. Cardiogenic shock: current concepts and improving outcomes. *Circulation.* 2008;117(5):686-697.

113. Bybee KA, Kara T, Prasad A, Lerman A, Barsness GW, Wright RS, Rihal CS. Systematic review: transient left ventricular apical ballooning: a syndrome that mimics ST-segment elevation myocardial infarction. *Ann Intern Med.* 2004;144(11):858-865.

114. Prasad A, Lerman A, Rihal CS. Apical ballooning syndrome (Tako-Tsubo or stress cardiomyopathy): a mimic of acute myocardial infarction. *Am Heart J.* 20205;155(3):408-417.

115. Kurowski V, Kaiser A, von Hof K, et al. Apical and midventricular transient left ventricular dysfunction syndrome (tako-tsubo cardiomyopathy): frequency, mechanisms, and prognosis. *Chest.* 2007;132(3):809-816.

116. Eitel I, et al. Clinical characteristics and cardiovascular magnetic resonance findings in stress (takotsubo) cardiomyopathy. *JAMA.* 2011;306(3):277-286.

117. Templin C. Clinical Features and Outcomes of Takotsubo (Stress) Cardiomyopathy. *N Engl J Med.* 2015;373(10):929-938.

Cardiac Arrhythmias and Hypertensive Emergencies

Candice Kim, MD, Melissa Dakkak, DO, Ronaldo Collo Go, MD, and Prakash Goutham Suryanarayana, MD

INTRODUCTION

Cardiac arrhythmias and hypertensive emergencies are not uncommon in the intensive care unit. This chapter will discuss basic cardiac electrophysiology, cardiac conduction, electrocardiography (ECG) interpretation, tachyarrhythmias, bradyarrhythmias, and hypertensive crisis.

BASIC CARDIAC ELECTROPHYSIOLOGY

Mechanisms of arrhythmia initiation, maintenance, and termination are best understood by reviewing the basic electrophysiologic properties of the cardiac cells. The resting cardiac transmembrane potential is normally –50 to –95 mV (depending on the type of cardiac cell) and is maintained by the electrochemical equilibration of the sodium (Na^+), potassium (K^+), calcium (Ca^{2+}), and chlorine (Cl^-) ions. From an electrophysiological standpoint, cardiac cells can be classified into fast-response (contractile cells) and slow-response (automatic) cells. Sinus node and atrioventricular (AV) node cells are considered slow response cells. The electrophysiological properties during diastole (resting phase) and systole (activation phase) are different.

The cardiac transmembrane action potential of fast response cells consists of 5 phases (Fig. 5-1):

- Phase 0: Rapid depolarization is caused by a sudden influx of Na^+ ions.
- Phase 1 (absent in slow-response cells): Early rapid repolarization due to inactivation of the inward Na^+ channels and simultaneous activation of outward K^+ channels, resulting in a net efflux of positive ions.
- Phase 2 (absent in slow-response cells): The plateau phase may last several hundred milliseconds and is mainly due to the outward K^+ and Cl^- ion current with an inward current of Na^+ and Ca^{2+}.
- Phase 3: Final rapid repolarization occurs due to opening of slow delayed rectifier K^+ channels and simultaneous closure of inward Na^+ and Ca^{2+} channels, resulting in a net efflux of positive ions.
- Phase 4: The resting membrane potential is reached. It is usually rectilinear in fast-response cells due to inward Na^+ and Ca^{2+} currents and outward K^+ currents.

- In slow-response cells, resting transmembrane potential is slightly less negative (around –60 mV) and is followed by gradual diastolic depolarization, which is responsible for the property of automaticity. Diastolic depolarization is caused predominantly by an inward current of both Na^+ and Ca^{2+} with slow/small outward current of K^+.

Different classes of antiarrhythmics have their effects on 1 or more phases (Table 5-1).

The Cardiac Conduction System

During normal antegrade conduction, an action potential is first generated in the sinoatrial (SA) node due to its automaticity. It is then conducted to the atrioventricular (AV) node, down the bundle of His and into the Purkinje fibers via cell-to-cell conduction facilitated by gap junctions.

The SA node is the natural pacemaker of the heart and is located epicardially, at the junction of superior vena cava and the right atrium. It is heavily innervated by vagal fibers, but also has a high concentration of β-adrenergic receptors, which makes the SA node susceptible to vagal inputs (decreasing automaticity) and circulating catecholamines (increasing automaticity).

The AV node is located within the Koch triangle, anterior to the coronary sinus ostium and just above the septal leaflet of the tricuspid valve. The AV node has pacemaker activity as well but at a slower automaticity than the SA node. Its main function is to cause a delay in the electrical activity between the atria and ventricles in order to coordinate atrial and ventricular contractions. Like the SA node, the AV node is also influenced by vagal inputs and circulating catecholamines.

The bundle of His is located in the membranous portion of interventricular septum and connects the AV node and bundle branches. The bundle of His branches off into right and left bundle branches at the level of the muscular intraventricular septum. The left bundle branch further divides into anterior and posterior fascicles. The ends of these branches then connect with the terminal Purkinje fibers, which form interweaving networks on the endocardial surface of both ventricles.

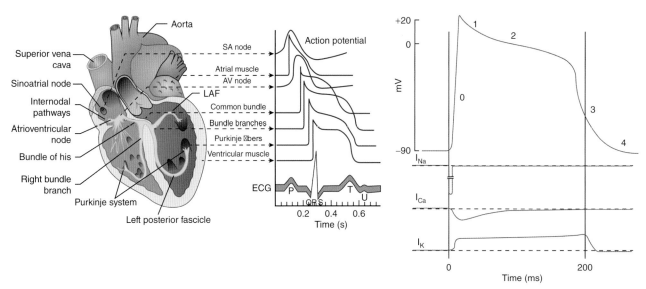

FIGURE 5-1 The conduction system of the heart and their action potentials. (Left panel: Data from Donahue JG, Choo PW, Manson JE, et al. The incidence of herpes zoster. *Arch Intern Med.* 155:1605-1609, 1995; Choo PW, Galil K, Donahue JG, et al. Risk factors for postherpetic neuralgia. *Arch Intern Med.* 1997;157:1217-1224. Right panel: Reproduced with permission from Elmoselhi A, Seif M. Electrophysiology of the Heart. In: Elmoselhi A. eds. *Cardiology: An Integrated Approach. New York,* NY: McGraw-Hill; 2018).

The Normal Electrocardiogram

The normal ECG is made up of a P wave, PR segment, QRS complex, ST segment, T wave, and QT interval. The P wave reflects atrial activation. The PR segment corresponds to the duration of atrioventricular conduction and is normally between 120 and 200 msec. The QRS complex represents the ventricular activation and is normally less than 100 msec. The ST segment and T wave reflect electrical ventricular recovery. The QT interval includes the total duration of ventricular activation and recovery and is normally less than 450 msec. Because the length of the QT interval is heart-rate dependent, a heart-rate adjusted value called QTc (corrected QT) is commonly used.

TABLE 5-1 Classes of Antiarrhythmics and Effects on Phases

Class	Effect on Phases	Example Drugs
Class Ia	Depress phase 0, prolong repolarization	Quinidine, procainamide, disopyramide
Class Ib	Depress phase 0, shorten repolarization	Lidocaine, phenytoin, mexiletine
Class Ic	Depress phase 0, minimal effect on repolarization	Flecainide, propafenone, moricizine
Class II	Decrease slope of phase 4	Propranolol, esmolol, timolol, metoprolol, atenolol
Class III	Prolong phase 3	Amiodarone, sotalol, ibutilide, dofetilide
Class IV	Prolong phase 2	Verapamil, diltiazem
Class V		Adenosine, digoxin, magnesium sulfate

In addition to class III, amiodarone can act as a class Ia, II, and IV drug.

TACHYARRHYTHMIAS

Tachycardia is defined as heart rate greater than 100 beats per minute (bpm). Sustained tachyarrhythmias are common in critically ill patients and occur at a frequency of approximately 12% in patients admitted to intensive care unit (ICU).[1] There are 3 mechanisms of tachyarrhythmias: abnormal automaticity, triggered activity, and reentry.[2] Normal automaticity originates in a normal pacemaker site of the heart (eg, sinus tachycardia), whereas abnormal automaticity results from a tissue that, under normal conditions, does not exhibit pacemaker properties but can become automatic under abnormal circumstances (eg, accelerated idioventricular rhythm). Triggered activity refers to spontaneous depolarization that occurs during or immediately after the cardiac action potential, giving rise to extrasystole, which can then precipitate tachyarrhythmias.[2] Reentrant tachyarrhythmias result from 2 electrically distinct pathways that connect to create a circuit.

Supraventricular Tachyarrhythmias

Sinus tachycardia is sinus rhythm at a heart rate greater than 100 bpm and usually reflects an underlying process such as hypovolemia. The management for sinus tachycardia is directed at treating the underlying cause.

Focal atrial tachycardia has a discrete origin within the atrium and will usually generate a regular rhythm ranging from 100 to 250 bpm[3] (Fig. 5-2). The P-wave axis on ECG will differ from that of sinus rhythm. Nonsustained focal atrial tachycardias are common and often do not require treatment.

Unlike focal atrial tachycardia, which has a discrete origin, multifocal atrial tachycardia is an irregular rhythm with at least 3 distinct P-wave morphologies on ECG, with a rate between 100 and 130 bpm.[3] The mechanism is unclear, but it is associated with underlying conditions, particularly

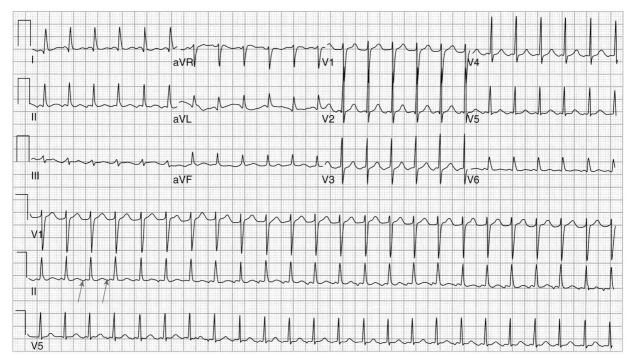

FIGURE 5-2 A 12-lead electrocardiogram tracing showing atrial tachycardia. Note the regular, narrow, complex tachycardia with negative P waves in lead II (*blue arrows*). This is an example of long RP tachycardia.

pulmonary disease, pulmonary hypertension, coronary artery disease, and valvular heart disease. First-line management is directed at treating the underlying condition. If needed, AV nodal blockers such as beta-blockers and calcium channel blockers (CCB) can be used to control the heart rate. Neither electrical cardioversion nor oral antiarrhythmics is useful for suppressing this arrhythmia.[3]

Atrial fibrillation (AF) is the most common sustained arrhythmia[4] and occurs when there are structural and/or electrophysiological abnormalities of the atrial tissue[5] (Fig. 5-3). It is associated most commonly with structural heart disease, advancing age, hypertension, heart failure, and coronary artery disease.[5] Atrial fibrillation can be classified by the duration of episodes. Paroxysmal atrial fibrillation resolves spontaneously or through intervention within 7 days, but episodes may reoccur. Persistent atrial fibrillation may persist for more than 7 days and is considered long-standing persistent AF if it persists for more than 12 months. Permanent atrial fibrillation occurs when attempts to restore to sinus rhythm are stopped. Nonvalvular AF occurs in the absence of rheumatic mitral stenosis, bioprosthetic or mechanical heart valve, or mitral valve repair.[5] The ECG will have no discernible P waves and the ventricular rhythm and rate can vary.

Treatment of AF is either to maintain sinus rhythm or to control the heart rate.[6] The Pharmacological Intervention in Atrial Fibrillation (PIAF) study showed that there was no difference in symptom improvement from either approach, and a sub-study showed no difference in quality of life.[7] The STAF study[8] showed no difference with primary endpoints of death, cardiopulmonary resuscitation, cerebrovascular event,

and systemic embolism, but more hospitalization in the rhythm-control group from repeated cardioversions and initiation of antiarrhythmic, and a tendency toward greater mortality in the rate-control group (2.5% vs 4.9%). The RACE study[9] showed no difference after a 2.3-year follow up for primary endpoints of death from cardiovascular causes, heart failure, thromboembolic complications, bleeding, pacemaker implantation, and adverse drug effects. The AFFIRM study[6] followed patients from a mean of 3.5 years to a maximum of 6 years, and 63% of the rhythm-control group were in normal sinus rhythm (NSR) compared to 34.6% of patients in the rate-control group. Despite this, there were 356 deaths (23.8%) in the rhythm-control group versus 310 deaths (21.3%) in the rate-control group, but these rates were not statistically significant.[6] Gillinov et al[10] showed that rate and rhythm controls were associated with similar days of hospitalization, complication rates, and persistent atrial fibrillation 60 days after onset in patients who develop postoperative atrial fibrillation after cardiac surgery. Rate control can be achieved via beta-blockers, digoxin, diltiazem, or verapamil for a left ventricular ejection fraction (LVEF) of 40% or greater, and beta-blockers or digoxin for LVEF less than 40% (Class of Recommendation [COR] I, Level of Evidence [LOE] B).[11] Amiodarone can be given in hemodynamically unstable patients or severely depressed EF (COR IIb, LOE B).[11] For rhythm control, flecainide and propafenone can be given if there is no structural heart disease; ibutilide can be given, but there is a risk of torsade de pointes; vernakalant can be given to patients with mild heart failure; and amiodarone can be given to patients with ischemic heart disease and heart failure.[11]

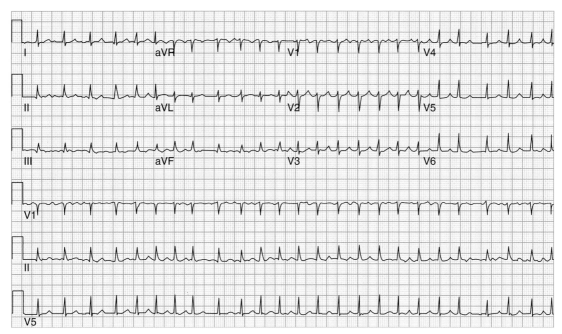

FIGURE 5-3 A 12-lead electrocardiogram tracing showing atrial fibrillation. It is irregularly irregular with no recognizable P waves. Differential diagnosis includes multifocal atrial tachycardia where P waves of at least 3 different morphologies are seen.

Thromboembolic risk management is an important part of AF management with the highest risk being advanced age and previous transient ischemic attack (TIA) or cerebrovascular accident (CVA).[11] The decision for no anticoagulation versus warfarin versus novel oral anticoagulants (NOAC) is complex and should be based on an individual's risk of stroke and bleed, which can be determined via CHA_2DS_2-VASc or CHADS2 scores or the presence of moderate to severe mitral valve stenosis and/or mechanical valves.[5] An increase in the stroke risk of approximately 2% with each 1-point increase in CHADS2 score has been shown in multiple non–valvular atrial fibrillation cohorts.[12] Compared to the CHADS2 score, the CHA_2DS_2-VASc score includes a larger number of risk factors. Based on this risk stratification scheme, women cannot achieve a score of 0.[5] A CHA_2DS_2-VASc score of 1 or more for men or 2 or more for women recommends anticoagulation (COR IIa, LOE B), NOAC preferred over vitamin K antagonists (VKA) (COR I, LOE A).[11] For moderate to severe mitral valve stenosis or mechanical valves, VKA is preferred for anticoagulation (COR I, LOE A).[11] Patients with contraindication to anticoagulation but who are at risk for CVA can opt to have left atrial appendage devices (COR IIb, LOE B).[11]

For patients who presents with TIA/CVA and new onset atrial fibrillation and after exclusion of hemorrhagic conversion, NOAC is started 1 day after TIA, 3 days after mild CVA (National Institutes of Health Stroke Score [NIHSS] < 8), 6 days after moderate CVA (NIHSS 8–15), and 12 days after severe CVA (NIHSS ≥16) (COR IIa, LOE C).[11] Aspirin is initiated until the appropriate time to start NOAC (COR IIa, LOE B). For intracranial hemorrhage, anticoagulants can be initiated 4 to 8 weeks after bleeding is controlled (COR IIb, LOE B).[11]

Patients who are in atrial fibrillation for more than 48 hours should be on oral anticoagulants for 3 weeks or more prior to cardioversion and continued for 4 weeks or more.

Atrial flutter is a macroreentrant atrial tachycardia that has a constant atrial rate but can have either a constant or a variable ventricular response, depending on the conduction through the AV node (Fig. 5-4). Typical flutter is the result of a reentrant circuit in the right atrium and traverses the cavotricuspid isthmus. It will have the classic "saw-tooth" waves on the ECG at a rate of 250 to 350 bpm. Counterclockwise flutter is characterized by negative flutter waves in the inferior leads with positive P waves in V_1; clockwise flutter will show the opposite pattern.[3] Atypical flutter is generally due to circuits around scar tissue or surgical incisions, and the cavotricuspid isthmus is not involved.[13] It will not have the classic saw-tooth pattern but will have a constant P wave morphology and a rate between 250 to 350 bpm. As with AF, management of atrial flutter is directed at either rate or rhythm control. Rate control is generally less effective in atrial flutter, so rhythm control may be preferred. Radiofrequency ablation is the preferred approach but electrical cardioversion may be utilized. If chemo-cardioversion is preferred, ibutilide is used.[14] Additionally, patients with atrial flutter share the same risk of thromboembolism as those with AF; therefore, the same anticoagulation recommendations apply.[3]

Atrioventricular nodal reentrant tachycardia (AVNRT) is a common, generally benign arrhythmia usually seen in young adults without structural or ischemic heart disease. Syncope is uncommon and sudden cardiac death is very rare[3] (Fig. 5-5).

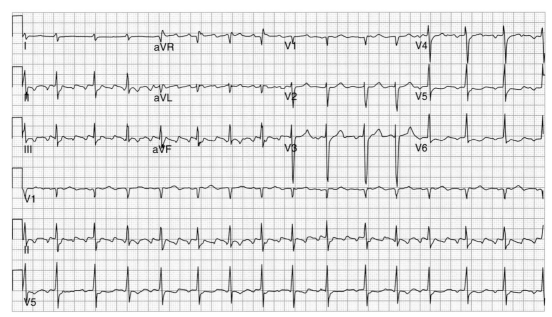

FIGURE 5-4 A 12-lead electrocardiogram tracing demonstrating atrial flutter. Note the saw-tooth pattern of the flutter waves.

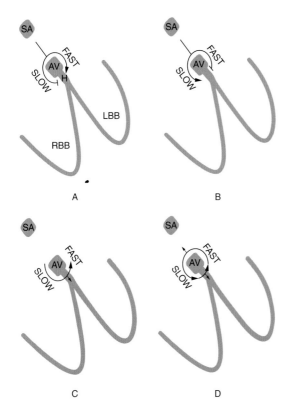

FIGURE 5-5 AV Nodal Conduction. In AV nodal conduction, there are two pathways, Slow Pathway with short refractory time, and Fast Pathway with long refractory time. In sinus rhythm (A), impulse are conducted through both but reach the bundle of His (H) only through the Fast Pathway. In B, due to the long refractory time of the Fast Pathway, a premature atrial impulse is carried through the Slow Pathway and into the bundle of His. In C and D, the impulse from the Slow Pathway may enter the Fast Pathway retrograde, if it has recovered and reentry. SA = Sinoatrial Node; AV = Atrioventricular Node; H = Bundle of His; RBB = Right Bundle Branch; LBB = Left Bundle Branch.

It appears to be due to a reentrant circuit within the AV node and perinodal tissues, and utilizes the fast and slow pathways[4] and the ventricular rate can range from 110 to 250 bpm.[3] "Typical" AVNRT accounts for more than 80% of AVNRT and is initiated by a premature beat, which conducts in an antegrade fashion to the ventricles via the slow pathway and conducts retrogradely to the atria via the fast pathway. This is represented as a negative P waves in the inferior leads and a short RP segment, usually less than 90 ms on the surface ECG.[3]

Atrioventricular reentrant tachycardia (AVRT) is dependent on an accessory pathway in addition to the AV node as part of the reentrant circuit[4] (Fig. 5-6). Ventricular rates can vary but are generally between 150 and 250 bpm. Unlike AVNRT, the RP segment in AVRT is usually greater than 90 ms.[4] Orthodromic AVRT is the most common type of AVRT. It is usually narrow complex, and the circuit consists of antegrade conduction from the atria to ventricles through the AV node and retrograde conduction from the ventricles to atria over the accessory pathway with completion of the circuit when the atria conduct back into the AV node.[3] Preexcited AVRT, including antidromic AVRT, is usually wide complex and uses the accessory pathway for antegrade conduction with retrograde conduction through the AV node. A preexcited QRS complex will have a short PR interval (< 120 ms) and a delta wave (slurred upstroke of the QRS complex). Atrial fibrillation can conduct antegradely via the accessory pathway leading to rapid, irregular, wide, and bizarre-looking QRS complexes.

The acute and long term treatment of supraventricular tachyarrhythmias are seen in Figures 5-7 and 5-8).

Preexcitation is due to simultaneous antegrade ventricular activation via the AV node and an accessory pathway (Fig. 5-9). The incidence of preexcitation on ECG is about 0.1% to 0.3% of the general population[15] with most cases

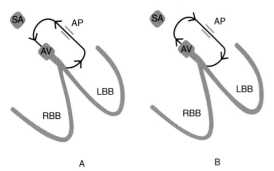

FIGURE 5-6 Accessory pathways. In A, orthodromic AVRT, the impulse is carried through the AV node (AV) and Bundle of His and exits through the Accessory Pathway (AP). This creates a normal QRS. In B, antidromic AVRT, the impulse is carried through the ventricle via the Accessory Pathway and exits via AV node. This creates a wide QRS. AV=Atrioventricular Node; SA=Sinoatrial Node; AP=Accessory Pathway; LBB = Left Bundle Branch; RBB = Right Bundle Branch.

occurring in healthy individuals with no organic heart disease; however, about 7% to 10% of patients have associated Ebstein anomaly.[4] When symptoms such as syncope or palpitations accompany preexcitation on ECG, a preexcitation syndrome is established, which has an increased risk of sudden cardiac death of up to 4% over a lifetime.[15] Therefore, catheter ablation should be considered for any patient who is at high risk or who has symptoms/tachycardia refractory to medical therapy.[4] Medical therapy aimed at slowing conduction through the accessory pathway is reasonable for those patients with high risk but no symptoms.[4] In patients with preexcitation and acute tachycardia, it is reasonable to use AV nodal blocking medications if the QRS is narrow. If the QRS is wide, it is unsafe to use AV nodal blocking agents, as this may cause preferential conduction through the accessory pathway leading to ventricular fibrillation. Beta-blockers, CCBs, digoxin, and adenosine are contraindicated. If tachycardia persists, synchronized direct current cardioversion (DCCV) is the treatment of choice.[4] Similarly, in those with accessory pathway and another type of supraventricular

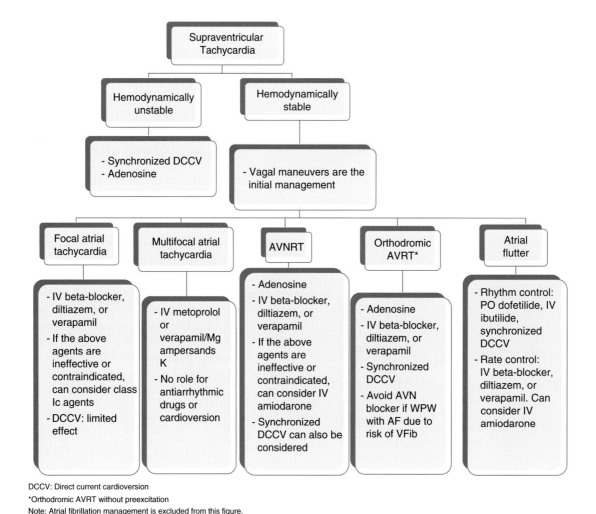

DCCV: Direct current cardioversion

*Orthodromic AVRT without preexcitation

Note: Atrial fibrillation management is excluded from this figure.

FIGURE 5-7 Acute treatment of supraventricular tachyarrhythmias. AVN = atrioventricular node; AVNRT = atrioventricular nodal reentrant tachycardia; AVRT = atrioventricular reentrant tachycardia; DCCV = direct current cardioversion; IV = intravenous; PO = oral; VFib = ventricular fibrillation; WPW = Wolff-Parkinson-White.

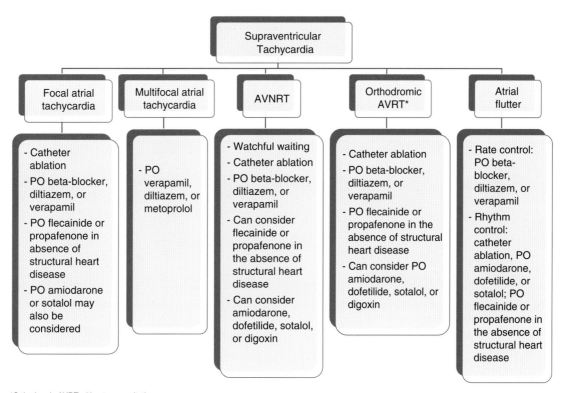

*Orthodromic AVRT without pre-excitation
Note: Atrial fibrillation management is excluded from this figure.

FIGURE 5-8 Long-term management of supraventricular tachyarrhythmias. AVNRT = atrioventricular nodal reentrant tachycardia; AVRT = atrioventricular reentrant tachycardia; DCCV = direct current cardioversion; PO = oral.

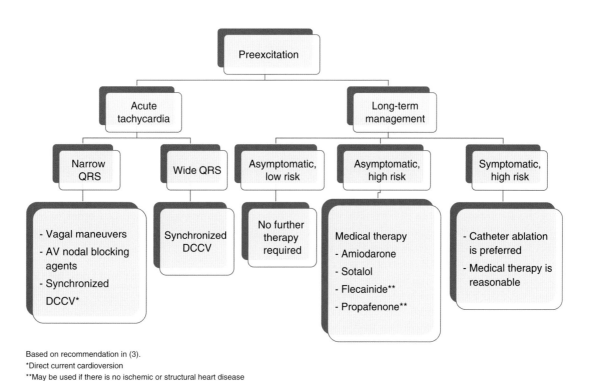

Based on recommendation in (3).
*Direct current cardioversion
**May be used if there is no ischemic or structural heart disease

FIGURE 5-9 Acute and ongoing management in preexcitation. DCCV = direct current cardioversion. (Data from Page RL, Joglar JA, Caldwell MA, et al. 2015 ACC/AHA/HRS guideline for the management of adult patients with supraventricular tachycardia: A Report of the American College of Cardiology/American Heart Association Task Force on Clinical Practice Guidelines and the Heart Rhythm Society. *Heart Rhythm.* 2016;13(4):e136-e221.)

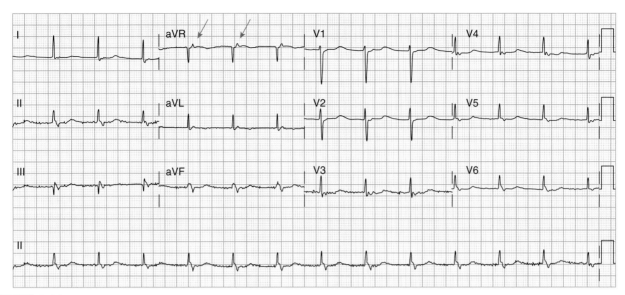

FIGURE 5-10 Electrocardiogram tracing of accelerated junctional rhythm. Note the retrograde P waves immediately following the QRS in lead aVR (shown by *blue arrows*). Unlike AVNRT, the rate here is less than 100/min. P waves may precede or follow, or sometimes are hidden within QRS complexes. If the junctional rhythm is secondary to slow sinus response, one may see evidence of atrioventricular dissociation but with more QRS than P waves.

tachycardia (SVT), such as atrial fibrillation, AV nodal blocking agents should be avoided.[15]

Accelerated junctional rhythm rises near the AV node and has an intrinsic rate between 30 and 60 beats/min (Fig. 5-10). This rhythm can be seen in around 10% of patients with acute myocardial infarction (most commonly in inferior myocardial infarctions). It is also not uncommon after valve surgery, cardiac catheterization, hyperkalemia, and other significant systemic disease processes. The ECG will demonstrate a narrow-complex QRS, unless there is an underlying bundle branch block, with or without evidence of AV dissociation. Unlike in a third degree AV block, the ventricular rate is faster than the atrial rate in junctional tachycardia. Therapy for accelerated junctional rhythm is usually directed at treating the underlying cause.[4]

Regular narrow QRS tachycardias can be grouped into 2 categories based on the position of the P waves relative to the QRS complexes. An R-R interval can be used to define the duration of the RP interval. If the P wave falls within the first half of the RR interval during tachycardia, it is considered short RP tachycardia, whereas when the P wave appears within the second half of RR interval, it is termed long RP tachycardia. In other words, tachycardias that have a shorter RP interval than PR interval are termed short RP tachycardias. On the other hand, those that have a longer RP interval than PR interval are termed long RP tachycardias. The RP interval gives a clue about the time taken for the retrograde (V→A) conduction. Typically, when the RP interval is short, the retrograde atrial activation occurs via a fast conducting pathway (fast pathway in AVNRT and accessory pathway in cases of AVNRT). The short RP interval, as seen in typical AVNRT, indicates that the antegrade conduction occurs through the AV-nodal slow pathway while the retrograde conduction occurs through the fast pathway. Therefore, the

P wave will occur within or shortly after the QRS. In contrast, when the retrograde conduction occurs via the AV node (in AVNRT) or slow pathway (in AVNRT), the retrograde conduction time would be longer and the RP interval would also be longer (Table 5-2).

List of vagal maneuvers and medications and their doses for supraventricular tachycardia can be found on Table 5-3.

Ventricular Tachyarrhythmias

Ventricular tachyarrhythmias account for up to 80% of sudden cardiac death and are divided into nonsustained and sustained.[16] Nonsustained ventricular arrhythmias consist of premature ventricular complexes (PVC) and nonsustained ventricular tachycardia (NSVT). Sustained ventricular arrhythmias consist of monomorphic ventricular tachycardia, polymorphic ventricular tachycardia, and ventricular fibrillation.

Premature ventricular complexes are very common and are generally benign with no known prognostic significance.[16] Echocardiogram may be useful in order to evaluate biventricular function and cardiac valves. Treatment is indicated

TABLE 5-2 Types of Short and Long RP Tachycardias

Short RP Tachycardias	Long RP Tachycardias
Typical AVNRT	Atypical AVNRT
Orthodromic AVRT	Antidromic AVRT
	Atrial tachycardia
	Permanent junctional reciprocating tachycardia
	Sinus node reentry tachycardia

AVNRT = atrioventricular nodal reentrant tachycardia; AVRT = atrioventricular reentrant tachycardia.

TABLE 5-3 List of Vagal Maneuvers, Medications, and Doses for Supraventricular Tachycardia

Treatment	Dose
Vagal maneuvers while supine	• Valsalva maneuver by bearing down against closed glottis for 10–30 min • Carotid massage after confirmation of no bruit by applying pressure on right or left sinus for 5–10 min • Diving reflex (ice-cold, wet towel to face)
Adenosine	• 6-mg intravenous (IV) bolus over 1–2 min; if no response after 1–2 min, 12-mg IV bolus; if still no response after 1–2 min, 12-mg IV bolus
Esmolol	• 500-µg/kg IV bolus over 1 min followed by 50–300 µg/kg/min infusion
Metoprolol	• 2.5- to 5-mg IV bolus over 2 min, and can repeat every 10 min × 3 doses
Propranolol	• 1 mg IV over 1 min, and can repeat every 2 min × 3 doses
Diltiazem	• 0.25-mg/kg IV bolus over 2 min followed by 5- to 15-mg/h infusion
Verapamil	• 5- to 10-mg IV bolus over 2 min; if no response 30 min after first dose, then 0.005 mg/kg/min
Digoxin	• Loading dose, 0.25-mg IV bolus, and repeat every 6–8 h with maximum loading dose, 1 mg in 24 h
Amiodarone	• 150 mg IV over 10 min and start infusion at 1 mg/min (360 mg) over 6 h, then 0.5 mg/min (540 mg) over 18 h
Ibutilide	• Contraindicated if QTc > 440 • 1 mg IV over 10 min if ≥ 60 kg or 0.01 mg IV if < 60 kg; can repeat after 10 min

if the patient has persistent symptoms related to PVCs or has decreased left ventricular systolic function with a high PVC burden. A trial of beta-blockers or non-dihydropyridine CCBs can be considered. Catheter ablation is also a consideration if medical therapy is ineffective or intolerable.

Nonsustained ventricular tachycardia is a rhythm originating from the ventricle that lasts between 3 and 30 beats and persists for less than 30 seconds.[17] Nonsustained ventricular tachycardia is relatively common and can be seen in healthy individuals. Exercise-related NSVT is also common and has no association with a poor cardiovascular outcome. However, the finding of NSVT should always prompt further investigation.[16] Patients with polymorphic NSVT should have an extensive evaluation for coronary ischemia regardless of symptoms.

In the absence of structural heart disease and inherited arrhythmogenic disorders, NSVT is considered benign, and treatment should be guided by symptoms. In the setting of myocardial infarction, NSVT within the first 24 to 48 hours is of no prognostic significance. However, if NSVT persists beyond 48 hours, there is an increased risk of sudden cardiac death, especially in the setting of left ventricular dysfunction. These patients should be treated with beta-blockers

unless contraindicated. Additionally, in patients with prior myocardial infarction, history of syncope, and left ventricular ejection fraction less than 40%, an electrophysiological study is recommended, with placement of an implantable cardiac defibrillator (ICD) if sustained VT is inducible[16] (Fig. 5-11).

Monomorphic ventricular tachycardia (VT) is defined as sustained when it lasts for more than 30 seconds or requires earlier intervention due to hemodynamic instability.[16] It is associated with a good prognosis in the absence of structural heart disease. However, majority of patients with sustained monomorphic VT have structural heart disease with the most frequent etiology being ischemic heart disease. Therefore, patients with a new presentation of sustained monomorphic VT should undergo ischemic evaluation.

Polymorphic VT is defined as a ventricular rhythm at a rate greater than 100 bpm with clearly defined QRS complexes that change from beat to beat.[16] When polymorphic VT occurs in the setting of a prolonged QT, the arrhythmia is called torsade de pointes and is strongly associated with drugs or electrolyte abnormalities. Ventricular fibrillation differs from polymorphic VT in that it is a chaotic tachycardia with no consistently identifiable QRS complexes. Following cardiopulmonary resuscitation in patients with VF or polymorphic VT, the initial step is to rule out an acute coronary syndrome or myocardial infarction. The primary therapy for ischemic-induced polymorphic VT or VF is coronary revascularization. In the absence of a myocardial infarction, an echocardiogram should be obtained. For patients with structural heart disease, acute coronary syndrome or old Q wave myocardial infarctions are the main cause of polymorphic VT/VF. Ventricular fibrillation or polymorphic VT in the absence of structural heart disease suggests an inherited arrhythmogenic syndrome.

As with most tachyarrhythmias, the treatment of a hemodynamically unstable patient with VT or VF is immediate DCCV. In VF or pulseless VT, the DCCV should be asynchronous. If the patient is conscious, synchronized DCCV is recommended. In the acute setting, IV amiodarone, lidocaine, procainamide, or beta-blockers may be given.[17] Amiodarone is the drug of choice in the setting of pulseless VT/cardiac arrest. Amiodarone and lidocaine are both indicated for patients with decreased left ventricular systolic function. Lidocaine is also effective when the etiology of VT is presumed to be ischemic. Procainamide can be used in stable monomorphic VT. Beta-blockers are preferred in acute coronary syndromes.[17] In the long term, all patients who have had sustained VT or VF with no reversible cause or one that is not fully reversible should be considered for ICD in addition to antiarrhythmic therapy.

A true medical emergency is VT/VF storm (also termed an *electrical storm*), which indicates a state of cardiac instability.[18] An electrical storm is defined in patients without an ICD as 2 or more hemodynamically unstable VT episodes within 24 hours, and in patients with an ICD as 3 or more VT episodes in 24 hours.[18] Triggers are rarely found, but it is important to evaluate for ischemia and electrolyte abnormalities. Patients who are unstable should undergo electrical

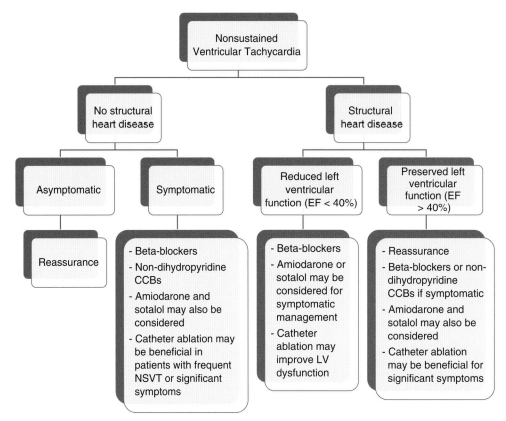

FIGURE 5-11 Treatment for nonsustained ventricular tachycardia. EF = ejection fraction; LV = left ventricle; NSVT = nonsustained ventricular tachycardia.

cardioversion. 300 mg IV amiodarone is given during a cardiac arrest from pulseless VT or VF or 150 mg IV amiodarone is given if patient has VT with a pulse. Intravenous lidocaine is relatively ineffective for terminating hemodynamically stable VT, and prophylactic use is associated with a higher mortality, so this is a third-line agent for short-term use. Catheter ablation should be considered within 48 hours in patients who continue to have recurrent shocks/VT despite therapy, if feasible.[16]

BRADYARRHYTHMIAS

Sinus Node Dysfunction

Sinus bradycardia is defined as a sinus node discharge rate of slower than 60 bpm with normal atrioventricular conduction. This can be a normal finding in athletes and young adults, and during sleep.[19] Sinus bradycardia is the most common rhythm in post-MI patients and can be due to medications, excessive vagal tone, or degenerative disease of the sinus node. It can also be due to hypothermia, myxedema, sepsis, and increased intracranial pressure. Treatment is unnecessary unless the bradycardia results in an inadequate cardiac output, which can manifest most as syncope. For patients with symptomatic sinus bradycardia, they can be treated acutely with IV atropine, temporary pacing, or isoproterenol as a bridge to pacemaker placement.[17] Indications for permanent pacemaker placement will be discussed in a separate section.

Sinus pause or sinus arrest is caused by a failure of the sinus node to discharge and can be due to acute myocardial infarction, degenerative changes, or excessive vagal tone.[19] Treatment is as above for sinus bradycardia. Permanent pacing is generally not indicated unless the patient is symptomatic or the sinus pause is greater than 3 seconds.[20]

Atrioventricular Node Dysfunction

Atrioventricular block is classified as a first, second, or third degree AV block.

First degree AV block is characterized on ECG by PR prolongation greater than 200 ms, but every atrial impulse is conducted to the ventricles.[19] No treatment is necessary, but it is recommended to minimize the use of agents that may slow AV node conduction, such as beta-blockers and CCBs.

Second degree AV block is further classified into type I and type II. Type I is characterized by progressive PR prolongation terminating in a nonconducted P wave (Fig. 5-12). The postpause PR interval will be decreased compared to the prepause PR interval. Type I second degree AV block generally does not require therapy, except to minimize AV nodal blocking agents. Type II is characterized by a constant PR interval with sudden nonconducted P waves. The indicated therapy is permanent pacing.[20] Atropine may be used as a bridge to pacemaker placement, but should be used with caution, as it may cause a paradoxical decrease in heart rate by increasing the atrial rate, which causes decreased conduction through the infranodal tissues.[17]

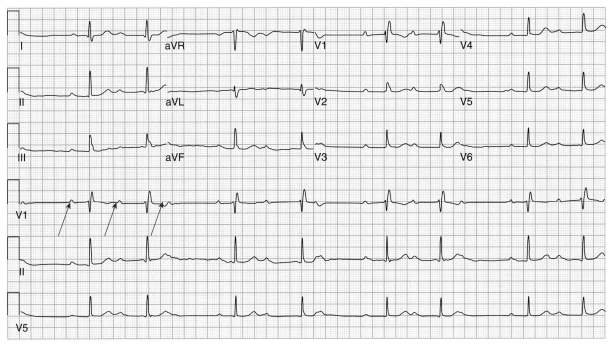

FIGURE 5-12 A 12-lead electrocardiogram tracing showing a Mobitz type I (Wenckebach) atrioventricular block. P waves are marked with *red arrows* in lead V1. Note the progressively prolonging PR intervals followed by dropped beat.

Third degree (complete) AV block occurs when no atrial activity is conducted to the ventricles.[19] There is complete dissociation of the atrial and ventricular electrical activities with an atrial rate that is faster than the ventricular rate.[17] Of note, third degree AV block is not the only cause of AV dissociation. Therapy for complete AV block is permanent pacing (Fig. 5-13).

HYPERTENSIVE CRISIS: URGENCIES AND EMERGENCIES

Hypertension is defined as a systolic blood pressure (SBP) greater than 140 mmHg or a diastolic blood pressure (DBP) greater than 90 mmHg.[10] Hypertensive crisis is defined as an SBP greater than 180 mmHg and/or a DBP greater than 120 mmHg and includes both hypertensive urgencies and emergencies. Hypertensive urgency is when SBP is greater than 180 mmHg or DBP is greater than 120 mmHg with an absence of or with minimal end-organ damage. Hypertensive emergency is an SBP greater than 220 mmHg and a DBP greater than 120 to 130 mmHg with end-organ damage. It may lead to acute myocardial infarction, hypertensive encephalopathy, intracranial hemorrhage, renal failure, and pulmonary edema.[21] The most common cause of hypertensive crisis is an acute exacerbation of chronic hypertension. Other causes include medication noncompliance or withdrawal, renal disease, drugs, collagen vascular disease, Cushing disease, pheochromocytoma, and postoperative state.[20] The exact pathophysiology remains unknown, but a sudden, severe increase in systemic vascular resistance seems to begin the cascade.

Hypertensive emergencies occur more commonly among the elderly, African Americans, and men.[22] The most common presentation of hypertensive emergency is that of a previously diagnosed hypertensive patient on treatment with poor control or noncompliance.

Hypertensive urgency can be managed with oral medications for gradual BP control with a goal BP of 160/100 mmHg over 24 to 48 hours. Hypertensive emergency requires admission to the intensive care unit for parenteral, titratable antihypertensive medications. The goal is to reduce the DBP by 10% to 15% (or to around 110 mmHg) within 1 hour.[23] Once the target has been reached, an oral antihypertensive regimen may be initiated. Aggressive lowering of the BP can worsen end-organ damage due to hypoperfusion, especially cerebral blood flow. Cerebral blood flow is regulated by the cerebral perfusion pressure and cerebrovascular resistance. The brain is able to maintain normal blood flow (or autoregulate) by adjusting cerebrovascular resistance.[24] The normal range for autoregulation is between 60 and 150 mmHg of mean arterial pressure. However, in chronically hypertensive patients, this range is shifted upward. Therefore, the systemic blood pressure required to maintain the lower limit of autoregulation will be higher,[24] which is why reducing the blood pressure rapidly is not recommended. An exception is in the setting of acute aortic dissection, where the goal is a rapid reduction in SBP to less than 120 mmHg and a mean arterial pressure (MAP) goal less than 80 mmHg within 5 to 10 minutes (Tables 5-4 and 5-5).

With regard to prognosis, the 1-year mortality for patients with untreated hypertensive emergencies is 79%. The 5-year survival rate for all patients who present with a hypertensive crisis is 74%.[24]

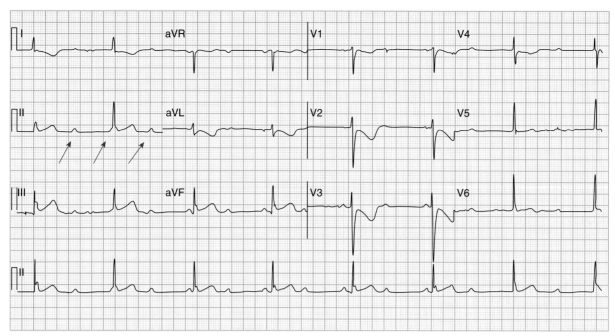

FIGURE 5-13 A 12-lead electrocardiogram tracing showing complete heart block. P waves are seen marching through the tracing, bearing no relationship whatsoever to QRS complexes (*red arrows*). There is atrioventricular dissociation (PP and RR intervals are constant but no constant PR relationship) with more Ps than QRSs. Also note ST elevation in inferior and lateral leads with ST depressions in I, aVL, V1→V4, suggestive of underlying RCA occlusion.

TABLE 5-4 Management of Hypertensive Emergency

Clinical Situation	Goal BP	Timing	Agent
Acute aortic dissection • **Type A: ascending aorta; treatment is surgery** • **Type B: descending aorta; treatment is BP and HR control ± surgery**	• SBP < 120 mmHg and MAP < 80 mmHg	20 min	• Esmolol, propranolol, or metoprolol • Alternative: verapamil or diltiazem • Nitroprusside if still hypertensive after beta-blockers
Ischemic stroke	• BP < 220/120–130 mmHg • Goal < 185/110 mmHg if candidate for thrombolytics • Goal ≤ 180/105 mmHg after thrombolytic therapy and BP measured every 15 min for 2 h, then every 30 min for 6 h, and then hourly for 16 h	Do not reduce BP by more than 15–20% in the first 24 h	• Labetalol, nicardipine, enalapril or enalaprilat, hydralazine
Hemorrhagic stroke	• If SBP > 200 mmHg or MAP > 150 mmHg, aggressive BP reduction is considered • Target BP 160/90 mmHg or MAP of 110 mmHg (if SBP > 180 mmHg or MAP > 130 mmHg without elevated ICP) • If SBP > 180 mmHg, MAP > 130 mmHg, and elevated ICP, keep cerebral perfusion pressure of 61–80 mmHg	Do not reduce BP by more than 15–20% in the first 24 h	• Labetalol, nicardipine, enalapril or enalaprilat, hydralazine
Hypertensive encephalopathy	• Reduce MAP by 10–15% in first hour and 20–25% in 24 h	1 h	• IV labetalol, nicardipine, fenoldopam, or clevidipine
Severe preeclampsia	• Goal: SBP of 120–160 mmHg/DBP 80–105 mmHg • Prior to delivery, maintain DBP > 90 mmHg to maintain uteroplacental perfusion	1 h	• Methyldopa, hydralazine, nicardipine, or labetalol
Cocaine toxicity or pheochromocytoma	• Reduce DBP by 10–15%	1 h	• Benzodiazepines • Phentolamine and nitroprusside are alternative agents • Avoid beta-blockers (including labetalol) due to unopposed α-adrenergic vasoconstriction
Perioperative/postoperative hypertension	• SBP < 140/90	24 h	• Any or prior antihypertensives
Acute pulmonary edema	• Reduce DBP by 10–15%	1 h	• Loop diuretics and nitroglycerin

BP = blood pressure; DBP = diastolic blood pressure; HR = heart rate; ICP = intracranial pressure; MAP = mean arterial pressure; SBP = systolic blood pressure

Reprinted from Varon J, Marik PE. The diagnosis and management of hypertensive crises. *Chest.* 2000;118(1):214-227.

TABLE 5-5 Drugs for Hypertensive Emergencies, Characteristics, and Doses

Drug	Characteristics and Doses
Nicardipine	• Second-generation CCB • Arterial vasodilation, particularly arterioles with small resistance • Crosses BBB • Does not increase ICP and maintains CBF • Acidic pH, therefore administered via central line, but if peripheral, rotate every 12 h • Contraindicated with advanced aortic stenosis • Initial: 5 mg/h with onset < 20 min; titrated by increments of 2.5 mg/h up to 30 mg/h • Achieve BP goals faster than labetalol after 30 min
Clevidipine (CLV)	• Third-generation CCB • Metabolized by ester hydrolysis and not affected by hepatic or renal function • Does not decrease CI • Drawback is that it is prepared in 20% phospholipid solution; therefore, not given in patients with abnormal lipid metabolism and requires calories to be calculated • Vial changed 4 h after puncturing to prevent infection • Initial infusion 1–2 mg/h with onset < 5 min and short half-time of 1 min • Same as nicardipine on BP control and better than nitroglycerine or sodium nitroprusside; mortality benefit compared to nitroprusside
Labetalol	• Alpha- and beta-blocker, 1:7 ratio IV and 1:4 ratio oral • Reduces HR without decreasing cardiac output • Does not decrease cerebral or renal blood flow and does not increase ICP • Intermittent IV with 20 mg followed by 20–80 mg every 10 min or constant infusion starting at 1 mg/min to total dose of 300 mg • Loading dose duration is 6–8 h
Esmolol	• IV beta-blocker with short half-life of < 10 min • Chronotropic control • Important in aortic dissection to decrease inotropy and avoid tachycardia • Loading dose 1 mg/kg followed by drip of 50 μg/kg/min
Enalaprilat	• Vasodilatory properties by reducing angiotensin II • Administered as intermittent IV doses of 0.625 mg or greater • Does not reduce BP within 60 min and peak effect up to 4 h and lasts up to 24 h • Contraindicated in third trimester • Useful in severe HTN associated with scleroderma and circulating angiotensin II
Sodium nitroprusside (NTP)	• Potent arteriolar and venous vasodilation that lowers BP quickly • 0.3 mcq/kg/min ideal body weight and titrated every 3-5 min • Induces coronary and cerebral steal syndromes and increased intracranial pressure, although this increase is of little clinical significance • No difference in incidence of MI, CVA, or renal dysfunction comparing clevidipine, nitroglycerine, or nicardipine • Mortality higher with nitroprusside (NTP) over clevidipine (CLV) • Can induce cyanide and thiocyanate toxicity although less likely to occur at recommended dose • Shortest half-life over all arteriolar vasodilators
Hydralazine	• Peripheral vasodilator with less predictability • 20-40 mg IM or IV and blood pressure decreases within 10-80 min • Induces reflex tachycardia, which is bad for aortic dissection and MI • Effective in preeclampsia and eclampsia • Immediate postoperative period patients
Captopril	• Fastest ACE inhibitor with onset 15 min and lasting 4–6 h; starting dose 6.25 mg
Clonidine	• A$_2$ agonist that decreases sympathetic tone • Can cause sedation • Drug and alcohol withdrawal • Starting dose, 0.1 mg/h • Rebound when discontinued and worsened with concomitant beta-blocker
Nifedipine	• Significant hypotension after administration with risk for major morbidity and mortality and short-acting form avoided in most circumstances • 30–60 mg PO daily • Advantages with severe preeclampsia

ACE = angiotensin-converting-enzyme; BBB = blood–brain barrier; BP = blood pressure; CBF = cerebral blood flow; CCB = calcium-channel blocker; CI = cardiac index; CHF = congestive heart failure; CVA = cerebrovascular accident; HR = heart rate; HTN = hypertension; ICP = intracranial pressure; IV = intravenous; MI = myocardial infarction.

Data from Van Gelder IC, Hagens VE, Bosker HA, et al. A comparison of rate control and rhythm control in patients with recurrent persistent atrial fibrillation. *N Engl J Med.* 2002;347(23):1834-1840; and Gage BF, Waterman AD, Shannon W, Boechler M, Rich MW, Radford MJ. Validation of clinical classification schemes for predicting stroke: results from the National Registry of Atrial Fibrillation. *JAMA.* 2001;285(22):2864-2870.

QUESTIONS

1. A 73-year-old man with prior history of type 2 diabetes mellitus, hypertension, dyslipidemia, and 3-vessel coronary artery bypass grafting (CABG) presented with dizziness, weakness, and shortness of breath. A 12-lead ECG was obtained at the time of arrival (Fig. 5-14). What is the diagnosis?

    A. Ventricular tachycardia
    B. SVT with aberrancy
    C. Preexcited tachycardia
    D. Pacemaker-mediated tachycardia

2. A 69-year-old patient is admitted to medical intensive care unit (MICU) for the management of chronic obstructive pulmonary disease (COPD) exacerbation. Chest radiograph shows multifocal pneumonia. He is toxic appearing and is unable to speak in complete sentences. Pulse is irregular and weak and pulse oximetry shows O_2 saturation of 84%. Blood pressure is 100/65 mmHg. Bedside cardiac monitor shows the following heart rhythm. ECG is obtained (Fig. 5-15). What is the diagnosis?

    A. Atrial fibrillation
    B. Atrial flutter with variable AV conduction
    C. Multifocal atrial tachycardia
    D. Sinus arrhythmia

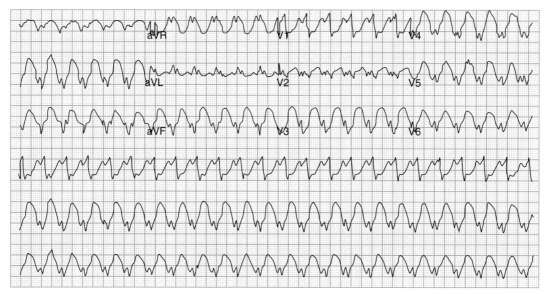

FIGURE 5-14 ECG obtained on arrival.

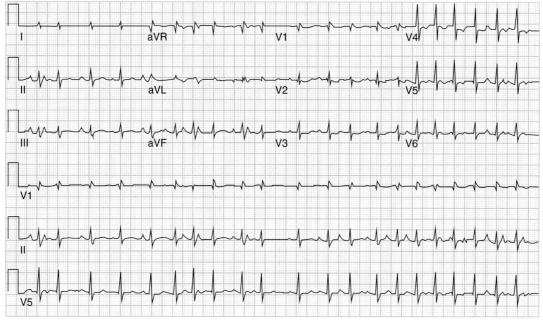

FIGURE 5-15 ECG obtained on arrival.

3. For the patient in question 3, how do you treat the condition?

   A. Direct-current cardioversion followed by anticoagulation
   B. Treatment of underlying condition, correction of hypoxia, IV magnesium sulfate, and if needed, IV calcium channel blockers
   C. IV beta-blockers
   D. IV amiodarone followed by anticoagulation

4. A 65-year-old woman is admitted with complaints of shortness of breath. Shortly after, she requires emergency intubation secondary to hypoxia. Her initial blood pressure was 220/140 mmHg. Chest x-ray shows pulmonary edema. A bedside echocardiogram shows preserved left ventricular (LV) systolic function with hyperdynamic LV. You make a diagnosis of hypertensive emergency with flash pulmonary edema. How do you treat the condition?

   A. IV nitroprusside, IV diuresis, and sedation, with the goal of reducing the mean BP by 10% to 15% in the first hour
   B. IV loop diuretics, sedation, and oral antihypertensive agents, with the goal of gradual reduction of blood pressure
   C. IV nitroprusside and sedation, with gradual reduction in blood pressure
   D. Loop diuretics and IV esmolol, with rapid reduction in blood pressure

5. A 55 year old man is seen in the emergency department for syncope. What is seen in this ECG (Fig. 5-16)?

   A. First degree AV block
   B. Second degree type I AV block
   C. Second degree type II AV block
   D. Third degree AV block

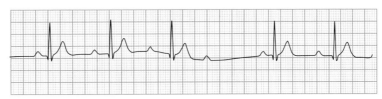

FIGURE 5-16 ECG upon arrival. Elmoselhi A, Seif M. Electrophysiology of the heart. (Reproduced with permission from Elmoselhi A, Seif M. Electrophysiology of the Heart. In: Elmoselhi A, ed. *Cardiology: An Integrated Approach.* New York, NY: McGraw-Hill; http://accessmedicine.mhmedical.com/content.aspx?bookid=2224&sectionid=171660003. Figure 4-30. Accessed February 13, 2018.)

6. A 27-year-old man presents with diabetes ketoacidosis. The admission ECG is shown below (Fig. 5-17). What is the ECG interpretation?

   A. Severe left ventricular hypertrophy
   B. Dextrocardia
   C. Old inferior myocardial infarction
   D. Preexcitation

7. The patient in question 6 starts complaining of severe palpitations. His BP drops to 70/40 mmHg. A repeat ECG (Fig. 5-18) was obtained and is shown below. What is your diagnosis?

   A. Ventricular tachycardia
   B. Wolff-Parkinson-White with atrial fibrillation
   C. Torsade de pointes
   D. Artifacts

8. A 55-year-old woman who had received orthotopic heart transplant 5 years ago presents with extreme weakness, fatigue, nausea, and vomiting. Her diuretics were recently changed from furosemide to spironolactone. Due to recent history of weight gain, she decides to take additional doses of spironolactone to achieve weight loss. Electrocardiogram at admission is shown below (Fig. 5-19). What is your diagnosis?

   A. Ventricular tachycardia
   B. Acute anterior ST-elevation myocardial infarction (STEMI)
   C. Preexcited tachycardia
   D. Hyperkalemia

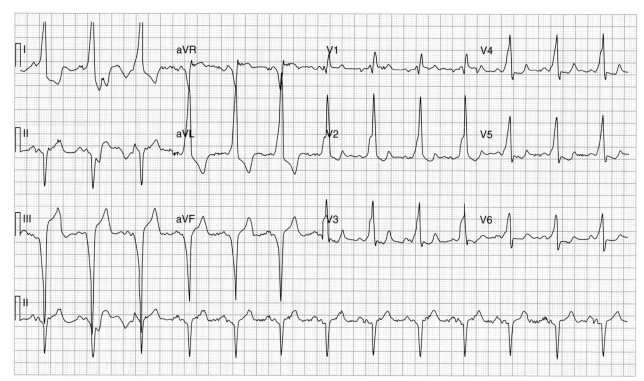

FIGURE 5-17 ECG on arrival.

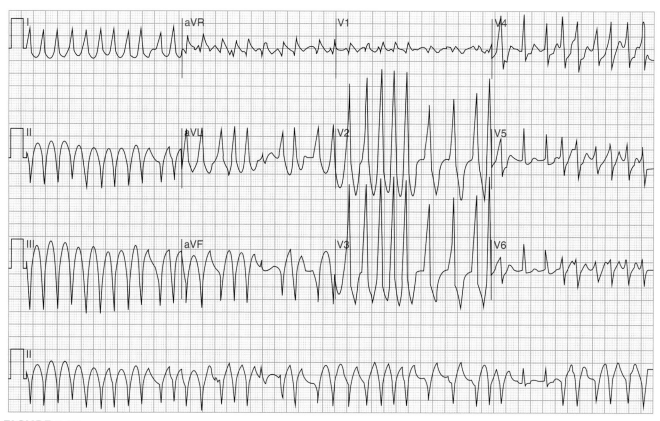

FIGURE 5-18 Repeat ECG.

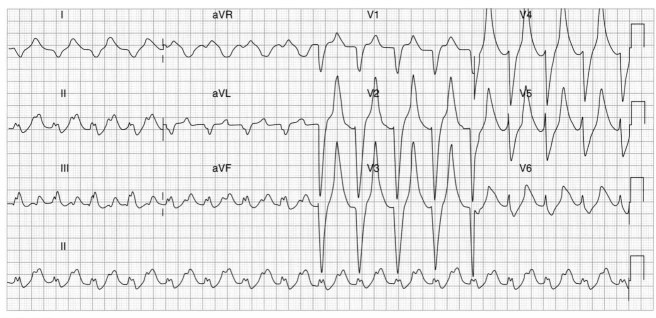

FIGURE 5-19 ECG on admission.

9. A 37-year-old woman presents with history of palpitations lasting for over an hour. She is anxious and claims that she has had similar palpitations several times in the past. Most of the previous episodes has resolved promptly with Valsalva maneuver. A 12-lead ECG is shown below (Fig. 5-20). What is the diagnosis?

   A. AVRT
   B. AVNRT
   C. Atrial tachycardia
   D. Atrial flutter with 1:1 conduction

10. For the patient in question 9, what is the drug of choice?

    A. IV amiodarone
    B. IV beta-blocker
    C. IV adenosine
    D. IV digoxin

11. Which of the following correctly identifies the pacemaker tracing (Fig. 5-21)?

    A. Failure to capture
    B. Pacemaker-mediated tachycardia
    C. Undersensing
    D. Oversensing

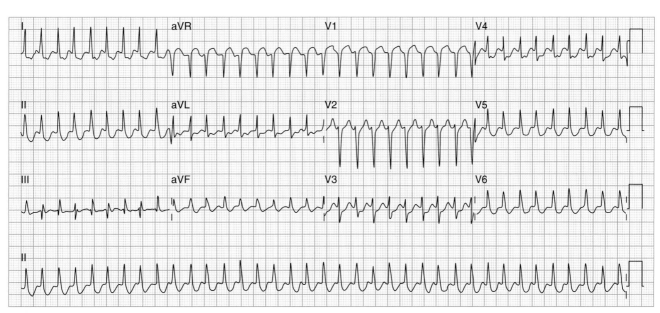

FIGURE 5-20 ECG on admission.

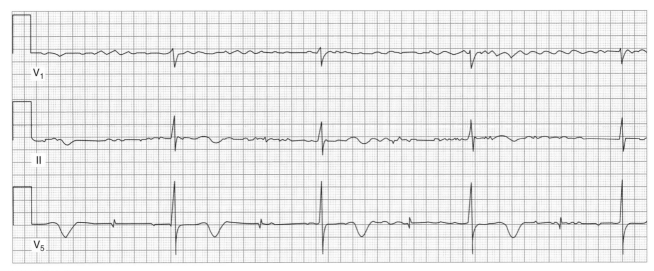

FIGURE 5-21 Pacemaker tracing.

12. For the problem identified in question 11, what is the next step?

   A. Perform chest radiograph, evaluate for electrolyte abnormalities, evaluate for infarction, check battery
   B. Change the rate
   C. Check for battery malfunction
   D. Perform chest radiograph

13. A 24-year-old woman was seen in the emergency department after she was found unresponsive at home. Her physical examination is remarkable for sensorineural hearing loss. She is not on any medications. She does not drink or smoke. Her current vital signs are the following: BP of 120/80 mmHg, HR of 80 beats/min, respiratory rate (RR) of 20 breaths/min, O_2 saturation of 95% on room air. Physical examination is otherwise unremarkable.

Labs:

Na	145 mEq/L
K	4 mEq/L
Cl	110 mEq/L
Mg	2 mEq/L
Phos	3 mEq/L
Creatinine	1.2 mg/dL

Her ECG is shown below (Fig. 5-22). What is your diagnosis?

   A. Jervell and Lange-Nielsen syndrome
   B. Romano-Ward syndrome
   C. Wolff-Parkinson-White syndrome
   D. Lown-Ganong-Levine syndrome

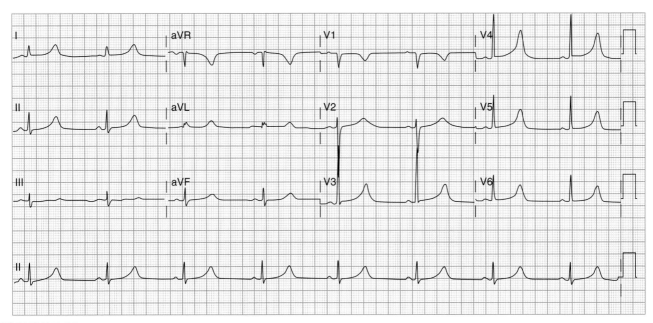

FIGURE 5-22 ECG on admission.

14. For the patient in question 13, what is your treatment?

    A. Beta-blocker
    B. Permanent pacemaker
    C. Automated implantable cardioverter-defibrillator
    D. Verapamil

15. Based on the ECG below (Fig. 5-23), what is the location of the lesion?

    A. Bundle of Kent
    B. Bundle of James
    C. Koch triangle
    D. Manhaim fibers

16. A 50-year-old man with history of hypertension is complaining of fever, abdominal pain, and hematuria. In the ED, he has an irregular heart rate of 90 to 130s beats/min, a respiratory rate of 23 breaths/min, blood pressure of 90/60 mmHg, and oxygen saturation of 94% on room air.

His physical examination is remarkable for scattered rhonchi and slightly tender abdomen on palpation.

Labs:

WBC	$18 \times 10^3/\mu L$
Platelets	$10 \times 10^4/\mu L$
Hgb	8 g/dL
Creatinine	0.9 mg/dL

He has a computed tomography (CT) scan of the abdomen, which shows right pyelonephritis with right ureterolithiasis. Electrocardiogram shows atrial fibrillation with rapid ventricular rate. What anticoagulation would you use?

    A. Heparin
    B. Enoxaparin
    C. Aspirin
    D. None

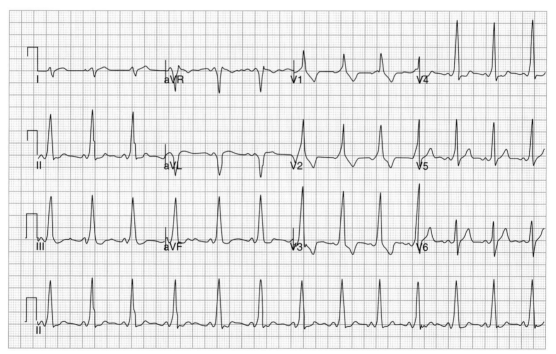

FIGURE 5-23 ECG on admission.

17. The patient suddenly complains of more pronounced shortness of breath and chest pain. His systolic blood pressure drops to the 70s and his heart rate increased to the 160s. Bedside ultrasound of his inferior vena cava (IVC) shows the IVC was 2.5 cm with no respiratory variation. What is the next step?

    A. Direct current cardioversion at 120 J
    B. Metoprolol 5 mg IV × 1
    C. Amiodarone 150 mg IV × 1
    D. Direct current cardioversion at 200 J

18. In the image below (Fig. 5-24), what does the red arrow represent?

    A. AV node
    B. Bundle of His
    C. SA node
    D. Atrium

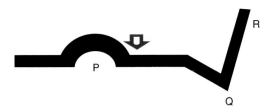

FIGURE 5-24 P-QR portion of ECG.

19. A 50-year-old man complains of light-headedness and is found to have the ECG below (Fig. 5-25). What is your diagnosis?

    A. SA block
    B. Sinus pause
    C. Second degree AV block, type II Mobitz
    D. Third degree heart block

20. Which of the following is true regarding symptomatic bradycardia?

    A. Atropine can be given at 1 mg IV every 5 to 10 minutes for 3 doses.
    B. In a nonemergent situation, the initial set rate for transcutaneous pacing is 50 BPM and output increased by 2 to 3 mA until QRS and T follows a pacer spike.
    C. Confirmation of transvenous pacemaker is through chest radiograph and right bundle branch block on ECG.
    D. Pacemakers have 5 positions.

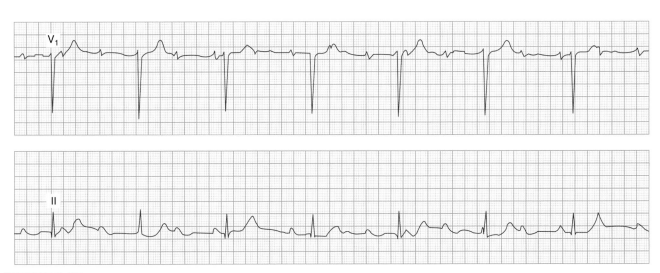

FIGURE 5-25 ECG on admission.

21. A 34-year-old man was involved in a head-on motor vehicle accident. His only complaints are left-sided chest pain. His vital signs are as follows: blood pressure of 220/120, heart rate of 120, a respiratory rate of 18, O_2 saturation of 98% on room air, and a temperature of 97.4°F. Physical examination includes some bruising on the anterior chest, clear breath sounds, and regular rate and rhythm. His abdomen is soft and nontender, his extremities show good pulses with no cyanosis or edema, and his neurologic examination is normal. His chest CT is shown below (Fig. 5-26).

The patient is complaining of worsening chest pain and his systolic blood pressure continues to be greater than 180 mmHg. Morphine and beta-blockers are increased with minimal improvement. What is the treatment of choice?

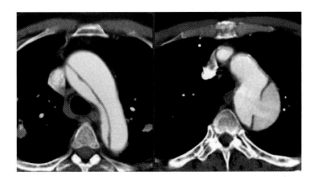

FIGURE 5-26 CT chest with IV contrast on admission. (Source: Berger F, Smithhuis R, van Delden O. "Classic Aortic Dissection". From Thoracic Aorta-the Acute Aortic Syndrome Aortic Dissection, Intramural Hematoma and Penetrating Ulcer. April 2006. Radiology Assistant. www.radiologyassistant.nl/en/p441baa8530e86/thoracic-aorta-the-acute-aortic-syndrome.html.).

A. Open surgery
B. Hydromorphone
C. Transition to nicardipine drip
D. Thoracic endovascular aortic repair (TEVAR)

22. A 24-year-old man is found on the street agitated and confused. He denies any headaches, dizziness, chest pain, shortness of breath, or any focal deficits. In the emergency department, he has a temperature of 100.4°F, a heart rate of 135 beats/min, a respiratory rate of 22 breaths/min, blood pressure of 240/120 mmHg, and O$_2$ saturation of 98% on room air. Physical examination is otherwise unremarkable. Chest radiograph is essential unremarkable. His ECG showed sinus tachycardia. His complete metabolic profile is unremarkable except for a magnesium level of 1.2 mg/dL. Urine toxicology is positive for cocaine. What is the next step?

A. Lorazepam
B. Nitroglycerin
C. Verapamil
D. Labetalol

23. A 35-year-old man is admitted for an abdominal aortic aneurysm repair. He has no known past medical history. He has had prior history of cocaine abuse. His current blood pressure is 240/120 mmHg. Urine toxicology is negative. He denies any pain and he does not appear anxious. What is the next step?

A. Labetalol
B. Lorazepam
C. Morphine
D. Do nothing

24. A 65-year-old man with diabetes mellitus and systolic heart failure was complaining of chest pain. In the ED, his blood pressure is 90/60 mmHg, his heart rate is 200 beats/min, his respiratory rate is 18 breaths/min, and his O$_2$ saturation is 92% on 2 L nasal cannula. Physical examination is otherwise unremarkable except for crackles at the bases of the lungs and lower extremity edema.

Labs:

WBC	$11 \times 10^3/\mu L$
Hgb	12 g/L
Magnesium	2 mEq/L
Potassium	3 mEq/L
Creatinine	1.4 mg/dL
Calcium	8.8 mg/dL

His electrocardiogram is below (Fig. 5-27). What is the next step?

A. Cardiopulmonary resuscitation
B. Sotalol
C. Amiodarone
D. Magnesium

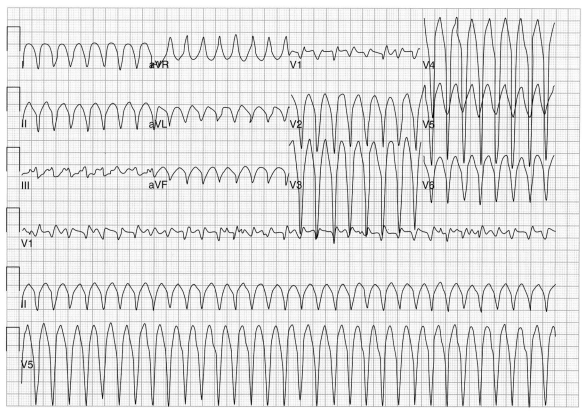

FIGURE 5-27 ECG on admission.

25. Which of the following does not reduce mortality from sudden cardiac death in patients with left ventricular dysfunction?

   A. Mineralocorticoid receptor antagonists
   B. ICD
   C. Cardiac resynchronization therapy
   D. Cardiac ablation

26. A 62-year-old woman presents 3 days after the placement of a dual chamber pacemaker for complete heart block. She complains of 2 episodes of syncope, chest pain, and shortness of breath in the last 24 hours. Chest x-ray obtained in the ED is shown below (Fig. 5-28). Her hemoglobin is now 9 g/dL, which is lower than the previous value of 13.2 g/dL, on the day of pacemaker placement. What is your diagnosis?

   A. Lead perforation with pericardial effusion
   B. Lead dislodgement
   C. Lead fracture
   D. Pneumothorax

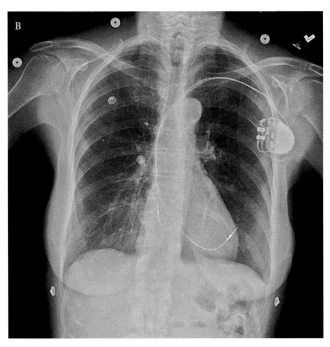

FIGURE 5-28 Chest radiograph on admission.

ANSWERS

1. A. Ventricular tachycardia

   The ECG shows ventricular tachycardia because of absence of classic right or left bundle branch, absence of RS complex in all precordial leads, and northwest axis. The morphology of the wide complex tachycardia is not consistent with a typical right or left bundle branch block;

therefore, it is not SVT with aberrancy (choice B). A negative QRS concordance in precordial leads and presence of AV dissociation are against the diagnosis of preexcited tachycardia (choice C). The ECG does not show pacemaker-mediated tachycardia because there are no pacer spikes preceding the QRS complex (choice D).

Differentiating between SVT and VT can be difficult when the QRS complexes are wide (Figs. 5-29 and 5-30). There are multiple criteria that can be used to differentiate between SVT with aberrancy and VT, the most common being the Brugada criteria. The Brugada criteria is a 4-step algorithm to differentiate between SVT and VT with a sensitivity of 98.7% and a specificity of 96.5%.[26]

A wide-complex tachycardia without any RS complexes is 100% specific for the diagnosis of VT (only QS, QR, or monophasic R complexes are observed). An RS interval greater than 100 ms is indicative of VT and is independent of the duration of the QRS complex. Atrioventricular dissociation was 100% specific for VT. A more simplified algorithm for distinguishing SVT from VT looks solely at lead aVR. This algorithm has a 96.5% sensitivity and a 94.6% specificity for VT diagnosis (Table 5-30).[27]

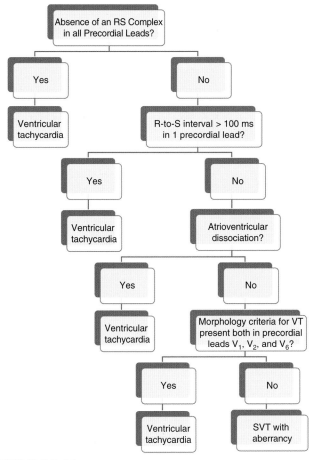

If any question is answered as "yes," the rhythm is VT.

FIGURE 5-29 Part 1. Algorithm to distinguish ventricular tachycardia from SVT with aberrancy.

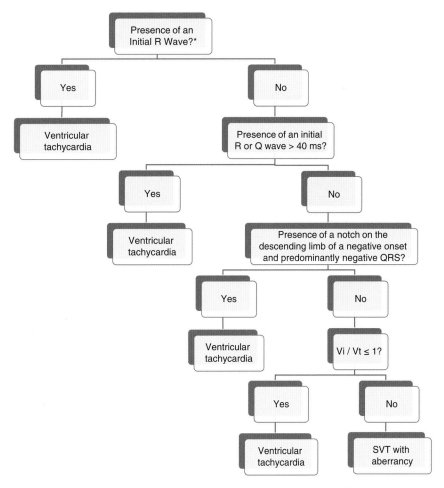

*Note: This is purely looking at lead aVR. Vi = voltage during initial 40 ms of QRS; Vt = voltage during terminal 40 ms of QRS.

FIGURE 5-30 Part 2. Algorithm to distinguish ventricular tachycardia from SVT with aberrancy.

2. C. Multifocal atrial tachycardia

Multifocal atrial tachycardia is the correct answer because there are at least 3 different P-wave morphologies, a heart rate over 100 beats/min, and an irregular rhythm. It is also commonly associated with lung disease. Respiratory rate intervals typically do not vary by more than 10% in sinus arrhythmia. Atrial fibrillation (choice A) is incorrect because there are multifocal P waves that precede every QRS. Atrial flutter (choice B) is incorrect because the P waves have different morphologies. Sinus arrhythmia (choice D) is incorrect because of the different P wave morphologies.

As mentioned previously, there are at least 3 distinct P-wave morphologies on ECG and the rhythm is usually irregular. Atrial fibrillation and atrial flutter with variable AV conduction are other differentials. In atrial fibrillation, only fibrillatory waves with irregular undulations are seen in between QRS complexes. Saw-tooth pattern of P waves with similar morphologies may be seen in between QRS

complexes in atrial flutter. Therefore, options A and B are wrong. P-wave morphology does not change in sinus arrhythmia. Respiratory rate intervals typically do not vary by more than 10% in sinus arrhythmia. Table 5-6 lists different types of supraventricular tachycardia.

TABLE 5-6 Examples of Regular and Irregular Supraventricular Tachycardia

Regular SVT	Irregular SVT
Sinus tachycardia	Atrial fibrillation
Focal atrial tachycardia	Multifocal atrial tachycardia
Atrial flutter	Atrial flutter with variable AV conduction
AVNRT	
AVRT	

AV = atrioventricular; AVNRT = atrioventricular nodal reentrant tachycardia; AVRT = atrioventricular reentrant tachycardia; SVT, supraventricular tachycardia.

3. B. Treatment of underlying condition, correction of hypoxia, IV magnesium sulfate, and if needed, IV calcium channel blockers

First-line treatment is to treat the underlying condition; if this fails, AV nodal blockers may be used. Neither oral antiarrhythmics nor electrical cardioversion is useful in suppressing this arrhythmia. Anticoagulation is not indicated. Only option B is correct.

4. A. IV nitroprusside, IV diuresis, and sedation, with the goal of reducing the mean BP by 10% to 15% in the first hour

Hypertensive emergency with acute pulmonary edema results from an acute increase in the left ventricular diastolic pressure. The initial treatment should be with loop diuretics in addition to easily titratable medications that reduce afterload, such as nitroprusside, nicardipine, fenoldopam, or nitroglycerin. Medications that acutely decrease cardiac contractility (such as beta-blockers, verapamil, diltiazem) should be avoided, as this may worsen the pulmonary edema. Reducing the blood pressure drastically in a short time may decrease cerebral perfusion and lead to neurologic damage in hypertensive crisis. Therefore, the goal blood pressure reduction is 10% to 15% within the first hour, followed by an additional 5% to 15% reduction in the subsequent 23 hours.

Intravenous loop diuretics, sedation, and oral antihypertensive agents, with the goal of gradual reduction of blood pressure (choice B) is incorrect because more gradual reduction of BP is appropriate in the setting of hypertensive emergency. Intravenous nitroprusside and sedation, with gradual reduction in blood pressure (choice C) is incorrect because IV diuretics are required in the setting of pulmonary edema. Loop diuretics and IV esmolol, with rapid reduction in blood pressure (choice D) is incorrect because esmolol is a selective β_1 antagonist and thus does not reduce BP effectively.

5. B. Second degree type I AV block

In a type I AV block, there is progressive prolongation of the PR interval followed by a drop beat. First degree AV block (choice A) is incorrect because the PR intervals are not constant. Second degree type II AV block (choice C) is incorrect because there is a progressive prolongation of the PR interval. Complete heart block (choice D) is not correct because there is an atrial ventricle association.

6. D. Preexcitation

Preexcitation is correct. The echocardiogram shows a short PR interval (< 120 ms), slurred onset (called a delta wave), and widening of the QRS (> 110 ms) is suggestive of preexcitation. In a preexcited ECG, the accessory pathway, by virtue of its ability to conduct quickly, activates a portion of the ventricle before the depolarization of the remaining part of the ventricle via the native conduction system. This results in a fusion beat leading to wide and often bizarre-looking QRS complex. Slurring at the beginning of the QRS is called a delta wave. The width of QRS depends on the relative contribution of the accessory pathway–mediated ventricular activation. The greater the myocardial activation is via the accessory pathway, the wider the QRS complex will be. Severe LVH (choice A) is incorrect. Left ventricular hypertrophy is diagnosed via several criteria: The Sokolow-Lyon index is S in V_1 plus R in V_4 or V_5 equal to 35 mm or more, and R in aVL equal to 11 mm or more. The Cornell criteria are S in V_3 plus R in aVL greater than 28 mm in men, and R in V_2 plus R in aVL greater than 20 mm in women. The Romhilt-Estes score must be greater than 5 points, or be 4 points of the following:

1) voltage criteria of R or S in limb leads ≥ 20 mm (3 points), S in V_1 or V_2 ≥ 30 mm (3 points), or R in V_5 or V_6 ≥ 30 mm (3 points);
2) ST-T abnormalities such as ST-T vector opposite to QRS (3 points) or ST-T vector opposite to QRS with digoxin (1 point);
3) negative terminal P mode in V_1 1 mm in depth and 0.04 sec (3 points);
4) left axis deviation (2 points);
5) QRS duration > 0.09 sec (1 point); and
6) delayed intrinsic inflection (1 point).

In the presence of preexcitation, diagnosis of LVH should not be made.

Dextrocardia (choice B) is suggested by global negativity (P, QRS, and T waves) will be seen in lead I and global positivity is seen in lead aVR. Absent R-wave progression is seen in precordial leads. Although negatively directed QS complexes in the inferior lead suggests old inferior MI (choice C), such a diagnosis cannot be made in the presence of preexcitation. This is called the pseudoinfarction pattern.

7. B. Wolff-Parkinson-White with atrial fibrillation

In patients with an accessory pathway who develop atrial fibrillation, the impulses are conducted to the ventricles both through the AV node and through the accessory pathway giving it a wide complex appearance. Ventricular tachycardia (choice A) is incorrect due to the irregularly irregular rhythm. Since the accessory pathway usually has a shorter refractory period, the ventricular rates can be rapid if the impulses are preferentially conducted through the accessory pathway leading to ventricular fibrillation. Therefore, AV nodal blocking drugs (adenosine, verapamil, diltiazem, amiodarone, beta-blockers, and digoxin) are contraindicated in the setting of preexcited atrial fibrillation, since this will promote conduction down the accessory pathway.

If the patient is hemodynamically unstable, then prompt electrical cardioversion is recommended. If the patient is hemodynamically stable, there is no first-line intravenous therapy for rhythm control. However, ibutilide and procainamide are both reasonable choices. Intravenous ibutilide slows conduction through both the AV node and the accessory pathway; however, caution should be used if there is concern for drug-induced QT prolongation and polymorphic VT. Intravenous procainamide does not affect the AV node and instead slows conduction through the ventricular myocardium and, therefore, the accessory pathway.

Once the patient is stabilized, it is reasonable to consider additional therapy, such as amiodarone, sotalol, flecainide, and propafenone, to maintain sinus rhythm. Catheter ablation is also a consideration for select patients.

Torsade de Pointe (choice C) is a type of polymorphic VT that demonstrates twisting of the QRS complexes around the isoelectric line. A clue to artifact (choice D) is the presence of spikes marching through the tracing that retain the basic cycle length of the preexisting RR intervals.

8 D. Hyperkalemia

Ventricular tachycardia (choice A) is incorrect with peaked T waves seen on ECG. The ECG does not show acute anterior STEMI (choice B). Preexcited tachycardia is incorrect. There are no delta waves present; therefore, it is not a preexcited tachycardia (choice C).

9. B. AVNRT

This ECG demonstrates rapid, regular, narrow complex tachycardia. Careful review of ECG shows P waves in the early part of the ST segment, especially in leads I, III, aVL, and V_4. This is suggestive of a short RP tachycardia due to AVNRT, which is the most common SVT and also is seen most commonly among younger women. The ECG in AVRT (choice A) due to an accessory pathway can be very fast and may demonstrate electrical alternans. Presence of very short RP is more typical of AVNRT than AVRT. Atrial tachycardia (choice C) is incorrect because it is typically an example of long RP tachycardia. Atrial flutter with 1:1 conduction (choice D) is incorrect because there is an isoelectric line following the QRS complex, which is not seen in atrial flutter.

10. C. IV adenosine

As with all supraventricular tachycardia (except multifocal atrial tachycardia and preexcitation syndromes), adenosine may be used to either convert or slow down the rhythm. Adenosine slows conduction through the AV node and interrupts AV reentrant pathways. This can help restore sinus rhythm in arrhythmias such as AVNRT and AVRT that are AV-node dependent. The typical dosing of adenosine is 6 mg intravenous; if ineffective, 12 mg IV may be given, followed by an additional 12 mg IV, if necessary. In patients currently on carbamazepine or dipyridamole or those who have heart transplants, adenosine should be given at half of the typical dose. By causing a transient AV nodal block, adenosine may help expose the underlying rhythm in focal atrial tachycardia, atrial flutter, and atrial fibrillation, but is generally not useful in converting these arrhythmias to sinus rhythm. There is no role for adenosine in multifocal atrial tachycardia. The use of adenosine in arrhythmias with preexcitation is extremely limited. Digoxin (choice D), beta-blockers (choice B), and amiodarone (choice A) are incorrect.

11. A. Failure to capture

Failure to capture is correct (Fig. 5-31). Electrical output is seen with pacer spikes but does not cause contraction secondary to increase in resistance at wire/myocardium interface, such as from fibrosis, ischemia, electrolyte abnormalities, and medications. Treatment is to increase power.

Pacemaker mediated tachycardia, as seen below (choice B) is incorrect because there is no evidence of tachycardia (Fig. 5-32).

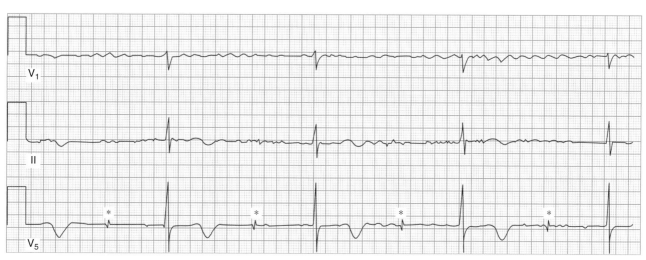

FIGURE 5-31   Failure to capture. Pacer spikes are seen, labeled as asterisks, but no contraction afterwards. (Reproduced with permission from Upadhyay GA, Singh JP. Pacemakers and defibrillators. In: Fuster V, Harrington RA, Narula J, Eapen ZJ, eds. *Hurst's The Heart.* 14th ed. New York, NY: McGraw-Hill; 2017.)

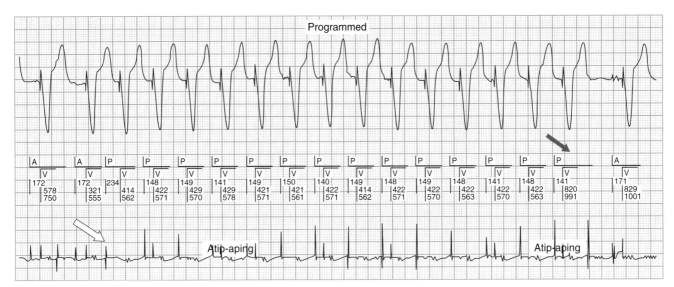

FIGURE 5-32 Pacemaker mediated tachycardia is a reentry tachycardia usually in dual chamber pacemakers where the pacemaker forms the anterograde limb and AV node is retrograde limb. This is secondary to (1) rate response being too sensitive; (2) tracking or interference of atrial noise; or (3) inappropriate rate response with pacemaker manipulation. (Reproduced with permission from Upadhyay GA, Singh JP. Pacemakers and Defibrillators. In: Fuster V, Harrington RA, Narula J, Eapen ZJ, eds. *Hurst's The Heart.* 14th ed. New York, NY: McGraw-Hill; 2017.)

Undersensing (choice C) is the failure to detect spontaneous depolarizing, resulting in asynchronous pacing (spikes regardless of P or QRS) (Fig. 5-33).

Oversensing (choice D) is the misinterpretation of electrical potential across sensing wires as endogenous depolarization, inhibiting a pacing spike (Fig. 5-34). In this situation, deep inspiration causes oversensing of diaphragmatic myopotentials, inhibiting ventricular output. Similar to oversensing, cross-talk occurs in dual chamber systems and is the misinterpretation of atrial pacemaker spike as ventricular depolarization, leading to inhibition of ventricular pacemaker output and, therefore, ventricular standstill. This can be treated by reducing atrial power and reducing ventricular sensitivity. Failure to pace can also be from output failure is secondary to lead malfunction or unstable connection between lead and pulse generator, insufficient power from battery, or misinterpretation.

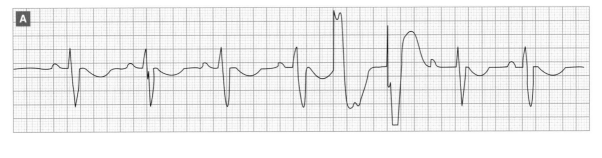

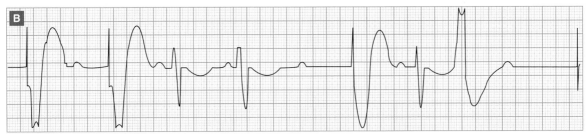

FIGURE 5-33 Undersensing. There is too many spikes and regardless of P or QRS complex. (Reprinted with permission from Garson A. Stepwise approach to the unknown pacemaker ECG. *Am Heart J.* 1990;119:924.)

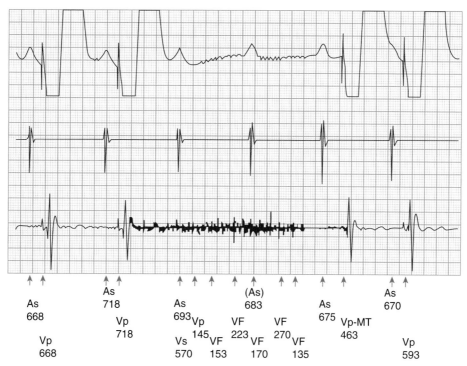

FIGURE 5-34 Oversensing results from pacemaker senses inappropriate signals, causing inhibition of a spike. (Reproduced with permission from Upadhyay GA, Singh JP. Pacemakers and defibrillators. In: Fuster V, Harrington RA, Narula J, Eapen ZJ, eds. *Hurst's The Heart*. 14th ed. New York, NY: McGraw-Hill; 2017.)

12. A. Perform chest radiograph, evaluate for electrolyte abnormalities, evaluate for infarction, check battery

    The above should be performed in order to elucidate the cause of the failure to capture. Changing the rate (choice B) will not affect the chances of successful capture. Battery malfunction (choice C) is not the only cause of failure to capture. Chest radiograph (choice D) alone may not provide you with the answer for the failure to capture.

13. A. Jervell and Lange-Nielsen syndrome

    Jervell and Lange-Nielsen syndrome is an autosomal recessive prolonged QT syndrome associated with sensorineural deafness. The normal value of QT is 0.44 to 0.46 and varies depending on age and sex. Typically, it is measured from lead II but can be measured in V_2 or V_3. Due to variability induced by heart rate, the corrected QTc is developed by Bazett:

    $$QTc = QT \text{ interval} \div \sqrt{RR \text{ interval (in sec)}}$$

    Normal values again vary by age and sex but typically are 0.37 to 0.44. If the end of T waves cannot be determined, U waves may sometimes be included with the measure if it occupies 50% or more of the T-U wave complex. Prolonged QT syndrome is also associated with T wave alternans and increased QT dispersion.

    Romano-Ward syndrome (choice B) is an autosomal dominant prolonged QT syndrome that is not associated with sensorineural deafness. Prolonged QT can be caused by hypokalemia, hypomagnesemia, hypocalcemia, hypothermia, increased intracranial pressure, postmyocardial infarction, congenital prolonged QT syndrome, and drugs. These drugs include chlorpromazine, haloperidol, quetiapine, olanzapine, amisulpride, thioridazine, quinidine, procainamide, disopyramide, flecainide, encainide, sotalol, amiodarone, amitriptyline, nortriptyline, desipramine, citalopram, escitalopram, bupropion, venlafaxine, mianserin, diphenhydramine, astemizole, loratadine, terfenadine, chloroquine, quinine, and macrolides.[28-30] Wolff-Parkinson-White syndrome (choice C) is incorrect because the ECG shows a narrow QRS and the PR interval is not short. Wolff-Parkinson-White also is not associated with a prolonged QT interval. Lown-Ganong-Levine syndrome (choice D) is incorrect because the ECG shows a normal PR interval, and it also is not associated with a prolonged QT interval.

14. A. Beta-blocker

    Beta-blockers decrease the catecholamine response and, therefore, reduce the incidence of syncope and sudden cardiac death. Permanent pacemaker (PPM; choice B) is indicated if symptomatic on beta-blockers, particularly if bradycardia triggers symptoms. An automated implantable cardioverter-defibrillator (choice C) is indicated if the patient is still symptomatic after PPM and beta-blockers. Verapamil (choice D) would only be an adjunct to the above pharmacological treatment.

15. A. Bundle of Kent

This is an ECG of WPW syndrome, a preexcitation syndrome, which is secondary to an accessory pathway that allows retrograde, anterograde, or bidirectional conduction that bypass the normal conduction from the atria to the ventricles via the AV node. It consists of a short PR interval, a delta wave, and a wide QRS. There are 2 types: Type A has a tall R wave in V_1–V_3 secondary to the left-sided tract, and type B has QS V_1–V_3 secondary to right-sided tract.[31] The accessory tract involved is the bundle of Kent and located in the AV ring or septum, most likely left-lateral.[31]

Bundle of James (choice B) is seen with Lown-Ganong-Levine (LGL) syndrome, which is also a preexcitation syndrome with a PR of 0.12 seconds or less and normal QRS. There is no delta wave, unlike in WPW. Koch triangle (choice C) is incorrect. It is located in the right atrium and is anatomically delineated by the tendon of Todaro, ostium of the coronary sinus, and the insertion of the septal leaflet of tricuspid valve. Inferiorly, it ends at the site of the ostium of the coronary sinus. It is a common site for catheter ablation procedures for SVT. Manhaim fibers (choice D) are another form of preexcitation syndrome. These are atriofascicular bypass tracts that connect the right atrium to the distal right bundle branch. They typically are present in the right ventricular free wall. Electrocardiograms typically have a normal or long PR interval and a wide QRS complex with a left-bundle appearance, which is not seen in this ECG.

16. D. None

The patient has a CHA$_2$DS$_2$-VASc score of 1. He also has hematuria and sepsis. Patient appears to be bleeding. Therefore, the risk of worsening his bleeding is higher than the risk of CVA.

In patients hospitalized with sepsis and atrial fibrillation, CVA risk does not differ between those who are on or off anticoagulants. CHA$_2$DS$_2$VASc poorly discriminated risk of ischemia stroke in patients with sepsis and atrial fibrillation. If the patient was a candidate for anticoagulation for atrial fibrillation, heparin (choice A) and enoxaparin (choice B) are preferred over aspirin (choice C). Approximately 20% to 30% of CVAs are secondary to atrial fibrillation (Table 5-7).[32]

A CHA$_2$DS$_2$-VASc score of 1 or greater in men or 2 or greater in women suggests a role for anticoagulation. The types of anticoagulation include vitamin K antagonists such as warfarin, non–vitamin K antagonist NOACs such as the direct thrombin inhibitor dabigatran and the factor Xa inhibitor apixaban, edoxaban, and rivaroxaban. A meta-analysis suggested that NOACs reduced stroke and systemic emboli by 19% and mortality by 10% compared to warfarin (relative risk, 0.81; 95% confidence interval, 0.73–0.91; $P < 0.0001$ and relative risk, 0.90; 95% confidence interval, 0.85–0.95; $P = 0.0003$, respectively).[33] Intracranial hemorrhage was decreased, but gastrointestinal bleeding was increased (relative risk, 0.48; 95%

TABLE 5-7 Comparison Between CHAD$_2$ and CHA$_2$DS$_2$-VASc. CHAD$_2$ was Expanded to Include Common Risk Factors for CVA, Which is Seen in CHA$_2$DS$_2$-VASc. CHA$_2$DS$_2$-VASc score ≥ 2 is Considered High CVA Risk. It Carries a 2% Stroke Risk Per Year, Particularly in Women; Therefore, Anticoagulation is Recommended. In Men, CHA$_2$DS$_2$-VASc = 1 Anticoagulation is Recommended

CHA$_2$DS$_2$-VASc	Score
Congestive heart failure	1
Hypertension	1
Age ≥ 75 y	2
Diabetes mellitus	1
Stroke/transient ischemic attack/thromboembolism	2
Vascular (prior myocardial infarction, peripheral artery disease, aortic plaque)	1
Age 65–74 y	1
Sex (female)	1
Max Score	9

confidence interval, 0.39–0.59; $P < 0.0001$ and relative risk, 1.25; 95% confidence interval, 1.01–1.55; $P = 0.04$).[33] Antiplatelet therapy was found inferior to VKA in stroke prevention with higher risk of bleeding.[34-36]

Despite these measures, acute CVA can occur, particularly in patients with advanced age and history of prior CVA or TIA. Thrombolytics can be given even if the international normalized ratio is less than 1.7, if the patient is on VKA or has a normal activated partial thromboplastin time, and if the last drug was given more than 48 hours previously if the patient is on dabigatran.[37-39] It has been postulated that triple therapy, dual antiplatelet and an OAC, might be initiated. However, a recent study showed that bleeding risk increased by 79% to 136%, while only marginally improving recurrent ischemic events. Triple therapy might be advocated in patients with recent stent placement for a short period of time.[40] When NOAC is used, it is recommended to use the lowest possible dose, and prasugrel or ticagrelor should not be substituted for clopidogrel, given the greater risk of bleeding.[41] A small trial suggested lower all-cause mortality (2.5% vs 6.4%) in patients with dual therapy without aspirin and triple therapy while having no effect on risk of myocardial infarction, CVA, revascularization, or stent thrombosis.[42]

This patient has sepsis from pyelonephritis. A recent retrospective cohort of 113,511 patients hospitalized with sepsis and atrial fibrillation showed that the CHA$_2$DS$_2$VASc score poorly discriminated the risk of ischemia stroke.[43] Rates of ischemic CVA did not differ between patients on and off anticoagulation (174 of 13,505 [1.3%] vs 185 of 13,505 [1.4%], respectively).[43] Bleeding was more significant in patients receiving parenteral anticoagulation (1163 of

13,505 [8.6%] vs 979 of 13,505 [7.2%]; relative risk, 1.21; 95% confidence interval, 1.10–1.32).[43]

17. **A. Direct current cardioversion at 120 J**

Direct current cardioversion at 120 J is correct. Direct current cardioversion is preferred in patients who are hemodynamically unstable (eg, with acute left heart failure, myocardial ischemia, or hypotension), since it can restore sinus rhythm more quickly and effectively. Metoprolol 5 mg IV (choice B) × 1 is incorrect. Beta-blocker use is not appropriate when the patient is hemodynamically unstable. Since DCCC is the quickest and most effective method for restoring sinus rhythm, amiodarone (choice C) is also

wrong.[44-46] The initial starting dose for DCCC is 120 J, and it can be increased to 200 J (choice D).

18. **A. AV node**

AV node is correct. Following depolarization of the atrium, the signal travels to the AV node. The bundle of His (choice B) is the purple portion. The SA node (choice C) is the green portion. The atrium (choice D) is the red portion.

19. **D. Third degree AV block**

Third degree complete heart block is complete disassociation between the atria and ventricles. See the table below for explanations for the other choices (Table 5-8).

TABLE 5-8 Types of Cardiac Blocks

Sinus pause (choice B) • > 3 sec warrants further investigation • Failure of SA node to discharge with no atrial activation	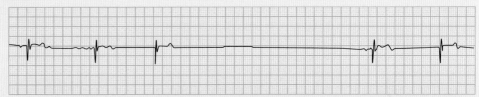 Vijayaraman P, Ellenbogen KA. Bradyarrhythmias. In: Fuster V, Harrington RA, Narula J, Eapen ZJ, eds. *Hurst's The Heart*. 14th ed. New York, NY: McGraw-Hill; http://accessmedicine.mhmedical.com/content.aspx?bookid=2046&sectionid=176564098. Figure 86-6. Accessed February 13, 2018.
SA Block (choice A) • SA node impulse generated but interference of delivery of impulse of SA node to atrium tissue • Pause duration is a muliple of prior PP interval	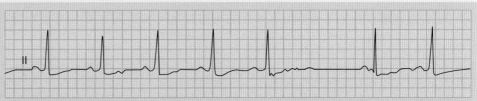 Vijayaraman P, Ellenbogen KA. Bradyarrhythmias. In: Fuster V, Harrington RA, Narula J, Eapen ZJ, eds. *Hurst's The Heart*. 14th ed. New York, NY: McGraw-Hill; http://accessmedicine.mhmedical.com/content.aspx?bookid=2046&sectionid=176564098. Figure 86-7. Accessed February 13, 2018.
Second degree AV block Mobtiz type II (choice C) • Constant PR interval followed by failure of P wave to be conducted to ventricles	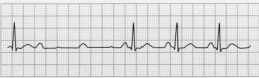 Elmoselhi A, Seif M. Electrophysiology of the heart. In: Elmoselhi A, eds. *Cardiology: An Integrated Approach*. New York, NY: McGraw-Hill; http://accessmedicine.mhmedical.com/content.aspx?bookid=2224&sectionid=171660003. Figure 4.30. Accessed February 13, 2018.
Third degree AV block (choice D) • No association between P and QRS • QRS is escape rhythm from junction or septum • Block in AV node with narrow QRS escape rhythm of 40–60 BPM (if no concommittant BBB) or block in His-Purkinje with wide QRS escape rhythm of 20–40 BPM	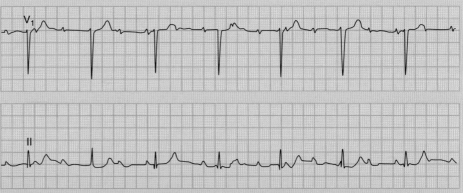 Vijayaraman P, Ellenbogen KA. Bradyarrhythmias. In: Fuster V, Harrington RA, Narula J, Eapen ZJ, eds. *Hurst's The Heart*. 14th ed. New York, NY: McGraw-Hill; http://accessmedicine.mhmedical.com/content.aspx?bookid=2046&sectionid=176564098. Figure 86-20. Accessed February 13, 2018.

20. D. Pacemakers have 5 positions.

Besides diagnostic ECG and labs, initial intervention for symptomatic bradycardia includes medications and a pacemaker. Medications include atropine 0.5 mg IV every 3 to 5 minutes with a maximum dose of 3 mg (choice A), dopamine greater than 5 μg/kg, dopamine 2 to 20 μg/kg/min, or epinephrine 2 to 10 μg/min. Transcutaneous pacemaker pads should be placed on the patient in lieu of the medications or in the event the medications do not work.

In a nonemergent situation, the initial set rate for transcutaneous pacing is 60 to 80 BPM or 10 to 30 BPM higher than the intrinsic beat and the output increased by 5 to 10 mA until QRS and T follows a pacer spike. In an emergent situation such as cardiac arrest, another approach would be to set the pacer at a maximum output until a pacer spike is followed by QRS and pulses are present. Transvenous pacing is more complicated. The preferred sites of insertion are the right internal jugular vein and left subclavian vein. A pacing catheter is inserted under sterile technique and a balloon is inflated with 1.5 mL once the catheter is advanced by 20 cm. The pacer is turned on with initial settings of 60 to 80 BPM with maximum output of 20 mA. Placement is confirmed via chest x-ray and a left bundle branch block (LBBB) pattern on ECG (choice C).

Permanent pacemakers are indicated only for a symptomatic sinus node block (> 3 second pause), symptomatic AV block, and asymptomatic second or third degree block with atrial fibrillation with greater than a 5-second pause or asystole greater than 3 seconds or HR less than 40. Complete heart block is a candidate for resynchronization therapy (CRT; choice D) is incorrect. Candidates for CRT include patients with chronic heart failure with LVEF of 35% or more in New York Heart Association (NYHA) functional class II, III, and IV, despite medical treatment, with (1) LBBB with QRS greater than 150 ms; (2) LBBB with QRS of 120 to 150 ms; (3) non-LBBB with QRS greater than 150; and (4) non-LBBB with QRS 120–150 ms.[47] In patients with atrial fibrillation, CRT is an option if patients have QRS greater than 120 ms and LVEF less than 35% and remain in NYHA functional class III to IV despite medical treatment, or patients with reduced LVEH who are candidates for AV junctional ablation.[47] Standard CRT consists of RV and LV pacing with sensed AV delay between 100 and 120 ms with LV lead in the lateral or posterolateral vein.

Compared to single chamber pacemakers, dual chamber pacemakers have lower rates of atrial fibrillation, stroke, decreased pacemaker syndrome symptoms (dyspnea, dizziness, palpitations, pulsations, and chest pain), and improved better performance.

Pacemakers usually have 5 positions (choice D): position I, paced chamber; position II, sensed chamber; position III, pacemaker response to sensed event; position IV, rate modulation; and position V, location or absence of multisite pacing. There are 2 groups of modes. The single chamber modes include VVI or VVIR for ventricular demand pacing but cannot maintain synchrony if there is AV block. The other single chamber mode is AAI or AAIR for sinus node dysfunction with intact AV node function. Dual chamber pacemaker modes include DDD, DDDR, DDI, DDIR, and DVI. Only the first 3 are relevant to temporary pacemakers (Table 5-9).

TABLE 5-9 5 Positions of Pacemaker

	Meaning	Options
Position I	Chamber paced	A (atrium), V (ventricle), D (dual)
Position II	Chamber sensed	A (atrium), V (ventricle), D (dual), O (absence)
Position III	How pacemaker responds to sensed event	I (inhibits output), T (trigger response), D (event in atrium inhibits atrial output but triggers ventricular output or event in ventricle inhibits ventricle output), O (no response to sensed input)
Position IV	Rate modulation	R (rate modulation in response to activity)
Position V	Location or absence of multisite pacing	O (multisite pacing), A (multisite in atrium), V (multisite in ventricle), D (dual multisite)

21. D. TEVAR

Aortic disease encountered in the intensive care unit include aortic aneurysm, aortic dissection, intramural hematoma, penetrating atherosclerotic ulcer, traumatic aortic injury, pseudoaneurysm, and inflammatory diseases.[48] The aorta is the body's main conduit, composed of 3 layers: intima, media, and adventitia. The aorta serves as a "second pump" via Windkessel function during diastole.[48] The normal diameter is 40 mm and tapers gradually, with a normal expansion of 0.9 mm in men and 0.7 mm in women. Acute aortic dissection results from an intimal tear into the media or the rupture of the vasa vasorum in the media. This causes the formation of a false and true lumen. It can mimic acute myocardial infarction with a dissecting flap obstructing coronary perfusion, mesenteric ischemia, CVA, renal ischemia, spinal ischemia, cerebrovascular accident, and encephalopathy.[49,50] It is categorized according to the DeBakey or the Stanford classification. DeBakey classification has 4 types: type I involves the ascending aorta, arch, and descending aorta and can involve abdominal aorta; type II is in the ascending aorta; type IIIa is in the descending thoracic aorta distal to the left subclavian artery and proximal to the celiac artery; and type IIIb is the thoracic and abdominal aorta distal to the left subclavian. Stanford classification has 2 types: type A involves the ascending aorta, which can include the arch and the thoracoabdominal aorta and can include DeBakey type I and type II. Stanford type B involves the descending thoracic or thoracoabdominal aorta distal to the left subclavian artery and can include DeBakey type IIIa and IIIb.

Stanford's type B is usually associated with hypertension, and Stanford type A is associated with hypotension, which can be accompanied with cardiac tamponade, rupture, or failure for aortic regurgitation.[49,50] Laboratory markers are nonspecific, and radiographic imaging is crucial for diagnosis. More than 80% of acute aortic dissection has a widening of the aortic silhouette on a chest radiograph.[49] Transthoracic echocardiography is limited to the proximal aortic segments and the aortic valve. The sensitivity and specificity are 77% to 80% and 93% to 96%, respectively.[51,52] Transesophageal echocardiography allows assessment from the aortic root to the descending aorta, but it has a small blind spot: a short segment of the distal ascending aorta, before the innominate artery.[48] The sensitivity is 99% and the specificity is 89%. Computed tomography is fast, visualizes the entire aorta, and is the preferred initial imaging study. The sensitivity is 93%, the specificity is 98%, and the accuracy is 96%.[53] An MRI has a sensitivity and specificity of 98%.[54] The false lumen has a higher signal intensity, whereas a true lumen has no signal. Aortography is less accessible.

Treatment for a type A aortic dissection is surgery, given that mortality is 50% in the first 48 hours if not operated and surgery reduces 1-month mortality from 90% to 30%; however, the patient has a type B aortic dissection (choice A).[55-57] Treatment for an uncomplicated type B aortic dissection includes pain management and heart rate and blood pressure control. This patient has been on increasing doses of pain and antihypertensives with no improvement in his blood pressure (choices B and C). For a complicated type B aortic dissection (symptomatic despite medication, uncontrolled hypertension, aortic expansion, malperfusion, or signs of rupture), TEVAR is the treatment of choice.[48] Thoracic endovascular aortic repair closes the tear and redirects blood to the true lumen and prompts thrombosis of the false lumen (choice D).

22. A. Lorazepam

Cocaine has 3 metabolites: benzoylecgonine, ecgonine methyl ester, and norcocaine. Benzoylecgonine is the metabolite tested in the urine and can be detected for more than 10 days. Cocaine has the following physiologic effects: (1) It blocks presynaptic uptake of amines at adrenergic receptors; (2) it stimulates α_1, α_2, β_1, and β_2 receptors, which causes vasoconstriction; (3) it blocks sodium channels, causing a slow Na^+ cardiac current and acts as a local anesthetic; and (4) increases the excitatory neurotransmitter glutamate and aspartate in the brain. Cocaine causes increased myocardial oxygen demand but decreases oxygen availability due to vasoconstriction, worsens myocardial performance, and is prothrombogenic and proarrhymic.[58] Cocaine can also be adulterated with levamisole, which can cause agranulocytosis, leukoencephalopathy, vasculitis, and cutaneous necrosis, and clenbuterol, which can cause hyperglycemia and hypokalemia.

Cocaine-induced hypertension can be treated initially with benzodiazepines (choice A).[59] If the use of lorazepam fails, nitroglycerin (choice B) has been shown to lower blood pressure and reverse cocaine-induced coronary vasospasm. Calcium channel blockers such as verapamil (choice C) have had conflicting data in cocaine-intoxicated animals, but verapamil has been shown to reverse cocaine-induced coronary artery vasoconstriction.[60] However, it is not the preferred agent. Beta-blockers such as labetalol (choice D) results in unopposed vasoconstriction and paradoxically increase blood pressure, and it has been suggested that labetalol does not reverse coronary vasoconstriction.[61]

23. A. Labetalol

Labetalol is correct. Postoperative hypertension can result from pain-induced sympathetic stimulation, emergence from anesthesia, hypercarbia, volume overload, and discontinuation of long-term antihypertensives.[62] Systolic blood pressure must be maintained at 100 to 150 mmHg to maintain cerebral perfusion pressure but, at the same time, minimizing risk of hematoma. Lorazepam (choice B) is incorrect. The patient is not anxious; therefore, anxiolytics would not be helpful. Morphine (choice C) is incorrect. The patient is not in pain; therefore, opioids would not be helpful. Doing nothing (choice D) is incorrect. This can increase the risk of hematoma and cardiovascular events.

24. C. Amiodarone

In the setting of cardiac arrest, management of ventricular tachycardia and ventricular fibrillation begins with 2-minute cycle of good quality cardiopulmonary resuscitation (CPR) followed by defibrillation, initially at 120 to 200 J for biphasic or 360 for monophasic (choice A). Good quality CPR is at rate of 100 or more per minute, with a depth of 2 inches or more. After defibrillation, 2 cycles of CPR, then epinephrine 1 mg IV/ intraosseous (IO) infusion and followed by amiodarone 300 mg IV. Lidocaine 1 to 1.5 mg/kg may be used in lieu of amiodarone or if the patient still has VT/VF after amiodarone is given.

However, this patient clearly is not in cardiac arrest. Evaluation of ventricular arrhythmias begins with 4 considerations: (1) sustained, which means 30 seconds or more, or less than 30 seconds with hemodynamic collapse, vs nonsustained, which means less than 30 seconds; (2) monomorphic, polymorphic, or fibrillation; (3) symptoms; and (4) intrinsic cardiac disease. Ventricular arrhythmias with no structural heart disease, monomorphic RV outflow tract (OT) or LVOT, and idiopathic left ventricular tachycardia generally carries a benign prognosis. Polymorphic VT may further be classified on normal QRS and abnormal QRS. Polymorphic VT with normal QRS is associated with (1) acute myocardial infarction and may present up to 11 days postinfarction with no evidence of recurrent ischemia and (2) nonischemic cardiomyopathy. Polymorphic QRS with abnormal QRS might suggest prolonged QT syndrome, torsade de pointes, and catecholaminergic polymorphic ventricular tachycardia.

The aim of rhythm control of ventricular tachycardia and ventricular fibrillation is to prevent sudden cardiac death. Beta-blockers are the first-line treatment of ventricular arrhythmias, but sotalol, a potassium current inhibitor with beta-blocker properties, has been shown as a proarrhythmic (choice B).[63-67] Magnesium levels are normal, so there is no need to replete (choice D). The best option would be amiodarone (choice C).

25. D. Ablation

The first step to reduce sudden cardiac death is to optimize pharmacologic therapy. Angiotensin-converting enzyme inhibitors, beta-blockers, and mineralocorticoid receptor antagonists (MRA) have been shown to reduce sudden cardiac death by 15% to 25%, 35%, and 20% to 25% respectively (choice A).[68-72] An ICD is recommended to reduced sudden cardiac death in NYHA class II to III, LVEF of 35% or less, and after 3 months or more of optimized medical therapy in patients expected to survive with good functional status for 1 year or more (LOE A; choice B). The SCD-Heft Trial showed ICD was associated with a 23% decreased risk of death (hazard ratio, 0.77; 95% confidence interval 0.62–0.96, $P = 0.008$) and 7% decrease in 5-year mortality.[73] In the MADIT II study, ICD showed a 31% decrease in all-cause mortality (hazard ratio, 0.69; 95% confidence interval, 0.51–0.93; $P = 0.016$).[74]

Cardiac resynchronization therapy (CRT) is recommended to prevent sudden cardiac death in NYHA class II to III, LVEF of 35% or less, and after 3 months or more of optimized medical therapy in patients expected to survive with good functional status for 1 year or more, and with QRS 150 ms or more (LOE A) and 120 to 150 ms (LOE B; choice C). The COMPANION trial showed that patients with QRS 120 to 149 ms and CRT reduced all causes of mortality by 26% (hazard ratio, 0.64; 95% confidence interval 0.48–0.85; $P < 0.002$).[75] The CARE-HF study showed CRT reduced sudden cardiac death by 46%

(hazard ratio, 0.54; 95% confidence interval, 0.35–0.84; $P = 0.0005$) and a reduction in total mortality of 40% (hazard ratio, 0.60; 95% confidence interval, 0.47–0.77; $P < 0.001$).[76] Ablation has been shown to decrease incidence of these arrhythmias but generally does not affect mortality (choice D).[77-82] Other interventions such as amiodarone do not affect mortality.

26. A. Lead perforation with pericardial effusion

Lead perforation with pericardial effusion is correct. Note that the tip of the RV lead is clearly outside the ventricle. The patient in question also had new onset of anemia after the recent implantation of a pacemaker, which should also give clue to the diagnosis of lead perforation into the pericardial space with resultant pericardial effusion. Lead dislodgement (choice B) is incorrect. A patient with lead dislodgement may have recurrence of original symptoms for which the pacemaker was implanted. Patients also may have symptoms of pacing at odd sites such as diaphragmatic stimulation. Sometimes the symptoms can be very subtle. Lead fracture (choice C) is incorrect. Failure to capture may be seen on ECG recording. Pneumothorax (choice D) is incorrect. Pneumothorax may go unnoticed if it is small. It may sometimes be seen on the x-ray obtained on the day after the procedure. Symptoms of pneumothorax are different and usually does not present after several days of lead implantation, as in this case.

REFERENCES

1. Annane D, Sebille V, Duboc D, et al. Incidence and prognosis of sustained arrhythmias in critically ill patients. *Am J Respir Crit Care Med.* 2008;178(1):20-25.
2. Antzelevitch C, Burashnikov A. Overview of basic mechanisms of cardiac arrhythmia. *Card Electrophysiol Clin.* 2011;3(1):23-45.
3. Page RL, Joglar JA, Caldwell MA, et al. 2015 ACC/AHA/HRS guideline for the management of adult patients with supraventricular tachycardia: a report of the American College of Cardiology/American Heart Association Task Force on Clinical Practice Guidelines and the Heart Rhythm Society. *Heart Rhythm.* 2016;13(4):e136-e221.
4. Zishiri E, Callahan T. Chapter 24: Atrial fibrillation. In: Griffin BP, Callahan TD, Menon V, Wu WM, Cauthen CA, Dunn JM. *Manual of Cardiovascular Medicine.* 4th ed. Philadelphia, PA: Lippincott, Williams, & Wilkins; 2012; 424-444.
5. January CT, Wann LS, Alpert JS, et al. 2014 AHA/ACC/HRS guideline for the management of patients with atrial fibrillation: executive summary. *J Am Coll Cardiol.* 2014;64(21):2246-2280.
6. Wyse DG, Waldo AL, DiMarco JP, et al. A comparison of rate control and rhythm control in patients with atrial fibrillation. *N Engl J Med.* 2002;347(23):1825-1833.
7. Hohnloser SH, Kuck KH, Lilienthal J. Rhythm or rate control in atrial fibrillation—Pharmacological Intervention in Atrial Fibrillation (PIAF): a randomised trial. *Lancet.* 2000;356(9244):1789-1794.
8. Carlsson J, Miketic S, Windeler J, et al. Randomized trial of rate-control versus rhythm-control in persistent atrial fibrillation:

the Strategies of Treatment of Atrial Fibrillation (STAF) study. *J Am Coll Cardiol.* 2003;41(10):1690-1696.

9. Van Gelder IC, Hagens VE, Bosker HA, et al. A comparison of rate control and rhythm control in patients with recurrent persistent atrial fibrillation. *N Engl J Med.* 2002;347(23): 1834-1840.

10. Gillinov AM, Bagiella E, Moskowitz AJ, et al. Rate control versus rhythm control for atrial fibrillation after cardiac surgery. *N Engl J Med.* 2016;374(20):1911-1921.

11. Kirchhof P, Benussi S, Kotecha D, et al. 2016 ESC Guidelines for the management of atrial fibrillation developed in collaboration with EACTS. *Eur Heart J.* 2016;37:2893-2962.

12. Gage BF, Waterman AD, Shannon W, Boechler M, Rich MW, Radford MJ. Validation of clinical classification schemes for predicting stroke: results from the National Registry of Atrial Fibrillation. *JAMA.* 2001;285(22):2864-2870.

13. Kalman JM, Olgin JE, Saxon LA, Lee RJ, Scheinman MM, Lesh MD. Electrocardiographic and electrophysiologic characterization of atypical atrial flutter in man. *J Cardiovasc Electrophysiol.* 1997;8(2):121-144.

14. Wellens HJ. Contemporary management of atrial flutter. *Circulation.* 2002;106(6):649-652.

15. Al-Khatib SM, Arshad A, Balk EM, et al. Risk stratification for arrhythmic events in patients with asymptomatic pre-excitation: a systematic review for the 2015 ACC/AHA/HRS guideline for the management of adult patients with supraventricular tachycardia. *Heart Rhythm.* 2016;13(4):e222-e237.

16. Pedersen CT, Kay GN, Kalman J, et al. EHRA/HRS/APHRS expert consensus on ventricular arrhythmias. *Heart Rhythm.* 2014;11(10):e166-e196.

17. Oommen SS. Chapter 22: Bradyarrthymias, atrioventricular block, asystole, and pulseless electrical activity. In: Griffin BP, Callahan TD, Menon V, Wu WM, Cauthen CA, Dunn JM. *Manual of Cardiovascular Medicine.* 4th ed. Philadelphia, PA: Lippincott, Williams, & Wilkins; 2012; 390-410.

18. Israel CW, Barold SS. Electrical storm in patients with an implanted defibrillator: a matter of definition. *Ann Noninvasive Electrocardiol.* 2007;12(4):375-382.

19. Miller JM, Zipes DP. Chapter 34: Diagnosis of cadiac arrthymias. In: Mann DL, Zipes DP, Libby P, Bonow RO, Braunwald E. *Braunwald's Heart Disease: A Textbook of Cardiovascular Medicine.* 10th ed. Philadelphia, PA: Elsevier-Saunders; 2014; 662-684.

20. Epstein AE, DiMarco JP, Ellenbogen KA, et al. 2012 ACCF/ AHA/HRS focused update incorporated into the ACCF/AHA/ HRS 2008 guidelines for device-based therapy of cardiac rhythm abnormalities: a report of the American College of Cardiology Foundation/American Heart Association Task Force on Practice Guidelines and the Heart Rhythm Society. *J Am Coll Cardiol.* 2013;61(3):e6-e75.

21. Rodriguez MA, Kumar SK, De Caro M. Hypertensive crisis. *Cardiol Rev.* 2010;18(2):102-7.

22. Bennett NM, Shea S. Hypertensive emergency: case criteria, sociodemographic profile, and previous care of 100 cases. *Am J Public Health.* 1988;78(6):636-640.

23. Varon J, Marik PE. The diagnosis and management of hypertensive crises. *Chest.* 2000;118(1):214-227.

24. Powers WJ. Acute hypertension after stroke: the scientific basis for treatment decisions. *Neurology.* 1993;43(3 Pt 1):461-467.

25. Rodriguez MA, Kumar SK, De Caro M. Hypertensive crisis. *Cardiol Rev.* 2010;18(2):102-107.

26. Brugada P, Brugada J, Mont L, Smeets J, Andries EW. A new approach to the differential diagnosis of a regular tachycardia with a wide QRS complex. *Circulation.* 1991;83(5):1649-1659.

27. Vereckei A, Duray G, Szenasi G, Altemose GT, Miller JM. New algorithm using only lead aVR for differential diagnosis of wide QRS complex tachycardia. *Heart Rhythm.* 2008;5(1): 89-98.

28. Schwartz PJ, Crotti L, Insolia R. Long-QT syndrome: from genetics to management. *Circ Arrhythm Electrophysiol.* 2012;5(4): 868-877.

29. Abrams DJ, MacRae CA. Long QT syndrome. *Circulation.* 2014;129(14):1524-1529.

30. Olen MM, Baysa SJ, Rossi A, Kanter RJ, Fishberger SB. Wolff-Parkinson-White syndrome: a stepwise deterioration to sudden death. *Circulation.* 2016;133(1):105-106.

31. Cohen MI, Triedman JK, Cannon BC, et al. PACES/HRS expert consensus statement on the management of the asymptomatic young patient with a Wolff-Parkinson-White (WPW, ventricular preexcitation) electrocardiographic pattern. *Heart Rhythm.* 2012;9(6):1006-1024.

32. Kirchhof P, Benussi S, Kotecha D, et al. 2016 ESC guidelines for the management of atrial fibrillation developed in collaboration with EACTS. *Eur Heart J.* 2016;37(38):2893-2896.

33. Ruff CT, Giugliano RP, Braunwald E, et al. Comparison of the efficacy and safety of new oral anticoagulants with warfarin in patients with atrial fibrillation: a meta-analysis of randomised trials. *Lancet.* 2014;383(9921):955-962.

34. ACTIVE Writing Group of the ACTIVE Investigators; Connolly S, Pogue J, Hart R, et al. Clopidogrel plus aspirin versus oral anticoagulation for atrial fibrillation in the Atrial fibrillation Clopidogrel Trial with Irbesartan for prevention of Vascular Events (ACTIVE W): a randomised controlled trial. *Lancet.* 2006;367(9526):1903-1912.

35. Connolly SJ, Pogue J, Eikelboom J, et al. Benefit of oral anticoagulant over antiplatelet therapy in atrial fibrillation depends on the quality of international normalized ratio control achieved by centers and countries as measured by time in therapeutic range. *Circulation.* 2008;118(20):2029-2037.

36. Investigators A, Connolly SJ, Pogue J, et al. Effect of clopidogrel added to aspirin in patients with atrial fibrillation. *N Engl J Med.* 2009;360(20):2066-2078.

37. Diener HC, Stanford S, Abdul-Rahim A, et al. Anti-thrombotic therapy in patients with atrial fibrillation and intracranial hemorrhage. *Expert Rev Neurother.* 2014;14(9):1019-1028.

38. Hankey GJ, Norrving B, Hacke W, Steiner T. Management of acute stroke in patients taking novel oral anticoagulants. *Int J Stroke.* 2014;9(5):627-632.

39. Xian Y, Liang L, Smith EE, et al. Risks of intracranial hemorrhage among patients with acute ischemic stroke receiving warfarin and treated with intravenous tissue plasminogen activator. *JAMA.* 2012;307(24):2600-2608.

40. Sarafoff N, Martischnig A, Wealer J, et al. Triple therapy with aspirin, prasugrel, and vitamin K antagonists in patients with drug-eluting stent implantation and an indication for oral anticoagulation. *J Am Coll Cardiol.* 2013;61(20):2060-2066.

41. Jackson LR 2nd, Ju C, Zettler M, et al. Outcomes of patients with acute myocardial infarction undergoing percutaneous coronary intervention receiving an oral anticoagulant and dual antiplatelet therapy: a comparison of clopidogrel versus prasugrel from the TRANSLATE-ACS study. *JACC Cardiovasc Interv.* 2015;8(14):1880-1889.

42. Dewilde WJM, Oirbans T, Verheugt FWA, et al. Use of clopidogrel with or without aspirin in patients taking oral anticoagulant therapy and undergoing percutaneous coronary intervention: an open-label, randomised, controlled trial. *Lancet*. 2013;381(9872):1107-1115.

43. Walkey AJ, Quinn EK, Winter MR, McManus DD, Benjamin EJ. Practice patterns and outcomes associated with use of anticoagulation among patients with atrial fibrillation during sepsis. *JAMA Cardiol*. 2016;1(6):682.

44. Van Gelder IC, Wyse DG, Chandler ML, et al. Does intensity of rate-control influence outcome in atrial fibrillation? An analysis of pooled data from the RACE and AFFIRM studies. *Europace*. 2006;8(11):935-942.

45. Groenveld HF, Crijns HJ, Van den Berg MP, et al. The effect of rate control on quality of life in patients with permanent atrial fibrillation: data from the RACE II (Rate Control Efficacy in Permanent Atrial Fibrillation II) study. *J Am Coll Cardiol*. 2011;58(17):1795-1803.

46. Ruff CT, Giugliano RP, Braunwald E, et al. Comparison of the efficacy and safety of new oral anticoagulants with warfarin in patients with atrial fibrillation: a meta-analysis of randomised trials. *Lancet*. 2014;383(9921):955-962.

47. Brignole M, Auricchio A, Baron-Esquivias G, et al. 2013 ESC guidelines on cardiac pacing and cardiac resynchronization therapy: the task force on cardiac pacing and resynchronization therapy of the European Society of Cardiology (ESC). Developed in collaboration with the European Heart Rhythm Association (EHRA). *Eur Heart J*. 2013;34(29):2281-2329.

48. Erbel R, Aboyans V, Boileau C, et al; ESC Committee for Practice Guidelines. 2014 ESC Guidelines on the diagnosis and treatment of aortic diseases: document covering acute and chronic aortic diseases of the thoracic and abdominal aorta of the adult. The task force for the diagnosis and treatment of aortic diseases of the European Society of Cardiology (ESC). *Eur Heart J*. 2014;35(41):2873-2926.

49. Hagan PG, Nienaber CA, Isselbacher EM, et al. The International Registry of Acute Aortic Dissection (IRAD). *JAMA*. 2000;283(7):897.

50. Braverman AC. Acute aortic dissection: clinician update. *Circulation*. 2010;122(2):184-188.

51. Mintz GS, Kotler MN, Segal BL, Parry WR. Two dimensional echocardiographic recognition of the descending thoracic aorta. *Am J Cardiol*. 1979;44(2):232-238.

52. Khandheria BK, Tajik AJ, Taylor CL, et al. Aortic dissection: review of value and limitations of two-dimensional echocardiography in a six-year experience. *J Am Soc Echocardiogr*. 1989;2(1):17-24.

53. Sommer T, Fehske W, Holzknecht N, et al. Aortic dissection: a comparative study of diagnosis with spiral CT, multiplanar transesophageal echocardiography, and MR imaging. *Radiology*. 1996;199(2):347-352.

54. Nienaber CA, von Kodolitsch Y, Nicolas V, et al. The diagnosis of thoracic aortic dissection by noninvasive imaging procedures. *N Engl J Med*. 1993;328(1):1-9.

55. Chiappini B, Schepens M, Tan E. Early and late outcomes of acute type A aortic dissection: analysis of risk factors in 487 consecutive patients. *Eur Heart J*. 2005;14(5):45.

56. Trimarchi S, Nienaber CA, Rampoldi V. Contemporary Results of Surgery in Acute Type A Aortic Dissection: The International Registry of Acute Aortic Dissection Experience. *ACC Curr J Rev*. 2005;26(2):180-186.

57. Perko MJ, Norgaard M, Herzog TM, Olsen PS, Schroeder TV, Pettersson G. Unoperated aortic aneurysm: a survey of 170 patients. *Ann Thorac Surg*. 1995;59(5):1204-1209.

58. Schwartz BG, Rezkalla S, Kloner RA. Cardiovascular effects of cocaine. *Circulation*. 2010;122(24):2558-2569.

59. Hollander JE. Cocaine intoxication and hypertension. *Ann Emerg Med*. 2008;51(3):S18-S20.

60. Negus BH, Willard JE, Hillis LD, et al. Alleviation of cocaine-induced coronary vasoconstriction with intravenous verapamil. *Am J Cardiol*. 1994;73(7):510-513.

61. Boehrer JD, Moliterno DJ, Willard JE, Hillis LD, Lange RA. Influence of labetalol on cocaine-induced coronary vasoconstriction in humans. *Am J Med*. 1993;94(6):608-610.

62. Varon J. Perioperative hypertension management. *Vasc Health Risk Manag*. 2008;(3)4:615-627.

63. Singh BN, Singh SN, Domenic JR. Amiodarone versus sotalol for atrial fibrillation. *ACC Curr J Rev*. 2005;14(8):53-54.

64. Lafuente-Lafuente C, Longas-Tejero MA, Bergmann JF, Belmin J. Antiarrhythmics for maintaining sinus rhythm after cardioversion of atrial fibrillation. *Cochrane Database Syst Rev*. 2012(5):CD005049.

65. Kühlkamp V, Mewis C, Mermi J, Bosch RF, Seipel L. Suppression of sustained ventricular tachyarrhythmias: a comparison of d,l-sotalol with no antiarrhythmic drug treatment. *J Am Coll Cardiol*. 1999;33(1):46-52.

66. Waldo AL, Camm AJ, deRuyter H, et al. Effect of d-sotalol on mortality in patients with left ventricular dysfunction after recent and remote myocardial infarction. The SWORD Investigators. Survival With Oral d-Sotalol. *Lancet*. 1996;348(9019):7-12.

67. Hohnloser SH, Dorian P, Roberts R, et al. Effect of amiodarone and sotalol on ventricular defibrillation threshold: the optimal pharmacological therapy in cardioverter defibrillator patients (OPTIC) trial. *Circulation*. 2006;114(2):104-109.

68. McMurray JJ, Adamopoulos S, Anker SD, et al. ESC Guidelines for the diagnosis and treatment of acute and chronic heart failure 2012: the task force for the diagnosis and treatment of acute and chronic heart failure 2012 of the European Society of Cardiology. Developed in collaboration with the Heart Failure Association (HFA) of the ESC. *Eur Heart J*. 2012;33(14):1787-1847.

69. Garg R, Yusuf S. Overview of randomized trials of angiotensin-converting enzyme inhibitors on mortality and morbidity in patients with heart failure. Collaborative Group on ACE Inhibitor Trials. *JAMA*. 1995;273(18):1450-1456.

70. Pitt B, Zannad F, Remme WJ, et al. The effect of spironolactone on morbidity and mortality in patients with severe heart failure. Randomized Aldactone Evaluation Study Investigators. *N Engl J Med*. 1999;341(10):709-717.

71. Zannad F, McMurray JJ, Krum H, et al. Eplerenone in patients with systolic heart failure and mild symptoms. *N Engl J Med*. 2011;364(1):11-21.

72. Bapoje SR, Bahia A, Hokanson JE, et al. Effects of mineralocorticoid receptor antagonists on the risk of sudden cardiac death in patients with left ventricular systolic dysfunction: a meta-analysis of randomized controlled trials. *Circ Heart Fail*. 2013;6(2):166-173.

73. Packer DL, Prutkin JM, Hellkamp AS, et al. Impact of implantable cardioverter-defibrillator, amiodarone, and placebo on the mode of death in stable patients with heart failure: analysis from the sudden cardiac death in heart failure trial. *Circulation*. 2009;120(22):2170-2176.

74. Goldenberg I, Moss AJ, McNitt S, et al. Time dependence of defibrillator benefit after coronary revascularization in the Multicenter Automatic Defibrillator Implantation Trial (MADIT)-II. *J Am Coll Cardiol*. 2006;47(9):1811-1817.

75. Bristow MR, Saxon LA, Boehmer J, et al. Cardiac-resynchronization therapy with or without an implantable defibrillator in advanced chronic heart failure. *N Engl J Med*. 2004;350(21):2140-2150.

76. Bardy GH, Lee KL, Mark DB, et al. Amiodarone or an implantable cardioverter-defibrillator for congestive heart failure. *N Engl J Med*. 2005;352(3):225-237.

77. Carbucicchio C, Santamaria M, Trevisi N, et al. Catheter ablation for the treatment of electrical storm in patients with implantable cardioverter-defibrillators: short- and long-term outcomes in a prospective single-center study. *Circulation*. 2008;117(4):462-469.

78. Calkins H, Epstein A, Packer D, et al. Catheter ablation of ventricular tachycardia in patients with structural heart disease using cooled radiofrequency energy: results of a prospective multicenter study. Cooled RF Multi Center Investigators Group. *J Am Coll Cardiol*. 2000;35(7):1905-1914.

79. Stevenson WG, Wilber DJ, Natale A, et al. Irrigated radiofrequency catheter ablation guided by electroanatomic mapping for recurrent ventricular tachycardia after myocardial infarction: the Multicenter Thermocool Ventricular Tachycardia Ablation Trial. *Circulation*. 2008;118(25):2773-2782.

80. Tanner H, Hindricks G, Volkmer M, et al. Catheter ablation of recurrent scar-related ventricular tachycardia using electroanatomical mapping and irrigated ablation technology: results of the prospective multicenter Euro-VT-study. *J Cardiovasc Electrophysiol*. 2010;21(1):47-53.

81. Reddy VY, Reynolds MR, Neuzil P, et al. Prophylactic catheter ablation for the prevention of defibrillator therapy. *N Engl J Med*. 2007;357(26):2657-2665.

82. Kuck KH, Schaumann A, Eckardt L, et al. Catheter ablation of stable ventricular tachycardia before defibrillator implantation in patients with coronary heart disease (VTACH): a multicentre randomised controlled trial. *Lancet*. 2010;375(9708):31-40.

CHAPTER

6

Acute Coronary Syndromes

Uschi Auguste, MD, and Yumiko Kanei, MD

INTRODUCTION

An acute coronary syndrome (ACS) encompasses a clinical spectrum of myocardial ischemia ranging from unstable angina (UA) and non–ST-segment elevation myocardial infarction (NSTEMI) to ST-segment elevation myocardial infarction (STEMI), and represents an acute phase of coronary atherosclerosis.[1-3] Early recognition, diagnosis, and prompt revascularization of the culprit lesion with percutaneous coronary intervention (PCI) is the contemporary management strategy for patients presenting with STEMI or high-risk NSTEMI.[1,2,4,5] Acute plaque rupture and subsequent atherothrombosis with consequent myocardial injury is the most common etiology for ACS; however, myocardial necrosis in the absence of unstable plaque may ensue in critically ill patients who are admitted for non–cardiac-related conditions, such as pulmonary embolism and septic shock. These patients pose a unique diagnostic and management challenge, as concomitant multiorgan failure, electrolyte derangements, and coagulopathy further complicate the clinical picture.[6-8] In this chapter, we will review the universal definition of myocardial infarction (MI) and the related patient presentations, risk stratification models, complications, and management strategies.

PATHOPHYSIOLOGY

Acute myocardial infarction is characterized by myocardial necrosis and is diagnosed in the setting of a rise or fall in cardiac biomarkers in conjunction with clinical symptoms of ischemia, new ischemic electrocardiography (ECG) changes, new regional wall motion abnormalities on imaging, or findings on coronary angiography.[9-11] Myocardial ischemia ensues when the supply of myocardial oxygen is insufficient relative to myocardial oxygen demand. The pathophysiology of ACS is similar in STEMI, NSTEMI, and UA, and involves a milieu of factors, including endothelial dysfunction, vulnerable plaque, plaque disruption, and atherothrombosis, as summarized in Figure 6-1. It is typically precipitated by rupture or erosion of atherosclerotic plaque within a coronary artery,

causing thrombosis and leading to an acute and commonly critical reduction in coronary blood flow.[1,12,13] This results in myocardial hypoperfusion, ischemia, diastolic dysfunction, systolic dysfunction, electrocardiographic changes, angina, and ultimately, necrosis.[12,14] ST-segment elevation myocardial infarctions usually represent complete occlusion of the coronary artery, while in NSTE-ACS (NSTEMI and UA), there is a critical reduction in flow.

The universal classification of myocardial infarction is summarized in Table 6-1. Patients with acute plaque rupture resulting in intraluminal thrombosis and decreased myocardial blood flow are classified as type 1 MI.[9,10] These patients need to be rapidly identified, as aggressive pharmacotherapy and immediate reperfusion are the most effective strategy for mitigating the sequelae related to myocardial infarction, including mechanical complications and death. Type 2 MI refers to myocardial injury with necrosis precipitated by an imbalance between myocardial oxygen supply and demand, or demand ischemia, as seen in tachyarrhythmias, anemia, respiratory failure, hypotension, and severe hypertension. This can occur even in normal coronaries, and is the common type of MI seen in critically ill patients.[7,9-11]

EPIDEMIOLOGY

Acute coronary syndromes represent an important cause of morbidity and mortality. According to the American Heart Association (AHA) heart disease and stroke statistics published in 2016, the overall rate of death attributable to cardiovascular disease was 222.9 per 100,000 Americans, and of those, 370,213 died of coronary artery disease (CAD).[12-15] While some patients have a history of stable angina, an ACS may be the initial presentation of CAD; however, not all patients with elevated troponin have ACS. Prospective studies report approximately 50% of critically ill patients to have elevated troponin, several of whom have no clinically unstable plaque or significant CAD.[16,17] In a single-center study performed in noncardiac critically ill patients, the prevalence of MI, defined as elevated troponin and ischemic ECG changes was 26% to 36%.[18]

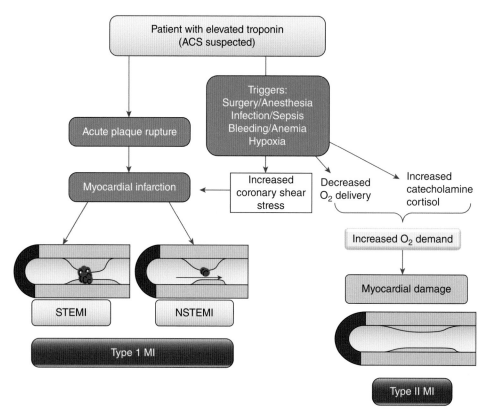

FIGURE 6-1 Summary of pathophysiology of myocardial ischemia: atherothrombosis secondary to spontaneous plaque rupture and demand ischemia (supply–demand mismatch). Pathophysiology of ACS is similar in STEMI, NSTEMI, and UA, and involves a milieu of factors, including endothelial dysfunction, atherothrombosis, vulnerable plaque, plaque disruption, and thrombosis secondary to rupture or erosion of atherosclerotic plaque. However, as commonly seen in critically ill patients, myocardial injury may ensue in the absence of plaque rupture in the setting of increased demand, such as tachyarrhythmias and anemia. ACS = acute coronary syndrome; MI = myocardial infarction; NSTEMI = non–ST-segment elevation myocardial infarction; STEMI = ST-segment elevation myocardial infarction; UA = unstable angina.

PATIENT PRESENTATION AND DIAGNOSIS

Chest pain is a frequent presenting concern for patients coming into the emergency room, and rapid identification and management of patients with an acute coronary syndrome is paramount to mitigate the sequela of myocardial necrosis. Patients in the critical care unit may not report chest pain since they are often sedated or incapacitated from other causes; therefore, other objective findings need to be utilized in the setting of strong clinical suspicion. In the absence of

TABLE 6-1 Universal Definition of Myocardial Infarction

Type I	Spontaneous MI: Plaque rupture with thrombus
Type 2	MI secondary to ischemic imbalance
Type 3	MI leading to sudden death
Type 4a	MI related to percutaneous coronary intervention
Type 4b	MI related to stent thrombosis
Type 5	MI related to CABG

CABG = coronary artery bypass graft; MI = myocardial infarction.

reported anginal symptoms, new clinical findings such as dynamic ECG changes, new ST-segment elevation, new regional wall motion abnormalities on echocardiography, or new moderate-to-severe mitral regurgitation, should prompt further investigation to rule out ACS. Nonsedated patients will likely express angina. Typical angina has 3 defining characteristics: (1) retrosternal chest pressure usually lasting more than 10 minutes that is (2) provoked by exertion or emotional stress, and (3) relieved by rest or nitroglycerin. Pain may be associated with radiation to the arm, jaw, and back, and furthermore, there may be associated diaphoresis, nausea, dyspnea, and occasionally syncope.[1,2,18,19]

There is a subset of patients with atypical presentations, including women, diabetics, chronic renal failure, and the elderly (> 75 years). These patients may report sharp pain, epigastric discomfort, progressively worsening dyspnea, or pleuritic chest pain. It is important to obtain a proper history to support the diagnosis of ACS and include association of symptoms with activity, and relief with nitrates or rest, and assess change in baseline angina. Risk factors for CAD also help stratify patients presenting with suspected ACS, and are summarized in Table 6-2.[1,2]

While ACS is an important cause of chest pain, the differential diagnosis of chest pain is fairly broad. It is also

TABLE 6-2 Risk Factors for Coronary Artery Disease

| **Nonmodifiable risk factors** |
| Age (> 45 y in men, > 55 y in women) |
| Family history of premature CAD (age < 55 y) |
| Gender (men) |
| **Modifiable risk factors** |
| Hypertension |
| Smoking |
| Dyslipidemia |
| Diabetes |
| **Nontraditional risk factors** |
| Lipoprotein (a) |
| Homocysteine |
| Small dense LDL-C particles |

CAD = coronary artery disease; LDL-C = cholesterol contained in low-density lipoprotein.

important to know life-threatening nonatherosclerotic conditions that may mimic acute coronary syndromes, and for which initiation of standard therapy for ACS may exacerbate the underlying condition (Table 6-3).

Electrocardiograms in Acute Coronary Syndrome

Interpretation of the ECG is an essential component of the initial diagnostic evaluation of patients with suspected ACS. In patients with high suspicion for ACS but with a nondiagnostic ECG, serial ECGs at 15- to 30-minute intervals during the

TABLE 6-3 Nonatherosclerotic Processes That Cause Chest Pain and Elevated Troponin (Acute Coronary Syndrome Mimic)

| **Cardiac** |
| Takotsubo cardiomyopathy |
| Myocarditis |
| Myopericarditis |
| Cardiogenic shock |
| Other etiologies of coronary artery disease: Kawasaki syndrome, ankylosing spondylitis, trauma, radiation |
| Severe aortic stenosis |
| Spontaneous coronary dissection |
| Anomalous coronary arteries |
| **Vascular** |
| Aortic dissection |
| Pulmonary emboli |
| Emboli to the coronaries: vegetation from endocarditis, mural thrombi, prosthetic valve thrombi, cardiac masses |
| Hypertensive emergency |
| Persistent hypotension |
| **Neurological** |
| Ischemic and embolic stroke |
| Intracranial hemorrhage |
| **Miscellaneous** |
| Cocaine |
| Infiltrative diseases: eg, sarcoidosis |
| Extreme endurance |
| Rhabdomyolysis |

first hour to evaluate dynamic ST change should be obtained. Supplemental electrocardiographic leads V_7 to V_9 to rule out posterior infarcts can also aid the diagnosis.[1,2,20,21] It should be noted that there is a myriad of nonischemic clinical scenarios that confound interpretation of the ECG, such as a left bundle branch block (LBBB), left anterior fascicular block, preexcitation, severe hyperkalemia, and left ventricular hypertrophy (LVH).[22,23]

Figure 6-2 summarizes common ECG findings in patients presenting with ACS.

Cardiac Biomarkers in Acute Coronary Syndrome

In addition to careful history taking and ECG analysis, myocardial injury with necrosis can be detected with biomarkers such as cardiac troponin (cTn) I or T, creatinine kinase (CL)–muscle/brain (MB) fraction. Cardiac biomarkers are invaluable in differentiating UA from NSTEMI and also help estimate the extent of myocardial necrosis. Troponin is a complex of 3 regulatory proteins, troponin C, troponin I, and troponin T, which integrate to the contraction apparatus in skeletal and cardiac muscle. Troponin is attached to tropomycin and lies within the groove of actin filaments in muscle tissue.

Cardiac troponin I and T are the preferred diagnostic tests for acute coronary syndromes because of the tissue-specific expression within the myocardium. Troponins are more specific and sensitive than CK, CK-MB (isoenzymes of CK), and myoglobin. In patients with STEMI, troponin begins to rise within 4 hours after onset of symptoms and may be persistently elevated for up to 2 weeks post-infarct.[24-26] The gains in sensitivity are offset with the decrease in specificity. While elevated troponin is indicative of myocardial injury, it does not discriminate etiology or mechanism of injury. Myocardial infarction is consistent with the presence of elevated cTn to at least the 99th percentile of the upper reference limit, with subsequent increase or decrease (> 3 standard deviations of variance) on serial blood draws in the context of appropriate clinical criteria for ischemia, dynamic ECG changes, or imaging evidence of myocardial injury.[9-11,24]

A positive troponin in a patient with low pretest probability for ACS may be suggestive of ACS; however, this result needs to be corroborated with ECG data and clinical presentation. Conversely, a negative troponin does not rule out ACS, and an emergent angiogram should not be delayed if there are electrocardiographic and clinical symptoms consistent with STEMI. Circulating cTnT or cTnI can be found in the plasma of patients with a transient ischemic attack (TIA) or inflammatory myocardial injury, as well as pulmonary embolus.[27] In addition to the absolute level of troponin, a critical component of the diagnosis of ACS is the cTn kinetics. Absolute cTn elevation is seen in multiple chronic cardiac and noncardiac conditions; however, a rise or fall in serial cTn levels supports acutely evolving cardiac injury, as seen with an acute coronary syndrome.[24,28-30]

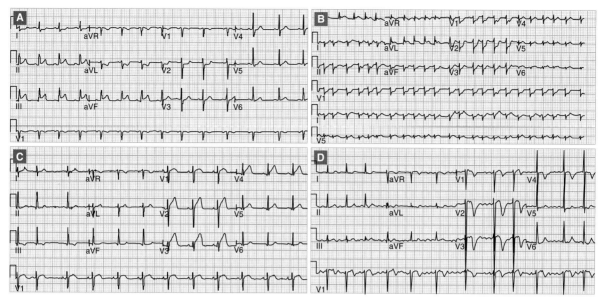

FIGURE 6-2 Samples of electrocardiograms (ECG) in patients presenting with acute coronary syndrome. ST-elevation is defined as more than 0.1 mV ST elevation at the J-point in 2 contiguous leads, except in V_2–V_3, where the cut off is 0.2 mV in men more than 40 years of age and 0.15 mV in women. (A) ECG with inferior STE and depressions in I and aVL, with suggestion of posterior involvement. (B) Underlying atrial fibrillation with rapid ventricular response with anterolateral STE and ST depressions anteriorly and inferiorly. (C) An anterior ST-segment elevation myocardial infarction (STEMI). (D) Atrial fibrillation with Wellens sign (symmetrical deep T-wave inversions in V_1–V_4), concerning for critical left anterior descending (LAD) coronary artery disease.

There is a high prevalence of coronary artery disease in patients with reduced glomerular filtration rate and in patients with end-stage renal disease (ESRD), and these patients tend to have worse clinical outcomes post-ACS.[31] Troponin T levels predict short-term prognosis regardless of level of creatinine.[32] Patients with advanced renal disease not yet on dialysis and presenting with STEMI should proceed to urgent angiogram, and post-procedure have close monitoring of urine output, creatinine, and electrolytes, to determine the need for dialysis, as the risk for contrast-induced nephropathy is high in this group. Additionally, acute renal insufficiency post-MI is associated with worse morbidity and mortality.[33,34]

Brain (B-type) natriuretic peptide (BNP) is a peptide that is synthesized and released predominantly from the ventricular myocardium secondary to myocyte stretch and is a well-established biomarker in patients with heart failure. In patients with ACS, it is useful for prognostication and assessment of the degree of left ventricular dysfunction.[35-37] In the current guidelines, it is a class IIb indication to use BNP to provide additional prognostic information.[1,2]

Risk Stratification

Prompt diagnosis of ACS is crucial to stratify patients who are at greatest risk for recurrent ischemic events and death. The HEART score uses elements of patient **H**istory, **E**CG, **A**ge, **R**isk factors, and **T**roponin to stratify the risk of patients presenting to the emergency department (ED)

with chest pain, and can be extrapolated to patients already admitted, such as in the critical care unit, who report chest pain, and for whom a definitive diagnosis of ACS has not been established.[38-40]

Table 6-4 summarizes the components of the heart score.

Patients with ACS are a heterogeneous group and have varied risks of death and recurrent cardiac events. Several well-validated clinical prediction tools have been developed to stratify patient risk for major complications related to their myocardial infarction. The Thrombolysis In Myocardial Infarction (TIMI) and Platelet glycoprotein IIb/IIIa in Unstable angina: Receptor Suppression Using Integrilin (PURSUIT) scores were developed from large clinical trials in patients with NSTE-ACS and predict short-term prognosis, whereas the Global Registry of Acute Coronary Events (GRACE) score was developed from a global registry and estimates in the hospital and from 6-month mortality in patients who present across the ACS spectrum.[41-44] Of note, compared to TIMI, PURSUIT and GRACE risk scores are better discriminators for in-hospital and 1-year mortality in patients presenting with NSTEMI or STEMI. The Killip classification system is used to assess the severity of heart failure in patients presenting with ACS and represents an independent predictor of all-cause mortality in patients with ACS.[45] More recently, a prospectively derived validated score for estimating 1-year mortality of STEMI at hospital discharge was proposed (Dynamic TIMI) using variables from the original TIMI risk score combined with index hospitalization clinical events that adversely affect mortality.[41,46]

TABLE 6-4 Components of the HEART Score

Components of HEART Score	Clinical Factor	Score
History	Highly suspicious	2
	Moderately suspicious	1
	Low suspicion	0
ECG	Slight ST depression	2
	Nonspecific ST-T changes	1
	Normal	0
Age	> 65 y	2
	45–65 y	1
	< 45 y	0
Risk factors	> 3 risk factors or known CAD	2
	1 or 2 risk factors	1
	No risk factors	0
Troponin	> 2× upper limit of normal	2
	1–2× upper limit of normal	1
	Normal	0

Risk factors: Smoking, HTN, dyslipidemia, family history of CAD, diabetes, and obesity

Risk score associated with major adverse cardiac events within 6 weeks of initial presentation

Score 0–3: 2.5%

Score 4–6: 20.3%

Score 7–10: 72.7% (high risk for cardiovascular events and would benefit from early invasive strategy)

A score of ≥ 7 points represents patients with high-risk NSTE-ACS and is associated with a risk of 72.7%; such patients would benefit from early aggressive strategies. Major cardiac events are defined as all-cause mortality, myocardial infarction, or coronary revascularization. CAD = coronary artery disease; HEART = history, ECG, age, risk factors, troponin; HTN = hypertension.

Table 6-5 summarizes the components of TIMI, Dynamic TIMI, PURSUIT, and GRACE scores.

MANAGEMENT OF PATIENTS PRESENTING WITH ACUTE CORONARY SYNDROME

Pharmacotherapy

In patients with ACS, the goal of therapy is the prevention of further myocardial ischemia/injury and death. In addition to obtaining serial ECGs and cardiac biomarkers, assessment of left ventricular function and initiation of the appropriate pharmacotherapy are paramount to the optimization of care.[1-3,47] Patients should be treated with antiplatelet, anticoagulation, and antianginal agents, and in clinically appropriate scenarios, β antagonists, angiotensin-converting enzyme inhibitors (ACEI), and nitrates. Ultimately, in patients with STEMI, prompt reperfusion should ensue in clinically appropriate settings, and in NSTE-ACS, the decision regarding early invasive strategy or an ischemia-guided strategy for coronary reperfusion needs to be established.[4,48-51]

Tables 6-6, 6-7, and 6-8 summarize the most current guideline recommended antiplatelet, anticoagulation, and adjunct medications used in patients presenting with ACS.

Reperfusion Therapy

Numerous studies have shown a reduction in mortality and recurrent ischemia after reperfusion; therefore, the goal is to rapidly restore myocardial blood flow. There is a myriad of factors to consider prior to selecting the appropriate reperfusion therapy in patients presenting with STEMI and NSTE-ACS. Coronary reperfusion with PCI is indicated in all eligible patients with STEMI with symptom onset within 12 hours.[1,2,4,19,47,52] If the patient is not at a PCI-capable institution, transfer should be initiated. However, if the time to transfer to the PCI capable institution results in a medical contact–to–balloon time greater than 120 minutes, fibrinolytic therapy should be administered within 30 minutes of hospital arrival in eligible patients (Fig. 6-3). In critically ill patients with severe electrolyte derangements, significant coagulopathy, and septic shock with progressive end-organ failure who have concurrent STEMI, coronary angiogram may need to be deferred until clinical stabilization. Interdisciplinary discussions involving the intensivist and cardiologist regarding prognosis and treatment goals are paramount to facilitating the care of such patients.

Of note, fibrinolytic therapy should not be administered to patients with NSTE-ACS, unless the ST depressions are consistent with posterior or inferolateral STEMI. According to data from the Estudio Multicéntrico Estreptoquinasa Repúblicas de América del Sur (EMERAS) trial, in patients who present 12 to 24 hours after the onset of symptoms, there is no benefit with the administration of fibrinolysis, unless there is persistent ST elevations and ongoing chest pain.[47,52-54] Contraindications to fibrinolytic therapy are summarized in Table 6-9. If there is failure to resolve ST elevations in the worst lead by at least 50% at 60 to 90 minutes, urgent coronary angiogram and "rescue" PCI should be performed.[2]

Early-Invasive Strategy Versus Ischemia-Guided Strategy in Patients With NSTE-ACS

In patients with NSTE-ACS, clinical assessment needs to be done to determine treatment strategy, which includes an early-invasive or an ischemia-guided approach. An ischemia-guided approach is typically employed for patients without high-risk features and with low-risk scores, whereas an early-invasive approach is preferred for patients with refractory angina, hemodynamic instability, sustained ventricular arrhythmia, and evidence of heart failure[4,48,49] (Fig. 6-4). In an early-invasive strategy, diagnostic angiogram is performed with intent to undergo revascularization within 24 hours of presentation, whereas an ischemia-guided approach would reserve diagnostic angiogram for individuals with objective evidence of ongoing myocardial ischemia or provocative stress testing.[1,4,49]

Demand Ischemia

There is a plethora of available guideline-based therapies for patients with STEMI and NSTEMI; however, patients with demand ischemia (type II MI) continue to represent a cohort

TABLE 6-5 Summary of the Various Components of Validated Clinical Prediction Tools

TIMI Risk Score [0–7]	Dynamic TIMI Score [0–29]	PURSUIT Risk Score [0–18]	GRACE Risk Score [0–258]
TIMI for NSTEMI	**Baseline TIMI for STEMI [0–14]**	**Separate point allocation for diagnosis**	• **Age (years)**
• **Age** > 65 y [1]	• **Age (years)**	• **Age/Decade** UA[MI]	< 40 [0]
• **> 3 risk factors for CAD** [1]	65–74 [2]	50 8[11]	40–49 [18]
• **ASA use** within 7 d [1]	> 75 [3]	60 9[12]	50–59 [36]
• **Known CAD** (stenosis >50%) [1]	• **Diabetes, hypertension, or angina** [1]	70 11[13]	60–69 [55]
• **> 1 anginal episode 24 h** [1]	• **Systolic BP** < 100 mmHg [3]	80 12[14]	70–79 [73]
• **ST-segment deviation** [1]	• **Heart rate** > 100 beats/min [2]	• **Sex**	80 [91]
• **Elevated cardiac markers** [1]	• **Killip class** II, III, or IV [2]	Male [1]	• **Heart rate (bpm)**
	• **Weight** < 65 kg [1]	Female [0]	< 70 [0]
Score Risk of Death	• **Anterior STEMI or LBBB** [1]	• **Worst CCS class in previous 6 wk**	70–89 [7]
Recurrent	• **Time to Rx** > 4 h [1]	No angina or CCS I/II [0]	90–109 [13]
MI day 14	**Additional index hospitalization events for dynamic score**	CCS III/IV [2]	110–149 [23]
[0–1] 5%	• **Recurrent myocardial infarction** [1]	• **Signs of heart failure** [2]	150–199 [36]
[2] 8%	• **Stroke** [5]	• **ST-depression on presenting ECG** [1]	> 200 [46]
[3] 13%	• **Major bleeding** [1]		• **Systolic BP (mmHg)**
[4] 20%	• **CHF or shock** [3]		< 80 [63]
[5] 26%	• **Arrhythmia** [2]		80–99 [58]
[6–7] 41%	• **Renal failure** [3]		100–119 [47]
			120–139 [37]
	Score 1-Year Mortality		140–159 [26]
	[0–1] 1.3%		160–199 [11]
	[2] 2.3%		> 200 [0]
	[3] 3.6%		• **Creatinine (mg/dL)**
	[4] 5.5%		0–0.39 [2]
	[5] 7.8%		0.4–0.79 [5]
	[6–7] 13.5%		0.8–1.19 [8]
	[≥ 8] 24.8%		1.2–1.59 [11]
			1.6–1.99 [14]
			2–3.99 [23]
			> 4 [31]
			• **Killip class**
			Class I [0]
			Class II [20]
			Class III [39]
			Class IV [59]
			Use of diuretic
			• **Elevated cardiac biomarkers [14]**
			• **ST-segment deviation [28]**
			• **Cardiac arrest [39]**
			Mortality Risk Score
			In hospital
			Low (<1%) [≤108]
			Inter. (1–3%) [109–140]
			High (>3%) [≥140]
			Mortality Risk Score
			6 months
			Low (<3%) [≤88]
			Inter. (3–8%) [89–118]
			High (>8%) [≥118]

CAD = coronary artery disease; CCS = Canadian Cardiovascular Society grading; CHF = congestive heart failure; ECG = electrocardiogram; GRACE = Global Registry of Acute Coronary Events; MI = myocardial infarction; NSTEMI = non–ST-segment elevation myocardial infarction; PURSUIT = Platelet glycoprotein IIb/IIIa in Unstable angina: Receptor Suppression Using Integrilin; STEMI = ST-segment elevation myocardial infarction; TIMI = Thrombolysis In Myocardial Infarction; UA = unstable angina.

without (1) clear strategies for differentiation from type I MI and (2) guidelines for in-hospital management, particularly in the intensive care unit (ICU). Troponin should not be routinely obtained in patients without clinical suspicion for myocardial ischemia. For patients with elevated troponin who have no cardiovascular risk factors and have low risk stratification scores, an alternative etiology for myocardial necrosis needs to be investigated. These patients should have the underlying precipitant of myocardial necrosis treated, and can obtain further risk assessment with stress testing once clinically stable. Elevated troponin may be the first presentation of underlying significant CAD in some patients.[55-57]

Figure 6-5 summarizes a possible diagnostic approach to patients in the ICU with elevated troponin.

TABLE 6-6 Antiplatelet Therapy for Patients With Acute Coronary Syndrome

	Drug	Indication	Management
Cyclooxygenase inhibitors	*Inhibit synthesis of thromboxane A$_2$ causing irreversible inhibition of platelet aggregation*		
	Aspirin	NSTE-ACS; STEMI **Invasive and conservative**	• 162–325-mg load on presentation and before primary PCI • 81-mg maintenance dose indefinitely unless contraindicated
ADP-P2Y$_{12}$–receptor antagonists	*Inhibits ADP-dependent activation of the platelet*		
Thienopyridine	**Clopidogrel**	NSTE-ACS; STEMI **Invasive and conservative**	• 300–600 mg as early as possible or at time of PCI • To support reperfusion with fibrinolytic therapy, 300-mg loading dose if age < 75 y, no loading if age > 75 y • 75 mg daily post-PCI for at least 1 y • Postfibrinolysis, 75 mg daily for at least 14 days and up to 1 y if no bleeding
	Prasugrel	NSTE-ACS; STEMI **Invasive**	• 60 mg at time of PCI • 10 mg daily post-PCI for at least 1 y • Contraindicated in patients with prior stroke/TIA
Nonthienopyridine	**Ticagrelor**	NSTE-ACS; STEMI **Invasive and conservative**	• 180 mg as early as possible or at time of PCI • 90 mg twice a day post-PCI for at least 1 y
GP IIb/IIIa inhibitors	*Inhibits the glycoprotein IIb/IIIa receptor, which is involved in the final pathway for platelet aggregation*		
	Eptifibatide *Contraindicated in patients on hemodialysis	NSTE-ACS; STEMI **Early invasive**	• 180-µg/kg IV bolus, then 2 µg/kg/min; a second 180-µg/kg bolus is administered 10 min after the first bolus (reduce dose by 50% in patients with CrCl < 50 mL/min) • At time of PCI if large thrombus burden or inadequate P2Y$_{12}$-receptor antagonist loading
	Tirofiban	NSTE-ACS; STEMI **Early invasive**	• 25-µg/kg IV bolus, then 0.15 µg/kg/min (reduce dose by 50% in patients with CrCl < 30 mL/min)
	Abciximab	NSTE-ACS; STEMI **Early invasive**	• 0.25-mg/kg IV bolus, then 0.125 µg/kg/min • If large thrombus burden or inadequate P2Y$_{12}$-receptor antagonist loading

Current guidelines recommends at least 1 year of dual antiplatelet therapy (DAPT) post-ACS regardless of the type of stent used; however, earlier discontinuation of a P2Y$_{12}$ inhibitor may be necessary if the risk of bleeding outweighs the benefit of DAPT. ACS = acute coronary syndrome; CrCl = creatinine clearance; GP = glycoprotein; IV = intravenous; NSTE = non–ST-elevation; PCI = percutaneous coronary intervention; STEMI = ST-elevation myocardial infarction; TIA = transient ischemic attack.

TABLE 6-7 Anticoagulation in Patients Presenting With Acute Coronary Syndrome

	Drug	Indication	Management
Indirect thrombin inhibitors	*Binds antithrombin and the resultant complex inhibits thrombin, factor Xa, and factor IXa*		
	Unfractionated heparin	NSTE-ACS; STEMI **Invasive/ conservative**	**In patients with STEMI for PCI** • 70- to 100-U/kg bolus to achieve therapeutic ACT **In patients with NSTE-ACS** • IV UFH for 48 h or until PCI is performed
	Low–molecular-weight heparin: enoxaparin	NSTE-ACS; STEMI **Invasive/ conservative**	• 1 mg/kg SC every 12 h (reduce dose to 1 mg/kg/d SC in patients with CrCl < 30 mL/min)
Direct thrombin inhibitors	*Binds to the active site as well as substrate recognition site thrombin and blocks its fibrin interaction*		
	Bivalirudin *Preferred over UFH with GP IIb/IIIa–receptor antagonist in patients at high risk of bleeding	STEMI; NSTEMI **Invasive**	• 0.75-mg/kg IV bolus, then 1.75–mg/kg/h infusion with or without prior treatment with UFH; additional bolus of 0.3 mg/kg may be given • If CrCl < 30 mL/min, decrease infusion
Factor Xa inhibitors	*Binds to the active site of Xa, both the free form and within the prothrombinase complex, and blocks its thrombin interaction*		
	Fondaparinux	NSTE-ACS; STEMI	• Not recommended as sole anticoagulant for PCI. An additional anticoagulant should be administered for PCI. • Contraindicated if CrCl is < 30 mL/min

In patients with ACS, anticoagulation, in addition to antiplatelet therapy, is recommended for all patients irrespective of initial treatment strategy. Fondaparinux is not recommended as sole anticoagulant for primary PCI because of the risk of catheter thrombosis. ACS = acute coronary syndrome; ACT = activated clotting time; CrCl = creatinine clearance; GP = glycoprotein; IV = intravenous; NSTE = non–ST-elevation; PCI = percutaneous coronary intervention; SC = subcutaneous; STEMI = ST-elevation myocardial infarction; UFH = unfractionated heparin.

TABLE 6-8 Additional Medications Used for Patients With Acute Coronary Syndrome

Medication Class	Indication	Caution
Morphine	• Pain • Anxiety • Pulmonary edema	• Lethargic or moribund patient • Hypotension • Bradycardia • Prior hypersensitivity
β-Receptor antagonists	• Oral: all patients without contraindication • IV: patients with refractory hypertension or ongoing ischemia without contraindication	• Signs of HF, particularly low-output state and cardiogenic shock • Prolonged first-degree or high-grade AV block • Uncontrolled reactive airway disease
ACE Inhibitors	• For patients with anterior infarction, post-MI LV systolic dysfunction (EF < 40%) • Ok for routine use in all patients without contraindication	• Hypotension • Renal failure • Hyperkalemia
ARB	• For patients intolerant of ACE inhibitors	• Hypotension • Renal failure • Hyperkalemia
Aldosterone antagonist eplerenone	• Added to optimal medical therapy in eligible patients with MI with EF < 40%, DM, or heart failure (creatinine < 2.5 mg/dL in men and < 2.0 mg/dL in women, K < 5.0 mEq/L)	• Renal failure • Hyperkalemia
Statins	• All patients without contraindications	• Prior hypersensitivity • Significant hepatic impairment
Calcium channel blocker	• Initiate therapy with nondihydropyridine CCBs with recurrent ischemia and contraindications to beta-blockers • Cocaine-induced coronary spasm if nitrates and benzodiazepines fail to treat chest pain and hypertension	• Patients with LV dysfunction and cardiogenic shock • Prolonged PR > 0.24 s • Second or third degree AV block without a pacemaker • Immediate-release nifedipine should not be administered
Nitrates: nitroglycerin	• Ongoing ischemia • Hypertension and HF • Cocaine-induced vasospasm, chest pain, and hypertension	• Avoid in suspected RV infarction • Avoid with SBP < 90 mmHg or if SBP < 30 mmHg below baseline • Avoid if recent (24 to 48 h) use of phosphodiesterase inhibitor
Oxygen	• Clinically significant hypoxemia (oxygen saturation < 90%) • HF • Dyspnea	• Caution with COPD and CO_2 retention

The benefit of beta-blockers for secondary prevention is greatest in patients with myocardial infraction (MI) complicated by heart failure (HF), left ventricle (LV) dysfunction and ventricular arrhythmias. Caution should be exercised in patients with evidence of low-output state, as administration of beta-blockers can precipitate cardiogenic shock. ACE = angiotensin-converting enzyme; AV = atrioventricular; ARB = angiotensin II receptor blocker; CCB = calcium channel blocker; COPD = chronic obstructive pulmonary disorder; DM = diabetes mellitus; EF = ejection fraction; RV = right ventricle; SBP = systolic blood pressure.

Echocardiography in Acute Coronary Syndrome

Echocardiography is a noninvasive and inexpensive modality that had diagnostic and prognostic value in diagnosing complications in acute coronary syndromes. It is now included in the universal definition of acute myocardial infarction; however, there is a paucity of recommendations regarding the timing of its use in the acute setting.[10,58-60] Echocardiography should be an adjunct and not an impediment to lifesaving therapy. A caveat to the use of transthoracic echocardiography (TTE) is that performing the study and adequately interpreting the images requires a level of competence and training, and should be supervised by an expert such as a cardiologist.

COMPLICATIONS OF MYOCARDIAL INFARCTION

There is a myriad of complications related to acute MI; however, with increased implementation of early reperfusion strategies post-STEMI, the incidence has decreased. In the reperfusion era, after cardiogenic shock and congestive heart failure, mechanical complications are the most common cause of early mortality after hospitalization for STEMI.[61-63]

Cardiogenic Shock

Cardiogenic shock complicates 5% to 10% of all patients presenting with acute MI and has a mortality rate of approximately 50%.

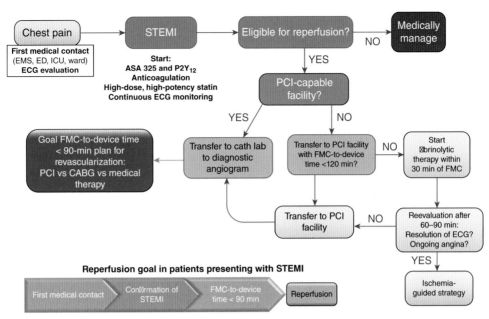

FIGURE 6-3 STEMI pathway. Summary of the pathway for patients with STEMI presenting to PCI-capable and non–PCI-capable facilities. ASA 325 = 325 mg aspirin; CABG = coronary artery bypass grafting; ECG = electrocardiography; ED = emergency department; EMS = emergency medical services; FMC = first medical contact; ICU = intensive care unit; PCI = percutaneous coronary intervention; STEMI = ST-elevation myocardial infarction.

Cardiogenic shock is characterized by persistent hypotension (< 90 mmHg), a need for vasopressors or inotropes to maintain blood pressure above 90 mmHg, a low cardiac index (< 2.2 L/min/m²), elevated filling pressure, and evidence of tissue hypoperfusion.[64-68]

The current STEMI guidelines recommend emergent revascularization in a suitable patient with cardiogenic shock due to pump failure based on results from the SHould we emergently revascularize Occluded Coronaries for Cardiogenic shocK (SHOCK) trial, which demonstrated significantly

lower mortality 6 and 12 months post-revascularization as compared to medical stabilization. The use of intra-aortic balloon pumps (IABP) is recommended for patients with cardiogenic shock after STEMI who do not rapidly stabilize with pharmacological therapy.[2,67-69]

Intra-aortic balloon pumps are the most commonly used mechanical assist device for support in hemodynamically unstable patients with cardiogenic shock. They provide

TABLE 6-9 Contraindications to Fibrinolytic Therapy

Absolute Contraindications to Fibrinolytic Therapy
History of intracranial hemorrhage
Any cerebral vascular lesion
Known intracranial malignancy (primary or metastatic)
Ischemic stroke within 3 mo EXCEPT ischemic stroke within 3 h
Suspected or known aortic dissection
Active bleeding/coagulopathy
Significant closed head trauma

Relative Contraindications
Ischemic stroke > 3 mo
Dementia
Other intracranial pathology
Malignant hypertension
History of severe hypertension
Recent internal bleeding (2–4 wk)
Noncompressive vascular access punctures
Traumatic or prolonged CPR
Pregnancy
Active peptic ulcer
Anticoagulant use
Allergic reaction to fibrinolytic agent or recent exposure

CPR = cardiopulmonary resuscitation.

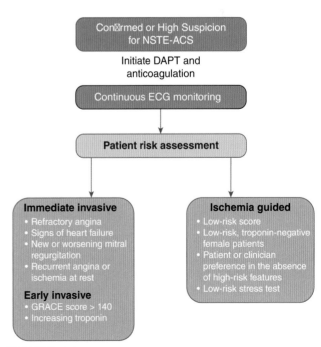

FIGURE 6-4 Early-invasive strategy versus ischemia-guided strategy in patients with NSTE-ACS.

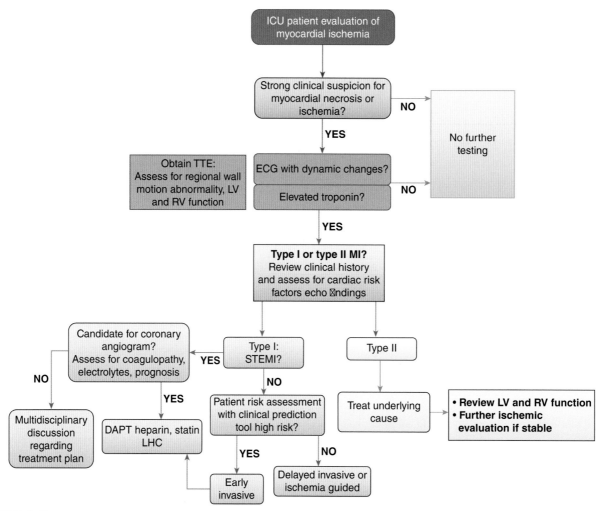

FIGURE 6-5 Proposed diagnostic and management approach to patients in the ICU with elevated troponin. ECG = electrocardiogram; ICU = intensive care unit; DAPT = dual antiplatelet therapy; LHC = left heart catheterization; LV = left ventricle; MI = myocardial infarction; RV = right ventricle; STEMI = ST-elevation myocardial infarction; TTE = transthoracic echocardiogram.

benefit by decreasing afterload and increasing coronary perfusion during diastole by inflating with diastole and deflating in systole. Intra-aortic balloon pump counterpulsation may be used to treat severe persistent or recurrent ischemia, despite maximal medical therapy[67,70-72] (Table 6-10). The Intra-Aortic Balloon Pump in Cardiogenic Shock II (IABP-SHOCK II) trial was a recent trial that randomized patients with acute MI and cardiogenic shock to IABP or no IABP. The study showed no difference in 30-day mortality; however, timing of insertion of IABP was not controlled and 86.6% of IABPs were placed post-PCI.[69] Furthermore, the sample size was small and patients had mild to moderate degrees of shock; therefore, the results may not be entirely generalizable to patients presenting with ACS and severe refractory shock. Intra-aortic balloon pump use in cardiogenic shock is currently a class IIa recommendation in the most recent guidelines.[2]

Left ventricle assist devices (LVAD) may provide superior hemodynamic support compared to IABP. Impella is a

TABLE 6-10 Indications, Contraindications, and Complications for Intra-Abdominal Balloon Pump Use in Patients With Acute Coronary Syndrome

Clinical Indications for IABP
Cardiogenic shock
Low cardiac output after cardiopulmonary bypass
Prophylactic use in high-risk or complicated PCI
Intractable myocardial ischemia awaiting further therapy
Refractory heart failure as a bridge to further therapy
Intractable ventricular arrhythmias as a bridge to further therapy

Complications of IABP
Vascular: limb ischemia, loss of peripheral pulse, local vascular injury, injury to renal artery from malposition, aortic dissection, compartment syndrome
Device complications: balloon rupture
Hematological: thrombocytopenia, hemolysis

Contraindications to IABP
Aortic regurgitation, aortic dissection, aortic stents
Severe sepsis, abdominal aortic aneurysm, severe peripheral vascular disease, major aortic surgery

IABP = intra-aortic balloon pump; PCI = percutaneous coronary intervention.

temporary percutaneous LVAD with a nonpulsatile axial flow pump that propels blood from the left ventricle into the ascending aorta, and its use has increased in recent years. In a small randomized trial comparing Impella 2.5 and IABP in patients with cardiogenic shock, Impella showed improved hemodynamic variables, but not improved mortality.[71,73,74] Additionally, extracorporeal membrane oxygenation (ECMO) can be employed for patients with severe cardiac or pulmonary failure. Venovenous ECMO use is more common for severe respiratory failure, but venoarterial ECMO can be used in severe cardiogenic shock.[75-77]

The indications for ECMO are summarized in Table 6-11.

Other Mechanical Complications

While the incidence of mechanical complications such as free wall rupture, ventricular septal rupture, papillary rupture, and ischemic mitral regurgitation are low, they portend high mortality. The pathophysiological mechanism for mechanical complications is reduced myocardial perfusion resulting in necrosis, neutrophilic infiltration, activation of matrix metalloproteinases and serine proteases causing disruption of the myocytes, increased wall stress, and disruption of the wall.[61,62] Immediate diagnosis of a mechanical complication in a hemodynamically compromised patient is paramount for initiation of the appropriate lifesaving intervention. Emergent 2-dimensional (2-D) transthoracic echocardiogram with color flow Doppler should be obtained to make a diagnosis.

Figure 6-6 demonstrates color flow Doppler in a patient with papillary muscle rupture and severe mitral regurgitation post–inferolateral MI.

Other sequelae include atrial and ventricular arrhythmia, pericarditis, LV thrombus, right ventricular (RV) infarction, LV aneurysm, LV pseudoaneurysm, and dynamic LV outflow tract obstruction causing hemodynamic collapse.[61,62,78-81] Table 6-12 summarizes these complications and their acute management.

TABLE 6-11 Summary of Cardiac Indications and Complications With the utilization of Venoarterial Extracorporeal Membrane Oxygenation for the Management of Cardiopulmonary Collapse

Indications for Venoarterial ECMO	Complications
Failure to wean post–cardiopulmonary bypass	Thrombosis
Short-term bridge to heart transplantation or ventricular assist device insertion	Bleeding and coagulopathy (5–79%)
Perioperative support in congenital heart disease	Limb ischemia (13–25%)
Support after heart transplantation	Infection (17–49%)
Cardiogenic shock resulting in tissue hypoperfusion • Myocardial infarction • Sepsis-induced myocardial depression • Fulminant myocarditis • Cardiomyopathy	Neurologic events (10–33%)
Extracorporeal CPR	
Assisted CPR during cardiac arrest	
Catecholamine crisis and circulatory collapse in pheochromocytoma	
Drug overdose	

CPR = cardiopulmonary resuscitation; ECMO = extracorporeal membrane oxygenation.

Arrhythmia

Arrhythmias are common in patients presenting with ACS and range from life threatening, such as ventricular fibrillation, to relatively benign, such as accelerated idioventricular rhythm seen postreperfusion (Table 6-13). Prehospital ventricular

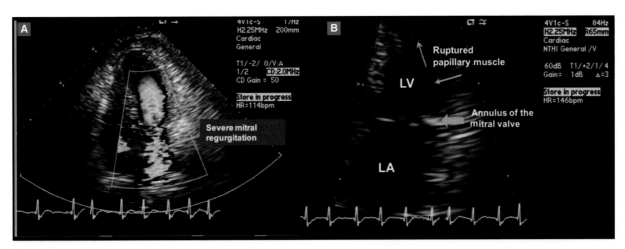

FIGURE 6-6 Color flow Doppler in a patient with papillary muscle rupture and severe mitral regurgitation post inferolateral MI (A) Severe mitral regurgitation. (B) Ruptured papillary muscle in a patient who presents late after acute occlusion of the left circumflex artery.

TABLE 6-12 Mechanical Complications in Patients With Acute Coronary Syndrome

	Incidence	Risk Factors	Presentation	Management
Cardiogenic shock	5–10%	• Extensive LV infarction • Mechanical complications, including papillary muscle rupture, VSD, free-wall rupture with tamponade • RV infarction	• Refractory hypotension • End-organ damage • Encephalopathy	• Revascularization with timely PCI or CABG • Hemodynamic support with inotropic agents • Mechanical support: IABP, Impella, ECMO
Left ventricular free wall rupture	0.5%	• Age • Female gender • Lack of LVH • Large transmural anterior infarct (usually > 20% myocardial involvement), first MI • Hypertension during the acute phase of STEMI, and lack of angina or prior MI • Q waves on ECG • Use of corticosteroids or NSAIDS, and administration of fibrinolytic • Late reperfusion	• Angina, pleuritic chest pain • Syncope • Cardiogenic shock • Tamponade	• Avoid steroids and NSAIDS • Hemodynamic stabilization • Surgical repair
Ventricular septal rupture	0.2%	• Age • Female • Anterior infarct • Tachycardia • Heart failure • Angiographic factors: fewer collaterals and low TIMI flow • Increased mortality in patients with inferior-basal defects than for those with anterior-apical defects	• Usually 3–7 d post-MI • May be initially asymptomatic • Rapid deterioration • Pulmonary edema and cardiogenic shock	• Hemodynamic support with IABP • Evaluation for surgical repair vs percutaneous repair
Papillary muscle rupture	0.26%	• Inferior MI	• Cardiogenic shock and pulmonary edema	• Surgical replacement and sometimes repair for acute papillary muscle or chordae rupture • Vasodilator therapy for acute severe MR

CABG = coronary artery bypass graft; ECG = electrocardiography; ECMO = extracorporeal membrane oxygenation; IABP = intra-aortic balloon pump; LV = left ventricle; LVH = left ventricle hypertrophy; MI = myocardial infarction; MR = mitral regurgitation; NSAIDS = nonsteroidal anti-inflammatory drugs; PCI = percutaneous coronary intervention; STEMI = ST-elevation myocardial infarction; TIMI = Thrombolysis in Myocardial Infarction score; VSD = ventricular septal defect.

TABLE 6-13 Summary of Common Arrhythmias in Patients Presenting With Acute Coronary Syndrome

Rhythm	Management
Accelerated idioventricular rhythm	Benign and well-tolerated reperfusion arrhythmia Does not usually require treatment
VT	Cardioversion for hemodynamically unstable VT Reperfusion Antiarrhythmic drug therapy in accordance with the Advanced Cardiac Life Support guidelines Nonsustained VT immediate post-MI is common and does not require specific treatment
VF	Immediate defibrillation Reperfusion Antiarrhythmic drug therapy in accordance with the Advanced Cardiac Life Support guidelines
Sinus bradycardia	Hemodynamically important sinus bradycardia should be treated with atropine or temporary pacing if not responsive
Complete heart block	Reperfusion Usually transient in inferior MI and can be management with temporary pacing Indications for permanent pacing for persistent AV block or bundle branch block after STEMI are reviewed in the ACC/AHA/HRS device-based therapy guidelines
Atrial fibrillation	Rate control Rhythm control especially in patients with hemodynamic instability; synchronized cardioversion may be required Indications for anticoagulation according to current guidelines

ACC = American College of Cardiology; AHA = American Heart Association; AV = atrioventricular; HRS = Heart Rhythm Association; MI = myocardial infarction; STEMI = ST-elevation myocardial infarction; VF = ventricular fibrillation; VT = ventricular tachycardia.

fibrillation continues to account for most out-of-hospital deaths in patients with acute MI.[82-84] In 2014, 356,500 people experienced out-of-hospital cardiac arrests in the United States, of which only 12% survived. Ventricular fibrillation is the most common shockable rhythm noted postarrest. Survival from out-of-hospital cardiac arrest is optimal when both CPR and defibrillation are initiated early in conjunction with therapeutic hypothermia for patients who remain comatose postresuscitation.[85-89] Emergent coronary angiogram is recommended when the initial ECG is consistent with STEMI. Patients whose initial rhythm is VF in an out-of-hospital cardiac arrest who survive to admission have a 60% rate of survival to hospital discharge after early PCI.[90]

QUESTIONS

1. A 64-year-old-man with a history of CAD with multiple PCI in the past and DM presents to the ED after becoming unresponsive while at a dinner party. Cardiopulmonary resuscitation is initiated by a guest, and when EMS arrives on the scene, he is found to the have the initial rhythm in Figure 6-7A. He is intubated and defibrillated several times, and achieves return of spontaneous circulation (ROSC) within 10 minutes. In the ED, he is unresponsive, and his physical exam is notable for normal S1 and S2 with an S3 gallop, jugular venous pressure (JVP) of 10 cm, rales in bilateral lower lung fields, and cool distal extremities.

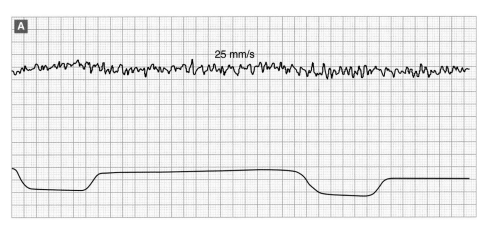

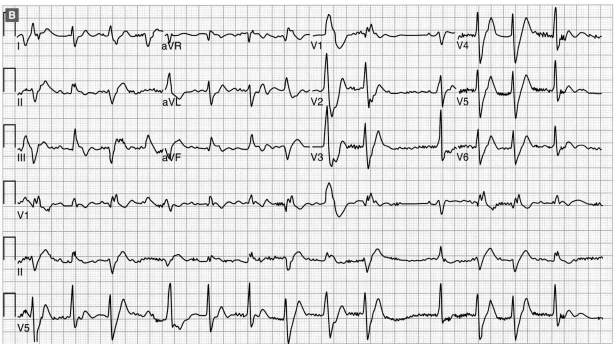

FIGURE 6-7 (A) Strip obtained by emergency medical services. (B) Electrocardiography strip from the emergency department.

While in the ED, he has an episode of pulseless ventricular tachycardia and is cardioverted immediately with ROSC within a minute. Intravenous amiodarone is initiated, as is norepinephrine for persistent hypotension. His vitals are as follows: BP of 80/60 mmHg, heart rate (HR) of 110 beats/min, respiratory rate (RR) of 18 breaths/min, blood oxygen saturation (SpO_2) of 90% on room air with a fraction of inspired oxygen (FiO_2) of 100%. The ECG obtained in the ED is shown in Figure 6-7B. A computed tomography (CT) scan of his head in the ED reveals no acute intracranial pathology. What is the next best step for the patient?

A. Initiate targeted temperature management
B. Urgent electrophysiology consult for arrhythmia management
C. Administer aspirin, ticagrelor, rosuvastatin, and heparin bolus, and activate cardiac catheterization laboratory
D. A and C

2. A patient on hypothermic protocol for cardiac arrest is noted to have a temperature of 30°C. While the team is adjusting the settings to increase his core temperature,

his telemetry reveals sustained ventricular tachycardia. What is the next best step for the patient?

A. Start bretylium (5 mg/kg)
B. Stop hypothermia protocol and immediately begin rewarming the patient
C. Synchronized cardioversion (2 J/kg)
D. B and C

3. A 75-year-old-man with no previous medical history is brought to the ED by his wife for increasing somnolence, which was preceded by several days of chest pain and worsening dyspnea with minimal exertion. She denies recent trauma. His cardiac exam is notable for a 4/6 holosystolic murmur at the apex, and lung auscultation reveals scattered rales in the left lung field. An ECG on arrival to the ED is shown in Figure 6-8A. His vitals are as follows: BP of 90/60 mmHg, HR of 120 beats/min, RR of 20 breaths/min, SpO_2 85% on 3 Liters nasal cannula (NC). Prior to urgent left heart catheterization, the patient undergoes a limited bedside transthoracic echocardiogram, which shows severe mitral regurgitation and flail mitral valve chordae. Color Doppler is shown in Figure 6-8B.

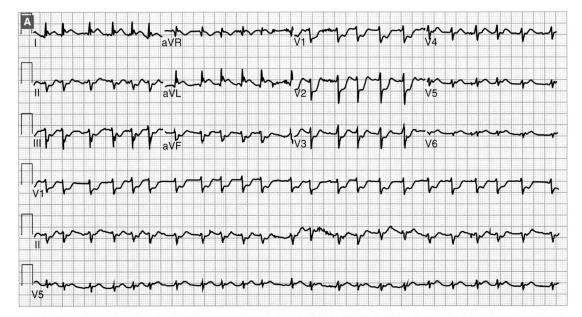

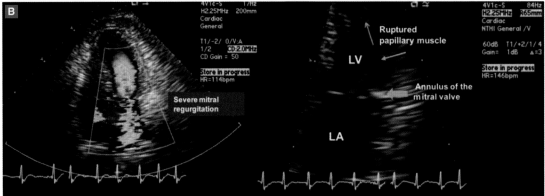

FIGURE 6-8 (A) Electrocardiography tracing. (B) Transthoracic echocardiogram with a 4-chamber view and color Doppler over the mitral valve.

What is the next best step for this patient?

A. Administer fibrinolytics while awaiting clinical stabilization

B. Proceed to left heart catheterization and cardiothoracic consultation

C. Stat bedside transesophageal echocardiogram

D. Intubation

4. A 63-year-old man with medical history of hypertension and peripheral vascular disease presents after an episode of syncope after having acute severe substernal chest pressure. His ECG is shown below (Fig. 6-9A). His vitals in the ED are as follows: BP of 90/60 mmHg and HR of 44 beats/min. On auscultation, there is variable intensity to S1 and examination of the neck veins reveals canon A waves and Kussmaul sign. His home medications are aspirin 81 mg, atorvastatin 20 mg, lisinopril 40 mg, and hydrochlorothiazide 25 mg. The patient is unable to recall when he last took his home medications and receives aspirin 325 mg by EMS en route to the ED. In the ED, he receives clopidogrel 600 mg, atorvastatin 80 mg, and a heparin bolus prior to transfer for emergent coronary angiogram. His angiogram is notable for extensive thrombus and decreased flow in the right coronary artery (Fig. 6-9B).

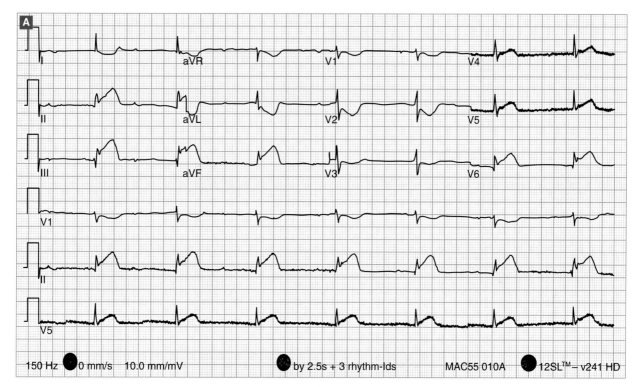

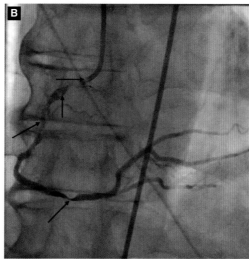

FIGURE 6-9 (A) Electrocardiography tracing. (B) Angiogram showing decreased flow (*black arrows*) in the right coronary artery.

Stat laboratory results obtained in the emergency room are notable for troponin T 0.5 µg/L (N < 0.04 µg/L) and serum creatinine of 1.5 mg/dL. What is the next best step for this patient?

A. Immediate implantation of a permanent pacemaker to maintain atrioventricular synchrony
B. Early reperfusion with primary PCI
C. Administration of beta-blockers
D. Stat transthoracic echocardiogram

5. In patients with right ventricular infarcts, all the following are false EXCEPT:

A. Sublingual nitroglycerin and metoprolol can safely be used for relief of angina.
B. In patients who survive hospitalization, long-term prognosis is poor.
C. Maintenance of atrioventricular synchrony and revascularization does not affect recovery of RV function.
D. The initial therapy for hypotension in patients with RV infarction is volume expansion, up to 2 Liters of normal saline intravenously, while maintaining right atrial pressure less than 18 mmHg.

6. A 61-year-old man with poorly controlled hypertension and medication nonadherence presents to the ED 2 hours after the acute onset of severe substernal chest pain radiating to the back. He also endorses profuse diaphoresis and nausea. He reports that his chest pain was initially stuttering, lasting 5 to 10 minutes and spontaneously resolving; however, for the last hour, he has had severe constant pain. On examination, his blood pressure is 180/60 mmHg, his heart rate is 100 beats/min, his respiratory rate is 18 breaths/min, and his Spo$_2$ is 95% on room air. Cardiac auscultation is notable for a soft S1, a low-pitched early diastolic murmur at the right sternal boarder, and an S3 gallop. Pulmonary exam reveals rales at bilateral bases. The remainder of the physical exam is unremarkable.

His ECG is notable for ST elevation in V$_1$-V$_2$, I, and aVL, and inferolateral ST depressions (Fig. 6-10A). The patient receives aspirin 81 mg, clopidogrel 600 mg, heparin 5000 U, and atorvastatin 80 mg prior to being taken emergently for left heart catheterization for management of his STEMI. Coronary angiogram demonstrates left main artery occlusion (Fig. 6-10B). Percutaneous coronary intervention of the left main artery is performed successfully, but chest pain does not improve and there is concern for a possible dissection flap in the aortic root,

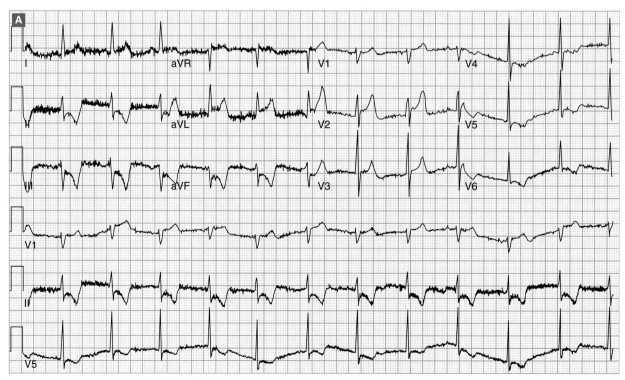

FIGURE 6-10 (A) Electrocardiogram on presentation. (B) Coronary angiogram showing left main obstruction. (C) Transesophageal echocardiography views of the short axis of the ascending aorta.

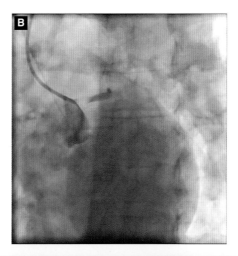

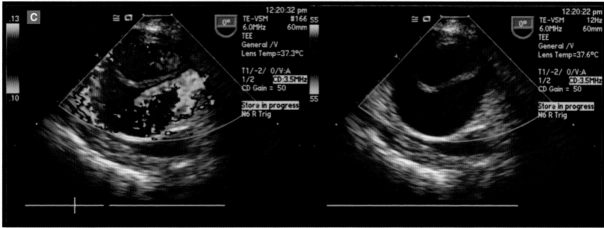

FIGURE 6-10 (*Continued*)

prompting stat transesophageal echocardiogram (TEE). The images are shown in Figure 6-10C.

Which is true regarding the abnormality seen in Figure 6-10C?

A. Surgical repair does not change morbidity and mortality.
B. Mortality exceeds 25% within the first 24 hours if there is no treatment.
C. Pulse deficit is more common in distal than in proximal aortic dissection.
D. Aortography is first line for diagnostic testing in the ED.

7. For the patient in question 6, what is the next best step?

A. Insertion of an IABP to improve hemodynamic status
B. Stat cardiothoracic surgery evaluation
C. Intravenous fluids
D. Confirmation of findings with computed tomography angiography (CTA)

8. An 89-year-old-woman with well-controlled hypertension and dyslipidemia presents with acute severe substernal chest pain that started after news of the death of her best friend. In the ED, she is noted to have an initial ECG with ST elevation anteriorly (Fig. 6-11A). She is taken emergently for coronary angiogram, which reveals no significant coronary artery disease. Her left ventriculogram and echocardiogram are shown in Figures 6-11B and 6-11C, respectively. Her echocardiogram is significant for a moderately reduced ejection fraction, an intracavitary gradient of 66 mmHg, mild mitral regurgitation, and systolic anterior motion of the mitral valve. Troponin T peaked at 3.36 µg/L (N < 0.04 µg/L). The patient is transferred to the coronary care unit for further management, where she develops sustained hypotension. What is the next best step for this patient?

A. Start dobutamine
B. Give intravenous fluids
C. Start norepinephrine
D. Place an intra-aortic balloon pump

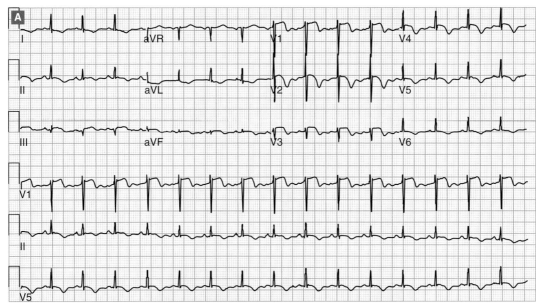

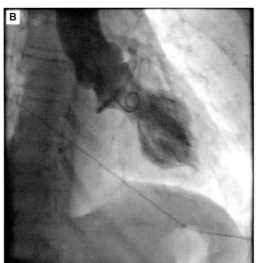

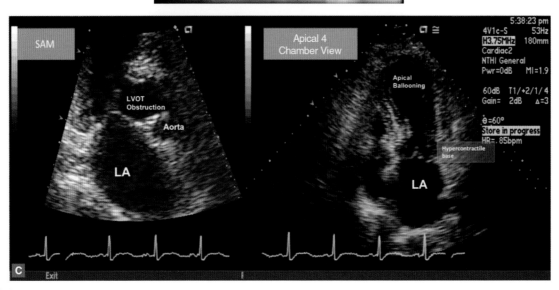

FIGURE 6-11 (A) Electrocardiogram with inferior ST elevations and diffuse T-wave inversion. (B) Left ventriculogram: systolic frame. (C) Transthoracic echocardiogram with systolic frames showing hypercontractile base and apical ballooning.

9. For the patient in question 8, the patient's hemodynamic status significantly improves. What is the next best step for her medical management?

   A. Continue DAPT and high-dose statin
   B. Start carvedilol and lisinopril
   C. Start verapamil
   D. Start disopyramide

10. A 66-year-old Hispanic woman with CAD with prior PCI to the distal LAD and proximal left circumflex artery, chronic arthritis, insulin-dependent diabetes, and hypertension is admitted to the general medicine service for management of right elbow cellulitis and 3 days' duration fever. Her blood cultures grow methicillin-resistant *Staphylococcus aureus* (MRSA). The patient is started on IV vancomycin. Of note, the patient underwent total right elbow replacement 6 months prior to presentation. On hospital day 2, she develops an episode of severe substernal chest pain at rest, associated with diaphoresis and nausea, lasting 10 minutes. Subsequent ECG is notable for diffuse ST depressions (Fig. 6-12A), which resolves when her chest pain diminishes. The patient is started on heparin drip, and aspirin and clopidogrel are continued. She is transferred to the cardiac care unit (CCU) for further management. Her

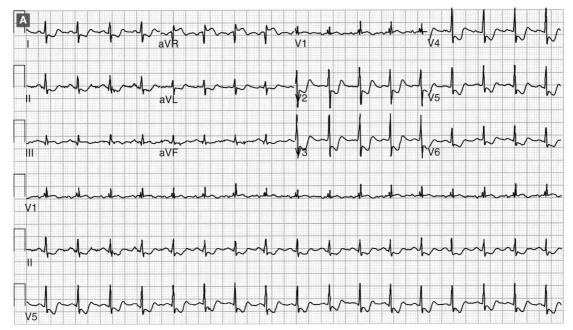

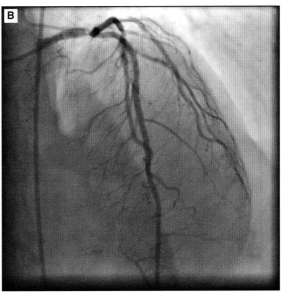

FIGURE 6-12 (A) Electrocardiogram with diffuse ST depression in a patient presenting with chest pain. (B) Coronary angiogram with distal left main lesion.

troponin T peaks at 0.06 μg/L (N < 0.04 μg/L). She develops a second episode of chest pain associated with diaphoresis and shortness of breath, and undergoes urgent coronary angiogram. Her angiogram is significant for severe distal left main stenosis, and multiple tandem obstructive lesions in the LAD (Fig. 6-12B). Cardiac surgery is consulted, but because of her active infection, the decision was made to proceed with PCI, and she subsequently undergoes Impella-assisted PCI. The following statements are true EXCEPT:

A. Morphine should be administered with caution in patients with unstable angina due to an association with increased mortality.
B. Transient ST-segment depression for less than 20 minutes is not considered NSTE-ACS.
C. Early invasive strategy is indicated for patients with NSTE-ACS who have elevated risk for clinical events and have no life-threatening comorbidity.
D. Early invasive strategy is indicated in NSTE-ACS in patients with ongoing chest pain or hemodynamic instability.

11. For the patient in question 10, she remains stable after PCI, and undergoes surgical debridement of a right elbow abscess 5 days after PCI. What is the next best step for the management of her antiplatelet therapy?

A. Continue aspirin and clopidogrel
B. Stop clopidogrel and continue aspirin only
C. Switch to prasugrel and clopidogrel
D. Change clopidogrel to eptifibatide

12. A 24-year-old-man presents to the ED with 2 days of intermittent severe constant substernal chest pain he describes as stabbing in nature, rated 7/10. He denies radiation, associated nausea, emesis or diaphoresis. He notes that his pain is worse with deep inspiration and does not change with position. He does endorse cocaine use on the evening prior to the onset of his pain. His physical exam is unremarkable and vital signs are as follows: BP of 190/80 mmHg, pulse of 100 beats/min, RR of 18 breaths/min, and Spo$_2$ of 98% on room air. His ECG is shown in Figure 6-13.

Laboratory results from the ED are notable for troponin T, 0.4 μg/L (N < 0.04 μg/L); creatine kinase (CK), 200 U/L (N = 0–200 U/L); aspartate aminotransferase (AST), 100 U/L (N = 0–40 U/L); D-dimer, 2.50 μg/mL FEU; and serum creatinine, 1.1 mg/dL. Chest x-ray reveals no acute pulmonary infiltrates. What is the next best step for the patient?

A. Contrast-enhanced CT chest dissection protocol
B. Start high-dose statin, aspirin 81 mg, and Plavix 75 mg
C. Start alprazolam
D. A and C

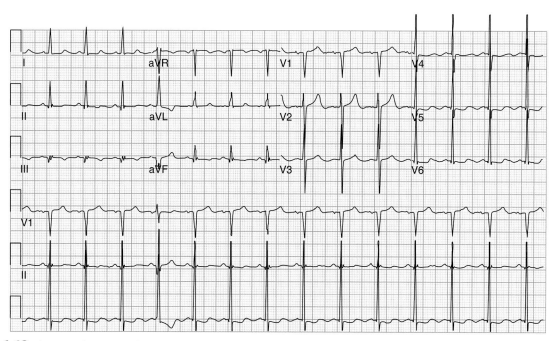

FIGURE 6-13 Electrocardiogram with normal sinus rhythm, left ventricle hypertrophy with early repolarization and inferior infarct age indeterminate.

13. For the patient in question 12, the troponin T peaked at 0.5 µg/L (N < 0.04 µg/L). Transthoracic echocardiogram performed reveals normal left and right ventricular size and function, no regional wall motion abnormalities, and no significant valvular disease. What is the next best step?

    A. Coronary angiogram
    B. Stress ECG
    C. TEE
    D. No further studies

14. A 26-year-old man with no significant past medical history presents to the emergency room with 4 hours of severe substernal chest pressure associated with dyspnea with minimal exertion. Additionally, he reports having had flu-like symptoms, including fever and malaise, 1 week prior to presentation. He denies recreational drug and alcohol abuse. Physical examination is notable for diaphoresis, 8-cm jugular vein distention, and rales to bilateral mid-lung fields. There is no lower extremity edema. An electrocardiogram is notable for inferolateral ST elevations (Fig. 6-14).

    A bedside transthoracic echocardiogram reveals global hypokinesis with severely reduced left ventricular systolic function. His initial troponin I is 4.9 µg/L. The patient undergoes urgent coronary angiogram, which reveals normal coronaries. What is the next best step for facilitating a diagnosis is this patient?

    A. Cardiac magnetic resonance (CMR) imaging to detect myocardial edema, and scattered, nonterritorial myocardial enhancement on late gadolinium
    B. TTE with contrast
    C. Endomyocardial biopsy
    D. Coronary computed tomography angiography (CCTA)

15. The patient in question 14 has an uneventful hospital course; however, a predischarge transthoracic echocardiogram reiterates a dilated left ventricle with severely reduced left ventricular systolic function. What is the next best step for the management of this patient?

    A. Start aspirin 81 mg, clopidogrel 75 mg, atorvastatin 80 mg, daily
    B. Start acyclovir 200 mg twice daily
    C. Start digoxin
    D. Start metoprolol succinate 100 mg daily, enalapril 10 mg twice daily, and spironolactone 25 mg daily

16. A 60-year-old man is admitted to the CCU post anterior wall myocardial infarction complicated by cardiogenic shock. The patient remains hypotensive despite escalating pressors; therefore, an intra-aortic balloon pump is placed. Which of the following does not affect the efficiency of the intra-aortic balloon pump?

    A. Timing of inflation and deflation
    B. Assist ratio
    C. Tachycardia
    D. Patient's age

17. A 55-year-old man presents with cardiogenic shock on IABP. He develops atrial fibrillation overnight. What adjustments need to be made to the programming of the IABP?

    A. No change is necessary
    B. Discontinue the balloon pump
    C. Change the assist ratio to 1:2
    D. Change to pressure trigger

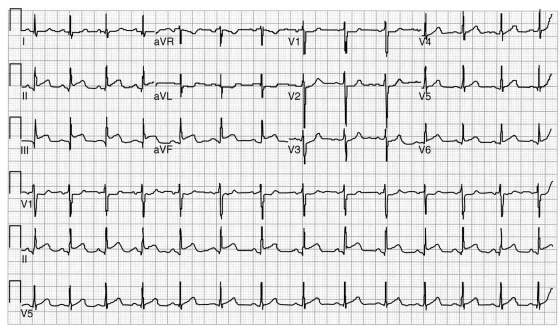

FIGURE 6-14 Electrocardiogram at presentation.

18. A 75-year-old man with no prior significant medical history presents to the ED with acute onset of substernal chest pressure associated with diaphoresis and nausea. He is found to have ST elevation in the anterior leads and is taken urgently for coronary angiogram after receiving ticagrelor 180 mg, atorvastatin 80 mg, and heparin 5000 U bolus in the ED. He is noted to have an acute thrombotic lesion to the mid LAD. Given the high thrombus burden, the patient receives a bolus of abciximab. Two hours after the procedure, an automated platelet count from ethylenediaminetetraacetic acid (EDTA) blood was $70 \times 10^3/\mu L$. Prior to the procedure, it was $270 \times 10^3/\mu L$. What is appropriate at this time?

A. Repeat platelet count in a non-EDTA tube
B. Repeat complete blood count
C. Rule out heparin-induced thrombocytopenia (HIT)
D. All of the above

19. A patient is admitted for STEMI and undergoes a coronary angiogram. The automated platelet count from EDTA blood is $75 \times 10^3/\mu L$. Prior to the procedure, it has been $300 \times 10^3/\mu L$. The patient's medication regimen while in the CCU includes ticagrelor 90 mg every 12 hours, aspirin 81 mg, atorvastatin 80 mg, and metoprolol succinate 25 mg. What is the best next step?

A. Discontinue DAPT and transfuse 1 unit of platelets
B. Discontinue aspirin only
C. Change ticagrelor to 90 mg 1 time daily because it is a potent antiplatelet agent
D. Continue aspirin 81 mg and ticagrelor 90 mg every 12 hours

20. A 22-year-old African American man with unknown medical history presents to the ED after having sudden loss of consciousness while playing basketball. A bystander finds him to be pulseless and initiates CPR. On arrival, EMS personnel find ventricular fibrillation for which he is defibrillated 3 times prior to return of spontaneous circulation. He also receives amiodarone 150 mg and is emergently intubated given his agonal breathing. His postarrest ECG is concerning for acute anterior infarct and diffuse ischemia (Fig. 6-15). What is the next best step?

A. Initiate therapeutic hypothermia
B. Order coronary angiogram to assess for anomalous coronaries, obstructive CAD, and coronary vasospasm
C. Order a toxicology screen
D. All of the above

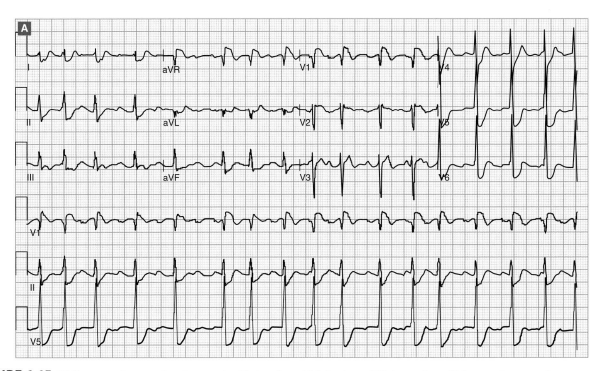

FIGURE 6-15 (A) Electrocardiogram showing anterior ST elevation with inferolateral ST depressions. (B) Repeat electrocardiogram at 5 minutes (atrial flutter with variable block and nonspecific ST-T changes).

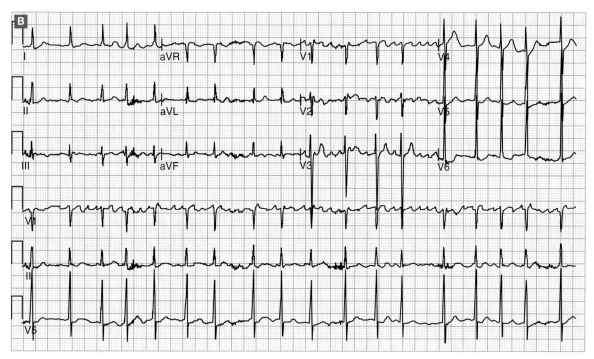

FIGURE 6-15 (*Continued*)

21. A patient is admitted for cardiac arrest. He undergoes a chest x-ray, which reveals pulmonary congestion and an enlarged cardiac silhouette. He has a coronary CT that shows a calcium score of 0 and no coronary artery disease, but does show the left coronary artery arising from the right aortic cusp with a retroaortic course. Additionally, his right ventricle is noted to be dilated with fatty infiltration.

    What is the most likely etiology of sudden cardiac death in this patient?

    A. Anomalous coronary artery
    B. Hypercoagulable state with arterial thrombus
    C. Arrhythmogenic right ventricular dysplasia
    D. Brugada syndrome

22. For an intra-aortic balloon pump, what type of timing error is seen on the arterial waveform below (Fig. 6-16)?

    A. Early inflation
    B. Early deflation
    C. Late inflation
    D. Late deflation

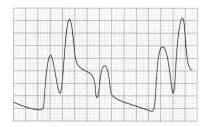

FIGURE 6-16 Aortic balloon pump tracing.

23. A 50-year-old man with anterior wall STEMI has had cardiac catheterization and stent placement in the LAD. He is still hypotensive, oliguric, and in cardiogenic pulmonary edema. He is intubated with pressors initiated and an intra-aortic balloon pump inserted. The patient's cardiac output is 2.5 L/min, urine output has improved 2 mL/kg/h, lactic acid has trended down from 5 to 1 mmol/L, and ECG changes have improved. The patient is still on dobutamine 5 μg/kg. How do you wean off the intra-aortic balloon pump?

    A. Slowly lower pressors and discontinue intra-aortic balloon pump
    B. Slowly go from 1:2 to 1:1
    C. Slowly decrease the balloon by 10% every 1 hour
    D. Abruptly discontinue intra-aortic balloon pump

24. A 40-year-old man has noticed progressive shortness of breath on exertion for the last 2 weeks. Today, he also experiences palpitations prior to syncope. Emergency medical services arrive and he is noted to be in ventricular fibrillation. He has cardioversion and he is started on amiodarone drip. He wakes up right after cardioversion and therefore is not intubated. He has remained in sinus rhythm. On physical examination, his vital signs are BP of 120/80 mmHg, HR of 90 beats/min, RR of 18 breaths/min, Spo₂ of 95%, and a temperature of 97.8°F. His physical examination is unremarkable except for a systolic murmur. An ECG shows LVH and no ST-T wave changes. An echocardiograph shows the left ventricular wall thickness is 30 mm in the basal anterior septum and there is

systolic anterior motion of the mitral valve. What is the next step?

A. Beta-blocker
B. Verapamil
C. Phenylephrine
D. Automated implantable cardioverter-defibrillator

ANSWERS

1. D. A and C

    The patient in the clinical scenario is presenting with ventricular fibrillation, and his post–cardiac arrest ECG is concerning for acute ischemia in the inferolateral coronary territory. The most appropriate next step for this patient is the initiation of hypothermic protocol, now referred to as targeted temperature management (TTM), and prompt coronary angiogram to facilitate revascularization. Therefore, both choices A and C are correct. The patient's initial rhythm on presentation is likely a result of his ischemia; therefore, Advanced Cardiac Life Support protocols should be followed for management of the patient's arrhythmia, and not urgent consultation of the electrophysiology service.

    In patients post–cardiac arrest, neurologic dysfunction and myocardial dysfunction are the major contributors to mortality. Post–cardiac arrest care involves optimization of cardiopulmonary function to maintain adequate organ perfusion as well as employing neuroprotective measures to improve outcomes. Several studies have demonstrated that in patients with out-of-hospital cardiac arrest due to VF, induced hypothermia improves neurological outcomes.[85-87,91] The prevention of neuronal death by employment of this strategy is thought to be pleiotropic, and includes reduction in cerebral edema, reduction in cerebral metabolism, reduction in cytokine release, and reduction in free radical formation.[85,87,92] The current recommendation for adult patients with out-of-hospital VF cardiac arrest who remain comatose is targeted temperature management to 32°C to 36°C for 12 to 24 hours to be initiated within 6 hours of ROSC. This recommendation also applies to comatose adults with ROSC post–out-of-hospital arrest or post in-hospital arrest from any non-VF rhythm, based on retrospective studies, which showed benefit of hypothermia in non-VF arrest.[90,92]

    Of note, the data to support TTM in patients presenting with nonshockable rhythms are derived from small studies. Additionally, there is emerging evidence that suggests that neuroprotection results from prevention of hyperthermia, rather than induction of hypothermia. In a study conducted by Nielsen et al, 950 adults with out-of-hospital cardiac arrest regardless of rhythm were randomly assigned to targeted temperature management at 32°C or 36°C for 36 hours. There was no difference in mortality or

neurological function between the 2 groups.[89] It remains unclear what the benefit of temperature management at 32°C to 34°C versus 36°C is, and whether specific patients benefit from mild hypothermia versus normothermia.[88,93,94] Furthermore, advances in critical care medicine further confound the data, and incremental benefit from targeted temperature management may not be as high. However, the in-hospital mortality post–cardiac arrest is high, therefore, employing a strategy that improves neurological outcomes should be adopted despite the low-quality evidence.

There are 3 phases of TTM that include induction, maintenance, and rewarming. The goal is to initiate surface cooling methods to achieve target temperature within 3 to 4 hours. Important contraindications to TTM include known bleeding diathesis, pre-existing coma prior to arrest or coma related to acute intoxication, sepsis, and major surgery within 14 days, given the increased infection and bleeding risk.[94]

Emergent coronary angiogram and primary PCI are recommended in patients with out-of-hospital cardiac arrest when the initial ECG is consistent with STEMI.[2,90] Given the high prevalence of coronary artery disease in patients with out-of-hospital cardiac arrest, even in patients without STEMI, urgent angiogram should be strongly considered in clinically appropriate scenarios. Figure 6-17 summarizes the approach to a patient presenting with ventricular fibrillation.

2. D. B and C

    The patient in the above clinical scenario has a core temperature lower than that recommended for therapeutic hypothermia, which increases the risk of complications. Important complications related to induced hypothermia include arrhythmias, hyperglycemia, electrolyte derangements, and coagulopathy. Therefore, monitoring of electrolytes, the complete blood count (CBC), and prothrombin time (PT)/partial thromboplastin time (PTT) are essential.[85,87] Starting bretylium (5 mg/kg) (choice A) is incorrect. Although bretylium used to be the most studied agent for management of refractory ventricular tachycardia in the setting of hypothermia, in a study conducted by Stoner et al with anesthetized dogs with induced hypothermic VF, there was no significant improvement in resuscitation rate with placebo, amiodarone, or bretylium.[95] Moreover, bretylium is currently not available in most of the world. The most appropriate next step for this patient is prompt rewarming and, if there is sustained arrhythmia and hemodynamic instability, prompt cardioversion.

3. D. Intubation

    The patient in the clinical scenario has a posterolateral STEMI. Additionally, he has a papillary muscle rupture as a complication to his acute MI, which is further complicated by cardiogenic shock secondary to left ventricular

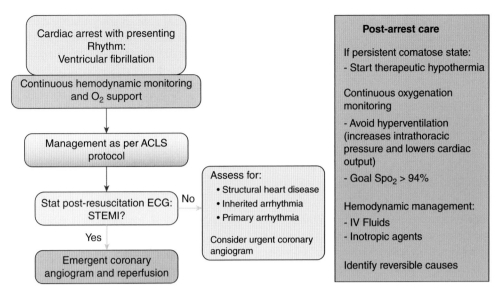

FIGURE 6-17 Management of ventricular fibrillation. ACLS = Advanced Cardiac Life Support; ECG = electrocardiography; IV = intravenous; Spo₂ = blood oxygen saturation; STEMI = ST-elevation myocardial infarction.

pump failure in the setting of myocardial ischemia and acute severe mitral regurgitation. The goal is to first acutely manage and stabilize the patient's hemodynamic and respiratory status; therefore, choice D, intubation, is the best next step.

Early reperfusion for the management of his STEMI and shock is an important next step; however, only after the patient is stabilized for the procedure. Of note, the use of fibrinolytics does not increase survival in patients with ongoing cardiogenic shock.[2,3,47,52] Fibrinolytics are ineffective in patients who are already in cardiogenic shock, as perfusion is significantly impaired, therefore choice A is incorrect.

Prior to proceeding to left heart catheterization to define his anatomy and plan a revascularization strategy, or heading to the operating room for mitral valve repair or replacement, he needs to be stabilized; therefore, choice B would not be the next best step. Transesophageal echocardiogram is not an appropriate next step in a patient with respiratory distress in whom a mechanical complication has already been confirmed; therefore, choice C is incorrect.

4. B. Early reperfusion with primary PCI

The patient is presenting with an acute inferior STEMI, which is complicated by complete heart block. In patients with inferior infarction, right sided ECGs (V₃R-V₆R) should be performed to assess for right ventricular involvement. An ST elevation in V₄R has a sensitivity of approximately 80% and specificity of 76% to 88% in the diagnosis of right ventricular MI.[20,22] In addition to repeat ECG, an echocardiogram is an invaluable, inexpensive, and widely available tool for further assessment of right ventricular function[81,96-98] An echocardiogram would be beneficial if done before an angiogram.

However, the angiogram already identifies the artery involved (choice D). Beta-blockers would make the heart block worse (choice C).

There is a high incidence of complete heart block (CHB) in patients presenting with inferior STEMI as opposed to other culprit lesions. The incidence of all patients with MI complicated by CHB is reported to be between 3% and 13%.[99] Patients presenting with STEMI who have a CHB have higher in-hospital mortality. Primary angioplasty significantly improves AV bock in patients presenting with acute inferior STEMI (choice B), therefore, emergent permanent pacemaker is not indicated as per the ACC/AHA/HRS practice guidelines (choice A).[100]

5. D. The initial therapy for hypotension in patients with RV infarction is volume expansion, up to 2 Liters of normal saline intravenously, while maintaining right atrial pressure less than 18 mmHg.

For patients with right ventricular infarcts, intravenous fluid should be administered, and nitrates should be avoided (choice A), as patients are preload dependent. Emergent primary PCI of the culprit lesion should be performed, since prompt intervention was associated with a higher recovery rate of RV function, atrioventricular synchrony, and 30-day mortality.[101-104] (choice D). In a patient with persistent shock despite the use of inotropic agents, intra-aortic balloon pump counterpulsation and more intensive mechanical support can be employed, including the use of ventricular assist devices (VAD). (choice C) While short-term prognosis in patients with RV infarct and hemodynamic instability is similar to patients with cardiogenic shock, patients who survive hospitalization have favorable outcomes (choice B).[81,97,98,103,104] The SHOCK study demonstrated that survival curves remained relatively stable with an annual mortality rate of 8 to 10 deaths per 100 patient-years, 1 year after revascularization.[98]

6. B. Mortality exceeds 25% within the first 24 hours if there is no treatment.

The patient in the clinical vignette has a type A dissection complicated by extension of the dissection flap into the ostium of the left main coronary artery. Compression or occlusion of the coronary ostia or frank propagation of the dissection process into the coronary vessel explains the STE seen on the ECG of a patient presenting with such complications.

Type A dissection is associated with life-threatening complications, including cardiac tamponade, acute aortic regurgitation, stroke, and myocardial infarction, and without surgical intervention, there is a 1% to 2% mortality rate per hour, making choice B correct. Myocardial ischemia and infarction may be present in 10% to 15% of patients with aortic dissection.[105-107]

While surgery is the first line intervention, it may be avoided in patients with concurrent comorbid conditions, such as advanced malignancy, which have a significant impact on 1-year survival or patients with hemorrhagic stroke (choice A). Choice C is incorrect because pulse deficits are more commonly seen in patients with proximal aortic dissections, as there is increased likelihood of compression of the true lumen of arterial side branches by an expanding hematoma or the dissection flap.

Digital subtraction angiography is historically the gold standard for evaluating a patient with high suspicion for aortic dissection; however, it has largely been replaced by CTA because of its noninvasive nature and the secondary information ascertained regarding distal complications, as well as delineation of the false lumen and assessment for intramural hematoma (choice D). Magnetic resonance imaging (MRI) also has high sensitivity and specificity for detecting aortic dissection and does not require intravenous iodinated contrast. Additionally, it detects and quantifies aortic regurgitation. Limitations associated with MRI include its limited availability emergently and the long time for image acquisition. Transesophageal echocardiogram is fast and portable and in unstable patients is the preferred study. It has 98% sensitivity and 95% specificity for the diagnosis of acute aortic regurgitation; however, it is semi-invasive and operator dependent. Additionally, there may be incomplete investigation of the distal ascending aorta and the proximal aortic arch with TEE.[59,108]

7. B. Stat cardiothoracic surgery evaluation

Acute type A dissection is a surgical emergency; therefore, choice B is correct. Severe aortic regurgitation as seen with this patient is a contraindication to the insertion of an intra-aortic balloon pump; therefore, choice A is incorrect. Type A dissection was confirmed with TEE; therefore,

additional confirmatory testing does not need to be performed unless there is concern for distal complications[105] (choice D). Intravenous fluid administration would be inappropriate in this patient, as he is hypertensive; therefore, choice C would be incorrect.

8. B. Give intravenous fluid

This patient has stress-induced cardiomyopathy, also referred to as Takotsubo cardiomyopathy or broken-heart syndrome. This was first described in Japan in 1990, and was characterized by chest pain with electrocardiographic evidence of ischemia, usually deep symmetrical T-wave inversions, transient apical ballooning with hypokinesis or regional wall motion abnormality in a noncoronary distribution, and absence of angiographic evidence of significant obstructive coronary artery disease or acute plaque rupture.[23,109,110] Patients also typically have recovery of their left ventricular systolic function within 3 to 6 months. It should be noted that this is a diagnosis of exclusion, and patients need to have an ischemia evaluation prior to definitive diagnosis of Takotsubo cardiomyopathy. The pathogenesis is not well understood and there is a myriad of proposed mechanisms for this phenomenon; however, the prevailing mechanism seems to be a catecholamine-mediated myocardial dysfunction.[110] In this patient, there is evidence of left ventricular outflow tract (LVOT) obstruction, given the hyperdynamic motion of the basal segments. Patients with LVOT gradients are susceptible to volume depletion, which can lead to hypotension. Administering IV fluids is the first option for management of hypotension with evidence of dynamic LVOT obstruction (choice B). Additional inotropic agents such as dobutamine (choice A) and norepinephrine (choice C) will increase the hypercontractility of the basal segments. This will worsen the dynamic LVOT obstruction. This is the same rationale for the cautionary use of inotropic agents in hypertrophic obstructive cardiomyopathy (HOCM) with systolic anterior motion of mitral valve (SAM). Inotropic agents will cause SAM to come closer to septum; therefore worsening the dynamic LVOT obstruction. Intra-aotic balloon pump (choice D) will decrease afterload and can worsen symptoms, particularly if there is SAM. It is not the first line of treatment for hypotension from LVOT.

9. B. Start carvedilol and lisinopril

Most patients with Takotsubo cardiomyopathy have concurrent CAD; however, if there is no post-angiography evidence of an acute thrombotic lesion, coronary dissection, coronary vasospasm, unstable plaque, or high-grade stenotic lesions, or even if there is no additional pathology to explain the left ventricular dysfunction, then the primary management strategy should focus on acute heart failure.[110] While there are no randomized trials regarding optimal medical management, patients are treated for heart failure with beta-blockers, ACEIs, or angiotensin II receptor blockers (ARBs) and diuretics as needed for volume overload states (choice B). Verapamil (choice C) and disopyramide (choice D) are not indicated for acute heart failure. In fact, verapamil's negative inotropy may further exacerbate acute heart failure. Dual antiplatelet therapy and statin (choice A) are of unknown benefit in Takotsubo cardiomyopathy.

10. B. Transient ST-segment depression for less than 20 minutes is not considered NSTE-ACS.

All the choices but choice B are correct. The patient in this vignette has a high-risk ECG, characterized by diffuse marked horizontal ST depressions. Given her prior history of CAD, coupled with her ongoing typical anginal symptoms, it is appropriate to pursue an early invasive strategy (choices C and D). The employment of risk stratification models would further support this decision (refer to the text). Figure 6-18 summarizes the early-invasive versus ischemia-guided strategies in NSTE-ACS. Morphine (choice A) has been suggested to increase mortality in NSTE-ACS and should be used with caution.[111]

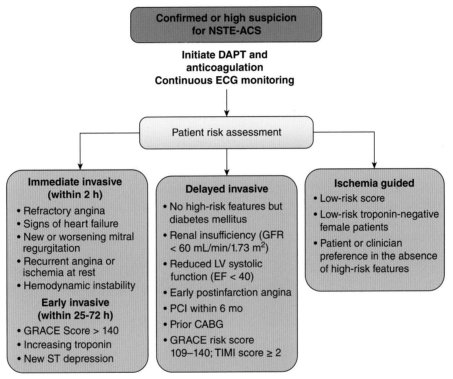

FIGURE 6-18 Early-invasive versus ischemia-guided strategies in non–ST elevation acute coronary syndrome (NSTE-ACS). CABG = coronary artery bypass graft; DAPT = dual antiplatelet therapy; ECG = electrocardiography; EF = ejection fraction; GFR = glomerular filtration rate; GRACE = Global Registry of Acute Coronary Events; LV = left ventricle; PCI = percutaneous coronary intervention; TIMI = Thrombolysis in Myocardial Infarction.

11. A. Continue aspirin and clopidogrel

For patients undergoing nonurgent surgical procedures, 60 days or more should elapse after a myocardial infarction before proceeding to noncardiac surgery. The postoperative MI rate decreases substantially as the length of time from MI to operation increases[112]:

- 0 to 30 days: 32.8%
- 31 to 60 days: 18.7%
- 61 to 90 days: 8.4%
- 91 to 180 days: 5.9%

In patients post–elective PCI, elective noncardiac surgery should be delayed optimally by 6 months after drug-eluting stent implantation and 1 month after bare metal stent implantation.[113] In post-PCI patients in whom noncardiac surgery is required, a consensus decision among treating clinicians as to the relative risks of surgery and discontinuation or continuation of antiplatelet therapy can be useful. Furthermore, if the risk of further delay is greater than the expected risks of ischemia and stent thrombosis, the patient may proceed to the planned surgical intervention. In this case, the patient is undergoing a wound debridement of the elbow and therefore should not have interruption of her DAPT, as this is a low risk procedure with a low risk of excessive bleeding (choice A).[1112-115] The risk for in-stent thrombosis is high if aspirin is continued but clopidogrel is discontinued, therefore choice B is wrong. There is no added benefit from switching aspirin to prasugrel (choice C). Integrilin (Eptifibatide) is given during percutaneous coronary intervention and is not indicated in this case (choice D).

12. **D. A and C**

Cocaine is a potent sympathomimetic agent that has multiple cardiovascular and hematologic effects that likely contribute to the development of myocardial ischemia. It is also a potent vasoconstrictor and therefore causes coronary spasm and decreases myocardial blood flow.[116-118] In a young patient presenting post–cocaine use with chest pain, cocaine-induced coronary spasm is a most likely diagnosis, but acute coronary syndromes, as well as other important vascular complications such as aortic dissection need to be considered (choice A). It is important to note that cocaine may also cause rhabdomyolysis, which increases myoglobin and total creatine kinase levels, which may further confound the diagnosis of cocaine-associated MI. Only 0.7% to 6% of patients with cocaine-associated chest pain have acute plaque rupture; therefore, the employment of risk stratification clinical tools helps minimize inappropriate invasive procedures and prolonged hospitalizations.[117-121]

Benzodiazepines (choice C) and nitroglycerin are the first-line therapies for cocaine-induced chest pain. For persistent hypertension, IV nitroglycerine and nitroprusside may be used. Calcium channel blockers may be used if nitroglycerine or nitroprusside fails to improve the hypertension.[120] Therefore, choice D is the most appropriate. High-dose statin, aspirin, and Plavix are of unproven benefit in this scenario (choice B).

13. **D. No further studies**

While the most likely etiology of the patient's chest pain and mild troponin elevation is coronary vasospasm secondary to cocaine use, it is not unreasonable to assess the patient for anomalous coronaries. However, obstructive CAD is highly unlikely in a 24-year-old-man without risk factors. An ischemic evaluation would be inappropriate for this patient (choices A and B), and TEE would not add additional information (choice C). Therefore, choice D would be most appropriate.

14. **A. Cardiac magnetic resonance (CMR) imaging to detect myocardial edema, and scattered, nonterritorial myocardial enhancement on late gadolinium**

Diagnosis of myocarditis is difficult owing to the lack of specific and sensitive diagnostic techniques. There is a myriad of infectious and noninfectious etiologies, including viruses, fungi, toxins, and bacteria; however, the underlying etiology is usually not identified.[122] Additionally, patients with myocarditis may have clinical and electrocardiographic evidence that is suggestive of an acute coronary syndrome, but they will have no evidence of acute plaque rupture on coronary angiography. Cardiac magnetic resonance provides both structural and function characterization of the myocardium including regional differences in tissue characteristics that TTE (choice B) and CCTA (choice D) do not. Late gadolinium enhancement coupled with T2 imaging help differentiate ACS from myocarditis.[122-126] Post-ACS, there is typically a subendocardial or transmural pattern of late enhancement; however, with myocarditis, late gadolinium enhancement is typically epicardial, mid-wall, or patchy.[127] According to a joint scientific statement from the AHA, the American College of Cardiology Foundation (ACCF), and the European Society of Cardiology (ESC), class I recommendation for endomyocardial biopsy is in patients with clinical heart failure who have (A) a normal sized or dilated left ventricle, less than 2 weeks of symptoms, and hemodynamic instability, or (B) a dilated ventricle, 2 weeks to 3 months of symptoms, new ventricular arrhythmias, or Mobitz type II second degree or third degree heart block[127] The patient in the scenario is hemodynamically stable without arrhythmia, therefore choice C is incorrect.

15. **D. Start metoprolol succinate 100 mg daily, enalapril 10 mg twice daily, and spironolactone 25 mg daily**

Patients with myocarditis who present with a dilated cardiomyopathy should receive standard treatment for heart failure, per the most recent guideline recommendations. For patients with a left ventricular ejection fraction less than 40%, ACE inhibitors and β-adrenergic blocking agents should be employed.[128] Antiplatelets and statins (choice A), acyclovir (choice B), and digoxin (choice C) have not been proven to be beneficial in myocarditis.

16. **D. Patient's age**

The IABP is a volume displacement device that uses the principle of counter-pulsation (inflation during diastole and deflation during systole) to increase coronary perfusion pressure, increase systemic perfusion pressure, decrease SVR, increase cardiac output, and reduce afterload.[67,70,72] Timing of inflation and deflation (choice A), assist ratio such as 1:1, 1:2, or 1:3 (choice B), and tachycardia (choice C) all have cardiogenic influences; therefore will affect the efficacy of the IABP. Age does not influence IABP.

17. **C. Change the assist ratio to 1:2**

The patient in the clinical scenario continues to be hypotensive and develops an arrhythmia, which is problematic because triggering the IABP is dependent on the patient's ECG tracing and can be impaired in the setting of arrhythmia or poor ECG tracing. Therefore, an intervention is necessary (choice A). Patient is still hemodynamically unstable, therefore, discontinuing the balloon pump would be inappropriate. (choice B) There are multiple strategies for atrial fibrillation with rapid ventricular response. These strategies include changing to atrial fibrillation trigger mode if available on the console and changing the assist ratio to 1:2 or 1:3 (choice C) given the variable R to R and tachycardia. Pressure trigger mode is not recommended in irregular rhythms (choice D).

18. **D. All of the above**

Exposure to antiplatelet and anticoagulation therapy post-PCI increases the risk of hematological complications, which include thrombocytopenia and bleeding. The incidence of thrombocytopenia post-PCI varies in reports (3–16.5%) and is related to increased morbidity and mortality. Pseudothrombocytopenia secondary to platelet aggregation with EDTA, lab error, and dilution after a massive RBC transfusion needs to be ruled out to avoid inappropriate cessation of antiplatelet therapy. Pseudothrombocytopenia should be distinguished from true thrombocytopenia by repeating a platelet count using blood anticoagulated with citrate or checking a peripheral blood smear (choice A).[129,130]

Another important cause of thrombocytopenia is heparin-induced thrombocytopenia (HIT; choice C), which typically occurs 5 to 10 days after initial heparin exposure, and can be complicated by arterial and venous thrombosis. Confirmation with serotine release assay should be done and anticoagulation should be replaced with direct thrombin inhibitors (DTI) lepirudin, argatroban, or bivalirudin.[131,132] Based on data from the Randomized Evaluation in PCI Linking Angiomax to Reduced Clinical Events 2 (Replace 2), Acute Catheterization and Urgent Intervention Triage strategY" Trial (ACUITY), Harmonizing Outcomes with Revascularization and Stents in Acute Myocardial Infraction study (HORIZONS-AMI), Bleeding with antithrombotic therapy (BAT) trials, for patients with STEMI and HIT who require stenting, bivalirudin is the preferred anticoagulant.[2,19] Another important cause of thrombocytopenia is post glycoprotein (GP) IIb/IIIa inhibitor use, especially abciximab (a modified chimeric monoclonal antibody). Multiple etiologies are proposed for GP IIb/IIIa inhibitor–induced thrombocytopenia, and include immune-mediated platelet consumption and pseudothrombocytopenia secondary to immune-mediated platelet clumping. Platelets should be checked 2 to 4 hours after administration of GP IIb/IIIa inhibitors, particularly abciximab.[133-136]

19. **D. Continue aspirin 81 mg and ticagrelor 90 mg every 12 hours**

Patients with moderate or high-risk ACS who develop thrombocytopenia post-PCI are at increased risk of mortality (choice A and B are wrong) and major bleeding as opposed to those who do not. The patient is several hours post–anterior wall STEMI and does not have severe thrombocytopenia or evidence of life-threatening bleeding; therefore, the patient should continue DAPT to prevent

stent thrombosis (choice A). Ticagrelor is dosed every 12 hours, therefore choice C would be inappropriate.

20. **D. All of the above**

Coronary artery disease is the most common etiology for sudden cardiac death; however, in young patients (18–35 years), the incidence of SCD-related atherosclerotic CAD is 0.7 per 100,000 person-years.[82] The most common causes of nonischemic sudden cardiac death are cardiomyopathies, including hypertrophic cardiomyopathy and arrhythmogenic right ventricular cardiomyopathy, as well as channelopathies.[82,84] The patient in the scenario has an out-of-hospital arrest with altered mental status; therefore, hypothermic protocol should be initiated (choice A). Additionally, acute intoxication should be ruled out (choice C). A coronary angiogram should be performed to assess for anomalous coronaries, obstructive CAD, and coronary vasospasm as potential inciting etiologies for the arrhythmia (choice B).

21. **C. Arrhythmogenic right ventricular dysplasia**

While the coronary CT findings are consistent with an anomalous coronary artery, there are no mentioned high-risk features, such as interarterial course or fish mouth ostium; therefore, it unlikely to the etiology of the patient's sudden cardiac death (choice A).[137] The patient's ECG on presentation is not consistent with Brugada syndrome. Brugada type 1 (choice D) is usually characterized by coved ST-segment elevation greater than 2 mm in more than 1 lead of V_1-V_3, and is referred to as the Brugada sign.[138-140] Additionally, the incidence is higher in South East Asian men.[139]

The right ventricular findings on the patient's CT is consistent with arrhythmogenic right ventricular dysplasia (ARVD), which is characterized by fibrofatty infiltration of the right ventricular myocardium and is associated with ventricular arrhythmias and sudden cardiac death. It is the second most common cause of sudden cardiac death after hypertrophic obstructive cardiomyopathy (HOCM) (choice C).[83,90,141-143]

22. **C. Late inflation**

An IABP is based on counterpulsation: a balloon inflation during diastole (middle of the T wave on ECG), which increases diastole pressure and deflation in early systole, which decreases LV afterload (the peak of the R wave), causing volume displacement in the aorta and improved coronary and systemic perfusion via the Windkessel effect (Fig. 6-19). It has 2 components: a double lumen catheter with a 25- to 50-mL balloon and a console with a pump to drive the balloon. The tip of the balloon should be 1 to 2 cm distal to the origin of the left subclavian artery by the second rib and the caudal end should be above the origin of the renal arteries by the first and second lumbar vertebral bodies.[144-146] In addition to monitoring IABP placement, there are 4 types of timing errors to troubleshoot.[144]

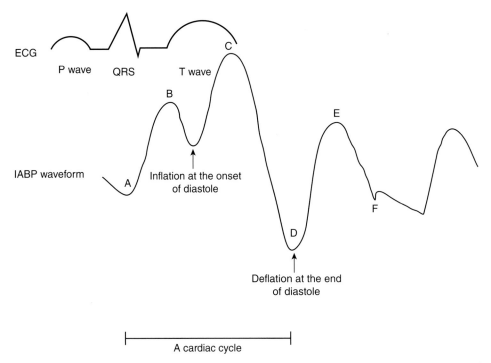

ECG

P wave   QRS   T wave

IABP waveform

Inflation at the onset
of diastole

Deflation at the end
of diastole

A cardiac cycle

FIGURE 6-19 (A) Unassisted aortic end-diastolic pressure. (B) Unassisted systolic pressure. At this point, the balloon inflates and improves coronary perfusion. (C) Diastolic augmentation causing peak diastolic pressure. At this point, the balloon deflates, decreasing afterload, cardiac work, and oxygen consumption. This improves cardiac output. (D) Reduced end-diastolic pressure. (E) This is the assisted peak systolic pressure. (F) This is the dicrotic notch.

Early balloon inflation occurs prior to aortic valve closure, causing an increase in LVEDP, LVEDV, wall stress, and oxygen demand. There is a pointed notch between Points B and C in Figure 6-19. This can be improved by setting inflation after the dicrotic notch (choice A).[145,146]

With early balloon deflation, the peak systolic pressure and assisted peak systolic pressure waves can appear similar or slightly less. Point B and Point E in Figure 6-19 would appear similar. This will not decrease afterload. This can be improved by balloon deflation before the onset of systole (choice B).[145,146]

Late balloon inflation occurs long after aortic valve closure, and the dicrotic notch precedes inflation, which can sometimes create a W shape between Point B and C in Figure 6-19. This has insufficient augmentation and is improved by inflating the balloon immediately after dicrotic notch (choice C).[145,146]

With late balloon deflation, peak systolic pressure exceeds the assisted peak systolic pressure or Point B exceeds Point E in Figure 6-19, with ejection against increased afterload. This is improved by deflation before the onset of systole (choice D).[145,146]

23. C. Slowly decrease the balloon by 10% every 1 hour

2 proposed 5-hour protocols suggest gradually decreasing the assist from 1:1 to 1:2 for 4 hours then to 1:3 for 1 hour, or 10% gradual deflation of the balloon for the next 5 hours

while monitoring hemodynamics, lactic acid, and urine output.[147-149] Abrupt cessation of IABP (choice D) or discontinuation of pressors (choice A) are not approaches used to wean off the IABP. The sequence in choice B is not correct.

24. A. Beta-blocker

The patient has hypertrophic obstructive cardiomyopathy (HOCM). This is caused by an autosomal dominant mutation on the following genes: beta myosin heavy chain, myosin binding protein C, troponin T, troponin I, alpha tropomyosin, regulatory light chain, and essential light chain. Genetic familial studies (Class of Recommendation [COR] I, Level of Evidence [LOE] B), ECG (COR I, LOE C), Holter monitor (COR I, LOE C), and transthoracic echocardiogram (Class I, LOE B) are used for the initial screening for HOCM.[150] On echocardiogram, there is left ventricular wall thickness of 15 mm or greater, most commonly in the basal anterior septum, and 30 mm or greater represents the highest risk for sudden cardiac death.[150] There is a systolic anterior motion of the mitral valve that can perpetuate the symptoms associated with HOCM. The gradient can appear normal at rest but when elicited with a stress test, it can be 30 mmHg or greater. Cardiac magnetic resonance can be obtained if diagnosis is nonocclusive.

Medical treatment for dyspnea consists of beta-blockers (COR I, LOE B)[150] (choice A) or verapamil (choice B) if beta-blockers are not improving symptoms (LOE B). Verapamil may be harmful if the patient is hypotensive or has severe dyspnea at rest (LOE B). If the patient is hypotensive, phenylephrine is the pressor of choice (COR I, LOE B) (choice C). Medically refractory HOCM can be treated with septal reduction surgery (COR I, LOE B) or surgical septal myectomy and alcohol septal ablation (COR II, LOE C).[150] An AICD is indicated prior to cardiac arrest, ventricular fibrillation, or unstable ventricle tachycardia (COR I, LOE B)[150] (choice D).

REFERENCES

1. Amsterdam EA, Wenger NK, Brindis RG, et al. 2014 AHA/ACC Guideline for the Management of Patients with Non-ST-Elevation Acute Coronary Syndromes: a report of the American College of Cardiology/American Heart Association Task Force on Practice Guidelines. *J Am Coll Cardiol.* 2014;64(24):e139-e228.

2. O'Gara PT, Kushner FG, Ascheim DD, et al; American College of Cardiology Foundation/American Heart Association Task Force on Practice Guidelines. 2013 ACCF/AHA guideline for the management of ST-elevation myocardial infarction: a report of the American College of Cardiology Foundation/American Heart Association Task Force on Practice Guidelines. *Circulation.* 2013;127(4):e362-e425.

3. Terkelsen CJ, Pinto DS, Thiele H, et al. 2012 ESC STEMI guidelines and reperfusion therapy: evidence base ignored, threatening optimal patient management. *Heart.* 2013;99(16):1154-1156.

4. McKay RG. "Ischemia-guided" versus "early invasive" strategies in the management of acute coronary syndrome/non–ST-segment elevation myocardial infarction. *J Am Coll Cardiol.* 2003;41(4 Suppl 1):S96-S102.

5. Yan AT, Yan RT, Tan M, et al. In-hospital revascularization and one-year outcome of acute coronary syndrome patients stratified by the GRACE risk score. *Am J Cardiol.* 2005;96(7):913-916.

6. Berlot G, Vergolini A, Calderan C, Bussani R, Torelli L, Lucangelo U. Acute myocardial infarction in non-cardiac critically ill patients: a clinical-pathological study. *Monaldi Arch Chest Dis.* 2010;74(4):164-171.

7. Lim W, Whitlock R, Khera V, et al. Etiology of troponin elevation in critically ill patients. *J Crit Care.* 2010;25(2):322-328.

8. Vasile VC, Chai H-S, Abdeldayem D, Afessa B, Jaffe AS. Elevated cardiac troponin T levels in critically ill patients with sepsis. *Am J Med.* 2013;126(12):1114-1121.

9. Sandoval Y, Smith SW, Schulz KM, et al. Diagnosis of type 1 and type 2 myocardial infarction using a high-sensitivity cardiac troponin I assay with sex-specific 99th percentiles based on the third universal definition of myocardial infarction classification system. *Clin Chem.* 2015;61(4):657-663.

10. Thygesen K, Alpert JS, Jaffe AS, Simoons ML, Chaitman BR, White HD. Third universal definition of myocardial infarction. *Circulation.* 2012:126(16):2020-2035.

11. White HD, Thygesen K, Alpert JS, Jaffe AS. Clinical implications of the third universal definition of myocardial infarction. *Heart.* 2014;100(5):424-432.

12. Liang M, Puri A, Devlin G. The vulnerable plaque: the real villain in acute coronary syndromes. *Open Cardiovasc Med J.* 2011;5:123-129.

13. Crea F, Liuzzo G. Pathogenesis of acute coronary syndromes. *J Am Coll Cardiol.* 2013;61(1):1-11.

14. Nesto RW, Kowalchuk GJ. The ischemic cascade: temporal sequence of hemodynamic, electrocardiographic and symptomatic expressions of ischemia. *Am J Cardiol.* 1987;59(7):C23-C30.

15. Mozaffarian D, Benjamin EJ, Go AS, et al; American Heart Association Statistics Committee; Stroke Statistics Subcommittee. Executive summary: heart disease and stroke statistics—2016 update: a report from the American Heart Association. *Circulation.* 2016;133(4):447-454.

16. Guest TM, Ramanathan AV, Tuteur PG, Schechtman KB, Ladenson JH, Jaffe AS. Myocardial injury in critically ill patients. A frequently unrecognized complication. *JAMA.* 1995;273(24):1945-1949.

17. Noble J, Reid A, Jordan L, Glen A, Davidson J. Troponin I and myocardial injury in the ICU. *Br J Anaest.* 1999;82(1):41-46.

18. Rennyson SL, Hunt J, Haley MW, Norton HJ, Littmann L. Electrocardiographic ST-segment elevation myocardial infarction in critically ill patients: an observational cohort analysis. *Crit Care Med.* 2010;38(12):2304-2309.

19. Levine GN, Bates ER, Bittl JA, et al. 2016 ACC/AHA guideline focused update on duration of dual antiplatelet therapy in patients with coronary artery disease: a report of the American College of Cardiology/American Heart Association Task Force on Clinical Practice Guidelines: an update of the 2011 ACCF/AHA/SCAI guideline for percutaneous coronary intervention, 2011 ACCF/AHA guideline for coronary artery bypass graft surgery, 2012 ACC/AHA/ACP/AATS/PCNA/SCAI/STS guideline for the diagnosis and management of patients with stable ischemic heart disease, 2013 ACCF/AHA guideline for the management of ST-elevation myocardial infarction, 2014 AHA/ACC guideline for the management of patients with non-ST-elevation acute coronary syndromes, and 2014 ACC/AHA guideline on perioperative cardiovascular evaluation and management of patients undergoing noncardiac surgery. *Circulation.* 2016;134(10):e123-e155.

20. Zalenski RJ, Rydman RJ, Sloan EP, et al. Value of posterior and right ventricular leads in comparison to the standard 12-lead electrocardiogram in evaluation of ST-segment elevation in suspected acute myocardial infarction. *Am J Cardiol.* 1997;79(12):1579-1585.

21. Mead NE, O'Keefe KP. Wellen's syndrome: an ominous EKG pattern. *J Emerg Trauma Shock.* 2009;2(3):206-208.

22. Brady WJ, Chan TC, Pollack M. Electrocardiographic manifestations: patterns that confound the EKG diagnosis of acute myocardial infarction—left bundle branch block, ventricular paced rhythm, and left ventricular hypertrophy. *J Emerg Med.* 2000;18(1):71-78.

23. Prasad A. Apical ballooning syndrome: an important differential diagnosis of acute myocardial infarction. *Circulation.* 2007;115(5):e56-e59.

24. Keller T, Zeller T, Ojeda F, et al. Serial changes in highly sensitive troponin I assay and early diagnosis of myocardial infarction. *JAMA.* 2011;306(24):2684-2693.

25. Hamm CW, Goldmann BU, Heeschen C, Kreymann G, Berger J, Meinertz T. Emergency room triage of patients with

acute chest pain by means of rapid testing for cardiac troponin T or troponin I. *N Engl J Med.* 1997;337(23):1648-1653.

26. Irfan A, Reichlin T, Twerenbold R, et al. Early diagnosis of myocardial infarction using absolute and relative changes in cardiac troponin concentrations. *Am J Med.* 2013;126(9):781-788.e2.

27. Kelley WE, Januzzi JL, Christenson RH. Increases of cardiac troponin in conditions other than acute coronary syndrome and heart failure. *Clin Chem.* 2009;55(12):2098-2112.

28. Antman EM, Tanasijevic MJ, Thompson B, et al. Cardiac-specific troponin I levels to predict the risk of mortality in patients with acute coronary syndromes. *N Engl J Med.* 1996;335(18):1342-1349.

29. Mahajan N, Mehta Y, Rose M, Shani J, Lichstein E. Elevated troponin level is not synonymous with myocardial infarction. *Int J Cardiol.* 2006;111(3):442-449.

30. Nagele P, Brown F, Gage BF, et al. High-sensitivity cardiac troponin T in prediction and diagnosis of myocardial infarction and long-term mortality after noncardiac surgery. *Am Heart J.* 2013;166(2):325-332.e1.

31. Baber U, Auguste U. Patients with chronic kidney disease/diabetes mellitus: the high-risk profile in acute coronary syndrome. *Curr Cardiol Rep.* 2013;15(8):386.

32. Pfortmueller CA, Funk G-C, Marti G, et al. Diagnostic performance of high-sensitive troponin T in patients with renal insufficiency. *Am J Cardiol.* 2013;112(12):1968-1972.

33. Narula A, Mehran R, Weisz G, et al. Contrast-induced acute kidney injury after primary percutaneous coronary intervention: results from the HORIZONS-AMI substudy. *Eur Heart J.* 2014;35(23):1533-1540.

34. Marenzi G, Lauri G, Assanelli E. Contrast-induced nephropathy in patients undergoing primary angioplasty for acute myocardial infarction. *J Am Coll Cardiol.* 2004;44(9):1780-1785.

35. de Lemos JA, Morrow DA, Bentley JH, et al. The prognostic value of B-type natriuretic peptide in patients with acute coronary syndromes. *N Engl J Med.* 2001;345(14):1014-1021.

36. Haaf P, Reichlin T, Corson N, et al. B-type natriuretic peptide in the early diagnosis and risk stratification of acute chest pain. *Am J Med.* 2011;124(5):444-452.

37. Saaby L, Poulsen TS, Diederichsen ACP, et al. Mortality rate in type 2 myocardial infarction: observations from an unselected hospital cohort. *Am J Med.* 2014;127(4):295-302.

38. Backus BE, Six AJ, Kelder JC, et al. Chest pain in the emergency room: a multicenter validation of the HEART score. *Crit Pathw Cardiol.* 2010;9(3):164-169.

39. Six A, Backus B, Kelder J. Chest pain in the emergency room: value of the HEART score. *Neth Heart J.* 2008;16(6):191-196.

40. Six AJ, Cullen L, Backus BE, et al. The HEART score for the assessment of patients with chest pain in the emergency department: a multinational validation study. *Crit Pathw Cardiol.* 2013;12(3):121-126.

41. Amin ST, Morrow DA, Braunwald E, et al. Dynamic TIMI risk score for STEMI. *J Am Heart Assoc.* 2013;2(1):e003269.

42. de Araújo Gonçalves P, Ferreira J, Aguiar C, Seabra-Gomes R. TIMI, PURSUIT, and GRACE risk scores: sustained prognostic value and interaction with revascularization in NSTE-ACS. *Eur Heart J.* 2005;26(9):865-872.

43. Pollack CV, Sites FD, Shofer FS, Sease KL, Hollander JE. Application of the TIMI risk score for unstable angina and non-ST elevation acute coronary syndrome to an unselected emergency department chest pain population. *Acad Emerg Med.* 2006;13(1):13-18.

44. Yan AT, Yan RT, Tan M. Risk scores for risk stratification in acute coronary syndromes: useful but simpler is not necessarily better. *Eur Heart J.* 2007;28(9):1072-1078.

45. El-Menyar A, Zubaid M, AlMahmeed W, et al. Killip classification in patients with acute coronary syndrome: insight from a multicenter registry. *Am J Emerg Med.* 2012;30(1):97-103.

46. Giugliano RP, Braunwald E. The year in acute coronary syndrome. *J Am Coll Cardiol.* 2014;63(3):201-214.

47. Ting HH, Rihal CS, Gersh BJ, et al. Regional systems of care to optimize timeliness of reperfusion therapy for ST-elevation myocardial infarction: the Mayo Clinic STEMI Protocol. *Circulation.* 2007;116(7):729-736.

48. Cannon CP, Weintraub WS, Demopoulos LA, et al; TACTICS (Treat Angina with Aggrastat and Determine Cost of Therapy with an Invasive or Conservative Strategy)—Thrombolysis in Myocardial Infarction 18 Investigators. Comparison of early invasive and conservative strategies in patients with unstable coronary syndromes treated with the glycoprotein IIb/IIIa inhibitor tirofiban. *N Engl J Med.* 2001;344(25):1879-1887.

49. Milosevic A, Vasiljevic-Pokrajcic Z, Milasinovic D, et al. Immediate versus delayed invasive intervention for non-STEMI patients: the RIDDLE-NSTEMI study. *JACC Cardiovasc Interv.* 2016;9(6):541-549.

50. Kereiakes DJ. Adjunctive pharmacotherapy before percutaneous coronary intervention in non-ST-elevation acute coronary syndromes: the role of modulating inflammation. *Circulation.* 2003;108(16 Suppl 1):III22-III27.

51. Park KL, Goldberg RJ, Anderson FA, et al; Global Registry of Acute Coronary Events Investigators. Beta-blocker use in ST-segment elevation myocardial infarction in the reperfusion era (GRACE). *Am J Med.* 2014;127(6):503-511.

52. Gershlick AH, Banning AP, Myat A, Verheugt FW, Gersh BJ. Reperfusion therapy for STEMI: is there still a role for thrombolysis in the era of primary percutaneous coronary intervention? *Lancet.* 2013;382(9892):624-632.

53. Bagai A, Dangas GD, Stone GW, Granger CB. Reperfusion strategies in acute coronary syndromes. *Circ Res.* 2014;114(12):1918-1928.

54. Paolasso E, San Martin E, Ravizzini G, Diaz R. Randomised trial of late thrombolysis in patients with suspected acute myocardial infarction. EMERAS (Estudio Multicéntrico Estreptoquinasa Repúblicas de América del Sur) Collaborative Group. *Lancet.* 1993;342(8874):767-772.

55. Sandoval Y, Smith SW, Thordsen SE, Apple FS. Supply/demand type 2 myocardial infarction: should we be paying more attention? *J Am Coll Cardiol.* 2014;63(20):2079-2087.

56. Korff S, Katus HA, Giannitsis E. Differential diagnosis of elevated troponins. *Heart.* 2006;92(7):987-993.

57. Favory R, Neviere R. Bench-to-bedside review: significance and interpretation of elevated troponin in septic patients. *Crit Care.* 2006;10(4):224.

58. Fleischmann KE. The role of echocardiographic evaluation in patients presenting with acute chest pain to the emergency. In: Otto C, ed. *Practice of Clinical Echocardiography.* 5th ed. Philadelphia, PA: Elsevier; 2016: 185.

59. Meredith EL, Masani ND. Echocardiography in the emergency assessment of acute aortic syndromes. *Eur J Echocardiogr.* 2009;10(1):i31-i39.

60. Parato VM, Mehta A, Delfino D, et al. Resting echocardiography for the early detection of acute coronary syndromes

in chest pain unit patients. *Echocardiography*. 2010;27(6): 597-602.

61. French JK, Hellkamp AS, Armstrong PW, et al. Mechanical complications after percutaneous coronary intervention in ST-elevation myocardial infarction (from APEX-AMI). *Am J Cardiol*. 2010;105(1):59-63.

62. Kutty RS, Jones N, Moorjani N. Mechanical complications of acute myocardial infarction. *Cardiol Clin*. 2013;31(4): 519-531.

63. Vlodaver Z, Wilson RF. Complications of acute myocardial infarction. In: Vlodaver Z, Wilson R, Garry D, eds. *Coronary Heart Disease*. Boston, MA: Springer; 2012: 321-347.

64. Unverzagt S, Wachsmuth L, Hirsch K, et al. Inotropic agents and vasodilator strategies for acute myocardial infarction complicated by cardiogenic shock or low cardiac output syndrome. *Cochrane Database Syst Rev*. 2014;(1):CD009669.

65. Sanborn TA, Sleeper LA, Webb JG, et al; SHOCK investigators. Correlates of one-year survival inpatients with cardiogenic shock complicating acute myocardial infarction: angiographic findings from the SHOCK trial. *J Am Coll Cardiol*. 2003;42(8):1373-1379.

66. Thiele H, Ohman EM, Desch S, Eitel I, de Waha S. Management of cardiogenic shock. *Eur Heart J*. 2015;36(20):1223-1230.

67. Thiele H, Zeymer U, Neumann F-J, et al. Intra-aortic balloon counterpulsation in acute myocardial infarction complicated by cardiogenic shock (IABP-SHOCK II): final 12 month results of a randomised, open-label trial. *Lancet*. 2013;382(9905): 1638-1645.

68. Werdan K, Gielen S, Ebelt H, Hochman JS. Mechanical circulatory support in cardiogenic shock. *Eur Heart J*. 2013:35(3): 156-167.

69. Zeymer U, Werdan K, Schuler G, et al. Impact of immediate multivessel percutaneous coronary intervention versus culprit lesion intervention on 1-year outcome in patients with acute myocardial infarction complicated by cardiogenic shock: Results of the randomised IABP-SHOCK II trial. *Eur Heart J Acute Cardiovasc Care*. 2016;6(7):601-609.

70. Anderson RD, Ohman EM, Holmes DR, et al. Use of intraaortic balloon counterpulsation in patients presenting with cardiogenic shock: observations from the GUSTO-I study. Global utilization of streptokinase and TPA for occluded coronary arteries. *J Am Coll Cardiol*. 1997;30(3):708-715.

71. O'Neill WW, Kleiman NS, Moses J, et al. A prospective randomized clinical trial of hemodynamic support with Impella 2.5 versus intra-aortic balloon pump in patients undergoing high-risk percutaneous coronary intervention: the PROTECT II study. *Circulation*. 2012;126(14):1717-1727.

72. Sjauw KD, Engström AE, Vis MM, et al. A systematic review and meta-analysis of intra-aortic balloon pump therapy in ST-elevation myocardial infarction: should we change the guidelines? *Eur Heart J*. 2009;30(4):459-468.

73. Maini B, Naidu SS, Mulukutla S, et al. Real-world use of the Impella 2.5 circulatory support system in complex high-risk percutaneous coronary intervention: The USpella Registry. *Catheter Cardiovasc Interv*. 2012;80(5):717-725.

74. Meyns B, Dens J, Sergeant P, Herijgers P, Daenen W, Flameng W. Initial experiences with the Impella device in patients with cardiogenic shock—Impella support for cardiogenic shock. *Thorac Cardiovasc Surg*. 2003;51(6):312-317.

75. Marasco SF, Lukas G, McDonald M, McMillan J, Ihle B. Review of ECMO (extra corporeal membrane oxygenation) support in critically ill adult patients. *Heart Lung Circ*. 2008;17(Suppl 4): S41-S47.

76. Lafçı G, Budak AB, Yener AÜ, Cicek OF. Use of extracorporeal membrane oxygenation in adults. *Heart Lung Circ*. 2014;23(1):10-23.

77. Sheu JJ, Tsai TH, Lee FY, et al. Early extracorporeal membrane oxygenator-assisted primary percutaneous coronary intervention improved 30-day clinical outcomes in patients with ST-segment elevation myocardial infarction complicated with profound cardiogenic shock. *Crit Care Med*. 2010;38(9):1810-1817.

78. Dai X, Kaul P, Smith Jr SC, Stouffer GA. Predictors, treatment, and outcomes of STEMI occurring in hospitalized patients. *Nat Rev Cardiol*. 2016;13(3):148-154.

79. Acker MA, Parides MK, Perrault LP, et al. Mitral-valve repair versus replacement for severe ischemic mitral regurgitation. *N Engl J Med*. 2014;370(1):23-32.

80. Lamas GA, Mitchell GF, Flaker GC, et al. Clinical significance of mitral regurgitation after acute myocardial infarction. Survival and Ventricular Enlargement Investigators. *Circulation*. 1997;96(3):827-833.

81. Kinch JW, Ryan TJ. Right ventricular infarction. *N Engl J Med*. 1994;330(17):1211-1217.

82. Myerburg R, Kessler K, Castellanos A. Sudden cardiac death. Structure, function, and time-dependence of risk. *Circulation*. 1992;85(1 Suppl):I2-I10.

83. Priori SG, Blomström-Lundqvist C, Mazzanti A, et al. 2015 ESC Guidelines for the management of patients with ventricular arrhythmias and the prevention of sudden cardiac death: The Task Force for the Management of Patients with Ventricular Arrhythmias and the Prevention of Sudden Cardiac Death of the European Society of Cardiology (ESC) Endorsed by: Association for European Paediatric and Congenital Cardiology (AEPC). *Europace*. 2015;17(11):1601-1687.

84. Wellens HJ, Schwartz PJ, Lindemans FW, et al. Risk stratification for sudden cardiac death: current status and challenges for the future. *Eur Heart J*. 2014;35(25):1642-1651.

85. Bernard S. Hypothermia after cardiac arrest: expanding the therapeutic scope. *Crit Care Med*. 2009;37(7 Suppl):S227-S233.

86. Palagiri A, Sadaka F, Lakshmanan R. Prognostication in post cardiac arrest patients treated with therapeutic hypothermia. In: Sadaka F, ed. *Therapeutic Hypothermia in Brain Injury*. London: Intechopen; 2013. https://www.intechopen.com/books/how-to-link/therapeutic-hypothermia-in-brain-injury Accessed July 15, 2017.

87. Scirica BM. Therapeutic hypothermia after cardiac arrest. *Circulation*. 2013;127(2):244-250.

88. Holzer M. Targeted temperature management for comatose survivors of cardiac arrest. *N Engl J Med*. 2010;363(13):1256-1264.

89. Nielsen N, Wetterslev J, Cronberg T, et al. Targeted temperature management at 33°C versus 36°C after cardiac arrest. *N Engl J Med*. 2013;369(23):2197-2206.

90. Pedersen CT, Kay GN, Kalman J, et al. EHRA/HRS/APHRS expert consensus on ventricular arrhythmias. *Europace*. 2014;16(9):1257-1283.

91. Bernard SA, Gray TW, Buist MD, et al. Treatment of comatose survivors of out-of-hospital cardiac arrest with induced hypothermia. *N Engl J Med*. 2002;346(8):557-563.

92. Lavonas EJ, Drennan IR, Gabrielli A, et al. Part 10: Special circumstances of resuscitation: 2015 American Heart Association Guidelines Update for Cardiopulmonary Resuscitation

and Emergency Cardiovascular Care. *Circulation.* 2015;132 (18 Suppl 2):S501-S518.

93. Beniga JG, Johnson KG, Mark DD. Normothermia for neuroprotection: it's hot to be cool. *Nurs Clin North Am.* 2014;49(3):399-413.

94. Rittenberger JC, Callaway CW. Temperature management and modern post–cardiac arrest care. *N Engl J Med.* 2013;369(23):2262-2263.

95. Stoner J, Martin G, O'Mara K, Ehlers J, Tomlanovich M. Amiodarone and bretylium in the treatment of hypothermic ventricular fibrillation in a canine model. *Acad Emerg Med.* 2003;10(3):187-191.

96. Candell-Riera J, Figueras J, Valle V, et al. Right ventricular infarction: relationships between ST segment elevation in V4R and hemodynamic, scintigraphic, and echocardiographic findings in patients with acute inferior myocardial infarction. *Am Heart J.* 1981;101(3):281-287.

97. Harjola VP, Mebazaa A, Čelutkienė J, et al. Contemporary management of acute right ventricular failure: a statement from the Heart Failure Association and the Working Group on Pulmonary Circulation and Right Ventricular Function of the European Society of Cardiology. *Eur J Heart Fail.* 2016;18(3):226-241.

98. Lala A, Guo Y, Xu J, et al. Right ventricular dysfunction in acute myocardial infarction complicated by cardiogenic shock: a hemodynamic analysis of the SHould we emergently revascularize Occluded Coronaries for Cardiogenic shocK (SHOCK) trial and registry. *J Card Fail.* 2016;22(8 Suppl):S39.

99. Harikrishnan P, Gupta T, Palaniswamy C, et al. Complete heart block complicating ST-segment elevation myocardial infarction: temporal trends and association with in-hospital outcomes. *JACC Clin Electrophysiol.* 2015;1(6):529-538.

100. Epstein AE, DiMarco JP, Ellenbogen KA, et al. 2012 ACCF/AHA/HRS focused update incorporated into the ACCF/AHA/HRS 2008 guidelines for device-based therapy of cardiac rhythm abnormalities: a report of the American College of Cardiology Foundation/American Heart Association Task Force on Practice Guidelines and the Heart Rhythm Society. *Circulation.* 2013;127(3):e283-e352.

101. Goldstein JA. Acute right ventricular infarction: insights for the interventional era. *Curr Probl Cardiol.* 2012;37(12):533-557.

102. Assali AR, Teplitsky I, Ben-Dor I, et al. Prognostic importance of right ventricular infarction in an acute myocardial infarction cohort referred for contemporary percutaneous reperfusion therapy. *Am Heart J.* 2007;153(2):231-237.

103. Cheung AW, White CW, Davis MK, Freed DH. Short-term mechanical circulatory support for recovery from acute right ventricular failure: clinical outcomes. *J Heart Lung Transplant.* 2014;33(8):794-799.

104. Inohara T, Kohsaka S, Fukuda K, Menon V. The challenges in the management of right ventricular infarction. *Eur Heart J Acute Cardiovasc Care.* 2013;2(3):226-234.

105. Hiratzka LF, Bakris GL, Beckman JA, et al. 2010 ACCF/AHA/AATS/ACR/ASA/SCA/SCAI/SIR/STS/SVM guidelines for the diagnosis and management of patients with thoracic aortic disease. A report of the American College of Cardiology Foundation/American Heart Association Task Force on Practice Guidelines, American Association for Thoracic Surgery, American College of Radiology, American Stroke Association, Society of Cardiovascular Anesthesiologists, Society for Cardiovascular Angiography and Interventions, Society of Interventional Radiology, Society of Thoracic Surgeons, and Society for Vascular Medicine. *J Am Coll Cardiol.* 2010;55(14):e27-e129.

106. Tsai T, Trimarchi S, Nienaber C. Acute aortic dissection: perspectives from the International Registry of Acute Aortic Dissection (IRAD). *Eur J Vasc Endovasc Surg.* 2009;37(2):149-159.

107. Tsigkas G, Kasimis G, Theodoropoulos K, et al. A successfully thrombolysed acute inferior myocardial infarction due to type A aortic dissection with lethal consequences: the importance of early cardiac echocardiography. *J Cardiothorac Surg.* 2011;6:101.

108. Baliga RR, Nienaber CA, Bossone E, et al. The role of imaging in aortic dissection and related syndromes. *JACC Cardiovasc Imaging.* 2014;7(4):406-424.

109. Singh K, Carson K, Shah R, et al. Meta-analysis of clinical correlates of acute mortality in takotsubo cardiomyopathy. *Am J Cardiol.* 2014;113(8):1420-1428.

110. Templin C, Ghadri JR, Diekmann J, et al. Clinical features and outcomes of takotsubo (stress) cardiomyopathy. *N Engl J Med.* 2015;373(10):929-938.

111. Meine TJ, Roe MT, Chen AY, et al; CRUSADE Investigators. Association of intravenous morphine use and outcomes in acute coronary syndromes: results from the CRUSADE Quality Improvement Initiative. *Am Heart J.* 2005;149(6):1043-1049.

112. Levine GN, Bates ER, Bittl JA, et al. 2016 ACC/AHA guideline focused update on duration of dual antiplatelet therapy in patients with coronary artery disease: a report of the American College of Cardiology/American Heart Association Task Force on Clinical Practice Guidelines. *Am Col Cardiol.* 2016;68(10):1082-1115.

113. Livhits M, Ko CY, Leonardi MJ, Zingmond DS, Gibbons MM, de Virgilio C. Risk of surgery following recent myocardial infarction. *Ann Surg.* 2011;253(5):857-864.

114. Fleisher LA, Fleischmann KE, Auerbach AD, et al. 2014 ACC/AHA guideline on perioperative cardiovascular evaluation and management of patients undergoing noncardiac surgery: a report of the American College of Cardiology/American Heart Association Task Force on Practice Guidelines. *Circulation.* 2014;130(24):e278-e333.

115. To AC, Armstrong G, Zeng I, Webster MW. Noncardiac surgery and bleeding after percutaneous coronary intervention. *Cir Cardiovasc Intervent.* 2009;2(3):213-221.

116. Maceira AM, Ripoll C, Cosin-Sales J, et al. Long term effects of cocaine on the heart assessed by cardiovascular magnetic resonance at 3T. *J Cardiovasc Magn Reson.* 2014;16:26.

117. Pozner CN, Levine M, Zane R. The cardiovascular effects of cocaine. *J Emerg Med.* 2005;29(2):173-178.

118. Weber JE, Chudnofsky CR, Boczar M, Boyer EW, Wilkerson MD, Hollander JE. Cocaine-associated chest pain: how common is myocardial infarction? *Acad Emerg Med.* 2000;7(8):873-877.

119. Finkel JB, Marhefka GD. Rethinking cocaine-associated chest pain and acute coronary syndromes. *Mayo Clin Proc.* 2011;86(12):1198-1207.

120. McCord J, Jneid H, Hollander JE, et al. Management of cocaine-associated chest pain and myocardial infarction: a scientific statement from the American Heart Association Acute Cardiac Care Committee of the Council on Clinical Cardiology. *Circulation.* 2008;117(14):1897-1907.

121. Paraschin K, De Andrade AG, Parga JR. Assessment of myocardial infarction by CT angiography and cardiovascular MRI

in patients with cocaine-associated chest pain: a pilot study. *Brit J Radiol.* 2012;85(1015):e274-e278.

122. Caforio AL, Marcolongo R, Basso C, Iliceto S. Clinical presentation and diagnosis of myocarditis. *Heart.* 2015;101(16):1332-1344.

123. Alsaileek A, Nasim M, Aljizeeri A, Alharthi M, Al-Mallah MH. The role of delayed contrast-enhanced cardiac magnetic resonance in differentiating myocarditis from myocardial infarction. *Eur H J Suppl.* 2014;16(Suppl B):B24-B28.

124. Basman C, Agrawal PR, McRee C, Saravolatz L, Chen-Scarabelli C, Scarabelli TM. Diagnostic approach to myocarditis mimicking myocardial infarction at initial presentation. *Cardiol Res.* 2016;7(6):209-213.

125. Caforio AL, Pankuweit S, Arbustini E, et al; European Society of Cardiology Working Group on Myocardial and Pericardial Diseases. Current state of knowledge on aetiology, diagnosis, management, and therapy of myocarditis: a position statement of the European Society of Cardiology Working Group on Myocardial and Pericardial Diseases. *Eur Heart J.* 2013;34(33):2636-2648.

126. Feldman AM, McNamara D. Myocarditis. *N Engl J Med.* 2000;343(19):1388-1398.

127. Cooper LT, Baughman KL, Feldman AM. The role of endomyocardial biopsy in the management of cardiovascular disease: a scientific statement from the American Heart Association, the American College of Cardiology, and the European Society of Cardiology Endorsed by the Heart Failure Society of America and the Heart Failure Association of the European Society of Cardiology. *Eur Heart J.* 2007;28(24):3076-3093.

128. Schultheiss H-P, Kühl U, Cooper LT. The management of myocarditis. *Eur Heart J.* 2011;32(21):2616-2625.

129. Shenoy C, Harjai KJ. Thrombocytopenia following percutaneous coronary intervention. *J Interv Cardiol.* 2011;24(1):15-26.

130. Shenoy C, Orshaw P, Devarakonda S, Harjai KJ. Occurrence, predictors, and outcomes of post-percutaneous coronary intervention thrombocytopenia in an unselected population. *J Interv Cardiol.* 2009;22(2):156-162.

131. Greinacher A. Heparin-induced thrombocytopenia. *N Engl J Med.* 2015;373(19):252-261.

132. Salter BS, Weiner MM, Trinh MA, et al. Heparin-induced thrombocytopenia: a comprehensive clinical review. *J Am Coll Cardiol.* 2016;67(21):2519-2532.

133. Fahdi IE, Saucedo JF, Hennebry T, Ghani M, Sadanandan S, Garza-Arreola L. Incidence and time course of thrombocytopenia with abciximab and eptifibatide in patients undergoing percutaneous coronary intervention. *Am J Cardiol.* 2004;93(4):453-455.

134. Lajus S, Clofent-Sanchez G, Jais C, Coste P, Nurden P, Nurden A. Thrombocytopenia after abciximab use results from different mechanisms. *Thromb Haemost.* 2010;103(3):651-661.

135. Merlini PA, Rossi M, Menozzi A, et al. Thrombocytopenia caused by abciximab or tirofiban and its association with clinical outcome in patients undergoing coronary stenting. *Circulation.* 2004;109(18):2203-2206.

136. Schell D, Ganti A, Levitt R, Potti A. Thrombocytopenia associated with c7E3 Fab (abciximab). *Ann Hematol.* 2002;81(2):76-79.

137. Cheezum MK, Liberthson RR, Shah NR, et al. Anomalous aortic origin of a coronary artery from the inappropriate sinus of Valsalva. *J Am Coll Cardiol.* 2017;69(12):1592-1608.

138. Braat SH, Brugada P, de Zwaan C, Coenegracht JM, Wellens H. Value of electrocardiogram in diagnosing right ventricular involvement in patients with an acute inferior wall myocardial infarction. *Br Heart J.* 1983;49(4):368-372.

139. Priori SG, Napolitano C, Gasparini M, et al. Natural history of Brugada syndrome: insights for risk stratification and management. *Circulation.* 2002;105(11):1342-1347.

140. Priori SG, Wilde AA, Horie M, et al. HRS/EHRA/APHRS expert consensus statement on the diagnosis and management of patients with inherited primary arrhythmia syndromes. *J Arrhythm.* 2014;30(1):1-28.

141. Basso C, Corrado D, Marcus FI, Nava A, Thiene G. Arrhythmogenic right ventricular cardiomyopathy. *Lancet.* 2009;373(9671):1289-1300.

142. Basso C, Thiene G, Corrado D, Angelini A, Nava A, Valente M. Arrhythmogenic right ventricular cardiomyopathy. Dysplasia, dystrophy, or myocarditis? *Circulation.* 1996;94(5):983-991.

143. Marcus F, Towbin JA, Zareba W, et al. Arrhythmogenic right ventricular dysplasia/cardiomyopathy (ARVD/C): a multidisciplinary study: design and protocol. *Circulation.* 2003;107(23):2975-2978.

144. Krishna M, Zacharowski. Principles of intra-aortic balloon pump counterpulsation. *CEACCP.* 2009;9(1):24-28.

145. Interpreting intra-aortic balloon pump waveforms. *Cardiac Insider.* 2009;39(2):9-10.

146. Haddad EV, Robertson CH. Intra-aortic balloon counterpulsation. *Medscape.* http://emedicine.medscape.com/article/1847715-overview#a5. Accessed August 23, 2017.

147. Onorati F, Santini F, Amoncelli E, et al. How should I wean my next intra-aortic balloon pump? Differences between progressive volume weaning and rate weaning. *J Thorac Cardiovasc Surg.* 2013;145(5):1214-1221.

148. Robers L, Cochrane E, Bundell D, Mustaa Z. What is the optimum method of weaning intra-aortic balloon pumps? *Interact Cardiovasc Thorac Surg.* 2016;23(2):310-313.

149. Webb CAK, Weyker PD, Flynn BC. Management of intra-aortic balloon pumps. *Semin Cardiothorac Vasc Anes.* 2015;19(2):106-121.

150. Gersh BJ, Maron BJ, Bonow RO, et al; American College of Cardiology Foundation/American Heart Association Task Force on Practice Guidelines; American Association for Thoracic Surgery; American Society of Echocardiography; American Society of Nuclear Cardiology; Heart Failure Society of America; Heart Rhythm Society; Society for Cardiovascular Angiography and Interventions; Society of Thoracic Surgeons. 2011 ACCF/AHA guideline for the diagnosis and treatment of hypertrophic cardiomyopathy: a report of the American College of Cardiology Foundation/American Heart Association Task Force on Practice Guidelines. *Circulation.* 2011;124(24):e783-e831.

151. Spirito P, Bellone P, Harris KM, et al. Magnitude of left ventricular hypertrophy and risk of sudden death in hypertrophic cardiomyopathy. *N Engl J Med.* 2000;342(24):1778-1785.

Congestive Heart Failure

Srikanth Yandrapalli, MD, Sohaib Tariq, MD, and Gregg M. Lanier, MD

INTRODUCTION

Heart failure (HF) is the inability of the heart to pump an adequate supply of blood to meet the demands of the body. It is an epidemic and is associated with significant morbidity, mortality, and healthcare expenditure. Heart failure has an estimated prevalence of 5.8 million in the United States, and affects over 23 million people worldwide.[1] The cost of HF in the United States was around $30 billion in 2012, a number that is projected to increase to around $70 billion by the year 2030.[2] Acute decompensated HF (ADHF) is the clinical syndrome of new onset or worsening HF symptoms and signs requiring urgent treatment.[3] In the United States, ADHF exacerbations result in about 1 million hospitalizations yearly and contribute largely to the overall HF healthcare expenditure.[2] Hospitalization for ADHF serves as a poor prognostic indicator with an approximate 30% and 50% readmission rate at 1 month and 6 months, respectively, and a 1-year all-cause mortality as high as 30%.[4,5]

TYPES, PATHOPHYSIOLOGY, AND CLINICAL MANIFESTATIONS

Patients with HF can either present to the hospital with symptoms for the first time or present with ADHF in the setting of having a diagnosis of chronic HF. Heart failure is classified based on the left ventricular ejection fraction (LVEF), as usually determined by echocardiography, into HF with reduced ejection fraction (EF) (HFrEF) with an LVEF less than 40%, or HF with preserved EF (HFpEF) with an LVEF 50% or greater.[6] An EF between 40% and 49% is considered a gray zone. Epidemiological data indicates that HFpEF and HFrEF contribute equally to the total HF population.[6] Patients with HFpEF have a similar postdischarge mortality risk and equally high rates of rehospitalization as patients with HFrEF.[7] The pathophysiology of HF is complex and involves intricate interactions between neurohormonal systems and hemodynamic abnormalities, resulting in abnormal myocardial remodeling and progressive myocardial, endothelial, valvular, and vascular dysfunction.[8]

Heart failure with reduced EF results from systolic dysfunction, which limits the ability of the contracting myocardium to effectively eject the preload of the failing myocardium. This results in backward failure, elevated end-diastolic pressure, and an inability to produce an adequate cardiac output. Heart failure with preserved EF results from abnormal or impaired myocardial diastolic relaxation, which causes elevated end-diastolic pressures and prevents an appropriate increase in the ejection fraction under conditions of stress. Regardless of the type of HF, symptoms of acute decompensation are from elevated left ventricular end-diastolic pressure (filling pressure) with resultant alveolar and interstitial edema causing pulmonary congestion and dyspnea. The backward transmission of elevated filling pressures and subsequent pulmonary venous hypertension increase pulmonary arterial and right heart pressures, causing systemic congestive symptoms.

Irrespective of the type of HF, the symptoms and signs of HF are due to either congestion or decreased cardiac output and tissue perfusion. The spectrum of presentation in ADHF ranges from dyspnea to overt cardiogenic shock with end-organ damage. Hospitalization for HF is more commonly for congestive symptoms than for low cardiac output states.[3] At presentation, approximately 25% patients are hypertensive (systolic blood pressure [SBP] > 160 mmHg), around 50% are normotensive, and less than 10% are hypotensive (SBP < 90 mmHg).[3]

CLASSIFICATION AND STAGING

The New York Heart Association (NYHA) functional classification of HF is based primarily on symptoms (Table 7-1). In this classification, functional class is dynamic and can suddenly worsen if the patient is in acute decompensation, or it can improve with treatment. The American College of Cardiology (ACC)/American Heart Association (AHA) staging system of HF recognizes the progressive nature of HF and emphasizes the fact that established risk factors and structural abnormalities are necessary for the development of HF (Table 7-2).[8] The Killip-Kimball system, which classifies decompensated HF in the post–acute myocardial infarction state, is highly predictive of 30-day mortality (Table 7-3).[9]

TABLE 7-1 New York Heart Association Functional Class

Class	Description
I	No limitations in physical activity
II	Slight limitations in physical activity
III	Marked limitations in physical activity
IIIA	Symptoms with less than ordinary activity
IIIB	Symptoms with minimal exertion
IV	Symptoms at rest

TABLE 7-3 Killip-Kimball System

Class	Description	Mortality
I	No clinical signs of heart failure	6%
II	Rales in the lungs, third heart sound (S3), and elevated jugular venous pressure	17%
III	Acute pulmonary edema	38%
IV	Cardiogenic shock or arterial hypotension (measured as systolic blood pressure < 90 mmHg), and evidence of peripheral vasoconstriction (oliguria, cyanosis, and diaphoresis)	81%

INITIAL EVALUATION AND DIAGNOSTIC CONSIDERATIONS

The initial evaluation of HF should focus on identifying the potential cause of new onset HF or the precipitants of ADHF in patients with chronic HF (Table 7-4). Etiologies of HF are manifold, with ischemic dilated cardiomyopathy being the most common cause of HFrEF, and hypertension being more commonly associated with HFpEF. Many cases of HFrEF are idiopathic. Other etiologies of HF include hypertrophic cardiomyopathy, restrictive cardiomyopathy, stress (Takotsubo cardiomyopathy), infection, inflammation, valvular heart disease and endocarditis, metabolic-nutritional, alcohol and toxins, chemotherapy-induced cardiomyopathy, connective tissue diseases including lupus, peripartum cardiomyopathy, and hereditary muscular dystrophies.

A focused history and physical examination is required to diagnose the syndrome of HF and identify probable etiologic/precipitating factors. Data from the Organized Program to Initiate Lifesaving Treatment in Hospitalized Patients With Heart Failure (OPTIMIZE-HF) registry showed that precipitating factors were independently associated with in-hospital and postdischarge outcomes.[10] Routine diagnostic investigations as recommended by the ACC/AHA, the Heart Failure Society of America (HFSA), and the European Society of Cardiology (ESC) supplement the history and physical exam to identify the cause of HF, and also provide valuable information about various prognostic markers.[11-13] These diagnostic investigations include the following:

1. The electrocardiogram (ECG) is a critical component in the initial diagnostic evaluation of HF. It can be used to rapidly identify the causes of ADHF, like myocardial ischemia/infarction and tachyarrhythmias. Prolonged QRS duration suggests ventricular dyssynchrony. The ECG can reveal conduction disease, evidence of prior myocardial infarction (MI), and left ventricular hypertrophy.

2. Several different laboratory tests are available to help in the diagnosis and management of ADHF. Initial laboratory testing should include a complete blood count, urinalysis, and a comprehensive metabolic panel. Anemia can precipitate HF in patients with advanced HF or underlying coronary artery disease. Severe anemia can cause high-output HF. In patients with NYHA class II and III HF and iron deficiency (ferritin < 100 ng/mL or 100–300 ng/mL if transferrin saturation is < 20%), intravenous (IV) iron replacement is reasonable for improving functional status and quality of life (Class of Recommendation [COR] IIb,

TABLE 7-2 American College of Cardiology/American Heart Association Heart Failure Staging System

Stage	Description
A	At risk for development of heart failure but no apparent structural abnormality of the heart
B	Structural abnormality of the heart without any previous or current symptoms
C	Structural heart disease with current or previous symptom of heart failure
D	End-stage symptoms of heart failure refractory to standard treatment

TABLE 7-4 Important Causes and Precipitants of Acute Decompensation of Heart Failure

1. Medication related
   a. Noncompliance
   b. Initiation or increase in a beta-blocker, nondihydropyridine calcium channel blockers, nonsteroidal anti-inflammatory agents, corticosteroids
   c. Sodium-containing medications in hospitalized patients (antibiotics like piperacillin-tazobactam)
   d. Thiazolidinediones
   e. Class I sodium channel blocking antiarrhythmic agents (such as mexiletine, disopyramide, flecainide), sotalol (class III antiarrhythmic, has beta-blocker effect)
2. Dietary nonadherence
3. Myocardial ischemia/infarction
4. Tachy- and bradyarrhythmias
5. Uncontrolled hypertension
6. Anemia, thyroid disease
7. Substance related: alcohol, drugs (eg, cocaine)
8. Acute valvular insufficiency
9. Noncardiac causes of acute decompensation: pulmonary disease (pneumonia, chronic obstructive pulmonary disease exacerbation, pulmonary embolism)
10. Renal failure
11. Infectious: myocarditis, endocarditis
12. Pregnancy and peripartum cardiomyopathy

Level of Evidence [LOE] B-R).[14] Leukocytosis can suggest an underlying infection. An elevated blood glucose level at presentation is associated with increased 30-day mortality independent of the patient's diabetic status.[15] Hyponatremia in HF is associated with a poorer prognosis.[16] Hypo- or hyperkalemia can be present if the patient was on diuretics or renin-angiotensin-aldosterone system inhibitors. Cardiorenal syndrome is an important consideration when acute kidney injury is present in the setting of HF. A variety of factors contribute to the reduction in glomerular filtration rate in setting of HF including neurohumoral adaptations. These adaptations include: (1) reduced stroke volume and cardiac output; (2) activation of sympathetic nervous system and renin-angiotensin system; (3) systemic vasoconstriction, salt and water retention; (4) increased reabsorption of urea; (5) reduced renal perfusion due to systemic vasoconstriction; (6) increased renal venous pressure; (7) and right ventricular dysfunction. A cholestatic pattern (disproportionate elevation in the serum alkaline phosphatase compared with the serum aminotransferases) and congestive hepatopathy (elevated liver biochemical tests due to passive hepatic congestion in setting of right-sided heart failure) can be seen. Ischemic hepatitis, also known as shock liver, also can be seen due to acute liver hypoperfusion from cardiogenic shock, leading to marked serum aminotransferase elevation. The frequency of monitoring the above laboratory tests should depend on the initial values and response to therapy. Hemoglobin A$_{IC}$ and a lipid panel can identify patients with metabolic syndrome. Other laboratory tests like thyroid function, iron studies with ferritin (for hemochromatosis), serum-free light chains (κ and λ, for amyloid light chain disease), antinuclear antibody (ANA), and rheumatoid factor (for autoimmune heart dysfunction) should be obtained based on clinical suspicion. Serum myocardium-specific troponin levels can be elevated in acute HF patients secondary to cardiac myocyte injury from decompensation or from infiltrative diseases. An elevated troponin level in patients with ADHF is a poor prognostic marker and mildly elevated levels are often seen in ADHF.[17] A significantly elevated troponin level should also raise a suspicion of acute coronary syndrome precipitating HF.

3. Both B-type natriuretic peptide (BNP) and N-terminal-proBNP (NT-proBNP) are very useful in addition to clinical criteria in the diagnosis of ADHF[18,19] (COR I, LOE A). proBNP cleavage produces biologically active BNP and NT-proBNP. B-type natriuretic peptide is a natriuretic hormone that is primarily released from the heart (mostly from the ventricles). Release of BNP is increased in HF due to ventricular wall stretching in response to high filling pressures. These hormones have a very high negative predictive value and can be used to rule out cardiac causes of dyspnea when they are in the normal range. The diagnostic levels of BNP and NT-proBNP for ADHF are shown in Table 7-5.[18,19] In patients taking LCZ696, an NT-proBNP level should be checked instead of BNP, as the sacubitril

TABLE 7-5 Diagnostic Levels of Natriuretic Peptides for Acute Decompensated Heart Failure

Test	HF Unlikely	HF Likely
BNP (pg/mL)	< 100	> 400
NT-proBNP, age < 50 y (ng/mL)	< 300	> 450
NT-proBNP, age 50–75 y (ng/mL)	< 300	> 900
NT-proBNP, age > 75 y (ng/mL)	< 300	> 1800

BNP = B-type natriuretic peptide; HF = heart failure; NT-proBNP = N-terminal-pro BNP.

(neprilysin inhibitor) component of LCZ696 can elevate circulating BNP levels. Levels of BNP can be either normal or only mildly elevated in HFpEF patients and in morbidly obese patients.[7,20] The levels of these hormones can be elevated with increasing age and renal dysfunction.[20] Natriuretic peptide level–guided management of ADHF is controversial. An elevated BNP is a significant predictor of in-hospital mortality in ADHF patients with either HFrEF or HFpEF.[21] Patients whose natriuretic peptide concentrations fall during admission have lower cardiovascular mortality and readmission rates at 6 months.[13] In patients without HF, BNP can be elevated in the presence of MI, arrhythmias, sepsis, cirrhosis, renal failure, hyperthyroidism, and pulmonary disease. Serial BNP measurements alone have not proven to be useful in guiding management of acute HF patients and should be used in conjunction with the clinical scenario. Atrial natriuretic peptide (ANP) is another hormone released from the atria in response to atrial stretching (volume expansion) in HF. Although higher levels of ANP are seen in HF, ANP assays are still under investigation to prove clinical utility and not widely used or available commercially.

4. Chest radiography must be obtained in suspected HF and is useful in evaluating the pulmonary parenchyma for the presence of vascular congestion and edema, possible infectious processes, and pleural effusions. Additionally, heart size can be evaluated.

5. Echocardiography provides the most useful information regarding the etiology and type of HF. It is a simple, noninvasive tool that provides both structural and functional assessment of the heart. It is essential in distinguishing between HFrEF and HFpEF, as it can estimate LVEF. Regional wall-motion abnormalities suggest an ischemic etiology of cardiomyopathy but can also be seen in cardiac sarcoidosis, nonischemic dilated cardiomyopathy (NICM), Chagas cardiomyopathy, focal myocarditis, and Takotsubo cardiomyopathy (typically hyperdynamic basal LV function with apical akinesis). Sepsis can cause myocardial depression and resultant global hypokinesis. Left ventricle end-diastolic dimensions inform on the chronicity of the disease process, with a greater level of dilation of the heart being consistent with chronic HF and LV remodeling. Valvular etiology of HF, pericardial effusion, tamponade physiology, and pulmonary arterial pressure estimates can

be assessed with echocardiography. Patterns of LV hypertrophy can suggest hypertrophic cardiomyopathy, restrictive cardiomyopathy (such as amyloidosis), or hypertensive LV hypertrophy, which is common in HFpEF.

6. Coronary angiography in indicated (a) in patients with ADHF and known coronary artery disease (CAD) without a clear precipitant, especially if the troponin is elevated; (b) with a high pretest probability of underlying ischemic cardiomyopathy in patients who are candidates for percutaneous or surgical revascularization; (c) before heart transplant or left ventricular assist device (LVAD) placement; (d) in HF secondary to postinfarction ventricular aneurysm or other mechanical complications of MI; or (e) in HFrEF in association with angina or regional wall-motion abnormalities and/or scintigraphic evidence of reversible myocardial ischemia when revascularization is being considered.[11-13]

Right heart catheterization (RHC) provides important information regarding filling pressures, cardiac output, and pulmonary vascular resistance. The routine use of invasive hemodynamic monitoring for managing ADHF did not decrease overall mortality or hospitalizations, and is not recommended in routine practice.[22] However, RHC can guide therapy in patients with refractory HF, unclear volume status, hemodynamic instability and hypotension, worsening renal function, or cardiogenic shock, or when evaluating patients for heart transplantation or mechanical circulatory support devices.[11,13]

7. Cardiac magnetic resonance (CMR) imaging is reasonable to assess left ventricular dimensions and EF when echocardiography is inadequate. Additional information about myocardial perfusion, tissue injury (inflammation in myocarditis or necrosis), viability, and fibrosis from CMR imaging can help identify HF etiology and assess prognosis. Cardiac magnetic resonance provides very high anatomical resolution and is very useful in assessing suspected congenital heart disease, myocardial infiltrative processes (such as hemochromatosis and amyloidosis), or scar burden.[11] It is also useful in the evaluation of rarer diseases such as sarcoidosis, arrhythmogenic right ventricular cardiomyopathy, and Chagas disease.

8. Endomyocardial biopsy can be considered in patients with rapidly progressive HF despite appropriate medical treatment, in patients with suspected infiltrative diseases (amyloidosis, sarcoidosis, hemochromatosis), or in patients with malignant arrhythmias rising a suspicion for giant cell myocarditis.[12,13]

TREATMENT

Acute Decompensated Heart Failure

Treatment is aimed at improving symptoms, reversing a low-output state (if present), optimizing volume status, restoring normal oxygenation, identifying etiology, including patients who would benefit from revascularization or device therapy,

and optimizing chronic medical therapy. Hospitalization is recommended in ADHF patients who present with hypotension, worsening renal or liver function, altered mentation, NYHA class IV symptoms, acute coronary syndrome, or hemodynamically significant arrhythmias. Evaluation and treatment of precipitating factors of ADHF such as myocardial ischemia, arrhythmias, thyroid disease, or uncontrolled hypertension should be considered. Blood pressure goal is less than 130/80 mmHg (COR I).[14] It is very important to assess end-organ perfusion at the time of initial presentation of ADHF patients classifying them into 1 of the 4 subsets (cold and wet, warm and wet, cold and dry, warm and dry). Prophylactic anticoagulation against venous thromboembolism should be considered in ADHF patients confined to bed rest.

After appropriate risk stratification, ADHF patients with congestive symptoms should be treated initially with loop diuretics, usually intravenous, to restore optimal volume status. Monitoring of daily weights, intake and output, serum electrolytes, renal function, and end-organ function is recommended. Based on findings from the Diuretic Optimization Strategies Evaluation (DOSE) study, the initial intravenous dose should be 2.5 times the patient's home equivalent diuretic dose, and intermittent boluses were as good as continuous loop diuretic infusion.[23] Patients were converted from their home dose of loop diuretic to an equivalent intravenous dose, using a dose conversion of oral furosemide 40 mg to oral torsemide 20 mg and oral bumetanide 1 mg. Oral bioavailability of furosemide is approximately 50% compared to 80% to 100% for bumetanide and torsemide. Both oral and intravenous preparations are available for furosemide and bumetanide, whereas torsemide is only available in an oral form. It is proposed that administration of albumin prior to loop diuretics will increase the diuretic delivery to the kidney by retaining furosemide within the intravascular space. Coadministration of furosemide and albumin failed to prove efficacy in hypoalbuminemic patients with liver cirrhosis.[24] The addition of thiazide diuretics (metolazone 2.5–5 mg by mouth, or chlorothiazide 250–500 mg IV) can be beneficial if diuretic resistance develops despite escalating doses of loop diuretics. The addition of low-dose dopamine to IV diuretics in patients with ADHF was not associated with any beneficial effects in terms of diuresis, dyspnea relief, or mortality.[25,26] Available evidence does not favor ultrafiltration (UF) over loop diuretics as first-line therapy in patients with ADHF. In the Cardiorenal Rescue Study in Acute Decompensated Heart Failure (CARRESS-HF) trial, no difference in weight loss or improvement in symptoms was observed between diuretic therapy and UF.[27] At this time, routine use of UF is not recommended and should be confined to patients with refractory congestion who fail to respond to diuretic-based strategies.[11,13] Ultrafiltration can be considered in patients with refractory volume overload: oliguria unresponsive to fluid resuscitation measures, severe hyperkalemia (potassium > 6.5 mmol/L), severe acidemia (pH < 7.2), serum urea level greater than 150 mg/dL, and serum creatinine greater than 3.4 mg/dL.[13]

Vasodilators are a useful adjunct to diuretics especially in ADHF patients with acute pulmonary edema and severe hypertension. Nitroglycerin and sodium nitroprusside can be used to provide rapid symptom relief in ADHF patients with pulmonary edema and hypertension. Vasodilators should only be used if the SBP is more than 110 mmHg. Nitroprusside should be used in combination with invasive arterial blood pressure monitoring. In the randomized, controlled, Vasodilator in the Management of Acute Heart Failure (VMAC) study, the addition of nesiritide to standard therapy significantly decreased pulmonary capillary wedge pressure and dyspnea score at 3 hours compared with standard therapy alone.[28] However, in the Acute Study of Clinical Effectiveness of Nesiritide in Decompensated Heart Failure (ASCEND-HF) trial, there was no significant difference between nesiritide and placebo in terms of early dyspnea relief, worsening renal function, or 30-day rehospitalization and mortality rates.[29] Based on available evidence, the role of nesiritide in ADHF patients is limited.

Current practice guidelines recommend consideration of the short-term use of inotropic agents (intravenous milrinone or dobutamine) to improve cardiac output and end organ perfusion in ADHF patients with hypotension (SBP < 90 mmHg) with hypoperfusion. Inotropic agents may also be considered in advanced HF patients awaiting heart transplant to maintain hemodynamic stability, as a bridge to decision, and palliative care. These agents are useful until a definite or escalated supportive therapy is planned, possibly including coronary revascularization or mechanical circulatory support. Continuous cardiac rhythm monitoring and frequent BP monitoring are recommended while on inotropes. One large randomized controlled trial evaluated the clinical outcomes in patients hospitalized with ADHF when intravenous milrinone was added to standard medical therapy.[30] Milrinone was associated with significant sustained hypotension, and no differences were seen in in-hospital mortality, 60-day mortality, or readmission. A small randomized trial comparing low-dose dobutamine to optimal medical therapy showed no difference in mortality or improvement in symptoms, but hospitalizations for HF exacerbations were lower in the dobutamine group.[31] Levosimendan is a newer inotrope which is recommended in the ESC HF guidelines to reverse the hypotension and subsequent hypoperfusion caused by beta-blockade.[13] Both milrinone and dobutamine are inodilators, which can worsen hypotension. Epinephrine is a potent inotrope and vasoconstrictor. Use of this agent should immediately trigger consideration of escalation to mechanical circulatory support.

To achieve hemodynamic stabilization and maintain end-organ perfusion in patients presenting with refractory cardiogenic shock, escalation of therapy to mechanical circulatory support must be considered until the underlying cause of shock has been reversed (bridge to recovery) or a definite decision can be made for a long-term therapy, such as LVAD or heart transplant (bridge to decision). Intra-aortic balloon pump (IABP) is a percutaneously placed device that improves coronary perfusion and unloads the LV by reducing the cardiac afterload. In a recent randomized multicenter trial, IABP support had no effect on 30-day or 12-month survival in patients with cardiogenic shock undergoing early revascularization and optimal medical therapy.[32] An IABP may not provide adequate cardiac output in fulminant cardiogenic shock patients with profoundly low cardiac output. An axial flow pump LVAD (eg, Impella) also is placed percutaneously via the femoral or axillary artery and can provide cardiac output of 2.5 to 5 L/min. Augmenting cardiac output improves BP and coronary and end-organ perfusion, while decreasing LV end-diastolic pressure and pulmonary edema. In a recent trial, Impella was not associated with a reduction in 30-day mortality in acute MI patients complicated by cardiogenic shock when compared to IABP.[33] Venoarterial extracorporeal membrane oxygenation (VA-ECMO) is effective in providing emergent mechanical circulatory support in refractory cardiogenic shock patients as a bridge to recovery or decision. There is paucity of data or randomized trials to support survival benefit with VA-ECMO in acute cardiogenic shock patients. In patients with severe respiratory failure coexisting with cardiogenic shock, VA-ECMO should be considered. Venoarterial ECMO is also very useful in biventricular HF, as it decreases preload to the right ventricle, reduces central venous pressure, and increases arterial blood pressure. A limitation to VA-ECMO is the potential for increase of afterload to the LV. Several centers use a strategy of concomitant IABP or Impella device with VA-ECMO to avoid the potential for high left ventricular pressures and pulmonary edema.

Before escalation to mechanical assistance, it is important to consider whether the patient is a candidate for advanced therapies such LVAD (COR IIa) or heart transplant (COR I).[14] In some cases, a multidisciplinary team may need to decide whether to escalate support in patients with prohibitive comorbidities, such as renal failure, advanced age, cognitive, or social limitations. Sometimes an approach considering hospice/palliation (COR I) is more appropriate and ethical than futile use of mechanical support.[14]

Chronic Heart Failure

Goals of therapy are to improve symptoms, to improve functional class, and to improve survival. Decreasing afterload in patients with HF with vasodilator drugs enhances stroke volume and EF. Nonpharmacological strategies have an important contribution in management of these patients. Dietary sodium restriction (2–3 g daily), fluid intake less than 2 Liters a day, weight loss, lipid control, treatment of underlying sleep apnea, and exercise training to improve functional capacity are recommended. Nonsteroidal anti-inflammatory drugs (NSAIDs) should be avoided. Pneumococcal and annual influenza vaccines are recommended. Patients with obstructive sleep apnea and cardiovascular disease might benefit from continuous positive airway pressure (CPAP) to improve sleep quality and daytime sleepiness (COR IIb, LOE B-R), but in patients with central sleep apnea and NYHA class II-IV HFrEF, adaptive servo-ventilation causes harm (COR III, LOE B-R).[14]

The renin-angiotensin-aldosterone system (RAAS) inhibition with angiotensin-converting enzyme inhibitors (ACEI), angiotensin receptor blockers (ARBs), and mineralocorticoid receptor antagonists (MRAs) have been shown to reduce morbidity and mortality in an NYHA class II-IV chronic HFrEF population in various landmark trials.[34-42] Angiotensin-converting enzyme inhibitors are the first-line cornerstone of therapy in symptomatic or asymptomatic HF patients with an LVEF of 40% or less (COR I, LOE A).[14] Angiotensin receptor blockers are recommended in patients who are intolerable to ACEI (COR I, LOE A).[14] Angiotensin-converting enzyme inhibitors and ARBs have their beneficial effects in HF by causing vasodilation resulting in reduction of preload and afterload, downregulating sympathetic adrenergic activity by blocking the effects of angiotensin II, promoting renal excretion of sodium and water, and inhibiting cardiac remodeling. Moderate renal insufficiency (serum creatinine < 3.0 mg/dL) should not be considered a contraindication to initiating ACEI or ARB therapy, and monitoring of serum potassium levels and creatinine are recommended.

β-adrenergic blocker (beta-blocker) therapy is recommended for HF patients with an LVEF of 40% or less. Beta-blockers downregulate sympathetic adrenergic activity, reduce arrhythmia burden, and inhibit cardiac remodeling. A marked beneficial effect was seen in large clinical trials among symptomatic HF patients with NYHA class II-IV, when carvedilol, extended-release metoprolol, or bisoprolol were added.[43-45] Beta-blockers should not be initiated during acute decompensation, as they have negative inotropy. Both beta-blockers and ACEI should be started at low doses and up-titrated gradually to achieve target doses shown to be beneficial in clinical trials.

Mineralocorticoid receptor antagonist (spironolactone and eplerenone) therapy is recommended in current or recent NYHA class II-IV HF patients with an LVEF of 35% or less, in addition to standard medical therapy (beta-blockers, ACEI) and diuretics (COR I).[14] Creatinine should be 2.5 mg/dL or lower in men or 2.0 mg/dL or lower in women, and potassium should be 5.0 mEq/L or lower. Careful monitoring of potassium, renal function, and diuretic dosing should be performed at initiation and closely followed thereafter to minimize risk of hyperkalemia and renal insufficiency.

A combination of hydralazine and isosorbide dinitrate is recommended in addition to standard medical therapy including beta-blockers and ACEI for African American patients with NYHA class III-IV HF and reduced LVEF[11,13,46] (COR I). This combination can also be used in HF patients intolerant to ACEI/ARBs or those having severe side effects.[11,13,47] Diuretic therapy should be used to maintain normal volume status in HF patients with signs and symptoms of fluid overload. Digoxin can also be considered in symptomatic HF patients with reduced LVEF in addition to beta-blockers and ACEI, although its use remains controversial. The Digitalis Investigation Group (DIG) trial showed that digoxin has no mortality benefit, but helps in reducing rehospitalization for heart failure exacerbation.[48]

A recently approved therapeutic agent for chronic HF is an ARB in combination with a neprilysin inhibitor (ANRI). In the Prospective Comparison of Angiotensin-Converting Enzyme Inhibitor to Determine Impact on Global Mortality and Morbidity in Heart Failure (PARADIGM-HF) trial, the ANRI, sacubitril/valsartan, was superior to enalapril in reducing the risk of death from cardiovascular causes and hospitalization for chronic symptomatic HFrEF patients.[49] Use of ARB/ANRI is now a Class I recommendation to replace an ACEI or ARB in chronic NYHA class II-III HF[11,13,14] (COR I, LOE B). An ANRI should not be administered concomitantly with an ACEI or within 36 hours of the last dose.[14]

Ivabradine is also one of the newer therapeutic agents that acts by inhibiting the I_f current in the sinoatrial node, thereby reducing the heart rate. Ivabradine has proven to be beneficial in reducing the composite endpoint of cardiovascular death or HF hospitalization in symptomatic patients (NYHA class II-IV) with chronic HFrEF (LVEF ≤ 35%) in sinus rhythm with a resting heart rate of 70 beats or more per minute, and on optimal medical therapy[50] (COR IIa, LOE B).[14]

Intravenous inotropic support can be used in patients awaiting heart transplant to maintain hemodynamic stability until a donor heart becomes available. In some cases, milrinone or dobutamine may also be used as a bridge to evaluation in potential candidates for heart transplantation or LVAD. In patients who are not eligible for advanced HF therapies, inotropic agents can be used for palliative therapy to improve quality of life.

Asymptomatic Patients With Structural Heart Disease

Structural heart diseases (stage B HF) is more prevalent than symptomatic HF.[51] Identifying patients with subclinical systolic and diastolic dysfunction is very important to prevent progression to symptomatic stage C and stage D HF. Management of stage A HF and stage B HF (see Table 7-2) is focused on controlling cardiovascular risk factors (hypertension, diabetes, obesity, dyslipidemia, coronary artery disease) and reducing ventricular remodeling. Regular exercise, smoking cessation, and alcohol abstinence should be advised, along with achieving optimal BP control. Angiotensin-converting enzyme inhibitor therapy is recommended in asymptomatic patients with an LVEF less than 40%, and ARBs are recommended in patients intolerable to ACEI. Beta-blocker therapy is recommended in post-MI patients with reduced LVEF, whereas data are limited regarding their use in asymptomatic nonischemic heart disease patients.

Heart Failure With Preserved Ejection Fraction

No pharmacological therapy has been shown to improve outcomes in HFpEF patients, and there is not sufficient evidence to recommend routine treatment with RAAS inhibitors or beta-blockers in HFpEF patients.[6] Angiotensin-converting enzyme inhibitors, ARBs, and beta-blockers can be used if indicated for other comorbidities, like hypertension, kidney disease, atrial fibrillation, and CAD. Evaluation for ischemic heart disease should be considered. Dietary sodium restriction and diuretic use for optimizing fluid status is important in HFpEF patients, as they are volume sensitive. Management of HFpEF patients should focus on aggressive management of hypertension (COR I, LOE B); diuretics for relief of symptoms and evidence of volume overload (COR I, LOE C); coronary revascularization if presenting with angina or myocardial ischemia (COR IIa, LOE C); beta-blockers, ACEI, or ARB reasonable to treat blood pressure (COR IIa, LOE C); aldosterone receptor antagonists to decrease hospitalization if EF is 45% or greater, elevated BNP or HF admission within 1 year, glomerular filtration rate greater than 30 mL/min, creatinine less than 2.5 mg/dL, and potassium less than 5.0 mEq/L (COR IIb, LOE B-R); ARBs to decrease hospitalization (COR IIb, LOE B); exercise training; and treatment of coexistent comorbidities such as obesity and sleep apnea.[14]

Right Heart Failure

Right HF (RHF) is a complex clinical syndrome that can result from any structural or functional cardiac disorder that impairs the ability of the right ventricle (RV) to fill or eject appropriately into the pulmonary circulation. Right HF is associated with a poor prognosis,[52-54] and can be acute or chronic. Left HF is the most common cause of RHF. Acute RHF and RHF in the intensive care unit (ICU) are common with LV failure, RV ischemia, acute pulmonary embolism, pulmonary hypertension, sepsis, acute lung injury, cardiac tamponade, post–cardiothoracic surgery states, arrhythmias, pericardial disease, congenital heart disease, and valvular heart disease.[52] Positive pressure ventilation can also impede RV preload by increasing intrathoracic pressure and reducing RV transmural filling pressure.[52] Chronic RHF is seen in chronic obstructive pulmonary disease, interstitial lung disease, pulmonary arterial hypertension, and sleep-related breathing disorders such as obstructive sleep apnea. Dyspnea on exertion, exertional syncope, exertional angina, and right upper quadrant discomfort due to liver congestion are common symptoms. Patients can have increased intensity of the pulmonic component of the second heart sound, a holosystolic murmur at the left lower sternal border due to tricuspid insufficiency, a left parasternal heave, an elevated jugular venous pressure with prominent V wave, peripheral edema, or ascites.

Diagnostic evaluation is similar between right and left heart failure. In acute RHF, goals of treatment include optimization of preload, reduction of pulmonic reduction, and improvement of contractility, in addition to treating the underlying insult.[52-54] Proper fluid management is critical for successful management of RV failure. Maintenance of sinus rhythm and heart rate control is important. Preload optimization in RHF depends on RV afterload. In the setting of reduced RV contractility and normal RV afterload (like in RV myocardial infarction), a higher preload is needed to maintain forward flow, and a moderately high RV diastolic filling pressure of 8 to 12 mmHg is optimal to maintain RV myocardial perfusion. In the setting of increased RV afterload, reducing excessive RV preload with diuretics or ultrafiltration reduces RV dilatation and free wall tension, thereby reducing RV ischemia and improving contractility.[52-54] Lung protective ventilation, using the lowest effective plateau pressure, tidal volume, and positive end-expiratory pressure, helps with optimizing both RV preload and pulmonic afterload.[52] Optimization of RV afterload can be achieved by pulmonary vasodilators in the setting of pulmonary arterial hypertension. In cases with confirmed pulmonary arterial hypertension with normal left-side pressure, pulmonary vasodilators such as inhaled nitric oxide at doses of 20 to 40 parts per million, intravenous epoprostenol or treprostinil, inhaled iloprost, or oral sildenafil or tadalafil may be considered.

Inotropy is indicated for acute RHF with low cardiac output. Dobutamine is more extensively studied in this population, and low-dose dobutamine is a preferred option.[55-57] Dopamine and milrinone can be used in hypotensive and tachycardic patients, respectively. In refractory cases, ECMO support can be considered for potentially reversible RHF due to severe hypoxemic respiratory failure and/or pulmonary hypertension. Venoarterial ECMO pumps enough blood from the venous to the arterial circulation to unload the RV while maintaining systemic pressure and oxygenation. In cases of advanced RHF, mechanical circulatory support like RV assist devices are usually used as a bridge to heart, lung, or heart-lung transplantation.[57]

Use of Devices in Heart Failure

Implantable cardioverter-defibrillators (ICD) are indicated for the primary prevention of sudden arrhythmic death in ischemic (40 days post-MI) and nonischemic cardiomyopathy patients on guideline-directed medical therapy (GDMT) with an LVEF of 35% or less, NYHA class II or III symptoms, and expected survival more than a year[11,13,58] (COR I). Cardiac resynchronization therapy (CRT), which involves simultaneous pacing of both right and left ventricles (biventricular pacing), has been shown to increase LVEF, decrease HF symptoms, and reduce mortality in HFrEF patients with ventricular dyssynchrony.[49-51] Cardiac resynchronization therapy is indicated in HF patients on GDMT, with an LVEF of 35% or less, NYHA class II-IV symptoms, and ventricular dyssynchrony (left bundle branch block with QRS duration > 150 msec)[11,13,59] (COR I). In patients with ADHF, low output, and a CRT or ICD device, temporarily increasing the lower pacing rate may help to increase the cardiac output and avoid the need to use inotropic drugs. After stabilization of HF, RV pacing should be minimized or avoided, as it may worsen HF in the long term.

Cardiac Transplantation

The process of evaluating patients for cardiac transplantation requires determining whether an indication exists for cardiac or combined organ transplantation (eg, heart-kidney transplantation), referral to a transplant center, assessing absolute or relative contraindications, and weighing risks and benefits of various treatment options.

The indications for cardiac transplantation include refractory cardiogenic shock requiring continuous intravenous inotropes or circulatory support (eg, intra-aortic balloon pump, left ventricular assist device), persistent NYHA class IV heart failure symptoms despite optimal medical therapy, intractable angina due to coronary artery disease not amenable to revascularization (percutaneous or surgical), life-threatening arrhythmias resistant to medical therapy or catheter ablation, severe symptoms in patients with adult congenital heart disease not amenable to corrective surgery, and restrictive or hypertrophic cardiomyopathies. Patients with end-stage heart disease along with irreversible liver or lung dysfunction can be considered for dual organ transplantation. Contraindications to transplant include fixed pulmonary hypertension, noncompliance, inadequate social support, active cancer (or prior treated cancer within 5 years with a risk of recurrence), peripheral vascular disease, uncontrolled diabetes, drug use including tobacco and alcohol, and cachexia or morbid obesity.

Bridging to Cardiac Transplantation

The gap between the number of patients being listed for cardiac transplantation and number of donor organs available is rising significantly. One of the main reasons for this increasing gap is that the number of donor hearts available in United States has remained constant, while the population with end-stage heart failure continues to grow. There are several medical or surgical options available to maintain adequate organ perfusion while these patients are awaiting heart transplantation. Continuous intravenous inotropes, mechanical circulatory support (IABP, VA-ECMO, LVAD), and total artificial heart are among various treatment options for bridging to transplantation. Detailed evaluation, discussion with patients and their family, and clinical judgment play an important role before selecting any of these treatment options.

QUESTIONS

1. A 61-year-old man with history of ischemic cardiomyopathy and prior myocardial infarction is admitted to the ICU with symptoms of worsening shortness of breath and lower extremity edema. He has had cardiac resynchronization therapy with an implantable cardiac defibrillator (CRT-ICD) implanted 1 year ago. His home medications include carvedilol 12.5 mg twice a day, lisinopril 5 mg daily, aspirin 81 mg daily, spironolactone 25 mg daily, furosemide 40 mg daily, and atorvastatin 40 mg daily. On examination, he is afebrile, his heart rate (HR) is 60 beats/min, his blood pressure (BP) is 110/59 mmHg, his jugular venous pressure is elevated, his lungs are clear, he has a 3/6 holosystolic murmur with S3, and his lower extremities are cool with

+2 pitting edema. Laboratory testing reveals sodium of 124 mmol/L, potassium of 4.6 mmol/L, blood urea nitrogen (BUN) of 51 mg/dL, and creatinine of 1.8 mg/dL. An ECG shows 100% atrioventricular paced rhythm. Which of the following statements is FALSE with respect to this patient's management?

A. Right heart catheterization may be indicated to assess filling pressures and cardiac output.
B. Hold or decrease the beta-blocker until the patient is hemodynamically stable.
C. Start intravenous furosemide.
D. Start low-dose dopamine to improve renal function.

2. Which of the following abnormalities is the most important predictor of hospital morbidity and mortality in acute decompensated heart failure in addition to low systolic blood pressure?

A. Serum creatinine
B. Heart rate
C. Serum sodium
D. Hematocrit

3. A 26-year-old woman with no prior medical history presents to the emergency department (ED) with progressively worsening dyspnea for 1 week. Her symptoms are preceded by 3 days of fever, rigors, and nasal congestion. She is afebrile with HR of 116 beats/min and BP of 92/70 mmHg. Physical examination reveals bilateral rales, elevated jugular venous pressure, 2/6 systolic murmur at the left lower sternal border, cool extremities, and 2+ bilateral lower extremity edema. Echocardiogram reveals LVEF of 20%, nondilated LV (LV end-diastolic diameter of 3.4 cm), global hypokinesis, mild mitral regurgitation, and a normal right ventricular function. Labs are significant for creatinine of 1.6 mg/dL, aspartate aminotransferase (AST) of 385 U/L, alanine aminotransferase (ALT) of 413 U/L, troponin I of 4.8 ng/mL, and serum lactic acid of 2.8 mmol/L. Intravenous diuretics and dobutamine are initiated. Within 24 hours of admission, the patient develops hypotension and worsening heart failure refractory to inotropes and vasopressors. Urine output is 125 cc in the last 6 hours. Which of the following is the best next step in her management to stabilize her?

A. Add milrinone
B. Percutaneous axial flow pump (Impella)
C. Add metolazone
D. Endomyocardial biopsy

4. What clinical feature suggests that the patient in question 3 has acute, new-onset LV dysfunction?

A. Normal LV size
B. Lactic acid 2.8 mmol/L
C. Cool extremities
D. Worsening dyspnea for 1 week

5. A 48-year-old man with familial nonischemic cardiomyopathy and a single chamber ICD presents with 2 weeks of severe dyspnea on exertion and worsening orthopnea. In the emergency department, he is found to be lethargic with cool hands and feet. He is sitting up in the bed and is unable to lie flat. He is afebrile, with BP of 90/67 mmHg, HR of 122 beats/min, respiratory rate (RR) of 29 breaths/min, and oxygen saturation (Sao_2) of 91% on 100% oxygen via nonrebreather. Physical exam reveals basilar crackles bilaterally, 2/6 systolic murmur at the left lower sternal border and apex, jugular venous pressure elevated up to the angle of the jaw, cool extremities, and 1+ bilateral lower extremity edema. Labs are significant for sodium of 129 mEq/L, creatinine of 1.9 mg/dL, AST of 463 U/L, ALT of 621 U/L, troponin of 0.3 ng/L (< 0.02 ng/L), NT-proBNP of 4850 pg/mL (normal < 300 pg/mL), and lactic acid of 7.9 mmol/L. Echocardiography reveals severe biventricular systolic dysfunction, LVEF of 10%, left ventricular end-diastolic dimension of 66 mm, severely reduced right ventricular function, and mild mitral and tricuspid regurgitation. The ECG shows sinus tachycardia with frequent premature ventricular contractions (PVCs). Right heart catheterization reveals a right atrial pressure of 18 mmHg, pulmonary artery pressure of 48/30 mmHg with a mean of 36 mmHg, pulmonary capillary wedge pressure of 24 mmHg, and pulmonary artery saturation of 48%. Cardiac output and index are calculated at 2.2 L/min and 1.1 L/min, respectively. Dobutamine is initiated and he is transferred to an intensive care unit. Four hours later, repeat blood work shows creatinine of 2.1 mg/dL, AST of 549 U/L, ALT of 731 U/L, and lactic acid of 7.8 mmol/L. What intervention would stabilize the patient in this scenario?

   A. Percutaneous axial flow pump (left ventricle to aorta, Impella)
   B. Add milrinone
   C. VA-ECMO
   D. Centrifugal flow pump, left atrial to femoral artery bypass pump (TandemHeart)

6. A 62-year-old man with history of renal cell carcinoma post-chemotherapy and surgery 3 years ago, dilated cardiomyopathy, and left ventricular ejection fraction of 25% presents to the ED complaining of orthopnea, leg swelling, and paroxysmal nocturnal dyspnea. Over the last 1 month, he has gained 13 pounds and is now sleeping in a recliner. Current medications include carvedilol 6.25 mg twice daily, valsartan/sacubitril 24 to 26 mg twice daily, furosemide 80 mg twice daily, and spironolactone 25 mg once daily. He is compliant with his medications and dietary restriction of salt and fluid. On examination, patient is awake and alert. His BP is 115/75 mmHg, HR is 94 breaths/min, and RR is 14 breaths/min. Pulse oximetry reveals oxygen saturation of 95% on room air. Jugular venous pressure is approximately 15 cm H_2O. Cardiac exam reveals regular rate and rhythm, and S3 with a holosystolic murmur. Breath sounds are decreased bilaterally at the bases. Lower extremities are warm to touch with 3+ edema up to the knees. Which of the following is the best initial strategy for volume management?

   A. Start intravenous furosemide at a dose of 60 mg twice daily
   B. Increase the dose of oral furosemide to 160 mg twice daily
   C. Start a continuous infusion of furosemide at 5 mg per hour
   D. Start intravenous furosemide at a dose of 80 to 100 mg twice daily

7. After significant diuresis, the patient in question 6 remains functional class III with significant limitation in usual activities. He is readmitted 3 more times in 1 month for acute HF and develops more hypotension and intolerance to standard HF medications. Which advanced HF treatment is one for which he is a candidate and one that also will improve and prolong his life?

   A. Continuous IV inotropy with milrinone as palliative care
   B. LVAD as a bridge to cardiac transplantation
   C. Continuous IV inotropy with milrinone as a bridge to cardiac transplantation
   D. LVAD as destination therapy

8. A 56-year-old woman presents to her primary care doctor for an annual physical examination. She is postmenopausal with no medical history. She is physically active and runs 40 minutes a day, 6 days a week, with no shortness of breath. On exam, a systolic murmur is heard. The remainder of the exam is normal. An echocardiogram is obtained and reveals an LVEF of 33% with global hypokinesis, mild mitral regurgitation, and mild aortic stenosis. Which of the following is the most appropriate next step in her management?

   A. Start ACE inhibitor and statin
   B. Start ACE inhibitor and beta-blocker
   C. Start ACE inhibitor, beta-blocker, and aldosterone antagonist
   D. Start sacubitril/valsartan and beta-blocker

9. Which of the following risk factors is a therapeutic target to improve survival in HF patients?

   A. Anemia
   B. Renal dysfunction
   C. Hyponatremia
   D. Wide QRS

10. A 73-year-old woman with a history of ischemic dilated cardiomyopathy with an ICD implanted 8 years ago presents to the emergency room with worsening dyspnea on exertion and minimal lower extremity edema. She has diabetes mellitus, peripheral vascular disease, chronic renal insufficiency, and a recent hospitalization with HF exacerbation 6 weeks ago. Her current medical regimen includes metoprolol succinate 25 mg daily, lisinopril 5 mg daily, torsemide 40 mg twice daily, and aspirin 81 mg daily. On examination, she is afebrile, with HR of 106 beats/min and BP of 80/59 mmHg, and appears euvolemic. She is admitted to the ICU and started on intravenous furosemide. On hospital day 2, her urine output remains 30 to 40 cc/h and her creatinine increased from 1.8 mg/dL to 2.7 mg/dL. She continues to have minimal lower extremity edema. Review of telemetry reveals frequent episodes of nonsustained ventricular tachycardia. What is the next best step in her management?

   A. Start intravenous dopamine at 2 μg/kg/min
   B. Perform right heart catheterization
   C. Start intravenous dobutamine at 5 μg/kg/min
   D. Perform ultrafiltration

11. Echocardiogram is performed on the patient in question 10, and it shows left ventricular ejection fraction of 20% and an apical thrombus. Which of the following percutaneous mechanical support devices is contraindicated in this patient?

   A. Intra-aortic balloon pump
   B. TandemHeart
   C. Impella
   D. VA-ECMO

12. A 55-year-old woman presents to the ED with severe orthopnea for the past 12 hours. She has a history of hypertension and borderline diabetes. Examination reveals irregular rate and rhythm, with a HR of 121 beats/min, BP of 190/100 mmHg, jugular pressure of 14 cm, and body mass index (BMI) of 38 kg/m². Chest auscultation shows bilateral rales, while the precordial exam reveals an irregular and rapid heart rate with distant heart sounds and no discernible gallop. The patient is given intravenous furosemide, diltiazem, and heparin, with prompt improvement in symptoms. Her transthoracic echocardiogram shows normal biventricular size and function, mild mitral regurgitation, and mild left atrial enlargement. The ECG shows atrial fibrillation and voltage criteria for LV hypertrophy. She is admitted to the hospital and placed on oral losartan, diltiazem, rivaroxaban, and furosemide. Her HR is now irregular at 70 beats/min, and her BP is 130/65 mmHg, but she still complains of moderate dyspnea on exertion. Which of the following is the best next step in her management?

   A. Holter monitor
   B. Change diltiazem to metoprolol
   C. Transesophageal echocardiogram–guided cardioversion
   D. Sleep study

13. Which the following therapies has been proven effective to reduce mortality from HFpEF?

   A. Beta-blockers
   B. Angiotensin-converting enzyme inhibitors
   C. Diuretics
   D. No therapy reduces mortality

14. A 62-year-old man presents to the ED with a 2-hour history of severe chest pain, dyspnea, and diaphoresis. An initial ECG shows ST elevation in leads V_2-V_6. He is taken immediately for coronary angiography, which reveals a 100% proximal left anterior descending artery stenosis. The lesion is successfully opened with angioplasty followed by stent implantation. Left ventriculogram shows an EF of 25% with anterior wall hypokinesis. He is hypotensive during the procedure, and an IABP is placed and he is admitted to the ICU. During change of shift, the nurse observes blood in the connecting tubing of the IABP. What is the best next step of management?

   A. Continue IABP support
   B. Add heparin
   C. Immediately stop and remove IABP
   D. Flush the tubing with normal saline

15. The patient in question 14 becomes hypotensive with significant pulmonary edema 1 hour after placement of the IABP. An echocardiography is performed. Which of the following is most likely the cause of his decompensation?

   A. Severe aortic insufficiency
   B. Mitral regurgitation
   C. Atrial myxoma
   D. LV thrombus

16. A 51-year-old woman with ankle edema, ascites, and clinical findings of right HF presents to you for the first time. She immigrated to the United States from India 15 years ago. Her medical history is significant for hypertension and family history of tuberculosis. The heart sounds are distant, and the lungs are clear. Chest radiography is normal. Her ECG shows low voltage in the limb leads. A transthoracic echocardiogram is inconclusive because of poor acoustical windows, and the pericardium appears echogenic with trivial pericardial effusion present. Which test will be most useful in establishing diagnosis?

A. Positron emission tomography (PET) scan
B. Cardiac biopsy
C. Cardiac computed tomography (CT) scan
D. Transesophageal echocardiography

17. The right atrial tracing from a right heart catheterization is shown below (Fig. 7-1). What is the most likely diagnosis?

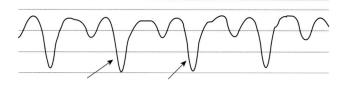

FIGURE 7-1 Right heart catheterization tracing.

A. Pulmonary hypertension
B. Constriction
C. Tricuspid regurgitation
D. Pericardial tamponade

18. A 52-year-old man with dilated nonischemic cardiomyopathy undergoes implantation of a continuous flow left ventricular assist device (CF-LVAD). He is postoperative day 6 in the ICU and is recovering well. What is his goal mean arterial pressure (MAP)?

A. 90–110 mmHg
B. 60–70 mmHg
C. 70–80 mmHg
D. 80–90 mmHg

19. The LVAD console for the patient in question 18 starts alarming. You observe a rise in the power, while the pulsatility index (PI) and pump speed are the same. What is the most likely cause of this presentation?

A. Arrhythmia
B. Hypertension
C. Inflow cannula obstruction
D. Device thrombus

ANSWERS

1. D. Start low-dose dopamine to improve renal function.

The role of low-dose dopamine in improving renal function is not well established. Neither low-dose dopamine nor low-dose nesiritide improved symptoms or renal function in acute decompensated HF patients presenting with renal dysfunction. Doses of intravenous furosemide (choice C) given either as continuous infusion or 12-hour bolus are equivalent in efficacy in acute decompensated heart failure patients. In patients with evidence of cardiogenic shock or low cardiac output, it is recommended to hold or decrease the beta-blocker (choice B). Right heart

catheterization is a useful test in some patients in guiding vasoactive medications including inotropes (choice A). Not listed as an option but something to consider is increasing the pacing rate of the CRT-ICD to provide a higher cardiac output (Heart Rate × Stroke Volume = Cardiac Output).

2. A. Serum creatinine

Clinical information obtained at the time of admission can help to predict outcomes during the hospitalization and following discharge. The ADHERE (Acute Decompensated Heart Failure National Registry) found that the single best predictor for mortality was an elevated blood urea nitrogen (≥ 43 mg/dL), followed by low SBP (< 115 mmHg), and high serum creatinine (≥ 2.75 mg/dL).[60] The OPTIMIZE-HF (Organized Program to Initiate Lifesaving Treatment in Hospitalized Patients With Heart Failure) registry also found SBP (≤ 100 mmHg) and serum creatinine (≥ 2.0 mg/dL) to be powerful predictors of in-hospital mortality.[5,7,10] Anemia and hyponatremia are common in patients with advanced HF and predict adverse outcomes in the long term and not in the short term; therefore serum sodium (choice C) and hematocrit (choice D) are wrong. Tachycardia (choice B) has not been shown to predict either in-hospital or postdischarge mortality in ADHF patients.

3. B. Percutaneous axial flow pump (Impella)

The patient has acute cardiogenic shock, likely from myocarditis, with isolated LV dysfunction and no significant valvular abnormalities. Impella pumps are axial-flow catheters that directly displace blood from the LV into the ascending aorta. The devices can be placed via the femoral artery in retrograde fashion across the aortic valve into the LV. Impella is a form of mechanical circulatory support and can provide adequate LV support. Its use is limited in biventricular failure, as it does not provide right ventricular support. An absolute contraindication to the Impella pumps is an LV thrombus and significant aortic regurgitation.

Adding milrinone (choice A) in acute cardiogenic shock patient with refractory hypotension and renal failure is relatively contraindicated. Continuing aggressive diuresis with metolazone (choice C) in patients with decreased perfusion to kidneys and significant pump failure is not beneficial. Delay in escalation of therapy in acute cardiogenic shock leads to worsening and permanent end-organ damage. Endomyocardial biopsy (choice D) to diagnose the etiology of underlying cardiomyopathy will not be helpful in the management of acute cardiogenic shock, although it may be helpful in establishing the etiology of the acute HF and possible subsequent treatment.

4. A. Normal LV size

Chronic LV dysfunction, by definition, occurs in a patient with remodeling, as seen on echocardiogram as LV dilation. A key finding of an acute, new-onset HF syndrome such as myocarditis is a nondilated LV, with the only main exceptions being restrictive HF, such as amyloidosis of hypertrophic cardiomyopathy. An elevated lactic acid (choice B) and cool extremities (choice C) reflect a low cardiac output syndrome, which can be present in both new-onset and chronic LV dysfunction. Similarly, worsening dyspnea for 1 week (choice D) may be seen in both entities.

5. C. VA-ECMO

Venoarterial ECMO is an effective tool in providing emergent mechanical circulatory support in patients with acute cardiogenic shock who are refractory to conventional therapy such as inotropes and vasopressors. Common etiologies of acute cardiogenic shock are acute decompensated systolic HF, myocardial infarction, and fulminant myocarditis. Extracorporeal membrane oxygenation is placed as a bridge to recovery, ventricular-assist device implantation, or heart transplant. Venoarterial ECMO should also be considered in patients who have severe respiratory failure coexisting with cardiogenic shock, similar to the patient described in this question. The patient described also has elements of right ventricular failure (high right atrial pressure), which VA-ECMO can support well by removing blood from the right atrium and pumping it continuously to the aorta (by cannulation either to the axillary or femoral artery). Adding milrinone (choice B) is relatively contraindicated due to worsening renal failure and in hypotension. Both Impella (choice A) and Tandem-Heart (choice D) will only provide isolated left ventricular support and will unlikely to provide him with adequate biventricular support for recovery.

6. D. Start intravenous furosemide at a dose of 80 to 100 mg twice daily

This patient presents with acute or chronic systolic HF and needs hospitalization. The best initial strategy to achieve effective diuresis in this patient is to increase the furosemide dose and administer it intravenously. As per 2013 ACC/AHA heart failure guidelines, HF patients presenting with signs and symptoms of volume overload should be treated promptly with intravenous loop diuretics to reduce morbidity. If these patients are already on oral loop diuretics, the initial intravenous dose should equal or exceed their chronic total oral daily dose and be given in the form of intermittent boluses or continuous infusion. Therefore, other choices given in the question are incorrect.

The Diuretic Optimization Strategies Evaluation (DOSE) trial failed to show any benefit of continuous infusion over intermittent bolus dosing.[23] This trial also compared high-dose diuretic strategy (total daily intravenous furosemide dose 2.5 times of daily equivalent of oral loop diuretic dose) to low-dose strategy (total intravenous furosemide dose equal to total daily oral loop diuretic dose). The high-dose strategy was associated with greater diuresis but also with transient worsening of renal function.[23]

7. D. LVAD as destination therapy

The patient in this vignette has progressive HF refractory to medical therapy and has several high-risk features such as hypotension, recurrent hospitalization, and continuous functional class III symptoms. Maintaining oral medical therapy will likely be insufficient to improve his symptoms of HF and prolong his life. Advanced therapies for HF include palliative inotropy, mechanical circulatory support with an LVAD (such as Heartmate II) as destination therapy or bridge to transplant, and orthotopic heart transplantation (OHT). This patient has recent cancer (within 5 years), meaning that he is not a candidate for heart transplant, and therefore, inotropy (choice C) and LVAD (choice B) as a bridge to transplant are not options. Continuous IV inotropy for palliation of symptoms (choice A) will likely improve his shortness of breath but will not prolong his life. An LVAD as destination therapy is a strategy of mechanical circulatory support that has been shown to improve symptoms of HF and prolong life in very sick patients that are not candidates for OHT. Should he have no recurrence of cancer for more than 5 years after treatment and remain at low risk for recurrence, then he could be re-evaluated for cardiac transplantation candidacy.

8. B. Start ACE inhibitor and beta-blocker

Neurohormonal therapy with an ACE inhibitor and beta-blocker is the cornerstone and first-line treatment for HF patients with reduced ejection fraction. Both medications should be started at low dosages and then up-titrated to a maximally tolerated dosage or to doses proven to be beneficial in clinical trials. There is no indication to start aldosterone antagonist (choice C) or sacubitril/valsartan (choice D) in an asymptomatic (functional class I) patient per the guidelines.[14]

9. D. Wide QRS

In patients with HF and left bundle branch block or QRS duration of 150 ms or greater, CRT, which involves simultaneous pacing of both right and left ventricles, is beneficial and improves survival. Treating, anemia (choice A), renal dysfunction (choice B), or hyponatremia (choice C) has not shown to improve survival in symptomatic HF patients. Treating anemia with intravenous iron may improve symptoms and functional class, but there is no evidence of a mortality benefit.

10. B. Perform right heart catheterization

Right heart catheterization is recommended to guide therapy in patients with acute decompensated HF who have unclear volume status, no response to a high dose of intravenous diuretics, worsening renal function, hemodynamic instability, and hypotension. Low-dose dopamine (choice A) has not been proven to improve renal function or symptoms.[61] In this patient, dobutamine (choice C) or other inotropic agents like milrinone can worsen the frequency of ventricular arrhythmias and can make her more hemodynamically unstable. Hypotensive patients are less likely to tolerate volume removal with venous ultrafiltration (choice D), but this can be an option in patients with cardiorenal syndrome and significant volume overload. The patient has minimal volume overload and possible low cardiac output. If the patient is hypovolemic, then ultrafiltration would further decrease preload and cause renal failure and hypotension.

11. C. Impella

The patient has an apical LV thrombus seen on echocardiography. Of the support devices listed, the Impella is placed in the LV via the femoral artery in retrograde fashion across the aortic valve into the LV, and therefore, may cause embolism of the LV thrombus. Intra-aortic balloon counterpulsation pumps are placed into the descending aorta and displace blood volume from the descending aorta by inflating during diastole and deflating during systole. An absolute contraindication to the IABP is moderate or severe aortic regurgitation (choice A). The Tandem-Heart device is an extracorporeal centrifugal pump that uses 2 percutaneously delivered cannulas to pump oxygenated blood from the left atrium to the systemic circulation via the femoral artery. An absolute contraindication to the TandemHeart device is left atrial thrombus (choice B). Venoarterial ECMO is placed via peripheral cannulas in the venous and arterial system. A contraindication to VA-ECMO is severe peripheral vascular disease (choice D).

12. C. Transesophageal echocardiogram–guided cardioversion

This is a typical presentation of hypertension with acute pulmonary edema in a woman with HFpEF. She presented in rapid atrial fibrillation, which may have precipitated the decompensation. These patients typically respond to blood pressure control. Atrial fibrillation is common in HFpEF, noted in 30% to 40% of patients. In contrast to HFrEF, there are no trials comparing rate versus rhythm control in HFpEF. There is an increased dependence on atrial systole in the setting of diastolic dysfunction. The ACC/AHA guideline recommends consideration of cardioversion for atrial fibrillation. A Holter monitor can be useful to determine adequate rate control, but this patient is symptomatic despite rate control (choice A). This patient likely has sleep apnea from a high BMI and will need an outpatient sleep study, especially as this can worsen HFpEF and increase the risk for atrial fibrillation (choice D), but conversion to sinus rhythm is the best initial step. There are no data to support use of metoprolol over diltiazem in patients with HFpEF (choice B). Diltiazem and verapamil are contraindicated in HFrEF, but this patient has HFpEF.

13. D. No therapy reduces mortality

As opposed to optimal medical therapy used in patients with HFrEF, all the clinical trials in patients with HFpEF have produced neutral results to date, and treatment is largely directed toward treatment of associated conditions and symptom improvement.

14. C. Immediately stop and remove IABP

Helium is commonly used for balloon inflation in IABP due to low density. It minimizes resistance, allowing rapid inflation and deflation. It is an inert gas and readily dissolves in blood, therefore reducing the risks of air emboli in case of balloon rupture. Presence of blood in helium tubing suggests balloon rupture. The IABP should be stopped immediately, and the helium line should be clamped and the balloon should be removed. It is an emergency; therefore, other options of conservative management are not correct (choices A, B, and D).

15. A. Severe aortic insufficiency

In patients with aortic regurgitation, IABP inflation during diastole will worsen the degree of regurgitation, increase myocardial wall stress, and may result in hypotension and pulmonary edema. For patients with known or suspected aortic dissections (ascending or descending), placement of IABP is also contraindicated. An IABP can also worsen left ventricular outflow tract obstruction and cause hypotension in such patients. Mitral regurgitation improves with IABP due to afterload reduction (choice B). Left ventricular thrombus and intra-cardiac tumors are not contraindications for IABP use (choices C and D).

16. C. Cardiac computed tomography (CT) scan

The patient has likely calcific constrictive pericarditis secondary to tuberculosis. Cardiac CT is good for visualizing the calcified pericardium. Cardiac MRI is another alternative test to visualize the pericardium and can identify other features of constriction, such as immobilization of the apex. Cardiac biopsy is a reasonable test for infiltrative diseases such as amyloidosis, which can cause right heart failure, but the transthoracic echocardiogram in the patient in this vignette suggests pericardial disease (choice B). Positron emission tomography (choice A) and transthoracic echocardiography (choice D) are not useful in visualizing the pericardium.

17. B. Constriction

In constrictive pericarditis, the right atrial (RA) pressure may be elevated, and the wave forms show steep X and Y descents. Right atrial pressure may be high in pulmonary hypertension, but a pulmonary artery measurement is needed to make this diagnosis (choice A). In the setting of tricuspid regurgitation, the RA tracing will demonstrate a large V wave during ventricular systole (choice C). In pericardial tamponade, a normal A wave, X descent, and V wave are seen, but the Y descent is blunted (choice D).

18. C. 70–80 mmHg

Current guidelines recommend a MAP goal of 70 to 80 mmHg for patients on LVAD support, as higher pressures are associated with an increase risk in stroke. Additionally, LVADs function optimally with a lower afterload. In high afterload states, the LVAD does not provide optimal LV unloading, and patients have increased shortness of breath. It is also recommended to initiate and titrate optimal HF medical therapy with beta-blockers, ACEIs, or ARBs in order to achieve optimal BP control. Blood pressure measurements in CF-LVAD patients is challenging as most of the patients do not have a palpable pulse; therefore, BP measurement by automated cuff or auscultation sometimes is not possible. In general, if an automated BP machine provides a BP measurement more than twice, it can be used as an accurate reading. If the automated BP machine is unable to provide a reading, then most likely the patient has minimal arterial pulsatility and the systolic BP approximates the MAP. In these patients, the Doppler BP (performed by identifying the brachial artery with a Doppler device and then inflating and deflating a BP cuff until the pulse is heard again) is taken as the MAP. A MAP of 80 to 110 mmHg is too high (choices A and D) and may result in an increase rate of stroke, and a MAP of 60 to 70 mmHg is likely too low and may result in dizziness (choice B).

19. D. Device thrombus

Left ventricular assist device thrombus can cause an increase in power consumption. Power is a direct measure of current and voltage applied to the motor of the device; therefore, any thrombus on the rotating components of the device will increase the pump power. These patients typically have features of hemolysis, such as an elevated lactate dehydrogenase (LDH), total bilirubin, low haptoglobin, and anemia. Additionally, they often have dyspnea, since the LVAD is not working optimally secondary to the thrombus in the LVAD. Arrhythmias (choice A), hypertension (choice B), and outflow/inflow obstruction (choice C) will lead to decrease in the power/flow.

Changes in various parameters of the LVAD and conditions associated with it are described as follows:

- ↓ power, ↓ PI, unchanged pump speed: hypertension, arrhythmia, outflow/inflow obstruction
- ↑ power, ↓ PI, unchanged pump speed: device thrombus, hypotension, vasodilation
- ↓ power, ↑ PI, fluctuating pump speed: suction event with decreased preload due to hypovolemia, overdiuresis, bleeding, right ventricular failure, or tamponade.

REFERENCES

1. Braunwald E. The war against heart failure: the Lancet lecture. *Lancet.* 2015;385(9970):812-824.
2. Mozaffarian D, Benjamin EJ, Go AS, et al; American Heart Association Statistics Committee; Stroke Statistics Subcommittee. Heart disease and stroke statistics—2016 update: a report from the American Heart Association. *Circulation.* 2016;133(4):e38-e360.
3. Gheorghiade M, Pang PS. Acute heart failure syndromes. *J Am Coll Cardiol.* 2009;53(7):557-573.
4. Rudiger A, Harjola VP, Müller A, et al. Acute heart failure: clinical presentation, one-year mortality and prognostic factors. *Eur J Heart Fail.* 2005;7(4):662-670.
5. Fonarow GC, Abraham WT, Albert NM, et al; OPTIMIZE-HF Investigators and Hospitals. Association between performance measures and clinical outcomes for patients hospitalized with heart failure. *JAMA.* 2007;297(1):61-70.
6. Redfield MM. Heart failure with preserved ejection fraction. *N Engl J Med.* 2016;375(19):1868-1877.
7. Fonarow GC, Stough WG, Abraham WT, et al; OPTIMIZE-HF Investigators and Hospitals. Characteristics, treatments, and outcomes of patients with preserved systolic function hospitalized for heart failure: a report from the OPTIMIZE-HF Registry. *J Am Coll Cardiol.* 2007;50(8):768-777.
8. Jessup M, Brozena S. Heart failure. *N Engl J Med.* 2003;348(20):2007-2018.
9. Killip T 3rd, Kimball JT. Treatment of myocardial infarction in a coronary care unit. A two year experience with 250 patients. *Am J Cardiol.* 1967;20(4):457-464.
10. Fonarow GC, Abraham WT, Albert NM, et al; OPTIMIZE-HF Investigators and Hospitals. Factors identified as precipitating hospital admissions for heart failure and clinical outcomes: findings from OPTIMIZE-HF. *Arch Intern Med.* 2008;168(8):847-854.
11. Yancy CW, Jessup M, Bozkurt B, et al; American College of Cardiology Foundation; American Heart Association Task Force on Practice Guidelines. 2013 ACCF/AHA guideline for the management of heart failure: a report of the American College of Cardiology Foundation/American Heart Association Task Force on Practice Guidelines. *J Am Coll Cardiol.* 2013;62(16):e147-e239.
12. Heart Failure Society of America; Lindenfeld J, Albert NM, Boehmer JP, et al. HFSA 2010 Comprehensive Heart Failure Practice Guideline. *J Card Fail.* 2010;16(6):e1-e194.
13. Ponikowski P, Voors AA, Anker SD, et al. 2016 ESC Guidelines for the diagnosis and treatment of acute and chronic heart failure: the Task Force for the diagnosis and treatment of acute and chronic heart failure of the European Society of Cardiology (ESC). Developed with the special contribution of the Heart Failure Association (HFA) of the ESC. *Eur J Heart Fail.* 2016;18(8):891-975.
14. Yancy CW, Jessup M, Bozkurt B, et al. 2017 ACC/AHA/HFSA focused update of the 2013 ACCF/AHA guideline for the management of heart failure: a report of the American College of Cardiology/American Heart Association Task Force on Clinical Practice Guidelines and the Heart Failure Society of America. *Circulation.* 2017;136(6):e137-e161.
15. Mebazaa A, Gayat E, Lassus J, et al; GREAT Network. Association between elevated blood glucose and outcome in acute heart failure: results from an international observational cohort. *J Am Coll Cardiol.* 2013;61(8):820-829.
16. Lee WH, Packer M. Prognostic importance of serum sodium concentration and its modification by converting-enzyme inhibition in patients with severe chronic heart failure. *Circulation.* 1986;73(2):257-267.
17. Wang TJ. Significance of circulating troponins in heart failure: if these walls could talk. *Circulation.* 2007;116(11):1217-1220.

18. McCullough PA, Nowak RM, McCord J, et al. B-type natriuretic peptide and clinical judgment in emergency diagnosis of heart failure: analysis from Breathing Not Properly (BNP) Multinational Study. *Circulation.* 2002;106(4):416-422.

19. Januzzi JL Jr, Camargo CA, Anwaruddin S, et al. The N-terminal Pro-BNP investigation of dyspnea in the emergency department (PRIDE) study. *Am J Cardiol.* 2005;95(8):948-954.

20. Gaggin HK, Januzzi JL Jr. Natriuretic peptides in heart failure and acute coronary syndrome. *Clin Lab Med.* 2014;34(1): 43-58, vi.

21. Fonarow GC, Peacock WF, Phillips CO, Givertz MM, Lopatin M; ADHERE Scientific Advisory Committee and Investigators. Admission B-type natriuretic peptide levels and in-hospital mortality in acute decompensated heart failure. *J Am Coll Cardiol.* 2007;49(19):1943-1950.

22. Binanay C, Califf RM, Hasselblad V, et al; ESCAPE Investigators and ESCAPE Study Coordinators. Evaluation study of congestive heart failure and pulmonary artery catheterization effectiveness: the ESCAPE trial. *JAMA.* 2005;294(13):1625-1633.

23. Felker GM, Lee KL, Bull DA, et al; NHLBI Heart Failure Clinical Research Network. Diuretic strategies in patients with acute decompensated heart failure. *N Engl J Med.* 2011;364(9):797-805.

24. Chalasani N, Gorski JC, Horlander JC Sr, et al. Effects of albumin/furosemide mixtures on responses to furosemide in hypoalbuminemic patients. *J Am Soc Nephrol.* 2001;12(5):1010-1016.

25. Triposkiadis FK, Butler J, Karayannis G, et al. Efficacy and safety of high dose versus low dose furosemide with or without dopamine infusion: the Dopamine in Acute Decompensated Heart Failure II (DAD-HF II) trial. *Int J Cardiol.* 2014;172(1):115-121.

26. Chen HH, Anstrom KJ, Givertz MM, et al; NHLBI Heart Failure Clinical Research Network. Low-dose dopamine or low-dose nesiritide in acute heart failure with renal dysfunction: the ROSE acute heart failure randomized trial. *JAMA.* 2013;310(23):2533-2543.

27. Bart BA, Goldsmith SR, Lee KL, et al; Heart Failure Clinical Research Network. Ultrafiltration in decompensated heart failure with cardiorenal syndrome. *N Engl J Med.* 2012;367(24):2296-2304.

28. Publication Committee for the VMAC Investigators (Vasodilation in the Management of Acute CHF). Intravenous nesiritide vs nitroglycerin for treatment of decompensated congestive heart failure: a randomized controlled trial. *JAMA.* 2002;287(12):1531-1540.

29. O'Connor CM, Starling RC, Hernandez AF, et al. Effect of nesiritide in patients with acute decompensated heart failure. *N Engl J Med.* 2011;365(1):32-43.

30. Cuffe MS, Califf RM, Adams KF Jr, et al; Outcomes of a Prospective Trial of Intravenous Milrinone for Exacerbations of Chronic Heart Failure (OPTIME-CHF) Investigators. Short-term intravenous milrinone for acute exacerbation of chronic heart failure: a randomized controlled trial. *JAMA.* 2002;287(12):1541-1547.

31. Oliva F, Latini R, Politi A, et al. Intermittent 6-month low-dose dobutamine infusion in severe heart failure: DICE multicenter trial. *Am Heart J.* 1999;138(2 Pt 1):247-253.

32. Thiele H, Zeymer U, Neumann FJ, et al; Intraaortic Balloon Pump in cardiogenic shock II (IABP-SHOCK II) trial investigators. Intra-aortic balloon counterpulsation in acute myocardial infarction complicated by cardiogenic shock (IABP-SHOCK II): final 12 month results of a randomised, open-label trial. *Lancet.* 2013;382(9905):1638-1645.

33. Ouweneel DM, Eriksen E, Sjauw KD, et al. Percutaneous mechanical circulatory support versus intra-aortic balloon pump in cardiogenic shock after acute myocardial infarction. *J Am Coll Cardiol.* 2017;69(3):278-287.

34. Konstam MA, Kronenberg MW, Rousseau MF, et al. Effects of the angiotensin converting enzyme inhibitor enalapril on the long-term progression of left ventricular dilatation in patients with asymptomatic systolic dysfunction. SOLVD (Studies of Left Ventricular Dysfunction) Investigators. *Circulation.* 1993;88(5 Pt 1):2277-2283.

35. Pitt B, Zannad F, Remme WJ, et al. The effect of spironolactone on morbidity and mortality in patients with severe heart failure. Randomized Aldactone Evaluation Study Investigators. *N Engl J Med.* 1999;341(10):709-717.

36. The CONSENSUS Trial Study Group. Effects of enalapril on mortality in severe congestive heart failure: results of the Cooperative North Scandinavian Enalapril Survival Study (CONSENSUS). *N Engl J Med.* 1987;316(23):1429-1435.

37. The SOLVD Investigators; Yusuf S, Pitt B, Davis CE, Hood WB, Cohn JN. Effect of enalapril on survival in patients with reduced left ventricular ejection fractions and congestive heart failure. *N Engl J Med.* 1991;325(5):293-302.

38. Cohn JN, Tognoni G; Valsartan Heart Failure Trial Investigators. A randomized trial of the angiotensin-receptor blocker valsartan in chronic heart failure. *N Engl J Med.* 2001;345(23):1667-1675.

39. Young JB, Dunlap ME, Pfeffer MA, et al; Candesartan in Heart failure Assessment of Reduction in Mortality and morbidity (CHARM) Investigators and Committees. Mortality and morbidity reduction with candesartan in patients with chronic heart failure and left ventricular systolic dysfunction: results of the CHARM low-left ventricular ejection fraction trials. *Circulation.* 2004;110(17):2618-2626.

40. Pitt B, Zannad F, Remme WJ, et al. The effect of spironolactone on morbidity and mortality in patients with severe heart failure. Randomized Aldactone Evaluation Study Investigators. *N Engl J Med.* 1999;341(10):709-717.

41. Pitt B, Remme W, Zannad F, et al; Eplerenone Post-Acute Myocardial Infarction Heart Failure Efficacy and Survival Study Investigators. Eplerenone, a selective aldosterone blocker, in patients with left ventricular dysfunction after myocardial infarction. *N Engl J Med.* 2003;348(14):1309-1321. Erratum in: *N Engl J Med.* 2003;348(22):2271.

42. Zannad F, McMurray JJ, Krum H, et al; EMPHASIS-HF Study Group. Eplerenone in patients with systolic heart failure and mild symptoms. *N Engl J Med.* 2011;364(1):11-21.

43. MERIT-HF Study Group. Effect of metoprolol CR/XL in chronic heart failure: Metoprolol CR/XL Randomised Intervention Trial in Congestive Heart Failure (MERIT-HF). *Lancet.* 1999;353(9169):2001-2007.

44. Packer M, Coats AJ, Fowler MB, et al; Carvedilol Prospective Randomized Cumulative Survival Study Group. Effect of carvedilol on survival in severe chronic heart failure. *N Engl J Med.* 2001;344(22):1651-1658.

45. CIBIS-II Investigators and Committees. The Cardiac Insufficiency Bisoprolol Study II (CIBIS-II): a randomised trial. *Lancet.* 1999;353(9146):9-13.

46. Taylor AL, Ziesche S, Yancy C, et al; African-American Heart Failure Trial Investigators. Combination of isosorbide dinitrate and hydralazine in blacks with heart failure. *N Engl J Med.* 2004;351(20):2049-2057.

47. Cohn JN, Archibald DG, Ziesche S, et al. Effect of vasodilator therapy on mortality in chronic congestive heart failure. Results of a Veterans Administration Cooperative Study. *N Engl J Med.* 1986;314(24):1547e52.

48. Digitalis Investigation Group. The effect of digoxin on mortality and morbidity in patients with heart failure. *N Engl J Med.* 1997;336(8):525-533.

49. McMurray JJ, Packer M, Desai AS, et al; PARADIGM-HF Investigators and Committees. Angiotensin-neprilysin inhibition versus enalapril in heart failure. *N Engl J Med.* 2014;371(11):993-1004.

50. Swedberg K, Komajda M, Böhm M, et al; SHIFT Investigators. Ivabradine and outcomes in chronic heart failure (SHIFT): a randomised placebo-controlled study. *Lancet.* 2010;376(9744):875-885. Erratum in: *Lancet.* 2010;376(9757):1988.

51. Goldberg LR, Jessup M. Stage B heart failure. *Circulation.* 2006;113(24):2851-2860.

52. Lahm T, McCaslin CA, Wozniak TC, et al. Medical and surgical treatment of acute right ventricular failure. *J Am Coll Cardiol.* 2010;56(18):1435-1446.

53. Ventetuolo CE, Klinger JR. Management of acute right ventricular failure in the intensive care unit. *Ann Am Thorac Soc.* 2014;11(5):811-822.

54. Skhiri M, Hunt SA, Denault AY, Haddad F. Evidence-based management of right heart failure: a systematic review of an empiric field. *Rev Esp Cardiol.* 2010;63(4):451-471.

55. Bardy GH, Lee KL, Mark DB, et al; Sudden Cardiac Death in Heart Failure Trial (SCD-HeFT) Investigators. Amiodarone or an implantable cardioverter-defibrillator for congestive heart failure. *N Engl J Med.* 2005;352(3):225-237.

56. Bristow MR, Saxon LA, Boehmer J, et al. Comparison of Medical Therapy, Pacing, and Defibrillation in Heart Failure (COMPANION) Investigators. Cardiac-resynchronization therapy with or without an implantable defibrillator in advanced chronic heart failure. *N Engl J Med.* 2004;350(21):2140-2150.

57. Moss AJ, Hall WJ, Cannom DS, et al; MADIT-CRT Trial Investigators. Cardiac-resynchronization therapy for the prevention of heart-failure events. *N Engl J Med.* 2009;361(14):1329-1338.

58. Goldenberg I, Kutyifa V, Klein HU, et al. Survival with cardiac-resynchronization therapy in mild heart failure. *New Engl J Med.* 2014;370(18):1694-1701.

59. Yancy CW, Jessup M, Bozkurt B, et al. 2017 ACC/AHA/HFSA focused update of the 2013 ACCF/AHA guideline for the management of heart failure: a report of the American College of Cardiology/American Heart Association Task Force on Clinical Practice Guidelines and the Heart Failure Society of America. *Circulation.* 2017;136(6):e137-e161.

60. Fonarow GC. The Acute Decompensated Heart Failure National Registry (ADHERE): Opportunities to improve care of patients hospitalized with acute decompensated heart failure. *Rev Cardiovasc Med.* 2003;4 (Suppl 7):S21-S30.

61. Lauschke A, Teichgraber UK, Frei U, Eckardt KU. Low dose dopamine worsens renal perfusion in patients with acute renal failure. *Kidney Int.* 2006;69(9):1669-1674.

8

Hypoxemic Respiratory Failure

Ronaldo Collo Go, MD, Maureen Dziura, MD, Hala El Chami, MD, and Imrana Qawi, MD

INTRODUCTION

Hypoxia occurs when tissues do not receive adequate oxygen to meet their metabolic demands. It is nonspecific and can mean reduced arterial partial pressure of oxygen (Pao_2; hypoxemic hypoxia), reduced hemoglobin for oxygen transportation (anemic hypoxia), decreased cardiac output or regional decrease in perfusion (stagnant hypoxia), disarray in cellular metabolism of oxygen such as in cyanide (histotoxic hypoxia), or mitochondrial dysfunction in sepsis (cytopathic dysoxia).[1]

Type 1 respiratory failure is defined as Pao_2 less than 60 mmHg with an equivalent arterial oxygen saturation (Sao_2) of 90% and normal or near or low arterial partial pressure of carbon dioxide ($Paco_2$). Type 2 respiratory failure involves hypercapnia and is defined as a $Paco_2$ of 46 mmHg or higher, regardless of oxygen saturation. Type 1 respiratory failure will be discussed in this chapter.

OXYGEN

Two percent of oxygen is dissolved in plasma (Pao_2) and 98% is bounded to hemoglobin (Sao_2). One gram of hemoglobin (Hgb) carries 1.34 mL O_2 per gram. Oxygen delivery is based on the formula $Do_2 = Cao_2 \times CO$, where Do_2 is the diffusing capacity of oxygen, Cao_2 is the arterial concentration of oxygen, and CO is cardiac output. Oxygen content is derived from the formula $Co_2 = (1.39 \times Hgb \times Sao_2/100) + (0.003 \times Po_2)$, where Co_2 is the concentration of oxygen, Hgb is the hemoglobin, Sao_2 is fraction of oxygen saturated hemoglobin over total hemoglobin, and Po_2 is the partial pressure of oxygen. Oxygen consumption is derived from the formula $\dot{V}o_2 = CO \times (Cao_2 - Cvo_2)$, where Cvo_2 is the venous concentration of oxygen. The alveolar–arterial (A-a) oxygen gradient is $Pao_2 - Pao_2$, where $Pao_2 = (Fio_2 \times [P_{ATM} - PH_2O]) - (Paco_2/R)$. In these formulas, Pao_2 is the alveolar oxygen tension; Pao_2 is the arterial pressure of oxygen; Fio_2 is the fraction of inspired oxygen, which is 0.21 on room air; P_{ATM} is atmospheric pressure, which is 760 mmHg at sea level, PH_2O is the partial pressure of water, which is 47 mmHg at 37°C; $Paco_2$ is arterial carbon dioxide tension; and R is 0.8 at steady state. The normal A-a gradient varies with age and is based on the formula $2.5 + 0.21 \times$ age in years.

A common, noninvasive way to measure oxygen bounded to hemoglobin is oxygen saturation via pulse oximetry. Based on the Beer-Lambert law, the principle states that light absorption of a given wavelength through a nonabsorbing solvent is directly proportional to the solute concentration, light path length, and extinct coefficient.[2] Deoxyhemoglobin absorbs light at a maximum of 600 to 750 nm, so light at 660 nm is optimal for its detection, and oxyhemoglobin absorbs light at a maximum of 850 to 1000 nm, so light at 940 nm is optimal for its detection.[3,4] In carbon monoxide poisoning, carboxyhemoglobin absorbs light at 660 nm and may cause a falsely normal or high O_2 saturation reading.[5,6] In methemoglobinemia, methemoglobin absorbs light at both 660 and 940 nm and may cause falsely low O_2 saturation.[7,8]

Another consideration is that the correlation of peripheral arterial oxygen saturation (Spo_2) with Sao_2 worsens when Spo_2 is less than 90%. Pulse oximetry also cannot detect hyperoxemia because large changes in Po_2 results in no change in oxygen saturation if it is almost 100% (Fig. 8-1).

MECHANISMS OF HYPOXEMIA

Hypoxemia refers to a decreased Pao_2. The 5 mechanisms of hypoxemia include reduced oxygen tension, hypoventilation, $\dot{V}/\dot{Q}$ mismatch, shunt, and diffusion abnormalities.[9,10] For a particular disease, these mechanisms are not necessarily mutually exclusive.

Reduction Oxygen Tension

The partial pressure of inspired oxygen (Pio_2), depends on Fio_2, P_{ATM} in mmHg, and PH_2O in mmHg according to the following equation: $Pio_2 = Fio_2 \times (P_{ATM} - PH_2O)$. For a person breathing room air at sea level and 37°C, the equation is $Pio_2 = 0.21 \times (760 - 47) = 150$ mmHg. This equation demonstrates that as the Fio_2 increases, the Pio_2 increases. Furthermore, as atmospheric pressure decreases (as it does at higher altitudes), the Pio_2 is lower. In the absence of diffusion abnormalities, the Pao_2 is determined via the Pio_2. If the Pio_2 is low enough, it will result in hypoxemia. Therefore, a decreased Fio_2 and increased altitude (lower P_{ATM}) can cause hypoxemia

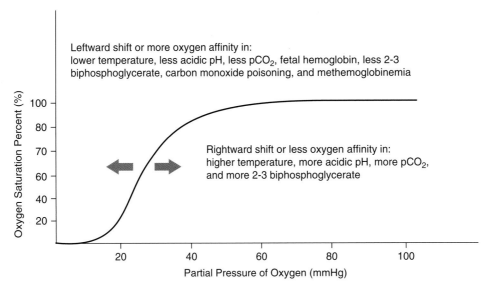

FIGURE 8-1 Oxygen-dissociation curve.

(decreased Pao_2). For example, for a person breathing room air at 37°C on Mount Everest (~29,500 ft, P_{ATM} = 231 mmHg) the equation is Pio_2 = 0.21 × (231 − 47) = 39 mmHg, and for a person breathing a 100% Fio_2 at sea level and 37°C, the equation is Pio_2 = 1.00 × (760 − 47) = 713 mmHg.

Hypoventilation

Inspired air is made up mostly of nitrogen (N_2) and O_2. When this air reaches the alveoli, it has mixed with water from the airways and CO_2 that was not expired on the last breath. The approximate partial pressures of gases in alveolar air are as follows: Po_2 = 100 mmHg, Pco_2 = 40 mmHg, P_{H_2O} = 47 mmHg, and P_{N_2} = 573 mmHg, for a total alveolar pressure of 760 mmHg. In the setting of hypoventilation, total alveolar pressure remains constant but the partial pressures change. Incomplete exhalation leads to poor clearance of CO_2 from the alveoli, but diffusion of CO_2 from blood to alveolus continues as long as a gradient still remains. The result is an increased partial pressure of CO_2 in the alveolus. Because the sum of all alveolar gases must remain constant, an increased partial pressure of CO_2 results in a decreased Pao_2. Decreased Pao_2 results in a lower Pao_2–Pao_2 gradient, causing decreased diffusion of oxygen across the alveolar-capillary membrane and a decreased Pao_2. Because the respiratory quotient is 0.8 (CO_2 produced/O_2 consumed), hypoventilation affects CO_2 levels more than O_2 levels.

V̇/Q̇ Mismatch

A $\dot{V}/\dot{Q}$ mismatch refers to ventilation and perfusion that are disproportionate to one another. In the ideal lung, ventilation would match the perfusion ($\dot{V}/\dot{Q}$ = 1) in all parts of the lung. However, even in healthy individuals, there is a small amount of $\dot{V}/\dot{Q}$ mismatch due to gravity and airflow resistance. Both ventilation and perfusion are increased in the bases of the lungs, but perfusion is affected more than ventilation is. The result is increased perfusion compared to ventilation ($\dot{V}/\dot{Q}$ < 1) in the lower portions of the lungs and increased ventilation compared to perfusion ($\dot{V}/\dot{Q}$ > 1) in the upper portions of the lungs. Diseased lungs have a greater degree of $\dot{V}/\dot{Q}$ mismatch due to areas of decreased ventilation, areas of decreased perfusion, or both.

In the scenario of high ventilation and low perfusion ($\dot{V}/\dot{Q}$ > 1), supplemental oxygen will improve hypoxemia because increased Fio_2 will increase the oxygen gradient from the alveolus to the blood and aid in diffusion. The extreme of this scenario, with ventilation but no perfusion ($\dot{V}/\dot{Q}$ = ∞) is called dead space. An example of dead space is the trachea, where ventilation is high but there is no pulmonary circulation to participate in gas exchange. There is both anatomic dead space and physiologic dead space. Anatomic dead space includes the oropharynx, trachea, and other non–gas exchanging airways, and is estimated at about 150 cc in a normal adult but varies based on height and anatomy. Physiologic dead space is pathologic and refers to a diseased area of the lung with normal (or increased) ventilation but no perfusion.

The extreme of the scenario of low ventilation and high perfusion ($\dot{V}/\dot{Q}$ < 1), with no ventilation and normal (or increased) perfusion, is shunt and will be discussed in further detail later.

Shunt

Shunt refers to blood flowing from the right to the left heart without participating in gas exchange. The result is deoxygenated blood returning to systemic circulation. If enough shunt is present, hypoxemia will result. Shunt fraction can be calculated using the following equation: $Q_s/Q_t = (Cc_{O_2} - Ca_{O_2})/(Cc_{O_2} - Cv_{O_2})$. Where Q_s/Q_t is the shunt fraction, Cc_{O_2} is the end-capillary oxygen content, Ca_{O_2} is the arterial oxygen content, and Cv_{O_2} is the mixed venous oxygen content. Shunt is an extreme form of $\dot{V}/\dot{Q}$ mismatch in which perfusion is present without ventilation ($\dot{V}/\dot{Q} = 0$). In its true form, supplemental oxygenation does not improve hypoxemia because there is no ventilation to deliver the oxygen to the alveolar-capillary membrane. Shunt can be either structural or physiologic. Structural shunts include a patent foramen ovale (PFO) or ventricular septal defect (VSD) with Eisenmenger syndrome. Physiologic shunts include pulmonary arteriovenous malformation (AVM) or alveolar-filling processes such as dense consolidation due to pneumonia or atelectasis.

Diffusion Abnormalities

Blood is oxygenated by diffusion of oxygen from the alveoli to the pulmonary capillaries. This diffusion is based on an oxygen gradient with higher concentrations of oxygen in the inspired alveolar air and lower concentration of oxygen in the venous blood returning to the lung. While carbon dioxide diffusion occurs very rapidly, oxygen diffusion requires a longer time to complete. Even so, a normal alveolar-capillary unit has enough surface area such that the blood passing by requires only about one-third of its contact time to fully equilibrate. When the alveolus or interstitium is disrupted by inflammation or fibrosis, the time for oxygen equilibration lengthens. With enough compromise of the alveolar-capillary membrane, oxygen diffusion time will lengthen to the point where full equilibration is not achieved by the time the blood has traversed the alveolus, resulting in hypoxemia. Hypoxemia due to diffusion abnormalities may be detected earlier in patients when testing includes pulse oximetry monitoring during exertion because as cardiac output increases, blood transit time across the alveolus decreases.

METHODS OF OXYGEN DELIVERY

Target oxygen saturation is 94% to 98%, but the elderly may have oxygen saturation less than 94% and remain clinically stable.[1] Nevertheless, exercise desaturation of 5% or more may be perceived as abnormal despite maintaining these target goals. Patients at risk for hypercapnia should have an oxygen saturation of 88% to 92%.[1] The method of oxygen supplementation is changed to meet these goals. Initial oxygen supplementation may be nasal cannula at 2 to 6 L/min, face mask at 5 to 10 L/min, or reservoir mask if So_2 less than 85, venturi mask 28% at 4 L/min for patients at risk for hypercapnia, or nonrebreather.[1]

A nasal cannula can deliver up to 6 L/min of oxygen. Flow higher than 6 L/min might increase patient discomfort or dryness, and increase the risk of epistaxis. It works primarily by washing out dead space in the nasal and oropharynx, thus increasing the oxygen content and decreasing the carbon dioxide content of inspired air. For every 1 L/min of oxygen delivered via nasal cannula, Fio_2 increases by 3% to 4%. Thus, a nasal cannula can deliver a maximum Fio_2 of about 45%. However, if the patient has limitations of airflow via the nasal passages or is breathing primarily through the mouth, the delivered Fio_2 will be lower than expected. In addition, if the patient is breathing rapidly, dead space washout will be suboptimal and the delivered Fio_2 will be lower.

A face mask can deliver up to 10 L/min of oxygen. It works in a similar manner to a nasal cannula in that it washes out nasal and oropharyngeal dead space. In addition, the mask acts as a reservoir of oxygen, which increases the amount of oxygen the patient initially inhales with each breath. The combination of the additional oxygen reservoir and increased flow rate increases the maximal delivered Fio_2 from 50% to 60%. Unlike the nasal cannula, the face mask covers the mouth, so patients who are breathing primarily through the mouth will still benefit from this method of oxygen delivery. However, as with nasal cannula, rapid breathing will exceed the ability of the apparatus to wash out dead space and fill the mask reservoir with oxygen, thus decreasing the delivered Fio_2. In addition, large tidal volumes will entrain room air through holes in side of the mask, thus decreasing the delivered Fio_2.

Nonrebreather masks require a minimum of 10 to 15 L/min to prevent inspiratory collapse of the reservoir bag. This bag increases the amount of oxygen the patient is breathing with each breath. One-way valves on the sides of the mask allow exhaled air to exit but inhibits room air from being entrained, thus increasing the guaranteed delivered Fio_2. Because the mask does not fit tightly, some room air may be entrained and dilute the Fio_2, especially with increased work of breathing. Maximum Fio_2 delivered is 80%.

Noninvasive ventilation (NIV) includes bilevel positive airway pressure (BPAP) and continuous positive airway pressure (CPAP). Both use positive pressure ventilation to deliver positive end-expiratory pressure (PEEP), which helps recruit alveoli and improve oxygenation. Bilevel positive airway pressure includes additional inspiratory positive pressure synched with the patient's breathing to aid ventilation. There are a variety of masks available to suit the needs and maximize comfort for each patient. An appropriately fitting mask will have minimal to no leak and thus can guarantee Fio_2 of 100%. Indications for NIV include chronic obstructive pulmonary disease (COPD) exacerbations, congestive heart failure (CHF) exacerbations, obstructive sleep apnea (OSA), and conditions that cause respiratory muscle weakness.

A high-flow nasal cannula is a large-bore nasal cannula that delivers heated and humidified air flows of up to 60 to 100 L/min. Because of the high flow, there is more dead space washout, which includes increased oxygen and decreased carbon dioxide. In addition, the high flow can generate up to 3 to 5 mmH_2O of PEEP, which helps with alveolar recruitment and oxygenation. Patients often find the mask and heated, humidified air more comfortable than NIV and can talk and clear secretions more easily.

DISEASES ASSOCIATED WITH HYPOXEMIA

The mechanisms of hypoxemia are not mutually exclusive and often coexist. Infections, trauma, cardiac causes of hypoxemia, acute respiratory distress syndrome (ARDS), and thromboembolic disease are discussed in other chapters of this book.

Interstitial Lung Diseases

Interstitial lung diseases (ILD) are a heterogeneous group of disorders that are classified together because of comparable clinical, radiographic, physiologic, and/or pathologic manifestations. The causes of hypoxemia are diffusion abnormalities and $\dot{V}/\dot{Q}$ mismatch. Identification of the type of ILD is important in terms of prognostication and response to immunosuppression. There are some types of interstitial lung diseases that can be diagnosed via computed tomography (CT), such as idiopathic pulmonary fibrosis. Often, the radiographic findings must correlate with histologic findings for diagnosis. Serologies may aid in the diagnosis of connective tissue associated interstitial lung disease. A diagnosis of an exacerbation of interstitial lung disease is often a diagnosis of exclusion. Ruling out underlying infection is paramount before immunosuppression via methylprednisolone 1 g intravenously (IV) for 3 days or cyclophosphamide or rituximab for scleroderma is initiated.

High-Altitude Illness

High-altitude illness is the result of hypobaric hypoxia, starting at altitude of 1500 meters, and symptoms include headaches, dizziness, nausea, vomiting, malaise, paresthesias, and insomnia. High-altitude pulmonary edema (HAPE) can manifest within 48 hours and can be accompanied by high-altitude cerebral edema (HACE). Treatment would include oxygen supplementation, rest, descent to 1000 to 3000 m, nifedipine or phosphodiesterase type 5 (PDE5) inhibitors for HAPE, and/or dexamethasone for HACE.[11-13] Hyperbaric treatment may be utilized. Prevention includes adequate rest before ascent, gradual ascent for altitudes more than 2800 m where the traveler spends one night at an intermediate level or stage ascent where traveler spends 5 to 7 days at intermediate level before proceeding higher, avoidance of alcohol and drugs, acetazolamide, nifedipine, tadalafil, or dexamethasone 24 hours prior to ascent.[11-13]

Pulmonary Hypertension

Pulmonary hypertension is classified into 5 groups, as seen in Table 8-1.[14] Early-stage pulmonary hypertension typically presents with dyspnea on exertion but can progress to being symptomatic at rest (see Table 8-1).[15] Physical examination is reflective of the underlying etiology and the severity of right heart failure, with an elevated jugular venous pressure (JVP) and increasing A wave due to loss of right ventricle (RV) compliance or elevated V wave from tricuspid regurgitation, a parasternal RV with palpable P2, a right-sided S4, increasing tricuspid regurgitation murmur, hepatomegaly, ascites, and lower extremity edema.[14]

Lab work, echocardiography, imaging studies such as $\dot{V}/\dot{Q}$ scan, pulmonary function tests (PFT), chest radiograph, and/or chest CT can suggest the presence of pulmonary hypertension and aid in diagnosing its etiology (COR I, LOE C). Pulmonary function tests may show a low diffusing capacity of carbon monoxide (DLCO). An echocardiogram (ECG) finding of a peak tricuspid regurgitation velocity greater than 3.4 m/s is highly suggestive of pulmonary hypertension.[16] A peak tricuspid regurgitation velocity of 2.9 to 3.4 m/s is also suggestive of pulmonary hypertension if: (1) right ventricle/left ventricle basal diameter ratio greater than 1 or a flattening of the interventricular septum; (2) right ventricular outflow Doppler acceleration time less than 105 msec and/or midsystolic notching, an early diastolic pulmonary regurgitation velocity greater than 2.2 m/sec, or a pulmonary artery

TABLE 8-1 Groups of Pulmonary Hypertension

Group	Causes
Group 1: Pulmonary arterial hypertension	Idiopathic, heritable (BMPR2, Alk-1, ENG, SMAD9, CAV1, KCNK3), drug and toxin induced, connective tissue disease, HIV, portal HTN, congenital heart diseases, PVOD, pulmonary capillary hemangiomatosis, persistent pulmonary hypertension of the newborn
Group 2: Pulmonary hypertension due to left ventricular disease (pulmonary venous hypertension)	Left ventricular systolic dysfunction, left ventricular diastolic dysfunction, valvular disease, congenital/acquired left heart inflow/outflow tract obstruction, congenital cardiomyopathies
Group 3: Pulmonary hypertension due to lung diseases or hypoxia	COPD, ILD, sleep disorders, alveolar hypoventilation disorders, chronic exposure to high altitudes, developmental lung diseases
Group 4: Chronic thromboembolic pulmonary hypertension	
Group 5: Pulmonary hypertension with unclear or multifactorial mechanisms	Chronic hemolytic anemias, myeloproliferative disorders, splenectomy, sarcoidosis, pulmonary histiocytosis, lymphangioleiomyomatosis, glycogen storage disease, Gaucher disease, thyroid disorders, tumor obstruction, fibrosing mediastinitis, chronic renal failure, segmental pulmonary HTN, neurofibromatosis

COPD = chronic obstructive pulmonary disease; HIV = human immunodeficiency virus; HTN = hypertension; ILD = interstitial lung disease; PVOD = pulmonary veno-occlusive disease.

TABLE 8-2 World Health Organization (WHO) Functional Classifications of Pulmonary Hypertension

WHO Classification	Description
Class I	No limitation with physical activity
Class II	Comfortable at rest, but ordinary activity causes fatigue, dyspnea, chest pain, or near syncope
Class III	Comfortable at rest but less than ordinary activity causes fatigue, dyspnea, chest pain, or near syncope
Class IV	Dyspnea or fatigue present at rest, signs of right heart failure

WHO = World Health Organization.

Data from Rich JD, S Rich. Clinical diagnosis of pulmonary hypertension. *Circulation.* 2014;130(20):1820-1830.

diameter greater than 25 mm; or (3) inferior cava diameter greater than 21 mm with decreased inspiratory collapse (< 50% with a sniff or < 20% with quiet inspiration) or an 18 cm^2 or greater right atrial area.[16] Right heart catheterization is needed to confirm the presence of pulmonary hypertension with the following measurements: pressures at end expiration revealing mean pulmonary artery pressure (PAPm) 25 mmHg or greater, pulmonary artery wedge pressure (PAWP) 15 mmHg or less, and pulmonary vascular resistance (PVR) greater than 3 WU (COR I, LOE C). If PAWP cannot be obtained, left ventricular end-diastolic pressure (LVEDP) should be obtained.[14] Table 8-1 lists the groups of pulmonary hypertension, and Table 8-2 lists the World Health Organization (WHO) functional classifications.

Patients with pulmonary arterial hypertension (group 1) from class I-III who have adequate cardiac output and are not hypotensive, vasoreactivity testing is advised (COR I, LOE C). Subtypes from connective tissue disease (CTD), human immunodeficiency virus (HIV), schistosomiasis, portal hypertension, and congenital heart disease are rarely vasoreactive. Nitric oxide, intravenous acetylcholine, tolazoline, epoprostenol, and adenosine are used in the test.[17-21] Acute vasoreactivity is defined as a fall in mPAP greater than 10 mmHg to an mPAP less than 40 mmHg with unchanged or increased cardiac output.[22] If vasoreactive, calcium channel blockers (CCB), amlodipine 20 to 30 mg/d, nifedipine 180 to 240 mg/d, or diltiazem 720 to 960 mg/d are advised (COR I, LOE C).[15]

For treatment-naïve WHO class II-III patients who are not candidates or for whom CCB treatment has failed, monotherapy with an endothelial receptor antagonist such as ambrisentan (COR I, LOE A), bosentan (COR I, LOE A), or macitentan (COR I, LOE B); a PDE5 inhibitor such as sildenafil (COR I, LOE A), or tadalafil (COR I LOE B); or the soluble guanylate cyclase stimulator riociguat (COR I, LOE B).[21] For treatment-naïve WHO class III patients, parenteral treatment with continuous IV epoprostenol (COR I, LOE A), IV treprostinil (COR IIa, LOE C), or subcutaneous treprostinil (COR I, LOE B) is advised.[15] For WHO class III patients with progression of symptoms despite being on 1 or more oral agents, IV epoprostenol, IV treprostinil, inhaled iloprost, or inhaled treprostinil should be added to their current regimen.[15] Treatment-naïve WHO class IV patients should be started with IV epoprostenol (COR I, LOE A), IV treprostinil (COR I, LOE C), or subcutaneous treprostinil (COR I, LOE B).[15,16]

Management of patients admitted to the ICU directly for an exacerbation of their pulmonary hypertension should include identifying the catalyst for the exacerbation, maximizing outpatient pulmonary hypertension medications, and/or treatment of right-sided heart failure.

Diffuse Alveolar Hemorrhage

Diffuse alveolar hemorrhage (DAH) is considered in a patient with diffuse bilateral opacities, and sequential aliquots of bronchoalveolar lavage (BAL) shows worsening hemorrhage. A finding of greater than 20% of 200 macrophages with hemosiderin helps confirm the diagnosis. Hemoptysis is absent in one-third of patients. Fever, cough, and associated anemia may be present. Causes are listed in Table 8-3.[23-25]

Management begins with stabilization via supportive care followed by etiology-focused treatment.

TABLE 8-3 Causes of Diffuse Alveolar Hemorrhage

Diseases	Iatrogenic	Drugs	Cardiac	Infections
Systemic lupus erythematosus	Radiation therapy	Cocaine	Mitral stenosis	*Staphylococcus aureus*
Goodpasture syndrome	Autologous bone marrow	Trimellitic anhydride	Subacute bacterial	Leptospirosis
Granulomatosis with polyangiitis	transplant	Isocyanates	endocarditis	Dengue
Eosinophilic granulomatosis with	Acute lung allograft	D-penicillamine		Anaerobic bacteria
polyangiitis	rejection	Warfarin		*Dirofilaria immitis*
Microscopic polyangiitis	Negative pressure	Nitrofurantoin		*Strongyloides*
Mixed cryoglobulinemia	pulmonary edema	Propylthiouracil		*Mycoplasma*
Behçet syndrome		Clopidogrel		*Legionella*
Scleroderma		Fibrinolytics		*Aspergillus*
Rheumatoid arthritis		Aspirin		Cytomegalovirus
Polymyositis		Amiodarone		Adenovirus
Mixed connective tissue disorder		Phenytoin		Influenza A
IgA nephropathy		Carbamazepine		Malaria
Ulcerative colitis		Methotrexate		
Multiple myeloma		Mitomycin C		
Lymphangioleiomyomatosis		Cytotoxic drugs		

QUESTIONS

1. A 72-year-old woman with history of Parkinson disease and diabetes presents to the emergency department (ED) complaining of nausea, vomiting, and abdominal pain. A CT scan revealed a small bowel obstruction secondary to a twist in the mesentery. She subsequently was intubated for exploratory laparotomy and lysis of adhesions. She continued to fail daily spontaneous breathing trials for the last 3 days. The chest radiograph below is the morning post breathing trial failure (Fig. 8-2).

   What is the next step?

   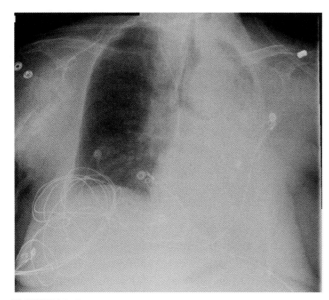

   FIGURE 8-2 Chest radiograph after third day of failing spontaneous breathing trial.

   A. Chest physiotherapy
   B. Acetylcysteine with bronchodilators
   C. Bronchoscopy
   D. Albuterol

2. A 30-year-old man decided to go hiking. After 48 hours, he has reached an altitude of 4000 feet. He decides to continue further when he suddenly complains of headache and shortness of breath. Then he starts to have fever and chills, and begins coughing up pinkish, frothy secretions. He starts to climb down where he encountered other hikers who managed to help him. What is the primary treatment?

   A. Descent and oxygen supplementation
   B. Nifedipine
   C. Sildenafil
   D. Dexamethasone

3. A 49-year-old man with a history of diabetes, alcohol abuse, and liver cirrhosis complains of shortness of breath that is alleviated when he is supine. His chest radiograph is below. What is the next step (Fig. 8-3)?

   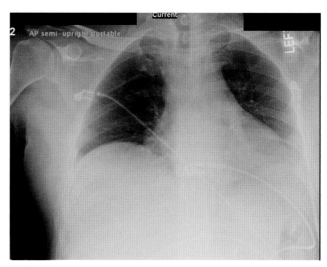

   FIGURE 8-3 Initial chest radiograph.

   A. Lung perfusion
   B. Contrast-enhanced transthoracic echocardiogram
   C. Right heart catheterization
   D. Pulmonary angiography

4. For the patient in question 3, what would increase the distribution of oxygen the most?

   A. Increase in cardiac output
   B. Increase in hemoglobin
   C. Increase in oxygen tension
   D. Decrease in hemoglobin

5. Which of the following can cause falsely elevated oxygen saturation?

   A. Ambient light
   B. Hypothermia
   C. Hypotension
   D. Black, green, and blue nail polish

6. A 60-year-old man presents to the ED complaining of progressive shortness of breath on exertion associated with low-grade fever and productive cough for the last 3 days. He recently traveled to California. He is married and lives at home with his wife. They have no pets. He currently smokes 2 packs per day for the last 30 years. He works in advertising. On physical examination, he is noted to have diminished breath sounds on bases. In the ED, a CT angiogram (CTA) of the chest shows no pulmonary embolism but showed fibrotic changes with traction bronchiectasis predominantly in the lower lobes. What is the next step?

A. Panculture
B. Solumedrol 1 g IV daily for 3 days
C. Pirfenidone 2403 mg by orally (PO) daily
D. Nintedanib 150 mg orally (PO) twice daily (BID)

7. A 60-year-old man with a history of hypertension and gastroesophageal reflux disease (GERD) complains of shortness of breath and dysphagia. On physical examination, he has telangiectasia on his face, crackles on auscultation of his chest, and discoloration of his hands to cold exposures. His chest radiograph shows bilateral patchy opacities. His chest CT shows bi-basilar lobe ground-glass opacities. His labs include the following:

White blood cells	$12 \times 10^3/\mu L$
Hemoglobin	15 g/dL
Platelets	$300 \times 10^3/\mu L$
Na	130 mEq/L
K	4 mEq/L
Cl	110 mEq/L
CO_2	27 mEq/L
Blood urea nitrogen	20 mg/dL
Creatinine	0.9 mg/dL
Ca	7.8 mg/dL
Glucose	110 mg/dL
B-type natriuretic peptide	100 pg/mL

Cultures were done and thus far negative. Connective tissue serologies were performed and showed the following:

Anti-ThRNP:	negative
Anti-PM-CL:	negative
Topoisomerase I:	negative
Fibrillin:	negative
Anti–RNP polymerase I and III:	positive
RF:	negative
ACCP:	negative
Anti-sSA:	negative
Anti-centromere:	negative
Aldolase:	negative
Anti-Jo-1:	negative
SSA/Ro:	negative
SSA/La:	negative

What is the next step?

A. Solumedrol 1 g IV for 3 days
B. Cyclophosphamide
C. Rituximab 50 mg/h IV and increased by 50 mg/h every 30 minutes up to 400 mg/h
D. Furosemide drip

8. A 50-year-old man, a current smoker with a history of diabetes mellitus and hypertension is complaining of progressive shortness of breath and subjective fevers and chills. He has recently traveled to the Middle East and is treated with oral antibiotics for 3 days but shows no improvement with his symptoms. After further inquiry, he also complains of hematuria. His BP is 130/70 mmHg, HR 98 beats/min, RR 18 breaths/min, temperature 99.4°F, and Spo$_2$ 90% on room air. Physical examination is remarkable for a saddle nose and diminished breath sounds on the right. His chest radiograph shows right upper lobe opacity. His labs include the following:

White blood cells	$15 \times 10^3/\mu L$
Hemoglobin	10 g/dL
Platelets	$250 \times 10^3/\mu L$
Na	140 mEq/L
K	4.2 mEq/L
Cl	111 mEq/L
CO_2	18 mEq/L
Blood urea nitrogen	50 mg/dL
Creatinine	4 mg/dL
Ca	8 mg/dL
Glucose	88 mg/dL

Urinalysis shows red cell casts, greater than 10 dysmorphic red blood cells, 2+ hematuria, and 2+ proteinuria. Cytoplasmic antineutrophil cytoplasmic antibodies (c-ANCA and PR3-ANCA) were positive. Renal biopsy was performed and showed necrotizing granulomatous inflammation of capillaries, venules, arterioles, arteries, and veins. What is your diagnosis?

A. Granulomatosis with polyangiitis
B. Eosinophilic granulomatosis with polyangiitis
C. Microscopic polyangiitis
D. Anti–glomerular basement membrane disease

9. A 34-year-old woman with history of asthma has decided to stop taking her high-dose inhaled corticosteroids with a long-acting β agonist while she is on vacations in the Caribbean for 2 weeks. Upon returning, she noted that she was feeling light headed, with shortness of breath, particularly on exertion, and some tingling sensation in her lower extremities. In the ED, she was noted to have a BP of 85/60 mmHg, an HR 130 beats/min, RR of 28 breaths/min, a temperature 100.1°F, and an oxygen saturation of 85% on room air. She was started on oxygen supplementation. Her chest radiograph shows bilateral patchy opacities. Her complete blood count (CBC) shows the following:

White blood cells	$14 \times 10^3/\mu L$
Eosinophils	20%
Hemoglobin	10 g/dL
Platelets	$140 \times 10^3/\mu L$
Troponin	2
Na	140 mEq/L
K	5 mEq/L
CO	18 mEq/L
Lactic acid	3 mmol/L
Creatinine	3 mg/dL

She was complaining of chest pain, which was temporarily relieved with sublingual nitroglycerin. Her shortness of breath progressed and she was intubated. Upon intubation, she was noted to bright red blood above the vocal cords. She had a bronchoscopy with sequential aliquots showing worsening hemorrhage. Cultures are negative. What is the next step?

A. Oral corticosteroid and oral cyclophosphamide
B. Antithymocyte globulin
C. IV corticosteroids (pulse dose)
D. IV corticosteroids (pulse dose) + IV cyclophosphamide ± plasma exchange

ANSWERS

1. A. Chest physiotherapy

Initial treatment for atelectasis include nonpharmacologic methods such as chest physiotherapy, postural drainage, incentive spirometry, humidification of oxygen supplementation, and early ambulation. There is debate on whether pharmacologic treatment such as albuterol and acetylcysteine (choice D and B) truly improve atelectasis.[26] Nebulized acetylcysteine can cause bronchoconstriction, and often, it is given with a bronchodilator. It has been suggested that acetylcysteine is truly beneficial with intrabronchial administration during bronchoscopy.[27] Bronchoscopy (choice C) maybe considered if the patient has persistent atelectasis after 24 hours of conservative treatment and/or to rule out intrabronchial etiology such as a neoplasm.

2. A. Descent and oxygen supplementation

High-altitude pulmonary edema is the result of a maladaptive response to reduced oxygen tension. There is poor ventilator response, increased sympathetic tone, heterogeneous vasoconstriction, inadequate production of nitric oxide, and overproduction of endothelin resulting in uneven disruption of the blood–gas barrier and the accumulation of plasma and red blood cells in the alveolar spaces. Risk factors include the following: male sex, cold weather, respiratory infection, altitude above 2500 m, pulmonary hypertension, PFO, atrial septal defect (ASD), and VSD.

High-altitude pulmonary edema rarely happens when the patient has been on a certain altitude for more than 7 days. Clinically, it presents with progressive shortness of breath followed by coughing up pink, frothy secretions within 2 to 4 days of ascent. It may be accompanied by low grade fever. Crackles are noted on auscultation. Diagnosis is based on history and physical examination. Treatment primarily involves descent to under 3000 m and oxygen supplementation. Adjunct treatment includes nifedipine (choice B).[28-33]

Tadalafil and sildenafil are used more for prophylaxis (choice C).[28-33] Dexamethasone is used for high-altitude cerebral edema and acute mountain sickness (choice D).[28-33]

3. B. Contrast-enhanced transthoracic echocardiogram

There are two types of pulmonary hypertension associated with liver cirrhosis: portopulmonary hypertension and hepatopulmonary syndrome. Portopulmonary hypertension is defined as the presence of portal hypertension and evidence of pulmonary hypertension via right heart catheterization. Signs and symptoms are nonspecific, and they can be related to complications of liver cirrhosis or pulmonary hypertension. Portopulmonary hypertension is histologically indistinguishable from idiopathic pulmonary arterial hypertension with the presence of intimal fibrosis, smooth muscle hypertrophy and fibroblasts, in situ thrombosis, and plexiform lesions from intraluminal endothelialization, or pulmonary arterioles with microaneurysm. Echocardiogram is often performed in cirrhosis patients for liver transplantation evaluation. Often, right ventricle systolic pressure of 50 mmHg or greater can suggest the presence of pulmonary hypertension. Right heart catheterization (choice C) is used to confirm pulmonary hypertension but with the hyperdynamic state in liver cirrhosis, systemic vascular resistance (SVR) is usually low. Therefore, some have suggested that a PVR greater than 120 dyn/s/cm³ should be a cutoff.[34] A mean pulmonary arterial pressure (Ppa) of 50 mmHg or higher and/or a PVR greater than 250 dyn/s/cm³ is a contraindication to liver transplantation due to the rate of 50% mortality postop.[34,35] Treatment is similar for group I pulmonary hypertension.

However, the presence of platypnea suggests that this cirrhotic patient might have hepatopulmonary syndrome. This occurs at any stage of liver disease and consists of arterial deoxygenation via a wide A-a gradient, and intrapulmonary vasodilatation. There is an increase in pulmonary nitric oxide, which causes these pulmonary dilatations at the capillary and precapillary level and more on the lower lobes. Their presence causes the symptoms of platypnea and orthodeoxia, and Pao₂ decreases by 4 mmHg or more, or 5% or more from supine to upright.[36] Contrast enhanced transthoracic echocardiogram can identify these pulmonary dilatations via opacification of left atrium more than 4 beats after the initial appearance of contrast in the right atrium. With a cardiac right-to-left shunt, opacification of the left atrium occurs 1 to 3 beats after its initial appearance in right atrium. Lung perfusion scan with macro-aggregated albumin (choice A) can quantify the severity of vasodilation via signal of Technetium-99m–radiolabeled micro-aggregated albumin outside of the lung.[34] Pulmonary angiography (choice D) may be used to discern type I hantavirus pulmonary syndrome (HPS) with normal or diffuse vascular dilatations from type II HPS with discrete arteriovenous communications. Treatment is lung transplantation, and hypoxia improves within months to years after transplantation. Type II HPS may not regress after transplantation but is amendable to embolization via coiling.

4. **A. Increase in cardiac output**

The delivery of oxygen is not as much affected by hypoxemia (choice C) or changes in hemoglobin (B and D), since the cardiac output can be altered to meet the oxygen demands.

5. **A. Ambient light**

Falsely elevated readings can be secondary to ambient light. Hypothermia, hypotension, and black, green, and blue nail polish can cause falsely low readings (choices B, C, and D). Hypothermia and hypotension can decrease blood flow to the periphery.[37-39] Black, green, and blue nail polish absorb light at 660 nm and/or 940 nm and therefore cause falsely low oxygen saturation.

6. **A. Panculture**

Diagnosis of usual interstitial pneumonia (UIP) via high-resolution CT has a 90% positive predictive value and a 100% negative predictive value if there is subpleural basal predominance, reticulation, honeycombing, and absence of atypical features (upper or middle lobe predominance, peri-bronchovascular manifestation, extensive ground glass, profuse micronodularity, discrete cysts, more than 3 lobes of diffuse mosaicism and air trapping, and consolidation).[40,41] Usual interstitial pneumonia is associated with connective tissue diseases, drug-induced lung disease, occupational lung diseases, and hypersensitivity pneumonitis. It is classified as idiopathic pulmonary fibrosis (IPF) after the other etiologies are ruled out. Idiopathic pulmonary fibrosis is less responsive to corticosteroids compared to other types of UIP. Antifibrotic agents such as pirfenidone (2403 mg by mouth daily; choice C) and nintedanib (150 mg orally twice daily; choice D) have been shown to delay the progression of the disease but have no role in acute exacerbations.[42,43]

Solumedrol 1 g IV daily for 3 days has been used to treat acute exacerbation of interstitial lung diseases (choice B). Before this is given, infection and cardiogenic pulmonary edema must be ruled out.

7. **B. Cyclophosphamide**

Scleroderma, or systemic sclerosis (SSc) is a heterogeneous disorder of excessive collagen deposition. Diagnosis is suggested by skin induration and presence of 1 or more of the following: heart burn or dysphagia, hypertension, renal insufficiency, dyspnea with or without radiographic findings, pulmonary hypertension, diarrhea, telangiectasia, erectile dysfunction, and digital infarcts.[44] Serologic testing include antitopoisomerase (anti-Scl70), antiendothelial cell

antibodies, anticentromere antibodies, and anti–RNA polymerase III antibodies.

The scleroderma lung study has suggested that cyclophosphamide can be used to treat SSc.[45,46] Corticosteroids with a dose greater than 15 mg/d is generally avoided to prevent development of renal crisis, particularly if positive for anti–RNP polymerase I and III antibodies (choice A). Rituximab may be considered in refractory causes.[47,48] (choice C). Patient is not volume overload with a low BNP so diuresis is not a good option (choice D).

8. **A. Granulomatosis with polyangiitis**

Antineutrophil cytoplasmic antibody (ANCA) promotes neutrophilic migration and release of metabolites on vascular wall.[49] Antineutrophil cytoplasmic antibody has been used to help diagnose a group of small-medium blood vessel vasculitis. These include microscopic polyangiitis, eosinophilic granulomatosis with polyangiitis, granulomatosis with polyangiitis, idiopathic pauci-immune pulmonary capillaritis, and anti–glomerular basement membrane disease. Most of these are considered pulmonary renal syndromes. However, there are other diseases associated with ANCA, such as drug-induced vasculitis (such as from propylthiouracil, methimazole, carbimazole, thiamazole, hydralazine, minocycline, penicillamine, allopurinol, procainamide, clozapine, phenytoin, rifampin, cefotaxime, isoniazid, indomethacin), rheumatologic diseases (systemic lupus erythematosus, Sjögren syndrome, rheumatoid arthritis, relapsing polychondritis, scleroderma, antiphospholipid syndrome), cocaine, and autoimmune gastrointestinal diseases (ulcerative colitis, primary sclerosing cholangitis, Crohn disease, and autoimmune hepatitis).[49] Therefore, biopsy, usually the lung or the kidney, is often needed to aide in the diagnosis.

There are 3 ANCA patterns that are screened by indirect immunofluorescence: cytoplasmic (c-ANCA), perinuclear (p-ANCA), and atypical (a-ANCA). The enzyme-linked immunosorbent assay test confirms the target antigen as PR3 or MPO. Combination of both provides sensitivity and specificity of 96% and 98.5%, respectively and helps with diagnosis[49] (Table 8-4).

9. **D. IV corticosteroids (pulse dose) + IV cyclophosphamide ± plasma exchange**

The patient has diffuse alveolar hemorrhage from eosinophilic granulomatosis with polyangiitis. Given the severity of her symptoms, the appropriate treatment would be IV corticosteroids (pulse dose) + IV cyclophosphamide ± plasma exchange. Table 8-5 lists the therapy according the severity of symptoms.[28,29,49] The other choices (A-C) would be insufficient.

TABLE 8-4 Types of ANCA Associated Vasculitis and How They are Diagnosed

ANCA-Associated Vasculitis	Diagnosis
Granulomatosis with polyangiitis	• 80–90% PR3-ANCA • 10–20% MPO-ANCA • 40% ANCA negative, particularly in pulmonary limited disease • Biopsy shows necrotizing granulomatous inflammation of capillaries, venules, arterioles, arteries, and veins
Microscopic polyangiitis (choice C)	• MPO-ANCA > PR3-ANCA • Biopsy is similar to polyarteritis nodosa, except vasculitis is restricted to venules, arterioles, and capillaries with some segmental necrosis and neutrophilic infiltration (choice C)
Eosinophilic granulomatosis with polyangiitis (choice B)	• MPO-ANCA > PR3-ANCA, although can be negative in the setting of pulmonary–cardiac disease Diagnosis based on 4 out of 6 of the following: • History of asthma or wheeze • > 10% eosinophils • Mono- or polyneuropathy • Transient pulmonary infiltrates • Paranasal sinus abnormalities • Biopsy of blood vessel with eosinophilic accumulation in extravascular space (choice B)
Anti–glomerular basement membrane (anti-GBM) disease (choice D)	• MPO-ANCA > PR3- ANCA • Renal biopsy shows immunoglobulin G (IgG; sometimes IgM or IgA) along glomerular capillaries and distal tubules[50] • Anti-GBM antibodies in serum needed since diabetic nephropathy and fibrillary glomerulonephritis can present with similar renal biopsy findings[50-52] (choice D)

TABLE 8-5 Severity of ANCA Vasculitis, Characteristics, and Medications

Severity	Characteristics	Medications
Limited	Isolated to upper airway disease, non–organ threatening	Topical medications, oral corticosteroids, and/or steroid-sparing agents such as methotrexate, azathioprine, or mycophenolate mofetil
Early generalized	Constitutional symptoms, end-organ involvement	Cyclophosphamide or methotrexate (better tolerated but longer to achieve remission and higher relapse rates) with alternatives such as azathioprine or mycophenolate mofetil
Generalized active	Constitutional symptoms, impaired and threatened organ function	Oral cyclophosphamide and oral corticosteroids (choice A) with alternative rituximab and anti-CD20
Severe	Organ failure including severe renal impairment (creatinine > 5.7 mg/dL), alveolar hemorrhage, central nervous system involvement, cardiomyopathy, gastrointestinal ischemia, or hemorrhage	IV corticosteroids (pulse dose or 1 mg/kg/d) + IV cyclophosphamide ± plasma exchange or IV corticosteroids (pulse dose or 1 mg/kg/d) + IV rituximab ± plasma exchange
Refractory	Failure to respond to treatment	Antithymocyte globulin (choice B), intravenous immunoglobulin, infliximab, deoxyspergualin
Remission		Transition from oral cyclophosphamide and oral corticosteroids in 3–6 mo to azathioprine, methotrexate, or mycophenolate mofetil for 18–24 mo

REFERENCES

1. O'Driscoll BR, Howard LS, Davison AG; British Thoracic Society. BTS guideline for emergency oxygen use in adult patients. *Thorax.* 2008;63(Suppl 6):vi1-vi68.
2. Bongard F, Sue D. Pulse oximetry and capnography in intensive and transitional care unit. *West J Med.* 1992;156(1):57-62.
3. Chan ED, Chan MM, Chan MM. Pulse oximetry: understanding its basic principles facilitates appreciation of its limitations. *Respir Med.* 2013;107(6):789-799.
4. Jubran A. Pulse oximetry. *Intensive Care Med.* 2004;30(11):2017-2020.
5. Hampson NB. Pulse oximetry in severe carbon monoxide poisoning. *Chest.* 1998;114(4):1036-1041.
6. Barker SJ, Tremper KK. The effect of carbon monoxide inhalation on pulse oximetry and transcutaneous PO₂. *Anesthesiology.* 1987;66(5):677-679.
7. Wright RO, Lewander WJ, Woolf AD. Methemoglobinemia: etiology, pharmacology, and clinical management. *Ann Emerg Med.* 1999;34(5):646-656.

8. Barker SJ, Tremper KK, Hyatt J. Effects of methemoglobinemia on pulse oximetry and mixed venous oximetry. *Anesthesiology.* 1989;70(1):112-117.

9. Rodriguez-Roisin R, Roca J. Mechanisms of hypoxemia. *Intensive Care Med.* 2005;31(8):1017-1019.

10. Pittman RN. Oxygen transport. In: *Regulation of Tissue Oxygenation.* San Rafael, CA: Morgan and Claypool Life Sciences; 2011: 23-36.

11. West JB. High-altitude medicine. *Am J Respir Crit Care Med.* 2012;186(12):1229-1237.

12. Bärtsch P, Swenson ER. Acute high-altitude illnesses. *New Engl J Med.* 2013;369(17):1666-1667.

13. Basnyat B, Murdoch DR. High-altitude illness. *Lancet.* 2003;361(9373):1967-1974.

14. Rich JD, S Rich. Clinical diagnosis of pulmonary hypertension. *Circulation.* 2014;130(20):1820-1830.

15. Taichman DB, Ornelas J, Chung L, et al. Pharmacologic therapy for pulmonary hypertension in adults. *Chest.* 2014;146(2):449-475.

16. Galiè N, Humbert M, Vachiery JL, et al. 2015 ESC/ERS guidelines for the diagnosis and treatment of pulmonary hypertension: The Joint Task Force for the Diagnosis and Treatment of Pulmonary Hypertension of the European Society of Cardiology (ESC) and the European Respiratory Society (ERS): Endorsed by: Association for European Paediatric and Congenital Cardiology (AEPC), International Society for Heart and Lung Transplantation (ISHLT). *Eur Heart J.* 2016;37(1):67-119.

17. Atz AM, Adatia I, Lock JE, Wessel DL. Combined effects of nitric oxide and oxygen during acute pulmonary vasodilator testing. *J Am Coll Cardiol.* 1999;33(3):813-819.

18. Dresdale DT, Schultz M, Michtom RJ. Primary pulmonary hypertension. I. Clinical and hemodynamic study. *Am J Med.* 1951;11(6):686-705.

19. Rudolph AM, Paul MH, Sommer LS, Nadas AS. Effects of tolazoline hydrochloride (priscoline) on circulatory dynamics of patients with pulmonary hypertension. *Am Heart J.* 1958;55(3):424-432.

20. Rubin LJ, Groves BM, Reeves JT, Frosolono M, Handel F, Cato AE. Prostacyclin-induced acute pulmonary vasodilation in primary pulmonary hypertension. *Circulation.* 1982;66(2):334-338.

21. Nootens M, Schrader B, Kaufmann E, Vestal R, Long W, Rich S. Comparative acute effects of adenosine and prostacyclin in primary pulmonary hypertension. *Chest.* 1995;107(1):54-57.

22. McLaughlin VV, Archer SL, Badesch DB, et al; ACCF/AHA. ACCF/AHA 2009 expert consensus document on pulmonary hypertension: a report of the American College of Cardiology Foundation Task Force on Expert Consensus Documents and the American Heart Association: developed in collaboration with the American College of Chest Physicians, American Thoracic Society, Inc, and the Pulmonary Hypertension Association. *Circulation.* 2009;119(16):2250-2294.

23. DeProst N, Parrot A, Cuquemelle E, et al. Diffuse alveolar hemorrhage in immunocompetent patients: etiologies and prognosis revisited. *Respir Med.* 2012;106(7):1021-1032.

24. von Ranke FM, Zanetti G, Hochhegger B, Marchiori E. Infectious diseases causing diffuse alveolar hemorrhage in immunocompetent patients: a state of the art review. *Lung.* 2013;191(1):9-18.

25. Lara AR, Schwarz MI. Diffuse alveolar hemorrhage. *Chest.* 2010;137(5):1164-1171.

26. Weiner AA, Steinvurzel B. Successful treatment of acute atelectasis with acetylcysteine. *NY State J Med.* 1966;66(11):1355-1357.

27. Mahmood N, Vargheses V, Aboeed A, Manickavel S, Khan MA. The role of intrabronchial mucolytics to treat atelectasis using fiberoptic bronchoscopy. *Am J Respir Crit Care Med.* 2013;187:A1419.

28. Stream JO, Grissom CK. Update on high-altitude pulmonary edema: pathogenesis, prevention, and treatment. *Wilderness Environ Med.* 2008;19(4):293-303.

29. Bärtsch P, Mairbäurl H, Maggiorini M, Swenson ER. Physiological aspects of high-altitude pulmonary edema. *J Appl Physiol (1985).* 2005;98(3):1101-1110.

30. Scherrer U, Allemann Y, Rexhaj E, Rimoldi SF, Sartori C. Mechanisms and drug therapy of pulmonary hypertension at high altitude. *High Alt Med Biol.* 2013;14(2):126-133.

31. Deshwal R, Iqbal M, Basnet S. Nifedipine for the treatment of high altitude pulmonary edema. *Wilderness Environ Med.* 2012;23(1):7-10.

32. Oelz O, Maggiorini M, Ritter M, et al. Prevention and treatment of high altitude pulmonary edema by a calcium channel blocker. *Int J Sports Med.* 1992;13 (Suppl 1):S65-S68.

33. Hackett PH, Roach RC. High-altitude medicine. In: Auerbach PS, ed. *Wilderness Medicine.* 6th ed. Philadelphia, PA: Mosby; 2012: 2.

34. Porres-Aguilar M, Altamirano JT, Torre-Delgadillo A, Charlton MR, Duarte-Rojo A. Portopulmonary hypertension and hepatopulmonary syndrome: a clinician-oriented review. *Eur Respir Rev.* 2012;21(125):223-233.

35. Krowka MJ, Plevak DJ, Findlay JY, Rosen CB, Wiesner RH, Krom RA. Pulmonary hemodynamics and perioperative cardiopulmonary-related mortality in patients with portopulmonary hypertension undergoing liver transplantation. Liver Transpl. 2000;6(4):443-450.

36. Gómez FP, Martínez-Pallí G, Barberà JA, Roca J, Navasa M, Rodríguez-Roisin R. Gas exchange mechanism of orthodeoxia in hepatopulmonary syndrome. *Hepatology.* 2004;40(3):660-666.

37. Ralston AC, Webb RK, Runciman WB. Potential errors in pulse oximetry. III: effects of interferences, dyes, dyshaemoglobins and other pigments. *Aneasthesia.* 1991;46(4):291-295.

38. Hinkelbein J, Genzwuerker HV, Fiedler F. Detection of a systolic pressure threshold for reliable readings in pulse oximetry. *Resuscitation.* 2005;64(3):315-319.

39. MacLeod DB, Cortinez LI, Keifer JC, et al. The desaturation response time of finger pulse oximeters during mild hypothermia. *Anaesthesia.* 2005;60(1):65-71.

40. Travis WD, Stabel U, Hansell DM, et al; ATS/ERS Committee on Idiopathic Interstitial Pneumonias. An official American Thoracic Society/European Respiratory Society Statement: update on the international multidisciplinary classification of the idiopathic interstitial pneumonias. *Am J Respir Crit Care Med.* 2013;188(6):733-748.

41. Souza CA, Müller NL, Flint J, Wright JL, Churg A. Idiopathic pulmonary fibrosis: spectrum of high-resolution CT findings. *AJR Am J Roentgenol.* 2005;185(5):1531-1539.

42. King TE, Bradford WZ, Castro-Bernardini S, et al; ASCEND Study Group. A phase 3 trial of pirfenidone in patients with idiopathic pulmonary fibrosis. *New Engl J Med.* 2014;370(22):2083-2092.

43. Richeldi L, Du Bois R, Raghu G, et al; INPULSIS Trial Investigators. Efficacy and safety of nintedanib in idiopathic pulmonary fibrosis. New Engl J Med. 2014;370(22):2071-2082.

44. Solomon JJ, Olson A, Fischer A, et al. Scleroderma lung disease. *Eur Respir Rev.* 2013;22(127):6-19.

45. Tashkin DP, Elashoff R, Clements PJ, et al; Scleroderma Lung Study Research Group. Cyclophosphamide versus placebo in scleroderma lung disease. *New Engl J Med.* 2006;354(25):2655-2666.

46. Hoyles RK, Ellis RW, Wellsbury J, et al. A multicenter prospective randomized double blinded, placebo-controlled trial of corticosteroids and intravenous cyclophosphamide followed by azathioprine for the treatment of pulmonary fibrosis in scleroderma. *Arthritis Rheum.* 2006;54(12):3962-3970.

47. Giuggioli D, Lumetti F, Colaci M, Fallahi P, Antonelli A, Ferri C. Rituximab in the treatment of patients with systemic sclerosis. Our experience and review of the literature. *Autoimmun Rev.* 2015;14(11):1072-1078.

48. Jordan S, Distler JH, Maurer B, et al. Effects and safety of rituximab in systemic sclerosis: an analysis from the European Scleroderma Trial and Research (EUSTAR) Group. *Ann Rheum Dis.* 2015;74(6):1188-1194.

49. Go R. Diffuse parenchymal lung diseases. In: *Pulmonary Diseases Examination and Board Review.* New York: McGraw-Hill; 2016: 121-156.

50. Borza DB, Chedid MF, Colon S, Lager DJ, Leung N, Fervenza FC. Recurrent Goodpasture's disease secondary to monoclonal IgA1-kappa antibody autoreactive with alpha1/alpha2 chains of type IV collagen. *Am J Kidney Dis.* 2005;45(2):397-406.

51. Burns AP, Fisher M, Li P, Pusey CD, Rees AJ. Molecular analysis of HLA class II genes in Goodpasture's disease. *QJM.* 1995;88(2):93-100.

52. Andres G, Brentjens J, Kohli R, et al. Histology of human tubulo-interstitial nephritis associated with antibodies to renal basement membranes. *Kidney Int.* 1978;13(6):480-491.

Hypercarbic Respiratory Failure

Sidney Braman, MD, and Steven H. Feinsilver, MD

INTRODUCTION

The main function of the lung is gas exchange: the elimination of carbon dioxide (CO_2) and the delivery of oxygen (O_2) to the tissues. When either function is impaired, the result is respiratory failure. Hypercarbic respiratory failure is a consequence of and is in direct proportion to a reduction of alveolar ventilation. Since the third major alveolar gas, nitrogen (N), is inert, any increase in CO_2 is accompanied by a reduction of O_2, unless supplemental oxygen is provided. When there is an acute or rapid reduction of alveolar ventilation, the result is acute respiratory acidosis. At other times, chronic respiratory failure can result from chronic lung disease, chest wall disease, or an abnormal respiratory control of ventilation. With such patients, there is often compensation of the hypercarbic respiratory failure and the acidosis may be corrected. This chapter will discuss the physiology of hypercarbic respiratory failure and describe clinical scenarios associated with hypercarbia and their associated management.

PHYSIOLOGY OF HYPERCARBIC RESPIRATORY FAILURE

Ventilation is the process of moving air from the atmosphere to the alveoli for the purpose of exchanging oxygen and carbon dioxide. Room air contains essentially no carbon dioxide. Mixed venous blood has a partial pressure of carbon dioxide (Pco_2) of approximately 46 mmHg. Alveolar Pco_2 ($Paco_2$) is approximately 40 mmHg, and there is no significant gradient between alveolar and arterial blood Pco_2 ($Paco_2$). Thus, $Paco_2$ is a nearly perfect indicator of alveolar Pco_2. An elevated $Paco_2$ indicates hypoventilation or hypercapnic respiratory failure.

Hypercapnic respiratory failure may exist in the presence of or independently of hypoxemia. As stated in Chapter 8, there are 5 mechanisms of hypoxemia: hypoventilation, ventilation/perfusion ($\dot{V}/\dot{Q}$) mismatch, shunt, diffusion abnormalities, and reduction in oxygen tension. As stated in Chapter 1, the alveolar–arterial (A-a) gradient may help determine which mechanism is involved.

Hypoventilation may be caused by a ventilatory drive problem ("won't do") or from a disease of the respiratory system ("can't do"). The $Paco_2$ is normally very carefully regulated by the brain, with even small changes resulting in almost immediate changes in ventilation. The normal ventilatory response to elevated $Paco_2$ is 1.5 to 2 L/min/mmHg. Normal resting minute ventilation is approximately 6 L/min. This indicates that the normal response to an elevated $Paco_2$ of only 43 mmHg would be to nearly double resting minute ventilation. The increase in ventilatory drive is normally perceived as dyspnea. Clinically, any patient with an elevated $Paco_2$ who does not appear dyspneic has a blunted ventilatory drive, either from a central nervous system (CNS) problem or from habituation. Hypoxic respiratory drive is much weaker, and patients who are hypoxic may not have symptoms of dyspnea. Hypoventilation due to decreased drive may be caused by a number of primary insults to the central nervous system, the best example being acute drug intoxication such as opiate use.

Even when ventilatory drive is not a problem, hypoventilation can be caused by problems in the spinal cord, nerves, respiratory muscles, or chest wall, without intrinsic lung disease. In all of these conditions, the A-a gradient would be expected to be normal. Only in the presence of intrinsic lung disease will the A-a gradient be elevated (Table 9-1).

SLEEP

Ventilatory drive is reduced during normal sleep, and $Paco_2$ rises slightly. This can lead to some respiratory instability during the initial few minutes of sleep as the $Paco_2$ level is "reset" about 2 to 6 mmHg higher. During deep nondreaming sleep (slow wave sleep), breathing becomes very regular, as there is little cortical influence. During rapid eye movement (REM; dreaming) sleep, ventilatory drive is further blunted and breathing becomes erratic. Muscle tone is decreased in REM sleep, and there is a greater dependence on diaphragmatic function, which becomes most apparent in neuromuscular disease states.

The upper airway maintains patency by a series of paired muscles, which are also respiratory muscles of inspiration. During sleep, muscle tone decreases in these muscles as well, leading to the potential for upper airway collapse (snoring and obstructive sleep apnea). Less common than obstructive

TABLE 9-1 Causes of Hypoventilation

Cause	Example
Reduced ventilatory drive	Narcotic overdose
Spinal cord	Trauma
Nerve, neuromuscular junction	Amyotrophic lateral sclerosis
Muscles	Polio
Ribcage	Scoliosis
Lung disease	Chronic obstructive pulmonary disease

sleep apnea is the obesity hypoventilation syndrome. These patients hypoventilate during sleep with little or no airway obstruction ("central" apneas). More severe cases will have evidence of hypoventilation during wakefulness and may benefit from respiratory support during sleep. A rare form of sleep related apnea called Ondine's Curse occurs when automatic ventilatory control is reduced further during sleep, so that patients can profoundly hypoventilate during sleep. This is the congenital central hypoventilation syndrome, and is now known to be a specific defect in the *PHOX2b* gene.

RECOGNITION OF RESPIRATORY FAILURE

Acute respiratory failure may be caused by a sudden catastrophic illness that overwhelms lung function and results in inadequate alveolar ventilation and hypercarbia. Extensive pneumonia, chest trauma, drowning, and drug overdose are common examples that can occur in patients with no underlying diseases. Other patients with acute respiratory failure may suffer from underlying conditions such as chronic obstructive pulmonary disease (COPD), asthma, or neuromuscular diseases such as kyphoscoliosis and muscular dystrophy. Early and mild stages of these diseases may not be advanced enough to cause chronic elevation of carbon dioxide. As the disease progresses, patients may develop and tolerate elevated levels of carbon dioxide for months to years. Renal compensation (retention of bicarbonate) will result in near-normal pH values, and the pulmonary symptoms of the underlying disease, such as dyspnea on exertion, predominate. However, because of limited respiratory reserves, an acute event such as infection can lead to an acceleration of the symptoms, with worsening shortness of breath and a struggle to maintain adequate ventilation. Those with an airway disease such as COPD, asthma, and bronchiectasis may also complain of increasing wheezing, cough, and sputum production. The sputum may change color from clear to yellow or green, and this reflects purulence from an acute bacterial bronchitis.

The pathophysiology of acute respiratory failure or an acute decompensation of chronic respiratory failure depends on the cause. Patients with underlying airway disease (COPD,

asthma, bronchiectasis) may show worsening airway wall edema and inflammation, bronchospasm, and plugging of the airway lumen with thick secretions. This increases airway resistance and the work of breathing, which in turn increases CO_2 production. Ventilation/perfusion mismatch occurs, causing further deficits in gas exchange and worsening hypercarbia and hypoxemia. Eventually, as the work of breathing continues to be excessive, respiratory muscle fatigue involving the diaphragm, chest wall, and accessory muscles occurs. This further reduces alveolar ventilation and causes the CO_2 to rise. If the rise of the CO_2 is rapid, renal compensation that takes many hours may not prevent a precipitous fall in the pH. In patients with chronic respiratory failure, preexisting buffering by renal compensation is somewhat protective and a less severe and precipitous fall in P_{CO_2} results.

Other causes of acute respiratory failure include conditions that result in alveolar flooding with edema, blood, or water. Acute pulmonary edema, diffuse alveolar hemorrhage, and drowning are examples of these 3 mechanisms. In such patients, alveolar ventilation can be so compromised that gas exchange and elimination of CO_2 is inadequate. In patients with chest wall trauma, pain, and splinting, minute ventilation and, hence, alveolar ventilation are compromised. Similarly, a large amount of blood (hemothorax) or air (pneumothorax) in the pleural space reduces the amount of functioning lung and can result in hypoventilation. One type of trauma-related severe chest wall deformity, with a high mortality rate of up to 40% when associated with lung contusion, is flail chest, defined as the fracture of 3 or more ribs in 2 or more places. In spontaneously breathing individuals, that diagnosis can be made by inspecting the chest wall. The flail segment is displaced inward rather than outward during inspiration. This paradoxical motion may not be seen in sedated, mechanically ventilated patients until positive pressure ventilation is discontinued.

In patients with acute life-threatening respiratory acidosis due to lung or chest wall causes, patients will complain of severe dyspnea, and the physical examination will show signs of respiratory distress. The patient may be diaphoretic and show nasal flaring, intercostal retractions, and the use of accessory and/or abdominal muscles of respiration. Tachypnea, tachycardia, hypertension, or hypotension may be present. Pursed lip breathing may be present, especially in patients with COPD. Patients may also show respiratory paradox, a sign of excessive respiratory load. This occurs when the chest wall and diaphragm are moving in the opposite directions. Inspection will show the abdominal wall moving in rather than out as the chest wall expands.

As a result of hypercarbia and acidosis, patients may develop CO_2 narcosis with mental status changes that range from confusion to frank coma. Terms that have been used to describe patients with CO_2 narcosis include disorientation, confusion, incoherence, somnolence, obstreperousness, combativeness, and bewilderment. Initially, patients show agitation and anxiety, and as respiratory distress increases, the level of alertness decreases. Apathy leads to drowsiness and then coma. Focal neurologic signs may also be present, and miosis, myoclonic jerks, sustained myoclonus, seizures, papilledema, and a flapping tremor of the hands (asterixis) can occur.

Patients with acute respiratory failure that results from excessive opioid and sedative use in the hospital setting, illicit drug use, and suicide attempts will not likely show signs of respiratory distress. Central nervous system respiratory center depression and slowing of the respiratory rate can result in hypercarbic respiratory failure and depressed mentation. This can lead to frank coma either from the drug or from respiratory acidosis. In patients who become apneic as a result of catastrophic CNS damage, the respiratory arrest and hypercarbic acidosis will demand immediate attention with respiratory support, and signs of respiratory failure are not relevant. Other causes of respiratory arrest that occur secondary to shock from sepsis, volume loss, or cardiac events are similar in this respect.

CLINICAL SYNDROMES

Acute Exacerbation of Chronic Obstructive Pulmonary Disease

Chronic obstructive pulmonary disease, characterized by progressive airflow obstruction due mainly to cigarette smoking and cooking with fossil fuels, is the third leading cause of death in the United States. It is projected to reach a similar level worldwide by 2020. An exacerbation of COPD is defined as an acute event characterized by worsening of the patient's symptoms (usually dyspnea, cough, and sputum production) that is beyond the normal day-to-day variation.[1] Mild exacerbation can be treated with short-acting bronchodilators; moderate exacerbation can be treated with short-acting bronchodilators, antibiotics, and/or oral corticosteroids; and severe exacerbation may require hospitalization or emergency visits, and may be associated with acute respiratory failure.[2] Exacerbation of COPD is the most common reason for admission to the hospital for hypercarbic respiratory failure. Often, the sputum becomes purulent, suggesting underlying bacterial infection. Approximately 70% to 80% of exacerbations can be attributed to respiratory infections, and coinfection with multiple organisms can worsen the outcomes. Viruses such as rhinovirus account for approximately 60% of acute exacerbations. Common bacteria that have been implicated include *Haemophilus influenzae*, *Streptococcus pneumoniae*, and *Moraxella catarrhalis*. The remaining causes are likely due to environmental exposures, but in many instances, the inciting event is unknown. The underlying pathophysiology of COPD is $\dot{V}/\dot{Q}$ mismatch, and during an exacerbation, this abnormality worsens. As a result, hypoxemia ensues, and with severe degrees of mismatch, hypercarbia results because of increased dead space ventilation. The respiratory failure of COPD is associated with a high risk for mortality with reported rates from 4% to 30%. Exacerbations are associated with poor long-term outcomes and a high risk of hospital readmission for those who survive.

Patients with COPD often have one or more comorbidities, such as congestive heart failure, coronary artery disease, diabetes mellitus, and gastrointestinal bleeding.[3] Exacerbations of COPD can be precipitated or caused by one of the comorbidities of COPD. In addition, COPD patients have a higher rate of bacterial pneumonia, especially those who are chronically using inhaled corticosteroids, one of the mainstays of treatments for severe COPD. Also, a high degree of suspicion for pulmonary embolic disease is necessary, especially when the clinical presentation lacks the typical infectious features of a COPD exacerbation, such as a viral prodrome or increased sputum production.[4] A reduction in previously elevated levels of $Paco_2$ could suggest pulmonary embolus rather than a COPD exacerbation.[5] A prior history of a COPD exacerbation within the last year is the best predictor of new exacerbation and the odds ratio of another exacerbation[6] grows rapidly with each subsequent attack.[7]

All patients with a COPD exacerbation should have a with admission chest radiograph.[8] New infiltrates may signify underlying pneumonia and findings of congestive heart failure may be present. The use of brain natriuretic peptide (BNP) or N-terminal pro BNP (NT-proBNP) can be helpful in identifying left ventricular dysfunction, and some studies have suggested it is a predictor of subsequent mortality,[9,10] and levels can help guide therapy.[11] Sputum Gram stain and culture are not recommended for routine use. However, for those who have had a recent hospitalization or who have failed outpatient antibiotic treatment, this study is indicated as Gram-negative organisms such as *Pseudomonas* are reported. Arterial blood gases (ABGs) are almost always needed, but in some hospitals, this test has been replaced by venous blood gas (VBG) analysis coupled with pulse oximetry.[12,13] Atrial and ventricular tachycardias should be anticipated, and atrial fibrillation and atrial flutter are also observed. Treatment of an acute exacerbation of COPD should target relief of symptoms, improvement in oxygenation, and reversal of respiratory acidosis, if present.[14] Supplemental oxygen can be offered with nasal prongs or a 24% or 28% venturi mask to assure controlled oxygen delivery to maintain the oxygen saturation (Spo_2) above 92% and the Po_2 above 55 mmHg. Limiting oxygen delivery to achieve these targets provides adequate tissue oxygenation and avoids the risk of worsening hypercarbia and respiratory acidosis, as high-flow oxygen therapy can induce hypercapnia in susceptible patients during exacerbations of COPD.[15] This can occur as a result of worsening $\dot{V}/\dot{Q}$ mismatch. Medical management should include a short-acting β agonist coupled with a short-acting anticholinergic, as some patients may achieve more benefit when both are offered together[8] (Level of Evidence [LOE] C).[2] Methylxanthines such as aminophylline and theophylline, once popular, are not helpful and potentially dangerous (LOE B).[2] Corticosteroids are indicated, as they improve lung function and may reduce length of stay and early treatment failure. Oral corticosteroids can be as effective as intravenous corticosteroids, if tolerated, and most patients can be treated with a short course of low-dose systemic corticosteroids, such as 40 mg of prednisone daily for 5 days[16,17] (LOE A).[2] High doses of corticosteroids (> 240 mg of methylprednisolone/day) in such critically ill patients have been associated with worse outcomes and more frequent adverse effects, such as diabetes and fungal infection, than lower doses (average daily dose of 96 mg/d).[18] Based on 1 study of ventilated patients in the intensive care unit (ICU), the use of antibiotics is important[18] (LOE B).[2] In that study, ofloxacin, 400 mg daily for 10 days, reduced the time on the ventilator, decreased the length of hospital stay, and improved overall mortality (number needed to treat [NNT] = 6; absolute risk reduction [ARR] 17.5%; 95% confidence interval [CI], 4.3–30.7; $P = 0.01$).[19]

In patients who have respiratory acidosis (pH < 7.35), or in those with severe respiratory distress induced by severe airflow obstruction and lung hyperinflation, mechanical ventilation is indicated. This can unload the respiratory muscles and decrease the excessive work of breathing, improve alveolar ventilation, reduce the P_{CO_2}, and with the use of a positive end-expiratory pressure (PEEP), reduce lung hyperinflation and improve the efficiency of the diaphragm and other respiratory muscles. The use of noninvasive positive-pressure ventilation (NIPPV) has been shown to achieve these objectives and avoid the complications of intubation and mechanical ventilation.

Noninvasive positive-pressure ventilation should be considered as first-line therapy for an acute exacerbation of COPD with hypercarbic respiratory failure, unless there is a contraindication to this form of therapy (Table 9-2) (LOE A).[2] Advantages of NIPPV for acute respiratory failure include avoiding the complications of intubation and invasive mechanical ventilation, such as upper airway trauma and ventilator-associated pneumonia, and better patient comfort, including the ability to speak and swallow. Lower mortality and length of hospital stay also have been demonstrated and improvement can be anticipated within the first hour of treatment. Noninvasive positive-pressure ventilation has been shown to reduce the rate of intubation and invasive ventilator support by as much as 50%. Failure with NIPPV, however, has been reported to be as high as 40% in some studies, and the training and experience of the clinicians partly determine whether the patient will succeed with NIPPV.[20] The best predictor of NIPPV success or failure is the degree of acidosis/academia at admission and the improvement after 1 hour on NIPPV.[21] It has been shown that severe acidosis (pH ≤ 7.25) in patients with a mean P_{aCO_2} of 87±22 mmHg

TABLE 9-2 Contraindications to Noninvasive Positive Pressure Ventilation

Pulmonary arrest
Cardiac arrest
Coma or severely impaired level of consciousness
Circulatory failure
Vomiting or high risk of aspiration
Excessive respiratory secretions
Severe craniofacial deformity
Facial surgery or trauma

can be successfully treated with NIPPV.[22] Mental status, overall severity of illness, and the presence of pneumonia have been found to be predictors of failure.[22,23] Bilevel positive airway pressure (PAP) is the usual initial modality, with inspiratory pressures starting at 10 to 15 cm H_2O and end-inspiratory pressures of 4 to 8 cm H_2O. Success can be measured by the patient's improvement of symptoms (reduced respiratory rate and subjective dyspnea) and the reduction of acidemia on repeat arterial blood gas determinations within 1 to 2 hours. Some patients do not tolerate the tight-fitting masks that are required with NIPPV, and some sedation may be necessary, although usually less than with invasive ventilation. Skin trauma to skin necrosis can occur with prolonged use of more than 1 to 2 days.

To monitor improvement with NIPPV, clinical and physiologic parameters can be followed. As arterial blood gases improve and respiratory acidosis is corrected, patients will experience less respiratory distress and dyspnea. Signs of respiratory muscle fatigue, worsening encephalopathy, or continued respiratory distress suggest NIPPV failure.

When this occurs, or there is a contraindication or lack of patient tolerance to NIPPV, intubation and mechanical ventilation should be immediately initiated. Strategies are required to improve gas exchange while avoiding high tidal volumes and excessive airway pressures that can lead to worsening hyperinflation and overdistention of alveoli.[24-26] One ventilator strategy that has been used for patients with COPD that avoids high volumes and ventilator pressures is permissive hypercapnia.[27,28] An elevated arterial P_{CO_2} is accepted to avoid ventilator-induced lung injury. Modest increases in arterial P_{CO_2} improve arterial P_{O_2} by reducing $\dot{V}/\dot{Q}$ heterogeneity and increasing lung compliance, thereby directing ventilation to underventilated areas. Also, elevations in alveolar P_{CO_2} have been shown to relax bronchial smooth muscle.

Obesity Hypoventilation Syndrome

The growing incidence of obesity, defined as a body mass index of more than 30 kg/m², has resulted in global challenges in healthcare. Obesity is associated with much comorbidity, such as obstructive sleep apnea (OSA), diabetes mellitus, metabolic syndrome, systemic hypertension, congestive heart failure, and pulmonary hypertension. Patients with extremes of obesity, called morbid obesity (body mass index [BMI] > 40 kg/m²), have a life expectancy that is reduced by 8 to 10 years compared to the nonobese. One syndrome associated with obesity is the obesity hypoventilation syndrome (OHS), a condition often associated with sleep apnea. Obesity hypoventilation syndrome is defined as obesity and daytime hypoventilation in the absence of other causes of hypoventilation such as pulmonary disease, neuromuscular weakness, chest wall disorders, or a metabolic explanation for hypoventilation.

As many as 1 in 5 patients admitted to the ICU is obese, and those with extreme obesity present unique challenges to the ICU staff, including bed positioning, skin care, transport within the hospital, vascular access, and physical therapy measures.[29]

One common presentation in such patients is acute respiratory failure, often complicating chronic OHS. This can be precipitated by excessive use of supplemental oxygen, overly vigorous diuresis that induces metabolic alkalosis, or excessive use of narcotics, anxiolytics, or sedatives.[30]

The mechanism involved in producing chronic carbon dioxide retention in the obese patient is likely multifactorial.[31,32] Lung volumes in obese patients are reduced, causing atelectasis and $\dot{V}/\dot{Q}$ mismatch. Excessive body mass produces an increase in the mechanical load on the respiratory system. This increases the work of breathing and carbon dioxide production. Why some obese patients develop chronic hypercapnia and others do not is not clear. In most OHS patients, OSA is a complicating factor. This is associated with increased upper airway resistance, evidence of an impaired chemoreceptor response to hypoxemia and hypercapnia, and leptin resistance. In obese patients, this resistance may result in hypercarbia, as the adipokine leptin enhances respiratory drive. Severe nocturnal hypoxemia has been demonstrated in OHS patients with obstructive sleep apnea; the mean oxygen nadir during sleep is lower and time spent with oxygen saturation less than 90% is increased. In 1 study, the mean oxygen nadir was 65%, with a mean of 50% of time with oxygen saturation less than 90%.[31] Although sleep apnea is common in patients with OHS, patients with obstructive sleep apnea alone are not expected to have chronic hypercarbia or hypoxemia while awake.

The clinical presentation of acute hypercarbic respiratory failure in patients with OHS is similar to patients with other causes. Patients will present with signs of respiratory acidosis, but the arterial blood gases will show pH levels of acute on chronic hypercarbia. Patients will usually show extreme obesity with large neck circumference and signs of cor pulmonale. If medical records are available, a previous serum bicarbonate can be useful, as levels less than 27 mEq/L have a 97% negative predictive value.[32] Also, hypoxemia during wakefulness may be seen with OHS. As OHS is a diagnosis of exclusion, other causes of chronic hypoventilation should be considered.

The management of hypercarbic respiratory failure in OHS patients includes supplemental oxygen, noninvasive and invasive ventilator support, diuresis, and investigation for common comorbidities.[34] If there are no contraindications to the use of bilevel PAP via a nasal or oronasal interface, it should be initiated immediately. This will rapidly eliminate the element of obstructive apnea likely to be present, but additional support with a timed back-up rate or NIPPV may be required. It should be anticipated that higher pressure levels and longer times will be needed to reduce the level of $Paco_2$ compared to nonobese patients.[35] Intubation and mechanical ventilation should be reserved for those who have a contraindication to NIPPV or who do not respond to initial use. As soon as the clinical condition of the patient stabilizes and the pH is within normal values, treatment is considered effective. Some patients will return their blood gases to normal values during the hospital admission, but many will have significant hypercapnia and hypoxemia on hospital discharge. With the use of NIPPV, oxygen therapy may not be needed. However, up to 50% of patients with OHS require oxygen to keep the oxygen saturation over 90%, even in the absence of hypopneas and apneas.[36] One retrospective cohort study found the need for daytime supplemental oxygen decreased from 30% to 6% in patients who were adherent to nocturnal treatment of OSA.[37]

In-hospital mortality is high among OHS patients. In 1 study, admission to the ICU was an independent predictor of hospital mortality, and an overall cumulative 3-year mortality for these patients was of 31.3%.[38] Plans for a vigorous posthospital discharge plan including NIPPV, dietary and other lifestyle interventions, and possible bariatric surgery need to be arranged.[38]

Status Asthmaticus

Approximately 2% to 4% of patients admitted to the hospital with severe asthma in the United States require mechanical ventilation.[39] Definition of severe asthma for 6 years of age or older include asthma that requires treatment with medications from Global Initiative for Asthma (GINA) guidelines steps 4 and 5 (high-dose inhaled corticosteroids and long-acting β agonist or leukotriene modifier/theophylline) for the last year, or systemic corticosteroids for 50% or more of the previous year.[40] Assessment of the severity of exacerbation may not be clinically apparent, and objective data for those who can perform the maneuvers are warranted. The most objective method to determine severe asthma exacerbation includes peak flow less than 200 L/min or peak flow percent less than 50%. Factors associated with asthma-related death include history of near-fatal asthma requiring intubation and mechanical ventilation; hospitalization or emergency visit for asthma in the past year; current or recent use of oral corticosteroids; no use of inhaled corticosteroids; overuse of short acting β agonists, especially more than 1 canister per month; psychiatric or psychosocial issues; poor adherence to medications or written asthma action plan; and food allergy.[41]

Triage of the asthma exacerbation begins with classification of its severity. Mild or moderate exacerbation is characterized by patients who can talk in phrases, prefer sitting to lying, are not agitated, and have an increased respiratory rate, a heart rate of 100 to 120 beats/min, no accessory muscles, oxygen saturation of 90% to 95% on room air, and peak expiratory flow (PEF) of more than 50% predicted or best.[41] Treatment includes short-acting $β_2$ agonists, ipratropium bromide, oral corticosteroids, and oxygen supplementation to maintain oxygen saturation greater than 92%.[41] Duration of corticosteroids is 5 to 7 days (LOE B).[41] High-dose inhaled corticosteroids (500–1600 μg beclomethasone dipropionate and hydrofluoroalkane [BDP-HFA] equivalent) is an equivalent dose to the oral corticosteroids (LOE A).[41] If symptoms do not improve within 1 hour and forced expiratory volume during the first second (FEV1) or PEF is less than 60%, consider the case to be severe asthma. If symptoms improve and

FEV1 or PEF is 60% to 80% of the patient's predicted or personal best, it is considered moderate and the patient can be discharged.[41] Severe exacerbation is characterized by patients who can only talk in words, who are agitated or hunched forward, or who have a respiratory rate greater than 30, a heart rate greater than 120 beats/min, oxygen saturation on room air less than 90%, accessory muscle use, and PEF of 50% or less of the predicted or best level.[41] Treatment is similar with moderate exacerbation, except for transition to intravenous (IV) corticosteroids and use of magnesium. Magnesium 2 g IV over 20 minutes reduces hospital admissions (LOE A).[41] Like in moderate exacerbation, reevaluation after treatment for severe exacerbation is warranted. If there is improvement, it can be recategorized as moderate exacerbation.[41]

As with COPD patients, severe airway obstruction results in both high $\dot{V}/\dot{Q}$ and low $\dot{V}/\dot{Q}$ mismatch and causes hypoxemia and carbon dioxide retention. The work of breathing is quite high with severe asthma, and carbon dioxide production increases. Respiratory muscle fatigue can be seen in a prolonged attack, and this results in worsening hypercarbic respiratory acidosis. The use of NIPPV can offer many advantages seen also with COPD: resting of the respiratory muscles, improving alveolar ventilation, and with positive end-expiratory pressures, reduction of auto-PEEP. Support for use of NIPPV comes from uncontrolled studies; it has been shown to be useful in acute, severe asthma and in the majority of patients reported, this avoids invasive mechanical ventilation.[42] For patients who are not responding to inhaled bronchodilators and either oral or IV corticosteroids, are still showing severe bronchospasm with a normal or elevated P_{CO_2}, and have no contraindication to NIPPV, this therapy should be initiated to avoid intubation and ventilator support (LOE B).[41,43] The use of low to medium levels of continuous positive airway pressure (CPAP) alone in acutely ill asthmatics has been shown to improve the sensation of dyspnea with the best levels at a CPAP of 5.3 ± 2.8 (standard deviation [SD]).[44] The advantages of ventilator support with bilevel positive pressures, especially in hypercarbic patients, makes CPAP alone less advantageous. The dangers and challenges of invasive ventilator support noted for patients with a COPD exacerbation hold true for patients with severe asthma and hypercarbic respiratory failure: dynamic hyperinflation and volutrauma.

Acute Pulmonary Edema

Left heart failure results in an elevation of pulmonary capillary wedge pressure (PCWP) and an increase in interstitial edema. A rapid increase in the PCWP may overwhelm the ability of lung lymphatics to remove the fluid, and flooding of the alveoli with low protein transudative fluid will occur. The result is acute pulmonary edema (APE), usually identified on the chest radiograph as bilateral alveolar infiltrates. In addition to hypoxemia, as many as one-half of the patients presenting with APE have hypercapnia on admission ($Pa_{CO_2} > 45$ mmHg).[45] Compared to normocapnic patients, those with

hypercapnia are more likely to be in the New York Heart Association class IV and have acute onset within 6 hours. While supplemental oxygen is necessary, NIPPV has been shown to more rapidly improve symptoms than oxygen alone.[46,47] Noninvasive ventilation offered as CPAP or bilevel pressure have shown similar results with APE. Both modalities rapidly improve gas exchange and reduce the need for invasive ventilator support.[46,48,49]

Drug Overdose

Narcotic and sedative agents are agents known to cause CNS respiratory depression by their effects on the medullary respiratory control center. Recently illicit drugs have become a common source of respiratory failure and respiratory arrest.[50] The physical exam often confirms the diagnosis as hypercarbia associated with a decreased respiratory rate (< 12/min) and tidal volume, altered mental status, and in the case of opioid intoxication (meperidine is an exception),[51] miotic pupils. The best predictor of opioid poisoning–induced respiratory depression is a response to naloxone.[52] Arterial blood gas analysis will show a normal A-a O_2 gradient when there is no underlying lung disease. Use of opioids with extended release and longer action formulations results in a higher risk of nonfatal overdose as compared to immediate release medications. This risk is greatest in the first 2 weeks of therapy.[53]

Neuromuscular Diseases

A number of causes of acute and chronic hypercarbic respiratory failure are due to problems in the spinal cord, nerves, respiratory muscles, or chest wall with or without intrinsic lung disease.[54] Further discussion is in Chapter 17.

QUESTIONS

1. A 63-year-old man is brought to the emergency department (ED) with a 3-day history of increasing dyspnea and increasing sputum production. He is a former cigarette smoker, 2 packs per day for 40 years, and quit 5 years ago. At baseline, he is short of breath on climbing 1 flight of stairs, and uses supplemental oxygen with sleep at 2 L/min. Medications include a long-acting anticholinergic drug and occasional use of a short acting β agonist. He has been given 2 L/min nasal oxygen in the ambulance.

   On physical exam, he is lethargic but arousable and able to follow simple commands. Respiratory rate is 16 breaths/min. Chest exam reveals increased anterioposterior (AP) diameter, low diaphragms, very decreased breath sounds, and no wheezing. His chest x-ray shows hyperinflation but no obvious infiltrate, and his lateral chest x-ray suggests right ventricular enlargement. Arterial blood gas shows pH of 7.32, P_{CO_2} of 69 mmHg, and P_{O_2} of 44 mmHg. Which of the following is your first step?

A. Intubation and mechanical ventilation
B. Noninvasive ventilation
C. Supplemental oxygen using a venturi mask
D. Computed tomography (CT) scan of the chest with CT angiogram

2. The patient in question 1 is admitted to the ICU with a diagnosis of acute COPD exacerbation. Which of the following explanations do you give to the medical student rounding with you?

A. Noninvasive positive pressure ventilation can be considered first-line therapy, although improvement may not be evident in the first 24 hours with this treatment.
B. Most exacerbations are attributed to respiratory infections.
C. Ventilation should aim to ensure a normal P_{CO_2}.
D. Antibiotics should not be administered without a clear infiltrate on chest x-ray.

3. A 20-year-old female college student has a negative past medical history except for asthma since early childhood. She presents to the hospital with a 3-day history of worsening asthma. She has been visiting her boyfriend's apartment at another college and reports exposure to cats. She is allergic to cats. She began to experience wheezing and had to return home, as she forgot to bring her asthma medications with her. Upon returning home, she began to use her albuterol inhaler and inhaled corticosteroid and slowly improved. However, the following day she developed an upper respiratory infection with nasal congestion, coryza, and a sore throat. Her wheezing again worsen despite using albuterol every 2 hours, and she presents to the hospital with extreme shortness of breath.

On examination, she is noted to be diaphoretic with wheezing and in extreme respiratory distress. She has a respiratory rate of 16 beats/min and a tachycardia of 110 beats/min. Her blood pressure (BP) is 120/70 mmHg, with a pulsus paradox of 25 mmHg. She is using accessory muscles of respiration and is unable to talk in full sentences. Her PEF is 150 L/min. An arterial blood gas is obtained on room air with the following results: P_{aO_2} of 55 mmHg, P_{aCO_2} of 42 mmHg, and pH of 7.46. Continuous 5 mg of nebulized albuterol is started and repeated every 20 minutes for a total of 3 doses, followed by continuous nebulized albuterol at 15 mg/h. In addition, 40 mg of intravenous methylprednisolone is started. Which of the following statements about this patient is correct?

A. The normal P_{aCO_2} of this patient is not reassuring and suggests impending respiratory failure.
B. The corticosteroid dose given should have been much higher.
C. The elevated pulsus paradoxus suggests underlying cardiac disease.
D. Antiviral therapy may hasten her improvement.

4. Which of the following additional treatments could you offer the patient in question 3, as it has convincingly shown improvement for patients with severe airflow obstruction?

A. Ipratropium bromide delivered by nebulization
B. Heliox
C. Repeated doses of magnesium sulfate IV
D. IV β agonist

5. A 57-year-old asbestos abatement worker has smoked regularly 1 pack of cigarettes a day since age 17. He was noted by his family to have a chronic productive cough and it was especially worse in the morning when he got up to go to work. He refused to see a physician for the cough stating it was just a "smoker's cough." A few days after Christmas, he developed a sore throat, cough, fever, and increasing breathing difficulties. Over 24 hours, he became so short of breath that he went to the ED. He was febrile and had labored breathing with expiratory wheezing. Pulse oximetry on admission to the ED was an S_{pO_2} of 82%. The house officer on call drew a VBG and called you with the results: pH of 7.30, P_{CO_2} of 59 mmHg, and bicarbonate (HCO_3) of 28 mEq/L. How do you interpret these results?

A. You feel this test is helpful and admit this patient with a COPD exacerbation to your ICU for acute respiratory failure.
B. You tell the house officer that venous samples are useless and he needs to immediately draw an arterial sample.
C. The P_{CO_2} is a valid number to follow and indicates need for immediate positive pressure ventilation.
D. The pH value suggests metabolic acidosis, so you should order an immediate lactate level.

6. A 46-year-old man comes to the ED with somnolence and respiratory failure. He is brought in by his family who report that he has had increasing sleepiness and complaints of shortness of breath on any exertion for the past 3 or 4 days. On exam, he responds only to pain. His blood pressure is 145/85 mmHg, his height is 71 inches, his weight is 266 pounds, and his BMI is 37.1 kg/m². He is morbidly obese with decreased breath sounds; his cardiac exam shows normal rhythm with no obvious murmur; pitting edema is seen of the lower extremities bilaterally. A venous blood gas shows a P_{CO_2} greater than 100 mmHg. He is intubated and mechanically ventilated and over the next few days improves, becomes more alert, and is extubated.

He is now able to give a history of daytime sleepiness (Epworth sleepiness score, 16), severe snoring, and witnessed apneas. He is a former cigarette smoker, but has never used inhaled bronchodilators. A sleep study was recommended years earlier, but not performed. Although he is responsive, when not stimulated he easily falls asleep. His venous P_{CO_2} is now 60 mmHg. Which of the following should be the next step in his management?

A. Intubation and mechanical ventilation
B. Ventilatory support with assisted servo-ventilation (ASV)
C. Ventilatory support with bilevel ventilation with inspiratory pressure of 15 cm H_2O and expiratory pressure of 5 cm H_2O (15/5)
D. CPAP with nasal or oronasal interface

7. An 80-year-old patient presents to the hospital on supplemental oxygen with the following arterial blood gas: pH of 7.24, P_{aCO_2} of 70 mmHg, and P_{aO_2} of 63 mmHg. He shows evidence of which of the following?

A. Acute metabolic acidosis
B. Acute respiratory acidosis
C. Acute-on-chronic respiratory acidosis
D. Acute respiratory and acute metabolic acidosis

8. A 65-year-old woman with a history of scoliosis since childhood is admitted for chest pain. Her initial lab work rules out myocardial infarction but includes a complete blood count (CBC) with a normal white blood cell (WBC) count but a hemoglobin of 18 g/dL; normal renal function; normal calcium, magnesium, and phosphorus; and electrolytes demonstrating a sodium of 142 mEq/L, potassium of 3.8 mEq/L, serum bicarbonate of 33 mEq/L, and a chloride of 97 mEq/L. Her pulse oximetry test shows a heart rate of 92 and an oxygen saturation of 89%. She has a temperature of 98.2°F, and her blood pressure is 110/63 mmHg. An arterial blood gas drawn with the patient breathing room air shows a pH of 7.33, P_{aCO_2} of 64 mmHg, and a P_{aO_2} of 53 mmHg. What is the A-a gradient of this 50-year-old woman?

A. 17 mmHg
B. 32 mmHg
C. 86 mmHg
D. 11 mmHg

9. A 23-year-old patient was admitted to the ICU for asthma exacerbation. She was on corticosteroids IV and continuous albuterol. Magnesium sulfate was added 2 hours later. Eight hours later, she was not improving. Her BP was 140/90 mmHg, her heart rate was 122/min, her respiratory rate was 20/min, and she was afebrile. A chest radiograph showed only hyperinflation. A metabolic panel revealed the following:

Sodium	**137 mEq/L**
Potassium	**3.9 mEq/L**
Chloride	**104 mEq/L**
Bicarbonate	**15 mEq/L**
Calcium	**9.8 mg/dL**
Glucose	**146 mg/dL**
Blood urea nitrogen	**10 mg/dL**
Creatinine	**0.5 mg/dL**
Anion gap	**18 mEq/L**
Lactic acid	**7 mmol/L**

Arterial blood gases 12 hours after admission revealed pH of 7.28, P_{aCO_2} of 34 mmHg, P_{aO_2} of 272 mmHg on oxygen 3 L/min, and bicarbonate of 15.6 mEq/L. Which of the following is the most likely cause of her deterioration?

A. Sepsis
B. Tissue hypoxia
C. Illicit drug use prior to hospitalization
D. A complication of treatment

ANSWERS

1. C. Supplemental oxygen using a venturi mask

   Neither intubation (choice A) nor noninvasive ventilation (choice B) is immediately mandatory. The patient is lethargic but responsive, and his arterial blood gas is consistent with mostly chronic hypoventilation. His pH is relatively normal despite significant hypercapnia. A CT scan of the chest looking for pulmonary embolism may often be useful, but would not be part of the initial orders (choice D).

   Oxygen administration is always appropriate for a patient who is severely hypoxemic. Although this can worsen hypercarbia, efforts need to be made to maintain oxygen saturation above about 92%, or a P_{aO_2} above 55 mmHg. It is thought that the mechanism of hypercarbia with oxygen therapy is actually worsening ventilation perfusion mismatch rather than reduction in ventilatory drive. If hypercapnia worsens or the patient's mental status worsens, ventilation may be required.

2. B. Most exacerbations are attributed to respiratory infections.

   Approximately 70% to 80% of exacerbations are attributed to respiratory infections. Viruses such as rhinovirus account for about 60% of acute exacerbations, the most common being rhinovirus.[55] Common bacteria that may be implicated include *Haemophilus influenzae*, *Streptococcus pneumoniae*, and *Moraxella catarrhalis*.[1] Exacerbation may also be due to environmental exposures. In many instances, the inciting event is not evident.

   Noninvasive ventilation may be first-line therapy, but improvement clinically should be evident in the first few hours (not 24 hours; choice A). The best predictor of success with noninvasive ventilation is the degree of acidosis on admission and improvement after 1 hour.[22] Altered mental status, increased overall severity of illness, and the presence of pneumonia have been found to be predictors of failure with noninvasive ventilation. Typically, bilevel positive airway pressure (bilevel PAP) is used, with inspiratory pressures of 10 to 15 cm H_2O and expiratory pressures of 5 cm H_2O.

   Ventilatory support should not aim for a normal P_{CO_2} (choice C). In a patient with chronic hypercapnia, this can lead to substantial metabolic alkalosis. A better goal is a normal pH, accepting hypercapnia if necessary to avoid ventilator-induced lung injury from high volumes and pressures. Modest increases in arterial P_{CO_2} may actually improve arterial P_{O_2} by reducing ventilation perfusion heterogeneity and increasing lung compliance, thereby directing ventilation to underventilated areas. Additionally, elevations and alveolar P_{CO_2} have been shown to relax bronchial smooth muscle.

Antibiotics are indicated for this patient even without evidence of infiltrate on radiographs (choice D). The Global Initiative for Obstructive Lung Disease (GOLD) guidelines recommend antibiotics be given to patients with a COPD exacerbation who have 3 cardinal symptoms: increasing dyspnea, increasing sputum volume, and increasing sputum purulence, or 2 of these symptoms if 1 is increased purulence of sputum, or in those who require invasive or noninvasive mechanical ventilation.[1]

3. A. The normal $Paco_2$ of this patient is not reassuring and suggests impending respiratory failure.

The usual acid–base finding on arterial blood gases in acute asthma is respiratory alkalosis. As the work of breathing is excessive, carbon dioxide production increases, and if the disease worsens, the severe $\dot{V}/\dot{Q}$ mismatch coupled with respiratory muscle fatigue that can result in hypoventilation leads to carbon dioxide retention and respiratory acidosis. A normal P_{CO_2}, rather than a low P_{CO_2}, should offer a warning that the patient may soon require ventilator support. Choice A is therefore correct. Choice B is not correct, as there is no evidence that larger doses of corticosteroids improve outcomes in acute asthma. Pulsus paradoxus is an exaggerated drop of more than 10 to 20 mmHg in systemic blood pressure during inspiration. It can be measured by a manually operated sphygmomanometer and not an automated blood pressure machine. If there is an indwelling arterial catheter, pulsus paradoxus can also be measured, and it can be observed by a respirophasic variation of the pulse oximetry waveform. Pulsus paradoxus primarily reflects the inspiratory decline in left ventricular stroke volume. It can be a sign of underlying cardiovascular disease. For example, among patients with pericardial effusion, the sensitivity of pulsus paradoxus for cardiac tamponade exceeds 80% and is higher than any other single physical finding.[56] Pulsus paradoxus is seen in approximately one-third of patients with constrictive pericarditis. However, in addition to pulsus paradoxus resulting from cardiac pathology, it can be seen in pulmonary as well as other noncardiac conditions.[57] Pulmonary conditions such as asthma, COPD, tension pneumothorax, pulmonary embolism, and bilateral pleural effusions can also cause pulsus paradox. Choice C is incorrect. Choice D would be correct if there was evidence of influenza infection. There was no evidence for this.

4. A. Ipratropium bromide delivered by nebulization

In patients who are not responding to the conventional first approach to a severe asthma exacerbation that includes oxygen, a β agonist, and a corticosteroid, an anticholinergic agent is a safe addition to induce smooth muscle relaxation in the larger airways.[58] Two meta-analyses have shown improvement when added to a β agonist in those with severe airflow obstruction.[59,60] However, a subsequent study showed that those who exhibited the most benefit from the addition of ipratropium were those who had consumed the least dose of inhaled β agonist before presentation, not those with the most severe asthma.[61]

The use of magnesium sulfate in acute asthma has been controversial. It is likely that magnesium produces bronchial smooth muscle relaxation by its action as a calcium antagonist or by its action on adenylyl cyclase activation.[62,63] The largest double trial of magnesium sulfate was a double-blind placebo-controlled study conducted on 1086 acute severe asthmatics in the United Kingdom.[64] Two grams of IV magnesium sulfate given over 20 minutes, nebulized magnesium sulfate (3 500-mg doses in 1 h), or placebo was administered in addition to standard therapy. Rates of admission for severe asthma to hospital or to the ICU, dyspnea measured on an analogue scale, lung function (peak flow rates), and the use of ventilatory support did not differ between groups. A Cochrane Review of 14 randomized trials of mainly a single dose of IV magnesium sulfate (1.2 or 2 g) compared to placebo concluded that hospital admissions can be avoided (a reduction of 7 hospital admissions for every 100 adults) and lung function can be improved.[63] Intravenous magnesium is a safe and effective treatment and may be considered in patients presenting with severe life-threatening asthma exacerbations (FEV1 < 25% of predicted value for those who are not improving with intensive conventional treatment).[65] However, repeated doses of magnesium sulfate have not proven beneficial (choice C).

The use of IV doses of β agonists would not be recommended, as it is a largely unproven treatment and there is a danger of myocardial toxicity[66] (choice D).

One additional modality is the use of heliox. Its use also has been a controversial subject in severe acute asthma. Helium is a low-density gas, and when combined with oxygen, it reduces turbulent flow and lowers the resistance of gas flow in larger airways. As it has higher viscosity, it may result in an increase in resistance on small airways where flow is more viscosity dependent. In theory, it should lower the work of breathing for asthmatics. However, there is a lack of evidence for its use in nonventilated patients.[67] As heliox has been shown to deliver nebulized inhaled particles deeper in to the airways, the use of heliox to deliver β agonists has gained wider use.[68] β-Agonist heliox-driven nebulization has been shown to improve bronchodilation and even can reduce the need for hospitalization for some[69] (choice B).

5. A. You feel this test is helpful and admit this patient with a COPD exacerbation to your ICU for acute respiratory failure.

Current international guidelines recommend obtaining an ABG in all patients admitted to hospital with a COPD exacerbation.[1] Sampling of arterial blood is often done by relatively inexperienced junior physicians with little prior training. Although a local anesthetic has been recommended, it is rarely used.[70] Technically, drawing an ABG is more difficult, more time consuming, and painful for the patient. Risks include bleeding, hematoma formation, and distal ischemia.[70,71] As a result, at many hospitals physicians have turned to a less invasive test of blood gas determination, the VBG.

How accurate is the venous blood sample? Can it help make judgments about clinical care of this COPD patient? Can VBG analysis combined with pulse oximetry replace ABG analysis in the initial assessment of COPD exacerbations? A meta-analysis of relevant articles evaluated the agreement between arterial and venous pH, Pco_2, and bicarbonate, and concluded that for Pco_2, it is poor.[72] The venous pressure of carbon dioxide ($Pvco_2$) cannot be relied upon as an absolute representation of $Paco_2$. However, a normal peripheral $Pvco_2$ was found to have a good negative predictive value for normal arterial C_2. The authors concluded that a normal $Pvco_2$ could be used as a screen to exclude hypercapnic respiratory disease.[77] They further found that venous and arterial pH and bicarbonate agree reasonably at all values, but the agreement was highest at normal values. The pooled mean difference (venous – arterial) for pH was –0.033 pH units (95% CI, –0.039 to 0.027) with narrow 95% limits of agreement, and for bicarbonate it was 1.03 mmol/L (95% CI, 0.56–1.50) with 95% limits of agreement ranging from –7.1 to 10.0 mmol/L. Results of another meta-analysis specifically on patients with an exacerbation of COPD also found good agreement for pH and HCO_3 values between arterial and peripheral VBG results in patients with COPD, but not for Pco_2.[73] A more recent prospective study of the usefulness of venous blood gas sampling in COPD patients with acute hypercarbic respiratory failure was reported on 234 patients evaluated in the ED.[13] There was good agreement between arterial and venous measures of pH and HCO_3 (mean difference, 0.03 and –0.04; limits of agreement, –0.05 to 0.11 and –2.90 to 2.82, respectively). They found that 96% of patients with an ABG pH of less than 7.35 also had a VBG pH of less than 7.35 and that only 2 patients were misclassified as having a normal venous pH but a low arterial pH. The authors speculated that it was difficult to fully exclude mixed arterial/venous stabs, which may explain why the sensitivities and specificities to predict an arterial pH of less than 7.35 were not 100%.

A patient with COPD exacerbation and a pH of less than 7.35 points to an episode of hypercarbic respiratory failure, and this should be followed by arterial sampling. An elevated HCO_3 on admission suggests underlying chronic hypercarbia. The study also showed good agreement between the arterial Po_2 and O_2 saturation determined by pulse oximetry if the O_2 was greater than 80%.

The answer to this question was choice A. It can be argued that the initial assessment of an acute COPD exacerbation can be based on a combined measurement of a VBG pH and Spo_2.[13] The VBG can be assessed with the same venipuncture sample for the CBC and blood chemistry analysis. If the initial pH is normal, arterial blood gases can be avoided, as respiratory acidosis is not likely present. This patient clearly showed evidence of acidosis and points to the need for intense observation and treatment. An arterial blood gas is indicated to confirm this finding and assess the correct level of Pco_2 and the Δ pH/Pco_2 to assess the chronicity of the CO_2 retention. Answer B, therefore, not correct. The venous sample was not entirely useless. Answer C is wrong, as the venous Pco_2 is not a reliable substitution for arterial Pco_2. The values do not give reliable information about the nature of the acidosis. Answer D, therefore, is not correct.

While venous blood gas analysis can assist in the initial evaluation of the acute exacerbation of COPD and avoid arterial sticks for many patients, unfortunately, use beyond this indication cannot be recommended, as there are no studies on how to use the test to guide clinical outcomes.

6. C. Ventilatory support with bilevel ventilation with inspiratory pressure of 15 cmH$_2$O and expiratory pressure of 5 cmH$_2$O (15/5)

This patient presents with respiratory failure, obesity, and symptoms suggesting obstructive sleep apnea (snoring, sleepiness). Hypoventilation implies at least an element of central sleep apnea (ie, obesity hypoventilation syndrome). Most patients with obesity hypoventilation will have at least some degree of obstructive sleep apnea as well. Bilevel PAP sets independent inspiratory and expiratory pressures. The difference between these 2 pressures represents pressure support. A pressure lower than 15/5 is likely to be too low for pressure support to be effective. Intubation and mechanical ventilation (choice A) would be effective, but is not indicated if the patient is alert and responsive. Assisted servo-ventilation (choice B) has been used for central sleep apnea, particularly in the setting of congestive heart failure, but recent evidence suggests that in patients with congestive heart failure, this may not be helpful or could even be harmful. It is designed to partially support respiration during central apneas, reducing the overall level of ventilation. This patient's problem is hypoventilation, and ASV would not be suitable. The use of CPAP (choice D) could be effective in eliminating the component of obstructive sleep apnea but would not improve his hypoventilation directly.

7. **C. Acute-on-chronic respiratory acidosis**

The patient clearly has acidosis. The increase in the $Paco_2$ shows it is a respiratory acidosis. Expected decrease in pH for acute acidosis in a patient with preexisting chronic respiratory acidosis is $0.05 \times$ (measured $Paco_2 - 40$)/10. A calculation for a pure acute respiratory acidosis would have caused a pH value of 7.16.

8. **A. 17 mmHg**

We can use the alveolar air equation $Pao_2 = Pio_2 - (Paco \times 1.2)$ and the equation $Pio_2 = (P_{ATM} - Ph_2o) \times Fio_2$, where Pio_2 is the inspiratory pressure of oxygen, P_{ATM} is atmospheric pressure, Ph_2o is the pressure of water, and Fio_2 is the fraction of inspired oxygen. We can determine that the Pio_{22} on room air is approximately 147 mmHg. The alveolar O_2 is therefore $147 - (64 \times 1.2)$, which is 70.2 mmHg. The alveolar–arterial oxygen difference (A-a gradient) is therefore $70.2 - 53 = 17.2$. The patient is 66 years old and the A-a oxygen gradient increases with age, and therefore must be corrected. The formula is A-a gradient corrected for age = $2.5 + (0.21 \times Age)$. The patient therefore has a normal A-a oxygen gradient and also signs of chronic compensated hypercarbic respiratory failure. This is likely due to her chest wall deformity, scoliosis, that has been long standing and may affect pulmonary function beginning in childhood.[74]

9. **D. A complication of treatment**

It is noted that this patient had an elevated lactate level. This is not an uncommon finding in acute severe asthma. One possible cause of an elevated serum lactate is vigorous respiratory muscle activity and respiratory muscle fatigue that results in lactate production. Using multiple regression to adjust for dyspnea and FEV1, it has been discovered that the total albuterol plasma concentration is a significant predictor of the serum lactate concentration in acute asthma.[75] In addition, this patient has a metabolic acidosis that is not always seen with hyperlactatemia. The acidosis is likely secondary to β-agonist toxicity. This patient has an anion gap acidosis. This can occur secondary to lactic acidosis, either type A, due to tissue hypoperfusion and hypoxia, or type B, secondary to other causes such as increased lactate due to excessive muscle exertion or a hyperadrenergic state that increases glycolysis. This patient did not have tissue hypoxia, signs of sepsis, or a history of liver disease or illicit drug use. Aggressive use of β agonists before she came to the hospital and on admission is the most likely cause (choice D).[76] It is thought that albuterol further potentiates the adrenergic state associated with asthma, thereby enhancing the rate of glycolysis and the production of pyruvate, and that concurrent lipolysis results in the production of intracellular free fatty acids, thereby inhibiting pyruvate dehydrogenase and promoting the conversion of pyruvate to lactate. Stimulation of $β_2$ receptors increases serum glucose, and this might increase the quantity of substrate available for glycolysis.[77] Choice B is unlikely, as there is adequate oxygenation shown on the arterial blood gas and no sign of impaired cardiac output. She has no signs of sepsis (BP and temperature are normal), and the history gives no evidence of drug abuse (choices A and C). This in itself would not be a cause of lactic acidosis without systemic effects (hypotension, severe respiratory depression).

REFERENCES

1. Vestbo J, Hurd SS, Agustí AG, et al. Global strategy for the diagnosis, management, and prevention of chronic obstructive pulmonary disease: GOLD executive summary. *Am J Respir Crit Care Med.* 2013;187(4):347-365.

2. Global Initiative for Chronic Obstructive Lung Disease. *Pocket Guide to COPD Diagnosis, Management, and Prevention. A Guide for Health Care Professionals. 2017 Edition.* Global Initiative for Chronic Obstructive Lung Disease; 2017. http://goldcopd.org/wp-content/uploads/2016/12/wms-GOLD-2017-Pocket-Guide.pdf. Accessed July 1, 2017.

3. Decramer M, Rennard S, Troosters T, et al. COPD as a lung disease with systemic consequences—clinical impact, mechanisms, and potential for early intervention. *COPD.* 2008;5(4):235-256.

4. Tillie-Leblond I, Marquette CH, Perez T, et al. Pulmonary embolism in patients with unexplained exacerbation of chronic obstructive pulmonary disease: prevalence and risk factors. *Ann Intern Med.* 2006;144(6):390-396.

5. Lippmann M, Fein A. Pulmonary embolism in the patient with chronic obstructive pulmonary disease. A diagnostic dilemma. *Chest.* 1981;79(1):39-42.

6. Hurst JR, Vestbo J, Anzueto A, et al; Evaluation of COPD Longitudinally to Identify Predictive Surrogate Endpoints (ECLIPSE) Investigators. Susceptibility to exacerbation in chronic obstructive pulmonary disease. *New Engl J Med.* 2010; 363(12):1128-1138.

7. Suissa S, Dell'Aniello S, Ernst P. Long-term natural history of chronic obstructive pulmonary disease: severe exacerbations and mortality. *Thorax.* 2012;67(11):957-963.

8. Bach PB, Brown C, Gelfand SE, McCrory DC; American College of Physicians-American Society of Internal Medicine; American College of Chest Physicians. Management of acute exacerbations of chronic obstructive pulmonary disease: a summary and appraisal of published evidence. *Ann Intern Med.* 2001;134(7):600-620.

9. Pavasini R, Tavazzi G, Biscaglia S, et al. Amino terminal pro brain natriuretic peptide predicts all-cause mortality in patients with chronic obstructive pulmonary disease: systematic review and meta-analysis. *Chron Respir Dis.* 2016;14(2):117-126.

10. Buchan A, Bennett R, Coad A, Barnes S, Russell R, Manuel AR. The role of cardiac biomarkers for predicting left ventricular dysfunction and cardiovascular mortality in acute exacerbations of COPD. *Open Heart.* 2015;2(1):e000052.

11. Brunner-La Rocca HP, Eurlings L, Richards AM, et al. Which heart failure patients profit from natriuretic peptide guided therapy? A meta-analysis from individual patient data of randomized trials. *Eur J Heart Fail.* 2015;17(12):1252-1261.

12. Hitchings AW, Baker EH. Avoiding unnecessary arterial blood sampling in COPD exacerbations: a stab in the right direction. *Thorax.* 2016;71(3):208-209.

13. McKeever TM, Hearson G, Housley G, et al. Using venous blood gas analysis in the assessment of COPD exacerbations: a prospective cohort study. *Thorax.* 2016;71(3):210-215.

14. Chow L, Parulekar AD, Hanania NA. Hospital management of acute exacerbations of chronic obstructive pulmonary disease. *J Hosp Med.* 2015;10(5):328-339.

15. Aubier M, Murciano D, Milic-Emili J, et al. Effects of the administration of O_2 on ventilation and blood gases in patients with chronic obstructive pulmonary disease during acute respiratory failure. *Am Rev Respir Dis.* 1980;122(5):747-754.

16. Leuppi JD, Schuetz P, Bingisser R, et al. Short-term vs conventional glucocorticoid therapy in acute exacerbations of chronic obstructive pulmonary disease: the REDUCE randomized clinical trial. *JAMA.* 2013;309(21):2223-2231.

17. de Jong YP, Uil SM, Grotjohan HP, Postma DS, Kerstjens HA, van den Berg JW. Oral or IV prednisolone in the treatment of COPD exacerbations: a randomized, controlled, double-blind study. *Chest.* 2007;132(6):1741-1747.

18. Kiser TH, Allen RR, Valuck RJ, Moss M, Vandivier RW. Outcomes associated with corticosteroid dosage in critically ill patients with acute exacerbations of chronic obstructive pulmonary disease. *Am J Respir Crit Care Med.* 2014;189(9):1052-1064.

19. Nouira S, Marghli S, Belghith M, Besbes L, Elatrous S, Abroug F. Once daily oral ofloxacin in chronic obstructive pulmonary disease exacerbation requiring mechanical ventilation: a randomised placebo-controlled trial. *Lancet.* 2001;358(9298):2020-2025.

20. Nava S, Ceriana P. Causes of failure of noninvasive mechanical ventilation. *Respir Care.* 2004;49(3):295-303.

21. Ambrosino N, Foglio K, Rubini F, Clini E, Nava S, Vitacca M. Non-invasive mechanical ventilation in acute respiratory failure due to chronic obstructive pulmonary disease: correlates for success. *Thorax.* 1995;50(7):755-757.

22. Masa JF, Utrabo I, Gomez de Terreros J, et al. Noninvasive ventilation for severely acidotic patients in respiratory intermediate care units: precision medicine in intermediate care units. *BMC Pulm Med.* 2016;16(1):97.

23. Hill NS. Where should noninvasive ventilation be delivered? *Respir Care.* 2009;54(1):62-70.

24. Williams TJ, Tuxen DV, Scheinkestel CD, Czarny D, Bowes G. Risk factors for morbidity in mechanically ventilated patients with acute severe asthma. *Am Rev Respir Dis.* 1992;146(3):607-615.

25. Brenner B, Corbridge T, Kazzi A. Intubation and mechanical ventilation of the asthmatic patient in respiratory failure. *Proc Am Thorac Soc.* 2009;6(2 Suppl):371-379.

26. Bergin SP, Rackley CR. Managing respiratory failure in obstructive lung disease. *Clin Chest Med.* 2016;37(4):659-667.

27. Darioli R, Perret C. Mechanical controlled hypoventilation in status asthmaticus. *Am Rev Respir Dis.* 1984;129(3):385-387.

28. Contreras M, Masterson C, Laffey JG. Permissive hypercapnia: what to remember. *Curr Opin Anaesthesiol.* 2015;28(1):26-37.

29. Pépin JL, Timsit JF, Tamisier R, Borel JC, Lévy P, Jaber S. Prevention and care of respiratory failure in obese patients. *Lancet Respir Med.* 2016;4(5):407-418.

30. Manthous CA, Mokhlesi B. Avoiding management errors in patients with obesity hypoventilation syndrome. *Ann Am Thorac Soc.* 2016;13(1):109-114.

31. Mokhlesi B. Obesity hypoventilation syndrome: a state-of-the-art review. *Respir Care.* 2010;55(10):1347-1362; discussion 1363-1345.

32. Sequeira TC, BaHammam AS, Esquinas AM. Noninvasive ventilation in the critically ill patient with obesity hypoventilation syndrome: a review. *J Intensive Care Med.* 2017;32(7):419-434.

33. Mokhlesi B, Tulaimat A, Faibussowitsch I, Wang Y, Evans AT. Obesity hypoventilation syndrome: prevalence and predictors in patients with obstructive sleep apnea. *Sleep Breath.* 2007;11(2):117-124.

34. Jones SF, Brito V, Ghamande S. Obesity hypoventilation syndrome in the critically ill. *Crit Care Clin.* 2015;31(3):419-434.

35. Gursel G, Aydogdu M, Gulbas G, Ozkaya S, Tasyurek S, Yildirim F. The influence of severe obesity on non-invasive ventilation (NIV) strategies and responses in patients with acute hypercapnic respiratory failure attacks in the ICU. *Minerva Anestesiol.* 2011;77(1):17-25.

36. Banerjee D, Yee BJ, Piper AJ, Zwillich CW, Grunstein RR. Obesity hypoventilation syndrome: hypoxemia during continuous positive airway pressure. *Chest.* 2007;131(6):1678-1684.

37. Mokhlesi B, Tulaimat A, Evans AT, et al. Impact of adherence with positive airway pressure therapy on hypercapnia in obstructive sleep apnea. *J Clin Sleep Med.* 2006;2(1):57-62.

38. Marik PE, Chen C. The clinical characteristics and hospital and post-hospital survival of patients with the obesity hypoventilation syndrome: analysis of a large cohort. *Obes Sci Pract.* 2016;2(1):40-47.

39. Pendergraft TB, Stanford RH, Beasley R, et al. Rates and characteristics of intensive care unit admissions and intubations among asthma-related hospitalizations. *Ann Allergy Asthma Immunol.* 2004;93(1):29-35.

40. Chung KF, Wenzel SE, Brozek JL, et al. International ERS/ATS guidelines on definition, evaluation, and treatment of severe asthma. *Eur Respir J.* 2014;43(2):343-373.

41. Global Initiative for Asthma. Global strategy for asthma management and prevention. 2017. www.ginasthma.org. Accessed July 30, 2017.

42. Leatherman J. Mechanical ventilation for severe asthma. *Chest.* 2015;147(6):1671-1680.

43. Camargo CA, Rachelefsky G, Schatz M. Managing asthma exacerbations in the emergency department: summary of the National Asthma Education and Prevention Program Expert Panel Report 3 guidelines for the management of asthma exacerbations. *Proc Am Thorac Soc.* 2009;6(4):357-366.

44. Shivaram U, Donath J, Khan FA, Juliano J. Effects of continuous positive airway pressure in acute asthma. *Respiration.* 1987;52(3):157-162.

45. Masip J, Páez J, Merino M, et al. Risk factors for intubation as a guide for noninvasive ventilation in patients with severe acute cardiogenic pulmonary edema. *Intensive Care Med.* 2003;29(11):1921-1928.

46. Gray A, Goodacre S, Newby DE, Masson M, Sampson F, Nicholl J; 3CPO Trialists. Noninvasive ventilation in acute cardiogenic pulmonary edema. *New Engl J Med.* 2008;359(2):142-151.

47. Peter JV, Moran JL, Phillips-Hughes J, Graham P, Bersten AD. Effect of non-invasive positive pressure ventilation (NIPPV) on mortality in patients with acute cardiogenic pulmonary oedema: a meta-analysis. *Lancet.* 2006;367(9517):1155-1163.

48. Masip J, Betbesé AJ, Páez J, et al. Non-invasive pressure support ventilation versus conventional oxygen therapy in acute cardiogenic pulmonary oedema: a randomised trial. *Lancet.* 2000;356(9248):2126-2132.

49. Keenan SP, Sinuff T, Burns KE, et al. Canadian Critical Care Trials Group/Canadian Critical Care Society Noninvasive Ventilation Guidelines Group. Clinical practice guidelines for the use of noninvasive positive-pressure ventilation and noninvasive continuous positive airway pressure in the acute care setting. *CMAJ*. 2011;183(3):E195-E214.

50. Johnson SR. The opioid abuse epidemic: how healthcare helped create a crisis. *Mod Healthc*. 2016;46(7):8-9.

51. Ghoneim MM, Dhanaraj J, Choi WW. Comparison of four opioid analgesics as supplements to nitrous oxide anesthesia. *Anesth Analg*. 1984;63(4):405-412.

52. Hoffman JR, Schriger DL, Luo JS. The empiric use of naloxone in patients with altered mental status: a reappraisal. *Ann Emerg Med*. 1991;20(3):246-252.

53. Harned M, Sloan P. Safety concerns with long-term opioid use. *Expert Opin Drug Saf*. 2016;15(7):955-962.

54. Howard RS. Respiratory failure because of neuromuscular disease. *Curr Opin Neurol*. 2016;29(5):592-601.

55. Ramaswamy M, Groskreutz DJ, Look DC. Recognizing the importance of respiratory syncytial virus in chronic obstructive pulmonary disease. *COPD*. 2009;6(1):64-75.

56. Roy CL, Minor MA, Brookhart MA, Choudhry NK. Does this patient with a pericardial effusion have cardiac tamponade? *JAMA*. 2007;297(16):1810-1818.

57. Swami A, Spodick DH. Pulsus paradoxus in cardiac tamponade: a pathophysiologic continuum. *Clin Cardiol*. 2003;26(5):215-217.

58. Fergeson JE, Patel SS, Lockey RF. Acute asthma, prognosis, and treatment. *J Allergy Clin Immunol*. 2017;139(2):438-447.

59. Stoodley RG, Aaron SD, Dales RE. The role of ipratropium bromide in the emergency management of acute asthma exacerbation: a metaanalysis of randomized clinical trials. *Ann Emerg Med*. 1999;34(1):8-18.

60. Rodrigo GJ, Castro-Rodriguez JA. Anticholinergics in the treatment of children and adults with acute asthma: a systematic review with meta-analysis. *Thorax*. 2005;60(9):740-746.

61. Garrett JE, Town GI, Rodwell P, Kelly AM. Nebulized salbutamol with and without ipratropium bromide in the treatment of acute asthma. *J Allergy Clin Immunol*. 1997;100(2):165-170.

62. Rodrigo GJ. Advances in acute asthma. *Curr Opin Pulm Med*. 2015;21(1):22-26.

63. Kew KM, Kirtchuk L, Michell CI. Intravenous magnesium sulfate for treating adults with acute asthma in the emergency department. *Cochrane Database Syst Rev*. 2014;(5):CD010909.

64. Goodacre S, Cohen J, Bradburn M, Gray A, Benger J, Coats T; 3Mg Research Team. Intravenous or nebulised magnesium sulphate versus standard therapy for severe acute asthma (3Mg trial): a double-blind, randomised controlled trial. *Lancet Respir Med*. 2013;1(4):293-300.

65. Camargo CA Jr, Rachelefsky G, Schatz M. Managing asthma exacerbations in the emergency department: summary of the National Asthma Education and Prevention Program Expert Panel Report 3 guidelines for the management of asthma exacerbations. *Proc Am Thorac Soc*. 2009;6(4):357-366.

66. Travers AH, Milan SJ, Jones AP, Camargo CA Jr, Rowe BH. Addition of intravenous beta(2)-agonists to inhaled beta(2)-agonists for acute asthma. *Cochrane Database Syst Rev*. 2012; 12:CD010179.

67. Rodrigo G, Pollack C, Rodrigo C, Rowe BH. Heliox for nonintubated acute asthma patients. *Cochrane Database Syst Rev*. 2006;(4):CD002884.

68. Rodrigo GJ, Castro-Rodriguez JA. Heliox-driven β2-agonists nebulization for children and adults with acute asthma: a systematic review with meta-analysis. *Ann Allergy Asthma Immunol*. 2014;112(1):29-34.

69. Kress JP, Noth I, Gehlbach BK, et al. The utility of albuterol nebulized with heliox during acute asthma exacerbations. *Am J Respir Crit Care Med*. 2002;165(9):1317-1321.

70. Okeson GC, Wulbrecht PH. The safety of brachial artery puncture for arterial blood sampling. *Chest*. 1998;114(3):748-751.

71. Bisarya K, George S, El Sallakh S. CASE REPORT acute compartment syndrome of the forearm following blood gas analysis postthrombolysis for pulmonary embolism. *Eplasty*. 2013;13:e15.

72. Bloom BM, Grundlingh J, Bestwick JP, Harris T. The role of venous blood gas in the emergency department: a systematic review and meta-analysis. *Eur J Emerg Med*. 2014;21(2):81-88.

73. Lim BL, Kelly AM. A meta-analysis on the utility of peripheral venous blood gas analyses in exacerbations of chronic obstructive pulmonary disease in the emergency department. *Eur J Emerg Med*. 2010;17(5):246-248.

74. Tsiligiannis T, Grivas T. Pulmonary function in children with idiopathic scoliosis. *Scoliosis*. 2012;7(1):7.

75. Lewis L, Ferguson I, House SL, et al. Albuterol administration is commonly associated with increases in serum lactate in patients with asthma treated for acute exacerbation of asthma. *Chest*. 2014;145(1):53-59.

76. Pourmand A, Dorwart K, Mazer-Amirshahi M, Nasser S, Shokoohi H. β Agonist-induced lactic acidosis, an evidence-based approach to a critical question. *Am J Emerg Med*. 2016; 34(3):666-668.

77. Dodda VR, Spiro P. Can albuterol be blamed for lactic acidosis? *Respir Care*. 2012;57(12):2115-2118.

Thromboembolic Disease

Ronaldo Collo Go, MD

INTRODUCTION

Thromboembolic disease is derived from Virchow's triad of alterations in blood flow, vascular endothelial injury, and alterations in constituents of the blood. Risk factors include antithrombin deficiency, protein C deficiency, protein S deficiency, factor V Leiden, prothrombin gene deficiency, non-O ABO blood group, dysfibrinogenemia, elevated factor VIII, elevated factor IX, elevated factor XI, hyperhomocysteinemia, cancer, antiphospholipid syndrome, infection, inflammatory disorders, nephrotic syndrome, obesity, smoking, trauma, surgery, immobilization, central venous catheter, pregnancy, hormonal therapy, and travel.[1]

PATHOPHYSIOLOGY

Acute pulmonary embolism (PE) causes physical obstruction of blood flow and release of humoral factors such as serotonin, thrombin, and histamine.[2] Hypoxic vasoconstriction leads to elevated pulmonary vascular resistance. Increased afterload consequently causes right ventricular dilation, hypokinesis, tricuspid regurgitation, and right heart failure.[2] Further dilation of the right ventricle causes leftward bowing of the intraventricular septum. This causes left diastolic dysfunction, with decreased left diastolic filling. Further dilation of the right ventricle causes cardiac ischemia due to decreased subendocardial perfusion.[2] Acute pulmonary embolism typically originates from deep venous thrombosis of the lower extremities. Locally, this thrombosis can progress and cause venous congestion and fluid sequestration. This can compromise oxygen delivery to the limb, causing edema, pain, and cyanosis.

ASSESSMENT

The increased use of computed tomography (CT) for evaluation of pulmonary embolism has not shown to improve outcomes and is not cost effective.[3-9] Therefore, decision-making tools have been developed to determine patients who will be benefit from additional testing (Table 10-1)[10-12].

Low to intermediate risk or probability warrant further testing with d-dimer (negative < 500 ng/mL) and adjusted for ages 50 years or older to maintain sensitivity greater than 97% and increase specificity.[3] Computed tomography angiography (CTA) or ventilation/perfusion ($\dot{V}/\dot{Q}$) scan is indicated for high risk or probability.

IMAGING STUDIES

Chest radiographs have been used as an initial investigation for dyspnea, although they are not helpful in confirming the presence of pulmonary embolism. As per Prospective Investigation Of Pulmonary Embolism Diagnosis (PIOPED) II, chest CTA has become the gold standard in diagnosis of acute pulmonary embolism with a sensitivity and specificity of 96% and 95%, respectively.[13] As per PIOPED I, $\dot{V}/\dot{Q}$ scan is typically reserved for patients who cannot tolerate chest CTA due to renal failure, obesity, or contrast allergy. It is best performed in patients with a normal chest radiograph and no underlying pulmonary disease. Ventilation/perfusion interpretation is shown in Table 10-2.[14]

Sensitivity is 40% and specificity is 98% for a high-probability $\dot{V}/\dot{Q}$ scan.[15] For a low-probability $\dot{V}/\dot{Q}$ scan, the sensitivity is 99% and specificity is 12%.[15] The positive predictive value of a high-probability $\dot{V}/\dot{Q}$ scan is 100% and the negative predictive value of a low-probability $\dot{V}/\dot{Q}$ scan is 94%.[15] The PIOPED III study suggested that magnetic resonance angiography (MRA) had a sensitivity of 78% and specificity of 96%, and MRA and magnetic resonance venography (MRV) had a sensitivity of 92% and specificity of 96%.[16] Due to technical difficulties, it is often reserved if CTA and $\dot{V}/\dot{Q}$ scan are negative and suspicion is still high. Pulmonary angiography's sensitivity and specificity have not been formally evaluated, but in addition to diagnosis, it can also be used to intervene. Lower extremity ultrasound can suggest the presence of thromboembolic disease, but cannot confirm the presence of pulmonary embolism.

TABLE 10-1 Predictive Criteria for Thromboembolic Disease

Modified Wells Criteria[10]		Geneva Criteria[11]		PERC[12]	
Clinical signs of DVT	3	Previous DVT/PE	3	Age < 50 y	Yes = 0/No = 1
Alternative diagnosis less likely	3	HR 75–94 bpm	3	Initial HR < 100 bpm	Yes = 0/No = 1
HR > 100 bpm	1.5	HR > 94 bpm	5	O_2 saturation > 94% RA	Yes = 0/No = 1
Immobilization (> 3 d) or surgery in the last 3 wk	1.5	Surgery or fracture within last month	2	No unilateral leg swelling	Yes = 0/No = 1
Previous DVT	1.5	Hemoptysis	2	No hemoptysis	Yes = 0/No = 1
Hemoptysis	1	Active cancer	2	No surgery or trauma within the last 4 wk	Yes = 0/No = 1
Cancer treated in last 6 mo	1	Unilateral lower extremity pain	3	No history of VTE	Yes = 0/No = 1
Total:		Pain on lower limb, deep venous palpation, and unilateral edema	4	No estrogen use	Yes = 0/No = 1
Low risk	0–1	Age > 65 y	1	**Total:**	Score 0 = pretest probability <1 %
Intermediate risk	2–6	**Total:**			
High risk	> 6	Low probability	0-3		
PE likely	> 4	Intermediate probability	4–10		
PE unlikely	≤ 4	High probability	≥ 11		

bpm = beats per minute; DVT = deep vein thrombosis; HR = heart rate; PE = pulmonary embolism; PERC = Pulmonary Embolism Rule-out Criteria; RA = room air; VTE = venous thromboembolism.

TREATMENT

Acute treatment is for 5 to 10 days. Long-term anticoagulation is for 3 months, and extended anticoagulation implies indefinite duration.[17] The decisions regarding whether or not to anticoagulate, which anticoagulation treatment to use, and the duration are dependent on the scenario, risk of bleeding, and individual comorbidities, as seen in Tables 10-1 to 10-3.[17-116] Table 10-3 shows different scenarios and their corresponding treatments of choice. As per the CHEST guidelines, quality of evidence is graded as high (Level A), moderate (Level B), and low (Level C) with the strength of recommendation as strong (Grade 1) and weak (Grade 2).[117] Table 10-4 shows factors that will affect the type of anticoagulation.

Risk factors for bleeding include age over 65 years, history of bleeding, cancer, renal failure, liver failure, previous cerebrovascular accident (CVA), thrombocytopenia, diabetes, anemia, antiplatelet therapy, poor anticoagulation control, reduced functional capacity, comorbidity, recent surgery, recurrent falls, alcohol use, and nonsteroidal anti-inflammatory drug (NSAID) use.[117] With no risk factors, there is a 0.8% annual risk of major bleeding with anticoagulation. With 1 risk factor, there is a 1.6% annual risk for major bleeding with anticoagulation.[117] With 2 risk factors, there is a 6.5% or higher annual risk of major bleeding with anticoagulation.[117]

Full anticoagulation precludes the use of catheter-directed thrombolytics, inferior vena cava (IVC) filter, or compression stockings. Patients who would benefit from catheter-directed thrombolytics for proximal lower extremity deep venous thrombosis have the following characteristics: iliofemoral deep vein thrombosis (DVT), fewer than 14 days of symptoms, good functional status, life expectancy of 1 year or more, and low risk of bleeding.[117] In full anticoagulation, IVC filters are not recommended due to a higher risk of DVT with no mortality benefit.[88,89]

Compression stockings were previously advocated to prevent post-thrombotic syndrome (PTS). A recent multicenter placebo-controlled study suggested that it does not prevent post-thrombotic syndrome but can be used to treat symptoms.[93]

TABLE 10-2 Interpretation of Ventilation/Perfusion Study

High Probability ≥ 80%	Intermediate Probability 20–79%	Low Probability < 20%	Normal
≥ 2 large mismatched segmental perfusion defects	1–2 large mismatched segmental perfusion defects	Nonsegmental perfusion defects such as cardiomegaly, enlarged aorta, enlarged hila, or elevated diaphragm	No perfusion defects

TABLE 10-3 Clinical Scenarios of Thromboembolic Disease, Treatment, and Considerations

Scenario	Treatment	Considerations\Rationale
Deep venous thrombosis or pulmonary embolism and no cancer-associated risk for at least 3 mo	• First choice: rivaroxaban, apixaban, or edoxaban (Grade 2B) • Second choice: vitamin K antagonist (Grade 2B)	• Similar risk reduction for recurrent VTE between NOAC vs VKA • Less bleeding with NOAC vs VKA • Similar risk reduction between VKA and LMWH in patients without cancer • LMWH expensive and burdensome
Deep venous thrombosis or pulmonary embolism with cancer risk	• First choice: LMWH (Grade 2B) • Alternatives: VKA, dabigatran, rivaroxaban, and apixaban (Grade 2C)	• Risk reduction for recurrent VTE greater for LMWH than for VKA • Unknown risk reduction for recurrent VTE between NOAC and LMWH
If patient has decided to stop anticoagulation for thromboembolic disease	• Aspirin over no aspirin (Grade 2B)	• Not a reasonable alternative to anticoagulation but better than no aspirin in reducing recurrent VTE
Acute isolated distal DVT of lower extremities without symptoms or risk factor for extension	• First choice: serial imaging for 2 wk over anticoagulation unless symptomatic (Grade 2C)	• Low risk for extension: soleus or gastrocnemius vein thrombosis • High risk for extension: positive d-dimer, > 5 cm length, > 7 mm in diameter, multiple veins, proximal veins, no reversible factors, active cancer, history of VTE, and inpatient status
Subsegmental pulmonary embolism without proximal pulmonary artery involvement or proximal DVT	• Low risk for recurrence: clinical surveillance (Grade 2C) • High risk of recurrence: anticoagulation (Grade 2C)	• High false positive • True positive if CTA good quality, multiple intraluminal defects, more proximal subsegment arteries, defects in more than 1 image or projection, defects surrounded by contrast, symptomatic, high clinical probability, and d-dimer elevated • High risk of recurrence if hospitalized or reduced mobility, active cancer, and no reversible risk factor for VTE
Acute pulmonary embolism with low risk of bleeding and hypotension	• First choice: thrombolytics (Grade 2B)	• Faster resolution of thromboembolism but mortality benefit uncertain • Higher risk of ICH compared to anticoagulation
Acute pulmonary embolism, low risk of bleeding, no hypotension, but with evidence of cardiopulmonary deterioration such as symptoms, tissue hypoperfusion, worsening gas exchange, or cardiac markers, or worsened after initial anticoagulation	• First choice: thrombolytics (Grade 2C)	
Acute pulmonary embolism with hypotension, high risk of bleeding and failed thrombolytics	• First choice: Catheter-assisted thrombus removal (Grade 2C)	
Upper extremity DVT involving axillary or more proximal vein	• First choice: anticoagulation (Grade 2C)	• Thrombolytics indicated for most of subclavian and axillary vein, symptoms < 14 d, good functional status, life expectancy > 1 y, and low risk of bleeding
Recurrent venous thrombosis on VKA, dabigatran, rivaroxaban, apixaban, or edoxaban	• First choice: LMWH (Grade 2C)	• LMWH associated with higher risk reduction in VTE compared to VKA
Recurrent venous thrombosis on LMWH	• First choice: increase LMWH by one-half to one-third (Grade 2C)	

CTA = computed tomography angiography; DVT = deep vein thrombosis; ICH = intracerebral hemorrhage; LMWH = low-molecular-weight heparin; NOAC = novel oral anticoagulants; VKA = vitamin K administration; VTE = venous thromboembolism

TABLE 10-4 Factors That May Influence Which Anticoagulant is Chosen for Initial and Long-Term Treatment for Venous Thromboembolism

Factor	Preferred Anticoagulant	Qualifying Remarks
Cancer	LMWH	More so if: just diagnosed, extensive VTE, metastatic cancer, very symptomatic; vomiting; on cancer chemotherapy
Parenteral therapy to be avoided	Rivaroxaban, apixaban	VKA, dabigatran, and edoxaban require initial parenteral therapy
Once daily oral therapy preferred	Rivaroxaban, edoxaban, VKA	
Liver disease and coagulopathy	LMWH	NOACs contraindicated if INR raised because of liver disease; VKA difficult to control and INR may not reflect antithrombotic effect
Renal disease and creatinine clearance < 30 mL/min	VKA	NOACs and LMWH contraindicated with severe renal impairment; dosing of NOACs with levels of renal impairment differ with the NOAC and among jurisdictions
Coronary artery disease	VKA, rivaroxaban, apixaban, edoxaban	Coronary artery events appear to occur more often with dabigatran than with VKA. This has not been seen with the other NOACs, and they have demonstrated efficacy for coronary artery disease. Antiplatelet therapy should be avoided if possible in patients on anticoagulants because of increased bleeding.
Dyspepsia or history of GI bleeding	VKA, apixaban	Dabigatran increased dyspepsia. Dabigatran, rivaroxaban, and edoxaban may be associated with more GI bleeding than VKA.
Poor compliance	VKA	INR monitoring can help to detect problems. However, some patients may be more compliant with an NOAC because it is less complex.
Thrombolytic therapy use	UFH infusion	Greater experience with its use in patients treated with thrombolytic therapy
Reversal agent needed	VKA, UFH	
Pregnancy or pregnancy risk	LMWH	Potential for other agents to cross the placenta
Cost, coverage, licensing	Varies among regions and with individual circumstances	

GI = gastrointestinal; INR = international normalized ratio; LMWH = low-molecular-weight heparin; NOAC = novel oral anticoagulants; UFH = unfractionated heparin; VKA = vitamin K administration; VTE = venous thromboembolism.

Reprinted with permission from Kearon C, Akl EA, Ornelas J, et al. Antithrombotic therapy for VTE disease. CHEST guideline and expert panel report. *Chest.* 2016;149(2):315-352.

QUESTIONS

1. A 45-year-old man is complaining of shortness of breath after travelling to Asia for business. He is accompanied by his wife. His blood pressure (BP) is 120/60 mmHg, his heart rate (HR) is 90 beats/min, his respiratory rate (RR) is 18 breaths/min, his O_2 sat is 98% on room air, and his physical examination is otherwise unremarkable except for a swollen right leg. His labs show the following:

White blood cells	$10 \times 10^3/\mu L$
Hemoglobin	14 g/dL
Hematocrit	45%
Platelets	$300 \times 10^3/\mu L$
Sodium	145 mEq/L
Potassium	4 mEq/L
Magnesium	2 mEq/L
Chloride	109 mEq/L

Carbon dioxide	28 mEq/L
Blood urea nitrogen	20 mg/dL
Creatinine	0.8 mg/dL
Lactic acid	0.8 mmol/L
B-type natriuretic peptide	40 pg/mL
Troponin	0.0 ng/mL

Ultrasound of his right lower leg is negative for deep vein thrombosis. The CTA of his chest shows a PE in the right lower lobe. His echocardiogram shows no wall motion abnormalities. His ejection fraction (EF) is greater than 60% and he has no diastolic dysfunction. His right ventricular systolic pressure (RVSP) is 15 mmHg. His right ventricle is not enlarged. Where should the patient be treated?

A. Outpatient
B. Medical-surgical
C. Progressive care unit (PCU)
D. Intensive care unit (ICU)

2. A 60-year-old woman with a history of lung non–small cell lung carcinoma developed deep venous thrombosis of her left femoral vein. She was started on low-molecular-weight heparin (LMWH). Three years later, she developed progressive left lower extremity pain associated with varicosities and ulceration. How would you prevent this complication?

   A. DVT prophylaxis for any hospitalization
   B. Elastic stockings
   C. Surgery
   D. Pentoxifylline

3. A 60-year-old man who was recently treated for pulmonary embolism with 3 months of NOAC presents to the emergency department (ED). He complains of persistent shortness of breath, particularly on exertion. What is the next step?

   A. V̇/Q̇ scan
   B. CTA
   C. Right heart catheterrization
   D. Magnetic resonance imaging (MRI)

4. A 50-year-old man was complaining of right leg pain. He was noted to have erythema, pain, and tenderness in his calf. Pulses are good, and there is good capillary refill. Ultrasound shows venous thrombosis. What is your diagnosis?

   A. Superficial phlebitis
   B. Superficial thrombophlebitis
   C. Phlegmasia alba dolens
   D. Phlegmasia cerulea dolens

5. A 76-year-old man was complaining of acute onset of shortness of breath. In the ED, he was noted to have oxygen saturation of 80% on room air. He had a CVA 2 months ago. He was transitioned to nonrebreather. His HR was 120 mmHg, his RR was 25/min, and his BP was 140/90 mmHg. His chest radiograph was unremarkable and a CTA was done (Fig. 10-1).

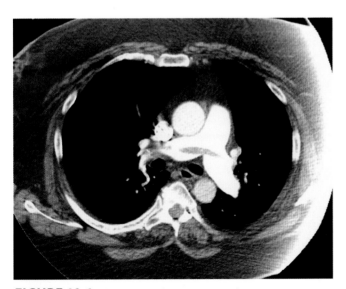

FIGURE 10-1 Chest CTA in the emergency department.

His blood pressure started to drop to 70/40 mmHg. A bedside ultrasound showed the IVC was 2.5 cm with no respiratory variation. What is the next step?

   A. Alteplase 15 mg bolus followed by 85 mg over 90 minutes
   B. Heparin drip
   C. Alteplase 50 mg bolus IV and repeated after 30 minutes
   D. Enoxaparin 1 mg/kg twice daily

6. In which of the following scenarios can you initiate prophylactic anticoagulation within 24 hours?

   A. Neurosurgery
   B. Abdominal aortic aneurysm repair
   C. Abdominal surgery
   D. All of the above

7. A 55-year-old man, who is 5 feet, 10 inches and weighs 360 pounds, is recently diagnosed with a pulmonary embolism. What is the appropriate initial dose of unfractionated heparin?

   A. 80 units/kg bolus (true body weight) then 18 units/kg/h
   B. 80 units/kg bolus (adjusted body weight) then 18 units/kg/h
   C. 80 units/kg bolus (true body weight) then 15 units/kg/h
   D. 80 units/kg bolus (adjusted body weight) then 10 units/kg/h

8. A 70-year-old woman with deep venous thrombosis has received 40,000 IU/d of heparin without reaching therapeutic partial thromboplastin time (PTT). Antithrombin activity was noted to be 50%. What is the next step?

   A. Fresh frozen plasma
   B. Re-bolus heparin
   C. Increase rate
   D. Initiate coumadin

ANSWERS

1. A. Outpatient

   Treatment for acute pulmonary embolism with novel oral anticoagulants (NOAC) does not require hospital admission. Candidates for outpatient PE treatment include (1) hemodynamic stability with good cardiopulmonary reserve; (2) no contraindications, such as recent bleed, severe renal disease, severe liver disease, and/or platelet count of less than 70,000/mm³; (3) compliance to medications; and (4) a patient who feels well enough to be treated at home.[17] Hospitalization, whether medical surgery, progressive care unit, or intensive care unit, is not necessary.

Stratification can be performed further with the pulmonary embolism severity index as seen in Table 10-5A and Table 10-5B.[1]

TABLE 10-5A Pulmonary Embolism Severity Index

Pulmonary Embolism Severity Index		30-Day Mortality
Predictors	Points	
Age	Age, in years	
AMS	60	
SBP < 100 mmHg	30	
Cancer	30	
Arterial O$_2$ sat < 90%	20	
Temp < 36°C	20	
RR ≥ 30	20	
HR ≥ 110 bpm	20	
Male	10	
History of heart failure	10	
History of chronic lung disease	10	
Classifications		
Class I (very low risk)	≤ 65	0 –1.6%
Class II (low risk)	66–85	1.7–3.5%
Class III (intermediate risk)	86–105	3.2–7.1%
Class IV (high risk)	106–125	4.0–11.4%
Class V (very high risk)	>125	10–24.5%

TABLE 10-5B Hestia Index

Hestia Index
Presence of any of the following precludes outpatient treatment:
• Hemodynamic instability (HR > 100 bpm, SBP < 100 mmHg)
• Thrombolysis or embolectomy
• High risk of bleeding
• Supplemental oxygen: need to keep O$_2$ sat > 90% for 24 h
• PE during anticoagulation therapy
• IV pain med > 24 h
• Medical or social reason for inpatient treatment > 24 h
• Creatinine clearance < 30 mL/min
• Severe liver impairment
• Pregnancy
• HIT

AMS = acute mountain sickness; HIT = heparin-induced thrombocytopenia; HR = heart rate; ICU = intensive care unit; IV = intravenous; PE = pulmonary embolism; RR = respiratory rate; SBP = systolic blood pressure.

Streiff MB, Agnelli G, Connors JM, et al. Guidance for the treatment of deep vein thrombosis and pulmonary embolism. *J Thromb Thrombolysis.* 2016;41(1):32-67.

Since the patient meets these criteria, he can be treated as an outpatient. Therefore, medical-surgical, the PCU, and the ICU are wrong (choices B, C, and D).

2. A. DVT prophylaxis for any hospitalization

PTS clinically presents with signs and symptoms of chronic venous insufficiency secondary to venous thrombosis. They range from swelling, pain, paresthesias, pruritus, varicose veins, telangiectasia, lipodermatosclerosis, edema, and ulceration.[117] Symptoms present months to 20 years after venous thrombosis diagnosis. Venous hypertension is central to this syndrome, and venous pressure is dependent on the weight of the column between the right atrium and the foot. Venous pressure is low when the patient is supine due to dynamic pressures from the pumping action of the heart, and increases when the patient is upright and motionless, up to 80 to 90 mmHg.[117,118] When walking, venous pressure reduces to a mean of 22 mmHg, and blood is ejected due to muscle contraction and competent venous valves.[118] In PTS, ambulatory venous hypertension is present as a result of thrombus or valvular incompetence.[119,120] There is no gold standard for diagnosis but the Villalta scale, Ginsberg measure, CEAP (clinical, etiology, anatomy, pathophysiology) classification, Venous Clinical Severity Score (VCSS), Widmer classification, and Brandjes scale are used.[117,120] Treatment consists of elastic compression stockings, pentoxifylline, and surgery[117] (choices B, D, and C).

3. A. $\dot{V}/\dot{Q}$ scan

Chronic thromboembolic pulmonary hypertension (CTEPH) is precapillary pulmonary hypertension as defined by right heart catheterization in the presence of chronic flow-limiting thrombus in elastic pulmonary arteries after at least 3 months of anticoagulation.[121,122] There is a permanent fibrotic organizing change, and this degree of obstruction is not directly correlated to the degree of hemodynamic derangement secondary to small vessel arteriopathy.[121] Chronic thromboembolic pulmonary hypertension should be considered for persistent dyspnea in a patient with a history of venous thromboembolic disease. Initial evaluation is with a $\dot{V}/\dot{Q}$ scan with a 96% sensitivity, compared to a 51% sensitivity with CT.[123] A normal $\dot{V}/\dot{Q}$ scan excludes CTEPH. If there are at least 1 to 2 large defects, then CTEPH is likely. If the $\dot{V}/\dot{Q}$ scan is indeterminate and CTEPH is likely, the next step would be right heart catheterization (choice C), then pulmonary angiography, MRI (choice D), or CT (choice B). Treatment is pulmonary thromboendarterectomy. For patients who are not surgical candidates, prior to surgery, or still symptomatic after surgery, medical management can be used. These include the guanylate cyclase stimulant riociguat, endothelin receptor antagonists such as bosentan, and prostanoids such as treprostinil or epoprostenol.

4. B. Superficial thrombophlebitis

See Table 10-6 for the descriptions of each presentation.

TABLE 10-6 Descriptions of Venous Thrombosis Syndromes and Treatment

Superficial Phlebitis (Choice A)	Superficial Thrombophlebitis (Choice B)	Phlegmasia Alba Dolens (Choice C)	Phlegmasia Cerulea Dolens (Choice D)
• Pain • Tenderness • Induration • Erythema around vein	• Pain • Tenderness • Induration • Erythema around vein • Ultrasound shows thrombosis in vein	• Edema • Pain • Blanching	• Edema • Pain • Cyanosis distal to proximal • Bleb and/or bullous • Venous gangrene
Treatment: • Supportive	Treatment: • Supportive if not extensive • Anticoagulation	Treatment: • Thrombolytics	Treatment: • Thrombolytics

5. A. Alteplase 15 mg bolus followed by 85 mg over 90 minutes

Massive pulmonary embolism, defined as a pulmonary embolism associated with SBP less than 90 mmHg for more than 15 minutes or requiring vasopressors, is a primary indication for thrombolytic therapy. However, thrombolytics are not without contraindications. See Table 10-7.[17]

TABLE 10-7 Contraindications for Thrombolytics

Absolute Contraindications	Relative Contraindications
• Structural intracranial disease • Previous intracranial hemorrhage • Ischemic CVA within 3 mo • Active bleeding • Recent brain or spinal surgery • Recent head trauma with fracture or injury • Bleeding diathesis	• SBP > 180 mmHg • DBP > 110 mmHg • Recent extracranial bleeding • Recent surgery < 2 wk • Recent invasive procedure • CVA > 3 mo • Currently on anticoagulation • Traumatic cardiopulmonary resuscitation • Pericarditis or pericardial fluid • Diabetic retinopathy • Pregnancy • Age > 75 y • Low body weight • Female • Black

CVA = cerebrovascular accident; DBP = diastolic blood pressure; SBP = systolic blood pressure.

Due to the recent ischemic CVA, age, and race, thrombolytics would not be a good option for this patient.

Administration of tissue plasminogen activator (TPA) is preferably through a peripheral IV. After the TPA infusion is finished, heparin drip is started to prevent recurrent thrombosis once the PTT decreases to less than twice the normal control value. Choice A is the alteplase dose for a massive PE, and choice C is the alteplase dose for a massive PE during a cardiac arrest. Other dosing regimens are seen in Table 10-8.[124]

Tissue plasminogen activators may also be considered in submassive pulmonary embolism (pulmonary embolism with evidence of right heart strain) if the patient continues to clinically deteriorate or is in massive or extensive deep venous thrombosis. Heparin drip (choice B) or Enoxaparin (choice D) are not ideal options for this situation unless the patient has contraindications to thrombolytics.

6. D. All of the above

See Table 10-9 for list of surgical interventions and recommendations for when it is appropriate to start pharmacologic DVT prophylaxis if there is no active bleeding.[1]

TABLE 10-8 Indications for TPA and Dosages

TPA During Cardiac Arrest for PE	TPA for Massive PE	TPA for Massive or Extensive DVT	TPA for Blocked Catheters
• Alteplase 100 mg IV bolus • Alteplase 50 mg IV bolus followed by another 50-mg IV bolus in 30 min • Alteplase 15 mg IV bolus followed by 85 mg over 90-120 min	• Alteplase 15 mg IV bolus followed by 85 mg over 90–120 min • Urokinase 4400 U/kg loading dose at 90 mL/h in 10 min followed by 4400 U/kg/h at 15 mL/h for 12 h • Streptokinase 250,000 U loading dose over 30 min followed by 100,000 U/h over 12–24 h • Reteplase 10 U IV and another 10 U IV 30 min later	• Alteplase 0.5–1.0 mg/h for 12–24 h • Urokinase 4400 U/kg IV bolus followed by 2200 U/kg/h for 1–3 d • Streptokinase 250,000 U bolus followed by 100,000 U/h for 1–3 d • Reteplase 1 U/h for 18–36 h	• Alteplase for patients ≥ 30 kg 2 mg in 2 mL saline and leave in catheter for 30–120 min then withdraw; dose may be repeated or can be infused 2 mg/50 mL over 4 h • Urokinase 5000 U in each lumen for 1–2 min • Streptokinase 250,000 U of streptokinase in 2-mL solution and leave in occluded port for 2 h, aspirate, flush with saline, and reconnect cannula

DVT = deep vein thrombosis; IV = intravenous; PE = pulmonary embolism; TPA = tissue plasminogen activator.

TABLE 10-9 Risk Stratification of Bleeding Risk With Anticoagulation Following Surgery

Bleeding Risk Category	Type of Surgery or Procedure	Anticoagulation Recommendation
Very high	Neurosurgical procedure (intracranial or spinal) Prostatectomy or partial nephrectomy, bladder surgery Heart valve replacement Coronary artery bypass grafting	Can initiate prophylactic dose Anticoagulation at 24 h Consider therapeutic dose anticoagulation no sooner than 72 h
High	Pacemaker or AICD placement Major cancer surgery Major vascular surgery (AAA repair, peripheral artery bypass) Reconstructive plastic surgery Renal or hepatic biopsy Bowel polypectomy (assume this will be part of a colonoscopy) Major orthopedic surgery	Can initiate prophylactic dose anticoagulation within 12–24 h Consider therapeutic dose anticoagulation no sooner than 48–72 h
Moderate	Major intra-abdominal surgery Major intra-thoracic surgery	Can initiate prophylactic dose anticoagulation within 12–24 h Consider therapeutic dose anticoagulation no sooner than 24–48 h
Low	Laparoscopic cholecystectomy or hernia repair Coronary angiography Arthroscopy Biopsy (prostate, bladder, thyroid, lymph node) Bronchoscopy ± biopsy Central venous catheter removal Multiple dental extraction or gum surgery	Can initiate prophylactic dose anticoagulation within 12 h Consider therapeutic dose anticoagulation 24–18 h
Very low	Minor denial procedures (single tooth extractions or root canals) Minor dermatologic procedures (excisions of basal and squamous cell carcinomas, actinic keratoses, and malignant or premalignant nevi) Cataract removal ECT Arthrocentesis Joint or soft tissue injections GI endoscopy without biopsy	Interruption of anticoagulation typically not necessary

AAA = abdominal aortic aneurysm; AICD = automated implantable cardioverter-defibrillator; ECT = electroconvulsive therapy; GI = gastrointestinal.

7. B. 80 units/kg bolus (adjusted body weight) then 18 units/kg/h

The typical normogram for intravenous unfractionated heparin infusion begins with an initial dose of 80 units/kg bolus then 18 units/kg/h. See Table 10-10.[125,126]

Obese patients have lower weight-based but higher heparin requirements relative to nonobese patients. To achieve therapeutic anticoagulation and avoid unnecessary delays or excessive anticoagulation, reduce the dose of heparin by 13–15 units/kg actual body weight per hour or use the adjusted dose weight (ADW): ADW = (Actual Body Weight – Ideal Body Weight] × 0.40, or 0.3 × Ideal Body Weight.[125-127]

Low-molecular-weight heparin should also be adjusted for weight. In patients with BMI greater than 40 kg/m² or weight greater than 200 kg, the dose is 0.75 mg/kg actual body weight with anti-factor Xa monitoring.[127]

TABLE 10-10 Unfractionated Heparin Normogram

aPTT (in seconds)	What to Do	When to Get Next aPTT
< 35 (< 1.2 × control)	80 units/kg bolus then increase rate to 4 units/kg/h	6 h
35–45 (1.2–1.5 × control)	40 units/kg bolus then increase rate by 2 units/kg/h	6 h
46–70 (15–2.3 × control)	No change	6 h and if 2 consecutive values therapeutic, next PTT in morning
71–90 (2.3–3 × control)	Decrease rate by 2 units/kg/h	6 h
> 90 (> 3.0 × control)	Hold infusion 1 h, then decrease rate by 3 units/kg/h	6 h

aPTT = activated partial thromboplastin time.

8. A. Fresh frozen plasma

Unfractionated heparin is a heterogeneous mixture of polysaccharides (5000-30,000 Da) derived from either bovine or porcine and only 1/3 carry the critical pentasaccharide sequence that can form the heparin/antithrombin/thrombin complex.[128-131] Heparin indirectly has anticoagulant effects by potentiating anticoagulant effects of antithrombin III (AT) through decreasing the half-life of coagulant enzymes and promoting binding to AT through conformational change and anticoagulant effects of heparin cofactor II.[128-131] The enzymes include thrombin and factor Xa. Heparin resistance is when high doses of unfractionated heparin (> 35,000 IU/d) is required to bring PTT and activated clotting time (ACT) within therapeutic range (ACT ≥ 450–480 seconds) and is usually seen in patients on extracorporeal membrane oxygenation (ECMO) or cardiopulmonary bypass. Heparin resistance can be from antithrombin deficiency either congenital or acquired from pretreatment with heparin. Heparin /antithrombin complex binds to thrombin which causes disassociation of heparin. The thrombin/antithrombin complex is removed from the body through the reticuloendothelial system.[128]

Other causes include increased heparin clearance, increased heparin-binding proteins, elevated fibrinogen and factor VIII, and medications such as aprotinin.[130-132]In addition to antithrombin, ACT may also be effected by hypothermia, hemodilution, medications such as warfarin, aprotinin, platelet inhibitors, direct thrombin inhibitors, protamine, fibrinogen, other factor deficiencies (II, V, VIII, XI, and XII), anticardiolipin, or antiphosphate antibodies.[133] Predictors of resistance includes platelets of 300,000 or greater, age 65 years or older, and antithrombin activity of 60% or less.[130-132] Treatment would consist of fresh frozen plasma or recombinant antithrombin (AT). Re-bolusing or increasing rate will have no effect in heparin resistance (choices B and C). Initiating coumadin is premature without a therapeutic PTT (choice D).

REFERENCES

1. Streiff MB, Agnelli G, Connors JM. Guidance for the treatment of deep vein thrombosis and pulmonary embolism. *J Thromb Thrombolysis.* 2016;41(1):32-67.

2. Goldhaber SZ, Elliott CG. Acute pulmonary embolism: part I. epidemiology, pathophysiology, and diagnosis. *Circulation.* 2003;108(22):2726-2729.

3. Raja AS, Greenberg JO, Qaseem A, Denberg TD, Fitterman N, Schuur JD; Clinical Guidelines Committee of the American College of Physicians. Evaluation of patients with suspected acute pulmonary embolism: best practice advice from the Clinical Guidelines Committee of the American College of Physicians. *Ann Intern Med.* 2015;163(9):701-711.

4. Boone JM, Brunberg JA. Computed tomography use in a tertiary care university hospital. *J Am Coll Radiol.* 2008;5(2):132-138.

5. Broder J, Warshauer DM. Increasing utilization of computed tomography in the adult emergency department, 2000–2005. *Emerg Radiol.* 2006;13(1):25-30.

6. Lee J, Kirschner J, Pawa S, Wiener DE, Newman DH, Shah K. Computed tomography use in the adult emergency department of an academic urban hospital from 2001 to 2007. *Ann Emerg Med.* 2010;56(6):591-596.

7. Larson DB, Johnson LW, Schnell BM, Salisbury SR, Forman HP. National trends in CT use in the emergency department: 1995–2007. *Radiology.* 2011;258(1):164-173.

8. Minges KE, Bikdeli B, Wang Y, et al. National trends in pulmonary embolism hospitalization rates and outcomes for Medicare beneficiaries, 1999–2010. *J Am Coll Cardiol.* 2013;61(10):E2070.

9. Feng LB, Pines JM, Yusuf HR, Grosse SD. U.S. trends in computed tomography use and diagnoses in emergency department visits by patients with symptoms suggestive of pulmonary embolism, 2001–2009. *Acad Emerg Med.* 2013;20(10):1033-1040.

10. Douma RA, Gibson NS, Gerdes VE, et al. Validity and clinical utility of the simplified Wells rule for assessing clinical probability for the exclusion of pulmonary embolism. *Thromb Haemost.* 2009;101(1):197-200.

11. Gal G, Righini M, Roy PM, et al, Prediction of Pulmonary Embolism in the Emergency Department: the Revised Geneva Score. *Ann Intern Med.* 2006;144(3):165-171.

12. Kline JA, Courtney DM, Kabrhel C, et al. Prospective multicenter evaluation of the pulmonary embolism rule-out criteria. *J Thromb Haemost.* 2008;6(5):772-780.

13. Stein PD, Fowler SE, Goodman LR, et al; PIOPED II Investigators. Multidetector computed tomography for acute pulmonary embolism. *N Engl J Med.* 2006;354(22):2317-2327.

14. PIOPED Investigators. Value of the ventilation/perfusion scan in acute pulmonary embolism. Results of the prospective investigation of pulmonary embolism diagnosis (PIOPED). *JAMA.* 1990;263(20):2753-2759.

15. Worsley DF, Alavi A. Comprehensive analysis of the results of the PIOPED Study. Prospective Investigation of Pulmonary Embolism Diagnosis Study. *J Nuc Med.* 1995;36(12):2380-2387.

16. Stein PD, Chenevert TL, Fowler SE, et al; PIOPED III (Prospective Investigation of Pulmonary Embolism Diagnosis III) Investigators. Gadolinium enhanced magnetic resonance angiography for pulmonary embolism: a multicenter prospective study (PIOPED III). *Ann Intern Med.* 2010;152(7):434-443.

17. Kearon C, Akl EA, Ornelas J, et al. Antithrombotic therapy for VTE disease. CHEST guideline and expert panel report. *Chest.* 2016;149(2):315-352.

18. Kearon C, Akl EA, Comerota AJ, et al. Antithrombotic therapy for VTE disease: antithrombotic therapy and prevention of thrombosis, 9th ed: American College of Chest Physicians Evidence-Based Clinical Practice Guidelines. *Chest.* 2012;141(2 Suppl):e419S-494S.

19. Schulman S, Kearon C, Kakkar AK, et al.; RE-COVER Study Group. Dabigatran versus warfarin in the treatment of acute venous thromboembolism. *N Engl J Med.* 2009;361(24):2342-2352.

20. Bauersachs R, Berkowitz SD, Brenner B, et al. Oral rivaroxaban for symptomatic venous thromboembolism. *N Engl J Med.* 2010;363(26):2499-2510.

21. van Es N, Coppens M, Schulman S, Middeldorp S, Buller HR. Direct oral anticoagulants compared with vitamin K antagonists for acute venous thromboembolism: evidence from phase 3 trials. *Blood.* 2014;124(12):1968-1975.

22. Castellucci LA, Cameron C, Le Gal G, et al. Clinical and safety outcomes associated with treatment of acute venous

thromboembolism: a systematic review and meta-analysis. *JAMA*. 2014;312(11):1122-1135.

23. Carrier M, Cameron C, Delluc A, Castellucci L, Khorana AA, Lee AY. Efficacy and safety of anticoagulant therapy for the treatment of acute cancer-associated thrombosis: a systematic review and meta-analysis. *Thromb Res*. 2014;134(6): 1214-1219.

24. Vedovati MC, Germini F, Agnelli G, Becattini C. Direct oral anticoagulants in patients with VTE and cancer: a systematic review and meta-analysis. *Chest*. 2015;147(2):475-483.

25. Di Minno MN, Ageno W, Dentali F. Meta-analysis of the efficacy and safety of new oral anticoagulants in patients with cancer-associated acute venous thromboembolism: comment. *J Thromb Haemost*. 2014;12(12):2136-2138.

26. Franchini M, Bonfanti C, Lippi G. Cancer-associated thrombosis: investigating the role of new oral anticoagulants. *Thromb Res*. 2015;135(5):777-781.

27. Bochenek T, Nizankowski R. The treatment of venous thromboembolism with low-molecular-weight heparins. A meta-analysis. *Thromb Haemost*. 2012;107(4):699-716.

28. Bloom BJ, Filion KB, Atallah R, Eisenberg MJ. Meta-analysis of randomized controlled trials on the risk of bleeding with dabigatran. *Am J Cardiol*. 2014;113(6):1066-1074.

29. Touma L, Filion KB, Atallah R, Eberg M, Eisenberg MJ. A meta-analysis of randomized controlled trials of the risk of bleeding with apixaban versus vitamin K antagonists. *Am J Cardiol*. 2015;115(4):533-541.

30. Abraham NS, Singh S, Alexander GC, et al. Comparative risk of gastrointestinal bleeding with dabigatran, rivaroxaban, and warfarin: population based cohort study. *BMJ*. 2015;350:h1857.

31. Kang N, Sobieraj DM. Indirect treatment comparison of new oral anticoagulants for the treatment of acute venous thromboembolism. *Thromb Res*. 2014;133(6):1145-1151.

32. Majeed A, Hwang HG, Connolly SJ, et al. Management and outcomes of major bleeding during treatment with dabigatran or warfarin. *Circulation*. 2013;128(21):2325-2332.

33. Kearon C, Ginsberg JS, Kovacs MJ, et al. Extended Low-Intensity Anticoagulation for Thrombo-Embolism Investigators. Comparison of low-intensity warfarin therapy with conventional-intensity warfarin therapy for long-term prevention of recurrent venous thromboembolism. *N Engl J Med*. 2003;349(7):631-639.

34. Schulman S, Kearon C, Kakkar AK, et al. Extended use of dabigatran, warfarin, or placebo in venous thromboembolism. *N Engl J Med*. 2013;368(8):709-718.

35. Agnelli G, Buller HR, Cohen A, et al. Apixaban for extended treatment of venous thromboembolism. *N Engl J Med*. 2013; 368(8):699-708.

36. Castellucci LA, Cameron C, Le Gal G, et al. Efficacy and safety outcomes of oral anticoagulants and antiplatelet drugs in the secondary prevention of venous thromboembolism: systematic review and network meta-analysis. *BMJ*. 2013;347:f5133.

37. Iorio A, Kearon C, Filippucci E, et al. Risk of recurrence after a first episode of symptomatic venous thromboembolism provoked by a transient risk factor: a systematic review. *Arch Intern Med*. 2010;170(19):1710-1716.

38. Boutitie F, Pinede L, Schulman S, et al. Influence of preceding length of anticoagulant treatment and initial presentation of venous thromboembolism on risk of recurrence after stopping treatment: analysis of individual participants' data from seven trials. *BMJ*. 2011;342:d3036.

39. Prandoni P, Noventa F, Ghirarduzzi A, et al. The risk of recurrent venous thromboembolism after discontinuing anticoagulation in patients with acute proximal deep vein thrombosis or pulmonary embolism. A prospective cohort study in 1,626 patients. *Haematologica*. 2007;92(2):199-205.

40. Prandoni P, Lensing AWA, Cogo A, et al. The long-term clinical course of acute deep venous thrombosis. *Ann Intern Med*. 1996;125(1):1-7.

41. Palareti G, Legnani C, Lee A, et al. A comparison of the safety and efficacy of oral anticoagulation for the treatment of venous thromboembolic disease in patients with or without malignancy. *Thromb Haemost*. 2000;84(5):805-810.

42. Baglin T, Douketis J, Tosetto A, et al. Does the clinical presentation and extent of venous thrombosis predict likelihood and type of recurrence? A patient-level meta-analysis. *J Thromb Haemost*. 2010;8(11):2436-2442.

43. Hansson PO, Sorbo J, Eriksson H. Recurrent venous thromboembolism after deep vein thrombosis: incidence and risk factors. *Arch Intern Med*. 2000;160(6):769-774.

44. Schulman S, Wåhlander K, Lundström T, Clason SB, Eriksson H; THRIVE III Investigators. Secondary prevention of venous thromboembolism with the oral direct thrombin inhibitor ximelagatran. *N Engl J Med*. 2003;349(18):1713-1721.

45. Napolitano M, Saccullo G, Malato A, et al. Optimal duration of low molecular weight heparin for the treatment of cancer-related deep vein thrombosis: the Cancer-DACUS Study. *J Clin Oncol*. 2014;32(32):3607-3612.

46. Couturaud F, Sanchez O, Pernod G, et al. Six months vs extended oral anticoagulation after a first episode of pulmonary embolism: the PADIS-PE randomized clinical trial. *JAMA*. 2015;314(1):31-40.

47. Kearon C, Gent M, Hirsh J, et al. A comparison of three months of anticoagulation with extended anticoagulation for a first episode of idiopathic venous thromboembolism. *N Engl J Med*. 1999;340(12):901-907.

48. Ridker PM, Goldhaber SZ, Danielson E, et al; PREVENT Investigators. Long-term, low-intensity warfarin therapy for prevention of recurrent venous thromboembolism. *N Engl J Med*. 2003;348(15):1425-1434.

49. Farraj RS. Anticoagulation period in idiopathic venous thromboembolism. How long is enough? *Saudi Med J*. 2004; 25(7):848-851.

50. Palareti G, Cosmi B, Legnani C, et al. D-dimer testing to determine the duration of anticoagulation therapy. *N Engl J Med*. 2006;355(17):1780-1789.

51. Schulman S, Granqvist S, Holmstrom M, et al. The duration of oral anticoagulant therapy after a second episode of venous thromboembolism. *N Engl J Med*. 1997;336(6):393-398.

52. Douketis J, Tosetto A, Marcucci M, et al. Risk of recurrence after venous thromboembolism in men and women: patient level meta-analysis. *BMJ*. 2011;342:d813.

53. Douketis J, Tosetto A, Marcucci M, et al. Patient-level meta-analysis: effect of measurement timing, threshold, and patient age on ability of D-dimer testing to assess recurrence risk after unprovoked venous thromboembolism. *Ann Intern Med*. 2010;153(8):523-531.

54. Palareti G, Cosmi B, Legnani C, et al. D-dimer to guide the duration of anticoagulation in patients with venous thromboembolism: a management study. *Blood*. 2014;124(2):196-203.

55. Kearon C, Spencer FA, O'Keeffe D, et al. D-dimer testing to select patients with a first unprovoked venous thromboembolism

who can stop anticoagulant therapy: a cohort study. *Ann Intern Med.* 2015;162(1):27-34.

56. Brighton TA, Eikelboom JW, Mann K, et al. Low-dose aspirin for preventing recurrent venous thromboembolism. *N Engl J Med.* 2012;367(21):1979-1987.

57. Becattini C, Agnelli G, Schenone A, et al. Aspirin for preventing the recurrence of venous thromboembolism. *N Engl J Med.* 2012;366(21):1959-1967.

58. Simes J, Becattini C, Agnelli G, et al. Aspirin for the prevention of recurrent venous thromboembolism: the INSPIRE collaboration. *Circulation.* 2014;130(13):1062-1071.

59. Bates SM, Jaeschke R, Stevens SM, et al. Diagnosis of DVT: antithrombotic therapy and prevention of thrombosis, 9th ed: American College of Chest Physicians Evidence-Based Clinical Practice Guidelines. *Chest.* 2012;141(2 Suppl):e351S-e418S.

60. Righini M, Paris S, Le Gal G, Laroche JP, Perrier A, Bounameaux H. Clinical relevance of distal deep vein thrombosis. Review of literature data. *Thromb Haemost.* 2006;95(1):56-64.

61. Masuda EM, Kistner RL. The case for managing calf vein thrombi with duplex surveillance and selective anticoagulation. *Dis Mon.* 2010;56(10):601-613.

62. Masuda EM, Kistner RL, Musikasinthorn C, Liquido F, Geling O, He Q. The controversy of managing calf vein thrombosis. *J Vasc Surg.* 2012;55(2):550-561.

63. De Martino RR, Wallaert JB, Rossi AP, Zbehlik AJ, Suckow B, Walsh DB. A meta-analysis of anticoagulation for calf deep venous thrombosis. *J Vasc Surg.* 2012;56(1):228-237.e221.

64. Spencer F, Kroll A, Lessard D, et al. Isolated calf deep vein thrombosis in the community setting: the Worcester Venous Thromboembolism study. *J Thromb Thrombolysis.* 2012;33(3):211-217.

65. Hughes MJ, Stein PD, Matta F. Silent pulmonary embolism in patients with distal deep venous thrombosis: systematic review. *Thromb Res.* 2014;134(6):1182-1185.

66. Kearon C. Natural history of venous thromboembolism. *Circulation.* 2003;107(23 Suppl 1):I22-I30.

67. Macdonald PS, Kahn SR, Miller N, Obrand D. Short-term natural history of isolated gastrocnemius and soleal vein thrombosis. *J Vasc Surg.* 2003;37(3):523-527.

68. Parisi R, Visona A, Camporese G, et al. Isolated distal deep vein thrombosis: efficacy and safety of a protocol of treatment. Treatment of Isolated Calf Thrombosis (TICT) Study. *Int Angiol.* 2009;28(1):68-72.

69. Palareti G. How I treat isolated distal deep vein thrombosis (IDDVT). *Blood.* 2014;123(12):1802-1809.

70. Galanaud JP, Sevestre MA, Genty C, et al. Incidence and predictors of venous thromboembolism recurrence after a first isolated distal deep vein thrombosis. *J Thromb Haemost.* 2014;12(4):436-443.

71. Schwarz T, Buschmann L, Beyer J, Halbritter K, Rastan A, Schellong S. Therapy of isolated calf muscle vein thrombosis: a randomized, controlled study. *J Vasc Surg.* 2010;52(5):1246-1250.

72. Elsharawy M, Elzayat E. Early results of thrombolysis vs anticoagulation in iliofemoral venous thrombosis. A randomised clinical trial. *Eur J Vasc Endovasc Surg.* 2002;24(3):209-214.

73. Enden T, Klow NE, Sandvik L, et al. Catheter-directed thrombolysis vs. anticoagulant therapy alone in deep vein thrombosis: results of an open randomized, controlled trial reporting on short-term patency. *J Thromb Haemost.* 2009;7(8):1268-1275.

74. Enden T, Sandvik L, Klow NE, et al. Catheter-directed Venous Thrombolysis in acute iliofemoral vein thrombosis—the CaVenT study: rationale and design of a multicenter, randomized, controlled, clinical trial (NCT00251771). *Am Heart J.* 2007;154(5):808-814.

75. Haig Y, Enden T, Slagsvold CE, Sandvik L, Sandset PM, Klow NE. Determinants of early and long-term efficacy of catheter-directed thrombolysis in proximal deep vein thrombosis. *J Vasc Interv Radiol.* 2013;24(1):17-26.

76. Enden T, Haig Y, Klow NE, et al. Long-term outcome after additional catheter-directed thrombolysis versus standard treatment for acute iliofemoral deep vein thrombosis (the CaVenT study): a randomized controlled trial. *Lancet.* 2012;379(9810):31-38.

77. Enden T, Resch S, White C, Wik HS, Klow NE, Sandset PM. Cost-effectiveness of additional catheter-directed thrombolysis for deep vein thrombosis. *J Thromb Haemost.* 2013;11(6):1032-1042.

78. Watson LI, Armon MP. Thrombolysis for acute deep vein thrombosis. *Cochrane Database Syst Rev.* 2004;(4):Cd002783.

79. Bashir R, Zack CJ, Zhao H, Comerota AJ, Bove AA. Comparative outcomes of catheter-directed thrombolysis plus anticoagulation vs anticoagulation alone to treat lower-extremity proximal deep vein thrombosis. *JAMA Intern Med.* 2014;174(9):1494-1501.

80. Engelberger RP, Fahrni J, Willenberg T, et al. Fixed low-dose ultrasound-assisted catheter-directed thrombolysis followed by routine stenting of residual stenosis for acute ilio-femoral deep-vein thrombosis. *Thromb Haemost.* 2014;111(6):1153-1160.

81. Decousus H, Leizorovicz A, Parent F, et al. A clinical trial of vena caval filters in the prevention of pulmonary embolism in patients with proximal deep-vein thrombosis. Prévention du Risque d'Embolie Pulmonaire par Interruption Cave Study Group. *N Engl J Med.* 1998;338(7):409-415.

82. PREPIC Study Group. Eight-year follow-up of patients with permanent vena cava filters in the prevention of pulmonary embolism: the PREPIC (Prevention du Risque d'Embolie Pulmonaire par Interruption Cave) randomized study. *Circulation.* 2005;112(3):416-422.

83. Stein PD, Matta F. Vena cava filters in unstable elderly patients with acute pulmonary embolism. *Am J Med.* 2014;127(3):222-225.

84. Stein PD, Matta F, Keyes DC, Willyerd GL. Impact of vena cava filters on in-hospital case fatality rate from pulmonary embolism. *Am J Med.* 2012;125(5):478-484.

85. Muriel A, Jimenez D, Aujesky D, et al. Survival effects of inferior vena cava filter in patients with acute symptomatic venous thromboembolism and a significant bleeding risk. *J Am Coll Cardiol.* 2014;63(16):1675-1683.

86. Prasad V, Rho J, Cifu A. The inferior vena cava filter: how could a medical device be so well accepted without any evidence of efficacy? *JAMA Intern Med.* 2013;173(7):493-495.

87. Girard P, Meyer G, Parent F, Mismetti P. Medical literature, vena cava filters and evidence of efficacy. A descriptive review. *Thromb Haemost.* 2014;111(4):761-769.

88. Mismetti P, Laporte S, Pellerin O, et al. Effect of a retrievable inferior vena cava filter plus anticoagulation vs anticoagulation alone on risk of recurrent pulmonary embolism: a randomized clinical trial. *JAMA.* 2015;313(16):1627-1635.

89. Brandjes DP, Buller HR, Heijboer H, et al. Randomised trial of effect of compression stockings in patients with symptomatic proximal-vein thrombosis. *Lancet.* 1997;349(9054):759-762.

90. Prandoni P, Lensing AW, Prins MH, et al. Below-knee elastic compression stockings to prevent the post-thrombotic syndrome: a randomized, controlled trial. *Ann Intern Med.* 2004;141(4):249-256.

91. Kahn SR, Comerota AJ, Cushman M, et al; American Heart Association Council on Peripheral Vascular Disease, Council on Clinical Cardiology, and Council on Cardiovascular and Stroke Nursing. The postthrombotic syndrome: evidence-based prevention, diagnosis, and treatment strategies: a scientific statement from the American Heart Association. *Circulation.* 2014;130(18):1636-1661.

92. Kahn SR, Shapiro S, Wells PS, et al. Compression stockings to prevent post-thrombotic syndrome: a randomised placebo-controlled trial. *Lancet.* 2014;383(9920):880-888.

93. Kahn SR, Shapiro S, Ducruet T, et al. Graduated compression stockings to treat acute leg pain associated with proximal DVT. A randomised controlled trial. *Thromb Haemost.* 2014;112(6):1137-1141.

94. Wiener RS, Schwartz LM, Woloshin S. When a test is too good: how CT pulmonary angiograms find pulmonary emboli that do not need to be found. *BMJ.* 2013;347:f3368.

95. Carrier M, Righini M, Wells PS, et al. Subsegmental pulmonary embolism diagnosed by computed tomography: incidence and clinical implications. A systematic review and meta-analysis of the management outcome studies. *J Thromb Haemost.* 2010;8(8):1716-1722.

96. Carrier M, Righini M, Le Gal G. Symptomatic subsegmental pulmonary embolism: what is the next step? *J Thromb Haemost.* 2012;10(8):1486-1490.

97. Stein PD, Goodman LR, Hull RD, Dalen JE, Matta F. Diagnosis and management of isolated subsegmental pulmonary embolism: review and assessment of the options. *Clin Appl Thromb Hemost.* 2012;18(1):20-26.

98. Costantino G, Norsa AH, Amadori R, et al. Interobserver agreement in the interpretation of computed tomography in acute pulmonary embolism. *Am J Emerg Med.* 2009;27(9):1109-1111.

99. Lucassen WA, Beenen LF, Buller HR, et al. Concerns in using multi-detector computed tomography for diagnosing pulmonary embolism in daily practice. A cross-sectional analysis using expert opinion as reference standard. *Thromb Res.* 2013;131(2):145-149.

100. Stein PD, Fowler SE, Goodman LR, et al. Multidetector computed tomography for acute pulmonary embolism. *N Engl J Med.* 2006;354(22):2317-2327.

101. Courtney DM, Miller C, Smithline H, Klekowski N, Hogg M, Kline JA. Prospective multicenter assessment of interobserver agreement for radiologist interpretation of multidetector computerized tomographic angiography for pulmonary embolism. *J Thromb Haemost.* 2010;8(3):533-539.

102. Pena E, Kimpton M, Dennie C, Peterson R, Le Gal G, Carrier M. Difference in interpretation of computed tomography pulmonary angiography diagnosis of subsegmental thrombosis in patients with suspected pulmonary embolism. *J Thromb Haemost.* 2012;10(3):496-498.

103. Le Gal G, Righini M, Parent F, van Strijen M, Couturaud F. Diagnosis and management of subsegmental pulmonary embolism. *J Thromb Haemost.* 2006;4(4):724-731.

104. Le Gal G, Righini M, Sanchez O, et al. A positive compression ultrasonography of the lower limb veins is highly predictive of pulmonary embolism on computed tomography in suspected patients. *Thromb Haemost.* 2006;95(6):963-966.

105. den Exter PL, van Es J, Klok FA, et al. Risk profile and clinical outcome of symptomatic subsegmental acute pulmonary embolism. *Blood.* 2013;122(7):1144-1149; quiz 1329.

106. Kearon C, Ginsberg JS, Hirsh J. The role of venous ultrasonography in the diagnosis of suspected deep venous thrombosis and pulmonary embolism. *Ann Intern Med.* 1998;129(12):1044-1049.

107. Otero R, Uresandi F, Jimenez D, et al. Home treatment in pulmonary embolism. *Thromb Res.* 2010;126(1):e1-e5.

108. Aujesky D, Roy PM, Verschuren F, et al. Outpatient versus inpatient treatment for patients with acute pulmonary embolism: an international, open-label, randomised, non-inferiority trial. *Lancet.* 2011;378(9785):41-48.

109. Piran S, Le Gal G, Wells PS, et al. Outpatient treatment of symptomatic pulmonary embolism: a systematic review and metaanalysis. *Thromb Res.* 2013;132(5):515-519.

110. Vinson DR, Zehtabchi S, Yealy DM. Can selected patients with newly diagnosed pulmonary embolism be safely treated without hospitalization? A systematic review. *Ann Emerg Med.* 2012;60(5):651-662.

111. Zondag W, Kooiman J, Klok FA, Dekkers OM, Huisman MV. Outpatient versus inpatient treatment in patients with pulmonary embolism: a meta-analysis. *Eur Respir J.* 2013; 42(1):134-144.

112. Chan CM, Woods C, Shorr AF. The validation and reproducibility of the pulmonary embolism severity index. *J Thromb Haemost.* 2010;8(7):1509-1514.

113. Jimenez D, Aujesky D, Moores L, et al. Simplification of the pulmonary embolism severity index for prognostication in patients with acute symptomatic pulmonary embolism. *Arch Intern Med.* 2010;170(15):1383-1389.

114. Moores L, Aujesky D, Jimenez D, et al. Pulmonary Embolism Severity Index and troponin testing for the selection of low-risk patients with acute symptomatic pulmonary embolism. *J Thromb Haemost.* 2010;8(3):517-522.

115. Kahn SR, Comerota AJ, Cushman M, et al; American Heart Association Council on Peripheral Vascular Disease, Council on Clinical Cardiology, and Council on Cardiovascular and Stroke Nursing. The postthrombotic syndrome: evidence-based prevention, diagnosis, and treatment strategies. *Circulation.* 2014;130(18):1636-1661.

116. Meissner MH, Moneta G, Burnand K, et al. The hemodynamics and diagnosis of venous disease. *J Vasc Surg.* 2007;46(Suppl S): 4S-24S.

117. Pollack AA, Wood EH. Venous pressure in the saphenous vein at the ankle in man during exercise and changes in posture. *J Appl Physiol.* 1949;1(9):649-662.

118. Meissner MH, Zierler BK, Bergelin RO, Chandler WL, Strandness DE Jr. Coagulation, fibrinolysis, and recanalization after acute deep venous thrombosis. *J Vasc Surg.* 2002;35(2):278-285.

119. Lang IM, Madani M. Update on chronic thromboembolic pulmonary hypertension. *Circulation.* 2014;130(6):508-518.

120. Lang IM, Pesavento R, Bonderman D, Yuan JX. Risk factors and basic mechanisms of chronic thromboembolic pulmonary hypertension: a current understanding. *Eur Respir J.* 2013;41(2):462-468.

121. Tunariu N, Gibbs SJ, Win Z, et al. Ventilation-perfusion scintigraphy is more sensitive than multidetector CTPA in detecting chronic thromboembolic pulmonary disease as a treatable cause of pulmonary hypertension. *J Nucl Med.* 2007;48(5):680-684.

122. Raschke RA, Reilly BM, Guidry JR, et al. The weight-based heparin dosing nomogram compared with a "standard care" nomogram. A randomized controlled trial. *Ann Intern Med.* 1993;119(9):874-881.

123. Garcia DA, Baglin TP, Weitz JI A, et al. Parenteral anticoagulants: antithrombotic therapy and prevention of thrombosis, 9th ed: American College of Chest Physicians Evidence-Based Clinical Practice Guidelines. *Chest.* 2012; 141(2 Suppl):e24S-e43S.

124. River-Bou WL, Cabanas JG, Villanueva SE. Thrombolytic therapy. http://emedicine.medscape.com/article/811234-overview#a4. Updated December 15, 2016. Accessed August 7, 2017.

125. Hohner EM, Kruer RM, Gilmore VT, Streiff M, Gibbs H. Unfractionated heparin dosing for therapeutic anticoagulation in critically ill obese adults. *J Crit Care.* 2015;30(2):395-399.

126. Myzienski AE, Lutz MF, Smythe MA. Unfractionated heparin dosing for venous thromboembolism in morbidly obese patients: case report and review of the literature. *Pharmacotherapy.* 2010;30(3):105e-112e.

127. LaLama JT, Feeney ME, Vandiver JW, et al. Assessing an enoxaparin dosing protocol in morbidly obese patients. *J Thromb Thrombolysis.* 2015;39(4):516-521.

128. Finley A, Greenberg C. Heparin sensitivity and resistance: Management during cardiopulmonary bypass. *Anesth Analg* 2013;116:1210-1222.

129. Spies BD. Treating heparin resistance with antithrombin or fresh frozen plasma. *Ann Thorac Surg.* 2008;85(6):2153-2160.

130. Ranucci M, Isgrò G, Cazzaniga A, Soro G, Mencicanti L, Frigiola A. Predictors for heparin resistance in patients undergoing coronary artery bypass grafting. *Perfusion.* 1999;14(6):437-442.

131. Ranucci M, Isgrò G, Cazzaniga A, et al. Different patterns of heparin resistance: therapeutic implications. *Perfusion.* 2002; 17(3):199-204.

132. Hirsh J, Bauer KA, Donati MB, Gould M, Samama MM, Weitz JI. Parenteral anticoagulants: American College of Chest Physicians Evidence-Based Clinical Practice Guidelines (8th edition). *Chest.* 2008;133(6 Suppl):141S-159S.

133. Uprichard J, Manning RA, Laffan MA. Monitoring heparin anticoagulation in the acute phase response. *Br J Haematol.* 2010;149(4):613-619.

Acute Respiratory Distress Syndrome

Oleg Epelbaum, MD, and Christian Becker, MD

INTRODUCTION

Acute respiratory distress syndrome (ARDS) is a diffuse inflammatory reaction of the lung to an insult and is characterized by increased pulmonary capillary permeability, lung edema, and atelectasis. The histological hallmark of ARDS is diffuse alveolar damage and its pathognomonic hyaline membranes. The associated radiographic feature is bilateral alveolar infiltrates.

The Berlin definition of ARDS published in 2012[1,2] has superseded the prior American-European Consensus Conference definition of 1994.[3] The Berlin criteria updated the diagnostic requirements for ARDS, classified its severity based on the ratio of the arterial pressure of oxygen (Pao_2) to the fraction of inspired oxygen (Fio_2) (P/F ratio), and eliminated the term *acute lung injury*. The diagnostic criteria mandate that all of the following conditions are met before the syndrome is diagnosed: (1) In patients without known ARDS risk factors, cardiogenic or hydrostatic pulmonary edema as well as other alternative causes of bilateral pulmonary infiltrates need to be excluded; patients with a known ARDS risk factor are no longer required to undergo echocardiography or right heart catheterization to rule out cardiogenic pulmonary edema; (2) respiratory symptoms are of acute onset or are worsening significantly within 1 week prior to diagnosis; (3) imaging (either chest x-ray or computed tomography [CT]) shows bilateral alveolar infiltrates; and (4) oxygenation is impaired, the degree of which determines ARDS severity: P/F ratio greater than 200 but less than or equal to 300 defines mild, greater than 100 but less than or equal to 200 defines moderate, and 100 or less defines severe ARDS.

The incidence of ARDS is estimated to be approximately 86 cases per 100,000 person-years, which results in about 190,000 cases in the US every year.[4] Both incidence and mortality are comparable to those of acute myocardial infarction.[5]

Acute respiratory distress syndrome is triggered by predisposing factors, with more than 60 possible insults having been identified. In clinical practice, the vast majority of cases are caused by pulmonary or extrapulmonary sepsis, aspiration, severe trauma or burns, or transfusion or drug reactions, or as a complication of hematopoietic stem cell transplantation.[6,7]

The pathobiology and pathophysiology of the syndrome are complex and evolving, and as a result are beyond the scope of this chapter. The reader is referred to several recent informative and well-written review articles on this topic.[8-10]

Low Tidal Volume Ventilation

It has been recognized for decades that mechanical ventilation is capable of causing or exacerbating lung pathology through mechanisms known collectively as ventilator-induced lung injury (VILI).[11] Gross barotrauma in the form of pneumothorax is the most clinically obvious example of VILI. On a microscopic level, multiple experimental models have demonstrated that ventilation with excessive tidal volumes, so-called *volutrauma*, produces inflammation and changes indicative of high-permeability pulmonary edema even in healthy lungs.[12] Structural distortion caused by injurious ventilation inflicts damage on lung epithelial cells as well as their cytoskeletal framework and, by extension, on the extracellular matrix. This mechanical cascade is then converted to chemical signals through the release of pro-inflammatory cytokines, which promote pulmonary and extrapulmonary organ dysfunction. The adverse inflammatory response triggered by such damaging ventilation is termed *biotrauma*.[13]

Concurrently, pioneering CT examinations of the lungs of ARDS patients revealed that the aerated lung volume in these patients is significantly smaller than that predicted by their body frame, leading to the adoption of the term "baby lung" when referring to this discrepancy.[14] Contrary to the diffuse infiltration apparent on plain radiography, on CT, the majority of patients exhibited lower-lobe predominant or patchy distribution of increased density.[15] Whether the opacities present on CT represent edema or compressive atelectasis remains a subject of debate,[16,17] but what seems clear is that there is great inhomogeneity in the degree of aeration among lung units in ARDS patients.[18] Substantiating the baby lung hypothesis is the finding that although the small functional size of the ARDS lung translates to a decreased overall compliance (Δ volume/Δ pressure), the specific compliance (ie, compliance normalized for lung volume) is similar to that of healthy lung.[19] From this concept, it follows that the administration of conventional tidal volumes to the small aerated component of the ARDS lung would result in excessive lung deformation or strain (tidal volume/initial lung volume) with each ventilator breath (ie, volutrauma), thereby risking barotrauma because of excessive force per unit of cross-sectional area, defined as stress and approximated by the following equation: Transalveolar Pressure (P_L) = Alveolar Pressure (PA) – pleural pressure (P_{pl}). Under conditions of zero flow, the end-inspiratory airway pressure or plateau pressure (P_{plat}) is assumed to represent PA. The demonstration that healthy lungs incur VILI at a much higher strain and resultant stress than damaged lungs do has been suggested as evidence of so-called "stress raisers" in the ARDS lung.[20,21] The now-classic experimental model proposed by Mead et al showed that the stress at the interface of open and collapsed spheres is significantly greater than the overall distending pressure applied to the structure containing those spheres.[22] This situation is theorized to correspond to the boundary between inhomogeneous alveoli of ARDS, thus predisposing the nonuniform baby lung to VILI. In fact, the normal specific compliance of the aerated lung zones does not necessarily imply intact structure and function as demonstrated by nuclear isotope studies showing increased extravascular lung water in those regions.[23]

The conceptual framework described above prompted a number of investigators in the late 1990s to compare ventilation with lower versus higher tidal volumes (TV) in ARDS patients, and the results were mixed. A notable proof-of-concept study showing benefit was that by Amato et al, in which a 28-day mortality reduction was seen in 29 subjects randomized to lung-protective ventilation with low tidal volumes (tolerating "permissive" hypercapnia) and higher positive end-expiratory pressure (PEEP) levels as compared to 24 conventionally ventilated controls.[24] The incidence of gross barotrauma was significantly reduced in the protective ventilation group despite higher PEEP, which was set based on the lower inflection point of the pressure-volume curve. Other investigators found a favorable effect of low TV ventilation on both lung and systemic proinflammatory cytokine levels in ARDS patients.[25] These findings paved the way for the ARDS Network's (ARDSNet) landmark ARMA multicenter randomized, controlled trial (RCT) of low (6 mL/kg predicted body weight [PBW]) versus high (12 mL/kg) TV ventilation in over 800 subjects with ARDS.[26] In the low-tidal volume (LTV) arm, a goal P_{plat} of 30 cm H_2O or less was targeted to limit stress in addition to limiting strain. Positive end-expiratory pressure was set according to a stepwise PEEP/Fio_2 oxygenation table. Significantly fewer patients in the LTV group died on the ventilator prior to hospital discharge (absolute risk reduction ~ 9%), which was the primary endpoint, despite lower mean PEEP/Fio_2 ratios early in their clinical course. Permissive hypercapnia was evident and well tolerated. In fact, it recently has been shown to have a potential attenuating effect on VILI in its own right.[27] Subsequent RCTs, real-world observational studies, and meta-analyses upheld the mortality benefit of LTV ventilation.[28-30] A later analysis demonstrated that survival improves with the LTV

strategy even in quartiles of P_{plat} below 30 cm H_2O, further emphasizing the importance of strain reduction even when stress is within traditionally accepted boundaries.[31,32] Additionally, several studies have shown that P_{plat} may be a suboptimal surrogate for lung stress and one for which a ceiling of 30 cm H_2O may not be universally applicable in ARDS ventilation.[33-35] It is worth recalling that P_{plat} is only 1 of the 2 components of the P_L calculation, which is the difference between P_{plat} and P_{pl}. Thus, the same P_{plat} may translate into very different magnitudes of stress depending on the P_{pl}, which could be much higher than average in patients with elevated chest wall elastance (reciprocal of compliance) and therefore P_{pl} (eg, morbid obesity, anasarca, chest wall trauma), and lower than average in patients with spontaneous respiratory effort. While it is not practical to measure pleural pressure directly at the bedside of ARDS patients, an estimate can be obtained using a balloon catheter to transduce an esophageal pressure (P_{es}), itself a flawed technique that has not reached widespread adoption. Even if the P_{plat} were an accurate estimate of P_L in a given patient, the actual stress on a tissue level may be higher than expected, especially in severe cases manifesting the highest degree of heterogeneity, and thereby stress amplification, as discussed above.[18] On the other end of the spectrum, low airway pressures carry their own price of potential recruitment failure if the high opening pressures of diseased ARDS lung units are not attained, though increasing the PEEP could mitigate the harm and in fact improve outcomes through lower driving pressure.[36]

An analogous caveat applies to the generalization that a TV of 6 mL/kg is associated with safe strain in all ARDS cases. Although it is adjusted for the patient's body frame with the use of predicted body weight (PBW), it does not take into account the patient's abnormal resting lung volume. This is significant because the same TV therefore could produce protective or injurious strain, depending on the size of that patient's baby lung. Terragni et al showed that even at a TV of 6 mL/kg PBW, many ARDS patients exhibit CT evidence of tidal hyperinflation, and it is more pronounced in those with a smaller aerated lung compartment.[37]

Interest in the so-called driving pressure (P_{plat}-PEEP) reflects the desire to refine the generic TV and P_{plat} criteria that have characterized lung protective ventilation strategies inspired by the ARMA trial. The appeal of this idea becomes apparent after rearrangement of the formula for the static compliance (C_{rs}) of the respiratory system (C_{rs} = TV / [P_{plat} – PEEP]) to solve for driving pressure, which yields the quotient TV/C_{rs} and can thus be considered a normalization of TV for compliance, which in ARDS is a function of the size of the baby lung. In a recent retrospective analysis of individual patient data from multiple randomized controlled trials of ARDS, Amato et al demonstrated that driving pressure predicted outcome independent of P_{plat} but that the converse is not true.[38] Additionally, these investigators showed that the benefit of LTV ventilation in those trials was mediated by the concurrent reduction in driving pressure rather than the assignment to the LTV arm per se. Although driving pressure has since been shown to correlate reasonably well with lung stress, it is still not universally used.[39]

Cressoni et al have shown in an animal model that VILI develops if the mechanical power—that is, the breathing work performed by the ventilator per unit of time—applied to the lungs during mechanical ventilation is exceedingly high.[40] Driving pressure, through its interconnection with respiratory system elastance, is one of the determinants of power in an exponential manner.[41] Other components of power, namely TV, inspiratory flow rate, and respiratory frequency, likewise have a direct logarithmic relationship with it. The role of TV in the development of VILI has been discussed earlier, but it is noteworthy that a contribution of both inspiratory flow and respiratory rate to VILI has also been proposed.[42,43] The concept of power is intriguing because of the potential that it represents the all-encompassing link between ventilator parameters and VILI in ARDS.[44]

The 2017 American Thoracic Society (ATS)/European Society for Intensive Care Medicine (ESICM)/Society of Critical Care Medicine (SCCM) Guidelines for Mechanical Ventilation in ARDS make a strong recommendation in favor of LTV ventilation, initially set at 6 mL/kg PBW (range 4–8 mL/kg), while targeting a plateau pressure of less than 30 cm H_2O.[45] This is a subtle departure from the ARDSNet recommendation of initially setting the TV at 8 mL/kg PBW and titrating down to 6 mL/kg[46] (Fig. 11-1).

Positive End-Expiratory Pressure

Concurrently with the realization that mechanical ventilation of healthy animal lungs with TVs above a certain threshold leads to pulmonary edema came the observation that VILI is attenuated by the application of PEEP.[47] It was subsequently shown that PEEP blunts the pro-inflammatory cytokine release associated with high-TV ventilation and reduces the histological stigmata of high-permeability edema.[48,49] These findings gave rise to the notion that cyclical opening and closing of inflamed, surfactant-depleted lung units—whether damaged by harmful ventilation themselves or by an antecedent insult—further propagates the injury by means of a type of VILI called *atelectrauma*. Additionally, by prevention of end-expiratory alveolar collapse, the application of PEEP can increase the number of lung units receiving the TV during the subsequent inspiration—a phenomenon known as recruitment—and thereby enlarge the size of the baby lung, making it less likely to undergo excessive strain (volutrauma). Recruitment also accounts for the improvement in oxygenation produced by PEEP thanks to the salutary effect on ventilation/perfusion ($\dot{V}/\dot{Q}$) matching that results from reduced shunting past nonparticipating alveoli.[50] Rounding out the central role of PEEP in VILI prevention is the greater lung homogeneity that it creates via recruitment, which can offset the stress amplification that occurs at interfaces of well-aerated and poorly aerated alveoli.

Along with the theoretical benefits of PEEP, its potential drawbacks must also be recognized. Computed tomography studies have demonstrated that usually only a fraction of the ARDS lung consists of readily recruitable alveoli.[51,52] In the case of the minimally recruitable patient, the PEEP-induced increase in end-expiratory lung volume risks disproportionally affecting the aerated lung zones, making them prone to overdistention (ie, excessive strain) and barotrauma during the inspiratory phase.[53] Hyperinflation and a proinflammatory cytokine profile were observed despite low TVs when the ARDSNet stepwise table was used to set PEEP as in the ARMA trial.[54] This is particularly salient in light of recent animal data suggesting a greater inflammatory response in the lung subjected to volutrauma as compared to atelectrauma.[55] Additionally, PEEP can raise intrathoracic pressure sufficiently to cause a reduction in venous return and therefore ventricular preload, which could create or exacerbate hemodynamic compromise. In fact, if the decrease in cardiac output related to PEEP is significant enough, it could lead a drop in oxygen delivery despite the favorable impact of PEEP on the oxygen content of arterial blood.[56]

When higher PEEP levels were incorporated into a so-called "open lung" approach in comparison to non–lung-protective strategies, survival favored the groups receiving higher PEEP.[24,28] Subsequently, when the control arm was ventilated according to the ARDSNet protocol from ARMA, a mortality difference was no longer seen.[57] Higher versus lower PEEP settings as isolated interventions have been the subject of 3 multicenter randomized controlled trials (ALVEOLI 2004,[58] LOVS 2008,[59] Express 2008[60]) and a patient-level meta-analysis (PLMA)[61] combining data from these 3 studies, which have a number of features in common. They were conducted in the post-ARMA era of LTV ventilation in ARDS, and the mean P/F ratio was less than 200 in all the study groups. Positive end-expiratory pressure was titrated according to a stepwise PEEP/Fio_2 oxygenation table analogous to the ARDSNet protocol in ALVEOLI and LOVS and maximized until reaching a P_{plat} ceiling of 28 to 30 cm H_2O in Express. Statistically significant separation in average PEEP values was achieved between the control and experimental groups in all 3 trials, though reaching the target difference in ALVEOLI required an in-study protocol adjustment. Each trial had a mortality-based endpoint as its primary outcome measure, which did not reach statistical significance in any of them. Oxygenation was better in the higher PEEP arm of all 3 studies, and improvements in other outcomes (eg, LOVS: death with refractory hypoxemia; Express: ventilator-free days, organ failure–free days) did reach statistical significance in favor of higher PEEP. From a safety perspective, higher PEEP did not increase the incidence of gross barotrauma; while it did increase the need for intravenous fluid administration, vasopressor use did not differ between the groups. The subsequent meta-analysis largely recapitulated the results of the individual trials, except that in the population with worse gas exchange (P/F ratio < 200; ie, ARDS by the American-European Consensus Conference definition) there was a reduction in hospital mortality

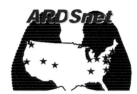

NIH NHLBI ARDS Clinical Network
Mechanical Ventilation Protocol Summary

OXYGENATION GOAL: PaO$_2$ 55-80 mmHg or SpO$_2$ 88-95%
Use a minimum PEEP of 5 cm H$_2$O. Consider use of incremental FiO$_2$/PEEP combinations such as shown below (not required) to achieve goal.

Lower PEEP/higher FiO2

FiO$_2$	0.3	0.4	0.4	0.5	0.5	0.6	0.7	0.7
PEEP	5	5	8	8	10	10	10	12

FiO$_2$	0.7	0.8	0.9	0.9	0.9	1.0
PEEP	14	14	14	16	18	18-24

Higher PEEP/lower FiO2

FiO$_2$	0.3	0.3	0.3	0.3	0.3	0.4	0.4	0.5
PEEP	5	8	10	12	14	14	16	16

FiO$_2$	0.5	0.5-0.8	0.8	0.9	1.0	1.0
PEEP	18	20	22	22	22	24

INCLUSION CRITERIA: Acute onset of
1. PaO$_2$/FiO$_2$ ≤ 300 (corrected for altitude)
2. Bilateral (patchy, diffuse, or homogenous) infiltrates consistent with pulmonary edema
3. No clinical evidence of left atrial hypertension

PART I: VENTILATOR SETUP AND ADJUSTMENT
1. Calculate predicted body weight (PBW)
   Males = 50 + 2.3 [height (inches) - 60]
   Females = 45.5 + 2.3 [height (inches) -60]
2. Select any ventilator mode
3. Set ventilator settings to achieve initial V$_T$ = 8 ml/kg PBW
4. Reduce V$_T$ by 1 ml/kg at intervals ≤ 2 hours until V$_T$ = 6ml/kg PBW.
5. Set initial rate to approximate baseline minute ventilation (not > 35 bpm).
6. Adjust V$_T$ and RR to achieve pH and plateau pressure goals below.

PLATEAU PRESSURE GOAL: ≤ 30 cm H$_2$O
Check Pplat (0.5 second inspiratory pause), at least q 4h and after each change in PEEP or V$_T$.
If Pplat > 30 cm H$_2$O: decrease V$_T$ by 1ml/kg steps (minimum = 4 ml/kg).
If Pplat < 25 cm H$_2$O and V$_T$< 6 ml/kg, increase V$_T$ by 1 ml/kg until Pplat > 25 cm H$_2$O or V$_T$ = 6 ml/kg.
If Pplat < 30 and breath stacking or dys-synchrony occurs: may increase V$_T$ in 1ml/kg increments to 7 or 8 ml/kg if Pplat remains ≤ 30 cm H$_2$O.

pH GOAL: 7.30-7.45
Acidosis Management: (pH < 7.30)
If pH 7.15-7.30: Increase RR until pH > 7.30 or PaCO$_2$ < 25 (Maximum set RR = 35).

If pH < 7.15: Increase RR to 35.
If pH remains < 7.15, V$_T$ may be increased in 1 ml/kg steps until pH > 7.15 (Pplat target of 30 may be exceeded).
May give NaHCO$_3$
Alkalosis Management: (pH > 7.45) Decrease vent rate if possible.

I: E RATIO GOAL: Recommend that duration of inspiration be ≤ duration of expiration.

PART II: WEANING
A. Conduct a SPONTANEOUS BREATHING TRIAL daily when:
1. FiO$_2$ ≤ 0.40 and PEEP ≤ 8 OR FiO$_2$ ≤ 0.50 and PEEP ≤ 5.
2. PEEP and FiO$_2$ ≤ values of previous day.
3. Patient has acceptable spontaneous breathing efforts. (May decrease vent rate by 50% for 5 minutes to detect effort.)
4. Systolic BP ≥ 90 mmHg without vasopressor support.
5. No neuromuscular blocking agents or blockade.

B. SPONTANEOUS BREATHING TRIAL (SBT):
If all above criteria are met and subject has been in the study for at least 12 hours, initiate a trial of UP TO 120 minutes of spontaneous breathing with FiO2 ≤ 0.5 and PEEP ≤ 5:
1. Place on T-piece, trach collar, or CPAP ≤ 5 cm H$_2$O with PS ≤ 5
2. Assess for tolerance as below for up to two hours.
   a.   SpO$_2$ ≥ 90: and/or PaO$_2$ ≥ 60 mmHg
   b.   Spontaneous V$_T$ ≥ 4 ml/kg PBW
   c.   RR ≤ 35/min
   d.   pH ≥ 7.3
   e.   No respiratory distress (distress= 2 or more)
      ➤ HR > 120% of baseline
      ➤ Marked accessory muscle use
      ➤ Abdominal paradox
      ➤ Diaphoresis
      ➤ Marked dyspnea
3. If tolerated for at least 30 minutes, consider extubation.
4. If not tolerated resume pre-weaning settings.

Definition of <u>UNASSISTED BREATHING</u>
(Different from the spontaneous breathing criteria as PS is not allowed)

1. Extubated with face mask, nasal prong oxygen, or room air, OR
2. T-tube breathing, OR
3. Tracheostomy mask breathing, OR
4. CPAP less than or equal to 5 cm H$_2$0 **without pressure support or IMV assistance.**

FIGURE 11-1 ARDSNet protocol. (Developed by the NIH-NHLBI ARDS Network as a part of a government research contract. www.ardsnet.org/files/ventilator_protocol_2008-07.pdf.)

of borderline statistical significance (adjusted risk ratio [RR], 0.90; 95% confidence interval [CI], 0.81–1.00).

In the ensuing years, there has been much speculation about the reasons why the convincing theory and experimental evidence behind the lung protective properties of PEEP has not translated into a clear-cut survival benefit in clinical trials. Among the hypotheses are the variability in ventilator settings at the time of application of ARDS criteria for enrollment and the lack of consistency in regard to recruitment maneuvers (RMs) (see "Nontraditional Mechanical Ventilation Modes").[57] Furthermore, as suggested by the meta-analysis, a possible

benefit to the patients with the most severe ARDS may have been masked by harm to those with milder disease. This notion is supported by CT data indicating that ARDS patients with the highest potential for recruitment are also those with the most lung involvement, the worst oxygenation, and greater mortality.[40] When the data from *LOVS* and Express were retrospectively analyzed, it was found that an improvement in oxygenation in response to raising PEEP—a marker of underlying recruitable lung—was associated with a lower risk of death.[62]

Perhaps the most controversial clinical question to emerge from this debate is whether the generic PEEP/Fio$_2$

table based entirely on oxygenation, as in ALVEOLI and LOVS, or the arbitrary P_{plat}-guided algorithm used in Express is the optimal approach to PEEP titration. To date, consensus on the best strategy for setting PEEP remains elusive, but there are many who favor basing the level on an individual patient's physiological parameters. Pointing to the success of the trials by Amato et al[24] and Villar et al,[28] proponents have advocated determining the lower inflection point of the pressure-volume (P-V) curve and setting the PEEP at a fixed point above that value to prevent deflation into the zone of derecruitment. In a different take on the same concept, Talmor et al compared P_{es}-guided PEEP settings to the ARDSNet table as a control, targeting PEEP levels that would yield a positive transalveolar pressure (PEEP-P_{pl}) at end-expiration, with P_{es} serving as a surrogate for P_{pl}.[33] Keeping the difference between PEEP and P_{pl} positive in principle ought to prevent end-expiratory derecruitment and minimize atelectrauma. In that study of 61 patients, despite higher average PEEP and P/F ratio in the P_{es}-guided arm, unadjusted mortality was no different in the 2 groups. A much larger multicenter EPVent-2 trial (Clinicaltrial.gov identifier NCT01681225) is further exploring this approach.

In clinical practice, constructing P-V curves and measuring P_{es} can be cumbersome tasks, and there is experimental evidence that recruitment (and consequently derecruitment) occurs along a continuum of pressure rather than as a threshold, all-or-nothing phenomenon demarcated by an abrupt P-V slope change.[63,64] Grasso et al have proposed the so-called stress index as an alternative, which is a measurement reflecting the behavior of the pressure-time (P-T) waveform during constant flow, volume-targeted ventilation.[65] A stress index less than 1 corresponds to a downward concavity of the curve, an indicator that effective elastance (the inverse of effective compliance) is decreasing with progressive inflation due to ongoing recruitment and increase in the size of the baby lung. Such a patient would be considered to have the potential for additional recruitment, and PEEP would be raised accordingly. On the opposite extreme is a stress index greater than 1, represented by an upward concavity in the P-T curve, that is indicative of a dynamically increasing elastance caused by overdistention. In this case, the PEEP would be reduced. The goal would be a linear P-T curve, signifying a constant elastance throughout TV delivery and therefore achievement of maximal possible recruitment without hyperinflation.

A study by Chiumello et al compares the ability of the above approaches to appropriately stratify the magnitude of PEEP according to the severity of ARDS.[66] Ironically, only the PEEP/Fio_2 table method ramped up the PEEP level in an incremental fashion across groups with mild, moderate, and severe ARDS.

The 2017 ATS/ESICM/SCCM Guidelines for Mechanical Ventilation in ARDS contain a conditional recommendation in favor of higher PEEP as opposed to lower PEEP for moderate or severe ARDS based on the mortality benefit in this subgroup, suggested by the PLMA discussed above.[45]

Nontraditional Mechanical Ventilation Modes

The use of unconventional modes of mechanical ventilation in ARDS has generally reflected the desire to achieve maximal safe mean airway pressure (mP_{aw}) in order to, in turn, maximize inspiratory alveolar recruitment and, thereby, oxygenation. A classic example of such a strategy is inverse ratio ventilation (IRV), in which inspiratory time is set to exceed expiratory time, an unnatural respiratory pattern requiring deep sedation and neuromuscular paralysis. Inverse ratio ventilation fell out of favor when it was recognized that the oxygenation benefit was likely related to intrinsic PEEP from the short expiratory time rather than to the high mP_{aw}, per se.[67] Airway pressure release ventilation (APRV) is a modification of the IRV concept that was first described about 30 years ago. It is characterized by cyclical inflations to a set peak airway pressure (P_{high}) separated by deflations to a much lower pressure (P_{low}) analogous to PEEP, but in practice frequently set to 0 cm H_2O. The duration of both P_{high} (T_{high}) and P_{low} (T_{low}) is determined by the clinician and programmed such that T_{high} greater than T_{low} to augment mP_{aw}. Carbon dioxide elimination occurs during the deflations and is proportional to their frequency and the accompanying pressure drop (ie, P_{high} − P_{low}). The unique feature of APRV in comparison to conventional IRV is that spontaneous patient breathing can be superimposed on ventilator activity at any point in the cycle. These efforts may or may not be pressure supported and, notably, they can have an additive effect on the TV generated by the ventilator. It is also important to recognize that without spontaneous respiration, APRV becomes indistinguishable from pressure-controlled IRV. Investigators have been able to demonstrate in animal[68] and human[69] studies that spontaneous breathing during APRV in ARDS leads to superior recruitment of dependent lung zones and V̇/Q̇ matching compared to APRV without spontaneous breathing. A recent observational study[70] showed a salutary effect of APRV on oxygenation, a parameter of questionable prognostic significance in ARDS, whereas a contemporary small prospective RCT[71] found no difference in ventilator-free days or mortality between APRV and synchronized intermittent mechanical ventilation. Robust clinical trial data supporting or refuting the utility of APRV in ARDS in the era of lung protective ventilation are not available.[72] On theoretical grounds, concerns about the use of this mode are primarily 2-fold. One concern is that control over the TV is not straightforward, especially when spontaneous breathing is present, and so violations of the LTV strategy are likely in clinical practice.[73] Average TVs in excess of 9 mL/kg PBW have been encountered in retrospective series of APRV use in the LTV era.[70,74] Secondly, the demonstration by Papazian et al of a survival benefit of early neuromuscular blockade in severe ARDS[75] has spurred inquiry into whether active patient effort is a contributor to lung injury and therefore mortality in ARDS.[76] In an animal model, forceful spontaneous breathing was injurious when coupled with moderate TVs (7–9 mL/kg) and protective in combination with low TVs (6 mL/kg).[77]

Proposed mechanisms for harm include large swings in P_L caused by drops in P_{pl} from vigorous negative-pressure efforts, as well as increased pendelluft), both of which are likely to be exacerbated by larger TVs.[78] Thus, the potentially liberal TVs associated with APRV, together with the permitted spontaneous breathing could act synergistically to exacerbate VILI in ARDS patients ventilated with this mode.

Another unconventional approach to protective, "open-lung" ventilation in ARDS is high-frequency oscillatory ventilation (HFOV), in which a fundamentally different mechanical ventilator pumps small, nonphysiologic TVs into the trachea at a rate that can exceed 300 times per minute. The oscillator continually pushes a column of gas down into the lower airways and then back up again and out through an outflow valve. The individual TVs are smaller than the anatomical dead space, yet carbon dioxide elimination takes place effectively, so gas exchange is believed to occur by a number of unique mechanisms.[79] One of them is pendelluft, which refers to the swinging back and forth of gas between adjacent lung units differing in their resistance and compliance (ie, having different time constants).[80] Other phenomena at play include collateral ventilation and turbulent flow facilitating diffusion (so-called Taylor dispersion).[81] Whereas the ultra-low TVs in theory minimize lung strain and thus risk of volutrauma, small-amplitude oscillations about a high mP_{aw} are thought to protect against both excessive stress and cyclical derecruitment. This unnatural mode of ventilation also presents practical challenges such as poor patient tolerance without paralysis and inadequate cardiac filling due to maintenance of a high intrathoracic pressure.[82] Not surprisingly, multiple animal experiments comparing VILI induced by HFOV to that of nonprotective conventional ventilation (CV) favored the former;[83] a subsequent comparison to protective CV yielded no difference in clinically measurable parameters.[84] Until recently, human clinical studies on the performance of HFOV in ARDS were limited to observational experience[85] and 2 flawed RCTs in which CV was not protective.[86,87] In aggregate, these data suggested an oxygenation benefit without an impact on mortality; a systematic review combining heterogeneous adult and pediatric studies available prior to 2010 resulted in a small survival advantage for HFOV that prompted further investigation.[88] Answers emerged in 2013 with the simultaneous publication of 2 multi-center RCTs, OSCILLATE[89] and OSCAR[90] comparing HFOV and CV that together enrolled nearly 1000 ARDS patients in the LTV era. OSCILLATE was halted prematurely due to significantly higher mortality in the HFOV arm (47% vs. 35%), and OSCAR showed no survival difference. High-frequency oscillatory ventilation reduced the incidence of refractory hypoxemia in OSCILLATE but had no effect on death following such episodes. No significant difference in oxygenation was observed in OSCAR. Although both trials have been subjected to criticism ranging from lack of experience with HFOV in many centers to suboptimal HFOV settings,[91] a number of subsequent meta-analyses have been performed,[92-94] and none has demonstrated improved survival with HFOV in ARDS contrary to the original systematic review. A major prevailing conclusion stemming from OSCILLATE and OSCAR is that HFOV offers no incremental benefit over CV in ARDS when the latter conforms to current standards of lung protection.[95]

Recruitment Maneuvers

The reason why the inspiratory and expiratory limbs of the lung's P-V curve are not superimposed is the presence of hysteresis, which is a property whereby the preceding inflation phase imparts a greater compliance to lung tissue for the subsequent deflation. This phenomenon results in a bigger lung volume associated with a given pressure on the expiratory limb compared to the inspiratory limb of the P-V curve. Theoretically, if the ARDS lung were to undergo an initial maximal tolerated inflation followed by the application of sufficient PEEP to prevent deflation back to the inspiratory limb, it would retain the higher aerated volume, and that would become the new, larger size of the baby lung. The expected benefit would then be improved oxygenation and lower risk of VILI. This is the principle behind so-called lung RMs: brief applications of a pressure that would be injurious if used consistently in order to achieve maximal alveolar opening in seconds to minutes and then consolidate the gains by raising the PEEP above the pre-RM level. An example of a commonly used RM is the application of a continuous positive airway pressure (CPAP) of 40 cm H_2O for 40 seconds in a passive patient.[96] A considerably longer version is the stepwise escalation of PEEP until a certain airway pressure ceiling is reached, followed by de-escalation from the peak to the new maintenance PEEP.[97] Based on animal experiments[98] and human CT data,[49,50] the latter approach may be more effective in opening the lung, while being less destructive. In the course of the sustained high CPAP, it has been shown that further recruitment is minimal after the first 10 seconds, beyond which the pressurized thorax begins to impact hemodynamics in the susceptible patient.[99] Despite the attractive physiological basis underlying RMs, the demonstration of improvement in gas exchange has been inconsistent at best.[100-104] As expected, failure to adjust the PEEP upward following the RM leads to rapid dissipation of any oxygenation gains.[105] Additionally, use of RMs later in the course of ARDS has been associated with failure to respond, probably because of progression to a more organized form of alveolar damage. Disappointing oxygenation data, however, do not necessarily negate a favorable impact of RMs on VILI, which could have survival implications. Markers of epithelial injury and inflammation have, in fact, been shown to decrease in ARDS subjects after an RM.[106,107] Perhaps the most challenging question surrounding RMs is whether they affect ARDS mortality, in part because most trials have studied them as part of a multifaceted ventilation strategy.[24,59,107] Studies in which RMs are an isolated variable are few and offer conflicting results.[94,95] Between the 2 most recent meta-analyses of RCTs, 1 showed lower hospital mortality,[108] while another showed lower ICU mortality but not hospital mortality.[109] When the available data on hypoxemia were pooled, the 2 meta-analyses diverged.

These reviews are handicapped by reliance on heterogeneous studies prone to bias. The totality of the evidence behind RMs in ARDS leaves room for provider discretion based on clinical circumstances; although, for both oxygenation and VILI reduction, delays in RM performance are likely to diminish utility.

The 2017 ATS/ESICM/SCCM Guidelines for Mechanical Ventilation in ARDS include a conditional recommendation in favor of RMs, with caution advised in patients who are hypovolemic or in shock.[45]

Prone Positioning

The observation that oxygenation can be improved by turning the patient with acute respiratory failure from the usual supine position (SP) to a prone position (PP) is not novel,[110] but only recently has PP joined the short list of ARDS interventions associated with a mortality benefit in an RCT.[111] Much of the research on this topic has focused on potential explanations for the salutary effect of PP on gas exchange. What has emerged is that the previously dependent degassed dorsal lung regions regain aeration in the PP, while the newly dependent ventral lung regions lose aeration.[112,113] The aggregate volume of well-aerated alveoli thereby increases due to the relatively larger dimensions of the dorsally oriented lung and the relief of pressure from the abdominal cavity and the heart in the PP.[114,115] Because of resultant improvement in lung geometry, the baby lung becomes not only functionally bigger but also more homogeneously inflated within the chest, thus attenuating the anteroposterior ventilation gradient normally present in the SP in ARDS.[113] In that regard, PP can be considered analogous to an RM when combined with high PEEP.[116] Concurrent gravitational redistribution of perfusion also occurs, but there is enough preservation of nondependent perfusion[117] such that $\dot{V}/\dot{Q}$ uniformity increases in the PP relative to the SP.[118] This mechanism of improved $\dot{V}/\dot{Q}$ matching is believed to underlie the oxygenation benefit of PP, which has been consistently present across animal and human studies.

As has been the case with PEEP and many other ARDS interventions, however, it has proven much more difficult to demonstrate a mortality reduction. None of the 4 initial RCTs[119-122] published between 2001 and 2009 showed an improvement in survival with PP, whether conducted in the LTV era or not, though lessons learned from them suggested that the benefits of this strategy may be maximal when subjects with the most severe ARDS are proned early and for an extended period of time. In 2 of the trials,[120,122] there was a significantly greater incidence of adverse events in the PP such as pressure ulcers and malpositioning of hardware. With this as background, Guérin and his experienced coinvestigators conducted the PROSEVA trial[111] enrolling 466 ARDS patients with a P/F ratio less than 150 mmHg within 36 hours of initiation of mechanical ventilation and within an hour of randomization. Patients were in a prone position for an average of 17 h/d. There was strict adherence to lung protective ventilation protocols and extensive use of neuromuscular blocking agents (NMBA). Mortality at 28 and 90 days was significantly lower in the PP arm, accompanied by an increase in ventilator-free days and with no difference in complications. Notably, a post-hoc analysis determined that although, as expected, PP increased the P/F ratio in PROSEVA, the effect on oxygenation could not account for the survival benefit.[123] This conclusion has prompted a closer look at the impact of PP on VILI reduction, which, as discussed, may be the thread linking all favorable ARDS interventions. In principle, the greater homogeneity of the baby lung afforded by PP should attenuate stress amplification while the greater overall aerated volume should reduce strain. These hypotheses are supported by animal studies of PP,[124,125] which, along with scant human data,[116,126] also demonstrate that PP mitigates against lung damage and inflammation caused by injurious ventilation.[127] In fact, PP may require synergy with lung protective ventilation to improve outcomes in ARDS as suggested by a post-PROSEVA meta-analysis that showed a mortality benefit only when analysis was restricted to trials employing LTV.[128] Another prism through which the role of PP in ARDS has been examined is that of cardiac performance, specifically as it relates to the right ventricle, whose function can be augmented by a PP-induced increase in preload and decrease in afterload.[129,130] Such optimization could play an important role in the clinical course of patients with ARDS complicated by acute cor pulmonale.

The 2017 ATS/ESICM/SCCM Guidelines for Mechanical Ventilation in ARDS contain a strong recommendation in favor of prone positioning for more than 12 h/d for severe ARDS.[45]

NONVENTILATORY STRATEGIES

Corticosteroids

Endogenous human corticosteroids (CS), cortisol being primary among them, are potent but nonspecific inhibitors of inflammation. They exert their effects in myriad ways, most notably by blocking the activity of a transcription factor known as nuclear factor-κB, which promotes the synthesis of numerous proinflammatory cytokines and has been implicated in the molecular biology of ARDS.[131] Although adrenal production of CS is expected to increase in response to the insult that triggered ARDS, hormone levels may be insufficient despite the increase, or their effect may be dampened by various mechanisms of tissue resistance to CS.[132] Therefore, supplementation with exogenous CS is a theoretically appealing option for abrogating the inflammatory cascade that drives lung injury in ARDS. Results of initial trials using high-dose therapy administered early in the course of ARDS and for brief periods (eg, methylprednisolone 30 mg/kg every 6 hours for 24 hours) were disappointing.[133,134] Subsequent investigations proposed that the inflammation fueling the exudative phase of ARDS can follow 2 distinct trajectories: reduction over the course of the first week with more favorable clinical outcome as opposed to persistence leading to fibroproliferation and eventual fibrosis with inferior outcome.[135,136] It was hypothesized that the transition to fibroproliferation and then to fibrosis is the consequence of protracted inflammation and the associated aberrant lung repair—a process that could be interrupted by CS.[137-139] This theory led to a reorientation of CS trials toward targeting "unresolving" ARDS with longer courses but lower doses (eg, methylprednisolone 0.5 mg/kg every 6 hours). In a small RCT predating universal LTV ventilation, Meduri et al reported improved short-term survival and oxygenation in the group randomized to a 32-day methylprednisolone taper for unresolving ARDS by day 7 compared to placebo.[140] ARDSNet then conducted a larger RCT in the LTV era that enrolled subjects with ARDS persisting 7 days or longer and randomized them to placebo or a 21-day course of methylprednisolone followed by a taper.[141] Although secondary short-term endpoints such as ventilator-free and ICU-free days favored the CS arm, 60- and 180-day mortality rates were similar. Importantly, receipt of CS conferred a higher mortality on those who entered the study 14 days or more after the onset of ARDS. The treatment group also suffered more adverse events attributable to neuromuscular dysfunction, which is a known side effect of CS therapy. In fact, this and other potential harms of CS may account for the discrepancy between the short-term benefits demonstrated by these trials and the lack of a survival advantage in the long run. Starting CS beyond 14 days may likewise have accentuated the drawbacks of CS because at that stage suppression of inflammation may no longer be beneficial or possibly may be detrimental. Meduri et al subsequently investigated the role of prolonged low-dose CS therapy (methylprednisolone 1 mg/kg/d) in early (≤ 72 hours) severe ARDS in a placebo-controlled RCT.[142] By day 7, there was a significant difference in the degree of lung injury and extubation rate favoring the CS arm. Other short-term outcome measures such as ICU stay and hospital mortality were also reduced. The extreme heterogeneity of the available CS RCTs has made the results of published meta-analyses difficult to interpret. Overall, they seem to parallel the 3 RCTs discussed above in showing improvement in 28-day metrics,[141] which then disappears when 60-day mortality is considered.[144] The systematic reviews support the notion, however, that CS can be administered to ARDS patients without an increase in adverse events such as new infections or neuromyopathy.[145,146] In addition to heterogeneity among studies, as a clinically defined entity, ARDS patients within a given trial invariably encompass a spectrum of pathology that includes not just diffuse alveolar damage but also other substrate that is more (eg, organizing pneumonia) or less (eg, influenza pneumonitis) responsive to CS therapy.[147,148] It is not difficult to envision how CS could have a differential effect on individual subjects within such a variable study population. Many questions about the efficacy of CS in ARDS remain unanswered. For example, should mortality be the dominant outcome measure or could protection against lung fibrosis and therefore eventual disability among survivors be viewed as a comparably important endpoint? Despite the uncertainty, CS is currently one of the most commonly used adjunctive therapies in the management of ARDS.[149]

Neuromuscular Blockade

The nondepolarizing NMBAs used for the postintubation management of mechanically ventilated patients, including those with ARDS, act by antagonizing the nicotinic acetylcholine receptor at the neuromuscular junction and fall into 2 categories: aminosteroids (eg, vecuronium, rocuronium) and benzylisoquinolines such as cisatracurium.[150] The latter compound has gained favor over the aminosteroids as the agent of choice for continuous neuromuscular blockade in critical care due to its metabolism via Hoffman elimination (temperature- and pH-dependent ester hydrolysis), which does not depend on renal or hepatic function, and its shorter recovery period.[151] Historically, enthusiasm for the use of NMBA has been tempered by a perceived association with neuromuscular dysfunction despite less supporting evidence of this—at least for short-term NMBA monotherapy—in comparison to CS.[152-154] Available RCT data of paralysis in ARDS are based exclusively on administration of 48-hour cisatracurium infusions to mechanically ventilated subjects with moderate to severe early ARDS. All 3 RCTs were performed in the LTV era by Papazian et al in France. The 2 initial smaller trials[155,156] examined the effect of paralysis on gas exchange and the proinflammatory cytokine response in the lung and serum. They found a significant and sustained improvement in P/F ratio in the NMBA group relative to the placebo arm as well as a significant difference in interleukin (IL)-6, IL-8, and IL-1β levels at 48 hours, favoring cisatracurium. The subsequent multicenter, double-blind RCT of 340 ARDS patients with P/F ratios of less than 150 designed to assess for an impact on survival showed a significant though delayed benefit in adjusted 90-day mortality as well as in secondary outcomes, such as ventilator-free days.[75] The survival advantage at 90 days was limited to the subgroup with a P/F ratio less than 120. From a safety perspective, episodes of gross barotrauma were less frequent in the NMBA arm, while the incidence of ICU-acquired weakness was not significantly different: It was present in about one-third of survivors to ICU discharge in each arm. Combining the results of these 3 RCTs into a meta-analysis largely recapitulated their already concordant findings.[157] The Prevention and Early Treatment of Acute Lung Injury (PETAL) network is currently recruiting a planned total of more than 1000 subjects across 48 sites as part of the Reevaluation of Systemic Early Neuromuscular Blockade (ROSE) trial (ClinicalTrials.gov identifier NCT02509078) with the goal of further defining the role of paralysis in the management of early ARDS. In the meantime, hypotheses are being proposed to explain the positive effects of cisatracurium reported thus far. One theory[158] suggests that neuromuscular blockade attenuates VILI in early ARDS by eliminating spontaneous patient efforts, which could lead to excessive TV and P_L, not only in the APRV mode as discussed above but also during synchronized conventional mechanical ventilation.[159] On the contrary, benefits of paralysis have been demonstrated even when the control group was sedated such that patient triggering was not observed.[156] Alternatively, an animal study has shown that cisatracurium may blunt VILI through a direct anti-inflammatory mechanism mediated by the nicotinic acetylcholine receptor.[160] This property of cisatracurium appears to be independent of any effect on patient-ventilator interaction because the same anti-inflammatory response was observed in an ex vivo lung model and an in vitro cell medium upon exposure to cisatracurium. The duration of paralysis may be a critical factor in determining the cost-benefit ratio of NMBA use in ARDS, since even 18 hours of passive ventilation can give rise to proteolytic atrophy of diaphragmatic myofibrils.[161]

Inhaled Pulmonary Vasodilators

Nitric oxide (NO) is the prototypical and best studied pulmonary vasodilator. It entered the ARDS armamentarium when a small series showed that continuous administration of inhaled NO (iNO) can improve oxygenation in ARDS by reducing the shunt fraction.[162] This effect is mediated by the diversion of pulmonary blood flow toward well-ventilated lung units, which received the bulk of the iNO, and away from poorly ventilated units that received relatively little iNO. The mean pulmonary artery pressure decreased without an associated fall in systemic vascular resistance (SVR). Intravenous infusion of prostacyclin, another pulmonary vasodilator, actually worsened oxygenation and shunt fraction with a drop in SVR, suggesting that generalized vasodilation is deleterious because it does not discriminate between aerated and nonaerated lung regions, and it may worsen systemic hemodynamics. With this physiological construct as background, a number of RCTs comparing iNO to placebo have been conducted,[163-165] demonstrating transient improvement in oxygenation that did not translate to meaningful clinical recovery or a survival advantage. The largest of the RCTs[165] administered iNO at a modest dose of 5 parts per million (ppm), and in fact, higher doses (eg, 10 ppm) have been associated with a relative blunting of effect over time.[164] Notably, the surviving subjects of that RCT were followed prospectively, and the resultant data collection yielded additional information. Analysis of that cohort revealed that iNO for ARDS has no impact on long-term survival, functional status, resource utilization, or overall treatment expense.[166] It did, however, result in higher total lung capacity at 6-month follow up,[167] though whether this improvement carries any clinical significance is currently unknown. Despite several meta-analyses echoing the major findings of the individual RCTs (fleeting oxygenation gains, no change in mortality),[168,169] the potential remained for a mortality benefit limited to the severe ARDS subgroup. A systematic review designed to address that question showed no survival difference even in the population with severe ARDS.[170] An important observation that has emerged regarding possible toxicity of iNO in ARDS is the association with increased incidence of acute kidney injury (AKI) leading to initiation of renal replacement therapy (RRT).[163] Aggregation of available data regarding AKI and RRT lends credence to such concerns.[169,171] The pathophysiological connection between iNO and kidney function remains speculative, but this adverse effect appears to be accentuated in ARDS patients receiving prolonged therapy. Despite unfavorable iNO study results, inhaled pulmonary vasodilation continues to be employed as part of salvage therapy for ARDS. The desire to avoid the high cost of iNO and its renal toxicity has generated comparisons to inhaled epoprostenol, which has been shown to produce a similar increase in the P/F ratio but at substantial savings.[172,173]

Conservative Fluid Management

Although the diagnosis of ARDS—a type of noncardiogenic pulmonary edema—requires exclusion of hydrostatic edema as the primary etiology of pulmonary infiltrates, the coexistence or eventual development of a hydrostatic component is a common occurrence.[174] The ARDS lung is rendered more vulnerable to hydrostatic edema than the healthy lung is, by its inherently increased endothelial permeability at the level of the capillary-alveolar interface, and additionally, ARDS patients frequently exhibit impaired ability to clear pulmonary edema fluid.[175] Early retrospective[176] and prospective[177] studies comparing lower versus higher pulmonary artery occlusion pressure (PAOP) and/or extravascular lung water in subjects with pulmonary edema showed improved outcomes in those with lower values. Subsequent therapeutic trials of the combination of furosemide and albumin targeting and achieving a more negative fluid balance relative to placebo produced a significant oxygenation benefit in nonshock ARDS patients.[178,179] Eventually, the issue of whether conservative or liberal fluid management is superior in ARDS was addressed by the pivotal ARDSNet RCT termed the Fluid and Catheter Treatment Trial (FACTT), which randomized 1000 patients to 1 or the other strategy to be applied during the nonshock phase of treatment.[180] Subjects were additionally co-randomized within each strategy to a protocol guided by either central venous pressure or PAOP, a part of the study that yielded no difference in outcomes. The cumulative difference in fluid totals between the 2 opposing management arms was about 7 Liters, due to significantly greater furosemide use in the conservative arm. While 60-day mortality was unaffected by the approach to fluid balance, the conservative group had significantly more ICU- and ventilator-free days with no increase in cardiovascular failure or AKI. In fact, a post-hoc analysis of this RCT demonstrated that positive fluid balance adversely affected the survival of those subjects who developed AKI following enrollment.[181] What FACTT also showed was an increased incidence in the conservative group of a somewhat nebulous phenomenon labeled *central nervous system failure*. In this regard, a concerning finding that emerged from a subsequent telephone contact study of FACTT survivors is that randomization to the conservative arm was an independent risk factor for neuropsychological impairment at 1 year.[182] Despite the absence of an overall survival difference between the 2 approaches to fluid in FACTT, investigators have understandably sought to retrospectively identify patient characteristics that may be associated with a differential outcome. For example, researchers have found that when *FACTT* subjects are stratified according to serum aldosterone level, survival of those in the lower half is significantly improved by a conservative fluid strategy.[183] Similarly, results of another post-hoc analysis suggest that ARDS patients whose presentation is characterized by hypotension and a proinflammatory blood biomarker profile have a mortality benefit from conservative fluid management, whereas patients lacking those features fare better with the liberal approach.[184] One of the criticisms of FACTT has been the rather cumbersome algorithm used to guide the conservative approach. Encouragingly, it has been shown that implementation of a considerably simpler alternative called FACTT Lite leads to comparable fluid balances and preservation of gains in ICU- and ventilator-free days over the liberal strategy.[185] The FACTT results, together with the observation that β_2-adrenergic agonists expedite resolution of edema in injured lungs,[186] prompted the study of these agents in ARDS both in aerosolized[187] and intravenous[188] forms. Whereas the aerosolized version had no impact on mortality, the intravenous formulation actually increased it, leading to the exclusion of these pharmaceuticals from the ARDS armamentarium.

Extracorporeal Support

The desire to ameliorate life-threatening hypoxemia in ARDS by oxygenating the blood by means of an extracorporeal apparatus akin to cardiopulmonary bypass dates back almost as far as the first description of the syndrome itself.[189] In the absence of circulatory failure, this can be accomplished by withdrawing deoxygenated blood via a large catheter inserted into the central venous system, pumping it through an oxygenator, and then returning it into the same or different central vein (venovenous ECMO). Alternatively, oxygenated blood can be returned into the arterial circulation in cases of cardiac pump failure (venoarterial ECMO) with the attendant risk of limb ischemia inherent in cannulating a major artery. These early applications of extracorporeal membrane oxygenation (ECMO) for ARDS were plagued by complications related to the catheters and circuit such as hemolysis, thrombosis, and bleeding, including catastrophic intracranial hemorrhage.[190] In that era, the patients were concurrently mechanically ventilated with TVs exceeding the modern standard of lung protection. Under these circumstances, ECMO failed to improve the dismal survival associated with severe respiratory failure at that time.[191] This technology has been refined since then, but use for ARDS had remained at a constant low level until 2009, when it surged in the midst of the H1N1 influenza pandemic as rescue therapy.[192] That year also saw the publication of the Conventional Ventilation or ECMO for Severe Adult Respiratory Failure (CESAR) trial conducted in the United Kingdom, to this day the dominant prospective RCT of ECMO for refractory hypoxemia in ARDS.[193] One hundred-eighty young adults, mostly with pneumonia as the etiology of severe ARDS (P/F ratio 75) and with a low burden of extrapulmonary organ failure, were randomized to conventional management at the admitting institution versus transfer to an ECMO-capable center for this possible additional intervention. Referral for consideration of

ECMO, which was actually performed in 68/90 (75%) of eligible transfers, resulted in a 16% absolute risk reduction of death or severe disability at 6 months (37% vs. 53%), which translates to a number needed to treat of 6 to 7. The rate of ECMO-related complications was very low. Importantly, because components of ARDS management apart from ECMO were not standardized across study sites, significant differences occurred between the referral center and the local hospitals with respect to duration of lung-protective ventilation and CS use, among others. The potential impact of this imbalance on the outcome of the trial raises legitimate concerns. Also worth noting is the fact that of the 22 severe ARDS patients transferred to the ECMO center but managed there conventionally, 16 (73%) improved without ECMO. Subsequent propensity score-matched cohort studies comparing the survival of ECMO recipients to that of nonrecipients from the 2009 H1N1 influenza pandemic in Europe have yielded conflicting results,[194,195] while meta-analyses are difficult to interpret in a situation in which a single RCT (CESAR) accounts for most of the data.[196,197] Eagerly awaited is the currently recruiting Extracorporeal Membrane Oxygenation for Severe Acute Respiratory Distress Syndrome (EOLIA) multicenter RCT (ClinicalTrials.gov identifier NCT01470703), which will add substantially to the current body of evidence. Regardless of the results of EOLIA, unanswered questions will continue to swirl around ECMO in ARDS, including the impact of a center's case volume on outcomes[198] and whether ECMO can be used as a substitute for, rather than an adjunct to, invasive mechanical ventilation.[199]

Extracorporeal support in ARDS can also be viewed from an angle other than rescue from refractory hypoxemia. As discussed earlier, the current TV (ie, $\leq$ 6 mL/kg PBW) and P_{plat} ($\leq$ 30 cm H_2O) thresholds for defining lung-protective ventilation are imperfect, and adherence to them does not preclude the occurrence of VILI.[31,37] Therefore, it is conceivable that reducing TV and P_{plat} farther than traditional norms as part of a so-called "ultra-protective" strategy could result in additional benefit. Interestingly, this notion of "lung rest" predates by many years the concept of VILI.[200] The limiting factor to the implementation of such an ultra-protective approach could be hypoxemia, but is more likely to be prohibitive respiratory acidosis.[198] Extracorporeal support technology that performs only carbon dioxide removal ($ECCO_2R$) has been available for many years, and the advantage of this variant is that the required extracorporeal flow is much lower than that of ECMO, allowing less invasive cannulation using much smaller catheters. Extracorporeal carbon dioxide removal has been shown to be effective at dampening respiratory acidosis during ultra-protective ventilation with a positive impact on lung inflammation and a favorable safety profile.[201,202] The 2 available RCTs of $ECCO_2R$ in severe ARDS were published in 1994[203] and 2013[204]—very different eras in ARDS management—and enrolled 40 and 80 patients, respectively. These small studies found no improvement in mortality or ventilator-free days, leaving this type of extracorporeal support, much like ECMO, in need of a larger trial, which is currently in the pilot phase (ClinicalTrials.gov Identifier NCT02282657).

Nutritional Interventions

The premise behind nutritional supplementation in ARDS is based on the synergistic anti-inflammatory properties of omega-3 fatty acids and γ-linolenic acid concurrently administered with antioxidants.[205,206] Indeed, initial small trials in human ARDS patients demonstrated improvement in relevant endpoints such as lung inflammation, compliance, oxygenation, and length of stay conferred by the administration of these supplements.[207,208] When subjected to more rigorous investigation in a multicenter RCT called OMEGA, supplementation with these agents was associated with worse outcomes in days free from all of the following: mechanical ventilation, ICU, and extrapulmonary organ failure.[209] These findings led to the early termination of this trial for futility. Combining OMEGA with all other relevant RCTs in a meta-analysis has reaffirmed lack of benefit in mortality and resource utilization in the general ARDS population.[210] Another intriguing dietary inhibitor of inflammation is the amino acid glutamine, which has yielded some promising animal data on lung injury attenuation and awaits further study in humans.[211,212] The ARDSNet EDEN RCT[213] tested the hypothesis that low-volume (so-called "trophic") enteral feeding of ARDS patients might be beneficial by reducing the frequency of gastrointestinal adverse events compared to full-calorie nutrition mediated by a favorable effect on ICU infections, specifically ventilator-associated pneumonia, as had been suggested by prior investigators.[214] Despite reducing the frequency of gastrointestinal intolerance, "trophic" feeding failed to improve not only mortality but also ventilator-free days and new infections. Given the absence of convincing benefit, specialized approaches to the nutritional support of ARDS patients are not currently advocated.

PROGNOSIS AND OUTCOMES

Although ARDS remains a lethal disease, with crude ICU mortality exceeding 40% for patients classified as severe according to the Berlin definition,[1,149] data extracted from RCTs[215] and death certificates[216] indicate that hospital survival is on the rise. Recent long-term survival figures are likewise encouraging,[217] though the first year postdischarge presents a challenge: It is characterized by significant functional impairment, residence in skilled care facilities, readmission, and substantial mortality.[166,218] In the course of that first year, there is a progressive increase but not normalization in 6-minute walk distance (6MWD)[215] paralleled by impaired though improving muscle strength.[216] Perception of physical well-being as measured by the Medical Outcomes Study 36-Item Short-Form Health Survey (SF-36), which is a health-related quality-of-life metric with both physical and mental domains, is below the expected level at 1 year[219] and its physical component remains subnormal out to 5 years despite further increase in 6MWD based on percent of predicted value.[220] The perceived physical disability reported by ARDS survivors has been shown to exceed that of critical illness survivors without ARDS.[221] Fewer than half of previously employed ARDS survivors return to work by 1 year, but at 5 years that number grows to more than three-quarters. Results of the mental component of the SF-36 demonstrate near-normal perceived well-being at 5 years in such areas as social functioning and emotional role, an encouraging finding in light of studies that have detected a high incidence of psychiatric conditions, including anxiety, depression, and post-traumatic stress disorder, among ARDS survivors at least out to 2 years.[222,223] Improved survival and greater recognition of sequelae impacting quality of life has prompted calls for a reorientation of ARDS trial outcomes toward morbidity rather than mortality endpoints, which is likely to impact study designs in the coming years.[224]

QUESTIONS

1. A 32-year-old man who was recently diagnosed with acute lymphoblastic leukemia and is currently undergoing induction chemotherapy is sent to the emergency department (ED) by his oncologist for fevers and shortness of breath of 4 days' duration. In the ED, he is found to be in moderate respiratory distress, hypotensive, and febrile to 39.4°C. His labs reveal leukopenia and neutropenia. His chest x-ray shows diffuse bilateral alveolar infiltrates. He is diagnosed with pneumonia complicated by ARDS, given intravenous fluids, intubated for severe hypoxemia, and started on volume-controlled ventilation in the ED with the following settings: respiratory rate (RR) of 25 breaths/min, TV of 420 mL (which translates to 6 mL/kg for his calculated PBW of 70 kg), PEEP of 5 cm H_2O and an Fio_2 of 1.0. A postintubation arterial blood gas (ABG) on these settings shows a pH of 7.30, a partial pressure of carbon dioxide (Pco_2) of 48 mmHg, and an arterial pressure of oxygen (Pao_2) of 46 mmHg. The peak airway pressure on the current ventilator settings is 25 cm H_2O, and the plateau pressure is measured as 23 cm H_2O. Which of the following ventilator interventions is the most appropriate next step to improve this patient's hypoxemia?

   A. Convert to HFOV
   B. Increase the RR to 30 breaths/min
   C. Increase the PEEP to 10 cm H_2O
   D. Increase the TV to 450 mL

2. Which of the following statements represents the likeliest outcome of the performance of a recruitment maneuver in this patient using sustained inflation with high CPAP?

   A. Sustained improvement in oxygenation regardless of subsequent PEEP adjustment
   B. Progressively greater benefit with prolonged application of high CPAP
   C. Reduced effective lung compliance
   D. Less improvement in oxygenation if repeated later in the course of his ARDS

3. A 59-year-old woman is admitted to the ICU for severe alcohol-induced pancreatitis. On ICU day 2, she develops ARDS and requires intubation and mechanical ventilation. Her body mass index (BMI) is 22 kg/m². She has a soft, nondistended abdomen. Her initial ventilator settings are as follows: RR of 15 breaths/min, TV of 300 mL (which translates to 6 mL/kg for her calculated PBW of 50 kg), PEEP of 12 cm H_2O, and Fio_2 of 0.8. The peak airway pressure on the current ventilator settings is 36 cm H_2O with plateau pressure of 34 cm H_2O. Her chest x-ray shows bilateral alveolar infiltrates without pleural effusions. A recent arterial blood gas shows a pH of 7.35 and a $Paco_2$ of 40 mmHg on the above ventilator settings. Her oxygen saturation is 97%. She is adequately sedated and is receiving neuromuscular blockade to achieve ventilator synchrony. Which of the following is the most appropriate next step in management?

    A. Increase the Fio_2
    B. Decrease the TV
    C. Increase the PEEP
    D. Decrease the RR

4. A 35-year-old man with acute respiratory failure from ARDS develops tense abdominal ascites and anasarca after fluid resuscitation. While receiving a TV of 4 mL/kg PBW, the plateau pressure is now 38 cm H_2O. The PEEP remains at 12 cm H_2O. An esophageal pressure catheter is inserted, and balloon position in the distal esophagus is confirmed. The pressure transduced through the esophageal catheter is 15 cm H_2O. Assuming that the esophageal pressure value is representative of the average pleural pressure, which of the following conclusions is best supported by the provided information?

    A. The transalveolar pressure is elevated (ie, ≥ 30 cm H_2O), and the PEEP level is sufficient to prevent end-expiratory alveolar collapse.
    B. The transalveolar pressure is elevated, and the PEEP level is insufficient to prevent end-expiratory alveolar collapse.
    C. The transalveolar pressure is not elevated, and the PEEP level is insufficient to prevent end-expiratory alveolar collapse.
    D. The transalveolar pressure is not elevated, and the PEEP level is sufficient to prevent end-expiratory alveolar collapse.

5. You are called by the nurse to evaluate a 75-year-old man in the ICU who has been receiving invasive mechanical ventilation for 14 days due to severe unresolving ARDS. Increasing levels of PEEP have been applied in an attempt to improve his oxygenation. His ventilator management currently consists of volume-controlled ventilation with a RR of 20 breaths/min, a TV of 420 mL (which translates to 6 mL/kg for his calculated PBW of 70 kg), a PEEP of 24 cm H_2O, and a Fio_2 of 1.0. When you arrive at the bedside, you notice that the ventilator is alarming because of high ventilator pressures. His peak airway pressure is 60 cm H_2O and invasive blood pressure monitoring indicates a blood pressure of 60/30 mmHg, which represents an acute drop from prior values. The patient is very tachycardic. On examination, you notice skin crepitus on the right side of the patient's chest extending into the right axilla, an absence of breath sounds over the right anterior hemithorax, jugular venous distention, and a deviation of the trachea to the left of midline. Which of the following is the most appropriate immediate next step in management?

    A. Obtain urgent chest x-ray
    B. Start catecholamine infusion
    C. Perform anterior chest needle decompression
    D. Decrease TV

6. Which of the following statements about the impact of individual ARDS interventions on the incidence of gross barotrauma is correct?

    A. Lower pneumothorax risk can be expected with the use of NMBAs.
    B. Lower pneumothorax risk can be expected with reduction of TV from 12 to 6 mL/kg PBW.
    C. Higher pneumothorax risk can be expected with the application of higher versus lower PEEP.
    D. Higher pneumothorax risk can be expected with the use of prone positioning.

7. A 57-year-old man is admitted to the ICU with ARDS. He is intubated and sedated upon arrival. His ventilator settings on volume-controlled ventilation include a RR of 20 breaths/min, TV of 420 mL (which translates to 6 mL/kg for his calculated PBW of 70 kg), PEEP of 20 cm H_2O, and Fio_2 of 1.0. Neuromuscular blocking with cisatracurium is initiated. Plateau pressures are between 26 and 29 cm H_2O with the patient paralyzed. He has a BMI of 27 kg/m². He is normotensive, his skin is warm, and there is no jugular venous distention. Breath sounds are coarse and symmetrical. The latest arterial blood gas shows a pH of 7.28, a $Paco_2$ of 52 mmHg, and a Pao_2 of 45 mmHg. For the use of NMB in this patient to be consistent with the parameters studied in the largest RCT of NMB published by Papazian et al in 2010, which of the following combinations of criteria would have to be fulfilled?

    A. Mild ARDS, early use of cisatracurium, 48-hour duration of NMB
    B. Severe ARDS, early use of cisatracurium, 48-hour duration of NMB
    C. Severe ARDS, late use of cisatracurium, 96-hour duration of NMB
    D. Mild ARDS, late use of cisatracurium, 48-hour duration of NMB

8. Which of the following strategies can be expected to improve not only a patient's oxygenation in ARDS but also survival based on data from a multicenter RCT in the era of lung-protective ventilation?

   A. Parenteral corticosteroids
   B. Prone positioning
   C. APRV
   D. Inhaled NO

9. Which is associated with improved survival in ARDS?

   A. Decrease in Δ pressure
   B. Increased $Paco_2$ with prone position
   C. Improvement in oxygenation with PEEP
   D. Improvement in oxygenation with reduction in tidal volume but no change in driving pressure

10. A 50-year-old man with a history of hypertension and diabetes was admitted for acute blood loss anemia from upper gastrointestinal bleeding. In the ED, he had hematemesis, and he aspirated, which required him to be intubated. Within 48 hours, he developed aspiration pneumonia, which progressed to ARDS. He had an endoscopy, which showed an ulcer with a clot. He has received 2 units packed red blood cells and was started on a pantoprazole drip, and his hemoglobin has been stable now for 24 hours. The patient still requires an Fio_2 of 80 with a PEEP of 10 cm H_2O. His hemoglobin is 9 g/dL, his albumin is 2.9 g/dL, his creatinine is 1 mg/dL, and his central venous pressure is 6 mm H_2O. Maintenance fluids have been decreased to keep the vein open. What is the next step?

    A. Furosemide
    B. Restart maintenance fluids
    C. Furosemide with albumin
    D. Dopamine

ANSWERS

1. C. Increase the PEEP to 10 cm H_2O

   The next immediate priority in management is to address the inadequate oxygenation in this patient with severe ARDS who is already receiving Fio_2 of 1.0. In addition to ensuring adequate oxygenation, ARDS mechanical ventilation principles are designed to limit VILI. The objective is to apply PEEP at a level that helps achieve adequate oxygenation through maintenance of alveolar recruitment while also rendering the baby lung less susceptible to VILI. PEEP is being underutilized in this patient with severe ARDS, so an increase is warranted and could be preceded by a recruitment maneuver. "Optimal" PEEP for a given patient would be that level that maximizes recruitment (or minimizes tidal derecruitment), while avoiding overdistention and its complications. The best method of determining optimal PEEP remains controversial. Although increasing the respiratory rate (choice B) or tidal volume (choice D)

could improve oxygenation, both maneuvers could also compromise lung-protective ventilation and promote barotrauma. Conversion to HFOV (choice A) may or may not produce an oxygenation benefit but cannot be advocated prior to exhaustion of conventional ventilatory strategies due to evidence for worsened survival with HFOV.

2. D. Less improvement in oxygenation if repeated later in the course of his ARDS

   Recruitment maneuvers are designed to produce short-term extreme lung inflation (ie, brief but sustained high CPAP) that exceeds the opening pressure of as many alveoli as is safely possible, thereby recruiting them to participate in gas exchange. This technique can improve oxygenation and increase the size of the baby lung, the latter also leading to an increase rather than a decrease (choice C) in effective lung compliance. Oxygenation gains following an RM are rapidly lost if PEEP is not subsequently increased to prevent derecruitment, so choice A is incorrect. It has been shown that recruitment plateaus after the first 10 seconds of a CPAP RM, so the application of CPAP for longer periods is unlikely to augment benefit. Therefore, choice B is incorrect. Recruitment maneuvers have been shown to lose effectiveness later in the course of ARDS presumably due to the more organized nature of the alveolar damage at that stage, making choice D the correct answer.

3. B. Decrease the TV

   Lung-protective ventilation includes low TV to limit volutrauma *and* a plateau pressure threshold of 30 cm H_2O or less to avoid barotrauma. This patient, while meeting the low-TV criterion of 6 mL/kg PBW, is violating the plateau pressure target. In such a case, TV reduction below 6 mL/kg PBW in order to reduce plateau pressure to 30 cm H_2O or less is the most appropriate management. The lower TV is likely to result in an increase in $Paco_2$, which is expected and tolerated as long as the pH remains within acceptable limits. If needed, the RR can be increased, rather than decreased (choice D) to dampen the worsening hypercapnia. It is also important to consider whether the plateau pressure could be over- or underestimating the transalveolar pressure (Plateau Pressure – Pleural Pressure) because of pleural pressure that is higher or lower than average. Higher than expected pleural pressure (and therefore a plateau pressure that overestimates transalveolar pressure or stress) is seen in the setting of stiff thoracoabdominal structures caused by obesity, anasarca, ascites, pleural effusion, and so on. None of these features is present in this patient. Conversely, exaggerated spontaneous breathing efforts can lead to drops in pleural pressure and thus an underestimation of transalveolar pressure if plateau pressure is used alone as an estimate. This is also not the case in this scenario, so conditions confounding interpretation of plateau pressure as a surrogate for transalveolar pressure are absent. Current oxygenation is adequate, so increasing the Fio_2 (choice A) or the PEEP (choice C) is not indicated.

4. C. The transalveolar pressure is not elevated, and the PEEP level is insufficient to prevent end-expiratory alveolar collapse.

Unlike the scenario in question 1, in this situation, the plateau pressure is a poor surrogate for transalveolar pressure (stress) because high thoracoabdominal elastance due to ascites and anasarca has led to a markedly elevated pleural pressure. When its value as estimated from esophageal manometry (15 cm H_2O) is subtracted from plateau pressure (38 cm H_2O), the difference, which is transalveolar pressure, is 23 cm H_2O, a magnitude well below the standard for excessive lung stress. Contrary to what interpretation of plateau pressure alone would suggest, calculation of transalveolar pressure actually indicates adherence to lung-protective ventilation in regard to barotrauma. The story is different at end-expiration, however, at which point pleural pressure exceeds the PEEP of 12 cm H_2O and net pressure is therefore in the direction of alveolar collapse with potential for atelectrauma and derecruitment. (Choices A, B, and D are wrong.)

5. C. Perform anterior chest needle decompression

This patient is at increased risk for gross barotrauma given the high PEEP and unresolving ARDS. He had a sudden decompensation with rapid development of obstructive shock caused by a clinically evident right tension pneumothorax. He is facing imminent cardiocirculatory arrest and therefore needs emergent anterior chest needle decompression. Waiting for radiographic confirmation (choice A) of pneumothorax would delay potentially life-saving management. Tension pneumothorax in this clinical setting is a clinical diagnosis. If immediately available, bedside thoracic ultrasound can complement clinical judgment in establishing the presence of pneumothorax when circulatory compromise is less severe. Starting a catecholamine infusion (choice B) or lowering the TV (choice D) would not correct the underlying obstructive shock physiology.

6. A. Lower pneumothorax risk can be expected with the use of NMBAs.

Of the options provided, NMB is the only intervention that has been shown in an RCT to affect the incidence of gross barotrauma (eg, pneumothorax), which was reduced. Barotrauma rates were not significantly different between subjects and controls in the landmark low-TV ventilation ARMA RCT (choice B), the 3 RCTs of higher versus lower PEEP and their meta-analysis (choice C), or in the PROSEVA RCT of prone positioning (choice D).

7. B. Severe ARDS, early use of cisatracurium, 48-hour duration of NMB

The groundbreaking study by Papazian et al of NMB in early (ie, within 48 hours of onset) ARDS compared cisatracurium infusion for a duration of 48 hours to placebo in moderate to severe ARDS (P/F ratio of ≤150).

As mentioned in the chapter, it found a significantly improved 90-day survival and increase in ventilator-free days. Importantly, the frequency of ICU-related neuromuscular weakness was not increased. Choices A, C, and D are wrong.

8. B. Prone positioning

This patient with severe ARDS is suffering from refractory hypoxemia despite advanced ventilator management. Of the choices provided, only prone positioning has been shown in a multicenter RCT (PROSEVA) by Guérin et al to improve both oxygenation and mortality. Although an oxygenation benefit has been reported with the use of corticosteroids (choice A), APRV (choice C), and inhaled NO (choice D), none of these interventions is associated with a conclusively demonstrated survival advantage.

9. A. Decrease in Δ pressure

A retrospective analysis has suggested that a decrease in driving pressure, also called Δ pressure, or Peak Pressure – PEEP, is associated with improved survival in ARDS.[223] This improvement in Δ pressure suggests an improvement in lung compliance also correlated with the improved survival in low tidal volume, improving inspiratory pressure, and PEEP.[226] Prospective studies are still needed. Increased $Paco_2$ with prone position is associated with poor prognosis (choice B).[227] Improvement in oxygenation with PEEP (choice C) and improvement in oxygenation with reduction in tidal volume (choice D) does not necessarily translate to improved survival unless there is decrease in driving pressure.[223,224,226]

10. A. Furosemide

Conservative fluid management for patients who are hemodynamically stable (mean arterial pressure > 65 mmHg and off pressors for at least 12 hours) have been shown to have better survival than liberal fluid management.[181,182] Diuretics may be implemented with a target CVP of 4 mm H_2O (normal range 2–6 mm H_2O).[228] Therefore, increasing maintenance fluids (choice B) is not the right answer. The use of albumin and diuretic will achieve a greater negative balance but might dehydrate the patient (choice C). There is no need to start dopamine in this patient (choice D).

REFERENCES

1. Force ADT, Ranieri VM, Rubenfeld GD, et al. Acute respiratory distress syndrome: the Berlin Definition. *JAMA*. 2012;307(23):2526-2533.

2. Ferguson ND, Fan E, Camporota L, et al. The Berlin definition of ARDS: an expanded rationale, justification, and supplementary material. *Intensive Care Med*. 2012;38(10):1573-1582.

3. Bernard GR, Artigas A, Brigham KL, et al. The American-European Consensus Conference on ARDS. Definitions,

mechanisms, relevant outcomes, and clinical trial coordination. *Am J Respir Crit Care Med.* 1994;149(3 Pt 1):818-824.

4. Rubenfeld GD, Caldwell E, Peabody E, et al. Incidence and outcomes of acute lung injury. *N Engl J Med.* 2005;353(16):1685-1693.

5. Angus DC, Linde-Zwirble WT, Lidicker J, Clermont G, Carcillo J, Pinsky MR. Epidemiology of severe sepsis in the United States: analysis of incidence, outcome, and associated costs of care. *Crit Care Med.* 2001;29(7):1303-1310.

6. Pepe PE, Potkin RT, Reus DH, Hudson LD, Carrico CJ. Clinical predictors of the adult respiratory distress syndrome. *Am J Surg.* 1982;144(1):124-130.

7. Hudson LD, Milberg JA, Anardi D, Maunder RJ. Clinical risks for development of the acute respiratory distress syndrome. *Am J Respir Crit Care Med.* 1995;151(2 Pt 1):293-301.

8. Gotts JE, Matthay MA. Sepsis: pathophysiology and clinical management. *BMJ.* 2016;353:i1585.

9. Mira JC, Gentile LF, Mathias BJ, et al. Sepsis pathophysiology, chronic critical illness, and persistent inflammation-immunosuppression and catabolism syndrome. *Crit Care Med.* 2017;45(2):253-262.

10. Laszlo I, Trasy D, Molnar Z, Fazakas J. Sepsis: from pathophysiology to individualized patient care. *J Immunol Res.* 2015;2015:510436.

11. Dreyfuss D, Saumon G. Ventilator-induced lung injury: lessons from experimental studies. *Am J Respir Crit Care Med.* 1998;157(1):294-323.

12. Dreyfuss D, Soler P, Basset G, Saumon G. High inflation pressure pulmonary edema. Respective effects of high airway pressure, high tidal volume, and positive end-expiratory pressure. *Am Rev Respir Dis.* 1988;137(5):1159-1164.

13. Curley GF, Laffey JG, Zhang H, Slutsky AS. Biotrauma and ventilator-induced lung injury: clinical implications. *Chest.* 2016;150(5):1109-1117.

14. Gattinoni L, Mascheroni D, Torresin A, et al. Morphological response to positive end expiratory pressure in acute respiratory failure. Computerized tomography study. *Intensive Care Med.* 1986;12(3):137-142.

15. Maunder RJ, Shuman WP, McHugh JW, Marglin SI, Butler J. Preservation of normal lung regions in the adult respiratory distress syndrome. Analysis by computed tomography. *JAMA.* 1986;255(18):2463-2465.

16. Gattinoni L, Marini JJ, Pesenti A, Quintel M, Mancebo J, Brochard L. The "baby lung" became an adult. *Intensive Care Med.* 2016;42(5):663-673.

17. Hubmayr RD. Perspective on lung injury and recruitment: a skeptical look at the opening and collapse story. *Am J Respir Crit Care Med.* 2002;165(12):1647-1653.

18. Cressoni M, Cadringher P, Chiurazzi C, et al. Lung inhomogeneity in patients with acute respiratory distress syndrome. *Am J Respir Crit Care Med.* 2014;189(2):149-158.

19. Gattinoni L, Pesenti A, Avalli L, Rossi F, Bombino M. Pressure-volume curve of total respiratory system in acute respiratory failure. Computed tomographic scan study. *Am Rev Respir Dis.* 1987;136(3):730-736.

20. Protti A, Cressoni M, Santini A, et al. Lung stress and strain during mechanical ventilation: any safe threshold? *Am J Respir Crit Care Med.* 2011;183(10):1354-1362.

21. Kolobow T, Moretti MP, Fumagalli R, et al. Severe impairment in lung function induced by high peak airway pressure during mechanical ventilation. An experimental study. *Am Rev Respir Dis.* 1987;135(2):312-315.

22. Mead J, Takishima T, Leith D. Stress distribution in lungs: a model of pulmonary elasticity. *J Appl Physiol.* 1970;28(5):596-608.

23. Kaplan JD, Calandrino FS, Schuster DP. A positron emission tomographic comparison of pulmonary vascular permeability during the adult respiratory distress syndrome and pneumonia. *Am Rev Respir Dis.* 1991;143(1):150-154.

24. Amato MB, Barbas CS, Medeiros DM, et al. Effect of a protective-ventilation strategy on mortality in the acute respiratory distress syndrome. *N Engl J Med.* 1998;338(6):347-354.

25. Ranieri VM, Suter PM, Tortorella C, et al. Effect of mechanical ventilation on inflammatory mediators in patients with acute respiratory distress syndrome: a randomized controlled trial. *JAMA.* 1999;282(1):54-61.

26. Brower RG, Matthay MA, Morris A, Schoenfeld D, Thompson BT, Wheeler A. The Acute Respiratory Distress Syndrome Network. Ventilation with lower tidal volumes as compared with traditional tidal volumes for acute lung injury and the acute respiratory distress syndrome. *N Engl J Med.* 2000;342(18):1301-1308.

27. Otulakowski G, Engelberts D, Gusarova GA, Bhattacharya J, Post M, Kavanagh BP. Hypercapnia attenuates ventilator-induced lung injury via a disintegrin and metalloprotease-17. *J Physiol.* 2014;592(20):4507-4521.

28. Villar J, Kacmarek RM, Perez-Mendez L, Aguirre-Jaime A. A high positive end-expiratory pressure, low tidal volume ventilatory strategy improves outcome in persistent acute respiratory distress syndrome: a randomized, controlled trial. *Crit Care Med.* 2006;34(5):1311-1318.

29. Sakr Y, Vincent JL, Reinhart K, et al. High tidal volume and positive fluid balance are associated with worse outcome in acute lung injury. *Chest.* 2005;128(5):3098-3108.

30. Putensen C, Theuerkauf N, Zinserling J, Wrigge H, Pelosi P. Meta-analysis: ventilation strategies and outcomes of the acute respiratory distress syndrome and acute lung injury. *Ann Intern Med.* 2009;151(8):566-576.

31. Hager DN, Krishnan JA, Hayden DL, Brower RG; ARDS Clinical Trials Network. Tidal volume reduction in patients with acute lung injury when plateau pressures are not high. *Am J Respir Crit Care Med.* 2005;172(10):1241-1245.

32. Hernandez LA, Peevy KJ, Moise AA, Parker JC. Chest wall restriction limits high airway pressure-induced lung injury in young rabbits. *J Appl Physiol (1985).* 1989;66(5):2364-2368.

33. Talmor D, Sarge T, Malhotra A, et al. Mechanical ventilation guided by esophageal pressure in acute lung injury. *N Engl J Med.* 2008;359(20):2095-2104.

34. Terragni PP, Filippini C, Slutsky AS, et al. Accuracy of plateau pressure and stress index to identify injurious ventilation in patients with acute respiratory distress syndrome. *Anesthesiology.* 2013;119(4):880-889.

35. Chiumello D, Carlesso E, Cadringher P, et al. Lung stress and strain during mechanical ventilation for acute respiratory distress syndrome. *Am J Respir Crit Care Med.* 2008;178(4):346-355.

36. Richard JC, Brochard L, Vandelet P, et al. Respective effects of end-expiratory and end-inspiratory pressures on alveolar recruitment in acute lung injury. *Crit Care Med.* 2003;31(1):89-92.

37. Terragni PP, Rosboch G, Tealdi A, et al. Tidal hyperinflation during low tidal volume ventilation in acute respiratory distress syndrome. *Am J Respir Crit Care Med.* 2007;175(2):160-166.

38. Amato MB, Meade MO, Slutsky AS, et al. Driving pressure and survival in the acute respiratory distress syndrome. *N Engl J Med.* 2015;372(8):747-755.

39. Chiumello D, Carlesso E, Brioni M, Cressoni M. Airway driving pressure and lung stress in ARDS patients. *Crit Care.* 2016;20:276.

40. Cressoni M, Gotti M, Chiurazzi C, et al. Mechanical power and development of ventilator-induced lung injury. *Anesthesiology.* 2016;124(5):1100-1108.

41. Gattinoni L, Tonetti T, Cressoni M, et al. Ventilator-related causes of lung injury: the mechanical power. *Intensive Care Med.* 2016;42(10):1567-1575.

42. Hotchkiss JR Jr, Blanch L, Murias G, et al. Effects of decreased respiratory frequency on ventilator-induced lung injury. *Am J Respir Crit Care Med.* 2000;161(2 Pt 1):463-468.

43. Protti A, Maraffi T, Milesi M, et al. Role of strain rate in the pathogenesis of ventilator-induced lung edema. *Crit Care Med.* 2016;44(9):e838-845.

44. Gattinoni L, Quintel M. How ARDS should be treated. *Crit Care.* 2016;20:86.

45. Fan E, Del Sorbo L, Goligher EC, et al; American Thoracic Society, European Society of Intensive Care Medicine, and Society of Critical Care Medicine. An Official American Thoracic Society/European Society of Intensive Care Medicine/Society of Critical Care Medicine clinical practice guideline: mechanical ventilation in adult patients with acute respiratory distress syndrome. *Am J Respir Crit Care Med.* 2017:195(9):1253-1263.

46. About the NHLBI ARDS Network. NIH-NHLBI ARDS Network Web site. http://www.ardsnet.org/. Accessed July 26, 2017.

47. Webb HH, Tierney DF. Experimental pulmonary edema due to intermittent positive pressure ventilation with high inflation pressures. Protection by positive end-expiratory pressure. *Am Rev Respir Dis.* 1974;110(5):556-565.

48. Tremblay L, Valenza F, Ribeiro SP, Li J, Slutsky AS. Injurious ventilatory strategies increase cytokines and c-fos m-RNA expression in an isolated rat lung model. *J Clin Invest.* 1997;99(5):944-952.

49. Muscedere JG, Mullen JB, Gan K, Slutsky AS. Tidal ventilation at low airway pressures can augment lung injury. *Am J Respir Crit Care Med.* 1994;149(5):1327-1334.

50. Borges JB, Okamoto VN, Matos GF, et al. Reversibility of lung collapse and hypoxemia in early acute respiratory distress syndrome. *Am J Respir Crit Care Med.* 2006;174(3):268-278.

51. Puybasset L, Gusman P, Muller JC, Cluzel P, Coriat P, Rouby JJ. Regional distribution of gas and tissue in acute respiratory distress syndrome III. Consequences for the effects of positive end-expiratory pressure. CT Scan ARDS Study Group. Adult Respiratory Distress Syndrome. *Intensive Care Med.* 2000;26(9):1215-1227.

52. Gattinoni L, Caironi P, Cressoni M, et al. Lung recruitment in patients with the acute respiratory distress syndrome. *N Engl J Med.* 2006;354(17):1775-1786.

53. Ranieri VM, Eissa NT, Corbeil C, et al. Effects of positive end-expiratory pressure on alveolar recruitment and gas exchange in patients with the adult respiratory distress syndrome. *Am Rev Respir Dis.* 1991;144(3 Pt 1):544-551.

54. Grasso S, Stripoli T, De Michele M, et al. ARDSnet ventilatory protocol and alveolar hyperinflation: role of positive end-expiratory pressure. *Am J Respir Crit Care Med.* 2007;176(8):761-767.

55. Guldner A, Braune A, Ball L, et al. Comparative effects of volutrauma and atelectrauma on lung inflammation in experimental acute respiratory distress syndrome. *Crit Care Med.* 2016;44(9):e854-865.

56. Chikhani M, Das A, Haque M, Wang W, Bates DG, Hardman JG. High PEEP in acute respiratory distress syndrome: quantitative evaluation between improved arterial oxygenation and decreased oxygen delivery. *Br J Anaesth.* 2016;117(5):650-658.

57. Kacmarek RM, Villar J, Sulemanji D, et al. Open lung approach for the acute respiratory distress syndrome: a pilot, randomized controlled trial. *Crit Care Med.* 2016;44(1):32-42.

58. Brower RG, Lanken PN, MacIntyre N, et al. Higher versus lower positive end-expiratory pressures in patients with the acute respiratory distress syndrome. *N Engl J Med.* 2004;351(4):327-336.

59. Meade MO, Cook DJ, Guyatt GH, et al. Ventilation strategy using low tidal volumes, recruitment maneuvers, and high positive end-expiratory pressure for acute lung injury and acute respiratory distress syndrome: a randomized controlled trial. *JAMA.* 2008;299(6):637-645.

60. Mercat A, Richard JC, Vielle B, et al. Positive end-expiratory pressure setting in adults with acute lung injury and acute respiratory distress syndrome: a randomized controlled trial. *JAMA.* 2008;299(6):646-655.

61. Briel M, Meade M, Mercat A, et al. Higher vs lower positive end-expiratory pressure in patients with acute lung injury and acute respiratory distress syndrome: systematic review and meta-analysis. *JAMA.* 2010;303(9):865-873.

62. Goligher EC, Kavanagh BP, Rubenfeld GD, et al. Oxygenation response to positive end-expiratory pressure predicts mortality in acute respiratory distress syndrome. A secondary analysis of the LOVS and ExPress trials. *Am J Respir Crit Care Med.* 2014;190(1):70-76.

63. Hickling KG. The pressure-volume curve is greatly modified by recruitment. A mathematical model of ARDS lungs. *Am J Respir Crit Care Med.* 1998;158(1):194-202.

64. Pelosi P, Goldner M, McKibben A, et al. Recruitment and derecruitment during acute respiratory failure: an experimental study. *Am J Respir Crit Care Med.* 2001;164(1):122-130.

65. Grasso S, Terragni P, Mascia L, et al. Airway pressure-time curve profile (stress index) detects tidal recruitment/hyperinflation in experimental acute lung injury. *Crit Care Med.* 2004;32(4):1018-1027.

66. Chiumello D, Cressoni M, Carlesso E, et al. Bedside selection of positive end-expiratory pressure in mild, moderate, and severe acute respiratory distress syndrome. *Crit Care Med.* 2014;42(2):252-264.

67. Shanholtz C, Brower R. Should inverse ratio ventilation be used in adult respiratory distress syndrome? *Am J Respir Crit Care Med.* 1994;149(5):1354-1358.

68. Wrigge H, Zinserling J, Neumann P, et al. Spontaneous breathing with airway pressure release ventilation favors ventilation in dependent lung regions and counters cyclic alveolar collapse in oleic-acid-induced lung injury: a randomized controlled computed tomography trial. *Crit Care.* 2005;9(6):R780-789.

69. Putensen C, Mutz NJ, Putensen-Himmer G, Zinserling J. Spontaneous breathing during ventilatory support improves ventilation-perfusion distributions in patients with acute respiratory distress syndrome. *Am J Respir Crit Care Med.* 1999;159(4 Pt 1):1241-1248.

70. Lim J, Litton E, Robinson H, Das Gupta M. Characteristics and outcomes of patients treated with airway pressure release ventilation for acute respiratory distress syndrome: A retrospective observational study. *J Crit Care.* 2016;34:154-159.

71. Varpula T, Valta P, Niemi R, Takkunen O, Hynynen M, Pettila VV. Airway pressure release ventilation as a primary ventilatory mode in acute respiratory distress syndrome. *Acta Anaesthesiol Scand.* 2004;48(6):722-731.

72. Jain SV, Kollisch-Singule M, Sadowitz B, et al. The 30-year evolution of airway pressure release ventilation (APRV). *Intensive Care Med Exp.* 2016;4(1):11.

73. Sasidhar M, Chatburn RL. Tidal volume variability during airway pressure release ventilation: case summary and theoretical analysis. *Respir Care.* 2012;57(8):1325-1333.

74. Gonzalez M, Arroliga AC, Frutos-Vivar F, et al. Airway pressure release ventilation versus assist-control ventilation: a comparative propensity score and international cohort study. *Intensive Care Med.* 2010;36(5):817-827.

75. Papazian L, Forel JM, Gacouin A, et al. Neuromuscular blockers in early acute respiratory distress syndrome. *N Engl J Med.* 2010;363(12):1107-1116.

76. Yoshida T, Fujino Y, Amato MB, Kavanagh BP. Fifty years of research in ARDS. Spontaneous breathing during mechanical ventilation. Risks, mechanisms, and management. *Am J Respir Crit Care Med.* 2017;195(8):985-992.

77. Yoshida T, Uchiyama A, Matsuura N, Mashimo T, Fujino Y. Spontaneous breathing during lung-protective ventilation in an experimental acute lung injury model: high transpulmonary pressure associated with strong spontaneous breathing effort may worsen lung injury. *Crit Care Med.* 2012;40(5):1578-1585.

78. Yoshida T, Torsani V, Gomes S, et al. Spontaneous effort causes occult pendelluft during mechanical ventilation. *Am J Respir Crit Care Med.* 2013;188(12):1420-1427.

79. Slutsky AS, Drazen JM. Ventilation with small tidal volumes. *N Engl J Med.* 2002;347(9):630-631.

80. Greenblatt EE, Butler JP, Venegas JG, Winkler T. Pendelluft in the bronchial tree. *J Appl Physiol (1985).* 2014;117(9):979-988.

81. Chang HK. Mechanisms of gas transport during ventilation by high-frequency oscillation. *J Appl Physiol Respir Environ Exerc Physiol.* 1984;56(3):553-563.

82. Chan KP, Stewart TE, Mehta S. High-frequency oscillatory ventilation for adult patients with ARDS. *Chest.* 2007;131(6):1907-1916.

83. Imai Y, Slutsky AS. High-frequency oscillatory ventilation and ventilator-induced lung injury. *Crit Care Med.* 2005;33(3 Suppl):S129-134.

84. Imai Y, Nakagawa S, Ito Y, Kawano T, Slutsky AS, Miyasaka K. Comparison of lung protection strategies using conventional and high-frequency oscillatory ventilation. *J Appl Physiol (1985).* 2001;91(4):1836-1844.

85. Mehta S, Granton J, MacDonald RJ, et al. High-frequency oscillatory ventilation in adults: the Toronto experience. *Chest.* 2004;126(2):518-527.

86. Derdak S, Mehta S, Stewart TE, et al. High-frequency oscillatory ventilation for acute respiratory distress syndrome in adults: a randomized, controlled trial. *Am J Respir Crit Care Med.* 2002;166(6):801-808.

87. Bollen CW, van Well GT, Sherry T, et al. High frequency oscillatory ventilation compared with conventional mechanical ventilation in adult respiratory distress syndrome: a randomized controlled trial [ISRCTN24242669]. *Crit Care.* 2005;9(4):R430-439.

88. Sud S, Sud M, Friedrich JO, et al. High frequency oscillation in patients with acute lung injury and acute respiratory distress syndrome (ARDS): systematic review and meta-analysis. *BMJ.* 2010;340:c2327.

89. Ferguson ND, Cook DJ, Guyatt GH, et al. High-frequency oscillation in early acute respiratory distress syndrome. *N Engl J Med.* 2013;368(9):795-805.

90. Young D, Lamb SE, Shah S, et al. High-frequency oscillation for acute respiratory distress syndrome. *N Engl J Med.* 2013;368(9):806-813.

91. Facchin F, Fan E. Airway pressure release ventilation and high-frequency oscillatory ventilation: potential strategies to treat severe hypoxemia and prevent ventilator-induced lung injury. *Respir Care.* 2015;60(10):1509-1521.

92. Gu XL, Wu GN, Yao YW, Shi DH, Song Y. Is high-frequency oscillatory ventilation more effective and safer than conventional protective ventilation in adult acute respiratory distress syndrome patients? A meta-analysis of randomized controlled trials. *Crit Care.* 2014;18(3):R111.

93. Maitra S, Bhattacharjee S, Khanna P, Baidya DK. High-frequency ventilation does not provide mortality benefit in comparison with conventional lung-protective ventilation in acute respiratory distress syndrome: a meta-analysis of the randomized controlled trials. *Anesthesiology.* 2015;122(4):841-851.

94. Sud S, Sud M, Friedrich JO, et al. High-frequency oscillatory ventilation versus conventional ventilation for acute respiratory distress syndrome. *Cochrane Database Syst Rev.* 2016;4:CD004085.

95. Malhotra A, Drazen JM. High-frequency oscillatory ventilation on shaky ground. *N Engl J Med.* 2013;368(9):863-865.

96. Fan E, Wilcox ME, Brower RG, et al. Recruitment maneuvers for acute lung injury: a systematic review. *Am J Respir Crit Care Med.* 2008;178(11):1156-1163.

97. Kacmarek RM, Villar J. Lung recruitment maneuvers during acute respiratory distress syndrome: is it useful? *Minerva Anesthesiol.* 2011;77(1):85-89.

98. Silva PL, Moraes L, Santos RS, et al. Impact of pressure profile and duration of recruitment maneuvers on morphofunctional and biochemical variables in experimental lung injury. *Crit Care Med.* 2011;39(5):1074-1081.

99. Arnal JM, Paquet J, Wysocki M, et al. Optimal duration of a sustained inflation recruitment maneuver in ARDS patients. *Intensive Care Med.* 2011;37(10):1588-1594.

100. Grasso S, Mascia L, Del Turco M, et al. Effects of recruiting maneuvers in patients with acute respiratory distress syndrome ventilated with protective ventilatory strategy. *Anesthesiology.* 2002;96(4):795-802.

101. Brower RG, Morris A, MacIntyre N, et al. Effects of recruitment maneuvers in patients with acute lung injury and acute respiratory distress syndrome ventilated with high positive end-expiratory pressure. *Crit Care Med.* 2003;31(11):2592-2597.

102. Meade MO, Cook DJ, Griffith LE, et al. A study of the physiologic responses to a lung recruitment maneuver in acute lung injury and acute respiratory distress syndrome. *Respir Care.* 2008;53(11):1441-1449.

103. Oczenski W, Hormann C, Keller C, et al. Recruitment maneuvers after a positive end-expiratory pressure trial do not induce sustained effects in early adult respiratory distress syndrome. *Anesthesiology.* 2004;101(3):620-625.

104. Xi XM, Jiang L, Zhu B; RM group. Clinical efficacy and safety of recruitment maneuver in patients with acute respiratory distress syndrome using low tidal volume ventilation: a multicenter randomized controlled clinical trial. *Chin Med J (Engl)*. 2010;123(21):3100-3105.

105. Farias LL, Faffe DS, Xisto DG, et al. Positive end-expiratory pressure prevents lung mechanical stress caused by recruitment/derecruitment. *J Appl Physiol (1985)*. 2005;98(1):53-61.

106. Hodgson CL, Tuxen DV, Davies AR, et al. A randomised controlled trial of an open lung strategy with staircase recruitment, titrated PEEP and targeted low airway pressures in patients with acute respiratory distress syndrome. *Crit Care*. 2011;15(3):R133.

107. Jabaudon M, Hamroun N, Roszyk L, et al. Effects of a recruitment maneuver on plasma levels of soluble RAGE in patients with diffuse acute respiratory distress syndrome: a prospective randomized crossover study. *Intensive Care Med*. 2015;41(5):846-855.

108. Suzumura EA, Figueiro M, Normilio-Silva K, et al. Effects of alveolar recruitment maneuvers on clinical outcomes in patients with acute respiratory distress syndrome: a systematic review and meta-analysis. *Intensive Care Med*. 2014;40(9):1227-1240.

109. Hodgson C, Goligher EC, Young ME, et al. Recruitment manoeuvres for adults with acute respiratory distress syndrome receiving mechanical ventilation. *Cochrane Database Syst Rev*. 2016;11:CD006667.

110. Douglas WW, Rehder K, Beynen FM, Sessler AD, Marsh HM. Improved oxygenation in patients with acute respiratory failure: the prone position. *Am Rev Respir Dis*. 1977;115(4):559-566.

111. Guerin C, Reignier J, Richard JC, et al. Prone positioning in severe acute respiratory distress syndrome. *N Engl J Med*. 2013;368(23):2159-2168.

112. Lamm WJ, Graham MM, Albert RK. Mechanism by which the prone position improves oxygenation in acute lung injury. *Am J Respir Crit Care Med*. 1994;150(1):184-193.

113. Pelosi P, Tubiolo D, Mascheroni D, et al. Effects of the prone position on respiratory mechanics and gas exchange during acute lung injury. *Am J Respir Crit Care Med*. 1998;157(2):387-393.

114. Gattinoni L, Taccone P, Carlesso E, Marini JJ. Prone position in acute respiratory distress syndrome. Rationale, indications, and limits. *Am J Respir Crit Care Med*. 2013;188(11):1286-1293.

115. Albert RK, Hubmayr RD. The prone position eliminates compression of the lungs by the heart. *Am J Respir Crit Care Med*. 2000;161(5):1660-1665.

116. Cornejo RA, Diaz JC, Tobar EA, et al. Effects of prone positioning on lung protection in patients with acute respiratory distress syndrome. *Am J Respir Crit Care Med*. 2013;188(4):440-448.

117. Wiener CM, Kirk W, Albert RK. Prone position reverses gravitational distribution of perfusion in dog lungs with oleic acid-induced injury. *J Appl Physiol (1985)*. 1990;68(4):1386-1392.

118. Henderson AC, Sa RC, Theilmann RJ, Buxton RB, Prisk GK, Hopkins SR. The gravitational distribution of ventilation-perfusion ratio is more uniform in prone than supine posture in the normal human lung. *J Appl Physiol (1985)*. 2013;115(3):313-324.

119. Gattinoni L, Tognoni G, Pesenti A, et al. Effect of prone positioning on the survival of patients with acute respiratory failure. *N Engl J Med*. 2001;345(8):568-573.

120. Guerin C, Gaillard S, Lemasson S, et al. Effects of systematic prone positioning in hypoxemic acute respiratory failure: a randomized controlled trial. *JAMA*. 2004;292(19):2379-2387.

121. Mancebo J, Fernandez R, Blanch L, et al. A multicenter trial of prolonged prone ventilation in severe acute respiratory distress syndrome. *Am J Respir Crit Care Med*. 2006;173(11):1233-1239.

122. Taccone P, Pesenti A, Latini R, et al. Prone positioning in patients with moderate and severe acute respiratory distress syndrome: a randomized controlled trial. *JAMA*. 2009;302(18):1977-1984.

123. Albert RK, Keniston A, Baboi L, Ayzac L, Guerin C, Proseva I. Prone position-induced improvement in gas exchange does not predict improved survival in the acute respiratory distress syndrome. *Am J Respir Crit Care Med*. 2014;189(4):494-496.

124. Santana MC, Garcia CS, Xisto DG, et al. Prone position prevents regional alveolar hyperinflation and mechanical stress and strain in mild experimental acute lung injury. *Respir Physiol Neurobiol*. 2009;167(2):181-188.

125. Perchiazzi G, Rylander C, Vena A, et al. Lung regional stress and strain as a function of posture and ventilatory mode. *J Appl Physiol (1985)*. 2011;110(5):1374-1383.

126. Chan MC, Hsu JY, Liu HH, et al. Effects of prone position on inflammatory markers in patients with ARDS due to community-acquired pneumonia. *J Formos Med Assoc*. 2007;106(9):708-716.

127. Park MS, He Q, Edwards MG, et al. Mitogen-activated protein kinase phosphatase-1 modulates regional effects of injurious mechanical ventilation in rodent lungs. *Am J Respir Crit Care Med*. 2012;186(1):72-81.

128. Beitler JR, Shaefi S, Montesi SB, et al. Prone positioning reduces mortality from acute respiratory distress syndrome in the low tidal volume era: a meta-analysis. *Intensive Care Med*. 2014;40(3):332-341.

129. Vieillard-Baron A, Charron C, Caille V, Belliard G, Page B, Jardin F. Prone positioning unloads the right ventricle in severe ARDS. *Chest*. 2007;132(5):1440-1446.

130. Jozwiak M, Teboul JL, Anguel N, et al. Beneficial hemodynamic effects of prone positioning in patients with acute respiratory distress syndrome. *Am J Respir Crit Care Med*. 2013;188(12):1428-1433.

131. Schwartz MD, Moore EE, Moore FA, et al. Nuclear factor-kappa B is activated in alveolar macrophages from patients with acute respiratory distress syndrome. *Crit Care Med*. 1996;24(8):1285-1292.

132. Meduri GU, Carratu P, Freire AX. Evidence of biological efficacy for prolonged glucocorticoid treatment in patients with unresolving ARDS. *Eur Respir J Suppl*. 2003;42:57s-64s.

133. Bernard GR, Luce JM, Sprung CL, et al. High-dose corticosteroids in patients with the adult respiratory distress syndrome. *N Engl J Med*. 1987;317(25):1565-1570.

134. Bone RC, Fisher CJ Jr, Clemmer TP, Slotman GJ, Metz CA. Early methylprednisolone treatment for septic syndrome and the adult respiratory distress syndrome. *Chest*. 1987;92(6):1032-1036.

135. Meduri GU, Headley S, Kohler G, et al. Persistent elevation of inflammatory cytokines predicts a poor outcome in ARDS. Plasma IL-1 beta and IL-6 levels are consistent and efficient predictors of outcome over time. *Chest*. 1995;107(4):1062-1073.

136. Meduri GU, Kohler G, Headley S, Tolley E, Stentz F, Postlethwaite A. Inflammatory cytokines in the BAL of patients with ARDS. Persistent elevation over time predicts poor outcome. *Chest.* 1995;108(5):1303-1314.

137. Meduri GU, Belenchia JM, Estes RJ, Wunderink RG, el Torky M, Leeper KV Jr. Fibroproliferative phase of ARDS. Clinical findings and effects of corticosteroids. *Chest.* 1991;100(4):943-952.

138. Meduri GU, Headley S, Tolley E, Shelby M, Stentz F, Postlethwaite A. Plasma and BAL cytokine response to corticosteroid rescue treatment in late ARDS. *Chest.* 1995;108(5):1315-1325.

139. Meduri GU, Tolley EA, Chinn A, Stentz F, Postlethwaite A. Procollagen types I and III aminoterminal propeptide levels during acute respiratory distress syndrome and in response to methylprednisolone treatment. *Am J Respir Crit Care Med.* 1998;158(5 Pt 1):1432-1441.

140. Meduri GU, Headley AS, Golden E, et al. Effect of prolonged methylprednisolone therapy in unresolving acute respiratory distress syndrome: a randomized controlled trial. *JAMA.* 1998;280(2):159-165.

141. Steinberg KP, Hudson LD, Goodman RB, et al. Efficacy and safety of corticosteroids for persistent acute respiratory distress syndrome. *N Engl J Med.* 2006;354(16):1671-1684.

142. Meduri GU, Golden E, Freire AX, et al. Methylprednisolone infusion in early severe ARDS: results of a randomized controlled trial. *Chest.* 2007;131(4):954-963.

143. Meduri GU, Bridges L, Shih MC, Marik PE, Siemieniuk RA, Kocak M. Prolonged glucocorticoid treatment is associated with improved ARDS outcomes: analysis of individual patients' data from four randomized trials and trial-level meta-analysis of the updated literature. *Intensive Care Med.* 2016;42(5):829-840.

144. Ruan SY, Lin HH, Huang CT, Kuo PH, Wu HD, Yu CJ. Exploring the heterogeneity of effects of corticosteroids on acute respiratory distress syndrome: a systematic review and meta-analysis. *Crit Care.* 2014;18(2):R63.

145. Tang BM, Craig JC, Eslick GD, Seppelt I, McLean AS. Use of corticosteroids in acute lung injury and acute respiratory distress syndrome: a systematic review and meta-analysis. *Crit Care Med.* 2009;37(5):1594-1603.

146. Meduri GU, Annane D, Chrousos GP, Marik PE, Sinclair SE. Activation and regulation of systemic inflammation in ARDS: rationale for prolonged glucocorticoid therapy. *Chest.* 2009;136(6):1631-1643.

147. Schwarz MI, Albert RK. "Imitators" of the ARDS: implications for diagnosis and treatment. *Chest.* 2004;125(4):1530-1535.

148. Brun-Buisson C, Richard JC, Mercat A, Thiebaut AC, Brochard L; REVA-SRLF A/H1N1v 2009 Registry Group. Early corticosteroids in severe influenza A/H1N1 pneumonia and acute respiratory distress syndrome. *Am J Respir Crit Care Med.* 2011;183(9):1200-1206.

149. Bellani G, Laffey JG, Pham T, et al. Epidemiology, patterns of care, and mortality for patients with acute respiratory distress syndrome in intensive care units in 50 countries. *JAMA.* 2016;315(8):788-800.

150. deBacker J, Hart N, Fan E. Neuromuscular blockade in the 21st century management of the critically ill patient. *Chest.* 2017;151(3):697-706.

151. Prielipp RC, Coursin DB, Scuderi PE, et al. Comparison of the infusion requirements and recovery profiles of vecuronium and cisatracurium 51W89 in intensive care unit patients. *Anesth Analg.* 1995;81(1):3-12.

152. Puthucheary Z, Rawal J, Ratnayake G, Harridge S, Montgomery H, Hart N. Neuromuscular blockade and skeletal muscle weakness in critically ill patients: time to rethink the evidence? *Am J Respir Crit Care Med.* 2012;185(9):911-917.

153. Wilcox SR. Corticosteroids and neuromuscular blockers in development of critical illness neuromuscular abnormalities: a historical review. *J Crit Care.* 2017;37:149-155.

154. De Jonghe B, Sharshar T, Lefaucheur JP, et al. Paresis acquired in the intensive care unit: a prospective multicenter study. *JAMA.* 2002;288(22):2859-2867.

155. Gainnier M, Roch A, Forel JM, et al. Effect of neuromuscular blocking agents on gas exchange in patients presenting with acute respiratory distress syndrome. *Crit Care Med.* 2004;32(1):113-119.

156. Forel JM, Roch A, Marin V, et al. Neuromuscular blocking agents decrease inflammatory response in patients presenting with acute respiratory distress syndrome. *Crit Care Med.* 2006;34(11):2749-2757.

157. Alhazzani W, Alshahrani M, Jaeschke R, et al. Neuromuscular blocking agents in acute respiratory distress syndrome: a systematic review and meta-analysis of randomized controlled trials. *Crit Care.* 2013;17(2):R43.

158. Slutsky AS. Neuromuscular blocking agents in ARDS. *N Engl J Med.* 2010;363(12):1176-1180.

159. Richard JC, Lyazidi A, Akoumianaki E, et al. Potentially harmful effects of inspiratory synchronization during pressure preset ventilation. *Intensive Care Med.* 2013;39(11):2003-2010.

160. Fanelli V, Morita Y, Cappello P, et al. Neuromuscular blocking agent cisatracurium attenuates lung injury by inhibition of nicotinic acetylcholine receptor-alpha1. *Anesthesiology.* 2016;124(1):132-140.

161. Levine S, Nguyen T, Taylor N, et al. Rapid disuse atrophy of diaphragm fibers in mechanically ventilated humans. *N Engl J Med.* 2008;358(13):1327-1335.

162. Rossaint R, Falke KJ, Lopez F, Slama K, Pison U, Zapol WM. Inhaled nitric oxide for the adult respiratory distress syndrome. *N Engl J Med.* 1993;328(6):399-405.

163. Lundin S, Mang H, Smithies M, Stenqvist O, Frostell C. Inhalation of nitric oxide in acute lung injury: results of a European multicentre study. The European Study Group of Inhaled Nitric Oxide. *Intensive Care Med.* 1999;25(9):911-919.

164. Gerlach H, Keh D, Semmerow A, et al. Dose-response characteristics during long-term inhalation of nitric oxide in patients with severe acute respiratory distress syndrome: a prospective, randomized, controlled study. *Am J Respir Crit Care Med.* 2003;167(7):1008-1015.

165. Taylor RW, Zimmerman JL, Dellinger RP, et al. Low-dose inhaled nitric oxide in patients with acute lung injury: a randomized controlled trial. *JAMA.* 2004;291(13):1603-1609.

166. Angus DC, Clermont G, Linde-Zwirble WT, et al. Healthcare costs and long-term outcomes after acute respiratory distress syndrome: a phase III trial of inhaled nitric oxide. *Crit Care Med.* 2006;34(12):2883-2890.

167. Dellinger RP, Trzeciak SW, Criner GJ, et al. Association between inhaled nitric oxide treatment and long-term pulmonary function in survivors of acute respiratory distress syndrome. *Crit Care.* 2012;16(2):R36.

168. Adhikari NK, Burns KE, Friedrich JO, Granton JT, Cook DJ, Meade MO. Effect of nitric oxide on oxygenation and mortality in acute lung injury: systematic review and meta-analysis. *BMJ.* 2007;334(7597):779.

169. Gebistorf F, Karam O, Wetterslev J, Afshari A. Inhaled nitric oxide for acute respiratory distress syndrome (ARDS) in children and adults. *Cochrane Database Syst Rev.* 2016(6): CD002787.

170. Adhikari NK, Dellinger RP, Lundin S, et al. Inhaled nitric oxide does not reduce mortality in patients with acute respiratory distress syndrome regardless of severity: systematic review and meta-analysis. *Crit Care Med.* 2014;42(2):404-412.

171. Ruan SY, Huang TM, Wu HY, Wu HD, Yu CJ, Lai MS. Inhaled nitric oxide therapy and risk of renal dysfunction: a systematic review and meta-analysis of randomized trials. *Crit Care.* 2015;19:137.

172. Torbic H, Szumita PM, Anger KE, Nuccio P, LaGambina S, Weinhouse G. Inhaled epoprostenol vs inhaled nitric oxide for refractory hypoxemia in critically ill patients. *J Crit Care.* 2013;28(5):844-848.

173. Ammar MA, Bauer SR, Bass SN, Sasidhar M, Mullin R, Lam SW. Noninferiority of inhaled epoprostenol to inhaled nitric oxide for the treatment of ARDS. *Ann Pharmacother.* 2015;49(10):1105-1112.

174. Gattinoni L, Cressoni M, Brazzi L. Fluids in ARDS: from onset through recovery. *Curr Opin Crit Care.* 2014;20(4):373-377.

175. Ware LB, Matthay MA. Alveolar fluid clearance is impaired in the majority of patients with acute lung injury and the acute respiratory distress syndrome. *Am J Respir Crit Care Med.* 2001;163(6):1376-1383.

176. Humphrey H, Hall J, Sznajder I, Silverstein M, Wood L. Improved survival in ARDS patients associated with a reduction in pulmonary capillary wedge pressure. *Chest.* 1990;97(5):1176-1180.

177. Mitchell JP, Schuller D, Calandrino FS, Schuster DP. Improved outcome based on fluid management in critically ill patients requiring pulmonary artery catheterization. *Am Rev Respir Dis.* 1992;145(5):990-998.

178. Martin GS, Mangialardi RJ, Wheeler AP, Dupont WD, Morris JA, Bernard GR. Albumin and furosemide therapy in hypoproteinemic patients with acute lung injury. *Crit Care Med.* 2002;30(10):2175-2182.

179. Martin GS, Moss M, Wheeler AP, Mealer M, Morris JA, Bernard GR. A randomized, controlled trial of furosemide with or without albumin in hypoproteinemic patients with acute lung injury. *Crit Care Med.* 2005;33(8):1681-1687.

180. National Heart, Lung, and Blood Institute Acute Respiratory Distress Syndrome Clinical Trials Network; Wiedemann HP, Wheeler AP, Bernard GR, et al. Comparison of two fluid-management strategies in acute lung injury. *N Engl J Med.* 2006;354(24):2564-2575.

181. Grams ME, Estrella MM, Coresh J, et al. Fluid balance, diuretic use, and mortality in acute kidney injury. *Clin J Am Soc Nephrol.* 2011;6(5):966-973.

182. Mikkelsen ME, Christie JD, Lanken PN, et al. The adult respiratory distress syndrome cognitive outcomes study: long-term neuropsychological function in survivors of acute lung injury. *Am J Respir Crit Care Med.* 2012;185(12):1307-1315.

183. Semler MW, Marney AM, Rice TW, et al. B-Type natriuretic peptide, aldosterone, and fluid management in ARDS. *Chest.* 2016;150(1):102-111.

184. Famous KR, Delucchi K, Ware LB, et al. Acute respiratory distress syndrome subphenotypes respond differently to randomized fluid management strategy. *Am J Respir Crit Care Med.* 2017;195(3):331-338.

185. Grissom CK, Hirshberg EL, Dickerson JB, et al. Fluid management with a simplified conservative protocol for the acute respiratory distress syndrome*. *Crit Care Med.* 2015;43(2): 288-295.

186. McAuley DF, Frank JA, Fang X, Matthay MA. Clinically relevant concentrations of beta2-adrenergic agonists stimulate maximal cyclic adenosine monophosphate-dependent airspace fluid clearance and decrease pulmonary edema in experimental acid-induced lung injury. *Crit Care Med.* 2004;32(7): 1470-1476.

187. National Heart, Lung, and Blood Institute Acute Respiratory Distress Syndrome Clinical Trials Network; Matthay MA, Brower RG, Carson S, et al. Randomized, placebo-controlled clinical trial of an aerosolized beta(2)-agonist for treatment of acute lung injury. *Am J Respir Crit Care Med.* 2011;184(5): 561-568.

188. Gao Smith F, Perkins GD, Gates S, et al. Effect of intravenous beta-2 agonist treatment on clinical outcomes in acute respiratory distress syndrome (BALTI-2): a multicentre, randomised controlled trial. *Lancet.* 2012;379(9812):229-235.

189. Hill JD, O'Brien TG, Murray JJ, et al. Prolonged extracorporeal oxygenation for acute post-traumatic respiratory failure (shock-lung syndrome). Use of the Bramson membrane lung. *N Engl J Med.* 1972;286(12):629-634.

190. Gattinoni L, Carlesso E, Langer T. Clinical review: extracorporeal membrane oxygenation. *Crit Care.* 2011;15(6):243.

191. Zapol WM, Snider MT, Hill JD, et al. Extracorporeal membrane oxygenation in severe acute respiratory failure. A randomized prospective study. *JAMA.* 1979;242(20):2193-2196.

192. Paden ML, Conrad SA, Rycus PT, Thiagarajan RR, ELSO Registry. Extracorporeal life support organization registry report 2012. *ASAIO J.* 2013;59(3):202-210.

193. Peek GJ, Mugford M, Tiruvoipati R, et al. Efficacy and economic assessment of conventional ventilatory support versus extracorporeal membrane oxygenation for severe adult respiratory failure (CESAR): a multicentre randomised controlled trial. *Lancet.* 2009;374(9698):1351-1363.

194. Noah MA, Peek GJ, Finney SJ, et al. Referral to an extracorporeal membrane oxygenation center and mortality among patients with severe 2009 influenza A(H1N1). *JAMA.* 2011;306(15):1659-1668.

195. Pham T, Combes A, Roze H, et al. Extracorporeal membrane oxygenation for pandemic influenza A(H1N1)-induced acute respiratory distress syndrome: a cohort study and propensity-matched analysis. *Am J Respir Crit Care Med.* 2013;187(3):276-285.

196. Munshi L, Telesnicki T, Walkey A, Fan E. Extracorporeal life support for acute respiratory failure. A systematic review and metaanalysis. *Ann Am Thorac Soc.* 2014;11(5):802-810.

197. Tramm R, Ilic D, Davies AR, Pellegrino VA, Romero L, Hodgson C. Extracorporeal membrane oxygenation for critically ill adults. *Cochrane Database Syst Rev.* 2015;1:CD010381.

198. Barbaro RP, Odetola FO, Kidwell KM, et al. Association of hospital-level volume of extracorporeal membrane oxygenation cases and mortality. Analysis of the extracorporeal life support organization registry. *Am J Respir Crit Care Med.* 2015;191(8):894-901.

199. Langer T, Santini A, Bottino N, et al. "Awake" extracorporeal membrane oxygenation (ECMO): pathophysiology, technical considerations, and clinical pioneering. *Crit Care.* 2016;20(1):150.

200. Gattinoni L, Pesenti A, Mascheroni D, et al. Low-frequency positive-pressure ventilation with extracorporeal CO_2 removal in severe acute respiratory failure. *JAMA.* 1986;256(7):881-886.

201. Terragni PP, Del Sorbo L, Mascia L, et al. Tidal volume lower than 6 mL/kg enhances lung protection: role of extracorporeal carbon dioxide removal. *Anesthesiology.* 2009;111(4):826-835.

202. Fanelli V, Ranieri MV, Mancebo J, et al. Feasibility and safety of low-flow extracorporeal carbon dioxide removal to facilitate ultra-protective ventilation in patients with moderate acute respiratory distress syndrome. *Crit Care.* 2016;20:36.

203. Morris AH, Wallace CJ, Menlove RL, et al. Randomized clinical trial of pressure-controlled inverse ratio ventilation and extracorporeal CO_2 removal for adult respiratory distress syndrome. *Am J Respir Crit Care Med.* 1994;149(2 Pt 1): 295-305.

204. Bein T, Weber-Carstens S, Goldmann A, et al. Lower tidal volume strategy (approximately 3 mL/kg) combined with extracorporeal CO_2 removal versus "conventional" protective ventilation (6 mL/kg) in severe ARDS: the prospective randomized Xtravent-study. *Intensive Care Med.* 2013;39(5):847-856.

205. Kumar KV, Rao SM, Gayani R, Mohan IK, Naidu MU. Oxidant stress and essential fatty acids in patients with risk and established ARDS. *Clin Chim Acta.* 2000;298(1-2):111-120.

206. Calder PC. n-3 fatty acids, inflammation, and immunity—relevance to postsurgical and critically ill patients. *Lipids.* 2004;39(12):1147-1161.

207. Gadek JE, DeMichele SJ, Karlstad MD, et al. Effect of enteral feeding with eicosapentaenoic acid, gamma-linolenic acid, and antioxidants in patients with acute respiratory distress syndrome. Enteral Nutrition in ARDS Study Group. *Crit Care Med.* 1999;27(8):1409-1420.

208. Singer P, Theilla M, Fisher H, Gibstein L, Grozovski E, Cohen J. Benefit of an enteral diet enriched with eicosapentaenoic acid and gamma-linolenic acid in ventilated patients with acute lung injury. *Crit Care Med.* 2006;34(4):1033-1038.

209. Rice TW, Wheeler AP, Thompson BT, et al. Enteral omega-3 fatty acid, gamma-linolenic acid, and antioxidant supplementation in acute lung injury. *JAMA.* 2011;306(14):1574-1581.

210. Li C, Bo L, Liu W, Lu X, Jin F. Enteral immunomodulatory diet (omega-3 fatty acid, gamma-linolenic acid and antioxidant supplementation) for acute lung injury and acute respiratory distress syndrome: an updated systematic review and meta-analysis. *Nutrients.* 2015;7(7):5572-5585.

211. Singleton KD, Beckey VE, Wischmeyer PE. Glutamine prevents activation of NF-kappaB and stress kinase pathways, attenuates inflammatory cytokine release, and prevents acute respiratory distress syndrome (ARDS) following sepsis. *Shock.* 2005;24(6):583-589.

212. Oliveira GP, de Abreu MG, Pelosi P, Rocco PR. Exogenous glutamine in respiratory diseases: myth or reality? *Nutrients.* 2016;8(2):76.

213. National Heart, Lung, and Blood Institute Acute Respiratory Distress Syndrome Clinical Trials Network; Rice TW, Wheeler AP, Thompson BT, et al. Initial trophic vs full enteral feeding in patients with acute lung injury: the EDEN randomized trial. *JAMA.* 2012;307(8):795-803.

214. Arabi YM, Haddad SH, Tamim HM, et al. Near-target caloric intake in critically ill medical-surgical patients is associated with adverse outcomes. *JPEN J Parenter Enteral Nutr.* 2010;34(3):280-288.

215. Erickson SE, Martin GS, Davis JL, Matthay MA, Eisner MD, NIH NHLBI ARDS Network. Recent trends in acute lung injury mortality: 1996-2005. *Crit Care Med.* 2009;37(5): 1574-1579.

216. Cochi SE, Kempker JA, Annangi S, Kramer MR, Martin GS. Mortality trends of acute respiratory distress syndrome in the United States from 1999 to 2013. *Ann Am Thorac Soc.* 2016;13(10):1742-1751.

217. Khandelwal N, Hough CL, Bansal A, Veenstra DL, Treggiari MM. Long-term survival in patients with severe acute respiratory distress syndrome and rescue therapies for refractory hypoxemia*. *Crit Care Med.* 2014;42(7):1610-1618.

218. Wang CY, Calfee CS, Paul DW, et al. One-year mortality and predictors of death among hospital survivors of acute respiratory distress syndrome. *Intensive Care Med.* 2014;40(3):388-396.

219. Herridge MS, Cheung AM, Tansey CM, et al. One-year outcomes in survivors of the acute respiratory distress syndrome. *N Engl J Med.* 2003;348(8):683-693.

220. Herridge MS, Tansey CM, Matte A, et al. Functional disability 5 years after acute respiratory distress syndrome. *N Engl J Med.* 2011;364(14):1293-1304.

221. Davidson TA, Caldwell ES, Curtis JR, Hudson LD, Steinberg KP. Reduced quality of life in survivors of acute respiratory distress syndrome compared with critically ill control patients. *JAMA.* 1999;281(4):354-360.

222. Bienvenu OJ, Colantuoni E, Mendez-Tellez PA, et al. Depressive symptoms and impaired physical function after acute lung injury: a 2-year longitudinal study. *Am J Respir Crit Care Med.* 2012;185(5):517-524.

223. Huang M, Parker AM, Bienvenu OJ, et al. Psychiatric symptoms in acute respiratory distress syndrome survivors: a 1-year national multicenter study. *Crit Care Med.* 2016;44(5): 954-965.

224. Spragg RG, Bernard GR, Checkley W, et al. Beyond mortality: future clinical research in acute lung injury. *Am J Respir Crit Care Med.* 2010;181(10):1121-1127.

225. Loring S, Malhotra A. Driving pressure and respiratory mechanics in ARDS. *N Engl J Med.* 2015;372(8):776-777.

226. Amato MB, Meade MO, Slutsky AS, et al. Driving pressure and survival in the acute respiratory distress syndrome. *N Engl J Med.* 2015;372(8):747-755.

227. Kallet RH, Zhuo H, Liu KD, Calfee CS, Matthay MA; National Heart Lung and Blood Institute ARDS Network Investigators. The association between physiologic dead-space fraction and mortality in subjects with ARDS enrolled in a prospective multi-center clinical trial. *Respir Care.* 2014;59(11):1611-1618.

228. Gattinoni L, Vagginelli F, Carlesso E, et al. Decrease in $Paco_2$ with prone position is predictive of improved outcome in acute respiratory distress syndrome. *Crit Care Med.* 2003;31(12):2727-2733.

229. The National Heart, Lung, and Blood Institute Acute Respiratory Distress Syndrome (ARDS) Clinical Trials Network; Wiedermann HP, Wheeler AP, Bernard GR, et al. Comparison of two fluid-management strategies in acute lung injury. *N Engl J Med.* 2006;354(24):2564-2575.

Mechanical Ventilation

Rania Esteitie, MD, Ronaldo Collo Go, MD, and Maher Tabba, MD

INTRODUCTION

This chapter will discuss the principles of mechanical ventilation, indications, modes of mechanical ventilation, weaning and spontaneous breathing trials, tracheostomy, complications of mechanical ventilation, special situations, and noninvasive mechanical ventilation.

DEFINITIONS

Proximal Airway Pressure, Alveolar Pressure, and Plateau Pressure

Proximal airway pressure applied by the ventilator (P_{vent}) is approximated during the expiratory phase in the inspiratory limb when flow is 0 and during the inspiratory phase in the expiratory limb when the flow is 0.[1] It uses the following equation[2]:

$$P_{vent} + P_{mus} = V_T/C_{RS} + R_{aw} \times V_I + PEEP + iPEEP + Inertance$$

In this equation, C_{RS} is respiratory system compliance, PEEP is peak end-expiratory pressure, iPEEP is intrinsic PEEP, P_{mus} is pressure from patient's inspiratory muscles, P_{vent} is proximal airway pressure from the ventilator, R_{aw} is airway resistance, V_I is the inspiratory volume, inertance (cm H_2O L^{-1} s^2) is pressure difference to cause change in rate of change in volume flow rate in time, and V_T is tidal volume. Alveolar pressure (P_A) during inspiration in volume control ventilation is V/C_{RS} + PEEP, and during inspiration in pressure control ventilation is $\Delta P \times (1 - e^{-t/T})$ + PEEP.[1] In this equation, t is the elapsed time after initiation of inspiration, and T is the time constant.

Due to R_{aw}, the presence of flow causes proximal airway pressure to be greater than P_A. Plateau pressure (P_{plat}) is determined by applying an end-inspiratory breath hold for 0.5 to 2 seconds, where the pressure equilibrates when the flow is 0. It is calculated via $P_{plat} = V_T/C_{RS}$ during passive inflation and via $P_{plat} = (V_T \times PIP) - (V_T \times PEEP)/(V_T + [T_E \times V_I])$ in spontaneous breathing modes.[1] In this equation, PIP is peak inspiratory pressure and T_E is the expiratory time constant. During end-inspiratory breath hold, the P_{plat} approximates P_A. Ideally, P_{plat} is less than 30 cm H_2O (Fig. 12-1).[1]

Understanding the relationship between peak and plateau pressures can help troubleshoot mechanically ventilated patients. PIP without increase in plateau pressure suggests an increase in airway resistance from a kinked or blocked endotracheal (ET) tube, bronchospasm, or increased secretions.[3] Increased PIP with increased plateau pressure suggests decreased compliance such as extrathoracic compression, bronchial intubation, atelectasis, pulmonary edema, pneumothorax, and hyperinflation.[3] Decreasing PIP, low tidal volumes, gurgling sounds, and stridor can indicate cuff leak.

When the difference between peak and plateau pressures is greater 5 cm H_2O, increased airway pressure can likely be attributed to increased airway resistance. Acute causes of elevated airway resistance are bronchospasm, ET tube obstruction, or ventilator circuit obstruction (eg, the ventilator tubing is kinked). If the difference between peak and plateau pressures is low, increased airway pressure is likely secondary to acute decrease of lung compliance and resultant increased elastic work. Acute causes of elevated elastic work are pneumothorax, tension pneumothorax, evolving pneumonia, pulmonary edema, acute respiratory distress syndrome (ARDS), and auto-PEEP caused by breath stacking.

Plateau pressure, low tidal volumes, and high PEEP are suggested to improve survival in ARDS but their relative relationship is uncertain. Driving pressure explores this relationship and is the amount of cyclic parenchymal deformation imposed on ventilated lung units. Driving pressure (change in P = V_T/C_{RS}) is calculated via P_{plat} − PEEP if there is no inspiratory effort.[4] Decreasing driving pressure is associated with better outcomes in ARDS.[4] The driving pressure limit varies, from 14 cm H_2O to 18 cm H_2O, but patients without ARDS have a driving pressure of 10.[5,6] One group of authors suggests limiting the driving pressure to 15 cm H_2O.[5] This relationship of driving pressure and mortality is not seen in nonARDS patients.[7]

Mean Airway Pressure

This is a major determinant of oxygenation. Airway pressure or P_{aw} that is too low can result in hypoventilation and atelectasis. A P_{aw} that is too high can result in barotrauma and

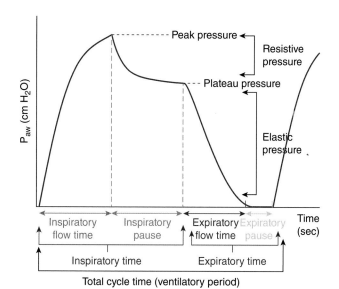

FIGURE 12-1 The relationship of pressure over time.

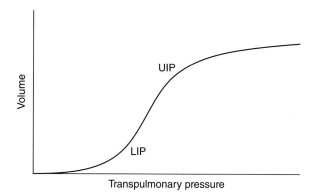

FIGURE 12-2 Volume and transpulmonary curve. LIP = lower inflection point. UIP = upper inflection point.

hemodynamic compromise. This can be calculated several ways. Flow-volume ventilation uses the following equation:

$$\text{Mean } P_{aw} = 0.5 \times (PIP - PEEP) \times (T_I/T_{tot}) + PEEP$$

where T_I is the inspiratory phase and T_{tot} is the total respiratory cycle. Pressure ventilation uses the following equation[1]:

$$P_{aw} = (PIP - PEEP) \times (T_I/T_{tot}) + PEEP$$

Transpulmonary Pressure and Esophageal Pressure

Transpulmonary pressure (TPP) is the pressure gradient between alveolar pressure and pleural pressure which drives the flow of air.[1,8,9] Atmospheric air is always constant so the dynamic changes in the lungs propels the flow of air. Due to hysteresis, the pressure required to generate inspiration is higher than expiration. To inflate the lung, pressure must overcome airway resistance, inertance (pressure gradient required to accelerate gas), and pressure required to overcome elastance.[9] When flow is zero, the transpulmonary pressure (alveolar pressure – pleural pressure) is the principle pressure maintaining the lung inflation.[9]

Esophageal pressure (P_{es}) is an indirect measure of pleural pressure. It is accomplished by inserting a thin catheter orally and nasally down to the esophagus (approximately 35–40 cm) and behind the heart. Identification of cardiac oscillations is used to determine accurate placement. Esophageal pressure is used to TPP.[1] It uses the following equation:

$$TPP = P_{aw} - P_{es}$$

Transpulmonary pressure is used to assess lung recruitability and usually kept below 25 cm H_2O.[10,11] The ideal TPP is obtained from observations from the volume and transpulmonary

pressure curve (Fig. 12-2). The lower inflection point (LIP) is the junction between the first and second portions of the curve or 20% decrease in steepest slope there is end of alveolar recruitment.[12-14] Amato's study suggested decreased mortality with pressure more than 2 cm above LIP and plateau less than 20 cm H_2O.[13] The upper inflection point (UIP) is 20% increase from the steepest slop and pressures above UIP are noted to cause overdistention and decreased alveolar recruitment. Based on these observations, it has been suggested that the pressures between LIP and UIP is where the lung has the highest compliance; alveoli is recruited throughout the inspiratory limb; and improved mortality is not solely dependent on PEEP which is an expiratory process.[14-19]

Esophageal pressure is used to titrate PEEP in ARDS as long as TPP between 0 to 25 cmH_2O.[1,11,20] In ARDS, there is a propensity for alveolar collapse. One single center randomized control study suggested that TPP are negative in ARDS due to flooding or atelectasis.[11] An esophageal directed ventilation with TPP goal of 0 to less than 25 cm H_2O improved mortality.[11]

Other roles of esophageal pressure is measurement of intrinsic PEEP and improve patient-ventilatory synchrony. Measurements of P_{aw} and flow mask true patient and ventilator asynchrony. Patients who are heavily sedated, respiratory muscles are actively contracting and going against ventilator support.[8,21-24] This is called reverse triggering or respiratory entrainment. Consequences are higher tidal volumes, erroneous plateau pressures, double inspiration, ineffective efforts, and prolonged mechanical ventilation (PMV).[8,21-24]

Intra-abdominal Pressure

Intra-abdominal hypertension (abdominal pressure > 12 mmHg) can cause cephalic displacement of the diaphragm leading to compression of pulmonary parenchyma and decreased lymphatic drainage.[25,26] This leads to atelectasis, decreased oxygenation, reduced carbon dioxide removal, reduced capillary blood flow, increased airway pressures, and reduced tidal volume and pulmonary compliance.[25,26] Intra-abdominal pressure is measured indirectly via bladder pressures. In mechanically ventilated patients, inhalation with diaphragmatic contraction

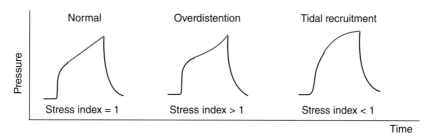

FIGURE 12-3 Pressure time waveforms and correlation with stress index. (Reprinted with permission from Hess DR. Respiratory Mechanics in Mechanically Ventilated Patients. *Respir Care*. 2014;59(11):1773-1794.)

increases the pressure. Subsequently, an increase in abdominal pressure decreases C_{RS} with flattening and rightward shift of the pressure-volume (PV) curve.[27-29]

Stress Index

Stress index (SI) is a parameter used to identify injurious mechanical ventilation. It is determined by the following equation:

$$P = aT_I^b + c$$

P is Pressure for P_{aw} or TPP, T is time interval from time 0—time 1, a is the slope of P_{aw}-time or TPP-time, b is the stress index and c is P_{aw} or TPP at time 0. It assesses the pressure-time curve during constant-flow volume control.[1] The SI is 1 if there is adequate requirement without overcompensation. An SI greater than 1 suggests overdistention and recommends a decrease of PEEP, VT, or both.[1] An SI less than 1 suggests the addition of PEEP[1] (Fig. 12-3).

Time Constant

The time constant (T) is a product of resistance and compliance and determines the rate of volume change that is passively inflated or deflated.[1] It is based on this equation: $V_t = V_i \times e^{-t/\tau}$, where V_t is the volume of a lung unit at time t, V_i is the initial volume of the lung unit, e is the base of the natural logarithm, and τ is the time constant.[1] For 1τ, there is a 63% volume change, 2τ there is 87% volume change, 3τ there is 95% volume change, 4τ there is 98% volume change, and 5τ there is more than 99% volume change.[1]

A higher resistance and compliance will have a longer time to fill and empty, and a lower resistance and compliance will have a shorter time to fill and empty.[1] For example, the value for a normal lung is 0.2 seconds, for asthmatic lungs is 0.4 seconds, and for fibrotic lungs is 0.1 seconds.[30]

Flow and Resistance

Flow ($\dot{V}$) can be turbulent or laminar. Transition from laminar to turbulent can be determined via Reynold's Number is greater than 2000. The equation for Reynold's number is 2rvd/η (r = radius of tube, v = velocity of flow, d = gas density, η = gas viscosity). Just like in fluid, radius is the major determinant in laminar flow as suggested by Poiseuille's law. Reduction of the radius by one-half with all the parameters constant will reduce flow by 1/16. The reduction of flow means higher resistance in smaller bronchi compared to larger bronchi. However, due to the large number of small bronchi, the area of greatest resistance is the intermediate bronchi between the 4th and 8th bifurcation.

Airway resistance (R_{aw}) is the change in pressure divided by the change in flow (PIP-P_{plat}/change in $\dot{V}$). The normal R_{aw} is 0.6 – 2.4 cm H_2O/L/sec. Factors that increase R_{aw} include increased airway diameter such as bronchodilation, decrease airway length, decrease viscosity, laminar flow, and increased volume. Factors that decrease R_{aw} include decrease airway diameter such as bronchoconstriction, increased airway length, increase viscosity, turbulent flow, and decreased volume.

Flow is monitored in the ventilator at the inspiratory valve and expiratory valve during volume-control ventilation.[1] During pressure control, inspiratory flow is determined via the following equation:

$$V_I = (\text{Change in P or Pressure Above PEEP}/R_{aw}) \times e^{-t/\tau}$$

τ is the time constant. t is time elapsed after inspiration. e is the base of natural algorithm. This value typically is positive.[1] Expiratory flow is typically negative and is determined via the following equation:

$$V = -(PA/R_{aw}) \times e^{-t/\tau}$$

It has been suggested that there is a maximum threshold for flow before respiratory rate increases. Inspiratory time is often increased to prolong expiration time in episodes of hypercapnia but there is a reflex increase in respiratory rate when the flow is increased from 60 L/min to 90 L/min.[31]

Lung Volumes and Capacities

Tidal volume (VT) is the volume during normal volume and typically is 500 mL. Inspiratory reserve volume (IRV) is the maximum volume that can be inhaled after normal inhalation. It can range from 1900 to 3300 ml. Expiratory reserve volume (ERV) is the maximum volume exhaled after normal exhalation. It can range from 700 to 1200 mL/breath. Residual volume (RV) is air left after exhalation. Maximum amount is 1200 mL/breath. Inspiratory capacity (IC) is the total amount of air inhaled and is the sum of VT and IRV. Functional residual capacity (FRC) is amount of air remaining in the lungs after exhalation and is the sum of RV and ERV. FRC has a direct correlation to PEEP. Vital capacity (VC) is the total exchangeable air and typically around 4800 mL. Total lung capacity (TLC) is the total of all volumes and is around 6000 mL.

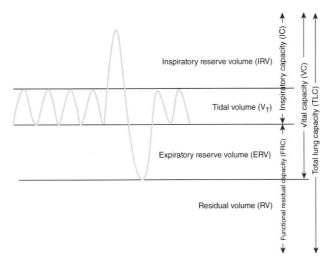

FIGURE 12-4 Types of volumes and capacities. Volumes include IRV =Inspiratory Reserve volume; VT= Tidal volume; ERV = Expiratory reserve Volume; RV = Residual volume. Capacities include: FRC = Functional residual capacity; IC = Inspiratory capacity; VC = Vital capacity; and TLC = Total lung capacity.

Respiratory System Compliance

Lung and chest wall compliance is determined via the following equation:

$$C_{RS} = \text{Change in Volume}/(P_{plat} - PEEP)$$

Acceptable values are 50 to 100 mL/cm H_2O. Respiratory system compliance also determines the slope of the PV curve. Chest wall compliance is determined via the following equation[1]:

$$C_{CW} = \text{Change in } V_T/\text{Change in } P_{es}$$

The normal value is 200 mL/cm H_2O, and is decreased in patients with obesity, abdominal compartment syndrome, chest wall abnormalities, and burns.[1] Lung compliance is determined via the following equation:

$$C_L = \text{Change in } V_T/\text{Change in TPP}$$

The normal value is 200 mL/cm H_2O, and is decreased in patients with ARDS, pulmonary edema, pneumothorax, fibrosis, bronchial intubation, and atelectasis, and it is increased in patients with emphysema.[1]

Work of Breathing

The work of breathing (WOB) is normally 4 to 8 J/min and is calculated via Volume × Pressure.

Minute Ventilation

Minute ventilation is the product of respiratory rate (RR) and tidal volume ($\dot{V}_E = RR \times V_T$). At rest, minute ventilation is 5 to 8 L/min. At mild exertion, minute ventilation can increase more than 12 L/min. There must be reciprocal changes between respiratory rate and tidal volume to meet the minute ventilation requirements for adequate carbon dioxide exchange.

Tension-Time Index and Pressure-Time Product

Both the tension-time index and the pressure-time product assess diaphragmatic fatigue. Tension-time index (TTI) = (Pdi/Pdimax)x Ti/Ttot) where Pdimax id maximum inhalation, Pdi/Pdimax is contractile force of diaphragm, and Ti/Ttot is contraction duration.1 A TTI > 0.15 predicts respiratory muscle fatigue. Work of breathing does not account for isometric phase and pressure-time product (PTP) account for energy expenditures during dynamic and isometric phases of respiration.

Auto-PEEP

Auto-PEEP occurs when air remains in the alveoli at the end of expiration, which increases the functional residual capacity (FRC). Auto-PEEP can be due to either flow restriction (as in chronic obstructive pulmonary disease), or insufficient time for lungs to return to FRC. Consequences of auto-PEEP include: (1) increased work of breathing because more work is required for inspiration; (2) worsening gas exchange; and (3) hemodynamic compromise due to increased intrathoracic pressure, decreased preload of right and left ventricle, and increased right ventricle afterload from increased pulmonary vascular resistance.[32-34]

Auto-PEEP can be recognized by: (1) delay between inspiratory effort and drop in airway pressure; (2) failure of peak airway pressure to change when external PEEP is applied; (3) reduction of plateau after prolonged exhalation; (4) static auto-PEEP via expiratory hold; (5) dynamic auto-PEEP via esophageal pressures; and (6) depiction on mechanical waveforms.[32-34] On a flow-volume loop, volume does not return to baseline (depicting volume still trapped in alveoli). On a flow-time scalar, expiratory flow does not return to baseline (depicting flow still trapped in alveoli). The less the return is, the greater the air-trapping is. The dashed line in Figure 12-5 depicts normal flow return to baseline.

Treatment strategies include the following: (1) decreasing respiratory rate/tidal volume or minute ventilation; (2) decreasing the inspiration-to-expiration (I:E) ratio or increase expiration time; (3) if with hemodynamic compromise remove from the ventilator; (4) if with dynamic hyperinflation and intrinsic expiratory flow limitation such as COPD apply PEEP by 75% to 85% of autoPEEP; and (5) heliox.[32-34] Heliox is a blend of helium and oxygen (usually at a 70:30 ratio), which is less dense than

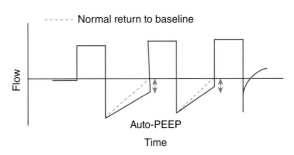

FIGURE 12-5 Flow-time scalar with auto-PEEP.

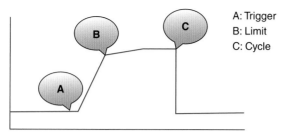

A: Trigger
B: Limit
C: Cycle

FIGURE 12-6 Three initiation phase variables on a waveform.

TABLE 12-1 Mode of Ventilation and Breath Types

Mode of Ventilation	Breath Types Available
Volume-assist control	Volume control, volume assist
Pressure-assist control	Pressure control, pressure assist
Volume SIMV	Volume control, volume assist, pressure support
Pressure SIMV	Pressure control, pressure assist, pressure support
Pressure support	Pressure support

SIMV = spontaneous intermittent mechanical ventilation.

air, theoretically permitting higher flow rates through a given airway segment for the same driving pressure, thereby alleviating dynamic hyperinflation. Several small studies have shown heliox reduce peak inspiratory pressure and arterial carbon dioxide tension, and improve oxygenation in mechanically ventilated patients by decreasing work of breathing, $Paco_2$, gas trapping, auto-PEEP, peak inspiratory pressures and plateau pressures, barotrauma, I:E ratio, and shunting.[35]

WAVEFORMS

The waveform of a ventilator cycle has 3 initiation phases variables (trigger, limit, and cycle)[36,37] (Fig. 12-6).

The trigger variable (point A), which causes inspiration to begin, can be a preset pressure variation (pressure triggering), a preset volume (volume triggering), a designated flow change (flow triggering), or an elapsed time (time triggering). The limit variable (point B) is the pressure, volume, or flow target that cannot be exceeded during inspiration. An inspiration thus may be limited when a preset peak airway pressure is reached (pressure limiting), when a preset volume is delivered (volume limiting), or when a preset peak flow is attained (flow limiting). Cycling (point C), refers to the factors that terminate inspiration. A breath may be pressure, volume, or time cycled when a preset pressure, volume, or flow as the time interval has been reached, respectively.

Three types of breath can be provided during mechanical ventilation, depending on whether the ventilator or the patient does the work and whether the ventilator or the patient

initiates (triggers) the breath. These types are mandatory, assisted, and spontaneous breaths (Table 12-1). Controlled breaths are machine cycled, trigger limited, and cycled by the ventilator. The patient is entirely passive, and the ventilator performs the work of breathing. Assisted breaths are like controlled breaths in that they are limited and cycled by the ventilator, but are triggered by the patient. Breathing work thus is provided partly by the ventilator and partly by the patient. Spontaneous breaths are triggered, limited, and cycled by the patient, who performs all the work of breathing.

The relationship between the various possible types of breath and the inspiratory phase variables just discussed is called a *mode of ventilation*. The different modes of ventilation differ in the trigger, limit, and cycle phase variables (Table 12-2).

Waveforms usually plot 1 of 3 parameters (pressure, flow, or volume) against time (Fig. 12-7). Time is plotted on the horizontal (*x*) axis and the other parameter is plotted on the vertical (*y*) axis. Flow-delivery waveforms are the next parameters to consider. Flow delivery can be set as square (rectangular), ascending ramp, descending ramp, sine (sinusoidal), or decay (exponential). See Figure 12-8.[1]

Loops are representations of pressure versus volume or flow versus volume. Expiration is typically depicted on the superior limb, and inspiration is on the inferior limb. A widened loop typically depicts increased airway resistance, whereas a narrowed loop typically depicts increased compliance (Fig. 12-9).[2]

TABLE 12-2 Mode of Ventilation and Their Trigger, Limit, and Cycle Phase Variables

Mode of Ventilation	Trigger	Limit	Cycle
Volume control	Ventilator or Patient	Volume	Volume/time
Pressure control	Ventilator or Patient	Pressure	Time
PRVC	Ventilator or Patient	Pressure	Time
Pressure support	Patient	Pressure	Flow
Volume support	Patient	Volume	Flow
CPAP	Patient	Pressure	Flow
SIMV	Ventilator or Patient	Volume, Pressure	Volume or time

CPAP = continuous positive airway pressure; PRVC = pressure-regulated volume control; SIMV = spontaneous intermittent mechanical ventilation.

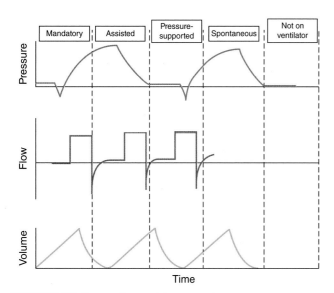

FIGURE 12-7 Waveforms of the types of breath.

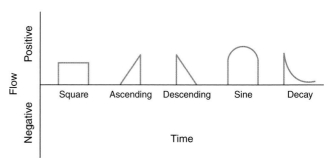

FIGURE 12-8 Types of flow.

MODES OF MECHANICAL VENTILATION

Mechanical ventilators are set to deliver a constant volume (volume cycled), a constant pressure (pressure cycled), or a combination of both with each breath. Modes of ventilation that maintain a minimum respiratory rate regardless of whether the patient initiates a spontaneous breath are referred to as assist-control (A/C) ventilation. Because pressures and volumes are directly linked by the pressure-volume curve, any given volume will correspond to a specific pressure, and vice versa, regardless of whether the ventilator is pressure or volume cycled.[3]

Each type of mechanical ventilation is a variation of ventilation and pressure; settings include respiratory rate, tidal volume, trigger sensitivity, flow rate, waveform, and inspiratory/expiratory (I/E) ratio. Each ventilation mode offers its own set of advantages and disadvantages.

Volume-Cycled Ventilation

Each breath delivers a preset tidal volume (volume control). The desired carbon dioxide removal is achieved via a fixed minute volume ($V_T \times RR$). This includes modes such as volume-controlled, volume-controlled spontaneous intermittent mechanical ventilation (SIMV), and volume-controlled continuous mandatory ventilation (Fig. 12-10A).

Spontaneous Intermittent Mechanical Ventilation

This mode is similar to A/C with 1 notable difference: Only the set breaths are fully supported. If the set rate is 6 and the

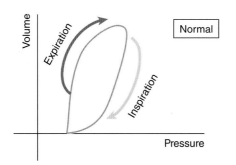

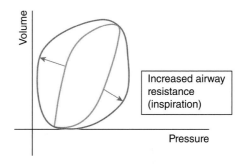

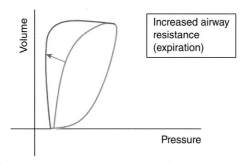

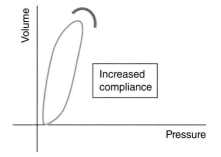

FIGURE 12-9 Variants of pressure versus volume loops.

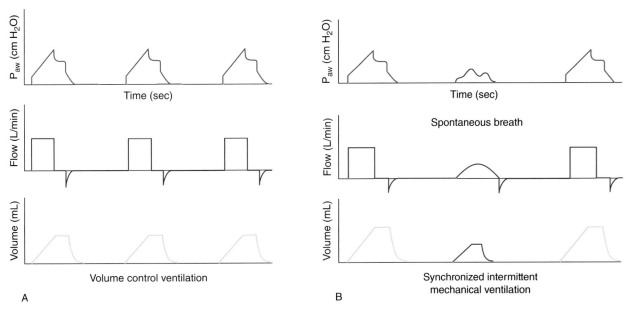

FIGURE 12-10 (A) Volume control ventilation. (B) Synchronized intermittent mechanical ventilation.

patient is breathing 12, then 6 of the breaths get the full set tidal volume and the other 6 get no support, pressure support, or volume support (Fig. 12-10B).

Pressure-Regulated Volume-Cycled Ventilation

Also known as VC+ on certain ventilators, pressure-regulated volume-cycled ventilation (PRVC) combines a pressure limit (pressure control) with volume assurance, thus guaranteeing a minimum minute ventilation. The ventilator adjusts the pressure from breath to breath, as the patient's airway resistance and respiratory system compliance changes to deliver the set tidal volume. The ventilator monitors each breath and compares the delivered tidal volume with the set tidal volume and adjusts the inspiratory pressure on the next breath appropriately (Fig. 12-11A).

Pressure-Cycled Ventilation

Parameters such as pressure and inspiratory time are set by the operator. Volume and flow are variable according to patient needs. The patient can breathe spontaneously during the inspiratory and expiratory phases of the PC mandatory breath cycle. This includes PCV, PC-SIMV, and APRV (Fig. 12-11B).

Airway Pressure Release Ventilation

This modified bilevel mode allows spontaneous breathing to occur at the upper pressure level (IRV), which is usually maintained throughout a long inspiratory phase. It is essentially the sum of continuous positive airway pressure (CPAP) and time-cycled pressure release.[38] Advantages include improved oxygenation and compliance secondary to spontaneous breathing,

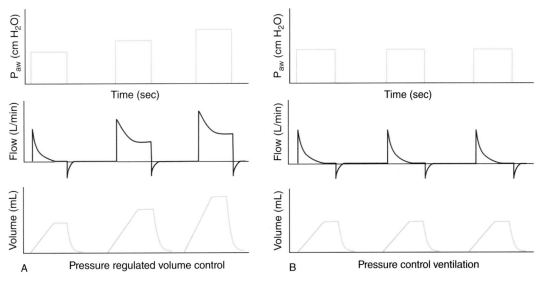

FIGURE 12-11 (A) Pressure regulated volume control. (B) Pressure control ventilation.

which improves $\dot{V}/\dot{Q}$ matching, increased cardiac output from improved venous return due to decreased intrathoracic pressure and right atrial pressure, improved perfusion to gastrointestinal tract and glomerular filtration rate, and decreased sedation and neuromuscular blockade use. The increased time at high pressures may improve recruitment. The pressure release feature allows for improved tidal volume (VT) for given ΔP by utilizing increased elastic recoil. There is less chance of overdistension given not "filling" lung but "emptying." The short release time does not allow significant derecruitment. Initial settings would include P_{high} at the P_{plat}, desired P_{mean} + 3 cm H_2O, or previous mean airway pressure, with a maximum of less than 35 cm H_2O; T_{high} at 4.5 to 6 seconds with respiratory rate of 8 to 12 beats/min; P_{low} at 0 cm H_2O; and T_{low} at 0.5 to 0.8 seconds with a target tidal volume of 4 to 6 mL/kg. The T_{low} is increased if VT is inadequate or shortened if VT is too high. (Fig. 12-12A).

High-Frequency Oscillatory Ventilation

High-frequency oscillatory ventilation (HFOV) provides adequate oxygenation and carbon dioxide clearance by breathing at small tidal volumes at or below dead space volumes, with exchange of fresh and old air in the airways and alveoli (Fig. 12-12). The very high respiratory rates (> 60 breaths/min) with small tidal volumes (also known as amplitudes) (1–4 mL/kg) are delivered at high frequencies (respiratory rate) of 3 to 15 Hertz (up to 900 breaths/min) by an oscillator pump. This rate is so fast that the airway pressure merely oscillates around a constant mean airway pressure. The constant mean airway pressure maintains alveolar recruitment, avoids low end-expiratory pressures, and avoids high peak airway pressures. A higher mean airway pressure is associated with better oxygenation. This method aims to prevent lung injury from overdistension and loss of recruitment (atelectrauma). Since the tidal volume is typically less than the dead space in this system, normal bulk flow of air would be deemed inadequate for effective gas exchange. It has been used in ARDS and bronchopleural fistula.

In conventional ventilation, gas mixing can be dependent on bulk convective flow, where tidal volumes must be an adequate size to fill anatomic dead space and the alveolar volume.[39] Inadequate tidal volumes lead to decreased clearance of carbon dioxide, development of atelectasisa, and reduction of mean airway pressure and oxygenation.[40]

In HFOV, there is improved gas exchanged at the alveolar level based on a few principles. There is an augmented longitudinal gas transport, since the velocity and concentration profile of oxygen is not homogenous, with higher concentrations at the core of the profile, and diffusion increases with velocity and tube diameter.[40] As forward movement occurs, there is continuous mixing of gas from the core to the periphery. Mixing is further enhanced by differences in inspiratory and expiratory profiles. This is called *coaxial flow*. The branching angles of the airways creates turbulent radial gas mixing from the center to the other layer.[40] There is also regional intra-alveolar inhomogeneity due to the difference in compliance and the resistance between neighboring alveoli, called *pendulluft*. There is further mixing of gases at the front of the flow called *Taylor dispersion*. Cardiac oscillations allow for cardiogenic mixing at the lungs adjacent to the heart, which serves as half of oxygen uptake in apneic patients.[40] Molecular diffusion also suggests that the slowing or cessation of flow causes instantaneous mixing of gases and appears to be more important in the periphery (see Fig. 12-12B).[39,40]

The initial HFOV settings include Fio_2 of 1, frequency between 5 and 10 Hz (with a suggestion of 8 Hz), mean airway pressure at 5 cm H_2O, and cycle volume at 170 mL if the frequency is 8 Hz, and base flow at 20 L/min.[39,40] An arterial blood gas is drawn after 15 to 30 minutes and settings are adjusted accordingly. Pao_2 is determined by P_{aw} and Fio_2.

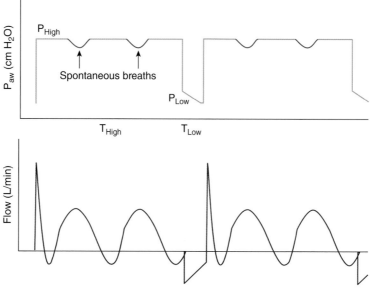

FIGURE 12-12A Airway pressure release ventilation. pressure high = P_{high}; pressure low = P_{low}; time high = T_{high}; time low = T_{low}. The spontaneous breaths seen are without pressure support, therefore appear concave. If with pressure support, the spontaneous breaths appear as convex.

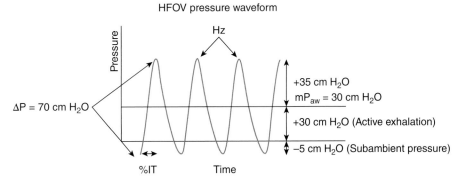

FIGURE 12-12B High Frequency Oscillatory Ventilation (HFOV). ΔP = oscillatory pressure amplitude; Hz = Hertz; *mPaw* = mean airway pressure; IT = inspiratory time. (Derdak S. High-frequency oscillatory ventilation for acute respiratory distress syndrome in adult patients. *Crit Care Med.* 2003;31:S317-S323. Reproduced with permission from Lippincott, Williams & Wilkins.)

$Paco_2$ is determined by oscillation frequency, amplitude, and inspiratory time. $Paco_2$ clearance is increased by increasing amplitude and decreasing frequency.

Advantages include decreased ventilator-induced lung injury, mobilization of secretions, and increased oxygenation. Disadvantages include heavy sedation/paralysis, higher risk of hemodynamic instability due to high mean airway pressures, and an active humidification requirement. Two studies, OSCILLATE[41] and OSCAR,[42] showed no evidence of benefit.

Proportional-Assist Ventilation

Proportional-assist ventilation (PAV) is another mode that attempts to overcome patient ventilator asynchrony and improve the work of breathing.[43-45] It is indicated for patient ventilator asynchrony and ventilator-dependent chronic obstructive pulmonary disease (COPD). Contraindications are deep sedation and bronchopleural fistulas. Most conventional modes of ventilation require pneumatic changes in flow or pressure to trigger a breath. Therefore, minimal respiratory effort might be required to trigger a breath, and the respiratory muscles are clinically silent during the second phase of inspiration.[43] However, this inspiration time might extend to the neural expiratory cycle of the patient's intrinsic breath cycle. This causes dyssynchrony and a paradoxically unnecessary burden on the respiratory muscles. Proportional-assist ventilation synchronizes the pressure assistance from the ventilator in direct proportion to the patient's inspiratory effort.[43] It determines the amount of assistance via the pressure out of respiratory muscles, which is the sum of elastance and all resistance forces[43-45]:

$$P_{musc} = (Flow \times Resistance) + (Volume \times Elastance)$$

Elastance is obtained via esophageal pressure monitoring or via the reciprocal of compliance. A comparison between PAV and pressure-support ventilation (PSV) is seen in Figure 12-13.[44] Note the wasted effort seen in PSV.

Neurally Adjusted Ventilation Assist

Neurally adjusted ventilation assist (NAVA) proportionally adjusts the level of assist depending on the diaphragmatic

muscle activity (EA_{di}) (Fig. 12-14). This is a surrogate for the neural respiratory drive and is measured via a transesophageal catheter. Diaphragmatic muscle activity is not captured in diaphragmatic hernia, central apnea without respiratory drive from brain damage or sedation, or phrenic nerve damage.[46-48]

Pressure-Support Ventilation

In spontaneously breathing patients, pressure support is delivered at a fixed pressure value. This partially replaces the patient's work of breathing and allows deeper breaths (Fig. 12-15).

Adaptive Support Ventilation

Adaptive support ventilation (ASV) is a positive pressure mode of mechanical ventilation that is closed-loop controlled, and automatically adjusts based on the patient's requirements. Closed-loop control involves a positive or negative feedback of the information on the respiratory mechanics of the patient. It is based on measurements made almost continuously that can be modified or adapted in a more physiological and individualized ventilatory support manner.[49] Adaptive support ventilation can be used as part of a lung protective strategy or as part of patient weaning.

There are 2 basic methods: (1) control between breaths (inter-breath), which refers to the setting of control between each breath, but keeping it constant throughout the breath cycle, and (2) intra breath control, which sets the control within the same breath.

In passive patients, ASV selects different tidal volume/respiratory rate combinations for normal lungs, COPD patients, and ARDS patients.[50] In active patients, ASV decreases work of breathing and improves patient-ventilator synchrony.[51] In the intensive care unit (ICU), ASV decreases the weaning duration in medical and surgical patients such as COPD adn postcardiac surgery.[52]

The basis for the adjustments is an equation that determines the respiratory rate that minimizes the work of inspiration at a given minute ventilation. This equation relies on an expiratory time constant, which can be obtained from

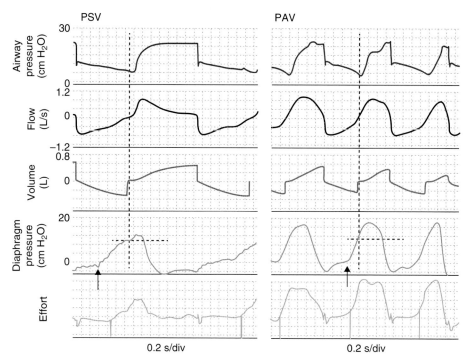

FIGURE 12-13 Comparison between Pressure Support Ventilation (PSV) and Proportional Assist Ventilation (PAV). The vertical dashed lines are the initiation of ventilator triggered breaths after generating 10 cm H20. In PSV, ventilator cycle extends beyond the expiration which can lead to ineffective efforts. The arrow is effort and delay to onset of breath is less with PAV. s = second; div = division. (Reproduced with permission from Younes M. Chapter 12. Proportional-assist Ventilation. In: Tobin MJ. eds. *Principles and Practice of Mechanical Ventilation*, 3e New York, NY: McGraw-Hill; 2013.)

the expiratory limb of the flow volume loop on a breath-by-breath basis.[53] Patients who have a long expiratory time constant (eg, COPD patients) receive a higher tidal volume and a lower respiratory rate when ventilated by ASV than patients with stiff lungs (eg, ARDS patients) or chest wall stiffness (eg, patients with kyphoscoliosis, morbid obesity, or a neuromuscular disorder) who expire quickly.

Automatic Tube Compensation

The endotracheal tube is the narrowest portion that connects the patient with the mechanical ventilator. The pressure flow curve of the endotracheal tube has a curvilinear pattern secondary to flow separation and turbulent flow greater than laminar flow.[54] At low flow states, flow is laminar but at high flow states, flow is turbulent. In a spontaneously breathing patient, there is great flow variability within the breath and between breaths and there is great variability within the flow dependent pressure drop in the endotracheal tube.[54] PSV is thought to overcome the resistance of the endotracheal tube via linear flow support. However, at low flow states, PSV overcompensates and at high flow states PSV undercompensates.[55-57] Automatic tube compensation (ATC) causes a nonlinear flow support by increasing pressure during inspiration and decreases pressure during expiration. This is calculated based on the size of the endotracheal tube. ATC can act as an adjunct mode of ventilation but has not been shown to be beneficial in weaning.[58,59]

INDICATIONS FOR WEANING AND SPONTANEOUS BREATHING TRIALS

Weaning implies the gradual reduction of ventilatory support once the patient appears to have improved. In acute respiratory failure, a daily spontaneous breathing test (SBT) for 30 to 120 minutes is associated with quicker extubation.[60] A spontaneous breathing trial can be performed via different modes such as SIMV and T-piece but PSV has been favored to be the best approach. It has been estimated that as much as 42% of the time that a patient spends on a mechanical ventilator is during the discontinuation process.[1]

Readiness for weaning includes the following:

- Adequate oxygenation: Pao_2 more than or equal to 60 mmHg on Fio_2 less than or equal to 0.4 (Pao_2/Fio_2 = 150–300) with PEEP less than or equal to 5 cm H_2O;
- hemodynamic stability or minimal pressor requirements such as norepinephrine 5 μg/kg/h;
- no myocardial ischemia or clinically significant hypotension;
- temperature less than 38°C;
- no significant acid–base disturbance (ie, absence of respiratory acidosis);
- hemoglobin more than or equal to 7–10 g/dL;
- patient arousable and can follow commands;
- stable metabolic status (eg, acceptable electrolytes);
- adequate cough; and
- able to initiate an inspiratory effort.

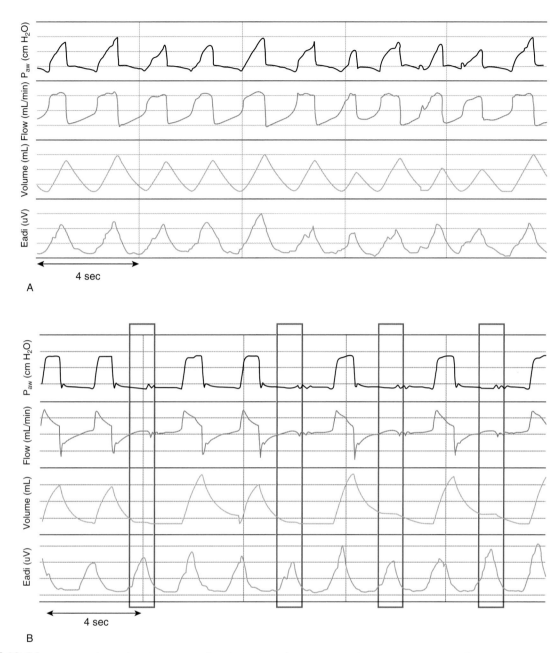

FIGURE 12-14 Example of recording during neurally adjusted ventilatory assist and pressure-support ventilation. (A) Neurally adjusted ventilatory assist using the neural trigger: No dysynchrony observed. (B) Pressure-support ventilation: wasted efforts are underscored. Each wasted effort is identified by a blue rectangle. EAdi is diaphragmatic electrical activity. (Source: Terzi N , Piquilloud L, Rozé H, et al. Clinical Review: Update on Neurally Adjusted Ventilatory Assist – Report of a Round Table Conference. *Critical Care.* 2012;16(225):1-13.)

A successful SBT is considered if the following parameters are met after 30 to 120 minutes:

- oxygen saturation (Sao_2) more than 90% or Pao_2 more than 60 mmHg on Fio_2 less than 0.4–0.5;
- increase in $Paco_2$ less than 10 mmHg or decrease in pH less than 0.10;
- respiratory rate less than 35 breaths/min;
- heart rate less than 135 or increased less than 20% from baseline; and
- systolic blood pressure more than 90 mmHg or change less than 20% from baseline.

Rapid shallow breathing index (RSBI) may be used to predict the likelihood of extubation failure. It is calculated as the respiratory rate (f) divided by tidal volume (V_T) in liters. An RSBI less than 105 is associated with a lower likelihood of extubation failure.[62] Rapid shallow breathing index (f/V_T) has a sensitivity 97%, specificity 64%, PPV 78%, and NPV 95%.[62] Accuracy is higher if measured after 30 minutes of spontaneous breathing.[63]

SBT and RSBI are not the only considerations for extubation. Patient's mental status, risks for tracheal edema such as prolonged extubation or traumatic intubation, worsening

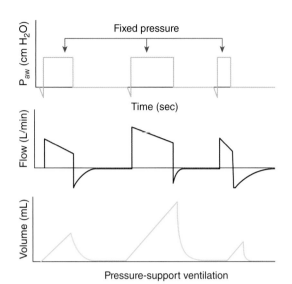

FIGURE 12-15 Pressure-support ventilation.

or new organ failure, and copious secretions should also be considered.

TRACHEOSTOMY

Tracheostomy is often considered in patients who have failed to be weaned after 7 days, have a functional or structural disorder of the upper airway (eg, maxillofacial trauma, neck surgery, angioedema, malignancy, subglottic stenosis, or vocal cord disease), and/or need airway protection (eg, in brain injury, neuromuscular diseases, or excessive respiratory secretion).[64]

Benefits

Prolonged translaryngeal intubation can lead to oral damage and ulceration, lip necrosis, dental damage, obstruction of sinus drainage, laryngeal trauma, cricoid cartilage damage, cuff-induced tracheal injury, and ventilator-associated pneumonia (VAP).[65] Tracheostomy placement has been shown to reduce dead space, airway resistance, and work of breathing, and facilitate weaning.[66,67] By preventing microaspiration of secretions, tracheostomy might reduce ventilator-associated pneumonia.[68] It also enables the healthcare provider to decrease the amount of sedation use, improve patient comfort, facilitate the weaning process, shorten ICU and hospital stay, give the patient more capability to communicate, facilitate performing a swallow study to evaluate the swallowing, allow for maintaining oral hygiene, and allow for easier and safer nursing care.[65]

Timing

Early (within 7–10 days of the intubation) versus late (more than 2–3 weeks) tracheostomy placement has shown conflicting data in respect to mortality, ventilator-associated pneumonia, and ventilator days.[68-70] Early tracheostomy is strongly suggested in patients when prolonged mechanical ventilation is predicted, such as in patients with neurologic disorders, muscular diseases, trauma, laryngotracheal pathology, and a slow healing

pulmonary disease such as advanced interstitial lung disease, COPD, or severe pneumonia with extensive lung damage.[71,72]

Types of Tracheostomy

There are 2 major techniques for tracheostomy placement: percutaneous dilatational tracheostomy (PDT) and surgical tracheostomy (ST). Percutaneous dilatational tracheostomy has been increasingly used as an alternative to ST because of the ease to perform by the bedside, minimize transportation, and decrease in the cost. Despite there is tendency for less bleeding and infection in PDT, there has been no difference in either technique in the outcome of the patients or complications rate.[73-77]

Complications

Complications of tracheostomy placement can be categorized into immediate, early, and late. Immediate complications usually are related to the technique of the procedure and the skills of the operator (bleeding, tracheal damage, or air embolism). Careful coordination should be taken to avoid aspiration, losing the airway, or gas exchange problems (hypoxemia, hypercapnia). Early complications include in addition to above, pneumothorax, pneumomediastinum, subcutaneous emphysema, stomal ulceration, accidental decannulation, and dysphagia.[78] Late complications include tracheal stenosis, granulation tissue formation, tracheomalacia, tracheoarterial fistula, ventilator-associated pneumonia, and aspiration.[79] Fatal complications and death is estimated to be 0.17%. Almost one-third occurs during the procedure and half of these complications occur within 7 days of the procedure. The main causes of death are hemorrhage (38.0%), airway complications (29.6%), tracheal perforation (15.5%), and pneumothorax (5.6%).[80]

PATIENT-VENTILATOR DYSSYNCHRONY

Patient-ventilator dyssynchrony occurs when the patient's demands are not met by the ventilator (Fig. 12-16).

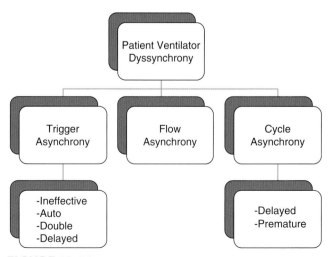

FIGURE 12-16 Patient-ventilator dyssynchrony.

TABLE 12-3 Types of Triggering, Description, Causes, and Intervention

Types	Description	Causes	Intervention
Ineffective triggering	Insensitive trigger setting, untriggered breaths	High iPEEP, weakness, incorrect vent settings	Apply PEEP, decrease RR/Vт, increase expiration time, reduce sedation, decrease trigger threshold
Inappropriate triggering	Patient inspires while the ventilator cycles to expiration	Short inspiratory time, low inspiratory flow rate, low tidal volume	Adjust trigger
Auto-triggering	Hiccups, coughing, cardiac oscillations, shivering, seizures, "rain out"	Hiccups, coughing, shivering, seizures, condensation in circuit, low trigger sensitivity	Adjust trigger setting

PEEP = positive end-expiratory pressure; RR = respiratory rate; Vт = tidal volume.

It is easiest to distinguish patient factors from ventilator factors. Patient factors include ventilator drive (inspiration), ventilator requirements (flow, volume), timing (I:E ratio). Ventilator factors include triggers on inspiration (flow, volume, pressure), delivery mechanisms (flow, volume, pressure), and cycling criteria.[81] Refer to Table 12-3 for types of triggering and management options.

VENTILATORY-INDUCED LUNG INJURY

Alveolar overdistension and cyclic atelectasis are the principal initiators of alveolar injury during positive pressure ventilation.[82] Alveolar overdistension is mitigated by using small tidal volumes, maintaining a low plateau pressure, and using pressure limited ventilation. Applied PEEP is the principal method used to keep the alveoli open and lessen cyclic atelectasis. Open lung ventilation is a ventilatory strategy that combines small tidal volumes (to lessen alveolar overdistension) and an applied PEEP above the low inflection point on the pressure-volume curve (to lessen cyclic atelectasis).[83]

SPECIAL CONSIDERATIONS

Cardiothoracic Surgery

Postoperative pulmonary dysfunction (PPD) is a frequent complication after cardiac surgery. Its pathogenesis is related to pulmonary inflammation, extracorporeal circulation (ECC), ischemia-reperfusion injury, and atelectasis.[84] Protective ventilation strategies can reduce the incidence of atelectasis and pulmonary infections in surgical patients. The open lung ventilation (OLA) strategy applies recruiting maneuvers and sufficient PEEP to increase transpulmonary pressure enough for opening the maximum possible number of alveoli with minimum delta pressure (P_{plat} – PEEP) to prevent pulmonary overdistension.[85]

Another complication is bronchopleural fistula. These patients come out of the operating room with a chest tube. The presence of a persistent air leak more than 24 hours after insertion of a chest tube is highly suggestive of a bronchopleural fistula (after exclusion of an external leak).

Weaning from positive pressure ventilation entirely is optimal. When not possible, it is important to select the strategy to minimize minute ventilation and intrathoracic pressure. Some strategies include the following:

- PSV may be preferable to full ventilation.
- Limit mean airway pressure and number of high pressure breaths.
- Avoid alkalosis; consider permissive hypercapnia.
- Minimize PEEP (intrinsic and extrinsic).
- Treat bronchospasm.
- Limit V_T to 6 to 8 mL/kg.
- Minimize inspiratory time (keep I:E ratio low, use high flows).
- Use the lowest chest tube suction that maintains lung inflation.

Neurologic/Neurosurgical

These patients can have ventilatory dysfunction that can lead to hypoxia and/or hypercapnia. Hyperventilation, head elevation, hypertonic saline, mannitol, and external ventricular drain placement are methods to help decrease intracranial pressure.

Neuromuscular Diseases

Expiratory muscles in muscular dystrophies are more impaired than inspiratory muscles. Weakened abdominal muscles reduce the ability to cough, as reflected by decreased peak expiratory flow rates. Indications for initiation of mechanical ventilation in neuromuscular diseases include the following:

- subjective symptoms (orthopnea, morning headaches, daytime somnolence, fatigue)
- cor pulmonale
- vital capacity less than 15–20 mL/kg (normal, 60–70 mL/kg), 60% predicted, 1 Liter, or 30–50% of prior measurement
- maximal inspiratory pressure (MIP) less negative than –30 cm H_2O;
- MEP less than 40 cm H_2O
- nasal "sniff" pressure less than 25 cm H_2O
- daytime Paco$_2$ more than 45 mmHg

- sustained nocturnal hemoglobin desaturation (> 5 minutes or > 10% of total study time)
- recurrent acute respiratory failure episodes requiring intervention; and
- failure to respond to continuous positive pressure.[86]

Noninvasive ventilation (NIV) is also an accepted support for people with neuromuscular and chest wall disorders. Improvements in ventilator modes, interfaces, and adjunctive secretion-removal techniques have facilitated care and increased the quality of life in such individuals.[87]

Pregnancy

During pregnancy, progesterone increases ventilation by increasing the respiratory center's sensitivity to carbon dioxide. Therefore, the tidal volume and minute ventilation are increased. The respiratory alkalosis is compensated by an increase in the excretion of bicarbonates by the kidneys, resulting in a normal pH. The plasma oncotic pressure falls during pregnancy, and the lung lymphatics may be affected by the smooth muscle relaxation seen in pregnancy. The gravid uterus causes a widened anteroposterior transverse diameter of the chest and an elevated diaphragm, which translates to an increased tidal volume, reduced functional residual capacity, and increased oxygen consumption.

Asthma and Chronic Obstructive Pulmonary Disease

One major cause of the morbidity and mortality arising during mechanical ventilation in patients with asthma and COPD is excessive dynamic pulmonary hyperinflation (DH) with intrinsic PEEP (or auto-PEEP). Dynamic hyperinsufflation appears when the pulmonary volume at the end of expiration is greater than the functional residual capacity as a consequence of insufficient emptying of the lung, by starting inspiration before completing the preceding expiration.[87,88] Hyperinsufflation increases the positive intrathoracic pressure, accentuating the decrease in venous return and increasing the pulmonary vascular resistances and, thus, right ventricle post-loading, causing hypotension.

Pneumothorax

Barotrauma from mechanical ventilation is a cause of iatrogenic pneumothorax, along with central venous catheters, thoracentesis, and transbronchial biopsies.[89,90] Papazian et al have suggested that the early administration of a neuromuscular blockade in ARDS, within 48 hours, has reduced the incidence of pneumothorax.[91] Treatment is emergent evacuation of air from pleural space. This can be accomplished via needle decompression and then tube thoracotomy or tube thoracotomy.[89] Needle decompression is reserved for tension pneumothorax or impending tension pneumothorax. It is performed by inserting a 14-guage to 16-guage needle in the second anterior intercostal space in the midclavicular line or in the fourth to fifth intercostal space in the midaxillary line. Small (10–14F) chest tubes are preferred over large (> 30F) chest tubes due to their high success rate and minimal complications.[91-93]

The tube thoracotomy is attached to a Pleur-evac. The Pleur-evac typically consists of 3 chambers: the collection chamber, the water seal, and the suction chamber. Fluid is typically filled up to the 2-cm mark for water seal. The suction source should be initially set at −80 mmHg at 20 Liters of air flow meter with a suction control setting of −20 cm H_2O.[94] Suction monitor bellows must expand. If it does not, check the settings to make sure there are no leaks or kinks in the system. For multiple tubes in 1 suction port, the suction source should be set more negative than −80 mmHg.

Bubbling in the water seal chamber may indicate an air leak. Investigation should begin with sequential clamping of the chest tube from proximal to distal to find the location of source of leak. If clamping of the chest tube at the proximal end resolves the leak, the most likely source is in the chest. This might be from the pneumothorax or bronchopleural fistula. If bubbling does not resolve by 5 to 7 days, cardiothoracic referral is warranted.[92,94] PEEP is typically contraindicated because it can make the pneumothorax worse, and if there is bronchopleural fistula, it will prevent it from healing.

Prolonged Mechanical Ventilation

When patients fail to be weaned from the ventilator and require mechanical ventilation for at least 21 days, they are considered to have prolonged mechanical ventilation (PMV). Barriers to mechanical ventilation are related to age, with associated anabolic resistance, comorbidities, and underlying cardiorespiratory disease.[95] These patients typically have a tracheostomy and can have a protocolized respiratory therapist–driven weaning protocol.

NONINVASIVE MECHANICAL VENTILATION

Noninvasive ventilation provides positive pressure ventilation delivered through a noninvasive interface (nasal mask, face mask, or nasal plugs). Candidates for noninvasive mechanical ventilation include acute COPD exacerbation with decompensated pH, cardiogenic pulmonary edema, respiratory failure in immunocompromised patients, palliative care, postoperative patients such as supradiaphragmatic, abdominal, and pelvic sugery, chest trauma, and post-extubation.[96] Clinical improvement is evident within 1 hour with improvement in vital signs such as blood pressure, respiratory rate, heart rate, oxygen saturation, and work of breathing. Ideally, an arterial blood gas should show an improvement with pH secondary to improvement in CO_2 and/or PO_2.

Contraindications include the following:

- cardiac or respiratory arrest;
- inability to cooperate, protect the airway, or clear secretions;

- severely impaired consciousness;
- nonrespiratory organ failure that is acutely life threatening;
- facial surgery, trauma, or deformity;
- high aspiration risk; and
- prolonged duration of mechanical ventilation anticipated.

Lack of improvement or indications and/or presence of contraindications should prompt for invasive mechanical ventilation. Delay in intubation is associated with high mortality.[96]

Interface

Patient-ventilator interfaces available for NIV include a full-face mask, oronasal mask, nasal mask, and nasal prongs. The efficacy of the various interfaces has been examined in a few studies. The face mask conferred the greatest physiologic improvement, but the nasal mask was best tolerated.[97]

Initiation

Based on these studies, the oronasal mask is generally preferred over a nasal mask or nasal prongs during the initiation of NIV. The primary disadvantage of the full face and oronasal masks is that monitoring for aspiration is more difficult.

Setting

Assist control requires that a tidal volume, respiratory rate, inspiratory flow rate, applied PEEP, and Fio_2 be set. To increase tidal volume, increase IPAP. To increase SpO_2/ineffective effort, increase EPAP this is synonymous with CPAP. Pressure support (PS) can be derived from IPAP-EPAP.

IPAP starts at 8 to 12 cm H_2O (maximum, 20–25 cm H_2O). EPAP starts at 3 to 5 cm H_2O (maximum, 10–15 cm H_2O). For persistent hypercapnea, increase IPAP in 2-cm H_2O increments (to a maximum of 20–25 cm H_2O), while maintaining the tidal volume at a maximum of 6 to 8 mL/kg. Predict required new minute ventilation (MV = Tidal Volume × Respiratory Rate). MVnew = (Paco2 now/Paco2 goal) × Mvcurrent where the Paco2 goal is 10 mmHg improved from the current level (eg, 60 mmHg instead of 70 mmHg). For persistent hypoxia, increase IPAP and EPAP in increments of 2-cm H_2O. Both IPAP and EPAP must be increased by the same amount to maintain the same tidal volume.

High-Flow Nasal Cannula

High-flow nasal cannula (HFNC) oxygen therapy comprises an oxygen blender, a humidifier, and a nasal cannula. It delivers adequately heated and humidified medical gas at up to 60 L/min of flow. It reduces anatomical dead space, has a PEEP effect, has a constant fraction of inspired oxygen, and provides good humidification.

For reduction of anatomic dead space, thoracoabdominal synchrony is better with HFNC than with face-mask delivery.

Breathing frequency is lower with HFNC, while $Paco_2$ and V_T (calculated from rib cage and abdominal measurements) remain constant.[98] Since V_T is constant and breathing frequency is reduced, minute ventilation is lower. It is also likely that alveolar ventilation, along with $Paco_2$, is constant. This evidence suggests that there is less dead space.[98]

High-flow nasal cannulas have been found to be effective for mild to moderate hypoxemic respiratory failure and were associated with significant reductions in breathing frequency, heart rate, dyspnea score, supraclavicular retraction and thoracoabdominal asynchrony, and significant improvement in Spo_2.[99] However, the FLORALI study, a small multicenter, open-label trial found that in patients with acute hypoxemic respiratory failure and without hypercapnia, treatment with high-flow nasal oxygen, standard face mask oxygen, or non-invasive ventilation did not result in significantly different intubation rates. There was a significant difference in favor of high-flow nasal oxygen in 90-day mortality.[100] Compared to high-flow face mask, HFNC as a preoxygenation device did not reduce the lowest level of desaturation in a randomized controlled trial (RCT).[100]

Humidification conditioning of the gas minimizes airway constriction and reduces the work of breathing. It improves mucociliary function, facilitates clearance of secretions, and is associated with less atelectasis, resulting in a good ventilation/perfusion ratio and better oxygenation. In other words, conditioning gases results in more effective delivery of oxygen to the lungs.[101]

Millar et al have reported the successful use of HFNC oxygen therapy to manage the hypercapnic respiratory failure of a patient unable to tolerate conventional NIV.[102] Bräunlich evaluated the effect of HFNC in healthy volunteers, COPD patients, and idiopathic pulmonary fibrosis (IPF) patients.[103] Tidal volume increased in the COPD and IPF groups, while it decreased in the healthy volunteers. Breathing frequency and minute volume decreased in all groups.[99]

QUESTIONS

1. A 75-year-old man is admitted to the ICU with COPD exacerbation, and he required invasive mechanical ventilation. The patient is started on intravenous corticosteroids and bronchodilators. The patient has been stable on A/C volume control mode with V_T of 500 mL, a rate of 12 breaths/min, a PEEP of 8 cm H_2O, and an Fio_2 of 50% with oxygen saturation of 98%. On his second day, the nurse notice sudden oxygen desaturation, agitation, and oral gurgling. Clinically, the patient seems agitated and uncomfortable. There are diminished breathing sounds bilaterally. There is no evidence of subcutaneous emphysema. The respiratory therapist also noticed a sudden change in his ventilator parameters. His ventilator parameters before and after the event are as follows:

Ventilator Parameters	Before	After
Peak pressure	35 cm H_2O	25 cm H_2O
Plateau pressure	25 cm H_2O	15 cm H_2O
Airway resistance	10 cm H_2O/L/sec	2 cm H_2O/L/sec
Respiratory rate	16 breaths/min	24 breaths/min
O_2 saturation	98%	85%
End-tidal CO_2	40 mmHg	20 mmHg
Exhaled tidal volume	450 mL	150 mL

What is the most likely diagnosis?

A. Pneumothorax
B. Rupture of the ET cuff
C. Exacerbation of the COPD
D. Pulmonary edema

2. A 65-year-old man with a past medical history of severe COPD and forced expiratory volume during the first second (FEV1) of 0.70 Liter is admitted with progressive dyspnea, wheezing, and excessive accessory respiratory muscle use due to an upper respiratory viral infection. The patient did not show any improvement on noninvasive ventilation and he required intubation and mechanical ventilation. Two hours later, his physical examination reveals the following:

Vital signs: temperature of 98.5°F, pulse of 125 beats/min, blood pressure (BP) of 80/45 mmHg, RR of 32 breaths/min

General: patient is awake, alert, and extremely agitated

Chest: diffuse bilateral wheezing with crackles

Cardiovascular: normal sinus rhythm with tachycardia

Abdomen: soft, not tender, and distended

Extremities: 2+ pitting edema bilaterally in the lower extremities

Peak pressure is 60 cm H_2O.

What is the most appropriate next step in managing this patient?

A. Prolong I:E ratio
B. Increase tidal volume
C. Increase respiratory rate
D. Disconnect the ET tube from the ventilator circuit for a few seconds

3. A 35-year-old obese man is admitted to the ICU with ARDS secondary to acute pancreatitis. The patient is intubated and on mechanical ventilation. The patient is synchronizing well with the ventilator and he has been hemodynamically stable.

The following are the mechanical ventilator setting and parameters:

Mode	Pressure Control Ventilation
Rate (ventilator)	20
Rate (patient)	20
Tidal volume	6 mL/kg
PEEP	10
Intrinsic PEEP	+5
Fio_2	100%
O_2 saturation	81%
Peak pressure	36
Plateau pressure	30
Minute ventilation	11

Fio_2 = fraction of inspired oxygen; PEEP = positive end-expiratory pressure.

If the transpulmonary pressure measured at the end of the inspiration is 10 cm H_2O, what is the next necessary change needing to be performed?

A. Increase PEEP
B. Decrease tidal volume
C. Increase respiratory rate
D. Increase inspiratory time

4. A 70-year-old man is admitted to the medical ICU with COPD exacerbation. The patient is started on noninvasive ventilation without success. The patient's respiratory status has continued to deteriorate, and he has required intubation and mechanical ventilation. The intensivist decides to start the patient on Adaptive Support Ventilation mode. Which of the following choices includes the required setting parameter(s)?

A. Driving pressure control
B. Respiratory rate and tidal volume (minute ventilation)
C. Lung compliance and airway resistance
D. Ideal body weight and desired minute ventilation

5. A 70-year-old man is admitted to the ICU with COPD exacerbation secondary to pneumonia. The patient requires intubation and mechanical ventilation. The ventilator graphics are noticed to have prolongation of the expiratory time of the flow and sometimes the absence of the patient's ventilator triggers, despite the patient's movement of the chest and abdominal wall muscles to initiate and trigger the next breath. What is the most appropriate next step in managing this patient?

A. Decrease sedation
B. Increase respiratory rate
C. Decrease the flow rate
D. Increase the PEEP Level

6. Match the following major mechanisms of the gas exchange in high-flow oscillator ventilation with their definition:

a) Pendelluft	I. Movement of new molecules to occupy space made available as old molecules are absorbed into the alveoli
b) Coaxial flow	II. Movement of gas from smaller alveoli to larger alveoli
c) Taylor dispersion	III. Movement of gas from central to the peripheral airway
d) Molecular diffusion	IV. Movement of central part of flow inside the airway and movement of peripheral part of flow outside of airway
e) Bulk convection flow	V. Movement of gas enhance by molecular collision

A. a) II; b) IV; c) III; d) V; e) I
B. a) I; b) II; c) III; d) IV; e) V
C. a) III; b) II; c) I; d) V; e) IV
D. a) I; b) II; c) IV; d) V; e) III

7. A 50-year-old obese man with history of obstructive sleep apnea (OSA), hypertension, and diabetes mellitus is admitted for ARDS and has been placed on APRV. The current arterial blood gas shows a pH of 7.00, a P_{CO_2} of 100 mmHg, a P_{O_2} 90 mmHg, and carbonate (CO_3) of 28 mEq/L. What adjustment is necessary to improve the hypercapnia?

A. Automatic tube compensation (ATC) turned off
B. T_{low} increased
C. T_{high} increased
D. P_{high} decreased

8. A 30-year-old woman with ARDS presumed to be triggered by a recent bout of influenza has been on APRV. Her F_{IO_2} is currently 40%. Her current settings are the following: P_{high} of 25 cm H_2O, P_{low} of 0 cm H_2O, T_{high} of 6 seconds, and T_{low} of 0.5 seconds. How is this patient weaned from the ventilator?

A. Decrease P_{high} and increase T_{high}
B. Increase P_{high} and decrease T_{high}
C. Transition to CPAP with PEEP of 10 cm H_2O and PS of 5 to 10 cm H_2O
D. Transition to CPAP with PEEP of 5 cm H_2O and PS of 5 to 10 cm H_2O

9. A 49-year-old man is admitted for asthma exacerbation. His current mechanical ventilation waveforms are below (Fig. 12-17). What mode is being used?

A. AC
B. PCV
C. SIMV
D. PRVC

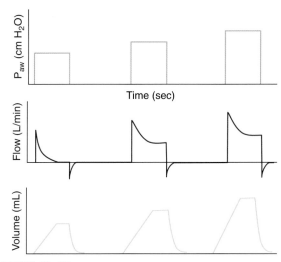

FIGURE 12-17 Mode of mechanical ventilation for patient admitted for asthma exacerbation.

10. Which of the following is the optimal pressure-volume plot?

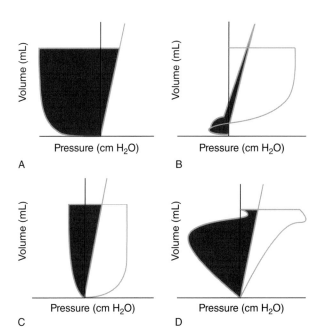

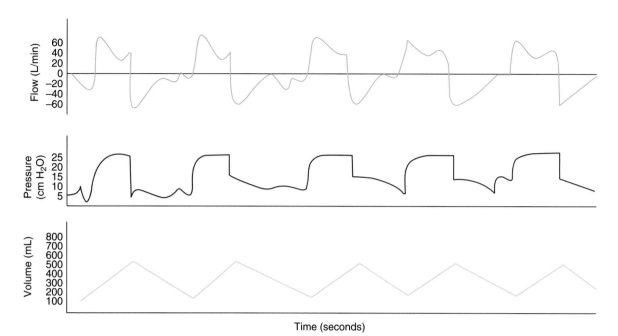

FIGURE 12-18 The ventilator waveform of a patient admitted for respiratory failure. (Adapted from deWit M. Monitoring of patient-ventilator interaction at the bedside. *Respir Care*. 2011;56(1):61-68.)

11. A patient with acute respiratory failure has the following ventilator waveforms. (Fig. 12-18). What is the cause of the asynchrony?

   A. Increased sedation
   B. Decreased tidal volume
   C. Decreased inspiratory time
   D. Cardiac oscillations

12. A 60-year-old man is admitted for respiratory failure with volume-controlled ventilation. The ventilator wave form is seen below (Fig. 12-19). What would be the next step?

   A. Increase flow
   B. Decrease flow
   C. Increase tidal volume
   D. Decrease tidal volume

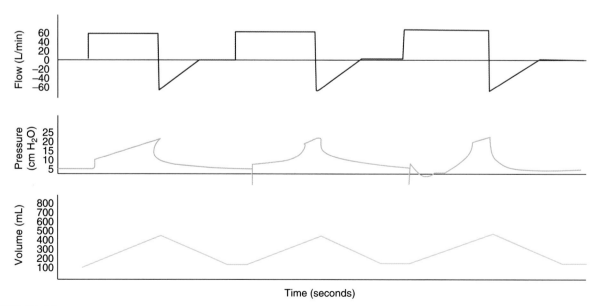

FIGURE 12-19 Volume controlled ventilation waveform for patient admitted for respiratory failure. (Adapted from Nilsestuen JO. Using Ventilator Graphics to Identify Patient-Ventilator Asynchrony. *Respir Care*. 2005;50(2):202-232.)

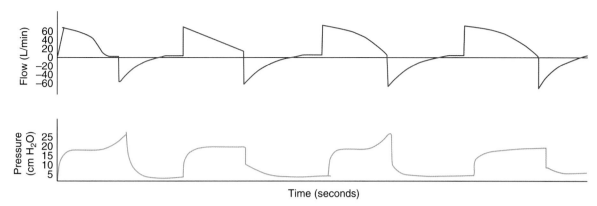

FIGURE 12-20 Ventilator waveform with dyssynchrony in PRVC. (Adapted from Nilsestuen JO. Using Ventilator Graphics to Identify Patient-Ventilator Asynchrony. *Respir Care.* 2005;50(2):202-232.)

13. In PRVC mode, what type of dyssynchrony is seen in Figure 12-20?

    A. Delayed termination
    B. Premature termination
    C. Rapid rise time
    D. Inadequate flow

14. A 50-year-old woman is admitted for asthma-COPD overlap exacerbation. She is hemodynamically stable. Her flow-time wave form is below (Fig. 12-21). What would be the next step?

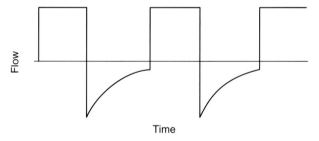

FIGURE 12-21 Flow-time scalar.

    A. Decrease expiratory time
    B. No change
    C. Increase tidal volume
    D. Increase PEEP

15. A 70-year-old man with chronic hypoxic and hypercapnic respiratory failure secondary to COPD is intubated for COPD exacerbation for the last 3 days. The patient has been on pressure support for 2 hours and the blood gas shows pH 7.35/pCO$_2$ 80 mmHg/pO$_2$ 60 mmHg/CO$_2$ 35 mmol/L. The patient is awake and following commands. His endotracheal secretions are moderate, and his cough reflex is weak. His RSBI is 85. What is the next step?

    A. Extubate the patient to noninvasive positive pressure ventilation (NIPPV)
    B. Extend the weaning trial for another hour
    C. Extubate the patient on nasal cannula
    D. Extubate the patient on oxymask

16. A 56-year-old man with a 30-pack-year smoking history, COPD, and peripheral vascular disease is admitted for right femoral popliteal bypass. Anesthesia has attempted to extubate him but he subsequently developed shortness of breath and hypoxia. Nebulizers, corticosteroids, and NIPPV are applied. Two hours later, the patient has increased work of breathing, and his oxygen saturation would intermittently drop to the 70s. His chest radiograph has shown a persistent infiltrate on the right lower lobe. On the second day, the chest radiograph shows no acute pulmonary disease. The patient is being liberated from the mechanical ventilator. What should be considered?

    A. Minimizing sedation
    B. Ventilator liberation protocol
    C. Protocolized rehabilitation toward early mobilization
    D. All of the above

17. A 42-year-old obese woman with OSA, diabetes mellitus, and hypertension is admitted for community-acquired pneumonia. After multiple attempts, she is emergently intubated with ET tube size 8.5. She has been intubated for 7 days and today she has tolerated the spontaneous breathing trial. What is the next step?

    A. Extubation to oxymask
    B. Cuff-leak test
    C. Tracheal ultrasound
    D. Solumedrol 40 mg IV

18. A 40-year-old woman with asthma exacerbation has been intubated for 3 days. She is on nebulizers and corticosteroids. She is on PRVC with a tidal volume of 400, a respiratory rate of 16 breaths/min, an Fio_2 of 40%, and PEEP of 5 cm H_2O. How is the RSBI calculated on this patient?

    A. Place the patient on a CPAP of 5 cm H_2O and calculate the respiratory rate over the tidal volume.
    B. Place the patient on a PEEP of 5 cm H_2O with a PS of 10 cm H_2O and calculate the respiratory rate over the tidal volume.
    C. Place the patient on a T-piece and calculate the tidal volume over the respiratory rate.
    D. Place the patient on a T-piece with a PS of 10 cm H_2O and calculate the tidal volume over the respiratory rate.

19. Which of the following is true regarding the role of an endotracheal tube in ventilator-associated pneumonia?

    A. A tracheal pressure of 20 to 30 cm H_2O is needed to prevent microaspiration.
    B. Transition to polyvinyl cuff and globular form is needed to prevent microaspiration.
    C. Oral chlorhexidine can be used to prevent oral colonization and, subsequently, VAP.
    D. Antibacterial adaptation to ET tubes is not possible.

20. A 65-year-old man with coronary artery disease and COPD is intubated for community-acquired pneumonia and COPD exacerbation. He has failed weaning trials and a tracheostomy is placed on day 14. He subsequently has a cardiac arrest secondary to non-ST-elevation myocardial infarction. He is unable to be weaned off from vasopressors and required hemodialysis. What is the mortality of this patient?

    A. 15%
    B. 50%
    C. 85%
    D. 97%

21. Which mode has the highest variation of breaths?

    A. VACV
    B. PACV
    C. PS
    D. Pressure SIMV

22. Which of the following scenarios has the highest recommendation for noninvasive positive pressure ventilation?

    A. Acute severe COPD exacerbation with pH less than 7.35
    B. Cardiogenic pulmonary edema on vasopressor support and active ischemia
    C. Asthma exacerbation
    D. Acute hypoxic respiratory failure in a bone marrow transplant recipient

23. A 60-year-old man with chronic hypoxic and hypercapnic respiratory failure secondary to COPD is admitted for COPD exacerbation. He has been given ipratropium-albuterol nebulizers every 6 hours and solumedrol 60 mg intravenously (IV) every 6 hours, and placed on bilevel positive airway pressure (BPAP). His initial blood gas showed the following: pH 7.15/PCO_2 100 mmHg/PO_2 mmHg 65/HCO_2 35 mmol/L. His chest radiograph shows hyperinflated lungs but no acute pulmonary disease. Which of the following is a predictor of the successful use of the BPAP?

    A. O_2 saturation of 94%
    B. Respiratory rate of 24 breaths/min
    C. Tidal volume of 400 mL
    D. Glasgow coma score (GCS) of 10

24. Which of the following is true?

    A. Asthma has a low compliance and a low resistance.
    B. COPD has a high compliance and a high resistance.
    C. ARDS has a low compliance and a low resistance.
    D. Obesity has a high compliance and a high resistance.

25. What is the transpulmonary pressure without and with spontaneous breaths in Figure 12-22?

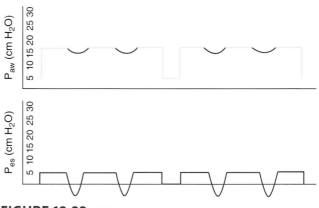

FIGURE 12-22 APRV mode.

A. Without spontaneous breath, TPP = 10 cm H_2O; with spontaneous breath, TPP = 25 cm H_2O

B. Without spontaneous breath, TPP = 15 cm H_2O; with spontaneous breath, TPP = 30 cm H_2O

C. Without spontaneous breath, TPP = 20 cm H_2O; with spontaneous breath, TPP = 20 cm H_2O

D. Without spontaneous breath, TPP = 25 cm H_2O; with spontaneous breath, TPP = 15 cm H_2O

26. In HFOV, which is the initial method for removing excessive CO_2?

    A. Cycle volume set to maximum
    B. Frequency set to minimum
    C. Mean airway pressure increased by 5 cm H_2O
    D. Bias flow increased

27. What determines the dampening of the pressure amplitude in HFOV?

    A. Low compliance
    B. Peripheral resistance
    C. Turbulent nature of flow
    D. All of the above

ANSWERS

1 B. Rupture of the ET cuff

The change in the ventilator parameters described in this patient is consistent only with ET tube cuff leak. The sudden decrease in the peak and plateau pressures and airway resistance is consistent with this problem. The sudden decrease in the end-tidal carbon dioxide and the oxygen desaturation represent reduction in the effective tidal volume. The large gradient between the inspired and exhaled tidal volumes supports the diagnosis. In pneumothorax and pulmonary edema (change in lung compliance), there is usually a sudden increase in the peak and plateau pressures (choices A and D, respectively). Choice C is not correct because, in a patient with COPD exacerbation and bronchospasm, there is usually an increase in the gradient between peak and plateau pressures.

2. D. Disconnect the ET tube from the ventilator circuit for a few seconds

Auto-PEEP is not uncommon in COPD on mechanical ventilation. Three causes include (1) dynamic hyperinflation with intrinsic expiratory flow limitation (eg, COPD); (2) dynamic hyperinflation without intrinsic expiratory flow limitation, such as in a high respiratory rate setting, high volume, prolonged inspiratory time, and increased flow resistance from the ventilator tubing; and (3) without dynamic hyperinflation, increased expiratory muscle activity. Consequences of auto-PEEP include increasing the work of breathing, which leads to patient-ventilator

asynchrony; worsening gas exchange, which leads to worsening hypoxemia and hypercapnia; and hemodynamic instability, which leads to tachycardia and hypotension.

The patient in this case develops increasing auto-PEEP secondary to COPD exacerbation and bronchospasm. The patient has been agitated with excessive use of respiratory accessory muscles and wheezing on physical examination. Because of the hemodynamic instability, the first adequate step in managing this patient is to disconnect the ET tube from the ventilator circuit to allow the exhalation of the trapped air and eliminate the dynamic hyperinflation. Other steps should be taken after that to prevent the recurrence of the auto-PEEP, for example adequate sedation or in some circumstances use of paralytics, ensuring adequate ET tube size, treating the patient with corticosteroids and bronchodilators to improve the bronchospasm and minimize the airway resistance, ensuring adequate ventilator rate and tidal volume, decrease inspiratory time and prolong expiration time, increasing the flow, and decreasing the patient's triggering effort by increasing the PEEP (waterfall phenomenon). Due to the hemodynamic instability, Choices A, B, and C are incorrect.

3. A. Increase PEEP

The patient is still hypoxic, so ventilator setting changes must be made. The pressure applied on the airway during mechanical ventilation (ie, the distending force) is intended to overcome the airway resistance and the lung/chest wall compliance to achieve the desired tidal volume. The airway pressure does not reflect the actual diseased lung mechanics because it does not take into account the effect of chest recoil. Managing a mechanically ventilated patient has been largely guided by using tidal volume, respiratory rate, PEEP, and airway pressure. Using the TPP can help this area.

Alveolar pressure is sometimes synonymous with plateau pressure, and it appears that it has reached the maximum allowed PEEP. However, evaluating the TTP can determine if additional PEEP can be placed to improve hypoxia.

Pleural pressure is measured indirectly as esophageal pressure via an esophageal monometer. The measurement is performed during a 5-second end-inspiratory or end-expiratory occlusion.

This patient has a TPP measured at the end of the inspiration of 10 (P_{plat} of 30 − P_{es} of 20). The PEEP can be increased to improve oxygenation. Decreasing tidal volume (choice B), increasing respiratory rate (choice C), and increasing inspiratory time (choice D) will not improve oxygenation.

4. D. Ideal body weight and desired minute ventilation

Adaptive support ventilation, a closed-loop mode, is an adaptive pressure-controlled ventilation in passive patients and switches to an adaptive pressure-support ventilation in spontaneously breathing patients. Adaptive support ventilation assumes that the adequate ventilation of normal subjects is 100 mL/min/kg of body weight. The minute ventilation (V̇E) is calculated as the ratio between the ventilation resulting from ideal body weight (IBW) and the minute ventilation (MinVol) percent set by the user: VE (L/min) = IBW (kg) × MinVol (%)/100. Then, ASV automatically selects the respiratory pattern in terms of respiratory rate (RR), VT, and I:E ratio for mandatory breathing, and reaches the respiratory pattern selected. The ASV can adjust the inspiratory pressure and the mandatory rate to reach the targets.

The ASV has been used in patients with normal lungs, postcardiac surgery, COPD, acute lung injury, restrictive lung disease, and others. Adaptive support ventilation could have future potential roles in impacting liberating patients from mechanical ventilators. There are more studies needed to evaluate mortality, patient interaction with the ventilator and comfort, and overall outcome.

5. **D. Increase the PEEP Level**

An intubated patient can trigger the mechanical ventilator to deliver the desired breath by decreasing the pressure (pressure trigger) or changing the flow (flow trigger) in the triggering circuit. There are 2 types of triggering dyssynchrony problems: (1) extra or double triggering, which occurs when there is excessive trigger sensitivity, or the ventilator cycles off before the patient's effort ceases and the persistent effort triggers another breath, or reverse triggering secondary to a patient's central respiratory control center reproducing an inspiratory effort, which triggers another breath, and (2) delay or missed triggers, which occurs when there is an inappropriate trigger setting, or intrinsic PEEP despite the presence of respiratory activity.

The patient shows delay or absence of triggers despite the chest and abdominal wall muscle effort to initiate the breath. Treatment usually involves increasing sedation to minimize the patient's spontaneous contributing effort to the respiratory cycle and not decreasing sedation (choice A), decreasing the tidal volume, decreasing the respiratory rate and not increasing respiratory rate (choice B), increasing the inspiratory flow and not decreasing the flow rate (choice C), decreasing the inspiratory time, or increasing the preset PEEP. Increasing PEEP causes the waterfall effect, which minimizes the patient's effort and triggers the ventilator.

6. **A. a) II; b) IV; c) III; d) V; e) I**

There are 5 physiologic mechanisms of gas exchange in high-frequency oscillator ventilation:

1. Bulk convection flow represents the movement of oxygen molecules to occupy the space available as oxygen molecules are absorbed into the alveoli

2. In pendelluft, the lung is consisting of heterogeneous alveoli with different compliances (different surface tensions). Alveoli with poor compliance have higher surface tension (small alveoli) compared with alveoli with good compliance, which have lower surface tension (large alveoli). Because of high surface tension, gas from the small alveoli travel into the larger alveoli with lower surface tension. This differences in compliance and inertance also causes regional differences in inflation and deflation times. Lung units that are deflating may receive gas from deflating lungs.

3. Taylor dispersion is the mechanism of the gas exchange between the central airway with higher Fio_2 and the peripheral and smaller airway with lower Fio_2, with the help of the force generated by the jet.

4. Coaxial flow describes the bidirectional flow in HFOV, in which the inner or the central part of the flow moving inside the airway (inspiratory) and the outer or the peripheral part of the flow moving outside of the airway (expiratory).

5. In molecular diffusion, the mechanical force produced by the oscillator enhances the diffusion of the gas through the airway (Brownian motion).

7   **B. T_{low} increased**

For worsening hypercapnia, such as in this patient, P_{high} can be increased while simultaneously decreasing T_{high} (choice C) to increase the rate of release to maintain mean airway pressure; T_{low} can be increased to allow for longer alveolar emptying, as long as peak expiratory flow rate is not less than 25%; or change to PCV.[104-106] For respiratory alkalosis, P_{high} can be decreased, T_{high} can be increased, or ATC is turned off[104-106] (choices D, C, and A). For worsening hypoxia, P_{high} can be increased at increments of 2 to 3 or P_{low} can be changed to closer to 75% peak expiratory flow rate.[104-106]

8. **A. Decrease P_{high} and increase T_{high}**

The drop-and-stretch method of weaning involves decreasing P_{high} by 2 to 3 cm H_2O and increasing T_{high} by 0.5 to 2 seconds every 2 to 3 hours until P_{high} is 10 to 16 cm H_2O and T_{high} is 12 to 15 seconds.[106] Choice B is wrong because it is the reverse. With her current settings, it is premature to start her on CPAP. Once the goal of P_{high} and T_{high} are met, she can be transitioned to CPAP with PEEP of 10 cm H_2O and PS of 5 to 10 cm H_2O (choices C and D).

9   **D. PRVC**

With pressure-regulated volume control, the mechanical ventilator adjusts the pressure via peak airway resistance and compliance from breath to breath to maintain a set tidal volume at the lowest possible pressure. There is usually a decelerating flow pattern.

Pressure control ventilation (choice B) provides a set pressure on a set respiratory rate. There is no variability with the pressure curve. Initial inspiratory pressure is the P_{plat} – PEEP.

The Fio₂, respiratory rate, and PEEP are the same as in other control modes. Inspiratory time and I:E ratio are determined by flow-time curves. Changing any of these parameters must be supplemented to changes in reciprocal parameters to maintain a certain tidal volume.

Assist control ventilation (choice A) shows that the target tidal volume is the same regardless of whether the breath is triggered by the patient or by the ventilator. There is a constant flow regardless of whether the breath was triggered by the patient or by the ventilator. The flow is either a square form for patients with obstructive disease or who need more exhalation time, or decelerating (ramp) form for patients who have heterogenous lung disease.[3] Assist control is flow limited, patient or time triggered, and volume cycled.[3]

Synchronized intermittent mandatory ventilation (choice C) is like AC in that it is flow limited, patient or time triggered, and volume cycled, but there are unassisted breaths in between the mandatory breaths.

10. C.

In a pressure-volume plot, pressures to the left of the diagonal line are generated by the patient and those to the right of the diagonal line are generated by the ventilator.[107] In choice C, the assistance provided by the mechanical ventilator causes the work pattern to appear normal. Choice A shows a patient with a high work of breathing without any mechanical ventilator support.[107] Choice B shows the patient does work only to trigger a breath and mechanical

ventilation does most of the work. Choice D shows unphysiologic workload for patient.[107]

11. A. Increased sedation

Trigger is dependent on pressure, pressure maximum, inspiratory time, time to return trigger pressure to baseline, and inspiratory delay time.[108] Trigger asynchrony is defined as patient effort without triggering the ventilation during the inspiratory phase.[108] Investigation into the mechanism of trigger asynchrony found that decreased patient respiratory effort, such as increased mechanical support, increased trigger asynchrony, and patient efforts during assisted breaths are carried over to mandatory breaths.[109] This leads to a shorter total breath cycle with a longer inspiratory time and a shorter expiratory time that leads to auto-PEEP.[108]

Trigger asynchrony types include ineffective trigger, double trigger, and trigger insensitivity.[108] This patient has ineffective trigger.[109]

There is a drop in pressure greater than 0.5 cm H₂O and an increase in flow. It is associated with auto-PEEP, improper threshold, deeper sedation, and difficult weaning[109-116] (choice A).

Double trigger is when the patient's inspiratory effort continues even after the ventilator's inspiratory time is finished.[110] This is secondary to small tidal volumes, short inspiratory times, or too-high flow-cycle threshold[110] (choices B and C) (Fig. 12-23).

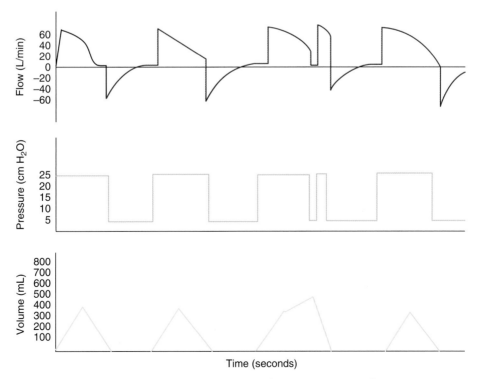

FIGURE 12-23 Double trigger. (Adapted from Robinson BR, Blakeman T, Toth P, Hanseman DJ, Mueller E, Branson RD. Patient-ventilator asynchrony in a traumatically injured population. *Respir Care.* 2013;58(11):1847-1855.)

Auto trigger is a delivered assisted breath that was not initiated by the patient.[110] This can be secondary to inappropriately sensitive trigger thresholds or cardiac oscillations as shown here.[110,111,117] (Fig. 12-24).

12. A. Increase flow

To unload the respiratory muscles and decrease the work of breathing, the patient should be able to trigger the ventilator.[110] However, respiratory muscle contraction continues after triggering the ventilator and flow is necessary to

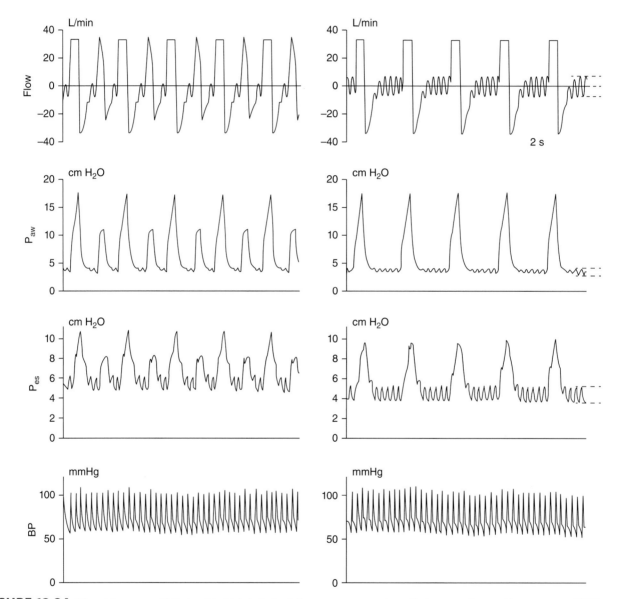

FIGURE 12-24 When trigger sensitivity is set to 1 L/min in the left, pressure-support ventilation was triggered between two SIMV breaths. When trigger sensitivity is set to 4 L/min on the right, pressure-support ventilation disappeared and marked cardiac oscillations noted between two SIMV breaths in flow, P_{aw} and P_{es}. BP = blood pressure; P_{es} = esophageal pressure; P_{aw} = mean airway pressure. (Reprinted with permisison from Imanaka H, et al. Autotriggering caused by cardiogenic oscillation during flow-triggered mechanical ventilation. *Crit Care Med.* 2000 Feb;28(2):402-407.)

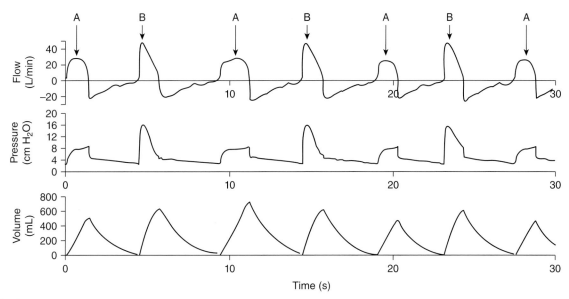

FIGURE 12-25 The ventilator mode is synchronized intermittent mandatory ventilation with pressure support. Breaths marked A are the pressure support breaths. In Breath A, there is tenting at the end of the pressure support breaths. This is delayed cycling, which can be corrected by changing to cycling sensitivity. Breaths marked B are volume controlled flow target breaths. In these breaths, flows are too high resulting in peak flow and peak pressure at the beginning of the breath. This can be corrected by decreasing peak flow. (Reprinted with permission from de Wit M. Monitoring of patient-ventilator interaction at the bedside. *Respir Care* 2011;56(1):61-68.)

prevent muscle fatigue. Rate and pattern of flow are chosen by the physician in flow-targeted breaths. Initial flow is set at 60 to 80 L/min and patterns are square, decelerating, accelerating, or sinusoidal. The patient's respiratory drive is strong. There is a dip in the pressure-time curve. This can shorten expiratory time leading to an ineffective trigger and auto-PEEP. The patient has ineffective flow, and treatment would be to increase the flow, change the pattern to decelerating, and transition from volume-control to pressure-control ventilation.[108,110] In Figure 12-25 of synchronized intermittent mechanical ventilation, the volume control breaths (choice B), has higher flows, causing early peaks in flow and pressure. This can be corrected by decreasing flow.

There is no role for changing the tidal volume in flow-related asynchrony (choices C and D).

13. B. Delayed termination

Delayed termination is an expiratory event in which the patient's neural timing precedes the ventilator's end of inflation. This is illustrated via a pressure spike toward the end of inspiration on the pressure-time waveform with a concurrent rapid decline in inspiratory on the flow-time waveform. This can lead to dynamic hyperinflation, trigger delays, and missed triggers.[109]

Premature termination (choice B) is also another expiratory event in which the patient has continued inspiratory effort despite the termination of the ventilator breath. This causes a drop or negative deflection in the flow-time, pressure-time, and esophageal pressure waveforms, as shown here [109] (Fig. 12-26).

Rapid rise time (choice C) shows the initial pressure is overshot, creating a pressure peak early in the breath, as seen below. This can lead to early termination (Fig. 12-27).

Inadequate flow (choice D) would have a scooped-out appearance on the pressure-time wave form, as shown below (Fig. 12-28).[109]

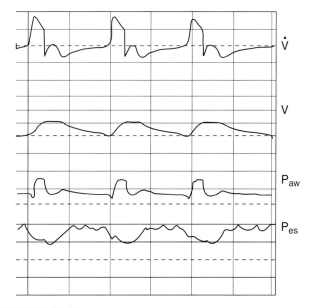

FIGURE 12-26 In premature termination, there is a continued patient effort despite termination of the ventilator breath, causing negative deflections in flow-time, pressure-time, and esophageal pressure wave forms. P_{es} = esophageal pressure; P_{aw} = mean airway pressure. (Reprinted with permission from Tokioka H, et al. The effect of breath termination criterion on breathing patterns and the work of breathing during pressure support ventilation. *Anesth Analg.* 2001 Jan;92(1):161-165..)

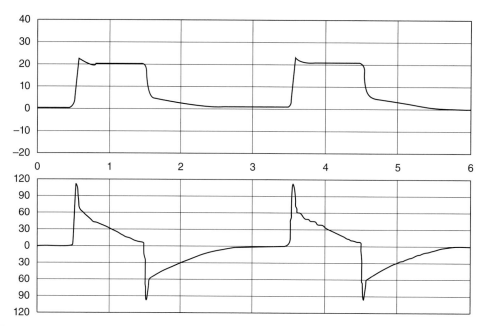

FIGURE 12-27 Early termination. (Reprinted with permission from Nilsestuen JO, Hargett KD. Using ventilator graphics to identify patient-ventilator asynchrony. *Respir Care.* 2005;50(2):202-232.)

14. D. Increase PEEP

Airflow obstruction is secondary to bronchospasm, interstitial edema, mucus, inflammatory cells, and/or dynamic airway collapse during expiration. Tidal volume and respiratory rate increase, causing a shorter expiratory time and inability for lungs to deflate back to baseline. This results in an increase in functional residual capacity, decrease in compliance, overstretching of respiratory muscles, and fatigue.[118,119] It leads to high pulmonary vascular resistance, decreased venous return, and decreased preload, increased WOB, disruption of synchrony, and barotrauma.[118,120] Treatment is aimed at decreasing respiratory rate, decreasing tidal volume, increasing expiratory time, and/or applying PEEP with the goal of P_{plat} less than 30 cm H_2O and intrinsic PEEP less than 10 cm H_2O. Applied PEEP, about 80% of intrinsic PEEP, improves inspiratory muscle effectiveness.[118] It has been suggested that the applied PEEP is only beneficial if tidal deflation is flow limited by decreasing the difference between alveolar and airway opening pressures without increasing lung volume, and if the patient can trigger the ventilator.[119,120] In pressure-targeted ventilation, adding additional PEEP beyond auto-PEEP will not increase V_T but paradoxically might decrease if it is due to stiffness of lung.[120] Dynamic hyperinflation is improved by

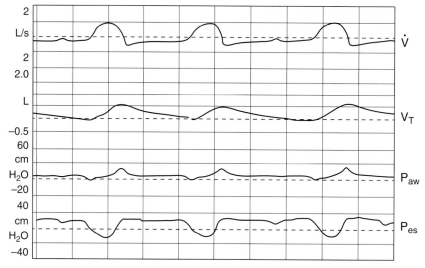

FIGURE 12-28 The rise time is 10%, showing a scooped out appearance in the Paw waveform. This suggest inadequate flow, delaying rise in airway pressure. P_{es} = esophageal pressure; P_{aw} = mean airway pressure. V_T = Tidal volume and $\dot{V}$ = Flow. (Reprinted with permission from Nilsestuen JO, Hargett KD. Using ventilator graphics to identify patient-ventilator asynchrony. *Respir Care.* 2005;50(2):202-232.)

decreasing minute ventilation through decreasing the tidal volume to shorten inspiratory time and decrease volume that needs to be exhaled, and decreasing respiratory rate to increase expiratory time, decrease trigger sensitivity, and increase inspiratory flow.[121,122] However, increasing inspiratory flow might paradoxically worsen bronchoconstriction if it is accompanied by bronchial hyperresponsiveness, and it has less effect with minute ventilation less than 10 L/min and can trigger spontaneous breaths.[121,122] Decreasing expiratory time (choice A), no change (choice B), or increasing tidal volume (choice C) might make the autoPEEP worse.

15. A. Extubate the patient to noninvasive positive pressure ventilation (NIPPV)

The decision to extubate is determined once the condition or disease that precipitated the need for mechanical ventilation has improved or resolved and the patient has passed a spontaneous breath trial. Needless to say, caution is still paramount, since extubation failure occurs in 10% to 20% of patients and can carry a mortality risk from 25% to 50%.[123] Successful extubation is the absence of ventilatory support for more than 48 hours. Risk factors for extubation failure include age greater than 65 years, underlying chronic cardiorespiratory disease, High Acute Physiology and Chronic Health Evaluation II (APACHE II) score, pneumonia, RSBI greater than 105, Pao_2/Fio_2 less than 200 mmHg, Glasgow Coma Scale less than 8, abundant endotracheal secretions, Pco_2 greater than 44 mmHg during a spontaneous breathing trial, weak or absent cough, hemoglobin less than 10 g/dL, increased B-type natriuretic peptide (BNP) during a spontaneous breathing trial, and a greater than 4.5% reduction in central venous saturation 30 minutes after spontaneous breathing trial initiation.[124-133] The current Liberation from Mechanical Ventilation in Critically Ill Adults Guidelines for American College of Chest Physicians (ACCP)/American Thoracic Society Clinical Practice Guideline (ATS) recommends prophylactic or preventive extubation to noninvasive ventilation in patients who are high risk for extubation failure. Their recommendation is based on clinical evidence from 5 randomized controlled trials that extubation to prophylactic or preventive noninvasive ventilation reduced re-intubation and mortality.[134-136] Extubating to nasal cannula or oxymask would place this patient at risk for re-intubation (choices C and D). There is no benefit in extending the weaning trial for another hour since the duration of a spontaneous breathing trial is 30 to 120 minutes (choice B).

16. D. All of the above

Although the strength of recommendation is conditional, the 2017 ACCP/ATS guidelines on Liberation from the Mechanical Ventilator in Critically Ill Adults includes the following: (1) patients who are ventilated for more than 24 hours should have a gradual decrease in sedation due to a trend toward shorter duration of mechanical ventilation,

shorter ICU length of stay, and lower short-term mortality; (2) patients who are ventilated for more than 24 hours should have a protocolized rehabilitation toward early mobilization due to shorter duration of mechanical ventilation, early ambulation, and shorter costs; and (3) for patients who are ventilated for more than 24 hours, ventilator liberation protocols showed shorter duration of mechanical ventilation but no effect on reintubation or mortality rates.[129,130]

17. B. Cuff-leak test

A cuff-leak test should be performed for patients who are at increased risk for post-extubation stridor. Risk factors include female, traumatic intubation, large endotracheal tube, more than 6 days' intubation, and reintubation after unplanned extubation.[129,130] Therefore, extubating her directly would be risky (choice A). A cuff-leak test begins with placing the patient on assist-control.[131-133] Inspiratory tidal volume and 6 expiratory tidal volumes were measured after the oropharynx is suctioned and endotracheal tube is deflated. The tidal volume between the inspiratory tidal volume and expiratory tidal volume and a leak of less than 110 mL or less than 10 to 15% is considered positive.[133-135] Cuff-leak test has a low sensitivity and low specificity.[134-138] The circumference is not the only parameter that effects the cuff-leak test. The respiratory compliance and inspiratory flow also affects the results. If a patient passes the other weaning parameters and has a positive leak test, systemic corticosteroids are needed at least 4 hours before extubation (choice D). Solumedrol 20 to 40 mg IV or dexamethasone 2 to 4 mg IV have been used.[139]

Ultrasound has been investigated as another method to assess the risk of laryngeal edema via measurement of air column width difference (ACWD) before and after endotracheal cuff deflation.[139,140] Larger scale studies are still needed (choice C).

18. A. Place the patient on a CPAP of 5 cm H_2O and calculate the respiratory rate over the tidal volume.

A rapid shallow breathing index less than 105 breaths/min/L is associated with a mild increase in weaning success but a moderate increase in weaning failure if the RSBI 105 is breaths/min/L or higher.[141-143] It is calculated by F/VT, where F is the respiratory rate and VT is tidal volume. This can be calculated via a T-piece or a CPAP of 5, although a CPAP of 5 tends to mitigate RSBI to a lower value.[141-143] Therefore, placing the patient on T-piece and calculating the respiratory rate over the tidal volume is another option. Choices B, C, and D are wrong.

19. C. Oral chlorhexidine can be used to prevent oral colonization and, subsequently, VAP.

The ET tube can be a conduit for ventilator-associated pneumonia due to microaspirations and biofilm formation.[144]

Endotracheal tube design adjustments have been made to counteract these mechanisms. It has been observed that to have a complete seal, the ET cuff must be inflated to a pressure of 60 cm H_2O [144,145] (choice A). At this pressure, there is high risk for tracheal mucosal necrosis. Recommended tracheal pressure is 20 to 30 cm H_2O.[145] The cuff material was changed from polyvinyl to polyurethane to prevent formation of folds or microchannels and from a globular to more cylindrical design[144] (choice B). Intermittent or continuous subglottic drainage of secretions have been shown to reduce mechanical ventilation, ICU stay, and incidence of VAP. Potential complications include increased VAP due to malfunction from tracheal mucosa suction and tracheal mucosal injury. The ET tube can be covered with biofilm from bacteria, particularly from oral flora, within a few hours after intubation. Methods to decrease bacterial colonization includes photodynamic therapy, silver-coated ET tubes, mucus shaver, and oral chlorhexidine[145-147] (choices C and D).

20. D. 97%

Prolonged mechanical ventilation is defined as requiring mechanical ventilation for 21 days or more for at least 6 h/d.[147] There is an increased respiratory load with diminished respiratory muscle strength. Patients have poor cognitive and physical quality of life. Mortality is 15% (choice A), but with the addition of age more than 50 years, vasopressors, thrombocytopenia, and hemodialysis on the 21st day can have 97% mortality.[148]

21. D. Pressure SIMV

Table 12-4 lists the variations of breath per mode of mechanical ventilation.

TABLE 12-4 Mode of Mechanical Ventilation and Variations of Breath

Mode	Variations of Breath
VACV	VC, VA
PACV	PC, PA
Volume SIMV	VC, VA, PS, spontaneous
Pressure SIMV	PC, PA, PS, spontaneous
PSV	PS, spontaneous

PA = proportional assist; PACV = pressure assist control ventilation; PC = pressure control; PS = pressure support; SIMV = spontaneous intermittent mechanical ventilation; VA = ventilator assist; VACV = ventilation assist control ventilation; VC = ventilator control.

22. A. Acute severe COPD exacerbation with pH less than 7.35

Noninvasive positive pressure ventilation was shown to reduce mortality and rate in intubation in severe exacerbation of COPD (pH < 7.35 with associated hypercapnia) (Grade 1A).[96,149-151] NIPPV or CPAP is also recommended for patients with cardiogenic pulmonary edema who are not on vasopressors or have ongoing ischemia since it decreases endotracheal intubation and hospital stay, and it trends toward a decrease mortality (Grade 1A)[96,149-151] (choice B). In immunocompromised patients, defined as solid organ transplant or BMT recipient or chemotherapy, 2 RCTs have shown reduction in endotracheal intubation and hospital mortality with the use of NIPPV but not CPAP (Grade 2B)[96,149-151] (choice D). Additional indications for the use of NIPPV include extubation to prophylactic NPPV for patients at high risk for extubation failure (Grade 2B), CPAP for respiratory failure after abdominal surgery (Grade 2C), and NIPPV for respiratory failure after lung resection (Grade 2C).[96,149-151] Although there are studies that have suggested the use of NIPPV in asthma, some clinicians are still reluctant to fully advocate their use in asthma exacerbations due to lack of large randomized control trials and the methods used in the smaller randomized trials[96,149-151] (choice C). Still, NIPPV has been used for asthma exacerbation, particularly in the emergency department.[152,153]

23. B. Respiratory rate of 24 breaths/min

After the patient is placed on a NIPPV, follow-up is recommended after 1 to 2 hours to determine if there is any benefit or if the patient needs to be intubated. The factors associated with successful use of NIPPV in the acute setting include synchronous breathing with the ventilator, less air leak, fewer secretions, respiratory rate less than 30/min, lower APACHE II score (< 29), pH greater than 7.30, GCS of 15, Pao_2/Fio_2 greater than 146 after the first hour, COPD, and cardiogenic pulmonary edema.[148] In COPD patients, the likelihood of success is 94% if RR are less than 30/min, APACHE II score is less than 29, pH is greater than 7.30, and the GCS is 15 at baseline, and the likelihood of success is 97% if all 4 are present after 2 hours of NIPPV.[96,148,151] Choices A, C, and D are wrong.

24. B. COPD has high compliance and high resistance

Compliance is the change in volume over the change in pressure. Static compliance is $V_T/(P_{plat} - PEEP_{total})$. Normal compliance is 50 to 100 mL/cm H_2O. It is low in pulmonary edema, interstitial disease, hyperinflation, and extrapulmonary conditions, such as pleural disease, obesity, and ascites. Compliance is high in COPD and asthma. Resistance is $R_{aw} = (PIP - P_{plat})/V_I$, and the normal value is less than 15 cm $H_2O/L/s$.

25. A. Without spontaneous breath, TPP = 10 cm H_2O; with spontaneous breath, TPP = 20 cm H_2O

To determine the true lung-distending pressure, the effects of pleural pressure must be subtracted. The esophageal pressure is an estimate of the pleural pressure. In the APRV mode, the P_{high} is set at 15 cm H_2O with the esophageal pressure at 5 cm H_2O. Therefore, without spontaneous breath, the TPP is 10 cm H_2O (15 − 5). During spontaneous breathing, there is a 10 cm H_2O drop (+5 to −5) in esophageal pressure; therefore, the TPP is 25 cm H_2O (15 cm H_2O − [−10 cm H_2O]).

26. A. Cycle volume set to maximum

If there is hypercapnia, and after endotracheal obstruction is ruled out, the amplitude or cycle volume is set to maximum (choice A); if this does not work, the frequency is set to minimum (5 Hz) (choice B). If there is hypoxemia, and Fio_2 is on maximum, mean airway pressure is increased by 5 cm H_2O every 30 minutes to a maximum of 45 to 55 cm H_2O (choice C). If there is a leak, such as suctioning of bronchopleural fistula, an increase in bias flow is need to maintain desired mean airway pressure (choice D).

27. D. All of the above

Unlike in conventional ventilation, the pressure amplitude progressively dampens from airway opening to alveoli. This is determined by the impedance to flow, as a consequence of low compliance, peripheral resistance due to obstruction of smaller airways and emphysema, and resistance on the tracheal tube and the large airway, due to the turbulent nature of flow.

REFERENCES

1. Hess DR. Respiratory mechanics in mechanically ventilated patients. *Respir Care*. 2014;59(11):1773-1794.
2. Hess DR, Medoff BD, Fessler MD. Pulmonary mechanics and graphics during positive pressure ventilation. *Int Anesthesiol Clin*. 1999;37(3):15-34.
3. Singer BD, Corbridge TC. Basic invasive mechanical ventilation. *South Med J*. 2009;102(12):1238-1245.
4. Amato MB, Meade MO, Slutsky AS. Driving pressure and survival in the acute respiratory distress syndrome. *New Engl J Med*. 2015;372(8):747-755.
5. Bugedo G, Retamal J, Bruhn A. Driving pressure: a marker of severity, safety limit or goal mechanical ventilation? *Crit Care*. 2017:21(199):1-7.
6. Neto AS, Hemmes SN, Barbas CS, et al. Association between driving pressure and development of postoperative pulmonary complications in patients undergoing mechanical ventilation for general anaesthesia: a meta-analysis of individual patient data. *Lancet Respir Med*. 2016;4(4):272-280.
7. Schmidt Marcello FS, Amaral ACKB, Fan E, et al. Driving pressure and hospital mortality in patients without ARDS. *Chest*. 2018;153(1):46-54.
8. Akoumianaki E, Maggiore SM, Valenza F, et al. The application of esophageal pressure measurement in patients with respiratory failure. *Am J Respir Crit Care Med*. 2914;189(5):520-531.
9. Slutsky AS, Ranieri VM. Ventilator-induced lung injury. *N Engl J Med*. 2013;369(22):2126-2136.
10. Cortes GA, Marini JJ. Two steps forward in bedside monitoring of lung mechanics: transpulmonary pressure and lung volume. *Crit Care*. 2013;17(2):219.
11. Talmor D, Sarge T, Malhotra A, et al. Mechanical ventilation guided by esophageal pressure in acute lung injury. *N Engl J Med*. 2008;359(20):2095-2104.
12. Grinnan DC, Truwit JD. Clinical review: respiratory mechanics in spontaneous and assisted ventilation. *Crit Care*. 2005;9(5):472-484.
13. Amato MB, Barbas CS, Medeiros DM, et al. Effect of a protective ventilation strategy on mortality in the acute respiratory distress syndrome. *N Engl J Med*. 1998;338:347-354
14. Marini JJ, Gattinoni L. Ventilatory management of acute respiratory distress syndrome: a consensus of two. *Crit Care*. 2004;32:250-255.
15. Mergoni M, Volpi A, Bricchi C, Rossi A. Lower inflection point and recruitment with positive end expiratory pressure in ventilated patients with acute respiratory failure. *J Appl Physiol*. 2001;91(1):441-450
16. Hickling KG. Reinterpreting the pressure-volume curve in patients with acute respiratory distress syndrome. *Curr Opin Critical Care*. 2002;8(1):32-38
17. Rotta AT. High versus low PEEP in ARDS [editorial]. *N Engl J Med*. 2004;351(20):2128-2129.
18. Harris RS, Hess DR, Venegas JG. An objective analysis of the pressure-volume curve in the acute respiratory distress syndrome. *Am J Resp Crit Care Med*. 2000;161(2 Pt 1):432-439.
19. Brower RG, Lanken PN, MacIntyre N, et al; National Heart, Lung, and Blood Institute ARDS Clinical Trials Network. Higher versus lower positive end-expiratory pressures in patients with the acute respiratory distress syndrome. *N Engl J Med*. 2004;351(4):327-333.
20. Gattinoni L, Pelosi P, Suter PM, Pedoto A, Vercesi P, Lissoni A. Acute respiratory distress syndrome caused by pulmonary and extrapulmonary disease. Different syndromes? *Am J Respir Crit Care Med*. 1998;158(1):3-11.
21. Akoumianaki E, Lyazidi A, Rey N, et al. Mechanical ventilation–induced reverse-triggered breaths: a frequently unrecognized form of neuromechanical coupling. *Chest*. 2013;143(4):927-938.
22. Simon PM, Zurob AS, Wies WM, Leiter JC, Hubmayr RD. Entrainment of respiration in humans by periodic lung inflations: effect of state and CO2. *Am J Respir Crit Care Med*. 1999;160(3):950-960.
23. Richard JC, Lyazidi A, Akoumianaki E, et al. Potentially harmful effects of inspiratory synchronization during pressure preset ventilation. *Intensive Care Med*. 2013;39(11):2003-2010.
24. de Wit M, Miller KB, Green DA, Ostman HE, Gennings C, Epstein SK. Ineffective triggering predicts increased duration of mechanical ventilation. *Crit Care Med*. 2009;37(20):2740–2745.
25. Pelosi P, Vargas M. Mechanical ventilation and intra-abdominal hypertension: 'Beyond Good and Evil.' *Critical Care*. 2012;16(6):187.
26. Papavramidi TS, Marinis AD, Pliakos I, Kesisoglou I, Papavramidou. Abdominal compartment syndrome – intraabdominal hypertension: defining, diagnosing, and managing. *J Emerg Trauma Shock*. 2011;4(2):279-291.
27. Malbrain ML, Deeren D, De Potter TJ. Intra-abdominal hypertension in the critically ill: it is time to pay attention. *Curr Opin Crit Care*. 2005;11(2):156-171.
28. Sindi A, Piraino T, Alhazzani W, et al. The correlation between esophageal and abdominal pressures in mechanically ventilated patients undergoing laparoscopic surgery. *Respir Care*. 2014;59(4):491-496.
29. Ranieri VM, Brienza N, Santostasi S, et al. Impairment of lung and chest wall mechanics in patients with acute respiratory distress syndrome: role of abdominal distention. *Am J Respir Crit Care Med*. 1997;156(4 Pt 1):1082-1091.

30. Melo e Silva CA, Ventura CE. A simple model illustrating the respiratory system's time constant concept. *Adv Physiol Educ.* 2006;30(3):129-130.

31. Corne S, Gillespie D, Roberts D, Younes M. Effect of inspiratory flow rate on respiratory rate in intubated ventilated patients. *Am J Resp Crit Care Med.* 1997;156(1):304-308.

32. Marini JJ. Dynamic hyperinflation and auto-positive end-expiratory pressure. *Am J Resp Crit Care Med.* 2011;184(7):756-762.

33. August A, Soriano JB. Dynamic hyperinfilation and pulmonary inflammation: A potential relevant relationship? *Eur Respir Rev.* 2006;15(100):68-71.

34. Mughal MM, Minai OA, Culver DA, Arroliga AC. Auto-positive end-expiratory pressure: Mechanisms and treatment. *CCJM.* 2005;72(9):801-809

35. Gluck EH, Onorato DJ, Castriotta R. Helium-oxygen mixtures in intubated patients with status asthmaticus and respiratory acidosis. *Chest.* 1990;98(3):693-698.

36. Schmidt GA. Ventilator waveforms: clinical interpretation. In: Schmidt GA, Hall JB, Kress JP, eds. *Principles of Critical Care.* 4th ed. New York, NY: McGraw Hill Publishers; 2015: 411-423.

37. Mellema MS. Ventilator waveforms. *Top Companion Anim Med.* 2013;28(3):112-123.

38. Lesnik I, Rappaport W, Fulginiti J, Witzke D. The role of early tracheostomy in blunt, multiple organ trauma. *Am Surg.* 1992;58(6):346-349.

39. Jarvis S, Burt K, English W. High frequency oscillatory ventilation. *Anaesthesia Tutorial of the Week.* 2012;261:1-11.

40. Pillow J. High frequency ventilation: theory and practical application. Draeger.com. https://www.draeger.com/Library/Content/hfov-bk-9102693-en.pdf. Updated September 2016. Accessed May 25, 2018.

41. Ferguson ND, Cook DJ, Guyatt GH, et al; the OSCILLATE Trial Investigators and the Canadian Critical Care Trials Group. High-frequency oscillation in early acute respiratory distress syndrome. *N Engl J Med.* 2013;368(9):795-805.

42. Young D, Lamb SE, Shah S, et al; OSCAR Study Group. High-frequency oscillation for acute respiratory distress syndrome. *N Engl J Med.* 2013;368(9):806-813.

43. Ambrosino N, Rossi A. Proportional assist ventilation (PAV): a significant advance or a futile struggle between logic and practice? *Thorax.* 2002;57(3):272-276.

44. Younes M. Proportional-assist Ventilation. In: Tobin MJ. eds. *Principles and Practice of Mechanical Ventilation,* 3e. New York, NY: McGraw-Hill; 2013. http://accessmedicine.mhmedical.com/content.aspx?bookid=520&sectionid=41692251. Accessed May 28, 2018.

45. Younes M. Proportional-assist ventilation. In: Tobin M, ed. *Principles and Practice of Mechanical Ventilation.* 2nd ed. New York, NY: McGraw-Hill; 2006: 335-364.

46. Kacmarek RM. Proportional assist ventilation and neurally adjusted ventilatory assist. *Respir Care.* 2011;56(2):140-152.

47. Verbrugghe W, Jorens PG. Neurally adjusted ventilatory assist: a ventilation tool or a ventilation toy? *Respir Care.* 2011;56(3):327-335.

48. Terzi N, Piquilloud L, Rozé H, et al. Clinical review: update on neutrally adjusted ventilatory assist—report of a round-table conference. *Crit Care.* 2012;16(255):1-13.

49. Fernández J, Miguelena D, Mulett H, Godoy J, Martinón-Torres F. Adaptive support ventilation: State of the art review. *Indian J Crit Care Med.* 2013;17(1):16-22.

50. Arnal JM, Wysocki M. Automatic selection of breathing pattern using adaptive support ventilation. *Intensive Care Med.* 2008;34(1):76-81.

51. Wu CP, Lin HI, Perng WC, et al. Correlation between the %MinVol setting and work of breathing during adaptive support ventilation in patients with respiratory failure. *Respir Care.* 2010;55(3):334-341.

52. Kirakli C, Ozdemir I, Ucar ZZ, Cimen P, Kepil S, Ozkn SA. Adaptive support ventilation for faster weaning in COPD: a randomized controlled trial. *Eur Respir J.* 2011;38(4):774-780.

53. Brunner JX, Laubscher TP, Banner MJ, Iotti G, Braschi A. Simple method to measure total expiratory time constant based on the passive expiratory flow-volume curve. *Crit Care Med.* 1995;23(6):1117-1122.

54. Guttman J, Haberthur C, Gmols G, Lichtwarck-Aschoff M. Automatic tube compensation (ATC). *Minerva Anestesiol.* 2002;68(5):369-377.

55. Brochard L, Rua F, Lorino H, Lemaire F. Inspiratory pressure support compensates for the additional work of breathing caused by the endotracheal tube. *Anesthesiology.* 1991;75(5):739-745.

56. Fiastro JF, Habib MP, Quan SF. Pressure support compensation for the additional work of breathing caused by the endotracheal tube. *Chest.* 1988;93(3):499-505.

57. Straus C, Louis B, Isabey D, Lemaire F, Harf A, Brochard L. Contribution of the endotracheal tube and the upper airway to breathing workload. *Am J Respir Crit Care Med.* 1998;157(1):23-30.

58. Burns KE, Lellouche F, Lessard MR, Friedrich JO. Automated weaning and spontaneous breathing trial systems versus non-automated weaning strategies for discontinuation time in invasively ventilated postoperative adults. *Cochrane Database Syst Rev.* 2014;(2). http://onlinelibrary.wiley.com/doi/10.1002/14651858.CD008639.pub2/abstract. Accessed September 3, 2018.

59. Figueroa-Casas JB, Montoya R, Arzabala A, Connery SM. Comparison between automatic tube compensation and continuous positive airway pressure during spontaneous breathing trials. *Respir Care.* 2010;55(5):549-554.

60. Esteban A, Frutos F, Tobin MJ, et al. A comparison of four methods of weaning patients from mechanical ventilation. Spanish Lung Failure Collaborative Group. *New Engl J Med.* 1995;332(6):345-350.

61. Esteban A, Alía I, Ibañez J, Benito S, Tobin MJ. Modes of mechanical ventilation and weaning. A national survey of Spanish hospitals. The Spanish Lung Failure Collaborative Group. *Chest.* 1994;106(4):1188-1193.

62. Yang KL, Tobin MJ. A prospective study of indexes predicting the outcome of trials of weaning from mechanical ventilation. *New Engl J Med.* 1991;324(21):1445-1450.

63. Chatila W, Jacob B, Guanglione D, Manthous CA. The unassisted respiratory rate–tidal volume ratio accurately predicts weaning outcome. *Am J Med.* 1996;101(1):61-67.

64. MacIntyre NR, Cook DJ, Ely EW Jr, et al; American College of Chest Physicians; American Association for Respiratory Care; American College of Critical Care Medicine. Evidence-based guidelines for weaning and discontinuing ventilatory support: a collective task force facilitated by the American College of Chest Physicians; the American Association for Respiratory Care; and the American College of Critical Care Medicine. *Chest.* 2001;120(6 Suppl):375S-396S.

65. Durbin CG, Perkins MP, Moores LK. Should tracheostomy be performed as early as 72 hours in patients requiring prolonged mechanical ventilation? *Respir Care.* 2010;55(1):76-87.

66. Pierson DJ. Tracheostomy and weaning. *Respir Care.* 2005;50(4):526-533.

67. Heffner JE. Timing of tracheotomy in mechanically ventilated patients. *Am Rev Respir Dis.* 1993;147(3):768-771.

68. Young D, Harrison DA, Cuthbertson BH, Rowan K. Effect of early vs late tracheostomy placement on survival in patients receiving mechanical ventilation: the TracMan randomized trial. *JAMA.* 2013;309(20):2121-2129.

69. Rumbak MJ, Newton M, Truncale T, Schwartz SW, Adams JW, Hazard PB. A prospective, randomized, study comparing early percutaneous dilational tracheotomy to prolonged translaryngeal intubation (delayed tracheotomy) in critically ill medical patients. *Crit Care Med.* 2004;32(8):1689-1694.

70. Möller MG, Slaikeu JD, Bonelli P, Davis AT, Hoogeboom JE, Bonnell BW. Early tracheostomy versus late tracheostomy in the surgical intensive care unit. *Am J Surg.* 2005;189(3):293-296.

71. Dunham CM, Cutrona AF, Gruber BS, Calderon JE, Ransom KJ, Flowers LL. Early tracheostomy in severe traumatic brain injury: evidence for decreased mechanical ventilation and increased hospital mortality. *Int J Burns Trauma.* 2014;4(1):14-24.

72. Lesnik I, Rappaport W, Fulginiti J, Witzke D. The role of early tracheostomy in blunt, multiple organ trauma. *Am Surg.* 1992;58(6):346-349.

73. Griggs WM, Myburgh JA, Worthley LI. A prospective comparison of a percutaneous tracheostomy technique with standard surgical tracheostomy. *Intensive Care Med.* 1991;17(5):261-263.

74. Park H, Kent J, Joshi M, et al. Percutaneous versus open tracheostomy: comparison of procedures and surgical site infections. *Surg Infect (Larchmt).* 2013;14(1):21-23.

75. Brotfain E, Koyfman L, Frenkel A, et al. Bedside percutaneous tracheostomy versus open surgical tracheostomy in non-ICU patients. *Crit Care Res Pract.* 2014;2014:156814.

76. Freeman BD, Isabella K, Lin N, Buchman TG. A meta-analysis of prospective trials comparing percutaneous and surgical tracheostomy in critically ill patients. *Chest.* 2000;118(5):1412-1418.

77. Cheung NH, Napolitano LM. Tracheostomy: epidemiology, indications, timing, technique, and outcomes. *Respir Care.* 2014;59(6):895-919.

78. Durbin CG Jr. Early complications of tracheostomy. *Respir Care.* 2005;50(4):511-515.

79. Epstein SK. Late complications of tracheostomy. *Respir Care.* 2005;50(4):542-549.

80. Simon M, Metschke M, Braune SA, Püschel K, Kluge S. Death after percutaneous dilatational tracheostomy: a systematic review and analysis of risk factors. *Crit Care.* 2013;17(5):R258.

81. Hill LL, Pearl RG. Flow triggering, pressure triggering, and autotriggering during mechanical ventilation. *Crit Care Med.* 2000;28(2):579-581.

82. Slutsky AS, Ranieri VM. Ventilator-induced lung injury. *N Engl J Med.* 2013;369(22):2126-2136.

83. International consensus conferences in intensive care medicine: ventilator-associated lung injury in ARDS. This official conference report was cosponsored by the American Thoracic Society, The European Society of Intensive Care Medicine, and The Societé de Réanimation de Langue Française, and was approved by the ATS Board of Directors, July 1999. *Am J Respir Crit Care Med.* 1999;160(6):2118-2124.

84. Weissman C. Pulmonary complications after cardiac surgery. *Semin Cardiothorac Vasc Anesth.* 2004;8(3):185–211.

85. Lachmann B. Open up the lung and keep the lung open. *Intensive Care Med.* 1992;18(6):319-321.

86. Lawn ND, Fletcher DD, Henderson RD, Wolter TD, Wijdicks EF. Anticipating mechanical ventilation in Guillain-Barré syndrome. *Arch Neurol.* 2001;58(6):893-898.

87. Kondili E, Alexopoulou C, Prinianakis C, Xirouchaki N, Georgopoulos D. Pattern of lung emptying and expiratory resistance in mechanically ventilated patients with chronic obstructive pulmonary disease. *Intensive Care Med.* 2004;30(7):1311-1318

88. Petrof BJ, Legaré M, Goldberg P, Milic-Emili J, Gottfried SB. Continuous positive airway pressure reduces work of breathing and dyspnea during weaning form mechanical ventilation in severe chronic obstructive pulmonary disease. *Am Rev Respir Dis.* 1990;141(2):281-289.

89. Yarmus L, Feller-Kopman D. Pneumothorax in the critically ill patient. *Chest.* 2012;141(4):1098-1105.

90. Baumann MH, Noppen M. Pneumothorax. *Respirology.* 2004;9(2):157-164.

91. Papazian L, Forel JM, Gacouin A, et al; ACURASYS Study Investigators. Neuromuscular blockers in early acute respiratory distress syndrome. *New Engl J Med.* 2010;363(12):1107-1116.

92. Macduff A, Arnold A, Harvey J; BTS Pleural Disease Guideline Group. Management of spontaneous pneumothorax. British Thoracic Society Pleural Disease Guideline 2010. *Thorax.* 2010;65(Suppl 2):ii18-ii31.

93. Lin YC, Tu CY, Liang SJ, et al. Pigtail catheter for the management of pneumothorax in mechanically ventilated patients. *Am J Emerg Med.* 2010;28(4):466-471.

94. A personal guide to managing chest tube. Maquet Web site. http://www.atriummed.com/EN/Chest_Drainage/Documents/ExpressHandbook-010138.pdf. Accessed June 10, 2017.

95. White AC. Long-term mechanical ventilation: management strategies. *Respir Care.* 2012;57(6):889-897.

96. Rochwerg B, Brochard RB, Elliott MW, et al. Official ERS/ATS Clinical Practice Guidelines: noninvasive ventilation for acute respiratory failure. *Eur Respir J.* 2017;50(2):1-20.

97. Navalesi P, Fanfulla F, Frigerio P, Gregoretti C, Nava S. Physiologic evaluation of noninvasive mechanical ventilation delivered with three types of masks in patients with chronic hypercapnic respiratory failure. *Crit Care Med.* 2000;28(6):1785-1790.

98. Itagaki T, Okuda N, Tsunano Y, et al. Effect of high-flow nasal cannula on thoraco-abdominal synchrony in adult critically ill patients. *Respir Care.* 2014;59(1):70-74.

99. Sztrymf B, Messika J, Bertrand F, et al. Beneficial effects of humidified high flow nasal oxygen in critical care patients: a prospective pilot study. *Intensive Care Med.* 2011;37(11):1780-1786.

100. Frat JP, Thille AW, Mercat A, et al; FLORALI Study Group; REVA Network. High-flow oxygen through nasal cannula in acute hypoxemic respiratory failure. *New Engl J Med.* 2015;372(23):2185-2196.

101. Vourc'h M, Asfar P, Volteau C, et al. High-flow nasal cannula oxygen during endotracheal intubation in hypoxemic patients: a randomized controlled clinical trial. *Intensive Care Med.* 2015;41(9):1538-1548.

102. Millar J, Lutton S, O'Connor P. The use of high-flow nasal oxygen therapy in the management of hypercarbic respiratory failure. *Ther Adv Respir Dis.* 2014;8(2):63-64.

103. Bräunlich J, Beyer D, Mai D, Hammerschmidt S, Seyfarth H-J, Wirtz H. Effects of nasal high flow on ventilation in volunteers, COPD and idiopathic pulmonary fibrosis patients. *Respiration.* 2013;85(4):319-325.

104. Doud EG. Airway pressure release ventilation. *Ann Thorac Med*. 2007:2(4):176-179.

105. Daoud EG, Farag HL, Chatburn RL. Airway pressure release ventilation: what do we know? *Respir Care*. 2012;57(2):282-292.

106. Modrykamien A, Chatburn RL, Ashton RW. Airway pressure release ventilation: an alternative mode of mechanical ventilation in acute respiratory distress syndrome. *Cleve Clin J Med*. 2011;78(2):101-110.

107. Gilstrap D, MacIntyre N. Patient-ventilator interactions. Implications for clinical management. *Am J Respir Crit Care Med*. 2013;188(9):1058-1068.

108. Nilsestuen JO, Hargett KD. Using the ventilator graphics to identify patient-ventilator asynchrony. *Respir Care*. 2005;50(2):202-232.

109. Leung P, Jubran A, Tobin J. Comparison of assisted ventilator modes on triggering, patient effort, and dyspnea. *Am J Respir Crit Care Med*. 1997;155(6):1940-1948.

110. de Wit M. Monitoring of patient-ventilator interaction at the bedside. *Respir Care*. 2011;56(1):61-68.

111. Thille AW, Rodriguez P, Cabello B, Lellouche F, Brochard L. Patient-ventilator asynchrony during assisted mechanical ventilation. *Intensive Care Med*. 2006;32(10):1515-1522.

112. de Wit M, Pedram S, Best AM, Epstein SK. Observational study of patient-ventilator asynchrony and relationship to sedation level. *J Crit Care*. 2009;24(1):74-80.

113. Vignaux L, Vargas F, Roeseler J, et al. Patient-ventilator asynchrony during non-invasive ventilation for acute respiratory failure: a multicenter study. *Intensive Care Med*. 2009;35(5):840-846.

114. Thille AW, Cabello B, Galia F, Lyazidi A, Brochard L. Reduction of patient-ventilator asynchrony by reducing tidal volume during pressure support ventilation. *Intensive Care Med*. 2008;34(8):1477-1486.

115. Leung P, Jubran A, Tobin MJ. Comparison of assisted ventilator modes on triggering, patient effort, and dyspnea. *Am J Respir Crit Care Med*. 1997;155(6):1940-1948.

116. Appendini L, Purro A, Patessio A, et al. Partitioning of inspiratory muscle workload and pressure assistance in ventilator-dependent COPD patients. *Am J Respir Crit Care Med*. 1996;154(5):1301-1309.

117. Imanaka H, Nishimura M, Takeuchi M, Kimball WR, Yahagi N, Kumon K. Autotriggering caused by cardiogenic oscillation during flow-triggered mechanical ventilation. *Crit Care Med*. 2000;28(2):402-407.

118. Blanch L, Bernabe F, Lucangelo U. Measurement of air trapping, intrinsic positive end-expiratory pressure, and dynamic hyperinflation in mechanically ventilated patients. *Respir Care*. 2005;50(1):110-124.

119. Marini JJ. Should PEEP be used in airflow obstruction? *Am Rev Respir Dis*. 1989;140(1):1-3.

120. Marini JJ. Dynamic hyperinflation and auto-positive end-expiratory pressure. *Am J Respir Crit Care Med*. 2011;184(7):756-762.

121. Ranieri VM, Giuliani R, Cinnella G, et al. Physiologic effects of positive end-expiratory pressure in COPD patients during acute ventilatory failure and controlled mechanical ventilation. *Am Rev Respir Dis*. 1993;147(1):5-13.

122. Leatherman JW, McArthur C, Shaprio RS. Effect of prolongation of expiratory time on dynamic hyperinflation in mechanically ventilated patients with severe asthma. *Crit Care Med*. 2004;32(7):1542-1545.

123. Thille AW, Richard JCM, Brochard L. The decision to extubate in the intensive care unit. *Am J Respir Crit Care Med*. 2013;187(12):1294-1302.

124. Vallverdú I, Calaf N, Subirana M, Net A, Benito S, Mancebo J. Clinical characteristics, respiratory functional parameters, and outcome of a two-hour T-piece trial in patients weaning from mechanical ventilation. *Am J Respir Crit Care Med*. 1998;158(6):1855-1862.

125. Epstein SK, Ciubotaru RL, Wong JB. Effect of failed extubation on the outcome of mechanical ventilation. *Chest*. 1997;112(1):186-192.

126. Thille AW, Harrois A, Schortgen F, Brun-Buisson C, Brochard L. Outcomes of extubation failure in medical intensive care unit patients. *Crit Care Med*. 2011;39(12):2612-2618.

127. Frutos-Vivar F, Ferguson ND, Esteban A, et al. Risk factors for extubation failure in patients following a successful spontaneous breathing trial. *Chest*. 2006;130(6):1664-1671.

128. Namen AM, Ely EW, Tatter SB, et al. Predictors of successful extubation in neurosurgical patients. *Am J Respir Crit Care Med*. 2001;163(3 Pt 1):658-664.

129. Mokhlesi B, Tulaimat A, Gluckman TJ, Wang Y, Evans AT, Corbridge TC. Predicting extubation failure after successful completion of a spontaneous breathing trial. *Respir Care*. 2007;52(12):1710-1717.

130. Khamiees M, Raju P, DeGirolamo A, Amoateng-Adjepong Y, Manthous CA. Predictors of extubation outcome in patients who have successfully completed a spontaneous breathing trial. *Chest*. 2001;120(4):1262-1270.

131. Smina M, Salam A, Khamiees M, Gada P, Amoateng-Adjepong Y, Manthous CA. Cough peak flows and extubation outcomes. *Chest*. 2003;124(1):262-268.

132. Chien JY, Lin MS, Huang YC, Chien YF, Yu CJ, Yang PC. Changes in B-type natriuretic peptide improve weaning outcome predicted by spontaneous breathing trial. *Crit Care Med*. 2008;36(5):1421-1426.

133. Teixeira C, da Silva NB, Savi A, et al. Central venous saturation is a predictor of reintubation in difficult-to-wean patients. *Crit Care Med*. 2010;38(2):491-496.

132. Schmidt GA, Girard TD, Kress JP, et al. Liberation from mechanical ventilation in critically ill adults: executive summary of an official American College of Chest Physicians/American Thoracic Society clinical practice guideline. *Chest*. 2017;151(1):160-165.

133. Ouellette DR, Patel S, Girard TD, et al. Liberation from mechanical ventilation in critically ill adults: an official American College of Chest Physicians/American Thoracic Society clinical practice guideline: inspiratory pressure augmentation during spontaneous breathing trials, protocols minimizing sedation, and noninvasive ventilation immediately after extubation. *Chest*. 2017;151(1):166-180.

134. Argalious MY. The cuff leak test: does it "leak" any information? *Respir Care*. 2012;57(12):2136-2137

135. Miller RL, Cole RP. Association between reduced cuff leak volume and postextubation stridor. *Chest*. 1996;110(4):1035-1040.

136. Jaber S, Chanques G, Matecki S, et al. Postextubation stridor in intensive care unit patients. Risk factors evaluation and importance of the cuff-leak test. *Intensive Care Med*. 2003;29(1):69-74.

137. De Bast Y, De Backer D, Moraine JJ, Lemaire M, Vandenborght C, Vincent JL. The cuff leak test to predict failure of tracheal extubation for laryngeal edema. *Intensive Care Med*. 2002;28(9):1267-1272.

138. Sandhu RS, Pasquale MD, Miller K, Wasser TE. Measurement of endotracheal tube cuff leak to predict postextubation stridor and need for reintubation. *J Am Coll Surg.* 2000;190(6):682-687.

139. Pluijm WA, van Mook WN, Wittekamp BHJ, Bergmans DC. Postextubation laryngeal edema and stridor resulting in respiratory failure in critically ill adult patients: updated review. *Crit Care.* 2015;19:295.

140. Prinianakis G, Alexopoulou C, Mamidakis E, Kondili E, Georgopoulos D. Determinants of the cuff leak test: a physiological study. *Crit Care.* 2005;9(1):R24-R31.

141. Patel KN, Ganatra KD, Bates JHT, Young MP. Variation in the rapid shallow breathing index associated with common measurement techniques and conditions. *Respir Care.* 2009;54(11):1462-1466.

142. Siegel MD. Technique and the rapid shallow breathing index. *Respir Care.* 2009;54(11):1449-1450.

143. Desair NR, Myers L, Simeone F. Comparison of 3 different methods used to measure the rapid shallow breathing index. *J Crit Care.* 2012;27(4):418e1-418e6.

144. Fernandez JF, Levine SM, Restrepo MI. Technologic advances in endotracheal tubes for prevention of ventilator-associated pneumonia. *Chest.* 2012;142(1):231-238.

145. Seegobin RD, van Hasselt GL. Endotracheal cuff pressure and tracheal mucosal blood flow: endoscopic study of effects of four large volume cuffs. *Br Med J (Clin Res Ed).* 1984;288(6422):965-968.

146. Biel MA, Sievert C, Usacheva M, et al. Reduction of endotracheal tube biofilms using antimicrobial photodynamic therapy. *Lasers Surg Med.* 2011;43(7):586-590.

147. MacIntyre NR, Epstein SK, Carson S, Scheinhorn D, Christopher K, Muldoon S; National Association for Medical Direction of Respiratory Care. Management of patients requiring prolonged mechanical ventilation: report of a NAMDRC consensus conference. *Chest.* 2005;128(6):3937-3935.

148. Carson SS, Kahn JM, Hough CL, et al; ProVent Investigators. A multicenter mortality prediction model for patients receiving prolonged mechanical ventilation. *Crit Care Med.* 2012;40(4):1171-1176.

149. Garpestad E, Brennan J, Hill NS. Noninvasive ventilation for critical care. *Chest.* 2007;132(2):711-720.

150. Hess DR. Noninvasive ventilation for acute respiratory failure. *Respir Care.* 2013;58(6):950-972.

151. Keenan SP, Sinuff T, Burns KE, et al; Canadian Critical Care Trials Group/Canadian Critical Care Society Noninvasive Ventilation Guidelines Group. Clinical practice guidelines for the use of noninvasive positive pressure ventilation and noninvasive continuous positive airway pressure in the acute care setting. *CMAJ.* 2011;183(3):E195-E214.

152. Mattu A. How to recognize and treat severe asthma in the emergency department. http://www.medscape.com/viewarticle/730504#vp_2. Accessed June 2, 2017.

153. Lazarus SC. Clinical practice: emergency treatment of asthma. *New Engl J Med.* 2010;363(8):755-764.

Airway Management

Joseph Cerminara, MD, Timothy Quinn, MD, Ronaldo Collo Go, MD,
and Ananda Dharshan, MD

INTRODUCTION

Securing the airway is an important task for treating critically ill patients. Indications for endotracheal intubation include surgical procedure, respiratory failure, cardiac arrest, airway protection (ie, coma), and airway obstruction (ie, anaphylaxis, airway burns, airway bleeding).

For any patient undergoing surgery, preoperative assessment includes American Society of Anesthesiologists Classification (ASA) which assesses the physiologic status to predict operative risk.[1] ASA 1 is a normal healthy patient with good exercise tolerance.[1] ASA 2 is patient with mild systemic disease that is well controlled and no functional limitation.[1] ASA 3 is a patient with severe systemic disease that is not life threatening with some functional limitation.[1] ASA 4 is severe disease with a constant threat to life.[1] ASA 5 is a patient with is not going to survive without surgery.[1] ASA 6 is a brain dead patient for organ harvest.[1]

For any patient requiring a secure airway, difficult intubation, defined as difficult facemask or supraglottic airway (SGA) ventilation, difficult supraglottic airway placement, difficult laryngoscopy, difficult tracheal intubation, or failed intubation attempts, should be anticipated.[2] Avoidance of "can't intubate can't oxygenate" situation or CICO is paramount. The ASA have released guidelines based on levels of evidence.[2] Recommendation for Category A has 3 levels: Level 1 has sufficient randomized control trials to conduct meta-analysis; Level 2 has multiple randomized control trials but not sufficient for meta-analysis; and Level 3 has a single randomized control trial.[2] Recommendation for Category B also has 4 levels: Level 1 has observational studies with clinical interventions for a specific outcome; Level 2 has observational studies with associative statistics; Level 3 has noncomparative observational studies with descriptive statistics; and Level 4 has case reports.[2] Based on the Fourth National Audit Project (4NAP), the following were associated with airway complications: human factors such as poor education and judgment; omission of airway assessment; poor planning; intubation failure managed with repeated attempts; obese patients; use of supraglottic devices on poor candidates such as obese patients or high risk for aspiration; delay for emergent front of neck airway;

unrecognized esophageal intubation; failure to use capnography; and recovery events such as blood in airway, tracheal edema, or postobstructive pulmonary edema (POPE).[3-5] The Royal Academy of Anesthesiologists and Difficult Airway Society Guidelines are stratified into 4 plans.[6,7] Plan A is preparation, oxygenation, induction, mask ventilation, and intubation.[6,7] Plan B is rescue airway via supraglottic device.[6,7] Plan C is final attempt at preoxygenation via facemask ventilation.[6,7] Plan D is emergent front of neck airway or eFONA.[6,7] These societies advocate the Vortex Approach where a maximum of 3 attempts at oxygenation via supraglottic airway (SGA), facemask, or tracheal intubation.[6] Further clinical deterioration or failure at all attempts mandates eFONA.[7]

Assessment

Initial airway assessment involves identifying patients who are difficult to ventilate or intubate. Factors associated with risk of difficult intubation include Mallampati class III or IV airway, inter-incisor distance of less than 3 cm, thyromental distance less than 6.5 cm, and decreased jaw or cervical spine range of motion.[2,7] A history of previous difficult intubations, previous head and neck surgery including decannulated tracheostomies, and radiation therapy should also be identified.[2,7] Factors associated with difficult bag-mask ventilation include facial hair, obesity, edentulous patients, advanced age, and obstructive sleep apnea. Scoring systems such as Mallampati and Cormack-Lehane should not be used alone but as adjunct to identify patients who are difficult to intubate (Fig. 13-1 and Table 13-1).[8-10] However, complete assessment is not always possible due to altered mental status and emergent need to secure the airway in the critical ill.

Preparation for Difficult Airway and Strategy for Intubation

The ASA, Royal Academy of Anesthesiologists, and Difficult Airway Society recommend having a preintubation strategy for intubation of a difficult airway.[2,6,7] The difficult airway algorithm from the ASA is shown in Figure 13-2, and it can be adapted to the individual situation. As with any medical

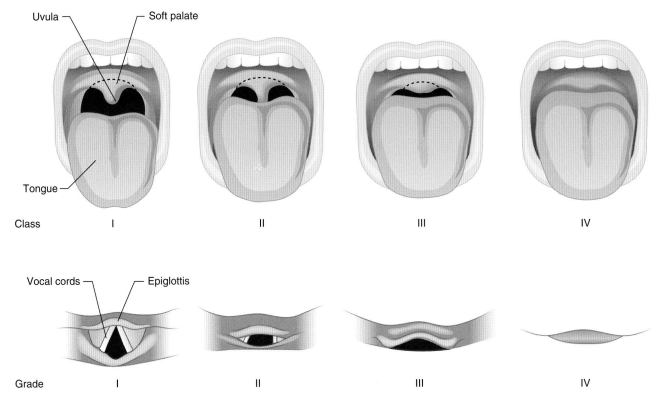

FIGURE 13-1 Mallumpati classes of oral opening and Grades of laryngeal view.

emergency, calling for expert help and consultation early may avoid unnecessary harm to the patient.

Difficult airway cart should be available which should include endotracheal tubes of various sizes, laryngoscopes and blades with various sizes, emergent cricothyrotomy and tracheostomy kits, supraglottic devices, video assisted laryngoscopy, light wands and tube exchangers, straps to secure endotracheal tubes, and end-tidal CO_2 detectors. Strategies for intubation include: (1) awake intubation via fiberoptic (Category B3) or blind tracheal intubation, supraglottic devices, and optically guided intubation (Category B4); (2) video assisted laryngoscopy (Category A1); (3) intubating stylets or tube changers (Category B3) with possible complications of lung laceration and gastric perforation; (4) supraglottic

TABLE 13-1 Advanced Airway Techniques for Intubation

Technique	Awake Fiber-Optic Intubation	Video Laryngoscopy	Intubating Stylet/ Tube-Changer	Supraglottic Airway	Intubating LMA	Light Wand
Advantages	88–100% success rates; spontaneous respirations	Improved laryngeal views, more successful in first-time intubations compared to direct laryngoscopy	Blind technique (advantage if bleeding or unable to visualize larynx)	Can be used to ventilate a patient who cannot be intubated	Can ventilate and attempt intubation through ILMA	96.8–100% success rates in observational studies on difficult airways
Disadvantages	Uncomfortable; nerve blocks or topicalization required; not feasible in an emergency	Usually larger than direct laryngoscopy (may not be able to pass tube next to video laryngoscope, or possible cuff damage)	Mucosal bleeding; lung/ esophageal perforation; blind technique	Nonsecure airway; risk of aspiration; risk of gastric insufflation	Sore throat, hoarseness, pharyngeal edema	"Blind technique"; risk of mucosal bleeding

ILMA = intubating laryngeal mask airway; LMA = laryngeal mask airway.

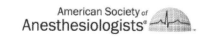

DIFFICULT AIRWAY ALGORITHM

1. **Assess the likelihood and clinical impact of basic management problems:**
   - Difficulty with patient cooperation or consent
   - Difficult mask ventilation
   - Difficult supraglottic airway placement
   - Difficult laryngoscopy
   - Difficult intubation
   - Difficult surgical airway access

2. **Actively pursue opportunities to deliver supplemental oxygen throughout the process of difficult airway management.**

3. **Consider the relative merits and feasibility of basic management choices:**
   - Awake intubation *vs.* intubation after induction of general anesthesia
   - Non-invasive technique *vs.* invasive techniques for the initial approach to intubation
   - Video-assisted laryngoscopy as an initial approach to intubation
   - Preservation *vs.* ablation of spontaneous ventilation

4. **Develop primary and alternative strategies:**

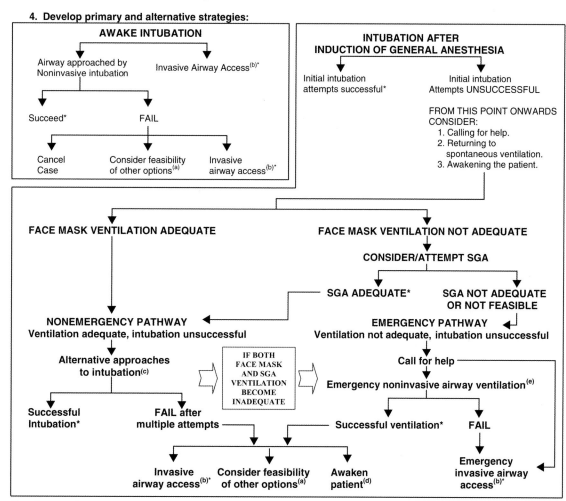

*Confirm ventilation, tracheal intubation, or SGA placement with exhaled CO_2.

a. Other options include (but are not limited to): surgery utilizing face mask or supraglottic airway (SGA) anesthesia (e.g., LMA, ILMA, laryngeal tube), local anesthesia infiltration or regional nerve blockade. Pursuit of these options usually implies that mask ventilation will not be problematic. Therefore, these options may be of limited value if this step in the algorithm has been reached via the Emergency Pathway.

b. Invasive airway access includes surgical or percutaneous airway, jet ventilation, and retrograde intubation.

c. Alternative difficult intubation approaches include (but are not limited to): video-assisted laryngoscopy, alternative laryngoscope blades, SGA (e.g., LMA or ILMA) as an intubation conduit (with or without fiberoptic guidance), fiberoptic intubation, intubating stylet or tube changer, light wand, and blind oral or nasal intubation.

d. Consider re-preparation of the patient for awake intubation or canceling surgery.

e. Emergency non-invasive airway ventilation consists of a SGA.

FIGURE 13-2 The American Society of Anesthesiologists Difficult Airway Algorithm. SGA = supraglottic airway. (Used with permission from Apfelbaum JL, Hagberg CA, Caplan RA, et al. Practice guidelines for the management of the difficult airway: an updated report by the American Society of Anesthesiologists Task Force on Management of the Difficult Airway. *Anesthesiology.* 2013;118(2):251-270.)

devices such as laryngeal mask airway (LMA) with possible complications of bronchospasm, difficulty in swallowing, respiratory obstruction, laryngeal nerve injury , edema, and hypoglossal nerve paralysis (Category B4); (5) intubating laryngeal mask airway (iLMA) with possible complications of sore throat, hoarseness, and pharyngeal edema (Category B3); (7) (6) fiberoptic guided intubation (Category B3) and with Mallampati 3-4 Scores (Category A2), and lighted stylets or wands (Category B3)[2] (see Table 13-1).

The most common laryngoscope blades in clinical practice are the Macintosh and Miller laryngoscope blades. The Macintosh blade is curved, and the tip is placed in the vallecula and lifted up and out at a 45-degree angle. This should allow for visualization of the vocal cords. The Miller blade is straight and usually thinner than the Macintosh blade. It is used first to move the tongue to the side, at which point the epiglottis can be visualized. The blade is then used to lift the epiglottis and reveal the vocal cords.

Video laryngoscopy has emerged as a reliable tool for intubation with increased first-pass success, even by critical care fellows who are relatively inexperienced with intubation.[1,6,7] An intubating bougie or tube changer is a rubber coated, medium-stiff wire with a slanted tip. A laryngoscope is used to move the tongue out of the way to obtain the view seen by direct laryngoscopy. The bougie is advanced on the posterior aspect of the epiglottis toward the laryngeal opening. The laryngeal opening can be approximated if no structures can be visualized. Once through the glottic opening in the trachea, the slanted tip will catch on the tracheal rings. After "tactile confirmation," an endotracheal tube is placed over the bougie and through the vocal cords.

Another technique in which the vocal cords are not directly visualized utilizes a lighted introducer or stylet. An endotracheal tube (ETT) with a stylet with a lighted tip is placed over the tongue, and the laryngeal opening is approximated. The light will make a particular midline circumscribed glow pattern when the stylet passes through the laryngeal opening into the trachea. An ETT can then be placed over the stylet. If the stylet enters the esophagus, the light will markedly dim.

Awake fiber-optic intubation remains the gold standard for management of a known difficult airway. It requires clinicians with advanced airway skills and other back-up plans in the event of complications. The procedure is a bit of a misnomer, as clinicians may use any combination of medications to relieve anxiety to facilitate the navigation of the bronchoscope loaded with an endotracheal tube past the vocal cords. The airway is prepared via antisialogues such as glycopyrrolate, atropine, or hyoscine, but the associated tachycardia might make it a less-desirable option.[11] Local anesthetics such as lidocaine, 1.5 mg/kg topical 3 minutes before intubation, can blunt the hypertensive response, airway reactivity, and incidence of dysarrthmias.[12,13] Zofran maybe given to blunt the gag reflex.[11] Some still advocate for mild sedation, such as with ketamine, midazolam, dexmedetomidine, remifentanil, and propofol.[11,12] Regardless of the individual technique, the goal is for the patient to maintain spontaneous ventilation throughout so that, at any point, the procedure may be aborted safely without any undo harm to the patient. The patient is induced with general anesthesia once the endotracheal tube is advanced into the trachea, confirmed with both fiber-optic visualization and capnography. Complications include trauma to the airway and laryngospasm.

Preoxygenation

It is important to optimize the conditions for successful intubation. Preoxygenation of the patient replaces nitrogen in the functional residual capacity (FRC) in the lung with oxygen, creating a reservoir of oxygen to avoid hypoxemia during a period of apnea and intubation attempts. Three minutes of facemask oxygenation helps to maintain significantly higher oxygen saturation compared to 1-minute facemask oxygenation (Category A2). When compared to 4 maximal breaths in 30 seconds, results are equivocal; however, time to desaturation is longer with 3 minutes of preoxygenation with mask and 100% fraction of inspired oxygen (Fio_2).[2]

Positioning

Proper positioning is required to improve visualization of the larynx under direct laryngoscopy. The 3-airway axis model of laryngoscopy was originally described in 1944 by Bannister and Macbeth.[13,14] In order to visualize the larynx, the clinician must align the oral, pharyngeal, and laryngeal axes. Placing a pillow under the head or using an intubation ramp helps align the pharyngeal and laryngeal axes. Subsequent neck extension will align the oral axis, allowing visualization through all 3 axes. See Figure 13-2.

Patients with cervical spine instability, fractures, neuropathies, or radiculopathies may have additional morbidities if extension of the neck occurs. In-line neck stabilization with close attention to not extend the neck, as well as the use of video laryngoscopy may be useful techniques for visualizing the larynx without stressing the cervical spine.

Cricoid Pressure

Also known as the Sellick maneuver, this is a manual compression of the cricoid cartilage (C6) to prevent gastroesophageal reflux during intubation. The rationale for its use is debatable, since some studies have suggested that it does not decrease the risk for reflux. It also increases the risk of esophageal rupture if the patient vomits because 90% the esophagus is lateral to the trachea, and it may further occlude the trachea.

Rapid Sequence Intubation

Rapid sequence intubation (RSI) has been synonymous with the administration of an induction agent and neuromuscular blockade (NMB). The rationale is that it decreases the risk of aspiration and secures the airway rapidly. It consists of the 6 Ps, which are seen in Table 13-2. *Preparation*, or identifying

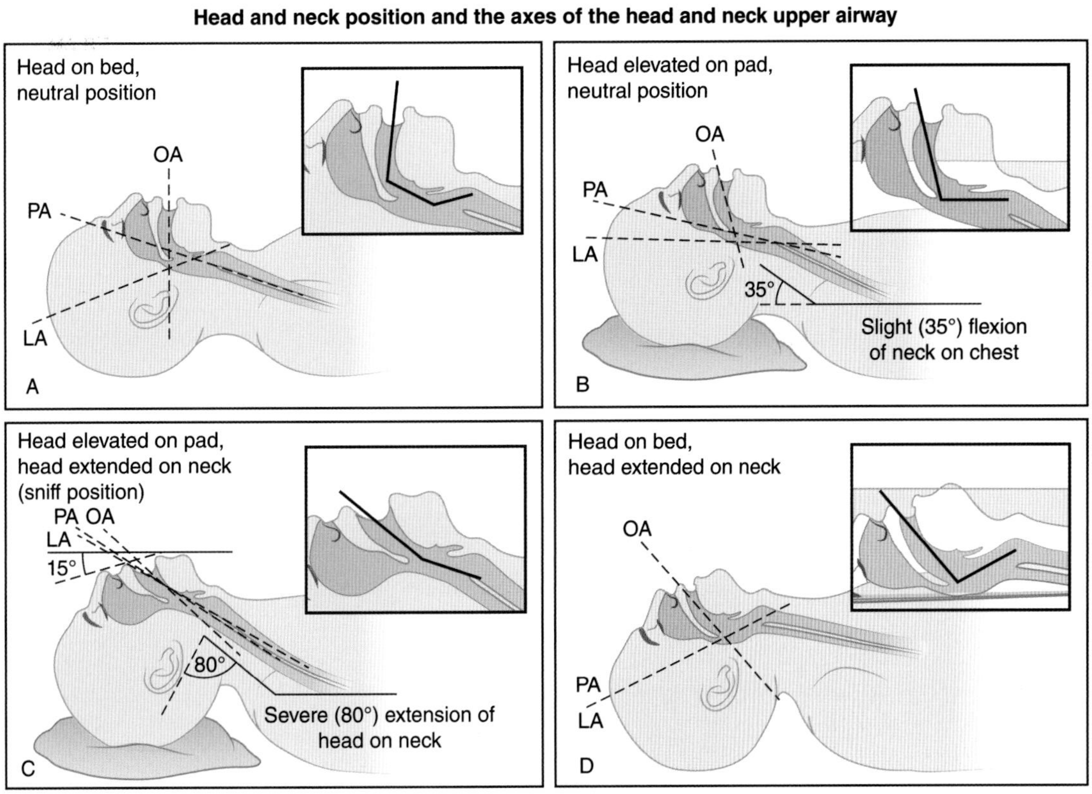

Head and neck position and the axes of the head and neck upper airway

FIGURE 13-3 The 3-airway axis model. LA = laryngeal axis; OA = oral axis; PA = pharyngeal axis. Each head position is accompanied by an *inset* that magnifies the upper airway (oral cavity, pharynx, and larynx) and superimposes *(bent bold line)* the continuity of these three axes within the upper airway. (A) The head is in the neutral position with a marked degree of nonalignment of the LA, PA, and OA. (B) The head is resting on a large pad that flexes the neck on the chest and aligns the LA with the PA. (C) The head is resting on a pad (which flexes the neck on the chest). Concomitant extension of the head on the neck brings all three axes into alignment (sniffing position). (D) Extension of the head on the neck without concomitant elevation of the head on a pad, which results in nonalignment of the PA and LA with the OA. (Reprinted with permission from Benumof JL, ed. *Airway Management: Principles and Practice.* St. Louis: Mosby; 1996: 263.)

the need for intubation, takes about 5 to 10 minutes.[13,15] *Preoxygenation*, or alveolar denitrogenation, creates a reservoir of oxygen and is performed via 100% nonrebreather (NRB) mask for 5 minutes. It avoids the need for ball-valve-mask ventilation and the risk of gastric aspiration. *Premedication* attenuates the physiologic response to intubation and provides sedation and analgesia. *Paralysis* has 2 components: induction medications and administration of NMBs. After the induction agent is given, the patient can be given either a depolarizing NMB or nondepolarizing NMB. After 45 seconds to 1 minute, the degree of paralysis is assessed via mandibular mobility. Neuromuscular blockade can be reversed by neostigmine, edrophonium, glycopyrrolate, atropine, or suggamex. The next P is *Passage*, which refers to the insertion of the endotracheal tube once paralysis is adequate. Visualization of the vocal cords may be improved by applying pressure on the thyroid. See Figure 13-3 for proper position or 3 airway axis model.

Delayed Sequence Intubation

Standard preoxygenation involves breathing high Fio_2 supplementation for more than 3 minutes or for 8 vital capacity breaths.[16,17] In healthy, nonobese patients, this provides a buffer of 8 minutes prior to saturations dropping to less than 90%.[2] This buffer diminishes in increased metabolism, lung disease, and abnormal habitus.[16] Adequate preoxygenation will allow oxygen saturations to be maintained at greater than 95% during apneic episode, such as when the patient being intubated.[18,19] Abandonment of preoxygenation can cause profound and immediate hypoxia after RSI medications are given.

As stated earlier, preoxygenation can be delivery via nonrebreather mask which can give Fio_2 65% to 80%, but other methods include bag-valve-mask device, which can deliver Fio_2 of 90%, or noninvasive positive-pressure ventilation (NIPPV), which can deliver Fio_2 of 100%.[16] Patients may not tolerate preoxygenation due to delirium; therefore, delayed sequence intubation (DSI) has been utilized. Ketamine 1 mg/kg IV is given and repeated at 0.5 mg/kg aliquots until dissociative state is induced.[20] The patient is placed in semi-Fowler position, and preoxygenation and denitrogenation are performed with high Fio_2 oxygen supplementation.[20] After 3 minutes, the patient is paralyzed and intubated, or sometimes the patient improves and there is no need for endotracheal intubation. This prospective observational multicenter study

TABLE 13-2 Rapid Sequence Intubation and the 6 "P"s

	Drugs	Dose	Onset	Duration	Notes
Preparation					
Preoxygenation					
Premedication	Fentanyl	2–3 μg/kg IV	Immediate	0.5–1 h	Blunts hypertension
	Esmolol	2 mg/kg IV	45–90 s	10–20 min	Blunts tachycardia
	Lidocaine	1.5 mg/kg IV	2–10 min	10–30 min	Diminish airway activity, decrease intracranial hypertension, and decrease incidence of dysrhythmias
Paralysis: Induction agent	Etomidate	0.15–0.3 mg/kg IV	30–60 s	3–5 min	Neuroprotective, hypnotic SE: adrenal insufficiency for 12 h, nausea, vomiting, myoclonus, seizures
	Propofol	0.5–2 mg IVP	9–50 s	3–10 min	Reduces ICP, hypnotic, greater degree of sedation SE: hypotension due to decreased SVR and decreased inotropy; avoid in soy and egg allergy; propofol infusion syndrome
	Ketamine	2 mg/kg IVP	1–2 min	5–15 min	Bronchodilator, hypnotic SE: hypertensive emergencies; can cause ischemic heart disease; emergence phenomena, which are attenuated with benzodiazepines; increased intracranial pressure; increased salivation and bronchorrhea; prevented by glycopyrrolate or scopolamine
	Scopolamine	0.2–0.4 mg IVP	10 min	2 h	Sedative and hypnotic SE: tachycardia
	Midazolam	0.3 mg/kg IVP	60–90 s	15–30 min	SE: respiratory depression, amnesia
	Thiopental	1.5–3 mg/kg IVP	30–60 s	5–30 min	Decrease intracranial pressure SE: laryngobronchospasm, hypersalivation
Paralysis: Depolarizing NMB	Succinylcholine	1.5 mg/kg IVP	30–60 s	5–15 min	MOA: Depolarizing: activates acetylcholine receptor Caution or avoid in hyperkalemia, history of malignant hyperthermia, denervation > 3 d, crush injury > 3 d, severe burns > 24 h, elevated CK, narrow angle glaucoma Other SE: dysrhythmias attenuated with atropine
Paralysis: Nondepolaring NMB	Rocuronium	1 mg/kg IVP	45–60 s	45–70 min	Eliminated primarily by liver
	Vecuronium	0.15 mg/kg IVP	2–3 min	45–60 min	Eliminated primarily by kidneys
	Cisatracurium	0.15–0.2 mg/kg IVP	2–3 min	28–50 min	Eliminated mostly by pH-dependent breakdown, followed by liver and kidneys
	Pancuronium	0.06–1 mg/kg IVP	2–3 min	35–45 min	SE: bronchospasm, hypotension, tachycardia
	Atracurium	0.4–0.5 mg/kg IV	1–4 min	20–35 min	
Passage					

ICP = intracranial pressure; IV = intravenous; IVP = IV push; MOA = mechanism of action; NMB = neuromuscular blockade; SE = side effects.

showed that this method is an alternative to rapid sequence intubation for those who do not tolerate preoxygenation, although further study is necessary to establish safety.[20]

Confirmation of Successful Intubation

Postintubation verification of endotracheal tube placement is a necessity. Capnography, auscultation, and chest radiographs are often needed to confirm placement of endotracheal tube. Continuous waveform capnography should be considered in patients undergoing chest compressions during cardiopulmonary resuscitation (CPR) as a way to confirm effect resuscitation (ie, CO_2 production) and ensure the endotracheal tube remains in the airway during compressions.[21] When in doubt, a flexible bronchoscope can be used to identify that the ETT is in the trachea. The tip of the ETT should be between 2 and 7 cm above the carina. The position of the ETT is influenced by the position of the neck. If the neck is flexed, the ETT will appear closer to the carina. If the neck is extended, the ETT will appear farther away from the carina.

Surgical Airways

If ventilation and intubation are unsuccessful, a definitive surgical airway can be a lifesaving technique. Needle cricothyrotomy with percutaneous ventilation is a relatively simple technique to provide oxygenation and ventilation in a difficult airway. It can be useful to provide more time to desaturation during difficult airway management. There are now various jet ventilation kits available commercially.

Retrograde intubation involves piercing the cricothyroid membrane with a needle and threading a wire through, cephalad toward the larynx. The wire is retrieved in the oropharynx often by an assistant with Magill forceps. The Cook medical retrograde intubation kit has an obturator, which is then placed over the wire. The wire is removed and an ETT can be placed over the obturator. Then, placement can be confirmed and the obturator removed.

A surgical cricothyrotomy can be done in an emergency by making a 2-cm transverse incision over the cricothyroid membrane. Another vertical incision is made in the middle of the transverse incision. An ETT or other breathing device can be placed and the balloon can be inflated, and then placement can be confirmed.

ANESTHESIA MONITORING

Capnography

Capnography measures end-tidal CO_2 during a breath (See Fig. 13-4). Time capnography measures CO_2 concentration during inspiration and expiration against time. Volume capnography consists of CO_2 plotted against the expiratory flow rate, allowing for the calculation of respiratory dead space and total CO_2 production.[22] Capnometry uses the acidic change in pH by CO_2.

Capnography has been used to determine ROSC and proper placement of an endotracheal tube. However, capnography tracing maybe present despite the endotracheal tube not being in the trachea in the following scenarios: (1) difficult bag-mask ventilation, pushing CO_2 in stomach; (2) recent ingestion of carbonated drinks or antacids; and (3) endotracheal tube elsewhere in the respiratory tract.[22] However, observational studies have shown that capnography has a sensitivity and specificity of 100% for endotracheal intubation, compared to auscultation, but this appears to be operator dependent.[22-24]

Other indications for capnography include monitoring during placement of tracheostomy, surgical procedures, mechanical ventilation, and measurement of metabolic rate.[22] In a patient with no underlying pulmonary disease, end-tidal CO_2 ($ETCO_2$) can correlate to $Paco_2$ (normal, 35–45 mmHg) with subtle variation of 2 to 5 mmHg. Larger variations are seen in pulmonary diseases or poor sampling. Since $ETCO_2$ does not always correlate with $Paco_2$, it is advised that routine evaluating of $Paco_2$ be performed, particularly in cases that monitor intracranial pressure.[22]

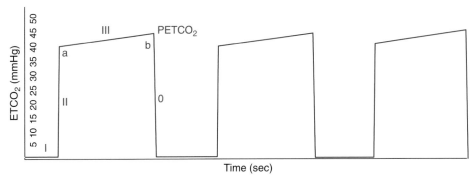

FIGURE 13-4 Capnography tracing during 3 breaths shows the expiratory component is normally divided into 3 phases: phase I is the start of the phase before CO_2 starts to appear in the breath, phase II shows the rapid increase in CO_2 as the expired breath now starts to contain breath from the alveoli, and phase III (plateau phase) represents the emptying of alveolar space. The angle (a) between phase II and phase III may be increased in bronchospasm. The angle (b) is the transition from phase III to inspiration. The end-tidal CO_2 ($PETCO_2$) is the highest concentration of CO_2 seen at the end of each breath.

Bispectral Index

Bispectral index (BIS) quantifies electroencephalogram (EEG) changes to monitor the degree of anesthesia and reduced patient awareness and recall. The 4 anesthetic-induced EEG changes include high-frequency activation of 14 to 30 Hz, low-frequency synchronization, periods of nearly suppressed EEG, and fully suppressed EEG.[25-28] A BIS greater than 97 indicates that the patient is awake, while the typical goal is 45 to 60. A BIS of 0 correlates with isoelectric EEG. Memory impairment begins with BIS less than 60.[29-31]

The BIS can be influenced by several factors. Factors that decrease values include NMB, hypovolemia, cardiac arrest, cerebral ischemia, hypoglycemia, hypothermia, dementia, postictal state, and brain injury. Factors that increase values include epilepsy, pacemakers, forced-air warmers, surgical navigation systems, shaver devices, electrocautery, ketamine, etomidate, halothane, isoflurane, and ephedrine. Its role in the intensive care unit (ICU) is still controversial.

Neuromuscular Monitoring

Indications for neuromuscular blockade include endotracheal intubation, mechanical ventilation for severe lung injury, raised intracranial pressure, shivering from hypothermia, status epilepticus, muscle spasms, and surgery. Complications include residual NMB, quadriplegic myopathy, corneal abrasions, decubitus ulcers, dysautonomia, bronchospasm, apnea, rash, malignant hyperthermia, atelectasis, and deep venous thrombosis.

Monitoring involves the use of a peripheral nerve stimulator, which contains 2 leads, the negative or black wire (distal) and the positive or red wire (proximal). If it is placed on the ulnar nerve, the thumb twitching (from the abductor pollicis muscle) is noted. If it is placed on facial nerve, eyebrow twitching (from the orbicularis oculi muscle) is noted. If it is placed on the posterior tibial nerve, flexion of the great toe (from the flexor hallucis brevis muscle) is noted. Muscular response can be determined visually and by touch, or by more objective means such as electromyography, acceleromyography, and mechanomyography.[32] Twitch patterns include single twitch, train of four (TOF), tetanus, and double burst stimulation.[32] Train of four monitoring measures NMB via TOF count and TOF (T4/T1) ratio. With the TOF button, 0.2-ms pulses are sent, 500 ms apart, every 10 seconds. The amplitude is started at 10 mA and slowly increased until 4 twitches are observed, which is the TOF count. The supramaximal stimuli occurs at the level at which 2 twitches are observed and typically is 25% of maximal stimulus.[33] Four twitches mean that 0% to 75% of receptors are blocked, 3 twitches mean that 75% of receptors are blocked, 2 twitches mean that 80% are blocked, 1 twitch means that 90% are blocked, and 0 twitches mean that 100% are blocked.

If there are no twitches, troubleshoot before assuming that the receptors are 100% blocked. Then consider holding bolus or decreasing infusion by 50% and repeating TOF after 15 to 30 minutes. Sometimes there is residual NMB even after induction blockade.[33-35] A TOF ratio greater than 0.9 is advocated to determine satisfactory recovery from NMB.

QUESTIONS

1. A 60-year-old woman with no past medical history was noted to have slurred speech and left-sided weakness after eating dinner. She was sent to the emergency department (ED). Her initial computed tomography (CT) scan shows no acute disease. Because the patient arrived in the ED within an hour and had no contraindications to thrombolytics, tissue plasminogen activator (TPA) was administered.

   During her hospitalization, she was noted to have become hypoxic and febrile. Her vitals are the following: blood pressure (BP) of 110/70 mmHg, heart rate (HR) of 120 beats/min (bpm), respiratory rate (RR) of 25 breaths/min, and O_2 saturation of 90% on NRB. Her laboratory studies show the following:

White blood cell count	14,000/μL
Sodium	145 mEq/L
Potassium	5.5 mEq/L
Chloride	109 mEq/L
CO_2	25 mEq/L
Blood urea nitrogen	25 mg/dL
Creatinine	1.5 mg/dL
Lactic acid	5 mmol/L
Glucose	105 mg/dL

   The chest radiograph shows no acute disease. The patient's hypoxia continues to progress, and now her work of breathing is more labored. The family and the patient have agreed to intubation. Inspection of her airway reveals Mallampati class I. For rapid sequence intubation, what medications would you use?

   A. Fentanyl, etomidate, and rocuronium
   B. Lidocaine, propofol, and rocuronium
   C. Fentanyl, etomidate, and succinylcholine
   D. Patient is not a candidate for NMB

2. A 37-year-old, 115-kg man presents to your hospital for an elective posterior cervical fusion. He has been in a vehicle crash and suffered massive head trauma that required a lengthy ICU stay, as well as a tracheostomy. He has several vertebral fractures and has limited range of motion of his cervical spine. He has recovered from his injuries and the tracheostomy was subsequently decannulated. Other past medical history includes mild asthma and depression. His medications include albuterol and paroxetine. What is the next step?

   A. Rapid sequence induction using propofol and rocuronium, and video assisted laryngoscopy
   B. Induction with ketamine and succinylcholine, and video assisted laryngoscopy
   C. Awake fiber-optic intubation
   D. Use of a supraglottic airway (laryngeal mask airway)

3. A 51-year-old woman has had thyroidectomy earlier this morning. She is on easy intubation with direct laryngoscopy. She suddenly has an acute onset of shortness of breath, with O_2 saturation at 85% on NRB. There is no change in her voice and she can talk in full sentences. With auscultation, there is no stridor noted in her neck and no adventitious breath sounds in her lungs. Her heart sounds are regularly regular and no murmur. Her electrocardiogram (ECG) shows normal sinus rhythm. What is the cause of her current presentation?

   A. Hypocalcemia
   B. Compressive hematoma
   C. Recurrent laryngeal nerve palsy
   D. Hypercalcemia

4. A 45-year-old man with history of diabetes mellitus and chronic obstructive pulmonary disease (COPD) is admitted for acute respiratory failure secondary to community-acquired pneumonia. He is placed on bilevel positive airway pressure (BPAP), but he is persistently dyssynchronous, and secretions are copious. The patient is still able to follow commands. The decision is made to place the patient on invasive mechanical ventilation. Propofol is given. After 2 attempts with a Mackintosh blade, intubation is unsuccessful. Epiglottis, false vocal cords, and true vocal cords are unable to be visualized. The patient's vital signs are as follows: O_2 saturation of 92%, HR of 90 beats/min, BP of 130/90 mmHg, and an RR of 16 breaths/min. What is the next step?

   A. Attempt tracheostomy
   B. Attempt retrograde intubation
   C. Place supraglottic airway
   D. Attempt intubation with tube changers

5. A 20-year-old man is undergoing emergent laparoscopic appendectomy under general anesthesia. He has no previous medical history and has had no previous surgeries. Because of a full stomach, the patient is induced with propofol, fentanyl, a defasciculating dose of rocuronium, and 100 mg of succinylcholine. Thirty minutes into the case the patient seems rigid. He becomes tachycardic. His end-tidal CO_2 is 55 mmHg and increasing. You increase the minute ventilation with hopes to normalize his hypercarbia. The patient's temperature also shows an increasing trend and is currently 38.3°C. What is the first step in treatment for this patient?

   A. Change mode of ventilation
   B. Apply cooling blankets
   C. Administer dantrolene 2.5 mg/kg IV
   D. Stop volatile anesthetics

6. A 72-year-old woman is undergoing hysterectomy for uterine cancer. Other past medical history is significant for obstructive sleep apnea, gastroesophageal reflux disease (GERD), osteoarthritis, COPD, smoking, and hypertension. During the case, you notice the capnograph shows decreasing $ETCO_2$ (Fig. 13-5). During this time, the patient also becomes tachycardic and hypotensive. What is the likely cause?

   A. Cardiac oscillations
   B. Pulmonary embolism
   C. Air leak
   D. Bronchospasm

7. What happens in hyperventilation in capnography?

   A. The O_2 saturation is normal, the $ETCO_2$ decreases, and the waveform's amplitude and width decrease.
   B. The O_2 saturation is normal or decreased, the $ETCO_2$ increases, and the waveform's amplitude and width increase.
   C. The O_2 saturation is normal, the $ETCO_2$ normal, and the waveform's amplitude and width vary.
   D. The O_2 saturation is normal or decreased, the $ETCO_2$ is absent, and the waveform's amplitude and width are absent.

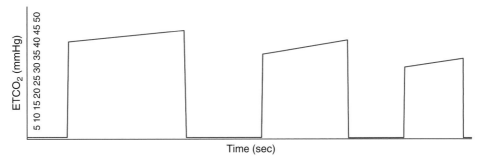

FIGURE 13-5 Capnography of a patient during surgery.

8. Which of the following is not a complication of tracheostomy within 7 days after the procedure?

   A. Bleeding
   B. Decannulation
   C. Bronchospasm
   D. Tracheoesophageal fistula

9. When is it appropriate to decannulate the tracheostomy?

   A. When the patient has tolerated the trach collar for 24 hours
   B. When the patient has tolerated the Passy Muir valve for 24 hours
   C. The patient is tolerating a decreased tracheostomy size
   D. It depends on the institution

10. A 25-year-old woman with a BMI of 25 kg/m^2 is complaining of a 2-day history of persistent cough, fever, chills, and shortness of breath. In the ED, she is noted to have an O$_2$ sat of approximately 70% on room air and a temperature of 102°F. Her chest radiograph shows bilateral patchy opacities. Influenza is positive and because of persistent hypoxia and increased work of breathing on BPAP, she is intubated. Two weeks later, she is unable to be weaned off the ventilator and her Po$_2$ was 65% on 100% Fio$_2$. Her family has decided to proceed with a tracheostomy. The nurse calls you because the patient was coughing, and it appears the tracheostomy popped out. What would be the next step?

    A. BPAP
    B. Endotracheal intubation
    C. Reinsert tracheostomy
    D. Reassess for decannulation

11. A 30-year-old man with no past medical history has been on mechanical ventilation for acute respiratory distress syndrome (ARDS) for 2 weeks. He still is not a candidate for weaning, and a tracheostomy was placed. Seventy-two hours after the tracheostomy is placed, high pressure bleeding is noted. The cuff is subsequently overinflated, but the bleeding continues. What is the next best step?

    A. Continued overinflation of the cuff
    B. Endotracheal intubation with digital compression
    C. Bronchoscopy
    D. Surgery

12. A 40-year-old woman with known anaphylaxis from peanut allergy is complaining of lip and tongue swelling. She has required invasive mechanical ventilation in the past and noted to have been a difficult airway. What do you want to do next?

    A. Rapid sequence intubation
    B. Awake intubation
    C. Solumedrol
    D. Fresh frozen plasma

13. The patient in question 12 has been placed on invasive mechanical ventilation. The nurse calls because she is noted to have a systolic blood pressure (SBP) between 80 and 90 mmHg, and she has diffuse wheezes on auscultation of her chest. What is your next step?

    A. Epinephrine
    B. Solumedrol
    C. Complement component 4 and tryptase levels
    D. Fresh frozen plasma

14. A 24-year-old man with no past medical history is admitted for biopsy of a smooth mass located near his spinal column. Rapid sequence intubation is performed with lidocaine, etomidate, and succinylcholine. An endotracheal tube size 7 is used. There are no hemodynamic abnormalities throughout the surgery. The patient is started on propofol through the intraoperative period. Postop, the patient's sedation is turned off, and he starts to wake up. He becomes agitated and bites on the endotracheal tube. His oxygen saturation drops and frothy pinkish secretions are suctioned. The patient is sedated, and his chest radiograph shows bilateral infiltrates. What is the mechanism of action?

    A. Mueller maneuver
    B. Elevated pleural pressures
    C. Biphasic response to acid fluid followed by neutrophilic inflammation
    D. Infection

ANSWERS

1. A. Fentanyl, etomidate, and rocuronium

   Rapid sequence intubation is performed to decrease the risk of aspiration. There are 3 pharmacologic components: pretreatment, induction, and neuromuscular blockade. Pretreatment is performed to minimize the physiologic responses to the presence of laryngoscopy and endotracheal tube. Medications used for pretreatment include the following: (1) atropine, which is used to blunt the muscarinic effects[36-41]; (2) lidocaine (1.5 mg/kg IV) 2–3 minutes before intubation may decrease airway resistance and increase intracranial pressure[42-48]; (3) fentanyl (3 μg/kg) may blunt the sympathetic response during RSI[48-51]; and (4) α-adrenergic via epinephrine (5–20 μg) or phenylephrine (50–200 μg) may prevent episodes of hypotension during intubation secondary to induction agents.

   Induction agents include etomidate, benzodiazepines, ketamine, propofol, and barbiturates. Etomidate (0.3 μg/kg) is an imidazole-derived sedative hypnotic that acts directly on the gamma-aminobutyric acid (GABA) complex. It also is a reversible inhibitor of 11β-hydroxylase causing adrenal suppression that might last 12 to 24 hours. Potential complications include myoclonus and adrenal insufficiency.[52-59] Benzodiazepines, usually midazolam (0.1–0.3 μg/kg IV) is an amnestic sedative that effects the GABA complex with anticonvulsant properties. In 10% to 25% of patients, it can cause hypotension and has no analgesic properties.[60,61] Ketamine (1–2 mg/kg IV) is a dissociative, amnestic sedative with analgesic properties. It effects the N-methyl-D-aspartate (NMDA) component of the GABA complex and opioid receptors, and stimulates the catecholamine receptors and releases catecholamines.[62-65] Therefore, it is known to cause hypertension and tachycardia. Despite no definitive evidence, the catecholamine release has been hypothesized to cause bronchodilation and is beneficial in asthmatics. Patients inducted with ketamine experience disturbing dreams, called the reemergence phenomenon. This is often mitigated with concomitant use of benzodiazepines.[66] Propofol (1.5–3 mg/kg IV) is a lipid-soluble alkylphenol derivative that is a sedative and amnestic but provides no analgesia. It reduces airway resistance and sympathetic discharge.[67-71] It does not prolong QTc. Barbiturates such as thiopental sodium (3–5 mg/kg IV) or methohexital (1–3 mg/kg IV) provide amnesia and sedation but no analgesia. Thiopental suppresses neuronal activity, can cause hypotension, and induces histamine release, creating bronchospasm.[72-74]

There are 2 types of NMB: depolarizing (succinylcholine 1.5 mg/kg IV), in which the agent binds to postsynaptic acetylcholine receptors causing fasciculating paralysis, and nondepolarizing (rocuronium 1 mg/kg IV, vecuronium 0.01-0.15 mg/kg IV, atracurium, and mivacurium), which competitively inhibits postsynaptic acetylcholine receptors. Succinylcholine is associated with complications such as hyperkalemia, rhabdomyolysis, malignant hyperthermia, and trismus. Despite causing muscular denervation, it has been suggested the succinylcholine is safe in myasthenia gravis.

Fentanyl, etomidate, and rocuronium is the best option. Fentanyl is indicated for pretreatment since etomidate has no analgesic properties. Etomidate is the most hemodynamically stable agent and it is indicated in hypotensive patients and severe sepsis. With the concern for myoclonus, it is brief and masked with NMB. Because of the potential for hypotension, which can worsen the cerebral perfusion pressure, propofol would not be a good option (choice B). The potassium is elevated; therefore, succinylcholine would be contraindicated (choice C). The patient does not have an absolute contraindication to rapid sequence intubation, such as total upper airway obstruction or loss of facial/oropharyngeal landmarks, or a relative contraindication, such as a difficult airway (choice D).

2. C. Awake fiber-optic intubation

In an otherwise healthy patient with anticipated difficult airway, an awake fiber-optic intubation is the best choice. This can be done via nasal or oral route. The nasopharynx should be prepared with decongestants such as oxymetazoline, phenylephrine, or glycopyrrolate.

Three nerves need to be blocked to facilitate awake intubation.[75] The glossopharyngeal nerve innervates the oropharynx, soft palate, posterior tongue, anterior epiglottis, and vallecula. It can be blocked with 5 mL of local anesthetic at the base of the tonsillar pillars. The superior laryngeal nerve innervates the base of the tongue, the posterior epiglottis, the aryepiglottic fold, and the arytenoids. It can be blocked by placing a small-gauge needle at the greater corner of the hyoid bone, bilaterally, and injecting 2 mL of local anesthetic. The recurrent laryngeal nerve provides sensory innervation to the vocal folds and trachea. It also provides motor innervation to all intrinsic muscles of the larynx except the cricothyroid muscle. The topical approach provides sensory analgesia while leaving motor function intact. Blocking the recurrent laryngeal nerve involves a transtracheal approach. The cricoid membrane is punctured. If an angiocatheter is used, the needle can be removed to help avoid tracheal or esophageal perforation during coughing. The sensory portion can be blocked by 4 mL of 4% lidocaine without affecting motor function of the recurrent laryngeal nerve (RLN). The superior and recurrent laryngeal nerves can be topicalized with inhalation of 4% nebulized lidocaine. For some patients, this does not provide enough comfort and the aforementioned regional techniques can be used to supplement. Rapid sequence intubation (choices A and B) is relatively contraindicated in a difficult airway. Use of a supraglottic airway (choice D) may temporize a situation in which a patient is unable to be intubated or bag-mask ventilated after induction, by allowing ventilation without an entirely secure airway.

3. B. Compressive hematoma

Postop thyroidectomy patients are at risk for hypoventilation due to obstruction.[76] In the first 24 hours, a compressive hematoma is the most likely cause of airway obstruction. In this situation, the wound needs to be explored and any hematoma evacuated. Incidence of compressive hematoma is 1%.

During the first 24 to 48 hours postoperatively, patients can have laryngeal dysfunction due to hypocalcemia (choice A). Normally, parathyroid glands are not all removed. If they are inadvertently damaged, hypocalcemia will result, leading to laryngeal dysfunction and possibly laryngospasm. The incidence of postoperative hypocalcemia is 6.2%.[77] Other signs of hypocalcemia include tetany, carpopedal spasm, seizure, QT prolongation, and cardiac arrest. Treatment is IV calcium.

There is a risk, due to the surgical area, of recurrent laryngeal nerve injury (choice C). If it is unilateral, it may lead to hoarseness, while bilateral recurrent laryngeal nerve injury can lead to stridor, aphonia, and devastating airway obstruction. The incidence of unilateral RLN injury is 0.77%, while bilateral RLN injury has an incidence of 0.39%.[77] Thyroidectomy is not associated with hypercalcemia (choice D).

4. **C. Place supraglottic airway**

   According to the ASA's Difficult Airway Algorithm, a supraglottic airway such as laryngeal mask airway should be placed.[1] This will enable the clinician to ventilate the patient while preparing for another attempt at intubation or a definitive surgical airway. It is also important to get additional help at this point and be sure equipment and personnel for a surgical airway are at ready. Attempting tracheostomy (choice A) would be reasonable if the patient is rapidly desaturating and/or if other techniques at securing the airway are unsuccessful. A retrograde intubation (choice B) may ultimately be required to intubate the patient; however, it is not the next best step. Although possible to insert without visualization of vocal cords, endotracheal tube changers (choice D) would not be an appropriate choice due to risk of gastric or lung perforation and a suitable alternative such as SGA.

5. **D. Stop volatile anesthetics**

   This patient may have malignant hyperthermia (MH), a pharmacogenetic disorder in which a hypermetabolic state occurs as a response to increased calcium release from the sarcoplasmic reticulum in skeletal muscles. This is caused by a mutation in the sarcoplasmic ryanodine receptor. This increase in myoplasmic calcium is triggered by volatile anesthetics and succinylcholine. Pathological release of calcium leads to the hypermetabolic state characterized by hyperthermia, muscle rigidity, acidosis, rhabdomyolysis, increased ATP consumption, increased carbon dioxide production, and increased oxygen consumption. Over 90 mutations have been identified in the human *RYR-1* gene, where at least 25 of these lead to MH.[78] These genetic abnormalities may be present in as many as 1 in 3000 people, whereas the incidence of MH is between 1:5000 and 1:100,000 anesthetics.[78] Malignant hyperthermia is often fatal if untreated.

   Treatment consists of the following steps: (1) stop any inhalational agent and/or succinylcholine, and continue anesthesia with non-MH triggering anesthetics; (2) increase minute ventilation; (3) call for help; (4) prepare and administer dantrolene at 2.5 mg/kg, and repeat until clinically stable; (5) begin cooling measures via ice pack to groin, axilla, neck; nasogastric lavage with iced solution; and administration of cold IV fluids if possible; and (6) treat arrhythmias as needed, and avoid calcium channel blockers. Labs should include blood gas, chemistry, creatinine kinase, myoglobin, coagulation profile, and should be checked every 6 to 12 hours.

   Applying cooling blankets (choice B) and administering dantrolene (choice C) are both therapies used in the treatment of MH. However, the triggering agent (in this case, a volatile anesthetic) should be discontinued. Changing the mode of ventilation (choice A) will not address MH.

6. **B. Pulmonary embolism**

   This patient shows decreasing $ETCO_2$ over time. This may be caused by a ventilation/perfusion mismatch due to an obstruction in the pulmonary artery, likely a pulmonary embolism. Figure 13-6 shows an air leak (choice C).

   A capnograph that shows cardiogenic oscillations (choice A) and the ripple effect would look like Figure 13-7.

   A capnograph that shows bronchospasm, COPD, emphysema, or an obstructed endotracheal tube (choice D), with slanting and a prolonged phase 2 and increased slope of phase 4, would look like Figure 13-8.

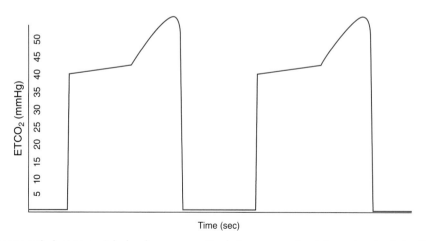

FIGURE 13-6 This capnograph depicts an air leak or loose connection between sampling tube such as in choice C.

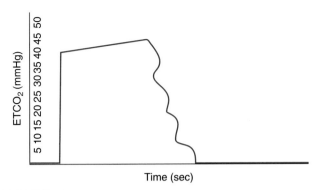

FIGURE 13-7 This capnograph that shows cardiogenic oscillations such as in choice A.

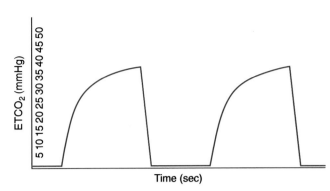

FIGURE 13-8 This capnograph shows bronchospasm such as in choice D.

7. A. The O_2 saturation is normal, the $ETCO_2$ decreases, and the waveform's amplitude and width decrease.

In hyperventilation, the O_2 saturation is normal, $ETCO_2$ decreases, and the waveform's amplitude and width decrease.[79] In hypoventilation, the O_2 saturation may be normal or decreased, and the $ETCO_2$, waveform amplitude, and width increase[79] (choice B). In physiologic variability, the waveform varies in the setting of normal O_2 saturation,

$ETCO_2$, and respiratory rate[79] (choice C). In complete airway obstruction, the O_2 saturation may be normal or decreased, and the $ETCO_2$, RR, and waveform are absent.[79] (choice D). Figures 13-9 to 13-12 show the capnographs of all four choices.

See monitoring section above for additional discussion on capnography waveforms and normal values.

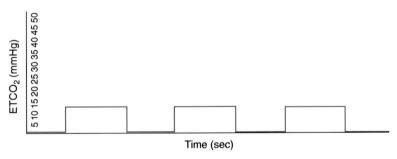

FIGURE 13-9 Capnograph in hyperventilation.

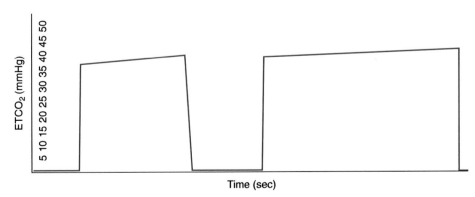

FIGURE 13-10 Capnograph in hypoventilation.

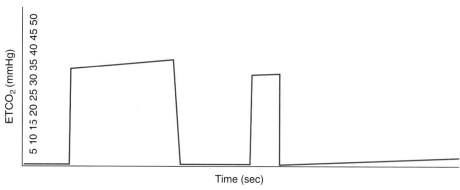

FIGURE 13-11 Capnograph in physiologic variability.

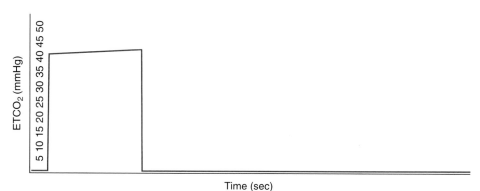

FIGURE 13-12 Capnograph in complete airway obstruction.

8. D. Tracheoesophageal fistula

The table below lists the early and late complications of tracheostomy.[80,81]

Early Complications (< 7 d): Stoma Not Mature	Late Complications (> 7 d): Stoma Mature
Hypoxemia	Tracheal stenosis
Bronchospasm	Tracheomalacia
Loss of airway	Tracheoinnominate artery erosion
Arrhythmias	
Cuff leak	Tracheoesophageal fistula
Decannulation	
Bleeding	Pneumonia
Barotrauma	Aspiration
Posterior tracheal wall injury	
Tracheal ring fracture	
Esophageal injury	
Thyroid injury	

9. D. It depends on the institution

Decannulation is the last step of tracheostomy, which can improve speech, swallowing, comfort, and physical appearance.[82] Candidates for decannulation include those with resolved condition, adequate consciousness, effective cough, ability to manage secretions, adequate oxygenation, good swallowing function, and tolerating tracheostomy tube occlusion.[82] It begins with increasing periods of spontaneous breathing trials via trach collar. Because upper airway obstruction is a complication of tracheostomy, patency can be performed by covering the tracheostomy hole while the cuff is deflated, allocating air into the upper airway for phonation, or manometry can be performed with a cap on the tube to measure airway pressures.[82-84] If the patient has stridor or shortness of breath, endoscopic evaluation is performed. In some cases, endoscopic evaluation is performed, even if the patient is asymptomatic. If airway patency is compromised by a physical obstruction such as stenosis, granulation tissue, or vocal cord paralysis, an ear, nose, and throat (ENT) specialist is consulted.[82-84] If no pathology is found, the tracheostomy can be replaced with a smaller tube.

Protocol is institution dependent, if patient has tolerated either capping or a Passy Muir valve for 48 hours.[85] Prior to capping, a cuff-leak test is performed by confirmation of air passage with deflated cuff. Avoid complete airway obstruction, such as with a capped nonfenestrated tube or a speaking valve, without deflating the cuff.[85] Once decannulated, a gauze is applied and the patient is monitored for 24 hours via telemetry. The voice will return to normal after 5 to 7 days, once the stoma heals via secondary intention.[85] Persistent tracheocutaneous fistula can occur and requires surgical correction.

Failure of decannulation can occur in 2% to 5% of patients and is apparent within 48 to 96 hours.[82,86] Interventions include long-term tracheostomy tube with inner cannula, sleep apnea tube, surgery, noninvasive ventilation with capped tracheostomy tube, or airway stent for tracheomalacia.[82]

10. B. Endotracheal intubation

It takes approximately 7 days for the stoma to mature. Before 7 days, if a tracheostomy is recannulated, it might be placed inadvertently into the anterior mediastinum (choice C). Therefore, it is generally advised to perform an endotracheal intubation for these patients. In some scenarios, fiber-optic reinsertion of tracheostomy can be performed.[82] After 7 days, the stoma has matured and the tracheostomy can be reinserted.[82] There is no role for BPAP in these situations (choice A), and the patient's degree of hypoxia makes him less likely to be a decannulation candidate (choice D).

11. B. Endotracheal intubation with digital compression

Tracheoinnominate fistula (TIF) has an incidence of 0.1% to 1%.[87] The tracheoinnominate artery supplies the right side of the head and neck and is the first branch of the aortic arch, and it has 2 branches: the right common carotid and the right subclavian artery.[87] It is 3 to 4 cm lateral to the trachea, behind the sternoclavicular joint.[87] Anterior to the tracheoinnominate artery are the left tracheoinnominate vein and the thymus, posterior are the sixth to tenth tracheal rings, posterior left is the left common carotid artery, and right posterior to tracheoinominate artery and the superior vena cava.[87] Risk factors for tracheoinnominate fistula include high cuff pressure, high-lying innominate artery in the thin and young, mucosal trauma, low tracheal incision, excessive neck movement, radiotherapy, and prolonged intubation.[87] Tracheal pressures are advised to be between 20 and 30 cm H_2O. A tracheal pressure greater than 30 cm H_2O results in compromised capillary perfusion, and a tracheal pressure greater than 50 cm H_2O results in complete occlusion of blood flow, which can lead to bleeding or rupture. Pressure less than 20 cm H_2O is an independent risk factor for ventilator-associated pneumonia.[88,89]

Since the mortality is high, there should be a high index of suspicion. Hemorrhage occurring at 48 hours or less is due to venous bleeding, coagulopathy, local trauma, or infection. Hemorrhage occurring after 48 hours is catastrophic, and suspicion for TIF is high, but other causes include pulmonary artery catheter induced arterial rupture, thoracic aneurysm rupture, or other vascular fistulas such as carotid or inferior thyroid.[89] Hemorrhage after 6 weeks is usually from granulation tissues, infection or inflammation, or malignancy.

Management begins with (1) tracheostomy cuff overinflation (choice A); (2) endotracheal intubation so that balloon lies distal through the stoma, and confirmation is via bronchoscopy followed by digital compression via insertion of a finger into the pretracheal space to tamponade the artery against the posterior manubrium; (3) and if that fails, slow withdrawal of the endotracheal tube with overinflation of the cuff. If bleeding stops and ventilation is adequate, proceed to surgery via median sternotomy[88-94] (choice D). Bronchoscopy is only an adjunct to confirm endotracheal intubation (choice C).

12. B. Awake intubation

Histamine-related angioedema may be associated with urticaria or anaphylaxis. Swelling usually lasts for 24 to 48 hours.[95] It may respond to corticosteroids, histamine-2 blockers, and epinephrine. Solumedrol can take a few hours to work and would need the airway to be secured (choice C).

Bradykinin-related angioedema may not respond to these medications and occurs secondary to decreased bradykinin degradation, such as that associated with angiotensin-converting enzyme inhibitors, or bradykinin overproduction, such as that from a dysfunctional C1 inhibitor as seen in hereditary angioedema type I and II. Bradykinin causes vasodilation which can lead to increased permeability and edema. There is a prodromal erythema marginatum, which should not be confused with urticaria because it is not raised or pruritic. Swelling lasts for 2 to 5 days, and there are case reports that support use of fresh frozen plasma and other potential treatments, including icatibant, ecallantide, and C1-inhibitor concentrate[95-105] (choice D). C1-inhibitor concentrate is approved for patients over 12 years of age at a dose of 20 U/kg.[101] Cinryze is another plasma-derived C1-inhibitor given at a dose of 1000 IU.[102,103] Ecallantide is a kallikrein inhibitor that reduces production of bradykinin. It is approved for patients over 16 years of age at a dose of 10 mg/mL for 3 doses (total dose, 30 mg).[104] Icatibant is a bradykinin-2 receptor antagonist that can be given to patients over 18 years of age as a 30-mg subcutaneous dose.[105]

Ishoo classification may be applied to decide if the patient can be discharged, admitted to inpatient unit, or admitted to the ICU.[95] Decision on whether to intubate is dependent on the patient's prior history of intubations and physical examination. Swelling of the lips to the larynx is random and noncontiguous. Signs that will suggest intubation include tongue swelling, particularly at the base, floor of mouth, or soft palate, and stridor, hoarseness, and drooling.[95]

Awake intubation via fiber-optic nasotracheal intubation or video-assisted laryngoscopy is preferred for patients who have a history of difficult intubation or angioedema to prevent suppression of intrinsic airway reflexes.[95] Local anesthetics with vasoconstrictors should be followed by glycopyrrolate to decrease secretions.[95] Rapid sequence intubation is contraindicated due to the difficulty of the intubation (choice A).

13. **A. Epinephrine**

Epinephrine at 0.01 mg/kg of 1:1000 solution to a maximum of 0.5 mg is preferred for airway edema, hypotension, and anaphylaxis.[95,106] Corticosteroids are effective for histamine-related angioedema but effects can take hours to days[106] (choice B). Low complement C4 is seen in patients with hereditary type I or II during acute attacks and elevated tryptase is seen in anaphylaxis or histamine-mediated angioedema[95] (choice C). Results might take a few days and can be helpful in diagnosis for future attacks.[95] There is no role of fresh frozen plasma in histamine-related angioedema[95] (choice D).

14. **A. Mueller maneuver**

Negative-pressure pulmonary edema (NPPE) or postobstructive pulmonary edema is suggested by the development of pulmonary edema after inspiration against an obstructive airway. Etiology includes upper airway infection, tumor, laryngospasm, foreign body, secretions, hiccup, goiter, temporomandibular joint arthroscopy, difficult intubation, Ludwig angina, desynchrony, and biting on the endotracheal tube.[107,108]

Pulmonary edema formation is dependent on the Starling equation for transcapillary fluid flux: $Qf = K([Pmv - Pi] - \sigma[\pi mv - \pi i])$ where Qf is net fluid flux from the capillary lumen to the interstitium, K is the coefficient of permeability, Pmv is the capillary lumen hydrostatic pressure, Pi is alveolar interstitial hydrostatic pressure, σ is the reflection coefficient, πmv is the microvascular osmotic pressure, and πi is the interstitial protein osmotic pressure.[107-109] The normal gradient is filtration of capillaries into the interstitium and into the lymphatics. When accumulation of fluid in the interstitium overwhelms the lymphatic drainage, pulmonary edema ensues. For most patients with NPPE, the ratio of pulmonary edema to plasma protein was less than 0.54, suggesting a hydrostatic cause, but some were higher, suggesting increased microvascular permeability.[110-113] Negative-pressure pulmonary edema has been found to be associated with diffuse alveolar hemorrhage.[114] The mechanism of edema formation is derived from the Muller maneuver which is negative thoracic pressure from inspiration against the obstructed glottis. There is a transient decrease in the ejection fraction during inspiration, which appears more pronounced in patients with known cardiac disease.[108,115] Negative-pressure pulmonary edema lasts for 24 to 48 hours and resolution is believed to be secondary to vectorial ion transport of sodium.[107] The osmotic gradient facilitates removal at a rate of 10% to 20% per hour, but in patients with high-permeability edema such as ARDS, this rate is far less. Treatment involves low tidal volume strategies, diuretics, and β agonists to help facilitate vectorial ion transport.[108]

Prolonged chest tube drainage (> 3 days) for large pneumothorax and removal of greater than 1.5 Liters of pleural effusion are risk factors for re-expansion pulmonary edema. The cause of the re-expansion pulmonary edema is secondary to increased permeability, inflammation, and high pleural pressures, more negative than –20 cm H_2O (choice B).[116-119] It is believed that chest pain during drainage from thoracentesis can suggest exceeding this threshold.[118]

Aspiration pneumonia is the inhalation of gastric contents, whether it is just gastric fluid or gastric fluid with food particles. There is a biphasic response of caustic reactions of the acidic fluid followed by neutrophilic inflammation 4 to 6 hours later[120] (choice C). This leads to increased vascular permeability with extravasation of the plasma and proteins into the alveolar space. This can lead to hypoxemia. One-third of patients with aspiration can lead to ARDS within 48 hours.[120]

It is premature to conclude that the patient has infection (choice D).

REFERENCES

1. Sankar A, Johnson SR, Beattie WS, Tait G, Wijeysundera DN, Myles PS. Reliability of the American Society of Anesthesiologists Physical Stats Scale in Clinical Practice. *Br J Anaesth.* 2914;113(3):424-432.

2. Apfelbaum JL, Hagberg CA, Caplan RA, et al. Practice guidelines for the management of the difficult airway: an updated report by the American Society of Anesthesiologists Task Force on Management of the Difficult Airway. *Anesthesiology.* 2013;118(2):251-270.

3. Cook TM, Woodall N, Harper J, Benger J; Fourth National Audit Project. Major complications of airway management in the UK: results of the Fourth National Audit Project of the Royal College of Anaesthetists and the Difficult Airway Society. Part 2: Intensive Care and Emergency Departments. *Br J Anaesth.* 2011;106(5):632-642.

4. Cook TM, Woodall N, Freck C; Fourth National Audit Project. Major complications of airway management in the UK: results of the Fourth National Audit Project of the Royal College of Anesthetits and the Difficult Airway Societ. Part 1: Anaesthesia. *Br J Anaesth.* 2011;106(5):617-631.

5. Cook TM. Strategies for the prevention of airway complications – narrative review. *Anaesthesia.* 2018;73(1):93-111.

6. Freck C, Mitchell VS, McNarry AF, et al. Difficult Airway Society 2015 guidelines for management of unanticipated difficult intubation in adults. *Br J Anaesth.* 2015;115(6):827-848.

7. Higgs A, McGrath BA, Goddard C, et al. Guidelines for the management of tracheal intubation in critically ill adults. *Br J Anaesth.* 2018;120(2):323-352.

8. Nickson C. Airway assessment. Life in the Fastlane website. https://lifeinthefastlane.com/ccc/airway-assessment/. February 19,2017. Accessed March 3, 2018.

9. Krage R, Rijn CV, van Groeningen D, Loer SA, Schwarte LA, Schober P. Cormack-Lehane Classification revisited. *Br J Anaesth.* 2010;105(2):220-227.

10. Lundstrom LH, Vester-Andersen M, Moller AM, Charuluxananan S, L'Hermite J, Wetterslev J. Poor prognostic value of the modified Mallampati score: a meta-analysis involving 177,088 patients. *Br J Anaesth.* 2011;107(5):659-667.

11. Leslie D, Stacey M. Awake intubation. *Con Ed Anaesth Crit Care Pain.* 2014;15(2):64-67.

12. Weingart S. Podcast 145 — Awake Intubation Lecture from SMACC. *EMCrit Blog.* March 16, 2015. Available at: https://emcrit.org/emcrit/awakeintubation/. Accessed June 21, 2017.

13. Reynolds SF, Heffner J. Airway management of the critically ill patient. *Chest*. 2005;127(4):1397-1412.

14. Bannister FB, Macbeth RG. Direct laryngoscopy and tracheal intubation. *Lancet*. 1944;244(6323):651-654.

15. Lafferty KA, Dillinger R. Rapid sequence intubation. March 23, 2017. https://emedicine.medscape.com/article/80222-overview. Accessed October 10, 2017.

16. Weingart S. Preoxygenation, reoxygenation, and delayed sequence intubation in the emergency department. *J Emerg Med*. 2011;40(6):661-667

17. Panditt JJ, Duncant T, Robbins PA. Total oxygen uptake with two maximal breathing techniques and tidal volume breathing technique: a physiologic study of preoxygenation. *Anesthesiology*. 2003;99(4):841-846.

18. Fruman MJ, Epstein RM, Cohen G. Apneic oxygenation in man. *Anesthesiology*. 1959;20:789-798.

19. Teller LE, Alexander CM, Frumin MJ, Gross JB. Pharyngeal insufflation of oxygen prevents arterial desaturation during apnea. *Anesthesiology*. 1988;69(6):980-982.

20. Weingart SD, Trueger ST, Wong N, Scofi J, Singh N, Rudolph SS. Delayed sequence intubation: a prospective observational study. *Ann Emerg Med*. 2015;65(4):349-355.

21. Berg RA, Hemphill R, Abella BS, et al. Part 5: adult basic life support: 2010 American Heart Association guidelines for cardiopulmonary resuscitation and emergency cardiovascular care. *Circulation*. 2010;122(18 Suppl 3):S685-S705.

22. Thomas AN, Harvey JR, Hurst T; Intensive Care Society. Capnography in the Critically ill Guidelines. 2016. www.ics.ac.uk/ICS/Guidelines_Standards/ICS/guidelines-and-standards.aspx?hkey=4ed20a1c-1ff8-46e0-b48e-732f1f4a90e2. Accessed October 15, 2017.

23. Grmec S. Comparison of three different methods to confirm tracheal tube placement in emergency intubation. *Intensive Care Med*. 2002;28(6):701-704.

24. Grmec S, Mally S. Prehospital determination of tracheal tube placement in severe head injury. *Emerg Med J*. 2004; 21(4):518-520.

25. Krauss B, Hess DR. Capnography for procedural sedation and analgesia in the emergency department. *Ann Emerg Med*. 2007;50(2):172-181.

26. Kelley S. *Monitoring Consciousness Using the Bispectral Index During Anesthesia*. 2nd ed. Boulder, CO: Covidien; 2010.

27. Sigl JC, Chamoun NG. An introduction to bispectral analysis for the electroencephalogram. *J Clin Monit*. 1994;10(6):392-404.

28. Rampil IJ. A primer for EEG signal processing in anesthesia. *Anesthesiology*. 1998;89(4):980-1002.

29. Gan TJ, Glass PS, Windsor A, et al. Bispectral index monitoring allows faster emergence and improved recovery from propofol, alfentanil, and nitrous oxide anesthesia. BIS Utility Study Group. *Anesthesiology*. 1997;87(4):808-815.

30. Ekman A, Lindholm ML, Lennmarken C, Sandin R. Reduction in the incidence of awareness using BIS monitoring. *Acta Anaesthesiol Scand*. 2004;48(1):20-26.

31. Myles PS, Leslie K, McNeil J, Forbes A, Chan MT. Bispectral index monitoring to prevent awareness during anaesthesia: the B-Aware randomised controlled trial. *Lancet*. 2004;363(9423):1757-1763.

32. Hughes S, Griffiths R. Anaesthesia monitoring techniques. *Anaeseth Intensive Care Med*. 2002:477-480.

33. McGrath CD, Hunter JM. Monitoring of neuromuscular block. *Con Ed Anaesth Crit Care Pain*. 2006;6(1):7-12.

34. Debaene B, Plaud B, Dilly MP, Donati F. Residual paralysis in the PACU after a single intubating dose of nondepolarizing muscle relaxant with an intermediate duration of action. *Anesthesiology*. 2003;98(5):1042-1048.

35. Baillard C, Gehan G, Reboul-Marty J, et al. Residual curarization in the recovery room after vecuronium. *Br J Anaesth*. 2000;84(3):394-395.

36. McCauley CS, Boller LR. Bradycardic responses to endotracheal suctioning. *Crit Care Med*. 1988;16(11):1165-1166.

37. Sorensen M, Engbaek J, Viby-Mogensen J, Guldager H, Molke Jensen F. Bradycardia and cardiac asystole following a single injection of suxamethonium. *Act Anaesthesiol Scand*. 1984;24(2):232-235.

38. Viby-Mogensen K, Wisborg K, Sorensen O. Cardiac effects of atropine and gallamine in patients receiving suxamethonium. *Br J Anaesth*. 1980;52(11):1137-1142.

39. Brandt MR, Viby-Mogensen J. Halothane anaesthesia and suxamethonium III. Atropine 30s before a second dose of suxamethonium during inhalation anaesthesia: effects and side effects. *Acta Anaesthesiol Scand Suppl*. 1978;67:76-83.

40. Greenan J, Dewar M, Jones CJ. Intravenous glycopyrrolate and atropine at induction of anaesthesia: a comparison. *J R Soc Med*. 1983;76(5):369-371.

41. Latorre F, Ellmauer S, Dick W. Atropine in the premedication of patients at risk. Its effect on hemodynamics and salivation during intubation anesthesia using succinylcholine. *Anaesthesist*. 1992;41(2):76-82.

42. Groeben H, Silvanus MT, Beste M, Peters J. Combined intravenous lidocaine and inhaled salbutamol protect against bronchial hyperreactivity more effectively than lidocaine or salbutamol alone. *Anesthesiology*. 1998;89(4):862-868.

43. Groeben H, Silvanus MT, Beste M, Peters K. Both intravenous and inhaled lidocaine attenuate reflex bronchoconstriction but at different plasma concentrations. *Am J Respir Crit Care Med*. 1999;159(2):530-535.

44. Robinson N, Clancy M. In patients with head injury undergoing rapid sequence intubation, does pretreatment with intravenous lignocaine/lidocaine lead to an improved neurological outcome? A review of the literature. *Emerg Med J*. 2001;18(6):453-457.

45. Butler J, Jackson R. Towards evidence based emergency medicine: best BETs from Manchester Royal Infirmary. Lignocaine premedication before rapid sequence induction in head injuries. *Emerg Med J*. 2002;19(6):554.

46. Brooks D, Anderson CM, Carter MA, et al. Clinical practice guidelines for suction in the airway of the intubated and non-intubated patients. *Can Respir J*. 2001;8(3):163-181.

47. Bachofen M. Suppression of blood pressure increases during intubation: lidocaine or fentanyl? *Anaesthesist*. 1988;37(3):156-161.

48. Samaha T, Ravussin P, Claquin C, Ecoffey C. Prevention of increase of blood pressure and intracranial pressure during endotracheal intubation in neurosurgery: esmolol versus lidocaine. *Ann Fr Anesth Reanim*. 1996;15(1):36-40.

49. Chung KS, Sinatra RS, Valevy JD, Paige D, Silverman DG. A comparison of fentanyl, esmolol, and their combination for blunting the haemodynamic responses during rapid sequence induction. *Can J Anaesth*. 1992;39(8):774-779.

50. Cork RC, Weiss JL, Hameroff SR, Bentley J. Fentanyl preloading for rapid-sequence induction of anesthesia. *Anesth Analg*. 1984;63(1):60-64.

51. Dahlgren N, Messeter K. Treatment of stress response to laryngoscopy and intubation with fentanyl. *Anaesthesia.* 1981;36(11):1022-1026.

52. Fuchs-Buder T, Sparr HJ, Ziegenfuss T. Thiopental or etomidate for rapid sequence induction with rocuronium. *Br J Anaesth.* 1998;80(4):504-506.

53. Guldner G, Schultz J, Sexton P, Fortner C, Richmond M. Etomidate for rapid-sequence intubation in young children: hemodynamic effects and adverse events. *Acad Emerg Med.* 2003;10(2):134-139.

54. Jellish WS, Riche H, Salord F, Ravussin P, Tempelhoff R. Etomidate and thiopental-based anesthetic induction: comparisons between differential titrated levels of electrophysiologic cortical depression and response to laryngoscopy. *J Clin Anesth.* 1997;9(1):36-41.

55. Zed PJ, Abu-Laban RB, Harrison DW. Intubating conditions and hemodynamic effects of etomidate for rapid sequence intubation in emergency department: an observation cohort study. *Acad Emerg Med.* 2006;13(4):378-383.

56. Oglesby AJ. Should etomidate be the induction agent of choice for rapid sequence intubation in the emergency department? *Emerg Med J.* 2004;1(6):655-659.

57. Jellish WS, Riche H, Salord F, Ravussin P, Tempelhoff R. Etomidate and thiopental-based anesthetic induction: comparisons between different titrated levels of electrophysiologic cortical depression and response to laryngoscopy. *J Clin Anesth.* 1997;9(1):36-41.

58. Kox WJ, von Heymann C, Heinze J, Prichep LS, John ER, Rundshagen I. Electroencephalographic mapping during routine clinical practice: cortical arousal during tracheal intubation? *Anesth Analg.* 2006;102(3):825-831.

59. Reddy RV, Moorthy SS, Dierdorf SF, Deitch RD Jr, Link L. Excitatory effects and electroencephalographic correlation of etomidate, thiopental, methohexital, and propofol. *Anesth Analg.* 1993;77(5):1008-1011.

60. Blumer JL. Clinical pharmacology of midazolam in infants and children. *Clin Pharmacokinet.* 1998;35(1):37-47.

61. Nordt SP, Clark RF. Midazolam: a review of therapeutic uses and toxicity. *J Emerg Med.* 1997;15(3):357-365.

62. Langsjo JW, Kaisti KK, Aalto S, et al. Effects of subanesthetic doses of ketamine on regional cerebral blood flow, oxygen consumption, and blood volume in humans. *Anesthesiology.* 2003;99(3):614-623.

63. Rogers R, Wise RG, Painter DJ, Longe SE, Tracey I. An investigation to dissociate the analgesic and anesthetic properties of ketamine using functional magnetic resonance imaging. *Anesthesiology.* 2004;100(2):292-301.

64. Hanouz JL, Persehaye E, Zhu L, et al. The inotropic and lusitropic effects of ketamine in isolated human atrial myocardium: the effect of adrenoceptor blockade. *Anesth Analg.* 2004;99(6):1689-1695.

65. Allen JY, Macias CG. The efficacy of ketamine in pediatric emergency department patients who present with acute severe asthma. *Ann Emerg Med.* 2005;46(1):43-50.

66. Grace RF. The effect of variable-dose diazepam on dreaming and emergence phenomena in 400 cases of ketamine-fentanyl anaesthesia. *Anaesthesia.* 2003;58(9):904-910.

67. Veselis RA, Reinsal RA, Feshchenko VA, Johnson R Jr. Information loss over time defines the memory defect of propofol: a comparative response with thiopental and dexmedetomidine. *Anesthesiology.* 2004;101(4):831-841.

68. Veselis RA, Feshchenko VA, Reinsel RA, Beattie B, Akhurst TJ. Propofol and thiopental do not interfere with regional cerebral blood flow response at sedative concentrations. *Anesthesiology.* 2005;102(1):26-34.

69. Eames WO, Rooke GA, Wu RS, Bishop MJ. Comparison of the effects of etomidate, propofol, and thiopental on respiratory resistance after tracheal intubation. *Anesthesiology.* 1996;84(6):1307-1311.

70. Conti G, Ferretti A, Tellan G, Rocco M, Lappa A. Propofol induces bronchodilation in a patient mechanically ventilated for status asthmaticus. *Intensive Care Med.* 1993;19(5):305.

71. Pivoz R, Brown RH, Weiss YS, et al. Wheezing during induction of general anesthesia in patients with and without asthma. A randomized blinded trial. *Anesthesiology.* 1995; 82(5):1111-1116.

72. Russo H, Ressolle F. Pharamacodynamics and pharmacokinetics of thiopental. *Clin Pharmacokinet.* 1998;35(2):95-134.

73. Reich DL, Hossain S, Krol M, et al. Predictors of hypotension after induction of general anesthesia. *Anesth Analg.* 2005;101(3):622-628.

74. Hirota K, Ohtomo N, Hashimoto Y, et al. Effects of thiopental on airway caliber in dogs: direct visualization method using a superfine fibreoptic bronchoscope. *Br J Anaesth.* 1998;81(2):203-207.

75. Butterworth JF, Mackey DC, Wasnick JD, Morgan GE, Mikhail MS, Morgan GE. Airway management. In: *Morgan and Mikhail's Clinical Anesthesiology.* 5th ed. New York, NY: McGraw-Hill; 2013: 309-341.

76. Christou N, Mathonnet M. Complications after total thyroidectomy. *Journal of Visceral Surgery.* 2013;150(4):249-256.

77. Bhattacharyya N, Fried MP. Assessment of the morbidity and complications of total thyroidectomy. *Arch Otolaryngol Head Neck Surg.* 2002;128(4):389-392.

78. Glahn KPE, Ellis FR, Halsall PJ, et al. Recognizing and managing a malignant hyperthermia crisis: guidelines from the European Malignant Hyperthermia Group. *Brit J Anaesth.* 2010;105(4):417-420.

79. Krauss B, Hess DR. Capnography for procedural sedation and analgesia in the emergency department. *Ann Emerg Med.* 2007;50(2):172-181.

80. Durbin Jr CG. Early complications of tracheostomy. *Respir Care.* 2005;50(4):511-515.

81. Epstein SK. Late complications of tracheostomy. *Respir Care.* 2005;50(4):542-549.

82. O'Connor HH, White AC. Tracheostomy decannulation. *Respir Care.* 2010;55(8):1076-1081.

83. Hess DR. Facilitating speech in the patient with a tracheostomy. *Respir Care.* 2005;50(4):519-525.

84. Johnson DC, Campbell SL, Rabkin JD. Tracheostomy tube manometry: evaluation of speaking valves, capping, and need for downsizing. *Clin Respir J.* 2008;3(1):8-14.

85. Engels PT, Bagshaw SM, Meier M, Brindley PG. Tracheostomy: from insertion to decannulation. *Can J Surg.* 2009;52(5):427-433.

86. Stelfox HT, Hess DR, Schmidt UH. A North American survey of respiratory therapist and physician tracheostomy decannulation practices. *Respir Care.* 2009;54(12):1658-1664.

87. Grant CA, Dempsey, Harrison J, Jones T. Tracheo-innominate artery fistula after percutaneous tracheostomy: three case reports and a clinical review. *Br J Anaesth.* 2006;96(1):127-131.

88. Mehta S, Myat HM. The cross-sectional shape and circumference of the human trachea. *Ann R Coll Surg Engl.* 1984;66(5):356-358.

89. Inada T, Kawachi S, Kuroda M. Tracheal tube cuff pressure during cardiac surgery using cardiopulmonary bypass. *Br J Anaesth.* 1995;74(3):283-286.

90. Allan JS, Wright CD. Tracheoinnominate fistulata: diagnosis and management. *Chest Surg Clin N Am.* 2003;13(2):331-341.

91. Nelems JM. Tracheo-innominate artery fistula. *Am J Surg.* 1981;14(5)1:526-527.

92. Bertelsen S, Jensen NM. Innominate artery rupture. A fatal complication of tracheostomy. *Ann Chir Gynaecol.* 1987;76(4): 230-233.

93. Courcy PA, Rodriguez A, Garrett HE. Operative technique for repair of tracheoinnominate artery fistula. *J Vasc Surg.* 1985;2(2):332-334.

94. Utley JR, Singer MM, Roe BB, Fraser DG, Dedo HH. Definitive management of innominate artery hemorrhage complicating tracheostomy. *JAMA.* 1972;220(4):577-579.

95. Moellman JJ, Bernstein JA, Lindsell C. A consensus parameter for the evaluation and management of angioedema in the emergency department. *Acad Emerg Med.* 2014;21(4): 469-484.

96. Bernstein JA, Moellman J. Emerging concepts in the diagnosis and treatment of patients with undifferentiated angioedema. *Int J Emerg Med.* 2012;5(1):39.

97. Bernstein JA, Moellman JJ. Progress in the emergency management of hereditary angioedema: focus on new treatment options in the United States. *Postgrad Med.* 2012;124(3): 91-100.

98. Lang DM, Aberer W, Bernstein JA, et al. International Consensus on hereditary and acquired angioedema. *Ann Allergy Asthma Immunol.* 2012;109(6):395-402.

99. Moellman JJ, Bernstein JA. Diagnosis and management of hereditary angioedema: an emergency medicine perspective. *J Emerg Med.* 2012;43(2):391-400.

100. Prematta M, Gibbs JG, Pratt EL, Stoughton TR, Craig TJ. Fresh frozen plasma for the treatment of hereditary angioedema. *Ann Allergy Asthma Immunol.* 2007;98(4): 383-388.

101. Craig TJ, Levy RJ, Wasserman RL, et al. Efficacy of Human C1 esterase inhibitor concentrate compared with placebo in acute hereditary angioedema attacks. *J Allergy Clin Immunol.* 2009;124(4):801-808.

102. Kreuz W, Rusicke E, Martinez-Saguer I, Aygoren-Pursun E, Heller C, Klingebiel T. Home therapy with intravenous human C1-inhibitor in children and adolescents with hereditary angioedema. *Transfusion.* 2012;52(1):100-107.

103. Wahn V, Aberer W, Eberl W, et al. Hereditary angioedema (HAE) in children and adolescents—a consensus on therapeutic strategies. *Eur J Pediatr.* 2012;171(9):1339-1348.

104. Cicardi M, Levy RJ, McNeil DL, et al. Ecallantide for the treatment of acute attacks in hereditary angioedema. *New Engl J Med.* 2010;363(6):523-531.

105. Cicardi M, Banerji A, Bracho F, et al. Icatibant, a new bradykinin-receptor antagonist, in hereditary angioedema. *New Engl J Med.* 2010;363(6):532-541.

106. Joint Task Force on Practice Parameters; American Academy of Allergy, Asthma and Immunology; American College of Allergy, Asthma and Immunology; Joint Council of Allergy, Asthma and Immunology. The diagnosis and management of anaphylaxis: an updated practice parameter. *J Allergy Clin Immunol.* 2005;115 (3 Suppl 2):S483-S523.

107. Bhattacharya M, Kallet RH, Ware LB, Matthay MA. Negative-pressure pulmonary edema. *Chest.* 2016;150(4):927-933.

108. Krodel DJ, Bittner EA, Abdulnour R, Brown R, Eikermann M. Case scenario: acute postoperative negative pressure pulmonary edema. *Anesthesiology.* 2010;113(1):200-207.

109. Staub NC. Pulmonary edema. *Physiol Rev.* 1974;54(3):678-811.

110. Fein A, Grossman RF, Jones JG, et al. The value of edema fluid protein measurement in patients with pulmonary edema. *Am J Med.* 1979;67(1):32-38.

111. Verghese GM, Ware LB, Matthay BA, Matthay MA. Alveolar epithelial fluid transport and the resolution of clinically severe hydrostatic pulmonary edema. *J Appl Physiol (1985).* 1999;87(4):1301-1312.

112. Ware LB, Fremont RD, Bastarache JA, Calfee CS, Matthay MA. Determining the aetiology of pulmonary oedema by the oedema fluid-to-plasma protein ratio. *Eur Respir J.* 2010; 35(2):331-337.

113. Fremont RD, Kallet RH, Matthay MA, Ware LB. Postobstructive pulmonary edema: a case for hydrostatic mechanisms. *Chest.* 2007;131(6):1742-1746.

114. Contou D, Voiriot G, Djibre M, Labbe V, Fartoukh M, Parrot A. Clinical features of patients with diffuse alveolar hemorrhage due to negative-pressure pulmonary edema. *Lung.* 2017;195(4):477-487.

115. Scharf SM, Woods BO, Brown R, Parisi A, Miller MM, Tow DE. Effects of the Mueller maneuver on global and regional left ventricular function in angina pectoris with or without previous myocardial infarction. *Am J Cardiol.* 1987;59(15):1305-1309.

116. Chen CL, Chen WC, Ho CF. Management and prevention of re-expansion pulmonary edema after tube thoracostomy for prolonged massive pneumothorax. *Chest.* 2010;138(4 Suppl):224A.

117. Kasmani R, Rani F, Okoli K, Mahajan V. Re-expansion pulmonary edema following thoracentesis. *CMAJ.* 2010;182(18):2000-2002.

118. Feller-Kopman D, Walkey A, Berkowitz D, Ernst A. The relationship of pleural pressure to symptom development during therapeutic thoracentesis. *Chest.* 2006;129(6):1556-1560.

119. Villena V, Lopez-Encuentra A, Pozo F, De-Pablo A, Martin-Escribano P. Measurement of pleural pressure during therapeutic thoracentesis. *Am J Respir Crit Care Med.* 2000;162(4 Pt 1): 1534-1538.

120. Raghavendran K, Nemzek J, Napolitano LM, Knight PR. Aspiration-induced lung injury. *Crit Care Med.* 2011;39(4):818-826.

Analgesia, Sedation, Delirium, and Coma

Maria Osundele, PharmD, CGP, BCPS, Ronaldo Collo Go, MD, Samer El Zarif, MD, Aamir Gilani, MD, and Murali G. Krishna, MD

INTRODUCTION

Pain, agitation, delirium, and coma are not uncommon in the intensive care unit (ICU). They are secondary to the patient's underlying disease or to the multiple interventions, such as medications, procedures, mechanical ventilation, wound care, and bed rest. They can also be a marker of critical illness, which is associated with catabolism, immune dysregulation, hypercoagulable states, increased myocardial workload, impaired wound healing, and ischemia.

An ideal individualized approach should be identification of pain, agitation, and alertness, followed by the use of nonpharmacologic and pharmacologic treatment. Nonpharmacological strategies to improve patient's comfort include lighting adjustment, music therapy, massage, verbal reassurance, optimized sleep hygiene, and involvement of family members in the care of the patient. Often, critically ill patients are unable to report pain, and the behavioral pain scale and critical care observation tool have been shown to have interrater reliability and best internal consistency.[1,2] Clinical scales have been used to evaluate the agitation or alertness and degree of sedation of critically ill patients regardless of their requirements for mechanical ventilation. These scales include Adaptation to the Intensive Care Environment (ATICE), the Minnesota Sedation Assessment Tool (MSAT), the Motor Activity Assessment Scale, and the Vancouver Interactive and Calmness Scale (VICS). The most commonly used are the Ramsey Sedation Scale, the Richmond Agitation Sedation Scale[1,2] (RASS; Table 14-1), and the Sedation Agitation Scale (SAS; Table 14-2).[3,4] All the scales have been validated, through correlations with other sedation scales, bispectral index (BIS), electrocardiography (EEG), actigraphy, and different investigators. According to the guidelines of the Society of Critical Care Medicine (SCCM), RASS and SAS are the most validated tools (Level of Evidence [LOE] B).[5-7]

MEDICATIONS

Nonopioids Versus Opioids

Uncontrolled pain can result in psychologic and physiologic consequences such as posttraumatic stress disorder; increased catecholamine leading to arteriolar vasoconstriction and impaired tissue perfusion; catabolic hypermetabolism leading to hyperglycemia, lipolysis, and muscle breakdown; impaired wound healing; suppression of natural killer cell activity; and chronic neuropathic pain.[8-13] Despite the availability of non-opiod analgesics, their safety profile has not been completely studied in critical care; therefore, opioids are the primary analgesics in the critically ill[5] (LOE). Non-opioid analgesics (Table 14-3) may be used as an adjunct or to decrease the amount of the opioid being administered.

Opioids are lipophilic, crossing the blood-brain barrier to act on μ, κ, and δ receptors in the central nervous system (CNS). Some, such as morphine, are hydrophilic in nature, thus exhibiting more peripheral effects (Table 14-4).

Fentanyl is 100 times more potent than morphine. It is considered as the first-line agent for pain management in the ICU, due to its quick onset, quick offset, easy titration, lack of an active metabolite, and less hemodynamic variability. Initial administration of fentanyl begins with a 25- to 50-μg bolus; this can be repeated every 15 to 30 minutes. If the patient requires more than 2 boluses within an hour, infusion at 25 to 700 μg/h or 0.7 to 10 μg/kg/h can be started. Dose adjustment is not required in renal impairment, but reduction should be considered in patients with severe hepatic impairment. Complications include stiff chest wall syndrome and serotonin syndrome when used with monoamine oxidase inhibitors (MAOI).

Remifentanil[14] is an ultra-rapid-acting opioid that binds to stereospecific μ-opioid receptors within the CNS, increasing the pain threshold, altering pain perception, and inhibiting ascending pain pathways. Recommended dosing is 1.5 μg/kg followed by 0.5 to 15 μg/kg/h.

Morphine is considered the gold standard among opioids when dose adjustment or opioid rotation is being considered. It can cause hypotension from histamine release, which causes nitric oxide–related vasodilatation. It is metabolized into active and inactive metabolites that depend on the renal system for elimination. One of its metabolites, morphine 3-glucuronide, can accumulate and cause seizures. Continuous infusion of morphine should be avoided in patients with severe renal impairment. Usual dose is 2 to 4 mg given every 3 to 4 hours with infusion ranging from 2 to 30 mg/h.[15]

TABLE 14-1 Richmond Agitation Sedation Scale[6,7]

Score	Description
+4	Combative: violent, immediate danger to staff
+3	Very agitated: pulls or removes tubes or catheters; aggressive
+2	Making frequent nonpurposeful movement, fighting ventilator
+1	Anxious, but movements not aggressive or vigorous
0	Alert and calm
−1	Drowsy: not fully alert but having sustained awakening, with eye-opening/eye contact to voice ≥ 10 s
−2	Light sedation: briefly awakens with eye contact to voice < 10 s
−3	Moderation sedation: movement or eye opening to voice but no eye contact
−4	Deep sedation: no response to voice, but movement or eye opening to physical stimulation
−5	Unarousable: no response to voice or physical stimulation

TABLE 14-2 Sedation Agitation Scale

Score	Description
7	Dangerous: pulls at endotracheal tube, removes catheters, climbs over bed rails, strikes staff, thrashes side to side
6	Very agitated: does not calm down despite frequent verbal reminders of limits, requires physical restraints, bites endotracheal tube
5	Agitated: anxious or mildly agitated, attempts to sit up, calms down with verbal instructions
4	Calm and cooperative: calm, awakens easily, follows commands
3	Sedated: difficult to arouse, awakens to verbal stimuli or gentle shaking but drifts off again, follows simple commands
2	Very sedated: arouses to physical stimuli but does not communicate or follow commands, may move spontaneously
1	Unarousable: minimal or no response to noxious stimuli, does not communicate or follow commands

Hydromorphone has a metabolite, 3-glucuronide, which can accumulate in renal impairment and cause neuroexcitation. It has a low volume of distribution, high water solubility, low protein binding, and low molecular weight; this suggests that it can be removed by hemodialysis. Doses range from 0.2 to 0.6 mg every 1 to 2 hours with continuous infusion at 0.5 to 3 mg/h.[15] Complications include serotonin syndrome with MAOIs and hypotension.

Opioid Conversion

Opioid rotation may be necessary in some patients due to the development of tolerance to the agent or due to changes in organ system and hemodynamic stability. The patient's level of comfort must be assessed and the steps below must be taken into consideration when converting from 1 opioid to another. Calculate the total dose in milligrams taken in the previous 24 hours (Table 14-4). If pain is controlled on the current opioid, reduce the new opioid daily dose by 25% to 50% to account for cross-tolerance, dosing-ratio variation, and inter-patient variability. If pain is uncontrolled on the current opioid, increase the opioid daily dose by up to 50% to 100%. Consider adjuvant therapy as needed. Titrate liberally and rapidly to analgesic effect during the first 24 hours. Monitor for adverse events and effectiveness.

A reversal agent for opioid toxicity is naloxone. It is an antagonist that blocks the μ and κ opioid receptors. It reverses

TABLE 14-3 Nonopiates and Characteristics

Nonopiates (Route)	Onset	Elimination Half-Life	Metabolic Pathway	Active Metabolites
Ketamine (IV)	30–40 s	2–3 h	N-demethylation	Norketamine
Acetaminophen (PO), acetaminophen (PR)	30–60 min variable	2–4 h	Glucuronidation, sulfonation	None
Acetaminophen (IV)	5–10 min	2 h	Glucuronidation, sulfonation	None
Ketorolac[a] (IM/IV)	10 min	2.4–8.6 h	Hydroxylation, conjugation/renal excretion	None
Ibuprofen (IV)	N/A	2.2–2.4 h	Oxidation	None
Ibuprofen (PO)	25 min	1.8–2.5 h	Oxidation	None
Gabapentin (PO)	N/A	5–7 h	Renal excretion	None
Carbamazepine immediate release (PO)	4–5 h	25–65 h initially, then 12–17 h	Oxidation	None

IM = intramuscular; IV = intravenous; max = maximum; N/A = not applicable; PO = orally; PR = rectally.

[a]For patients more than 65 y or less than 50 kg, 15 mg IV/IM every 6 h to a maximum dose of 60 mg/d for 5 days.

Used with permission from Barr J et al. Clinical practice guidelines for the management of pain, agitation, and delirium in adult patients in the intensive care unit. *Crit Care Med.* 2013;41(1):263-306.

TABLE 14-4 Selected Opioids

Opioid	Equivalent Dose: IV/PO	Onset (IV/PO)	Half-Life
Morphine	10 mg/30 mg	5–10 min/ 15-60 min	3–4 h
Fentanyl	0.1 mg/NA	1–2 min/NA	2–4 h
Hydromorphone	1.5 mg/ 7.5 mg	5–15min/ 30 min	2–3 h
Oxycodone (IR)	NA/20 mg	NA/10–30 min	3–5 h
Codeine	NA/200 mg	NA/15–30 min	4 h
Hydrocodone	NA/30–45 mg	NA/10–30 min	3–5 h
Oxymorphone	1 mg/10 mg	NA/15 min	3–6 h

IM = intramuscular; IV = intravenous; IR = immediate release; N/A = not applicable.

lipophilic opiates more readily than it does hydrophilic opioids (eg, fentanyl). The initial dose is 0.4 mg to 2 mg every 2 to 3 minutes, depending on the type and duration of action of the opioid used. For patients on long-acting opioids, a continuous infusion of naloxone may be needed for optimal response, since the half-life of the drug is relatively short. The onset of action is approximately 2 minutes with a duration of 30 to 120 minutes, depending on the route of administration. It is also used in patients with opioid-induced pruritus, although this is not a US Food and Drug Administration (FDA)-approved indication. Patients being treated for this condition should be monitored carefully for pain control. Commonly observed side effects with naloxone include abdominal cramps, vomiting, hypertension, tachycardia, seizures, chest pain, and arrhythmia. In certain patients, such as those with acute respiratory distress syndrome (ARDS) or congestive heart failure (CHF), naloxone can provoke pulmonary edema; this is likely a result of opiate-induced pulmonary vascular smooth muscle relaxation.

Complications and Treatment of Opioids

Opioid use is associated with side effects such as esophageal motility disorders, nausea and vomiting, gastroparesis, sphincter of oddi dysfunction, constipation, and narcotic bowel syndrome.[16] The μ-opioid receptors are the principal mediators of analgesia but also cause sedation, dependence, respiratory depression, and bowel dysfunction.[16,17] Tolerance develops with these receptors secondary to desensitization. In the gastrointestinal (GI) tract, differential tolerance occurs so that all organs except the colon develop tolerance.[16] Opioid induced constipation is defined as new or worsening symptoms of constipation, with initiation or change of opioid therapy, including 2 or more of the following: (1) straining during greater than one-third of bowel movements; (2) lumpy or hard stools; (3) sensation of incomplete evacuation; (4) sensation of anorectal obstruction/blockage with greater than one-third of defecations; (5) manual maneuvers to facilitate more than 25% of defecations; and/or (6) less than 3 spontaneous bowel movements per week.[16] For constipation

prophylaxis, patients should receive a bowel regimen consisting of a, laxatives and bowel stimulant (e.g. miralax, senna, bisacodyl) (Table 14-5).[16–20] The peripherally-acting μ-opioid antagonists (PAMORA) such as methylnaltrexone (subcutaneous or oral), naloxegol (oral), and naldemidine (oral) are indicated for the treatment of opioid-induced constipation (OIC) in patients when laxative therapy has produced insufficient response. It is recommended to discontinue all maintenance laxatives prior to starting these agents and re-initiate as needed if the response is suboptimal. Dose reduction is recommended in patients with renal impairment. Use of PAMORA is contraindicated in patients with known or suspected gastrointestinal obstruction due to the potential for GI perforation.[18] The most common adverse drug events associated with PAMORAs include abdominal pain, diarrhea, headaches, abdominal distension, hyperhidrosis, anxiety, muscle spasms, rhinorrhea, and chills. These agents should be re-evaluated once the patient is no longer receiving opioids.

Stiff chest wall syndrome is more common in pediatrics and with lipophilic synthetic opioids such as fentanyl, alfentanil, remifentanil, and sufentanil. This rigidity decreases chest wall compliance and may result in ineffective spontaneous ventilation and impairs the effective use of ventilator support. Risk factors include neurological diseases, metabolic disorders, and medications modifying dopamine levels. Early recognition is imperative, and management with the use of ventilatory support and prompt reversal with either naloxone or a short-acting neuromuscular blocking agent should be implemented as soon as possible.

Opioid-induced hyperalgesia is increased nociceptive sensitization secondary to opioids. The type of pain may be similar to or different from initial sensation. Several mechanisms have been proposed, including the activation of N-methyl-D-aspartate (NMDA) receptors on the postsynaptic nerve terminal. Ways to manage this effect include adequate hydration, opioid dose reduction, addition of adjuvant medication, and opioid rotation to agents with effect on the NMDA receptors, such as methadone or ketamine.[21]

Benzodiazepines

The benzodiazepines act by stimulating specific receptors in the CNS. Stimulation of this receptor potentiates the inhibitory effects of gamma-aminobutyric acid (GABA) on GABA-A receptors, resulting in chloride influx, hyperpolarization, and decreased ability of the neuron to reach an action potential, thereby producing sedation and anxiolysis. They produce amnesia, have anticonvulsant activity but lack analgesic properties. The addition of benzodiazepines to opioids may potentiate the effect of opioids through the inhibition of opioid metabolism.[22,23] Benzodiazepines are weak competitive inhibitors of cytochrome P450 3A4 (CYP3A4). They are a pregnancy category D. Patients with renal failure may experience propylene glycol toxicity[24] from lorazepam infusion or a high dose of diazepam. Flumazenil is a benzodiazepine antidote. It is given in increments of 0.2 mg titrated to effect with a

TABLE 14-5   Common Prophylaxis and Treatment Opioid Induced Constipation[16-20]

Medication	Class/Route	Mechanism of Action	Comment
Docusate (Colace)	Stool softener/oral, rectal, liquid, enema	Decreases the surface tension to lubricate and soften fecal matter	50–300 mg PO daily or PO divided doses Onset of effect: 12–72 h
Sennoside (Senokot), bisacodyl	Stimulants/oral tablets, oral liquid (sennoside); rectal, oral tablet (bisacodyl)	Increases electrolyte transport into the bowel and stimulates intestinal motility; inhibits water resorption and stimulates secretion and motility of small intestine and colon through the sensory nerve endings of colon mucosa	8.6–25 mg PO daily or PO divided doses not to exceed 70–100 mg/daily Onset of effect: 8–12 h
Polyethylene glycol	Hyperosmolar agent/oral	Osmotically increases intraluminal fluid	17 g (1 heaping tablespoon) PO daily for < 1 wk (powder) in 8 ounces of water Onset of effect: 24–96 h
Lactulose	Hyperosmolar agent, Oral or rectal	Bacterial degradation of lactulose resulting in acidic pH, prevents diffusion of NH_3 to blood, enhances diffuse of NH_3 from blood to colon, and causes osmotic diarrhea	10 g/15 mL or 20 g/30 mL Onset of effect: 8–48 h
Methylnaltrexone (Relistor)	PAMORA, oral or subcutanous	Blocks μ opioid receptor peripherally in the gastrointestinal tract	Opioid induced constipation in chronic noncancer pain: 12 mg SQ daily or 450 mg PO daily Or Opioid induced constipation in palliative care: 38–62 kg: 8 mg SC every other day 62–114 kg: 12 mg SC every other day <38 kg or >114 kg 0.15 mg/kg/dose SC every other day Dose further adjusted in renal and hepatic impairment
Naloxegol (Movantik)	PAMORA, oral	Blocks μ opioid receptor peripherally in the gastrointestinal tract	25 mg daily on empty stomach ≥1 h before or 2 h after the first meal of the day
Naldemidine	PAMORA, oral	Blocks μ opioid receptor peripherally in the gastrointestinal tract	0.2 mg PO daily
Alvimopan	PAMORA, oral	Blocks μ opioid receptor peripherally in the gastrointestinal tract For post bowel resection	12 mg PO 30 min to 5 h preoperative then 12 mg PO every 12 h until discharge for maximum of 7 d
Oxycodone/naloxone	Opioid/ opioid antagonist, oral	In OIC, naloxone displaces oxycodone from μ opioid receptors in GI tract but not in systemic circulation, so analgesic effects preserved	10 mg/5 mg PO every 12 h not to exceed (80 mg/40 mg daily)
Lubiprostone	Fatty acid derived from prostaglandin E	Increase fluid secretion via cystic fibrosis transmembrane regulator and type 2 chloride channels	24 mcq PO every 12 h

total dose of 1 mg in adults. The onset is within 1 to 2 minutes with peak effects within 10 minutes. Caution should be exercised in patients receiving long-term benzodiazepine therapy, as it may precipitate acute withdrawal and seizures. Its use is contraindicated in patients with known hypersensitivity to the drug or to benzodiazepines, and also in those who are receiving benzodiazepines to control a potentially life-threatening condition such status epilepticus or intracranial pressure. Further discussion on benzodiazepines is in Chapter 16.

Propofol

Propofol is an alkylphenol derivative compound prepared in a 10% lipid emulsion. It has sedative and amnestic properties but no analgesic properties. It has a rapid onset of action of less than 1 minute and a short duration of action (approximately 10 minutes, but it is dose dependent). Clearance of the drug is not affected by renal or hepatic dysfunction, and it is devoid of any active metabolites. Hypotension is a major cardiovascular effect in which a reduction in mean arterial pressure may occasionally exceed 30%; caution should be exercised when used in patients with hemodynamic instability, hypovolemia, or abnormally low vascular tone. It is administered as a continuous infusion starting at 5 to 10 µg/kg/min and then titrated to effect. Daily interruption with retitration or a light target level of sedation is recommended to minimize prolonged sedative effects. The dose ranges from 25 to 80 µg/kg/min.[25-27]

Propofol-related infusion syndrome (PRIS) can occur with prolonged infusions greater than 48 hours and doses greater than 80 µg/kg/min. Propofol-related infusion syndrome is a potentially fatal condition and must be recognized early to avert detrimental outcomes.[28] It is associated with metabolic acidosis, cardiac failure, arrhythmias (eg, bradycardia), cardiac arrest, rhabdomyolysis, hyperkalemia, hypertriglyceridemia, refractory hypotension, and kidney failure. All patients should have a baseline triglyceride level, and this should be monitored every 3 to 7 days thereafter. A triglyceride level of 400 mg/dL or more is associated with increased risk of PRIS and pancreatitis; therefore, alternate sedative should be sought. A commonly observed effect from propofol infusion is the presence of green-colored urine, which usually resolves approximately 6 hours after the discontinuation of the drug. The main metabolic pathway of propofol is oxidation, reduction, and hydrolysis by cytochrome P450 and glucuronate conjugation in liver microsomes. The glucuronate conjugates propofol-glucuronide, 4-(2,6-diisopropyl-1,4-quinol)-sulphate, and 4-(2,6-diisopropyl-1,4)-glucuronide are thought to produce the urine discoloration.[29]

Propofol is contraindicated in patients with allergies to soybeans or eggs. It has antiseizure properties. It is highly protein bound, approximately 97% to 99%, and metabolized to inactive sulfate and glucuronide conjugates. Propofol can be used safely in renally and hepatically impaired patients. Calories supplied by propofol should be taken into consideration when determining a patient's nutritional needs, as it supplies 1.1 kcal/mL.

Phenylpiperidine

Ketamine is a phenylpiperidine derivative structurally related to phencyclidine, and an NMDA receptor antagonist; it has amnestic effects, readily crosses the blood-brain barrier, relaxes bronchial smooth muscles causing bronchodilatation, and is useful in patients experiencing opioid-induced hyperalgesia.[21,30] Despite a negative inotropic effect, dose-dependent stimulation of the CNS sympathetic outflow causes an increase in heart rate, blood pressure, cardiac output, and myocardial oxygen consumption. The recommended dose is 1 to 2 mg/kg intravenously (IV), although lower doses can be used. Possible adverse effects or overdose may lead to panic attacks, hallucinations, aggressive behavior, seizures, increased intracranial pressure, and cardiac arrest. Alternative sedatives should be employed in patients at risk for these conditions. The emergence reaction, such as a hallucination-developing recovery from the dissociative state, is more severe in adults and can be attenuated with the administration of a benzodiazepine before recovery.

Dexmedetomidine

Dexmedetomidine is an α_2-adrenoceptor agonist with 8 times more affinity to the α_2 receptor compared to clonidine.[31,32] It is an anxiolytic and can potentiate the analgesic properties of opioids. Dexmedetomidine infusion has been shown to reduce the prevalence and duration of confusion and delirium when compared with the use of morphine and midazolam.[33,34] It has also been used to wean patients unable to wean off the ventilator secondary to agitation, or to prevent intubation of acutely agitated, delirious patients.[22] Side effects include bradycardia and hypotension. Dosing is based on a continuous infusion of 0.2 to 1.4 µg/kg/min; although doses up to 2.5 µg/kg/min have been used in some studies.[35] Doses greater than 1.4 µg/kg/min have not been shown to produce additional clinical efficacy.[34] An initial loading dose of 1 µg/kg over 10 minutes may be omitted if the patient is being converted from another sedative, is adequately sedated, or is at risk for hemodynamic instability. Abrupt cessation of α_2 agonists after prolonged infusion can cause a withdrawal syndrome. An approach to prevent this is the use of clonidine to wean patients off dexmedetomidine.[36,37]

Two phase 3 multicenter, randomized, double-blinded trials were to determine the efficacy of dexmedetomidine versus midazolam (MIDEX) and dexmedetomidine versus propofol (PRODEX) in reducing the duration of mechanical ventilation and enhancing patient comfort and interaction with clinicians.[33] Median duration of mechanical ventilation was shorter with dexmedetomidine (123 hours [interquartile range, 67–337]) versus midazolam (164 hours [interquartile range, 92–380]; $P = 0.03$) but not with dexmedetomidine (97 hours [interquartile range, 45–257]) versus propofol (118 hours [interquartile range, 48–327]; $P = 0.24$).[32] Patients' interactions were improved with dexmedetomidine (estimated score difference vs midazolam, 19.7 [95% confidence interval, 15.2–24.2]; $P < 0.001$; and vs propofol, 11.2 [95% confidence interval, 6.4–15.9]; $P < 0.001$).[32] Length of ICU and hospital stay and mortality were similar. Dexmedetomidine versus midazolam patients had more hypotension (51/247 [20.6%] vs 29/250 [11.6%]; $P = 0.007$)[32,38] and bradycardia (35/247 [14.2%] vs 13/250 [5.2%]; $P < 0.001$). An economic evaluation of the PRODEX and MIDEX trials was conducted by Turunen et al, and they concluded that dexmedetomidine appears to be a preferable option compared with standard sedatives for providing light to moderate ICU sedation exceeding 24 hours due to the potential savings primarily from shorter time to extubation.[39]

Another study, a meta-analysis by Cruickshank et al,[40] on the comparative effects of $α_2$ agonists and propofol or benzodiazepines in mechanically vented adult ICU patients concluded that dexmedetomidine may be effective in reducing ICU length of stay and time to extubation in critically ill ICU patients. Risk of bradycardia but not of overall mortality is higher among patients treated with dexmedetomidine. Well-designed RCTs are needed to assess the use of clonidine in ICUs and to identify subgroups of patients that are more likely to benefit from the use of dexmedetomidine.

SEDATION AND ISSUES WITH MECHANICAL VENTILATION

Assessment of sedation quality and depth is dependent on the RASS or the SAS.[1,41] The bispectral index provides objective data and has been shown to correlate well with RASS in monitoring sedation in mechanically ventilated patients, although it is generally reserved for monitoring in the operating room.[42,43]

Light Sedation Over Deep Sedation

A randomized trial of light versus deep sedation suggested that deep sedation was associated with more posttraumatic stress disorder ($P = 0.7$), more trouble remembering events (37% vs 14%; $P = 0.02$), and more disturbing memories of the ICU (18% vs 4%; $P = 0.05$).[44] This study suggested that deep sedation is associated with prolonged mechanical ventilation and longer ICU days.[44] It has been hypothesized that the development of posttraumatic stress disorder is from recall of memories from the ICU.[45] A randomized controlled trial by Girard et al on patients with an intervention group having spontaneous daily awakening trials combined with spontaneous breathing trials showed that intervention had better outcomes, with more days without breathing assistance (14.7 days

vs 11.6 days; mean difference, 3.1 days; 95% confidence interval [CI], 0.7–5.6; $P = 0.02$), shorter ICU stays (9.1 days vs 12.9 days; $P = 0.01$), and shorter hospital stays (median time in the hospital 14.9 days vs 19.2 days; $P = 0.04$).[46] The interventional group had more self-extubations but the number of re-intubations after self-extubations were similar to total reintubation rates. A randomized trial by Strom et al of mechanically ventilated patients receiving no continuous IV sedation had fewer mechanically ventilated days compared with IV sedation (propofol or midazolam) with daily interruptions.[47] Shehabi Y et al showed that patients with early deep sedation (RASS –3 to –5) delayed extubation and increased mortality.[48] The goal of sedation is RASS of 0 to –2 or SAS of 3 to 4 (LOE B).[5]

Nonbenzodiazepines Over Benzodiazepines

Current SCCM guidelines favor nonbenzodiazepine sedation over benzodiazepine sedation (LOE 2B).[5] Klompas et al sought to find associations among different sedatives and ventilator-associated events (VAEs), length of stay, and mortality in patients who were mechanically ventilated over a 7-year period in a large academy center.[23] A total of 9603 consecutive episodes of mechanical ventilation were evaluated. Hazard ratios (HRs) were compared for VAEs, hospital discharge, and hospital death among patients receiving benzodiazepines, propofol, and dexmedetomidine. Both benzodiazepines and propofol were associated with VAE risk compared with dexmedetomidine. Propofol and dexmedetomidine were associated with less time to extubation compared with benzodiazepines (HR, 1.4; 95% CI, 1.3–1.5) versus (HR, 1.7; 95% CI, 1.4–2.0), respectively. Relatively few dexmedetomidine exposures were available for analysis. There were no differences between any 2 agents for HRs for hospital discharge or mortality.

DELIRIUM

Delirium is a syndrome characterized by an acute and reversible alteration of consciousness and cognitive functions[49] lasting for hours or days. Predisposing factors include age, dementia, parkinsonism, impaired vision, impaired hearing, depression, functional status, male sex, alcohol abuse, electrolyte abnormalities, fecal or urinary retention, sepsis, surgery, medication, inadequate pain control, critical illness, and change in environment.[49,50] Delirium affects between 38% and 87% of all patients admitted to surgical and medical ICUs.[51] The incidence of delirium among mechanically ventilated patients is estimated to be between 60% and 80%.[51] The pathophysiology of delirium is associated with altered levels of neurotransmitters, such as reduced cholinergic function; excess release of dopamine,

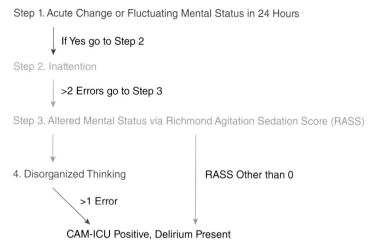

Step 1. Acute Change or Fluctuating Mental Status in 24 Hours

If Yes go to Step 2

Step 2. Inattention

>2 Errors go to Step 3

Step 3. Altered Mental Status via Richmond Agitation Sedation Score (RASS)

4. Disorganized Thinking   RASS Other than 0

>1 Error

CAM-ICU Positive, Delirium Present

FIGURE 14-1 Confusion Assessment Method for the Intensive Care Unit (CAM-ICU). (Adapted from www.icudelirium.org/docs/CAM-ICU-training-manual-2016-08-31_Final.pdf. Accessed March 15, 2018.)

norepinephrine, and glutamate; and altered serotonergic and GABA activity.[52,53]

Delirium is associated with prolongation of mechanical ventilation, prolonged length of ICU and hospital stay, increased costs, and increased morbidity[5,54] (LOE A). Prospective studies of patients with delirium have shown a significant decline in cognitive abilities and quality of life.[55,56] Two prospective cohort studies similarly revealed that each additional day with delirium was independently associated with a 10% increased risk of death at 6 months (HR, 1.10; 95% CI, 1.0–1.3) and 1 year (HR, 1.10; 95% CI, 1.0–1.2).[51,56]

Subtypes

There are 3 main types of delirium: hyperactive, hypoactive, and mixed delirium. The hyperactive form is characterized by psychomotor agitation, hallucinations, and considerable restlessness and agitation, whereas the hypoactive form, which is more difficult to identify, presents a lethargic clinical picture, in which the person remains disconnected from his or her surroundings. The mixed form fluctuates between the 2 types. Hyperactive delirium has a prevalence of about 1.6%, hypoactive delirium has a prevalence of 43.5%, and mixed delirium has a prevalence of 54.1%.[57] Hyperactive delirium (also known as "ICU psychosis") is known to have the best prognosis.[58] Hypoactive delirium carries a worse prognosis and generally is underdiagnosed in clinical settings.[59]

Management

The Confusion Assessment Method for the ICU (CAM-ICU) and the Intensive Care Delirium Screening Checklist (ICDSC) are used to screen for delirium[5] (LOE A). The CAM-ICU tool assesses 4 features: (1) acute change or fluctuation in mental status from baseline, (2) inattention, (3) altered level of consciousness, and (4) disorganized thinking (Fig. 14-1). The ICDSC tool is based on a screening checklist of 8 items based on *Diagnostic and Statistical Manual of Mental Disorders* (DSM) criteria and features of delirium. When these tools were compared with each other in critically ill patients, CAM-ICU was better able to predict the hospital length of stay and mortality in the ICU and the hospital when compared with ICDSC.[60]

Often, the delirium screening methods are incorporated in a protocolized bundle. This approach is preferred in several studies. First, a multicenter study explored the experience of both physicians and nurses caring for patients with delirium and found discrepancies in delirium recognition and management.[50] Second, a Swedish study focused on improving staff education for delirium assessment, prevention, and treatment and on caregiver-patient interaction showed a statistically significant decrease in the duration of delirium in the intervention group as compared to the control group (n = 37/62 [59.7%] vs n = 19/63 [30.2%] P = 0.001).[57] The mean length of hospital stay ± standard deviation was significantly lower on the intervention ward then on the control ward (9.4 ± 8.2 vs 13.4 ± 12.3 days, P < 0.001) especially for the delirious patients (10.8 ± 8.3 vs 20.5 ± 17.2 days, P < 0.001).[23]

One such bundle is the ABCDE (awakening and breathing coordination, choice of sedation, delirium monitoring, and exercise/early mobility) bundle.[46] In a prospective study, critically ill patients managed with the ABCDE bundle spent 3 more days breathing without assistance, experienced less delirium, and were more likely to be mobilized during their ICU stay than patients treated with usual care.[61]

The ABCDE bundle is a daily multidisciplinary checklist of known risk factors for delirium. It is an approach to setting daily goals for sedation and pain control, including daily review of appropriate selection of type and dosage of medications for sedation and analgesia. The ABCDE bundle also emphasizes the need for minimizing the use of these medications and executing daily awakening (SAT) and breathing trials (SBT) of patients on mechanical ventilation. In one study, SATs coordinated with daily SBTs decreased adverse cognitive outcomes, reduced hospital length of stay (LOS) by 4 days, and reduced death at 1 year by 14%.[22] The last component of ABCDE is focused on early mobility of critically ill patients. Current Clinical Practice Guidelines for the Management of Pain, Agitation, and Delirium in Adult Patients in the Intensive Care Unit recommend early mobilization of adult ICU patients whenever feasible to reduce the incidence and duration of delirium.[62] In addition, early physical therapy has been shown to independently reduce hospital LOS up to 3 days, reduce delirium incidence, and increase return to independent functioning.[63]

In a recent study, screening for delirium every 4 hours detected 55% more days of delirium than once-daily testing.[64] An earlier diagnosis of delirium can prompt clinicians to make necessary changes to the management plan to reduce the duration and intensity of delirium.

Nonpharmacologic Management of Delirium

Nonpharmacologic management includes avoidance of sleep deprivation, early mobilization, daily interruption of sedation and early liberation from mechanical ventilation, and consideration for environmental variables.[46,65,66] Environmental variables include minimizing the number of room changes, the presence of a clock or watch, access to reading glasses, presence of a family member, and absence of medical or physical restraints.[67]

Pharmacologic Management of Delirium

Pharmacologic management begins with review of the patient's current medications to determine if there is a medication that is associated with delirium (Table 14-6).

There is limited data to support the use of pharmacological agents for delirium management (Table 14-7).[68-70] In a recent review of literature, Neufeld and colleagues identified 19 studies looking at the efficacy of antipsychotics to treat delirium.[71] In all 19 studies, antipsychotic use was not associated with change in delirium duration, severity, or hospital or ICU length of stay.[71] First-generation antipsychotics such as haloperidol have shown limited benefit for delirium patients, but have shown differences in duration of delirium, length of stay, and delirium rating scores. Second-generation antipsychotics are also known for better efficacy and limited side effect profiles, but there is also limited data to support the use of second-generation antipsychotic agents to treat delirium. These include olanzapine, risperidone, ziprasidone, quetiapine, and aripiprazole.

COMA

Coma is a deep state of unconsciousness secondary to underlying disease and/or medications. Medically induced coma is a

TABLE 14-6 Medications Associated With Delirum and Preferred Alternative

Commonly Associated With Delirium	Preferred Alternative
Antihistamines (diphenhydramine)	Second-generation antihistamine (eg, loratadine)
Antiparkinsonians (benztropine, trihexyphenidyl)	Levodopa
Histamine-2 receptor agonists (cimetidine, ranitidine)	Proton pump inhibitors
Antispasmodics (oxybutynin)	Tolterodine
Low-potency antipsychotics (thioridazine, chlorpromazine)	Haloperidol, atypical antipsychotics
Antidepressants (tertiary tricyclic antidepressants)	Trazodone, selective serotonin reuptake inhibitors, secondary amine tricyclic antidepressants
Antiemetics (metoclopramide)	Ondansetron
Corticosteroids	Taper systemic, consider inhalation
High dose of opioid	Manage constipation, utilize multimodal pain management scheme, avoid meperidine
Benzodiazepines	Taper off, consider alternative sedatives
Certain antimicrobials (quinolone, high-dose beta-lactam antimicrobials, metronidazole)	Adjust dose, consider alternatives, discontinue once desired end point is reached
Diuretics, beta-blockers, clonidine, digoxin, theophylline, methyldopa, lithium	Adjust dose, close therapeutic monitoring

reversible intervention in which a controlled dose of sedatives causes a deep state of unconsciousness. This is a last resort in an attempt to protect the brain from swelling by reducing cerebral blood flow and the metabolic process of brain tissue. Indications include refractory seizures, traumatic brain injury, a low Glasgow Coma Scale (GCS) score, and protection of the brain during major neurosurgery. The RASS goal for medically induced patients is usually −3 or −4. Electroencephalogram is also used to monitor the brain waves while medication is administered until a certain pattern indicating a deep state of unconsciousness is seen. Duration of medically induced coma really depends on the nature of the injury, whether it is a brain injury or seizures, and the patient's clinical improvement. Medications that are used include opiates, benzodiazepines, propofol, and barbiturates. Barbiturates such as pentobarbital depress the sensory cortex and decrease motor activity, producing sedation, drowsiness, and hypnosis. It possesses a quick onset of 10 to 15 minutes and is up to 70% protein

TABLE 14-7 Agents for Delirium

Antipsychotic Agent	Dosage Form	Half-Life Metabolism	Dosages (mg)	Max Dose (mg/d)	QTc Prolongation Potential Dose-Related Effect	Sedation	Dopamine D$_2$ Receptor Affinity/ Extrapyramidal Symptoms	Anticholinergic Effects	Orthostatic Hypotension
Haloperidol (Haldol)	Tab, IV injection	14–26 h; hepatic	0.5–10 mg q 15–30 min, then q 6 h	35	Low	Low	High	Low	Low
Quetiapine (Seroquel)	Tab	6 h; hepatic	50 mg BID	400	Moderate	Moderate	Low	Moderate	High
Risperidone (Risperdal)	Tab, ODT, solution (1 mg/mL)	20 h; hepatic	1–2 mg daily	4–8	Moderate	Low	High	Low	Moderate
Aripiprazole (Abilify)	Tab, solution (5 mg/ mL), IM injection	75 h; hepatic	10–15 mg	30	Low	Low	Low	Low	Low
Ziprasidone (Geodon)	Capsule IM	2–5 h; hepatic	10 mg q 2 h	40	High	Low	High	Low	Moderate
Olanzapine (Zyprexa)	Tab, ODT, IM injection	30 h; hepatic	5	20	Low	Moderate	Low	Moderate	low

BID = twice daily; IM = intramuscular; IV = intravenous; ODT = orally disintegrating tablet; q = every; tab = tablet.

TABLE 14-8 Glasgow Coma Score

Eye Opening (E):	
• Spontaneous	4
• To voice	3
• To pain	2
• None	1
Verbal Response (V):	
• Normal conversation	5
• Disoriented conversation	4
• Incoherent words	3
• Sounds	2
• None	1
Motor Response (M):	
• Normal	6
• Localizes to pain	5
• Withdraws to pain	4
• Decorticate posture (rigidity, clenched fists, legs held out straight, arms bent inward toward body with wrists and fingers bent and held to chest)	3
• Decerebrate posture (arms and legs straight out, toes pointing down, and head and neck arched back)	2
• None	1

bound, with an effect lasting up to 4 hours after discontinuation. While these drugs (eg, pentobarbital) appear to reduce brain swelling like propofol does, one study on pentobarbital was not able to demonstrate improved patient mortality after 30 days. A pentobarbital loading dose of 30 to 40 mg/kg infused over 4 hours followed by a maintenance infusion of 1.8 to 3.3 mg/kg/h, and a mid-level loading dose of 10 mg/kg over 30 minutes followed by a maintenance infusion of 5 mg/kg/h have been used.

The Glasgow Coma Scale is used to examine and determine the depth of consciousness, track the patient's progress, and predict outcome. It estimates the extent of brain injury, and scores vary from 3 (severe brain injury and death) to 15 (mild to no brain injury) (Table 14-8).[72] It is often used in quantifying a patient's reaction, such as eye opening, movement, and verbal response. Coma is defined as GCS of 8 or less.

The GCS cannot assess patients who are on invasive mechanical ventilation. The Full Outline of UnResponsiveness (FOUR) score is a 17-point clinical grading scale used in the assessment of patients with an impaired level of consciousness with or without endotracheal intubation. It assesses 4 areas of neurological function: eye responses, motor responses, brainstem reflexes, and breathing pattern. The FOUR score has been validated with reference to the Glasgow Coma Scale in several clinical contexts; overall, the FOUR score has better biostatistical properties than the Glasgow Coma Scale in terms of sensitivity, specificity, accuracy, and positive predictive value. It has been found to have good interrater reliability; the predictive power of poor neurologic outcome via modified Ranke Scale had an area under the curve (AUC) of 0.75 for FOUR score and an AUC 0.76 for GCS, and a FOUR score of 0 had a mortality rate of 89% compared to a GCS of 3, which had a mortality rate of 71%.[73]

QUESTIONS

1. A 48-year-old man is admitted to the ICU with community-acquired pneumonia. He is mechanically ventilated and started on a midazolam infusion for sedation. He develops ARDS, and a continuous neuromuscular blockade is started. On day 11, the intensivist determines that the patient is ready for weaning since the fraction of inspired oxygen (Fio_2) has been lowered to 40% and the positive end-expiratory pressure (PEEP) to 5 mmH$_2$O. The midazolam infusion is stopped, but the patient does not have improvement in his mental status and his RASS remains at −4. The patient requires a tracheostomy at day 14 of mechanical ventilation. Which of the following sedation strategies would have lowered the possibility of tracheostomy in this patient?

   A. Slow titration of midazolam infusion to avoid withdrawal
   B. Avoidance of neuromuscular blocker
   C. Use of alternative sedation strategy with fentanyl, propofol, or dexmedetomidine
   D. Use of the Ramsay Sedation Scale rather than the RASS

2. Which of the following statements is NOT true with regard to the use of benzodiazepine infusions for sedation in the ICU?

   A. Diazepam can cause thrombophlebitis.
   B. Midazolam, lorazepam, and diazepam infusion can cause hemolysis, hypotension, soft tissue necrosis, seizure, and coma.
   C. Benzodiazepines are considered the drug of choice for the treatment of seizures.
   D. Benzodiazepines accumulate in patients with renal and hepatic failure and cause a prolonged sedative effect.

3. A 36-year-old man undergoes an emergent exploratory laparotomy for a gunshot wound and requires resection of the ileum. He is brought to the surgical ICU intubated and on mechanical ventilation. The patient is currently on a propofol infusion at 25 μg/kg/h. The patient is agitated and difficult to sedate, requiring 2-point restraints. The patient is dyssynchronous with the ventilator requiring 1 dose of vecuronium. Which of the following would be the next best step in the management of this patient?

   A. Ask the nurse to increase the dose of propofol to 50 μg/kg/min.
   B. Ask the nurse to start an infusion of midazolam.
   C. Ask the nurse to start an infusion of fentanyl.
   D. Ask the nurse to start an infusion of vecuronium.

4. A 36-year-old man is admitted for alcohol withdrawal. The patient is initially treated with lorazepam injection as needed based on the Clinical Institute Withdrawal Assessment (CIWA) scale but develops respiratory depression, requiring transfer to the ICU and mechanical ventilation. To treat the symptoms of withdrawal, the patient was started on fentanyl infusion, midazolam infusion, and propofol infusion. Attempts to lower the sedation were met with extreme agitation and dyssynchrony with the ventilator. After 5 days, dexmedetomidine was introduced. A few hours later, the patient became bradycardic and hypotensive. A crystalloid bolus was started. The electrocardiogram (ECG) shows a second degree heart block. Laboratory analysis shows the following:

White blood cells	$14 \times 10^3/\mu L$
Hemoglobin	10 g/L
Potassium	6 mEq/L
Creatinine	3 mg/dL
Lactic acid	5 mmol/L
Triglycerides	1000 mg/dL
Creatine kinase	110,000 U/L

Additionally, his serum osmolality gap is elevated. Which is the responsible medication?

A. Fentanyl
B. Midazolam
C. Propofol
D. Dexmedetomidine

5. A 63-year-old man undergoes coronary artery bypass grafting for triple vessel coronary artery disease. His postoperative course is complicated by cardiogenic shock, necessitating the use of inotropic support and causing an inability to wean from an intra-aortic balloon pump. He also develops sepsis related to hospital-acquired pneumonia resulting in ARDS and requiring paralysis with a continuous infusion of neuromuscular blockers. He is placed on continuous video-electroencephalography for suspected nonconvulsive status epilepticus. Which of the following is a contraindication to spontaneous awakening trial and spontaneous breathing trial?

A. Persistent hypoxemia secondary to ARDS on neuromuscular blockade
B. Intra-aortic balloon pump
C. Nonconvulsive status epilepticus
D. All of the above

6. Which of the following suggests that the patient in question 5 passed the spontaneous breathing trial?

A. A rapid shallow breathing index of less than 105
B. An absent cuff leak
C. A negative inspiratory force measured at –20 cm H_2O
D. A ratio of partial pressure of oxygen (Po_2) to Fio_2 less than 150

7. A 26-year-old man develops traumatic brain injury after a motor vehicle accident. He was intubated in the field and required emergent craniotomy for a traumatic epidural hematoma with a 6-mm midline shift. He is admitted to the surgical ICU postoperatively. He undergoes a sedation vacation. He is restless and opens his eyes to pain. He straightens his arms and legs and arches his head and neck backward. What is the GCS score of this patient?

A. 3T
B. 5
C. 4T
D. 8

8. A 50-year-old-woman with history of COPD and anxiety disorder is admitted and intubated for acute hypoxic and hypercapnic respiratory failure from COPD exacerbation secondary to community acquired pneumonia. Despite being on fentanyl and propofol, she is able to open her eyes to voice and tactile stimuli. She subsequently appears to become anxious but she is not dyssynchronous with the ventilator. What is her RASS score?

A. +2
B. –1
C. 0
D. +1

9. Pain treatment is which part of the ABCDEF bundle?

A. A
B. B
C. C
D. D

ANSWERS

1. C. Use of alternative sedation strategy with fentanyl, propofol, or dexmedetomidine

As recommended by the SCCM, pain, agitation, and delirium (PAD) guidelines, analgosedation should be attempted first. Fentanyl is preferred due to its quick onset and offset, lack of dependence on the renal system for elimination, and lack of an active metabolite. In the ICU, critically ill patients are often hemodynamically unstable and have either hepatic or renal impairment. Propofol or dexmedetomidine may be added if fentanyl provides inadequate sedation.

A multicenter double-blinded study showed that neuromuscular blockers have improved adjusted 90-day survival and time away from mechanical ventilator[74] (choice B). Midazolam should be weaned off slowly rather than being stopped abruptly in order to avoid withdrawal symptoms (choice A). However, the drug has an active metabolite that accumulates with prolonged infusion, especially in the presence of renal and hepatic impairment. This makes weaning the patient off midazolam a challenge. The use of the RASS or the SAS has been recommended as validated and reliable tools for monitoring sedation in adult patients compared to the Ramsay Sedation Scale.[1] In 2012, Riessen et al investigated whether the RASS allowed a better monitoring of sedation depth than the Ramsay score in measuring depth of sedation in ICU patients receiving analgosedation and concluded that the Ramsay score performed poorly compared to the RASS[34] (choice D).

2. B. Midazolam, lorazepam, and diazepam infusion can cause hemolysis, hypotension, soft tissue necrosis, seizure, and coma.

Only lorazepam or diazepam continuous infusion has a risk of propylene glycol toxicity. The clinical manifestations include hemolysis, skin necrosis, arrthymias, seizures, hypotension, and coma. In patients with clinical deterioration due to propylene glycol toxicity, levels ranging from 55 to 144 mg/dL have been found, with the lower end being associated with metabolic abnormalities and an increased anion gap, and the higher end associated with renal toxicity coupled with cardiovascular collapse. Surrogate diagnosis is based on the osmolality gap. Benzodiazepines have been shown to prolong ICU sedation, therefore leading to prolonged ventilation days and increased ICU length of stay, in part secondary to accumulation from poor hepatic and renal clearance[1,48] (choice D). While benzodiazepines remain the drug of choice for the management of seizures (choice C), patient selection, appropriate dosing, and careful titration are necessary to optimize clinical benefit while reducing unwanted adverse effects from the drug. Diazepam has been shown to cause thrombosis and phlebitis at the injection site[75] (choice A).

3. C. Ask the nurse to start an infusion of fentanyl.

Analgosedation is recommended as the initial step in sedating patients. This is even more important in postoperative patients. Increasing the infusion rate of propofol (choice A), or starting midazolam (choice B) or vecuronium (choice D) infusion will not provide optimal comfort for the patient, as these agents are devoid of analgesic properties, which is the underlying cause of this patient's discomfort. It is imperative to optimize sedation by providing analgesics and sedatives to patients prior to paralyzing them with neuromuscular blockers when indicated.

4. CD. Propofol

The diagnosis of propofol infusion syndrome requires a high index of suspicion. The dose of greater than 4 mg/kg/h for over 48 hours increases the risk, but propofol infusion syndrome has occurred with lower doses or shorter duration, hence this strategy does not completely eliminate risk. There have been reports of propofol infusion syndrome developing in patients after 1- to 5-hour high-dose infusions.[47] Other predisposing factors include exogenous

catecholamine, glucocorticoids, inadequate carbohydrate intake, and subclinical mitochondrial disease. Pathophysiology involves a disruption of the mitochondrial fatty acid oxidation resulting in increased malonylcarnitine, C5 acylcarnitine, creatine kinase, troponin T, lactate, and myoglobinemia.[28,76] Early markers of propofol infusion syndrome include elevated lactic acid, hypertriglyceridemia, and Brugada-type ECG. The severity of the clinical manifestations is dose dependent, and they include hypotension, rhabdomyolysis, bradycardia/cardiac arrhythmias, metabolic/lactic acidosis, and hypertriglyceridemia. The hypotension may be refractory to fluid resuscitation and pressors. Carnitine supplementation in patients with propofol infusion syndrome has been considered to have theoretical benefit; there are no trials to support this practice. More importantly, there is no data to support the use of carnitine supplementation in patients on propofol infusion to reduce the incidence of propofol infusion syndrome.

There are associated case reports of rhabdomyolysis from fentanyl, but that is not associated with hypertriglyceridemia (choice A). Propylene toxicity is not associated with midazolam (choice B). Dexmedetomidine (choice D) is associated with hypotension and bradycardia but not with abnormal laboratory findings.

5. D. All of the above

In the clinical vignette described above, the patient has multiple contraindications to a spontaneous breathing trial. Neuromuscular blockade (choice A), presence of intra-aortic balloon pump (choice B), and nonconvulsive status epilepticus (choice C) all pose significant barriers to the safe extubation of this patient.

6 A. A rapid shallow breathing index of less than 105

The rapid shallow breathing index is a well-studied and validated index for assessment of readiness of extubation. A cutoff threshold of 105 or lower has been established. An absent cuff leak, negative inspiratory force, and the ratio of Po_2 to Fio_2 are all useful measures in the assessment of readiness for extubation. An absent cuff leak (choice B) is the incorrect answer, as it would actually pose a barrier to extubation, as it may indicate edema in the airway. A negative inspiratory force (NIF) measured at -20 cm H_2O (choice C) would also be incorrect, since a low NIF indicates the possibility of diaphragmatic weakness, which may also pose a barrier to extubation. Similarly, a ratio of Po_2 to Fio_2 (PF) less than 150 (choice D) is incorrect, since a low PF ratio indicates the presence of hypoxic respiratory failure, which may pose a barrier to extubation.

7. C. 4T

In the clinical vignette described, the patient opens his eyes to pain and has an extensor response to pain. Opening eyes to pain is scored for eye opening as 2. Verbal response cannot be assessed since the patient is intubated; hence, the letter T is used. Maximum score is 10T and minimum score is 2T. For motor response, extensor response to pain is scored as 2; hence, the correct answer is a total score of 4T.

8. D. +1

The patient in this clinical vignette is restless but not dysynchronous with the ventilator or have frequent nonpurposeful movements, therefore has RASS score of +1. A patient with a RASS score of 0 is alert and calm (choice C). RASS score of +2 is agitated with frequent nonpurposeful movements and/or patient-ventilator dyssynchrony which is not seen in this patient (choice A). RASS score of – 1 is drowsy, but has sustained awakening more than 10 seconds with eye contact or voice (choice B).

9. A. A

The ABCDEF bundle consists of A for assessment, prevention, and management of pain; B for both spontaneous awakening trial and spontaneous breathing trial (choice B); C for choice for analgesia and sedation (choice C); and D for delirium assessment and prevention (choice D).

REFERENCES

1. Sessler CN, Gosnell MS, Grap MJ, et al. The Richmond Agitation-Sedation Scale: validity and reliability in adult intensive care unit patients. *Am J Respir Crit Care Med.* 2002;166(10):1338-1344.
2. Sessler CN. Sedation in ICU. *Chest.* 2004;126(6):1727-1730.
3. De Jonghe B, Cook D, Griffith L, et al. Adaptation to the Intensive Care Environment (ATICE): development and validation of a new sedation assessment instrument. *Crit Care Med.* 2003;31(9):2344-2354.
4. Devlin JW, Boleski G, Mlynarek M, et al. Motor Activity Assessment Scale: a valid and reliable sedation scale for use with mechanically ventilated patients in an adult surgical intensive care unit. *Crit Care Med.* 1999;27(7):1271-1275.
5. Barr J, Fraser GL, Puntillo K, et al; American College of Critical Care Medicine. Clinical practice guidelines for the management of pain, agitation, and delirium in adult patients in the intensive care unit. *Crit Care Med.* 2013;41(1):263-306.
6. Ely EW, Truman B, Shintani A, et al. Monitoring sedation status over time in ICU patients: the reliability and validity of the Richmond Agitation Sedation Scale (RASS). *JAMA.* 2003; 289(22):2989-2991.
7. Straker DA, Shapiro PA, Muskin PR. Aripiprazole in the treatment of delirium. *Psychosomatics.* 2006;47(5):385-391.
8. Jones J, Hoggart B, Withey J, Donaghue K, Ellis BW. What the patients say: a study of reactions to an intensive care unit. *Intensive Care Med.* 1979;5(2):89-92.
9. Gélinas C. Management of pain in cardiac surgery ICU patients: have we improved over time? *Intensive Crit Care Nurs.* 2007;23(5):298-303.
10. Schelling G, Richter M, Roozendaal B, et al. Exposure to high stress in the intensive care unit may have negative effects on health-related quality-of-life outcomes after cardiac surgery. *Crit Care Med.* 2003;31(7):1971-1980.
11. Granja C, Gomes E, Amaro A, et al; JMIP Study Group. Understanding posttraumatic stress disorder-related symptoms after critical care: the early illness amnesia hypothesis. *Crit Care Med.* 2008;36(10):2801-2809.
12. Akça O, Melischek M, Scheck T, et al. Postoperative pain and subcutaneous oxygen tension. *Lancet.* 1999;354(9172):41-42.
13. Hedderich R, Ness TJ. Analgesia for trauma and burns. *Crit Care Clin.* 1999;15(1):167-184.
14. Noly V, Riechebe P, Guignard B, et al. Remifentanil-induced postoperative hyperalgesia and its prevention with small dose of ketamine. *Anesthesiology.* 2015;103(1):147-155.
15. Anesthesiologists Task Force on Sedation and Analgesia by Non-Anesthesiologists. Practice guidelines for sedation and analgesia by non-anesthesiologists. *Anesthesiology.* 2002;96(4): 1004-1017.
16. Camilleri M, Lembo A, Katzka DA. Opioids in gastrointenterology: treating adverse effects and creating therapeutic benefits. *Clin Gastroenterol and Hepatol.* 2017;15(5):1338-1349.
17. Camilleri M. Opioid-Induced Constipation: Challenges and Therapeutic Opportunities. *Am J Gastroenterol* 2011;106(5): 835-842.
18. Katakami N, Harada T, Murata T, et al. Randomized phase III and extension studies of naldemedine in patients with opioid-induced constipation and cancer. *J Clin Oncol.* 2017; 35(34):3859-3866
19. Nelson AD, Camilleri M. Opioid-induced constipation: advances and clinical guidance. *Ther Adv Chronic Dis.* 2016; 7(2):121-134.
20. Tarumi Y, Wilson M, Szafran O, et al. Randomized, double-blind, place-controlled trial of oral docusate in the management of constipation in hospice patients. *J Pain Symptom Manage.* 2013;45(1):2-12.
21. Maieke N, Martini C, Dahan A, et al. Ketamine for chronic pain: risks and benefits. *Br J Clin Pharmacol.* 2014;77(2):357-367.
22. Klein Klowenberg PM, Zaal IJ, Spitonj C, et al. The attributable mortality of delirium in critically ill patients: prospective cohort study. *BMJ.* 2014;349:g6652.
23. Klompas M, Li L, Kleinman K, Szumita PM, Massaro AF. Associations between ventilator bundle components and outcomes. *JAMA Intern Med.* 2016;176(9):1277-1283.
24. Yaucher NE, Fish JT, Smith HW, Wells JA. Propylene glycol-associated renal toxicity from lorazepam infusion. *Pharmacotherapy.* 2003;23(9):1094-1099.
25. Bassett KE, Anderson JL, Pribble CG, Guenther E. Propofol for procedural sedation in children in the emergency department. *Ann Emerg Med.* 2003;42(6):773-782.
26. Frazee BW, Park RS, Lowery D, Baire M. Propofol for deep procedural sedation in the ED. *Am J Emerg Med.* 2005;23(2):190-195.
27. Miner JR, Burton JH. Clinical practice advisory: emergency department procedural sedation with propofol. *Ann Emerg Med.* 2007;50(2):182-187, 187.e1.
28. Kam KCA, Cardone D. Propofol infusion syndrome. *Anaesthesia.* 2007;62(7):690-701.
29. Juneg-Sam L, Hyun-Soo J, Byeong-Jay P. Green discoloration of urine after propofol infusion. *Korean J Anesthesiol.* 2013;65(2):177-179.
30. Mehta S, McIntyre A, Dijkers M, et al. Gabapentinoids are effective in decreasing neuropathic pain and other secondary outcomes after spinal cord injury: a meta-analysis. *Arch Phys Med Rehabil.* 2014;95(11):2180-2186.
31. Venn M, Newman J, Grounds M. A phase II study to evaluate the efficacy of dexmedetomidine in the medical intensive care unit. *Intensive Care Med.* 2003;29(2):201-207.

32. Jakob SM, Ruokonen E, Grounds RM, et al. Dexmedetomidine vs midazolam or propofol for sedation during prolonged mechanical ventilation: two randomized controlled trials. *JAMA.* 2012;307(11):1151-1160.

33. Riker RR, Shehabi Y, Bokesch PM, et al; SEDCOM (Safety and Efficacy of Dexmedetomidine Compared With Midazolam) Study Group. Dexmedetomidine vs midazolam for sedation of critically ill patients: a randomized trial. *JAMA.* 2009;301(5):489-499.

34. Riessen R, Pech R, Tränkle P, Blumenstock G, Haap M. Comparison of the RAMSAY score and the Richmond Agitation Sedation Score for the measurement of sedation depth. *Crit Care.* 2012;16(Suppl 1):P326.

35. Gagnon DJ, Riker RR, Glisic EK, Kelner A, et al. Transition from dexmedetomidine to enteral clonidine for ICU sedation. An observational pilot study. *Pharmacotherapy.* 2015;35(3):251-259.

36. Haenecour A, Goodwin A, Seto W, et al. Prolonged dexmedetomidine infusion and drug withdrawal in critically ill children. *Crit Care.* 2015;19(Suppl 1):p484.

37. Taylor DM, O'Brien D, Ritchie P, Pasco J, Cameron PA. Propofol versus midazolam/fentanyl for reduction of anterior shoulder dislocation. *Acad Emerg Med.* 2005;12(1):13-19.

38. Gerlach AT, Dasta JF. Dexmedetomidine: an updated review. *Annals of Pharmacology.* 2007;41(2):245-252.

39. Turunen H, Jakob SM, Ruokonen E, et al. Dexmedetomidine versus standard care sedation with propofol and midazolam in intensive care: an economic evaluation. *Crit Care.* 2015;19:67.

40. Cruickshank M, Henderson L, Maclennan G, et al. Alpha-2 agonists for sedation of mechanically ventilated adults in intensive care units: a systematic review. *Health Technol Assess.* 2016;20(25):v-xx, 1-117.

41. Riker RR, Picard JT, Fraser GL. Prospective evaluation of the Sedation-Agitation Scale for adult critically ill patients. *Crit Care Med.* 1999;27(7):1325-1329.

42. Ebersoldt M, Sharshar T, Annane D. Sepsis-associated delirium. *Intensive Care Med.* 2007;33(6):941-950.

43. Karamchandani K, Rewari V, Trikha A, et al Bispectral index correlates well with Richmond agitation sedation scale in mechanically ventilated critically ill patients. *J Anesth.* 2010;24(3):394-398.

44. Treggiari MM, Romand JA, Yanez ND, et al. Randomized trial of light versus deep sedation on mental health after critical illness. *Crit Care Med.* 2009;37(9):2527-2534.

45. Vasilevskis EE, Ely EW, Speroff T, Pun BT, Boehm L, Dittus RS. Reducing iatrogenic risks: ICU-acquired delirium and weakness—crossing the quality chasm. *Chest.* 2010;138(5):1224-1233.

46. Girard TD, Kress JP, Fuchs BD, et al. Efficacy and safety of a paired sedation and ventilator weaning protocol for mechanically ventilated patients in intensive care (Awakening and Breathing Controlled trial): a randomized controlled trial. *Lancet.* 2008;371(9607):126-134.

47. Strom T, Maritnussen T, Toft P. A protocol of no sedation for critically ill patients receiving mechanical ventilation: a randomised trial. *Lancet.* 2010;375(9713):475-480.

48. Shehabi Y, Bellomo R, Reade MC, et al. Early intensive care sedation predicts long-term mortality in ventilated critically ill patients. *Am J Respir Crit Care Med.* 2012;186(8):724-731.

49. Jackson P, Khan A. Delirium in critically ill patients. *Crit Care Clin.* 2015;31(3):589-603.

50. Palacios-Ceña D, Cachón-Pérez JM, Martínez-Piedrola R, Gueita-Rodriguez J, Perez-de-Heredia M, Fernández-de-las-Peñas C. How do doctors and nurses manage delirium in intensive care units? A qualitative study using focus groups. *BMJ Open.* 2016;6(1):e009678.

51. Pisani MA, Kong SY, Kasl SV, Murphy TE, Araujo KL, Van Ness PH. Days of delirium are associated with 1-year mortality in an older intensive care unit population. *Am J Respir Crit Care Med.* 2009;180(11):1092-1097.

52. Grap MJ, Borchers CT, Munro CL, et al. Actigraphy in the critically ill: correlation with activity, agitation and sedation. *Am J Crit Care.* 2005;14(1):52-60.

53. Maldonado JR. Neuropathogenesis of delirium: review of current etiologic theories and common pathways. *Am J Geriatr Psychiatry.* 2013;21(12):1190-1222.

54. Lundstrom M, Edlund A, Karlsson S, Brannstrom B, Bucht G, Gustafson Y. A multifactorial intervention program reduces the duration of delirium, length of hospitalization, and mortality in delirious patients. *J Am Geriatr Soc.* 2005;53(4):622-628.

55. Mu JL, Lee A, Joynt GM. Pharmacologic agents for the prevention and treatment of delirium in patients undergoing cardiac surgery: systematic review and meta-analysis. *Crit Care Med.* 2015;43(1):194-204.

56. Horikawa N, Yamazaki T, Miyamoto K, et al. Treatment for delirium with risperidone: results of a prospective open trial with 10 patients. *Gen Hosp Psychiatry.* 2003;25(4):289-292.

57. Peterson JF, Pun BT, Dittus RS, et al. Delirium and its motoric subtypes: a study of 614 critically ill patients. *J Am Geriatr Soc.* 2006;54(3):479-484.

58. Meagher DJ, Trzepacz PT. Motoric subtypes of delirium. *Semin Clin Neuropsychiatry.* 2000;5(2):75-85.

59. Morrison RS, Magaziner J, Gilbert M, et al. Relationship between pain and opioid analgesics on the development of delirium following hip fracture. *J Gerontol A Biol Sci Med Sci.* 2003;58(1):M76-M81.

60. Tomasi CD, Grandi C, Salluh J, et al. Comparison of CAM-ICU and ICDSC for the detection of delirium in critically ill patients focusing on relevant clinical outcomes. *J Crit Care.* 2012;27(2):212-217.

61. Balas MC, Vasilevskis EE, Olsen KM, et al. Effectiveness and safety of the awakening and breathing coordination, delirium monitoring/management, and early exercise/mobility bundle. *Critical Care Medicine.* 2014;42(5):1024-1036.

62. Gelinas C, Puntillo KA, Joffe AM, Barr J. A validated approach to evaluating psychometric properties of pain assessment tools for use in nonverbal critically ill adults. *Semin Respir Crit Care Med.* 2013;34(2):153-168.

63. Needham DM, Korupolu R, Zanni JM, et al. Early physical medicine and rehabilitation for patients with acute respiratory failure: a quality improvement project. *Arch Phys Med Rehabil.* 2010;91(4):536-542.

64. Meagher DJ. Delirium: optimising management. *BMJ.* 2001; 322(7279):144-149.

65. Morris PE, Goad A, Thompson C, et al. Early intensive care unit mobility therapy in the treatment of acute respiratory failure. *Crit Care Med.* 2008;36(8):2238-2243.

66. Schweickert WD, Pohlman MC, Pohlman AS, et al. Early physical and occupational therapy in mechanically ventilated, critically ill patients: a randomized controlled trial. *Lancet.* 2009;373(9678):1874-1882.

67. Pandharipande P, Cotton BA, Shintani A, et al. Prevalence and risk factors for development of delirium in surgical and trauma intensive care unit patients. *J Trauma.* 2008;65(1): 34-41.

68. Breitbart W, Marotta R, Platt MM, et al. A double-blind trial of haloperidol, chlorpromazine, and lorazepam in the treatment of delirium in hospitalized AIDS patients. *Am J Psychiatry.* 1996;153(2):231-237.

69. Kalisvaart KJ, de Jonghe JF, Bogaards MJ, et al. Haloperidol prophylaxis for elderly hip-surgery patients at risk for delirium: a randomized placebo-controlled study. *J Am Geriatr Soc.* 2005;53(10):1658-1666.

70. Schwartz TL, Masand PS. The role of atypical antipsychotics in the treatment of delirium. *Psychosomatics.* 2002;43(3):171-174.

71. Neufeld KJ, Yue J, Robinson TN, Inouye SK, Needham DM. Antipsychotic medication for prevention and treatment of delirium in hospitalized adults: a systematic review and meta-analysis. *J Am Geriatr Soc.* 2016;64(4):705-714.

72. Teasdale G, Jennett B. Assessment of coma and impaired consciousness. A practical scale. *Lancet.* 1974;2(7872):81-84.

73. Iyer VN, Mandrekar JN, Danielson RD, Zubkov AY, Elmer JK, Wijdicks EFM. Validity of the FOUR score coma scale in the medical intensive care unit. *Mayo Clin Proc.* 2009;84(8):694-701.

74. Papazian L, Forel JM, Gacouin A, et al; ACURASYS Study Investigators. Neuromuscular blockers in early acute respiratory distress syndrome. *New Engl J Med.* 2010;363(12):1107-1116.

75. Weir I, Holmes HI, Young ER. Venous sequelae following venipuncture and intravenous diazepam administration. Part one: etiological factors. *Oral Health.* 1996;86(5):9-17.

76. Krajcova A, Waldauf P, Andel M, Duska F. Propofol infusion syndrome: a structured review of experimental studies and 153 published case reports. *Crit Care.* 2015;19(398):1-9.

Stroke

Mais N. Al-Kawaz, MD, and Alexander E. Merkler, MD

INTRODUCTION

Stroke is defined as a neurologic deficit caused by a focal injury to the central nervous system secondary to vascular disease, and includes ischemic stroke, intracerebral hemorrhage (ICH), and subarachnoid hemorrhage (SAH).[1] Each year, approximately 800,000 new people develop a stroke in the United States.[2] Stroke is the fifth leading cause of death in the United States and a leading cause of major disability in adults.[2] Furthermore, the risk of recurrent stroke is as high as 20% at 5 years.[3] There are 2 major types of stroke: ischemic and hemorrhagic stroke. Approximately, 87% of stroke in the United States is ischemic and the remaining is hemorrhagic.[3] Hemorrhagic stroke can be further divided into ICH and SAH.[4] This chapter aims to outline the current understanding of common stroke presentations, risk factors, pathophysiology, complications, and treatment.

ACUTE STROKE PRESENTATION

Acute stroke should be suspected in a presentation of acute neurologic deficits that could be attributed to a vascular distribution. The knowledge of stroke is intertwined with typical clinical presentation syndromes associated with large or small vessel occlusions. Anterior cerebral artery (ACA) lesions typically present with leg weakness or numbness, aphasia, and apraxia, while middle cerebral artery (MCA) lesions manifest as face or arm weakness more than leg weakness, with aphasia (left side involvement) and, at times, neglect (right side involvement). Posterior circulation strokes present with cranial nerve deficits such as diplopia and often with cerebellar features such as ataxia, nausea, and nystagmus. Presence of alteration in mental status, headache, nausea, and vomiting is usually more indicative of increased intracranial pressure (ICP) and hemorrhagic strokes.[5]

ISCHEMIC STROKE

Risk Factors

Modifiable risk factors and nonmodifiable vascular risk factors result in disparities in ischemic stroke risk factors between different populations. Age and sex are known to be strong nonmodifiable indicators of ischemic stroke risk. The risk of stroke increases by 9% every year for men and 10% for women.[6] Men are at higher risk of ischemic strokes in the young and middle-aged groups; however, women have a higher ischemic stroke risk in their lifetime and tend to have worse mortality and morbidity outcomes.[7]

Ethnicity is another significant nonmodifiable risk factor for ischemic stroke. Blacks have a higher risk of ischemic stroke risk, especially in the young middle-aged group (between 45 and 54 years of age) with a black-to-white incidence ratio of 4.02.[8] The risk remains higher in the older age group but becomes more attenuated. Another nonmodifiable risk factor is a family history of strokes. The Framingham study showed that history of parental stroke before the age of 65 increases risk 3-fold.[9] Other hypercoagulable conditions have been linked to increased risk of ischemic stroke, including hereditary diseases such as sickle cell disease, Fabry disease, and homocystinuria,[10] and acquired hypercoagulable conditions such as the antiphospholipid syndrome.[11]

Modifiable stroke risk factors include hypertension, physical activity, obesity, diet and nutrition, diabetes, dyslipidemia, smoking, drug use, atrial fibrillation (AF), congestive heart failure, valvular disease, chronic obstructive pulmonary disease (COPD), and peripheral vascular disease.

Stroke Mechanism

Several different stroke etiological systems exist. The TOAST criteria (Trial of Org 10172 in Acute Stroke Treatment) includes 5 different ischemic stroke subtypes: large-artery atherosclerosis including large artery thrombosis and artery-to-artery embolization, cardioembolism, small-vessel occlusion, stroke of other determined cause, and stroke of undetermined cause.[12] Outlined below are the subtypes of ischemic strokes commonly utilized in clinical practice.

Large-Artery Atherosclerosis

Large-artery atherosclerosis refers to disease of the common and internal carotid arteries, the vertebral artery, and the major vessels of the circle of Willis. Typically, atherosclerosis leads to either extracranial stenosis at the proximal cervical internal carotid artery or intracranial atherosclerosis within the circle of Willis. Large vessel disease accounts for around 30% of all strokes.[13]

Cardioembolism

Cardioembolic stroke refers to an arterial embolism originating from the heart. The most common cause of cardioembolism is AF, although other causes include bacteria (infective endocarditis), tumor cells (marantic endocarditis), congestive heart failure, recent myocardial infarction, atrial myxoma, or mechanical heart valve. Cardioembolic sources of stroke account for 20% to 30% of total strokes.[14]

Small-Vessel Occlusion

Occlusion of small penetrating vessels is another common stroke mechanism accounting for approximately 25% of all strokes.[12] This mechanism results in lacunar stroke syndromes. It is pathologically associated with hypertension, diabetes, and hyperlipidemia. All three lead to lipohyalinosis and microatheroma formation.

Other Determined Cause

Other determined cause refers to other known stroke mechanism not able to be categorized into cardioembolism, large-artery disease, or small-vessel disease. Examples of other mechanisms of stroke include arterial dissection, vasculitis, sickle cell disease, or mitochondrial encephalomyopathy, lactic acidosis, and stroke-like episodes (MELAS).

Cryptogenic

Cryptogenic stroke refers to stroke without any known mechanism or stroke with more than 1 potential mechanism and accounts for up to 23% to 40% of all strokes. They occur more frequently in younger patients and have a higher risk of recurrence.[15] Cryptogenic strokes represent a diagnostic dilemma, as a more detailed and technologically advanced workup is recommended to identify an underlying mechanism.

Types of lacunar syndromes and large vessel stroke syndromes are seen in Tables 15-1 and 15-2.[16,17]

Pathophysiology

Ischemia within affected neurons occurs through a series of complex cellular processes. Neuronal cell death occurs predominantly through necrosis, or nonprogrammed cell death, and apoptosis, or programmed cell death. In conjunction with cell death, cytotoxic edema plays an important role in evolution of disease. Water influx intracellularly occurs as a result of calcium buildup in the cytoplasm, as well as buildup of sodium and chloride. Delayed edema results in increased intracranial pressure, herniation, and vascular compression. Other pathological processes that further exacerbate cerebral ischemia include acidosis, peri-infarct depolarization, and free radical formations.[18]

On a macrocellular scale, ischemia results in compartmentalization of brain tissue, with 1 compartment irreversibly affected (the ischemic core) and another that is structurally intact but becomes functionally impaired and is thus potentially salvageable (the penumbra). The extent of ischemia depends not only on duration of vessel occlusion, but also on cerebral perfusion pressure, which relies on multiple factors including extent of collaterals and systemic arterial pressure. Evidence suggests that there is temporal evolution of the ischemic stroke on the expense of the penumbra, thus warranting intervention within a certain time period.[18]

Diagnosis

Identification of an ischemic stroke event requires an acute neurologic deficit that could correlate to a vascular territory, small or large. The first step in diagnosis includes identifying a last known normal and performing a physical exam. The physical exam should focus on establishing a National Institute of Health Stroke Scale (NIHSS) score, which is an approximation of stroke severity. The scale must be used with caution, as it is biased toward dominant—often left-sided—MCA strokes, thus underestimating posterior circulation and cerebellar strokes. The scale contains 11 items including level of consciousness, orientation, visual fields, gaze preference, language fluency and comprehension, speech, motor strength, ataxia, neglect, and sensory loss.[19]

A noncontrast computed tomography (CT) scan then is obtained to primarily rule out intracranial hemorrhage, but

TABLE 15-1 Lacunar Syndromes

Syndrome/Signs	Vessel	Localization
Pure motor/contralateral hemiparesis	Lenticulostriate vessels from MCA or perforating arteries from basilar artery	Posterior limb of internal capsule or corona radiata or basis pontis
Pure sensory/contralateral hemisensory loss	Lenticulostriate vessels from MCA or thalamoperforators off the posterior cerebral artery	Ventroposterior lateral nucleus of the thalamus
Sensorimotor/contralateral weakness and sensory loss	Lenticulostriate vessels from MCA	Thalamus and adjacent posterior limb of internal capsule
Dysarthria-clumsy hand syndrome	Slurred speech and fine motor weakness of the contralateral hand	

MCA = middle cerebral artery.

TABLE 15-2 Large-Vessel Stroke Syndromes

Large Vessel	Symptoms
Internal carotid artery	Combined anterior and middle cerebral artery ischemic symptoms, intermittent ipsilateral visual disturbances due to central retinal artery occlusion (amaurosis fugax)
Anterior cerebral artery	Contralateral leg weakness and numbness, transcortical aphasia (left), ipsilateral or contralateral ideomotor apraxia
Middle cerebral artery	Contralateral face/arm > leg weakness and numbness, aphasia (left), gaze preference toward side of lesion, contralateral neglect (right), agraphesthesia/astereognosis (right)
Posterior cerebral artery (PCA)	Contralateral partial or complete homonymous hemianopia, alexia without agraphia, Weber syndrome if with midbrain involvement[a]
Superior cerebellar artery	Ipsilateral limb and gait ataxia
Anterior inferior cerebellar artery	Vertigo, ipsilateral deafness, facial weakness, and ataxia
Posterior inferior cerebellar artery/lateral medulla	Wallenberg syndrome: ipsilateral face and contralateral body pain and temperature sensory loss; ipsilateral seventh nerve palsy; ipsilateral palatal weakness; dysphagia; dysarthria; nystagmus; vomiting/nausea; ipsilateral Horner syndrome; skew deviation
Basilar artery	Locked-in syndrome with bilateral pontine infarcts: intact vertical eye movement, anarthria, quadriplegia
Brainstem stroke syndromes	
Deep penetrating arteries from PCA/medial midbrain	Weber syndrome: ipsilateral III nerve palsy, contralateral hemiparesis (including face)
Deep penetrating arteries from PCA/ventral midbrain	Benedikt syndrome: ipsilateral III nerve palsy, contralateral involuntary movements
Deep penetrating arteries from PCA/superior cerebellar peduncle	Nothnagel syndrome: ipsilateral III nerve palsy, contralateral dysmetria
Pontine perforators off the basilar artery/caudal pons	Foville syndrome: ipsilateral III and VI nerve palsy with or without contralateral hemiparesis
Paramedian pontine perforators off the basilar artery/paramedian pons	One-and-a-half syndrome: ipsilateral VI nerve palsy, bilateral intranuclear ophthalmoplegia
Vertebral artery or anterior spinal artery/medial medulla	Dejerine syndrome: ipsilateral tongue weakness and contralateral hemiparesis ± contralateral loss of vibration and position sensation

[a]Weber's syndrome: ipsilateral III nerve palsy with mydriasis and contralateral hemiparesis.

it can also help identify early signs of ischemia (hypoattenuation or loss of gray white differentiation) (Class of Recommendation [COR] I, Level of Evidence [LOE] A). Findings may influence decision to administer thrombolytic medications, namely intravenous (IV) tissue plasminogen activator (tPA), and may denote a certain hemorrhagic risk of administration depending on presence and size of visualized early hypoattenuation. The most sensitive and specific modality for ischemic stroke remains the diffusion-weighted imaging (DWI) sequence in magnetic resonance imaging (MRI), with a sensitivity ranging between 88% and 100% and a specificity ranging between 95% and 100%, within minutes of symptom onset. However, there are limiting factors to obtaining an MRI within the acute clinical presentation: high cost, prolonged duration of the test, and limited availability.[20]

In the acute setting, CT angiography (CTA) can be used to detect a large-vessel occlusion with an accuracy approaching that of angiography. A CTA has a high positive predictive value for large-vessel occlusions (91–100%), with a sensitivity

raging between 92% and 100% and a specificity ranging between 82% and 100%.[21]

Time-of-flight magnetic resonance (MR) angiography can also be obtained; however, it remains limited by availability and duration and has a lower sensitivity for occlusions, ranging from 60% and 85% for stenoses and from 80% to 90% for occlusions.[21]

Acute Management of Stroke

The first step in the management of acute stroke is prompt recognition of the event followed by a decision regarding emergent therapies, including IV tPA and mechanical thrombectomy. Thrombolysis using IV tPA has been shown to improve functional outcomes at 3 months with a number needed to treat of 3.[22] The more quickly a patient receives IV tPA, the greater chance is of functional improvement.[23] Once clinical stroke is suspected, a quick history and examination, including the NIHSS, should be performed. A noncontrast head CT is necessary to rule out hemorrhage and large completed areas of infarction. Once hemorrhage is ruled out, IV tPA should be administered if the last known well time is within 4.5 hours (COR I, LOE A). Beyond this time window, IV tPA is not effective and the risk of causing hemorrhage increases. Intravenous tPA was approved following a landmark National Institute of Neurological Disorders and Stroke (NINDS) trial in 1995 in which neurologic recovery or NIHSS improvement by more than 4 points was achieved within 24 hours following IV tPA therapy.[24] The major risk of treatment with IV tPA remains intracerebral hemorrhage with a risk of 6.4% when compared to 0.6% in patients who received placebo.[24]

Endovascular Therapy

Recently, 5 randomized clinical trials have proven the effectiveness of mechanical thrombectomy in cases of large-vessel occlusion. In any patient with suspected stroke due to large-vessel occlusion (typically NIHSS > 6), vessel imaging, preferably with CTA should be obtained (COR I, LOE A).

Perfusion imaging, MR or CT, can also be obtained to delineate penumbral tissue that can be potentially salvaged with intervention.[25]

For patients with proximal middle cereral artery or internal carotid artery occlusion and a region of tissue that is ischemic and not infarcted, or there is a mismatch between clinical deficit and infarct, mechanical thrombectomy is an option up to 24 hours from the time the patient was known to be well (COR I, LOE A).[25-27] Endovascular therapy should be offered to patients with basilar occlusion despite these guidelines, given the catastrophic outcomes if left untreated. Patients eligible for IV tPA should be given IV tPA regardless of consideration for endovascular therapy (COR I, LOE A).[25] Mechanical thrombectomy leads to greater chance of functional recovery at 3 months. Success is dependent upon multiple factors, including time to recanalization, extent of recanalization, and amount of salvageable tissue.[25]

Role for Hemicraniectomy

Up to 10% of ischemic strokes are large enough to lead to significant cerebral edema resulting in herniation, which, if left untreated, is associated with a mortality rate of up to 78%.[28] Hemicraniectomy involves removal of the skull and dura of the side of the large ischemic stroke in order to allow for external rather than internal herniation. A pooled analysis of 3 landmark European studies including Decompressive craniectomy in malignant middle cerebral artery infarcts (DECIMAL), Decompressive surgery for the treatment of malignant infarction of middle cerebral artery (DESTINY), and Hemicraniectomy after middle cerebral artery infarction with life-threatening edema trial (HAMLET) showed that patients who underwent surgical intervention had improved survival and functional outcomes. The number needed to treat for an outcome with a modified Rankin Scale (mRS) of 4 or less was 2 and the number needed to treat for an outcome with an mRS of 3 or less was 4.[29] However, a favorable functional outcome in these studies was defined by an mRS of 3, which indicates moderate disability and may be viewed differently by patients and families.

Follow-up studies have included patients over 60 years of age and indicated that hemicraniectomy was associated with better survival, but all patients were left with at least moderate disability (defined as an mRS of 3 or higher).[30] Given the above data, hemicraniectomy is typically reserved for patients less than 60 years of age and within 48 hours of presentation (COR I, LOE B).[31]

Workup

Following acute presentation and the decision-making process regarding thrombolytic and mechanical thrombectomy, further workup is warranted to identify the stroke mechanism. Vascular imaging, including MR or CT angiography, can be utilized to identify carotid artery disease and intracranial disease. Decision regarding secondary prevention with single or dual antiplatelet therapy (aspirin and clopidogrel) can be based on vascular imaging findings and whether the current event can be attributed to stenosis or occlusion.

The remaining workup includes echocardiography and telemetry to investigate a cardioembolic mechanism. Cryptogenic strokes require monitoring for a longer period of time than standard telemetry. Two large randomized trials have shown that prolonged cardiac monitoring is most beneficial in cryptogenic strokes. The Cryptogenic Stroke and Underlying AF (CRYSTAL AF) trial identified the underlying mechanism to be AF in 8.9% of stroke patients at 6 months and 30% of patients at 3 years.[32] The 30-Day Cardiac Event Monitor Belt for Recording Atrial Fibrillation after a Cerebral Ischemic Event (EMBRACE) trial showed that longer monitoring with an event monitor for 30 days was superior to the standard 24-hour telemetry, with a detection rate of 16.1% versus 3.2% in the control group.[33]

Secondary Stroke Prevention

Secondary stroke prevention with antiplatelets for ischemic stroke and transient ischemic attack (TIA) has long shown benefit in preventing recurrent events. Aspirin was found to have a minimal but real reduction of death and recurrent stroke when administered within 24 to 48 hours of symptoms (COR I; LOE A).[34] A combination of other antiplatelet agents (eg, clopidogrel) plus aspirin has mostly shown benefit in patients with intracranial atherosclerosis as concluded by recent trials, including SAMMPRIS[35] and VISSIT,[36] which revealed superiority of medical management over stenting for recurrent strokes in patients with intracranial atherosclerosis. Guidelines recommend dual antiplatelets for TIAs and minor strokes secondary to large-artery stenosis identified on vessel imaging (COR IIb, LOE B). For TIAs or minor ischemic strokes occurring due to severe stenosis, treatment with aspirin/clopidogrel for 90 days has shown to decrease risk of recurrent stroke by 32%.[37]

Hypertension is the most common modifiable risk factor in the United States, affecting blacks more than whites and men more than women. Recent Joint National Committee (JNC) guidelines recommended patients over the age of 60 years be treated for a blood pressure (BP) goal of less than 150/90 mmHg, while patients less than 60 years of age be treated for a BP goal of less than 140/90 mmHg. Patients with diabetes mellitus or chronic kidney disease should be treated for a BP goal of less than 130/80 mmHg, regardless of age (COR IIb, LOE B).[38] It should be noted that the Systolic Blood Pressure Intervention Trial (SPRINT), which investigated outcomes in patients with tight systolic BP control below 120 mmHg, rather than the commonly set goal of less than 140 mmHg, was stopped prematurely due to the significantly reduced risk of cardiovascular events and stroke in patients with strict control of systolic BP below 120 mmHg.[39] However, since that trial excluded patients with prior strokes and showed no difference in stroke events at follow-up, most neurologists follow American Heart Association (AHA)/American Stroke Association (ASA) guidelines, which recommend lowering the BP to below 140/90 mmHg in stroke patients without diabetes (COR I, LOE B).[1]

Management of dyslipidemia is also critical in secondary prevention with a goal low-density lipoprotein (LDL) of less than 70 mg/dL. In addition to their lipid lowering potential, statins have been found to exert a neuroprotective effect on the endothelium and cerebral blood flow.[40] A large randomized prospective controlled trial showed that 80 mg of atorvastatin, a high-dose statin, reduces the risk of recurrent strokes and cardiac events in patients with coronary artery disease or an LDL of 100 to 190 mg/dL.[41] Thus, ASA/AHA guidelines recommend initiating moderate to high statin therapy in patients with stroke and an LDL over 190 mg/dL, an LDL over 70 mg/dL and diabetes mellitus, an LDL less than 70 mg/dL and a 10-year atherosclerotic cardiovascular risk of 7.5% or higher, or atherosclerotic disease (COR I, LOE B). Metabolic syndrome, diabetes, and prediabetes (hemoglobin A1c, 5.7–6.4%) are independently associated with approximately a 60% risk of recurrent stroke in the elderly.[42]

Smoking has been identified to have a double risk of stroke within the general population, with the risk being dose dependent. This risk seems to be even higher when coupled with hypertension and returns back to baseline with abstinence in 10 years.[43] Smoking cessation should be encouraged in any patients with a stroke (COR I, LOE C).

Atrial fibrillation is a common cause of ischemic stroke and is the most common cause of cardioembolic stroke. Patients with AF face a heightened stroke risk, and an estimated 15% of all ischemic strokes are attributed to AF.[44] The CHA_2DS_2-VASc can be used as a stroke risk predictive tool in patients with AF, with higher scores indicative of a higher stroke risk.[45] Given the elevated associated risk, AF management has been an important topic in secondary stroke prevention, and multiple studies have indicated a risk reduction for stroke of approximately two-thirds in patients taking anticoagulation.[46] AHA/ASA guidelines recommend anticoagulation for patients with AF with the choice of agents tailored depending on age, medical history, and other associated risk factors (COR IIa, LOE B).

Carotid revascularization was shown to be superior to medical therapy alone in patients with moderate-to-severe symptomatic (ipsilateral) cervical carotid disease (50–99%) on vascular imaging.[47] The decision regarding stenting versus an endarterectomy is based on the patient's age, risk factors, and past medical history. Patients younger than 70 years of age are generally offered carotid artery stenting, while patients older than 70 years of age were shown to have a higher benefit from an endarterectomy.[48] Notably, carotid artery stenting was found to be associated with a higher periprocedural rate of stroke than carotid endarterectomy but a lower rate of periprocedural myocardial infarction (MI), and thus patients' prior medical history needs to be considered when making the decision regarding choice of intervention (COR IIa, LOE B).[48]

In summary, all patients with ischemic stroke should be evaluated for symptomatic cervical carotid artery disease and cardioembolic causes of stroke, namely AF, as these findings significantly alter secondary preventative strategies. Instead of antiplatelet therapy, patients with symptomatic cervical carotid disease should be offered carotid revascularization, and patients with AF should be placed on anticoagulation.

INTRACEREBRAL HEMORRHAGE

Though less common than ischemic strokes, intracerebral hemorrhage is associated with a higher mortality and morbidity, and a quicker clinical deterioration than ischemic strokes.[49] The annual incidence ranges between 16 and 33 cases per 100,000 yearly.[50] The primary brain injury following ICH usually occurs due to ruptured vessels, resulting in displacement of tissue, disruption of the parenchyma due to mass effect, and increased intracranial pressure. Vessels become compromised due to different mechanisms, including lipohyalinosis in long-standing hypertension and amyloid deposits in cerebral amyloid angiopathy (CAA). Secondary injury occurs due to inflammation, perihematomal edema, and necrosis and results in additional damage reaching a maximum volume at 12 days, with the fastest growth period being within the first 48 hours.[51]

Secondary brain injury was also found to impact disease course, possibly contributing to disappointing results despite clot evacuation surgeries. Studies indicated the presence of an ongoing injury following the initial hematoma formation for which the underlying pathophysiology is not entirely clear, but has been thought to be secondary to blood-brain barrier breakdown, release of excitotoxic amino acids following disruption of blood flow and ischemia, and thrombin-induced activation of the inflammatory cascade.[52]

Once a hematoma is formed, there is a significant risk of hematomal expansion within the first 24 hours. This risk increases with large hematomal size, sustained increased blood pressure, anticoagulant use, and evidence of extravasation on CT scan.[53] Extravasation on CT, or the "spot sign," has been specifically linked to increased hospital mortality and poor outcomes among survivors.[54] Expansion of the ICH into the intraventricular space occurs in 40% to 60% of patients and also is associated independently with death and poor outcomes.[55]

Risk Factors

Hypertension is one of the most common modifiable risk factors resulting in deep cortical hemorrhages over lobar hemorrhages.[56] Other risk factors have been outlined through a large population study and include advanced age, cerebral amyloid angiopathy, African American ethnicity, and increased alcohol intake.[57] Chronic kidney disease and intake of selective serotonin reuptake inhibitors (SSRIs) have also been invariably reported as ICH risk factors. Anticoagulation, particularly warfarin use, has been found to increase ICH risk up to 5-fold and result in worsening outcomes and hematomal expansion.[58] While aspirin intake increases ICH risk only minimally, dual antiplatelet therapy was found to increase ICH risk 2-fold.[59]

Clinical Presentation

Patients with ICH may present with focal neurological deficits, including unilateral weakness or numbness, and are often associated with headache, nausea, and vomiting. Meningismus and neck stiffness may be present if the hematoma expands into the intraventricular space. Seizures occur in up to 29% of patients, mostly in lobar hemorrhages, and are more likely to be nonconvulsive.[60] Stupor and coma may develop if the hematoma size is significant and may be the presenting symptoms in thalamic bleeds as well. Outlined in Table 15-3 are the most common locations for ICH, along with location-dependent presenting symptoms.

Clinical Evaluation

A noncontrast head CT should be the initial step to identify the presence of ICH, hematoma location, and extension into

TABLE 15-3 Clinical Presentation of Intracerebral Hemorrhage

Location	Symptoms
Putamen	Hemiplegia, hemisensory loss, homonymous hemianopsia, gaze palsy, stupor, and coma
Cerebellar	Gait imbalance, vomiting, occipital headache, neck stiffness, stupor with impending brainstem herniation
Thalamus	Hemiparesis and hemisensory loss
Lobar	Vary depending on location, more commonly associated with seizures
Pons	Deep coma, paralysis, pinpoint pupils, absent horizontal eye movements facial weakness, dysarthria, and hearing loss if patient is awake

TABLE 15-4 Intracerebral Hemorrhage Appearance on Magnetic Resonance Imaging

Hematomal Age	T2	T1
Hyperacute	Hyperintense	Isointense
Acute (1–2 d)	Hypointense	Isointense
Early subacute (2–7 d)	Hypointense	Hyperintense
Late subacute (7–14 d)	Iso to hyperintense	Hyperintense
Chronic intracerebral hemorrhage	Center: hyperintense; periphery: hypointense	Center: isointense; periphery: hypointense

T1 = T1 weighted images; T2 = T2 weighted images.

the ventricular space, and it can indicate an underlying etiology (COR I, LOE A).[61] The presence of a patchy appearance of hyperdense blood products within a larger hypodense ischemic area is often indicative of a hemorrhagic conversion of an ischemic stroke rather than a primary ICH. Hematomal size can be computed using the hematomal largest diameter (A) on CT imaging, the largest diameter perpendicular to A (B), and the number of 10-mm head CT slices on which the hemorrhage is visualized (C). The hematomal size can be then calculated using the formula $(A \times B \times C)/2$.

Acutely, MRI is not indicated to identify hemorrhage. A noncontrast CT is excellent to identify ICH.[62] However, MRI can be particularly useful in identifying a possible underlying etiology, including lobar microbleeds indicative of cerebral amyloid angiopathy, vascular malformation, aneurysms, or malignancy. Table 15-4 lists the appearances of ICH on MR imaging.

Etiology

One of the most common etiologies for ICH is hypertension. Hypertensive vasculopathy–related ICH occurs generally within the deep perforator vessel territory, including the pontine, midbrain perforators, thalamoperforators, and lenticulostriate arteries. The underlying pathophysiology is deemed to be secondary to a wear-and-tear pattern and subsequent tear within the vessel wall.[63]

Lobar ICH is commonly associated with cerebral amyloid angiopathy within the elderly population and is the second most common cause of spontaneous ICH. Cerebral amyloid angiopathy hemorrhages typically occur within the posterior lobes (occipital and temporal), in patients over the age of 65. They can present with superficial siderosis, microbleeds, and SAHs with less frequency.[64] The prognosis of lobar hemorrhages associated with CAA depends on the hematoma location, size, and Glasgow coma score at presentation. Recurrence rate in CAA-associated hemorrhages is significantly higher than hypertension-associated ICH and is reported to be 21% at 2 years.[65]

Intracerebral hemorrhages can also be associated with underlying tumors, vascular malformation, coagulopathies, anticoagulation use, central nervous system vasculopathy, aneurysms, and illicit drug use.

Management

Initial medical management of ICH focuses on BP management, ICP monitoring, and anticoagulation reversal. AHA/ASA guidelines recommend reversal of anticoagulation in patients taking warfarin with vitamin K and prothrombin complex concentrate (PCC) (COR I, LOE C). One antidote has been approved for novel anticoagulants: Idarucizumab is the treatment of choice for ICH in a patient using dabigatran.[66] These two agents are still not approved: Andexanet alfa, a reversal agent for factor Xa inhibitors and enoxaparin, and ciraparantag, a reversal agent for factor Xa inhibitors, factor IIa inhibitors, unfractionated heparin, and low molecular weight heparin. No effective reversal method has been identified for antiplatelet therapy with platelet transfusions falling out of favor following the PATCH trial (Platelet Transfusion Versus Standard Care After Acute Stroke Due to Spontaneous Cerebral Haemorrhage Associated With Antiplatelet Therapy), which revealed that platelet transfusion was inferior to standard medical therapy in patients presenting with ICH.[67]

Reduction in blood pressure is another therapeutic goal during acute presentation. Although a lower BP goal would prevent hematomal growth, aggressively lowering mean arterial pressure previously had been thought to lower cerebral perfusion pressure and increase the ischemic area surrounding the hematoma; however, this theory was unsupported by perfusion studies that showed that BP reduction does not affect oxygen delivery to the perihematomal tissue.[68] In clinical practice, studies have favored a lower BP goal. The second Interpretation and Implementation of Intensive Blood Pressure Reduction in Acute Cerebral Hemorrhage Trial (INTERACT II) showed that acute lowering of SBP below 140 mmHg in hypertensive patients presenting with ICH is safe and results in improved disability in survivors, with no significant reduction in death.[69] However, reducing SBP to below 140 mmHg as compared to below 180 mmHg was not supported by the second Antihypertensive Treatment of Acute Cerebral Hemorrhage (ATACH II) trial which showed no significant difference in death or major disability in the strict BP goal group.[70] Currently, guidelines state that for patients resenting with an SBP between 150 and 220 mmHg, acutely lowering SBP to lower than 140 mmHg is safe (COR I, LOE A).[61]

External ventricular drainage is required for patients with hydrocephalus due to intraventricular hemorrhage (COR IIa, LOE B). Drainage should allow for control of elevated ICP and a goal cerebral perfusion pressure of 50 to 70 mmHg should be maintained during the acute presentation (COR IIb, LOE C).[61] Aggressive ICP management is recommended with elevation of the head of the bed greater than 30 degrees, sedation, hyperosmotic agents such as mannitol, and sometimes barbiturate coma or hypothermia.

Surgical interventions are only recommended for patients with cerebellar hemorrhages larger than 3 cm in size with quick neurologic deterioration (COR I, LOE B). Current guidelines do not recommend surgery for supratentorial hemorrhages (COR IIb, LOE A). This recommendation is based on the International Surgical Trial in Intracerebral Haemorrhage (STICH) and STICH2 trials, which showed no significant difference in mortality or functional outcome in patients who underwent surgical intervention of supratentorial hemorrhages.[71,72]

SUBARACHNOID HEMORRHAGE

Etiology

Five percent of all strokes are caused by nontraumatic subarachnoid hemorrhages. Although the rate of mortality decreased by 15% between 1960 and 1995,[73,74] up to 25% of patients die within the first 24 hours, with a 30-day case fatality ranging from 36% to 50%.[75,76] The risk of permanent disability in survivors is approximately 50%. Aneurysmal SAH is the most common cause of spontaneous nontraumatic SAH, accounting for 75% to 80%. The remaining etiologies are listed in Table 15-5.[73]

Risk factors for aneurysm formation include hypertension, smoking, chronic alcohol abuse, family history of aneurysms, female sex, and genetic causes, including polycystic kidney disease and connective tissue diseases including Marfan syndrome, Ehlers-Danlos syndrome, and fibromuscular dysplasia.[76]

International Study of Unruptured Intracranial Aneurysms (ISUIA) is a large retrospective population study that aimed to identify the natural course of unruptured aneurysms and risk of intervention of unruptured aneurysms.[77] The study identified that the location and type of aneurysms are the 2 most important factors in determining risk of rupture. Saccular aneurysms account for about 90% of aneurysms, and their rupture is the most common cause of spontaneous SAH. Fusiform aneurysms account for the other 10% of aneurysmal SAH. As for location, posterior circulation aneurysms are more likely to rupture, although they accounted for 12%

TABLE 15-5 Causes of Nonaneurysmal Hemorrhage

Perimesencephalic hemorrhage
Trauma
Intracranial dissection
Dural AVM
Cervical AVM
Trauma
Mycotic aneurysm
Cocaine abuse
Sickle cell disease
Pituitary apoplexy
Coagulation disorder

AVM = arteriovenous malformation.

of all aneurysms in the ISUIA study.[77] Size of the aneurysm also accounts for a significant risk factor for rupture and subsequent SAH. The ISUIA study found a 0.05% yearly risk of rupture for aneurysms smaller than 10 mm. This risk escalates for giant aneurysms larger than 2.5 cm, with a cumulative risk of 40% for anterior circulation aneurysms and 50% for posterior circulation aneurysms.[77]

Presentation

The most common presenting feature of an aneurysmal SAH is the "worst headache ever" or a "thunderclap headache." The headache can be associated with nausea, vomiting, neck rigidity, and photophobia. Approximately 30% to 40% of patients also report a mild headache weeks prior, indicative of a sentinel headache due to a minor leak.

Severe SAH can present also with alteration in mental status, focal neurologic symptoms, and coma. Other unlikely accompanying symptom with SAH include vitreous hemorrhages (Terson syndrome). Although Terson syndrome is rather uncommon, documented in 3% of patients in 1 systemic review, it is predictive of increased mortality.[78] Aside from SAH, aneurysms can present with focal neurologic symptoms depending on location. The symptoms are detailed in Table 15-6.

Several scales have been proposed to assess the severity of presenting symptoms, which are eventually reflective of prognosis and outcomes. The Hunt and Hess scale (Table 15-7), which is widely used, was initially proposed to identify patients at a higher risk for surgical intervention but now is used as a general representation of the severity of presentation and to predict mortality.[79]

Diagnosis

Diagnosis of SAH is via noncontrast head CT or via lumbar puncture. The sensitivity of CT scans within the first 6 hours reaches 100% and deteriorates over the next few days, reaching 58% at 5 days.[80] If the CT scan is negative, guidelines recommend obtaining a lumbar puncture if the clinical suspicion

TABLE 15-6 Common Clinical Presentations of Intracranial Aneurysms

Location of Aneurysm	Clinical Manifestations
Anterior communicating artery	Bilateral temporal hemianopsia, bilateral lower extremity weakness
Posterior communicating artery	Third nerve palsy
Intercavernous internal carotid artery	Orbital or facial pain, progressive vision loss and ophthalmoplegia, epistaxis
Posterior circulation	Brainstem dysfunction

TABLE 15-7 Hunt and Hess Scale

Grade 1: asymptomatic patients and patients with minimal HA and nuchal rigidity
Grade 2: patients with severe HA and nuchal rigidity but no focal neurologic symptoms
Grade 3: patients who are confused and drowsy, and with focal neurologic symptoms
Grade 4: stuporous patients or patients with moderate to severe hemiparesis
Grade 5: patients with coma and decerebrate posturing

HA = Headache.

is high enough, especially if the CT is obtained in a delayed fashion (COR I, LOE B).[81] A positive lumbar puncture for SAH will often reveal failure to clear RBCs between tubes 1 and 4, and xanthochromia.

Obtaining a CT angiogram is the next step in identifying a possible aneurysm or vascular malformation that could have resulted in nontraumatic SAH. Aneurysms smaller than 3 mm may be better detected with digital subtraction angiography (DSA), as sensitivity for CTA gradually decreases for smaller aneurysms, reaching 91% for aneurysms smaller than 3 mm in size when compared to 96.5% sensitivity of DSA in detecting aneurysms of all sizes.[82] Therefore, if a CTA is unremarkable, a DSA should be performed (COR IIb, LOE C). Due to obscurations secondary to vasospasm, hematoma, or thrombosis, up to 24% of patients with SAH have a false-negative DSA. It is thus recommended that for patients with a negative DSA, a repeat angiogram is preformed within 4 to 14 days.

Management

Blood pressure control is medically advisable upon initial presentation until obliteration of aneurysm is established. No specific cutoffs have been firmly established, but guidelines recommend generally lowering SBP to below 160 mmHg until aneurysm obliteration is established (COR IIa, LOE C). Aneurysmal SAHs are then managed with surgical clipping versus endovascular coiling as soon as possible (COR I, LOE B). The International Subarachnoid Aneurysm Trial (ISAT) showed that patients who undergo coiling are at a lower risk of disability at 1 year when compared to patients who underwent surgical clipping.[84] However, the decision regarding coiling versus clipping should be done in a multidisciplinary team between surgeons and interventionalists, depending on patients' and aneurysms' characteristics (COR I, LOE C). Table 15-8 lists nonaneurysmal causes of subarachnoid hemorrhage.

External ventricular drainage (EVD) or lumbar drainage can be offered to patients who develop acute hydrocephalus. Current guidelines recommend placing an EVD in patients with hydrocephalus with a decreased level of consciousness (COR IIa, LOE B).[61] An EVD can assist in monitoring ICP and providing pressure relief in patients with hydrocephalus.

TABLE 15-8 Causes of Nonaneurysmal Subarachnoid Hemorrhage

Cause	Characteristics
Vascular malformation	Intracranial: arteriovenous malformations, dural arteriovenous fistula, cavernous malformation (occult to angiography), venous angioma (occult to angiography), capillary telangiectasias (occult to angiography), spinal dural arteriovenous fistula (cervical cord or at the cranio-cervical junction)
Intracranial dissection	Bleeding often devastating; high rebleeding risk of 40–60%.[83]
Cerebral venous sinus thrombus	Bleeding is usually superficial, confined to 1 area, and slow in presenting
Sickle cell disease	Mostly in children, low risk of rebleeding
Pituitary apoplexy	Presenting symptoms usually include visual loss and extraocular muscle movement dysfunction; thick subarachnoid blood may mask the underlying pituitary adenoma
Cerebral amyloid angiopathy	Bleeding usually localized to 1 area, superficial siderosis and microbleeds usually also visualized
Rare reported cases	Spinal aneurysms, moyamoya disease, tumor, RCVS, PRES, cerebral hyperperfusion syndrome after carotid endarterectomy

PRES = posterior reversible encephalopathy syndrome; RCVS = reversible cerebral vasoconstriction syndrome.

Complications

Acute

The risk of rebleeding is highest within the first 24 hours but remains elevated for the first month after SAH. The risk of rebleeding is 4% within the first 24 hours and approximately 1% per day for the next 30 days. Rebleeding is generally associated with a dismal outcome in mortality and functional outcomes in 3 months.[85] Independent predictors of bleeding were reported to be maximal aneurysm diameter, Hunt and Hess grade on admission, delayed obliteration of aneurysm, early external ventriculostomy placement, a higher initial BP on admission, and the presence of sentinel headaches. To avoid rebleeding, blood pressure is typically tightly controlled until an aneurysm is secured (obliterated) via coiling or clipping.[81] Thus, once a ruptured aneurysm is identified and the patient is medically stabilized, an aneurysm should be obliterated by surgical clipping or endovascular coiling as soon as possible to prevent rebleeding (COR I, LOE B).

Acute hydrocephalus occurs in 15% to 87% of SAH patients, 13.2% of which are usually symptomatic.[86] Clinical symptoms could entail deterioration in mental status (and coma), and in some miosis and impaired upward gaze. Approximately 8.9% to 48% of patients eventually become shunt dependent. Factors predictive of shunt dependence have not been reliably identified. However, a few studies have suggested that clipping rather than coiling aneurysms is associated with lower shunt dependence, although this was disputed in other studies.[87]

Subacute

Vasospasm resulting in delayed cerebral ischemia (DCI) was reported to occur in 12% to 30% of patients with aneurysmal SAH.[88] Delayed cerebral ischemia manifests with worsening mental status or focal neurologic deficit depending on the vessel involved and the degree of collaterals present. Vasospasm usually occurs within 4 to 14 days from the initial event, but earlier vasospasm has been reported in 10% of SAH patients and is predictive of infarctions, neurologic deterioration, and worse outcome at 3 months.[89] The risk of vasospasm increases with SAH proximal to major vessels and the circle of Willis, thick clot, and a higher value on the modified Fisher scale, which takes into account clot size, thickness, and intraventricular hemorrhage.[90]

Seizures have been reported in 6% to 18% of patients with SAH.[91] Factors predictive of seizures in SAH include a middle cerebral artery aneurysm, thick clot, rebleeding, infarctions, low Glasgow coma score, and patients treated with clipping rather than endovascular coiling.[81,84] Patients who develop nonconvulsive status epilepticus were found to have higher rates of morbidity; however, the impact of seizures on outcomes in patients with SAH has not been settled yet.[92] Although most physicians treat seizures prophylactically for a short term in SAH patients, no clinical evidence is present to dictate and support initiating prophylactic antiepileptics in SAH patients (COR IIb, LOE B).

Hyponatremia secondary to hypothalamic injury is a known complication following SAH. Hypothalamic injury results in release of natriuretic peptides and subsequent cerebral salt wasting syndrome. This mechanism eventually results in hyponatremia secondary to natriuresis.[93]

Several cardiac abnormalities have been reported in SAH patients, including ST segment depression, T wave inversion, U waves, and acute troponin leaks.[94] In addition, Takotsubo cardiomyopathy is frequently encountered in patients with SAH. Takotsubo cardiomyopathy often results in apical ballooning and is associated with transiently depressed ejection fraction, which causes poor cardiac outflow.

Other common complications of SAH include fever, pulmonary edema in up to 23% of patients, hepatic dysfunction in up to 24%, and thrombocytopenia.[95]

QUESTIONS

1. A 79-year-old right handed man with a history of hypertension and diabetes presents to emergency department (ED) with sudden onset right-sided hemiplegia and aphasia. His NIHSS is 17. After establishing a last known normal and a brief history, what is the best next step?

   A. Obtain a noncontrast CT of the head
   B. Administer IV tPA
   C. Obtain carotid ultrasound
   D. Perform mechanical thrombectomy

2. A 69-year-old man with a history of prior strokes and atrial fibrillation on coumadin presents with sudden onset lethargy and left hemiplegia. Noncontrast head CT reveals a large intraparenchymal hemorrhage. What is the next best step?

   A. Administer mannitol
   B. Obtain CT angiography
   C. Place external ventricular drain (EVD) for hydrocephalus
   D. Administer prothrombin complex concentrate

3. An 88-year-old man with a history of hypertension, hypercholesterolemia, s/p whipple procedure 5 years ago, diabetes presents to the emergency department with sudden onset of left sided hemiplegia. He regularly takes aspirin. Which of the following is true regarding tPA administration?

   A. tPA is contraindicated given aspirin use.
   B. tPA is contraindicated given the history of malignancy.
   C. tPA is contraindicated given the presentation beyond the time window.
   D. tPA is contraindicated given the history of surgical resection 5 years prior.

4. A 34-year-old man with a past medical history of an intracranial aneurysm that was incidentally discovered on imaging and is being closely managed with follow-up imaging presents to the emergency room after waking up with a sudden onset severe headache. A noncontrast head CT is unremarkable. Which of the following is the next best step?

   A. Perform an MRI of the head
   B. Perform vessel imaging of the head
   C. Discharge patient on migraine medications
   D. Perform a lumbar puncture

5. A 65-year-old woman with a history of diabetes who presents with sudden onset thunderclap headache and was found to have a Hunt and Hess grade 3 subarachnoid hemorrhage without intraventricular extension or hydrocephalus, and a 5-mm ruptured posterior communicating aneurysm is identified on imaging. What is the next best step?

   A. Perform an MRI of the brain
   B. Perform surgical clipping or endovascular coiling of the aneurysm
   C. Place an EVD
   D. Administer prothrombic complex concentrate

6. The modified Fisher scale is used to do predict which of the following?

   A. Risk of vasospasm
   B. Severity of SAH
   C. Mortality
   D. Neurologic outcome

7. A 75-year-old woman with atrial fibrillation on warfarin presents with new onset aphasia and right hemiparesis. Her caregiver states she was normal 2 hours prior at breakfast. She took warfarin the night prior. A head CT is performed as is unremarkable, and a CTA shows no proximal artery occlusion. What is the best next step in management?

   A. Administer IV tPA
   B. Obtain labs
   C. Administer aspirin
   D. Administer intra-arterial tPA

8. A 36-year-old man with no medical history presents with sudden onset left-sided weakness and headache while working out at the gym. He denies trauma and he takes no medications. His NIHSS is 8 for right-sided weakness and numbness. A noncontrast head CT reveals a moderate-sized right frontal hemorrhage. What is the next best step?

   A. Administer 1 unit of platelets
   B. Intubate stat for airway protection
   C. Obtain CTA
   D. Perform Permissive hypertension to 220/110 mmHg

9. A 56-year-old man with hypertension presents within 4 hours of new onset right-sided weakness. His NIHSS is 5 for pure hemiparesis. He takes no medications except for hydrochlorothiazide. A noncontrast CT of the head is unremarkable. Administration of IV tPA occurs 4 hours and 20 minutes after his last-known normal. Forty-five minutes later, he complains of headache, worsening weakness, and difficulty getting words out. What is the next best step?

   A. Repeat noncontrast head CT stat
   B. Administer prothrombic complex concentrate
   C. Intubate stat for airway protection
   D. Administer aspirin

10. A 62-year-old woman with no medical history presents with confusion and right-sided weakness. Her husband states that 20 minutes ago, she was normal when they were taking a walk and all of sudden, she collapsed. Her NIHSS is 18. A noncontrast head CT is unremarkable. Which of the following is the next best step?

    A. Obtain stat MR perfusion
    B. Begin IV tPA administration and obtain CT angiography for possible mechanical thrombectomy
    C. Obtain CT angiography for possible mechanical thrombectomy
    D. Administer IV tPA and, if no clinical improvement, obtain CT angiography for possible mechanical thrombectomy

ANSWERS

1. A. Obtain a noncontrast CT of the head

   The next step after establishing a brief history is obtaining a noncontrast CT of the head to evaluate for an acute hemorrhage or early signs of ischemic stroke. Administering IV tPA (choice B) without a noncontrast head CT is not indicated given the possibility of a hemorrhage. A carotid ultrasound (choice C) is sometimes performed to identify an underlying mechanism and should not be performed during the acute presentation. If the head CT is negative and the patient presented to the hospital within 4.5 hours of initiation of symptoms, IV tPA should still be given regardless of whether a patient is a candidate for mechanical thrombectomy (choice D). Intravenous tPA should not be delayed or deferred while deciding on whether to perform mechanical thrombectomy.

2. D. Administer prothrombin complex concentrate

   Reversal of an existing coagulopathy or an anticoagulation agent is the first step in management of patients presenting with an ICH after ensuring stability of airway, breathing, and circulation. Administering mannitol (choice A) can be considered if there is clinical or radiographic signs of impending herniation. An EVD (choice C) can be considered if there is evidence of hydrocephalus on imaging. A CT angiogram (choice B) can identify an underlying vascular malformation resulting in ICH but should not be a priority during the acute presentation.

3. C. tPA is contraindicated given the presentation beyond the time window.

   Intravenous tPA can only be delivered within 4.5 hours of the last known well time. All other listed options are not absolute contraindications (choices A, B, and D). Major abdominal surgery within the last 14 days is considered a relative contraindication; however, tPA is generally considered safe beyond that time period.

4. D. Perform a lumbar puncture

   Negative imaging with a CT or MRI does not definitively rule out the presence of SAH. The sensitivity of CT scans within the first 6 hours reaches 100% and deteriorates over the next few days, reaching 58% at 5 days. Guidelines generally recommend proceeding with an LP to rule out SAH if there is strong clinical suspicion despite negative imaging, as the presence of xanthochromia is highly sensitive and specific for SAH. The history of an aneurysm and thunderclap headache is highly suspicious of SAH, which should be investigated with a lumbar puncture. Discharging a patient maybe unsafe (choice C). Magnetic resonance imaging (choice A) and vessel imaging (choice B) might have the same diagnostic yield as a CT.

5. B. Perform surgical clipping or endovascular coiling of the aneurysm

   Following initial stabilization, surgical clipping or endovascular coiling is the most effective measure to prevent rebleeding in patients with aneurysmal SAH. An MRI (choice A) can be performed if the underlying cause is elusive; however, the identification of a ruptured aneurysm in this case obviates the need for further imaging. The patient is not on anticoagulation and thus reversal with prothrombic complex concentrate (choice D) would not be useful. An EVD is not yet needed in this case given the lack of hydrocephalus on imaging (choice C).

6. A. Risk of vasospasm

   The modified Fisher scale is based upon the amount of blood on noncontrast head CT. Both the thickness of the blood and the existence of intraventricular extension are considered in the modified Fisher scale. The modified Fisher scale is used to predict the risk of vasospasm after aneurysmal SAH. The Hunt and Hess scale is based upon clinical severity and predicts mortality (choices B and C).

7. B. Obtain labs

   The international normalized ratio must be checked prior to administration of IV tPA in a patient taking warfarin. The risk of intracranial hemorrhage is higher in patients with preexisting coagulopathy who receive IV tPA administration for acute ischemic stroke. The patient meets the 4.5-hour window to give tPA, which has been shown to improve functional outcomes, so choice C is wrong. Intravenous tPA is preferred over intra-arterial tPA if the patient meets the criteria.

8. C. Obtain CTA

   The patient presents with a nontraumatic intracerebral hemorrhage. As he takes no medications, no reversal agent is indicated. Given his young age and absence of obvious risk factors for intracerebral hemorrhage, a CTA should be performed to evaluate for an underlying vascular malformation. His blood pressure should be kept below 180 mmHg. Permissive hypertension (choice D) is allowed in acute ischemic stroke, but not in intracerebral hemorrhage. In the absence of obtundation or coma, the presence of ICH does not necessitate intubation (choice B). There is no mention of antiplatelet therapy or thrombocytopenia that might warrant transfusion with platelets (choice A).

9. A. Repeat noncontrast head CT stat

An acute change in neurologic status following administration of IV tPA is concerning for hemorrhagic conversion of the ischemic stroke and should be evaluated with an emergent noncontrast head CT. Reversal is not necessary unless a large active bleed is identified (choice B). Intubation for airway protection (choice C) should be performed if the mental status starts deteriorating. Aspirin (choice D) is recommended for secondary prevention and should not be administered within 24 hours of IV tPA administration, given the elevated risk of hemorrhage.

10. B. Begin IV tPA administration and obtain CT angiography for possible mechanical thrombectomy

The patient is a candidate for IV tPA given her clinical syndrome consistent with ischemic stroke and the fact that she presents less than 4.5 hours after her last known well time. Obtaining CT angiography (choice C) to evaluate for a possible thrombectomy should not delay IV tPA administration, and IV tPA administration does not remove the need for thrombectomy (choice D). In this case, IV tPA should be administered as a CTA is obtained to evaluate for mechanical thrombectomy. Ordering MR perfusion does not preclude the use of IV tPA (choice A).

REFERENCES

1. Kernan WN, Ovbiagele B, Black HR, et al. Guidelines for the prevention of stroke in patients with stroke and transient ischemic attack: a guideline for healthcare professionals from the American Heart Association/American Stroke Association. *Stroke.* 2014;45(7):2160-2236.

2. Mozzafarian D, Benjamin EJ, Go AS, et al., on behalf of the American Heart Association Statistics Committee and Stroke Statistics Subcommittee. Heart disease and stroke statistics— 2016 update: a report from the American Heart Association. *Circulation.* 2016;133(4):e38-e60.

3. Mozaffarian D, Benjamin EJ, Go AS, et al. Heart disease and stroke statistics—2015 update: a report from the American Heart Association. *Circulation.* 2015;131(4):e29-e32.

4. Krishnamurthi RV, Feigin VL, Forouzanfar MH, et al. Global and regional burden of first-ever ischaemic and haemorrhagic stroke during 1990-2010: findings from the Global Burden of Disease Study 2010. *Lancet Glob Health.* 2013;1(5):e259-e281.

5. Andersen KK, Olsen TS, Dehlendorff C, Kammersgaard LP. Hemorrhagic and ischemic strokes compared: stroke severity, mortality, and risk factors. *Stroke.* 2009;40(6):2068-2072.

6. Asplund K, Karvanen J, Giampaoli S, et al. Relative risks for stroke by age, sex, and population based on follow-up of 18 European populations in the MORGAM Project. *Stroke.* 2009;40(7):2319-2326.

7. Seshadri S, Beiser A, Kelly-Hayes M, et al. The lifetime risk of stroke: estimates from the Framingham Study. *Stroke.* 2006;37(2):345-350.

8. Howard VJ, Kleindorfer DO, Judd SE, et al. Disparities in stroke incidence contributing to disparities in stroke mortality. *Ann Neurol.* 2011;69(4):619-627.

9. Seshadri S, Beiser A, Pikula A, et al. Parental occurrence of stroke and risk of stroke in their children: the Framingham study. *Circulation.* 2010;121(11):1304-1312.

10. Janssen AW, de Leeuw FE, Janssen MC. Risk factors for ischemic stroke and transient ischemic attack in patients under age 50. *J Thromb Thrombolysis.* 2011;31(1):85-91.

11. Nencini P, Baruffi MC, Abbate R, et al. Lupus anticoagulant and anticardiolipin antibodies in young adults with cerebral ischemia. *Stroke.* 1992;23(2):189-193.

12. Kolominsky-Rabas PL, Weber M, Gefeller O, Neundoerfer B, Heuschmann PU. Epidemiology of ischemic stroke subtypes according to TOAST criteria: incidence, recurrence, and long-term survival in ischemic stroke subtypes: a population-based study. *Stroke.* 2001;32(12):2735-2740.

13. Smith WS, Lev MH, English JD, et al. Significance of large vessel intracranial occlusion causing acute ischemic stroke and TIA. *Stroke.* 2009;40(12):3834-3840.

14. Kamel H, Healey JS. Cardioembolic stroke. *Circ Res.* 2017; 120(3):514-526.

15. Putaala J, Metso AJ, Metso TM, et al. Analysis of 1008 consecutive patients aged 15 to 49 with first-ever ischemic stroke: the Helsinki young stroke registry. *Stroke.* 2009;40(4):1195-1203.

16. Fisher CM. Lacunar strokes and infarcts: a review. *Neurology.* 1982;32(8):871-876.

17. Southerland AM. Clinical evaluation of the patient with acute stroke. *Continuum (Minneap Minn).* 2017;23(1, Cerebrovascular Disease):40-61.

18. Caplan LR, Liebeskind DS. Chapter 2: Pathology, anatomy, and pathophysiology of stroke. In: Caplan LR. *Caplan's stroke: a clinical approach.* 5th edition. New York, NY; Cambridge: 2016: 19-54.

19. Brott T, Adams HP Jr, Olinger CP, et al. Measurements of acute cerebral infarction: a clinical examination scale. *Stroke.* 1989;20(7):864-870.

20. Albers GW, Lansberg MG, Norbash AM, et al. Yield of diffusion-weighted MRI for detection of potentially relevant findings in stroke patients. *Neurology.* 2000;54(8):1562-1567.

21. Hirai T, Korogi Y, Ono K, et al. Prospective evaluation of suspected stenoocclusive disease of the intracranial artery: combined MR angiography and CT angiography compared with digital subtraction angiography. *AJNR Am J Neuroradiol.* 2002;23(1):93-101.

22. Lansberg MG, Schrooten M, Bluhmki E, Thijs VN, Saver JL. Treatment time-specific number needed to treat estimates for tissue plasminogen activator therapy in acute stroke based on shifts over the entire range of the modified Rankin Scale. *Stroke.* 2009;40(6):2079-2084.

23. Hacke W, Kaste M, Bluhmki E, et al. Thrombolysis with alteplase 3 to 4.5 hours after acute ischemic stroke. *N Engl J Med*. 2008;359(13):1317-1329.

24. National Institute of Neurological Disorders, Stroke rt-PA Stroke Study Group. Tissue plasminogen activator for acute ischemic stroke. *N Engl J Med*. 1995;333(24):1581-1587.

25. Powers WJ et al. 2018 Gruidelines for the early management of patients with acute ischemic stroke: a guideline for heatlhcare professionals from the American Heart Association/American Stroke Association. *Stroke*. 2018;49(3):e46-e110.

26. Nogueira RG et al. Thrombectomy 6 to 24 hours after Stroke with a Mismatch between Deficit and Infarct. *N Engl J Med*. 2018;378(1):11-21.

27. Albers GW et al. Thrombectomy for Stroke at 6 to 12 hours with Selection by Perfusion Imaging. *N Engl J Med*. 2018;378(8):708-718.

28. Moulin DE, Lo R, Chiang J, Barnett HJ. Prognosis in middle cerebral artery occlusion. *Stroke*. 1985;16(2):282-284.

29. Vahedi K, Hofmeijer J, Juettler E, et al. Early decompressive surgery in malignant infarction of the middle cerebral artery: a pooled analysis of three randomised controlled trials. *Lancet Neurol*. 2007;6(3):215-222.

30. Juttler E, Unterberg A, Woitzik J, et al. Hemicraniectomy in older patients with extensive middle-cerebral-artery stroke. *N Engl J Med*. 2014;370(12):1091-1100.

31. Wijdicks EF, Sheth KN, Carter BS, et al. Recommendations for the management of cerebral and cerebellar infarction with swelling: a statement for healthcare professionals from the American Heart Association/American Stroke Association. *Stroke*. 2014;45(4):1222-1238.

32. Sanna T, Diener HC, Passman RS, et al. Cryptogenic stroke and underlying atrial fibrillation. *N Engl J Med*. 2014;370(26):2478-2486.

33. Gladstone DJ, Spring M, Dorian P, et al. Atrial fibrillation in patients with cryptogenic stroke. *N Engl J Med*. 2014;370(26):2467-2477.

34. The International Stroke Trial (IST): a randomised trial of aspirin, subcutaneous heparin, both, or neither among 19435 patients with acute ischaemic stroke. International Stroke Trial Collaborative Group. *Lancet*. 1997;349(9065):1569-1581.

35. Chimowitz MI, Lynn MJ, Derdeyn CP, et al. Stenting versus aggressive medical therapy for intracranial arterial stenosis. *N Engl J Med*. 2011;365(11):993-1003.

36. Zaidat OO, Fitzsimmons BF, Woodward BK, et al. Effect of a balloon-expandable intracranial stent vs medical therapy on risk of stroke in patients with symptomatic intracranial stenosis: the VISSIT randomized clinical trial. *JAMA*. 2015;313(12):1240-1248.

37. Wang Y, Wang Y, Zhao X, et al. Clopidogrel with aspirin in acute minor stroke or transient ischemic attack. *N Engl J Med*. 2013;369(1):11-19.

38. Abel N, Contino K, Jain N, et al. Eighth Joint National Committee (JNC-8) guidelines and the outpatient management of hypertension in the African-American population. *N Am J Med Sci*. 2015;7(10):438-445.

39. Group SR, Wright JT Jr, Williamson JD, et al. A randomized trial of intensive versus standard blood-pressure control. *N Engl J Med*. 2015;373(22):2103-2116.

40. Elkind MS, Sacco RL, MacArthur RB, et al. The neuroprotection with statin therapy for acute recovery trial (NeuSTART): an adaptive design phase I dose-escalation study of high-dose lovastatin in acute ischemic stroke. *Int J Stroke*. 2008;3(3):210-218.

41. Amarenco P, Bogousslavsky J, Callahan A 3rd, et al. High-dose atorvastatin after stroke or transient ischemic attack. *N Engl J Med*. 2006;355(6):549-559.

42. Kaplan RC, Tirschwell DL, Longstreth WT Jr, et al. Vascular events, mortality, and preventive therapy following ischemic stroke in the elderly. *Neurology*. 2005;65(6):835-842.

43. Shah RS, Cole JW. Smoking and stroke: the more you smoke the more you stroke. *Expert Rev Cardiovasc Ther*. 2010;8(7):917-932.

44. Friberg L, Rosenqvist M, Lindgren A, Terent A, Norrving B, Asplund K. High prevalence of atrial fibrillation among patients with ischemic stroke. *Stroke*. 2014;45(9):2599-2605.

45. Lip GY, Nieuwlaat R, Pisters R, Lane DA, Crijns HJ. Refining clinical risk stratification for predicting stroke and thrombo-embolism in atrial fibrillation using a novel risk factor-based approach: the euro heart survey on atrial fibrillation. *Chest*. 2010;137(2):263-272.

46. Hart RG, Pearce LA, Aguilar MI. Meta-analysis: antithrombotic therapy to prevent stroke in patients who have nonvalvular atrial fibrillation. *Ann Intern Med*. 2007;146(12):857-867.

47. North American Symptomatic Carotid Endarterectomy Trial Collaborators; Barnett HJM, Taylor DW, Haynes RB, et al. Beneficial effect of carotid endarterectomy in symptomatic patients with high-grade carotid stenosis. *N Engl J Med*. 1991;325(7):445-453.

48. Brott TG, Hobson RW 2nd, Howard G, et al. Stenting versus endarterectomy for treatment of carotid-artery stenosis. *N Engl J Med*. 2010;363(1):11-23.

49. Qureshi AI, Mendelow AD, Hanley DF. Intracerebral haemorrhage. *Lancet*. 2009;373(9675):1632-1644.

50. Sacco S, Marini C, Toni D, Olivieri L, Carolei A. Incidence and 10-year survival of intracerebral hemorrhage in a population-based registry. *Stroke*. 2009;40(2):394-399.

51. Venkatasubramanian C, Mlynash M, Finley-Caulfield A, et al. Natural history of perihematomal edema after intracerebral hemorrhage measured by serial magnetic resonance imaging. *Stroke*. 2011;42(1):73-80.

52. Lee KR, Kawai N, Kim S, Sagher O, Hoff JT. Mechanisms of edema formation after intracerebral hemorrhage: effects of thrombin on cerebral blood flow, blood-brain barrier permeability, and cell survival in a rat model. *J Neurosurg*. 1997;86(2):272-278.

53. Ohwaki K, Yano E, Nagashima H, Hirata M, Nakagomi T, Tamura A. Blood pressure management in acute intracerebral hemorrhage: relationship between elevated blood pressure and hematoma enlargement. *Stroke*. 2004;35(6):1364-1367.

54. Delgado Almandoz JE, Yoo AJ, Stone MJ, et al. The spot sign score in primary intracerebral hemorrhage identifies patients at highest risk of in-hospital mortality and poor outcome among survivors. *Stroke*. 2010;41(1):54-60.

55. Maas MB, Nemeth AJ, Rosenberg NF, Kosteva AR, Prabhakaran S, Naidech AM. Delayed intraventricular hemorrhage is common and worsens outcomes in intracerebral hemorrhage. *Neurology*. 2013;80(14):1295-1299.

56. Martini SR, Flaherty ML, Brown WM, et al. Risk factors for intracerebral hemorrhage differ according to hemorrhage location. *Neurology*. 2012;79(23):2275-2282.

57. Sturgeon JD, Folsom AR, Longstreth WT Jr, Shahar E, Rosamond WD, Cushman M. Risk factors for intracerebral hemorrhage in a pooled prospective study. *Stroke*. 2007;38(10):2718-2725.

58. Flibotte JJ, Hagan N, O'Donnell J, Greenberg SM, Rosand J. Warfarin, hematoma expansion, and outcome of intracerebral hemorrhage. *Neurology.* 2004;63(6):1059-1064.

59. Amin AP, Bachuwar A, Reid KJ, et al. Nuisance bleeding with prolonged dual antiplatelet therapy after acute myocardial infarction and its impact on health status. *J Am Coll Cardiol.* 2013;61(21):2130-2138.

60. Claassen J, Jette N, Chum F, et al. Electrographic seizures and periodic discharges after intracerebral hemorrhage. *Neurology.* 2007;69(13):1356-1365.

61. Hemphill JC 3rd, Greenberg SM, Anderson CS, et al. Guidelines for the management of spontaneous intracerebral hemorrhage: a guideline for healthcare professionals from the American Heart Association/American Stroke Association. *Stroke.* 2015;46(7):2032-2060.

62. Fiebach JB, Schellinger PD, Gass A, et al. Stroke magnetic resonance imaging is accurate in hyperacute intracerebral hemorrhage: a multicenter study on the validity of stroke imaging. *Stroke.* 2004;35(2):502-506.

63. Aguilar MI, Brott TG. Update in intracerebral hemorrhage. *Neurohospitalist.* 2011;1(3):148-159.

64. Greenberg SM, Rebeck GW, Vonsattel JP, Gomez-Isla T, Hyman BT. Apolipoprotein E epsilon 4 and cerebral hemorrhage associated with amyloid angiopathy. *Ann Neurol.* 1995;38(2):254-259.

65. O'Donnell HC, Rosand J, Knudsen KA, et al. Apolipoprotein E genotype and the risk of recurrent lobar intracerebral hemorrhage. *N Engl J Med.* 2000;342(4):240-245.

66. Syed YY. Idarucizumab: a review as a reversal agent for dabigatran. *Am J Cardiovasc Drugs.* 2016;16(4):297-304.

67. Baharoglu MI, Cordonnier C, Al-Shahi Salman R, et al. Platelet transfusion versus standard care after acute stroke due to spontaneous cerebral haemorrhage associated with antiplatelet therapy (PATCH): a randomised, open-label, phase 3 trial. *Lancet.* 2016;387(10038):2605-2613.

68. Kate MP, Hansen MB, Mouridsen K, et al. Blood pressure reduction does not reduce perihematoma oxygenation: a CT perfusion study. *J Cereb Blood Flow Metab.* 2014;34(1):81-86.

69. Anderson CS, Heeley E, Huang Y, et al. Rapid blood-pressure lowering in patients with acute intracerebral hemorrhage. *N Engl J Med.* 2013;368(25):2355-2365.

70. Qureshi AI, Palesch YY, Barsan WG, et al. Intensive blood-pressure lowering in patients with acute cerebral hemorrhage. *N Engl J Med.* 2016;375(11):1033-1043.

71. Mendelow AD, Gregson BA, Fernandes HM, et al. Early surgery versus initial conservative treatment in patients with spontaneous supratentorial intracerebral haematomas in the international surgical trial in intracerebral haemorrhage (STICH): a randomised trial. *Lancet.* 2005;365(9457):387-397.

72. Mendelow AD, Gregson BA, Mitchell PM, et al. Surgical trial in lobar intracerebral haemorrhage (STICH II) protocol. *Trials.* 2011;12:124.

73. Rinkel GJ, van Gijn J, Wijdicks EF. Subarachnoid hemorrhage without detectable aneurysm. A review of the causes. *Stroke.* 1993;24(9):1403-1409.

74. Hop JW, Rinkel GJ, Algra A, van Gijn J. Case-fatality rates and functional outcome after subarachnoid hemorrhage: a systematic review. *Stroke.* 1997;28(3):660-664.

75. Ingall T, Asplund K, Mahonen M, Bonita R. A multinational comparison of subarachnoid hemorrhage epidemiology in the WHO MONICA stroke study. *Stroke.* 2000;31(5):1054-1061.

76. Sandvei MS, Mathiesen EB, Vatten LJ, et al. Incidence and mortality of aneurysmal subarachnoid hemorrhage in two Norwegian cohorts, 1984-2007. *Neurology.* 2011;77(20):1833-1839.

77. International Study of Unruptured Intracranial Aneurysms Investigators. Unruptured intracranial aneurysms—risk of rupture and risks of surgical intervention. *N Engl J Med.* 1998;339(24):1725-1733.

78. McCarron MO, Alberts MJ, McCarron P. A systematic review of Terson's syndrome: frequency and prognosis after subarachnoid haemorrhage. *J Neurol Neurosurg Psychiatry.* 2004;75(3):491-493.

79. Hunt WE, Hess RM. Surgical risk as related to time of intervention in the repair of intracranial aneurysms. *J Neurosurg.* 1968;28(1):14-20.

80. Perry JJ, Stiell IG, Sivilotti ML, et al. Sensitivity of computed tomography performed within six hours of onset of headache for diagnosis of subarachnoid haemorrhage: prospective cohort study. *BMJ.* 2011;343:d4277.

81. Connolly ES Jr, Rabinstein AA, Carhuapoma JR, et al. Guidelines for the management of aneurysmal subarachnoid hemorrhage: a guideline for healthcare professionals from the American Heart Association/American Stroke Association. *Stroke.* 2012;43(6):1711-1737.

82. Lu L, Zhang LJ, Poon CS, et al. Digital subtraction CT angiography for detection of intracranial aneurysms: comparison with three-dimensional digital subtraction angiography. *Radiology.* 2012;262(2):605-612.

83. Santos-Franco JA, Zenteno M, Lee A. Dissecting aneurysms of the vertebrobasilar system. A comprehensive review on natural history and treatment options. *Neurosurg Rev.* 2008;31(2):131-140; discussion 140.

84. Molyneux AJ, Kerr RS, Yu LM, et al. International subarachnoid aneurysm trial (ISAT) of neurosurgical clipping versus endovascular coiling in 2143 patients with ruptured intracranial aneurysms: a randomised comparison of effects on survival, dependency, seizures, rebleeding, subgroups, and aneurysm occlusion. *Lancet.* 2005;366(9488):809-817.

85. Naidech AM, Janjua N, Kreiter KT, et al. Predictors and impact of aneurysm rebleeding after subarachnoid hemorrhage. *Arch Neurol.* 2005;62(3):410-416.

86. Graff-Radford NR, Godersky JC. Symptomatic congenital hydrocephalus in the elderly simulating normal pressure hydrocephalus. *Neurology.* 1989;39(12):1596-1600.

87. Mura J, Rojas-Zalazar D, Ruiz A, Vintimilla LC, Marengo JJ. Improved outcome in high-grade aneurysmal subarachnoid hemorrhage by enhancement of endogenous clearance of cisternal blood clots: a prospective study that demonstrates the role of lamina terminalis fenestration combined with modern microsurgical cisternal blood evacuation. *Minim Invasive Neurosurg.* 2007;50(6):355-362.

88. Kreiter KT, Mayer SA, Howard G, et al. Sample size estimates for clinical trials of vasospasm in subarachnoid hemorrhage. *Stroke.* 2009;40(7):2362-2367.

89. Baldwin ME, Macdonald RL, Huo D, et al. Early vasospasm on admission angiography in patients with aneurysmal subarachnoid hemorrhage is a predictor for in-hospital complications and poor outcome. *Stroke.* 2004;35(11):2506-2511.

90. Frontera JA, Rundek T, Schmidt JM, et al. Cerebrovascular reactivity and vasospasm after subarachnoid hemorrhage: a pilot study. *Neurology.* 2006;66(5):727-729.

91. Rhoney DH, Tipps LB, Murry KR, Basham MC, Michael DB, Coplin WM. Anticonvulsant prophylaxis and timing of seizures after aneurysmal subarachnoid hemorrhage. *Neurology.* 2000;55(2):258-265.

92. Little AS, Kerrigan JF, McDougall CG, et al. Nonconvulsive status epilepticus in patients suffering spontaneous subarachnoid hemorrhage. *J Neurosurg.* 2007;106(5):805-811.

93. Nakagawa I, Hironaka Y, Nishimura F, et al. Early inhibition of natriuresis suppresses symptomatic cerebral vasospasm in patients with aneurysmal subarachnoid hemorrhage. *Cerebrovasc Dis.* 2013;35(2):131-137.

94. Coghlan LA, Hindman BJ, Bayman EO, et al. Independent associations between electrocardiographic abnormalities and outcomes in patients with aneurysmal subarachnoid hemorrhage: findings from the intraoperative hypothermia aneurysm surgery trial. *Stroke.* 2009;40(2):412-418.

95. Solenski NJ, Haley EC Jr, Kassell NF, et al. Medical complications of aneurysmal subarachnoid hemorrhage: a report of the multicenter, cooperative aneurysm study. Participants of the multicenter cooperative aneurysm study. *Crit Care Med.* 1995;23(6):1007-1017.

Status Epilepticus

Margaret Huynh, DO, and Brandon Foreman, MD

INTRODUCTION

Acute seizures are common and are defined as a transient occurrence of signs and/or symptoms due to abnormal excessive or synchronous neuronal activity in the brain.[1] Intrinsically, the brain has mechanisms in place to terminate excessive electrical activity. The mean duration of a secondarily generalized tonic-clonic (GTC) seizure is 53 to 62 seconds, and rarely lasts longer than 2 minutes.[2,3] However, some seizures do not stop and progress to status epilepticus (SE), which may be convulsive (CSE), with clinically apparent motor (clonic) rhythmic jerking and/or (tonic) stiffening, or nonconvulsive (NCSE), with seizure activity on electroencephalography (EEG), and subtle or no obvious clinical signs. Status epilepticus is a neurological emergency often requiring management in the intensive care unit (ICU) for causes or complications of SE, or both.

DEFINITION AND CLASSIFICATIONS

In 2015, the International League Against Epilepsy (ILAE) proposed a conceptual definition that applies to all types of SE: (1) SE starts as a condition resulting from failure of seizure-termination mechanisms or the initiation of pathological mechanisms that likely lead to continuous seizure activity, and (2) SE creates long-term consequences that begin to occur after the onset of SE, including neuronal death, neuronal injury, and alteration of neuronal networks. This definition hinges on the identification of the *semiology* of SE: the clinical manifestations of seizure activity (Table 16-1). Specifically for generalized CSE, criterion 1 is defined when seizures last longer than 5 minutes and criterion 2 occurs at the point that long-term consequences begin to appear, around 30 minutes.[1] Convulsive SE is also defined as *recurrent* seizures between which there is incomplete recovery of consciousness.[4]

The point at which focal seizures or nonconvulsive seizures become SE (criterion 1) and create long-term consequences (criterion 2) is less clear. Current proposed definitions suggest that focal CSE *with impairment of consciousness* is defined at 10 minutes with long-term injury developing at greater than 60 minutes.[1] In contrast, the diagnosis of NCSE relies on EEG. The Salzburg criteria is a unified, validated set of rules to define NCSE on EEG with a diagnostic accuracy of 92.5%.[5-7] An NCSE is defined on EEG as epileptiform discharges at a periodicity of greater than 2.5 Hz, or

TABLE 16-1 Semiologic Classification of Status Epilepticus

With Prominent Motor Symptoms	Without Prominent Motor Symptoms

Convulsive (CSE)
• **Generalized**
 • **Clonic**
 • **Tonic**
 • **Tonic-clonic**
• **Focal (partial) onset ± secondary generalization**
 • **Repeated focal motor (Jacksonian)**
 • **Epilepsia partialis continua**
 • **Oculoclonic**
 • **Adversive**
 • **Ictal paresis**
• **Myoclonic**
 • **With coma**
 • **Without coma**
• **Tonic**
• **Hyperkinetic**
	Nonconvulsive SE (NCSE)
	• **NCSE with coma**
	• **NCSE without coma**
	 • **Generalized**: typical absence, atypical absence, myoclonic absence
	 • **Focal**
	  • Without impairment of consciousness (awake):
	   • Positive: aura, tactile sensory, visual, olfactory, gustatory, auditory, emotional (laughter, crying, agitation), psychosis, delusions, perseveration, echolalia
	   • Negative: mutism, anorexia, lethargy
	  • Aphasic (language impairment)
	   • With impaired consciousness: Subtle nystagmus or ocular movements, facial twitching, oral movements, confusion/amnesia, staring
	 • **Autonomic** (unknown whether focal or generalized phenomenon): episodic/paroxysmal desaturations, apnea, heart range and blood pressure changes, nausea/emesis

Adapted from Trinka E, Cock H, Hesdorffer D, et al. A definition and classification of status epilepticus—Report of the ILAE Task Force on Classification of Status Epilepticus. *Epilepsia*. 2015;56(10):1515-1523; and Jirsch J, Hirsch LJ. Nonconvulsive seizures: developing a rational approach to the diagnosis and management in the critically ill population. *Clin Neurophysiol*. 2007;118(8):1660-1670.

if discharges are slower, a clear evolution of the pattern over time or space, clinical or electrographic improvement with antiseizure drugs (ASDs), or subtle convulsive movements. The duration of time to fulfill criterion 1 is typically considered 10 minutes of continuous ictal activity or, for intermittent nonconvulsive seizures, more than 50% of a 1-hour EEG recording.[6]

BACKGROUND AND SIGNIFICANCE

Status epilepticus is associated with high mortality and morbidity and imposes a high financial burden on society. The annual incidence of SE is 10 to 41 per 100,000 people[8-13] and exhibits a U-shaped distribution across years of life, peaking both under 10 years of age and over 50 years of age.[14] The annual costs of SE are estimated to be $4 billion.[15] The overall mortality rate is approximately 20%.[14,16] Scoring systems have been devised to estimate outcome, including the Epidemiology-Based Mortality Score in Status Epilepticus and the Status Epilepticus Severity Score (STESS; Table 16-2).[17,18] The STESS is a validated scoring system,[19-22] with an overall sensitivity of 94% and a negative predictive value of 97%. It includes predictors of poor outcome, such as older age (> 65 years), impairment of consciousness, NCSE, and de novo onset of SE as underlying etiology. Other factors that have been reported to be associated with poor outcome include focal neurological signs, seizure duration, use of anesthetics for seizure control, injury severity scores such as the Acute Physiologic Assessment and Chronic Health Evaluation (APACHE), and other medical complications.[23-27]

Early diagnosis and urgent high-quality treatment are essential to reduce the morbidity and mortality associated with prolonged status epilepticus, and to maximize the efficacy of medication treatment.[28]

Status epilepticus itself is associated with multiple systemic complications (Table 16-3) and prognosis worsens

TABLE 16-2 Status Epilepticus Severity Score

Consciousness	Score
Alert or somnolent/confused	0
Stuporous or comatose	1
Seizure Type	
Simple partial, complex partial, absence, myoclonic	0
Generalized convulsive	1
Nonconvulsive status epilepticus	2
Age	
< 65 y	0
≥ 65 y	2
History of Seizures	
Yes	0
No	1

TABLE 16-3 Systemic Effects of Generalized Convulsive Status Epilepticus

Immediate/Early Status Epilepticus	Prolonged Status Epilepticus
Hypertension	Hypotension
Tachycardia	
Cardiac arrhythmias	Potential for cardiomyopathy (reversible left ventricular stunning)
Ischemia: troponin elevation, ischemic electrocardiography changes	
Hypoxia (due to apnea, upper airway obstruction, aspiration, mucous plugging)	Pulmonary edema
Acidosis (respiratory > metabolic) and lactic acidosis	Worsening acidosis
Hyperglycemia	Hypoglycemia
Hyperpyrexia	Worsening hyperpyrexia
Leukocytosis from demargination	Rhabdomyolysis with acute renal failure

with duration of time from seizure onset to treatment.[24,29-32] In humans, seizure activity lasting greater than 30 minutes is associated with significantly greater mortality than seizures lasting from 1 to 29 minutes (19% vs 2.6%).[24] Neuronal loss is observed after 40 minutes of seizure activity in animal models.[33] This early timeframe also affects treatment success as time-dependent pharmaco-resistance and self-perpetuation of SE occur after 15 to 30 minutes of seizure activity.[34] In fact, the duration of SE prior to treatment is one of the most important determinants of successful medical control of SE.[35] This is likely due to maladaptive changes that take place after sufficient stimulatory activity initiates SE. Within seconds to minutes, receptor trafficking, specifically internalization of synaptic γ-aminobutyric acid A ($GABA_A$) receptors and synaptic expression of N-methyl-D-aspartate (NMDA) and α-amino-3-hydroxy-5-methyl-4-isoxazolepropionic acid (AMPA) receptors occurs.[36-38] Further changes in inhibitory and excitatory neuropeptides occur within minutes to hours and later gene expression alteration maintains this abnormal electrical circuitry.[39] As SE proceeds and become self-sustaining, GABAergic drugs like benzodiazepines and barbiturates lose effectiveness in time- and dose-dependent manners, while NMDA antagonists are usually more effective even late in the course of status epilepticus.[40,41] In an animal model, diazepam readily stopped seizure when given 10 minutes after SE onset, while its potency decreased by 20 times when given 30 minutes after SE. Phenytoin (PHT) also showed a similar time-dependent relationship.[42,43] The pathophysiology also illustrates the importance of appropriate drug choice and dosing. Inadequate drug dosing and/or route of administration significantly contribute to ineffective termination of SE and even mortality.[44,45] Overall quality of treatment is crucial for SE control.

PRACTICAL MANAGEMENT CONCEPTS

Given the importance of timely and appropriate treatment and the high mortality associated with generalized CSE, guidelines propose algorithms for management. The most recent one, by the American Epilepsy Society proposes a 3-phase treatment: (1) a "stabilization phase" that should occur within 5 minutes of seizure onset and includes initial first aid and assessments; (2) an "initial therapy phase" that should occur in less than 20 minutes of onset and includes appropriate medical intervention; (3) a "second therapy phase" (20–40 minutes of seizure activity) when response to initial therapy should be apparent and a second-line agent should be administered, usually an intravenous (IV) formulation for rapid bioavailability; and (4) a "third therapy phase" (greater than 40 minutes of seizure activity), for which there is no clear guidance on treatment and includes either an anesthetic or another second-line therapy agent. The guideline also found strong evidence that the second therapy is often less effective than initial therapy.[46]

Such timelines serve as guidance. Throughout management, the provider should be astutely monitoring the patient, anticipating the next step, and ready to quickly treat seizures (ie, having medication readily available). Effective seizure termination by an antiseizure drug is usually defined as cessation of electrical and/or clinical seizure activity within 20 minutes from time of administration without recurrence within 60 minutes.[47]

Early Status Epilepticus: Primary Evaluation, Initial Management, and Therapy

The goals of initial SE management are to stop the seizures emergently, and to screen and treat for potentially life-threatening underlying causes of SE. These steps should take place quickly, whether in the prehospital, emergency department (ED), or ICU setting. As with any medical emergency, management begins by evaluating the patient's airway, breathing, circulation, and IV access. A brief neurological assessment should focus on the patient's mental status and any focal neurological deficits. Intubation for SE should be based on this clinical assessment. Laboratory studies should be sent concurrently, and a fingerstick glucose should be obtained (Table 16-4).

Benzodiazepines have Level A recommendation as first-line agent for SE.[4,46] An early in-hospital, randomized, double-blind control study compared lorazepam, diazepam plus

TABLE 16-4 Initial Diagnostic Workup for Status Epilepticus

Labs
Fingerstick glucose: *If glucose is low, administer thiamine 100 mg IV followed by 50 mL of D50*
Complete blood count with differential, comprehensive metabolic panel (including magnesium, calcium, phosphate, hepatic panel), antiseizure drug levels (if appropriate), blood gas, troponin, urinalysis, comprehensive toxicology screen (urine or blood), human chorionic gonadotropin (female of reproductive age), lactate

Imaging
Stat head CT without contrast, *as soon as patient is stabilized without clinical seizures*; may not be indicated in patients with a history of epilepsy with a clear precipitant for seizure exacerbation (ie, missed AED, systemic infection)
MRI brain with and without contrast, *in patients without a clear etiology or in whom EEG patterns lie on the ictal-interictal continuum*

Lumbar Puncture
If there is any concern for infectious or inflammatory process, lumbar puncture should be done following head imaging

AED = automated external defibrillator; CT = computed tomography; D50 = dextrose 50%; EEG = electroencephalography; IV, intravenous; MRI = magnetic resonance imaging.

phenytoin, phenytoin, and phenobarbital (PHB) as first-line treatment for status epilepticus and showed that lorazepam was superior.[47] Subsequently, 2 prehospital studies confirmed the role of benzodiazepine in the initial management of SE. In the first, lorazepam and diazepam aborted seizures in 59% and 42%, respectively, compared to 21% by placebo.[9] In the second, intramuscular (IM) midazolam aborted seizures in 73.4% compared to 63.4% in the intravenous lorazepam group; midazolam was faster and statistically noninferior.[48] Lorazepam is recommended IV at a dose of 2 mg for children and adults less than 40 kg or 4 mg for adults more than 40 kg.[48,49] Intravenous lorazepam and IV diazepam have no significant difference (Level of Evidence [LOE] A).[46] Intravenous diazepam can be administered at a dose of 0.2 to 0.3 mg/kg for children or adults less than 40 kg or 10 mg for adults more than 40 kg. If IV access is not available, IM midazolam is recommended over IV lorazepam (LOE A) as a 5-mg dose for children and adults less than 40 kg or 10 mg for adults more than 40 kg. Rectal diazepam 15 to 20 mg is an alternative if IM midazolam is not immediately available; it similarly reduces the risk of progression to established SE compared to placebo (risk ratio [RR], 0.43). Benzodiazepines are associated with hypotension and respiratory depression, leading to the underdosing of these critical medications. However, in 1 randomized controlled trial, administration of lorazepam 4 mg IV led to a *lower* rate of complications (eg, hypotension, cardiac arrhythmia, respiratory depression requiring bag-valve mask or attempt at intubation) compared to patients treated with placebo (10% vs 22%; LOE A).[9,46]

After seizures stop, further diagnostic studies may be indicated to identify the underlying etiology of the SE or its modifying factors. Up to two-thirds of SE identified in the ED occurs in patients with a history of epilepsy, and half have issues with their home medications.[50] Status epilepticus in patients who are hospitalized, on the other hand, usually results from an *acute symptomatic cause*, meaning that SE is provoked by either brain injury or a systemic illness occurring within 7 days of onset. Examples of acute symptomatic SE include stroke, traumatic brain injury, or hypoxic ischemic injury. Overall, acute symptomatic causes account for 48% to 63% of all hospitalized SE cases.[10,11,14] Although stroke is the most common cause of SE in the adult population, a growing proportion of SE is recognized as having an immune-mediated cause and manifestations may be subacute, or less clearly defined.[51]

Established Status Epilepticus: Starting a Second-Line Agent

Benzodiazepines fail to control SE in 35% to 45% of patients, which defines established SE.[47] If seizures persist or recur, a second-line agent should be administered immediately. Second-line ASDs are typically used to maintain seizure control if they are effective at terminating SE. Table 16-5 lists commonly used ASDs, including phenytoin/fosphenytoin (fPHT), valproic acid (VPA), levetiracetam (LEV), brivaracetam (BRV), lacosamide (LCS), and phenobarbital (PHB). Currently there is no high-quality data to support the use of 1 agent over another. Phenytoin/fPHT, VPA, and LEV are the most frequently used and recommended by

TABLE 16-5 Second-Line Antiseizure Medication

Phenytoin (PHT)/Fosphenytoin (fPHT)	
MOA:	Antagonist of voltage-gated sodium channel in the fast inactivated state
Loading dose:	PHT, 15–20 mg/kg at 50 mg/min; fPHT, 15–20 mg/kg IV at 150 mg/min, up to 1500 mg; obtain a postload drug level in 1 (PHT) or 2 (fPHT) h
Maintenance dose:	4–10 mg/kg/d in 2 divided doses per day
Therapeutic levels:	10–20 µg/mL total, 1–2 µg/mL free
Protein binding:	80–95%
*Approximate efficacy:	44–90%[24,54]
SE/monitoring:	Hypotension, arrhythmia, respiratory depression; IV PHT can cause subcutaneous and vessel injury with fast infusions ("purple glove syndrome") Monitor drug levels: Highly protein bound (correct total level for albumin, obtain free [active] level), zero-order kinetics (narrow therapeutic/toxic range) Contains propylene glycol and high phosphate load (caution in renal failure)
Drug Interactions:	Toxic levels can cause seizures, coma, death Decreases levels/effects of carbamazepine, lamotrigine, felbamate, oxcarbazepine Level/effect decreased by phenobarbital, carbamazepine Level/effect increased by valproic acid
Valproic Acid (VPA)	
MOA:	Voltage-gated sodium channel antagonist, T-type calcium channel antagonist, GABA agonist
Loading dose:	20–40 mg/kg IV bolus at 6 mg/kg/min, up to 3000 mg
Maintenance dose:	10–20 mg/kg every 6 h
Therapeutic levels:	50–125 µg/mL
Protein binding:	80–90%
*Approximate efficacy:	60–88%[24,54,55]
SE/monitoring:	Thrombocytopenia, increased bleeding risk (related to decreased platelet activation),[56] hepatotoxicity, hyperammonemia (related to beta-oxidation defect), pancreatitis; cardiac arrhythmias and hypotension are rare
Drug interactions:	Decreases levels/effects of oxcarbazepine Increases levels/effects of carbamazepine, barbiturates, ethosuximide, PHT, lamotrigine Level/effect decreased by carbamazepine, barbiturates, ethosuximide, PHT Level/effect increased by felbamate, topiramate Note: carbapenems, rifampin, and protease inhibitors decrease VPA concentrations; therefore, consider antiepileptic therapy modification
Levetiracetam (LEV)[57]	
MOA:	Related to synaptic vesicle protein 2A (SV2A) and effect on GABA, AMPA[58]
Loading dose:	30–60 mg/kg, 2000–4500 mg IV over 15 min
Maintenance dose:	1500–3000 mg divided every 12 h
Protein binding:	< 10%
*Approximate efficacy:	50–68%[59-61]
SE/monitoring:	Sedation, dizziness, agitation; low potential for interactions due to minimal hepatic metabolism and low plasma protein binding
Drug Interactions:	None

(Continued)

TABLE 16-5 Second-Line Antiseizure Medication (Continued)

Phenobarbital (PHB)	
MOA:	Agonist at the GABA$_A$ receptor, increasing Cl⁻ channel open time and burst duration; use-dependent sodium channel block
Loading dose:	20 mg/kg at 100 mg/min up to 700 mg
Maintenance dose:	1500–3000 mg divided every 12 h
Protein binding:	20–40%
*Approximate efficacy:	24–73.6%[47,61]
SE/monitoring:	Sedation, hypotension, respiratory depression, arrhythmias, propylene glycol toxicity
Drug interactions:	Similar to PHT/fPHT
Lacosamide (LCS)[62-64]	
MOA:	Selectively enhances slow inactivation of sodium channels
Loading dose:	200–400 mg IV < 5 min[65]
Maintenance dose:	200–800 mg divided every 12 h
Effectiveness:	~70%
SE/monitoring:	PR prolongation, arrhythmias, hepatotoxicity, confusion, vertigo, ataxia (SE dose dependent), angioedema reported[66]; some IV formulations include propylene glycol; therefore, monitor for potential toxicity
Drug interactions:	None
Brivaracetam (BRV)[67-69]	
MOA:	Highly selective and reversible SV2A ligand
Loading dose:	100 mg IV bolus as 2-min bolus or 15-min infusion
Maintenance dose:	25–1 mg PO or IV daily or BID
SE/monitoring:	Sinus bradycardia and first degree AVB higher in IV bolus, headache, somnolence, dizziness, and fatigue; low incidence of irritability (3%), injection/infusion site pain, rash
Drug interactions:	None

AMPA = α-amino-3-hydroxy-5-methyl-4-isoxazolepropionic acid; GABA = γ-aminobutyric acid; IV = intravenous; MOA = mechanism of action; SE = side effects

*Denotes effectiveness in obtaining seizure cessation within 20 minutes[61]

current guidelines.[4,46] The most recent American Epilepsy Society guidelines include the following: "There is no difference in efficacy between IV lorazepam followed by IV phenytoin, IV diazepam plus phenytoin followed by IV lorazepam, and IV phenobarbital followed by IV phenytoin (Level A). Intravenous valproic acid has similar efficacy to IV phenytoin or continuous IV diazepam as second therapy after failure of a benzodiazepine (Level C). Insufficient data exist in adults about the efficacy of levetiracetam as either initial or second therapy (Level U).[46] A single-center prospective randomized control pilot study of 150 patients compared PHT, VPA, and LEV following lorazepam and showed that the 3 agents are safe and equally effective, controlling seizures in 71% overall.[52] A multicenter randomized, controlled, blinded study comparing the effectiveness of fPHT, VPA, and LEV in established SE is currently being conducted.[53] Newer agents such as LCS and BRV will need to be compared in the future.

Phenytoin/Fosphenytoin

Historically, PHT has been used for SE since the 1960s.[70] Fosphenytoin, its water-soluble prodrug, can be administered at a faster rate and with fewer side effects (notably subcutaneous tissue injury and pain, and cardiovascular effects) than standard PHT, which is administered with propylene glycol. Fosphenytoin requires approximately 15 minutes to undergo conversion to its active form; therefore, the overall timing of efficacy is similar. As a general rule, sodium channel blockers such as PHT, carbamazepine, and oxcarbazepine are effective for focal seizures; however, they can *exacerbate* primarily generalized seizures. Despite this, fPHT is currently recommended over PHT as second-line ASD for established SE. In patients with a history of primary generalized epilepsy, VPA is preferred.[4]

Valproic Acid

Valproic acid, or valproate, is a safe and well-tolerated drug with a lower risk of cardiovascular side effects than PHT, even in unstable or elderly patients.[71,72] A randomized controlled study of 100 patients showed both VPA and PHT to be effective after diazepam failure in controlling SE (84% and 88%, respectively).[24] A meta-analysis and systematic review confirmed similar efficacy of VPA and PHT.[49,73] Valproic acid is oxidized in hepatic mitochondria in addition to being glucuronidated and metabolized by the cytochrome P450 system. Valproic acid should be avoided in patients with mitochondrial or hepatobiliary disease.

Levetiracetam/Brivaracetam

Levetiracetam is commonly used due to minimal protein binding, nearly 100% bioavailability, no known drug-drug interactions, and renal rather than hepatic metabolism. No significant cardiorespiratory side effects have been noted with IV loading doses up to 4000 mg.[57] In a small multicenter retrospective study of 40 patients, early treatment appeared to be more effective than late (78% vs 46%).[74] However, others have observed that LEV may be less effective at terminating SE than VPA or PHT.[59]

Brivaracetam, a recently approved medication similar to LEV, has a 20-fold higher affinity for the synaptic vesicle protein 2A (SV2A) ligand compared with LEV, and is now available in IV formulation.[75] Highly lipophilic, experimental data shows that it enters and acts faster in the brain than LEV.[69,76] Brivaracetam can be safely administered as 100 mg IV 2-min bolus or 15-minute infusion. Clinically insignificant electrocardiography (ECG) changes (sinus bradycardia, first degree AV block) have been observed with bolus therapy.[69] Brivaracetam is both hydrolyzed and metabolized by the cytochrome P450 system, and therefore, dosage adjustments are required for those with hepatic disease. Brivaracetam has not been studied in SE to date.

Lacosamide

Lacosamide is a novel agent that acts on sodium channels in a distinct way by enhancing their slow inactivation. Lacosamide is similar to LEV in its lack of drug-drug interactions and clinically relevant cardiopulmonary side effects using infusions of up to 400 mg under 5 minutes.[77] A dose-dependent prolongation in the PR interval on ECG and atrial arrhythmias has been reported.[64,78] Therefore, caution should be used in patients with preexisting arrhythmias, conduction block, or those on dromotropic agents. Lacosamide has not been systematically compared to fPHT, VPA, or LEV, although anecdotally its efficacy is similar.

Refractory Status Epilepticus

If a patient continues to have seizures despite a load of a second-line agent, SE is considered refractory (RSE). Most patients with *generalized* RSE require intubation,[79] and the use of sedatives and paralytics often used for induction masks ongoing motor activity. Importantly, almost *half* of those with clinical control of generalized SE exhibit seizures on EEG, suggesting electromechanical dissociation of SE that favors the development of NCSE in this context. Patients with generalized SE who do not stop seizing or those who remain comatose despite a second-line agent require continuous IV anesthetic (cIV) agents, such as midazolam, propofol, or pentobarbital (Table 16-6). In 2 systematic reviews, no treatment was found to be superior to another.[80,81] Continuous IV anesthetic dosing is titrated to cessation of electrographic seizures, or in some cases burst suppression, based largely on clinical preference. Generally, 24 to 48 hours of seizure control is recommended prior to cIV anesthetic weaning.[4]

New-onset refractory status epilepticus (NORSE) is a distinctive entity characterized by new, persistent seizures without a readily identifiable cause in otherwise healthy individuals. Recently, retrospective case series observed that although half of cases remain cryptogenic, the most frequent etiologies among those with a final diagnosis were autoimmune and paraneoplastic disorders (44/63 [70%]).[51] Patients with NORSE warrant cerebrospinal and serum autoimmune and paraneoplastic testing in many cases. Refractory SE may be refractory to second- and third-line therapies, and immunomodulatory therapy such as intravenous immunoglobulin or plasma exchange may be appropriate.

Semiology is crucial in determining an optimal approach to treating RSE. Although the use of cIV anesthetics and therapeutic coma is appropriate in generalized RSE and in some cases of NCSE with impaired consciousness, *careful consideration is required before using anesthetics to treat SE without an impairment in level of consciousness.* Therapeutic coma for RSE has been practiced historically, but is based on little evidence. In fact, data suggests that the use of cIV anesthetic for RSE and NORSE acts independently to *worsen* outcome.[51,84] A recent prospective study found that despite higher use in the United States compared to Europe (25% vs 9.75%), the use of therapeutic coma in RSE does not appear to affect mortality (15%) after controlling for demographics, SE severity, refractoriness, and comorbidities.[85] *In patients with focal SE or NCSE without impairment in level of consciousness, nonsedative ASDs should be maximized to avoid the potential morbidity associated with the use of therapeutic coma where possible.*[85]

In all cases of refractory status epilepticus—both CSE and NCSE—continuous monitoring of EEG is crucial to detect nonconvulsive seizures, which comprise the majority of seizures observed in these patients. Serial routine EEG (rEEG) may be used if needed in environments without continuous EEG (cEEG) monitoring capabilities; in the United States, transfer to regional centers with cEEG capabilities may be appropriate to adequately guide the need for and therapeutic success of cIV anesthetics.

INTRODUCTION TO ELECTROENCEPHALOGRAPHY

Electroencephalography is a tool that is used to observe cerebral activity. As a general rule, cEEG, versus routine EEG, is indicated in most ICU patients. In hospitalized patients, a single routine EEG misses around half of nonconvulsive seizures.[86] However, rEEG may be appropriate to screen for background abnormalities in a patient who has fully recovered to the baseline level of functioning. Background abnormalities that may indicate an increased risk for seizures include interictal epileptiform discharges, and clues to focal brain dysfunction (eg, prior stroke) may be observed as focal slowing. Routine EEG is most often performed in the outpatient setting.

Continuous EEG has become an invaluable tool for the diagnosis and management of seizures in the ICU and is broadly indicated, particularly in patients admitted to the ICU (Table 16-7). In a large cross-sectional sample of hospitalized patients, cEEG was associated with lower in-hospital mortality (odds ratio [OR], 0.63) without significant difference

TABLE 16-6 Third-Line Anti-Seizure Medication: Intravenous Anesthetics

Midazolam (MDZ)	
MOA:	GABA$_A$ receptor effect, increased permeability of chloride ions
Loading dose:	0.2 mg/kg IV at 2 mg/min
CI dose:	start at 0.2 mg/kg/h; 0.4 mg/kg/h more effective than low dose 0.2 mg/kg/h[82]
Titration/breakthrough:	0.1–0.2 mg/kg bolus, increase CI rate by 0.05–0.1 mg/kg/h every 3–4 h
SE/monitoring:	Respiratory depression, hypotension
Metabolism/excretion:	Renal
Note:	Lowest rate of withdrawal seizures and therapy failure due to SE (< 1%) compared to barbiturate and propofol; also the lowest mortality rate, at 2%[81]
Propofol (PRO)	
MOA:	GABA$_A$, NMDA-antagonist
Loading dose:	1–2 mg/kg
CI dose:	start at 20 µg/kg/min
CI range:	30–200 µg/kg/min
Titration/breakthrough:	increase rate by 5–10 µg/kg/min every 5 min or 1 mg/k bolus plus titration
*Success rate:	68%
SE/monitoring:	Hypotension, propofol infusion syndrome (PIS): arrhythmias, metabolic acidosis, rhabdomyolysis, hypertriglyceridemia, renal failure, adjust daily caloric intake
Notes:	Prolonged use of large doses associated with significant morbidity and mortality; higher risk of PIS in children and with comedication with steroids; higher risk > 48 h on infusion; contraindicated in young children
Metabolism:	hepatic
Pentobarbital (PTB)	
MOA:	GABA$_A$ agonist
Loading dose:	5–15 mg/kg at rate of 50 mg/min
CI initial dose:	0.5–5 mg/kg
Maintenance:	0.5–5 mg/kg/h
Titration/breakthrough:	Bolus 5 mg/kg, increase CI rate by 0.5–1 mg/kg/h every 12 h
*Success rate:	64%
SE/monitoring:	Hypotension, paralytic ileus, hepatic and pancreatic toxicity, immunosuppression, propylene glycol toxicity, lingual edema; long half-life
Note:	PTB has lower frequency of short-term treatment failure, breakthrough seizures, and change to a different cIV compared to MDZ or PRO, but higher frequency of hypotension[80]; higher death during therapy in PTB/THP group in systematic review but usually used after PRO/MDZ failed[81]
Ketamine	
MOA:	NMDA receptor antagonist
Dose:	Range used 0.06–7.5 mg/kg/h
Success rate:	82%*, 64%[83]
SE/monitoring:	no side effects observed in a retrospective study of 42 patients[83]
Notes:	Not typically used as third-line; used in super-refractory SE, usually as adjunct; only case reports and retrospective studies

CI = continuous infusion; GABA = γ-aminobutyric acid; MOA = mechanism of action; NMDA = N-methyl-D-aspartate; SE = side effects; VG = voltage gated

*Defined by completely controlled SE without breakthrough or withdrawal seizures, or discontinuation due to side effects, or death during the therapy based on a systematic review[81]

in hospitalization duration and costs compared to the use of routine (~ 45-minute) EEG in mechanically-ventilated ICU patients.[87] Continuous EEG is useful for monitoring the effect of antiseizure medication regimen (medication choice, dose adjustments) and titration and weaning of cIV anesthetics used to treat RSE. In fact, a retrospective study of 287 patients found that cEEG monitoring led to ASD changes in 52% of patients.[88] Another important utility is screening for or treating nonconvulsive seizures (eg, in patients who have known or history of nonconvulsive seizures or clinical seizure without return to baseline, who have stereotyped subtle clinical events, who are comatose or have depressed level of consciousness, or who have a neurologic or medical condition that places the patient at high risk for nonconvulsive seizures [Table 16-7].

In the largest retrospective series of hospitalized patients undergoing cEEG, 27% had nonconvulsive seizures. Of those, only 58% manifested their first seizure within 30 minutes of cEEG monitoring.[94] In patients who are not comatose, the sensitivity of cEEG to detect nonconvulsive seizures reaches 90% within 24 hours; in those who are comatose, the sensitivity is 88% at 48 hours.[90] For patients in whom the initial 2 hours of recording lacks epileptiform abnormalities, the probability of developing nonconvulsive seizures within 72 hours falls below 5%.[94] This can be useful when resources are limited or for patients in whom ongoing seizures should be ruled out prior to further care, as in the case of patients who present with seizures due to an aneurysmal subarachnoid hemorrhage undergoing urgent operative intervention.

TABLE 16-7 Indications for Continuous Electroencephalography

Indication/Setting	Rationale
Recent clinical seizure without return to baseline	**Convulsive seizures/SE can transition to nonconvulsive seizures/ NCSE after treatment in 20–48%.**[47,89]
Screening for NCSz or NCSE in at-risk patients: • History of epilepsy, acute brain injury (SAH, TBI, ICH), brain tumor, recent CSE, fluctuating mental status, and paroxysmal events that are concerning for seizures, comatose patient, anoxic, ICU patient	NCSz/NCSE are prevalent in the critically ill and need EEG to detect. • In 570 patients, seizures occurred in 19% of altered patients placed on cEEG; almost all of the seizures were nonconvulsive (92%).[90] • In surgical and medical ICUs, approximately 10% of encephalopathic and comatose patients placed on cEEG have NCSE.[91,92] • In the neuroscience ICU, as many as one-third of patients have NCSE.[93]
Monitoring and treatment of known nonconvulsive seizures	**Characterization and quantification of events to adjust treatment**
Abnormal routine EEG • Epileptiform discharges or periodic discharges	Higher risk of seizures
Loss of reliable exam in setting of clinical concerns above (eg, comatose, anoxic) • Patient on continuous anesthetic infusion (eg, for refractory SE) • Paralytic	Electro-clinical dissociation; EEG will be the primary mean to detect seizures

cEEG = continuous EEG; CSE, continuous status epilepticus; EEG = electroencephalography; ICH = intracerebral hemorrhage; ICU = intensive care unit; NCSE = nonconvulsive status epilepticus; NCSz = nonconvulsive seizures; SAH = subarachnoid hemorrhage; SE = status epilepticus; TBI = traumatic brain injury.

How Continuous Electroencephalography Is Interpreted

Raw EEG refers to the display of real-time waveforms arranged topographically on the screen (Fig. 16-1). A typical display is arranged in a bipolar montage, meaning that each electrode is recorded in reference to a nearby electrode. Electrodes are named per their location (eg, F represents frontal, C is central); even numbers are located on the right side of the head, while odd numbers are on the left. Technologists are trained to arrange electrodes on the scalp in the same way by following the International 10-20 System of measurement using increments of 10 cm and 20 cm based on common skull-based landmarks.

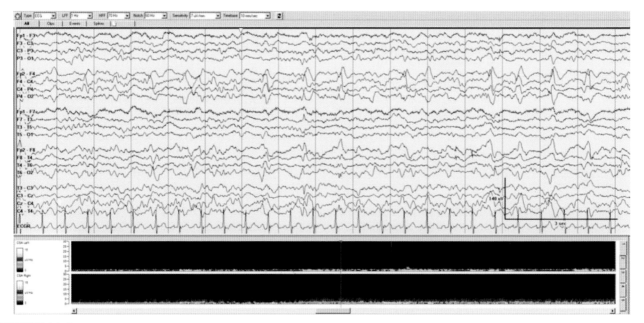

FIGURE 16-1 A representative continuous electroencephalography (cEEG) screen. On the top of the screen are standard filters used to clean the EEG for review and remove frequencies that are not typically used for interpreting clinical cEEG. The channel definitions are listed on the left side of the screen. Letters denote location (eg, F for frontal, C for central, P for parietal, O for occipital) and the numbers denote the hemisphere, with even numbers representing the right side and odd numbers representing the left. On the bottom of the screen are 2 panels representing quantitative EEG—the compressed spectral array (CSA). The top bar represents the left hemisphere and the bottom represents the right hemisphere. The y-axis represents frequency, and the power at each frequency is represented by color. The raw EEG is displaying 16 seconds of EEG with a 1-Hz lateralized periodic discharge pattern seen maximally in the right frontal region. The CSA is demonstrating 6 hours of EEG with an increase in the color over the right hemisphere representative of increased EEG power in the lower frequency range.

Quantitative EEG employs mathematical algorithms to create a numerical representation of this raw EEG, most commonly by displaying the power of each frequency in the raw EEG waveform across time, called the compressed spectral array, seen in Figure 16-1 at the bottom of the screen. Other measures commonly used include suppression ratios and asymmetry indices, which may be displayed on additional screens. Both raw and quantitative EEG may be available for review at bedside and remotely.

Raw cEEG data is ultimately interpreted by a skilled electroencephalographer with specialty training, and a detailed guide to EEG interpretation is beyond the scope of this brief chapter.

A provider in the ICU should know basic EEG terminologies and concepts (Table 16-8). A normal person generates an alpha posterior dominant rhythm and cycles through states of wakefulness, drowsiness (theta and delta), and sleep (theta and delta; sleep architecture: vertex and spindle waves, which are not shown). Encephalopathy typically refers to reversible change in brain function that manifests clinically as attentional impairment, sleep-wake cycle disturbances, deficits in memory and data processing, and changes in arousal. EEG monitoring can confirm generalized or focal cerebral dysfunction and provide a relative degree of dysfunction. However, it is not specific, and clinical correlation is important in its application.

TABLE 16-8 Commonly Encountered Electroencephalography Patterns

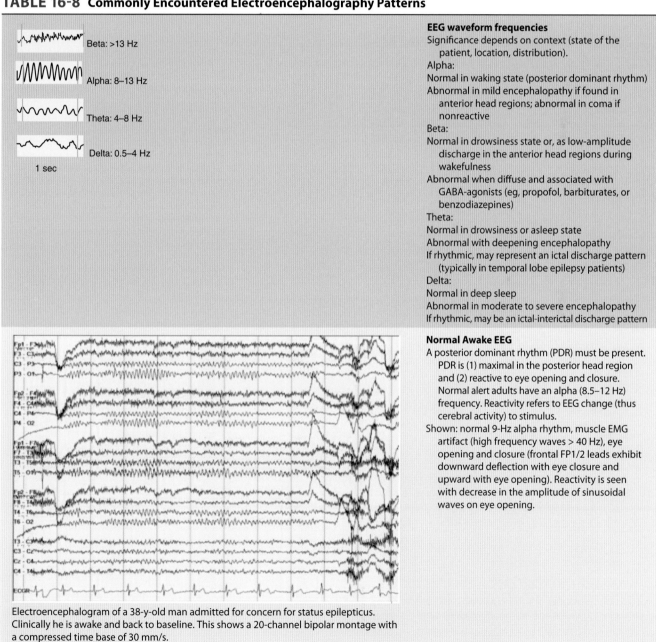

Beta: >13 Hz

Alpha: 8–13 Hz

Theta: 4–8 Hz

Delta: 0.5–4 Hz

1 sec

EEG waveform frequencies

Significance depends on context (state of the patient, location, distribution).

Alpha:

Normal in waking state (posterior dominant rhythm)

Abnormal in mild encephalopathy if found in anterior head regions; abnormal in coma if nonreactive

Beta:

Normal in drowsiness state or, as low-amplitude discharge in the anterior head regions during wakefulness

Abnormal when diffuse and associated with GABA-agonists (eg, propofol, barbiturates, or benzodiazepines)

Theta:

Normal in drowsiness or asleep state

Abnormal with deepening encephalopathy

If rhythmic, may represent an ictal discharge pattern (typically in temporal lobe epilepsy patients)

Delta:

Normal in deep sleep

Abnormal in moderate to severe encephalopathy

If rhythmic, may be an ictal-interictal discharge pattern

Normal Awake EEG

A posterior dominant rhythm (PDR) must be present. PDR is (1) maximal in the posterior head region and (2) reactive to eye opening and closure. Normal alert adults have an alpha (8.5–12 Hz) frequency. Reactivity refers to EEG change (thus cerebral activity) to stimulus.

Shown: normal 9-Hz alpha rhythm, muscle EMG artifact (high frequency waves > 40 Hz), eye opening and closure (frontal FP1/2 leads exhibit downward deflection with eye closure and upward with eye opening). Reactivity is seen with decrease in the amplitude of sinusoidal waves on eye opening.

Electroencephalogram of a 38-y-old man admitted for concern for status epilepticus. Clinically he is awake and back to baseline. This shows a 20-channel bipolar montage with a compressed time base of 30 mm/s.

(Continued)

TABLE 16-8 Commonly Encountered Electroencephalography Patterns (Continued)

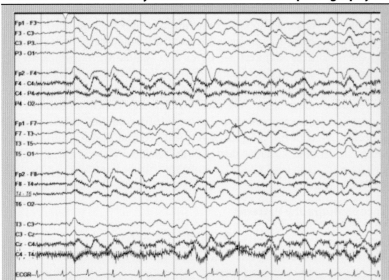

Electroencephalogram of a 71-y-old woman with end-stage renal disease who is awake but encephalopathic. This shows a 20-channel bipolar montage with a compressed time base of 30 mm/s.

Frontal Intermittent Delta Activity (FIRDA)

A transient rhythmic slow wave pattern over anterior EEG leads, FIRDA, has a nonspecific pattern that is associated with structural brain lesions as well as toxic, infectious, and metabolic disorders (anemia, electrolyte imbalance, hyperglycemia, hepatic dysfunction, renal dysfunction).

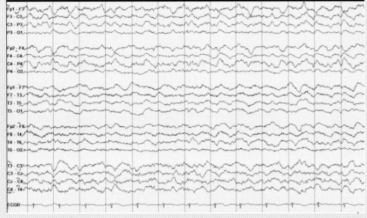

Electroencephalogram of a 45-y-old man with NSTEMI placed on ECMO who is comatose. This shows a 20-channel bipolar montage with a compressed time base of 30 mm/s.

Moderate to Severe Diffuse Slowing

Shown is majority of a recording comprising delta activity, thus generalized slowing. In a comatose or encephalopathic patient, this is a sign of generalized cerebral dysfunction. In a normal person, this could represent drowsiness/sleep. Generalized slowing is a nonspecific finding consistent with a generalized disturbance such as toxic, metabolic, or structural abnormalities that are multifocal or diffuse.

If focal slowing is observed, the finding is consistent with a focal disturbance of cerebral function, and an underlying structural lesion should be considered.

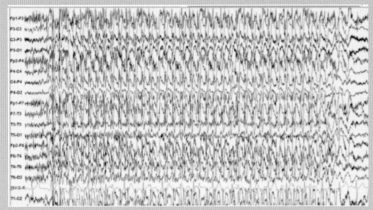

Electroencephalogram of a 19-y-old woman with spells of unresponsiveness who is otherwise awake and normal. This shows a 20-channel bipolar montage with a compressed time base of 30 mm/s.

Generalized Seizure

This EEG shows onset of spike and wave discharges in all EEG leads. It can be primary generalized or secondarily generalized. If it is convulsive, the recording would be contaminated by significant EMG muscle artifact.

(Continued)

TABLE 16-8 Commonly Encountered Electroencephalography Patterns (Continued)

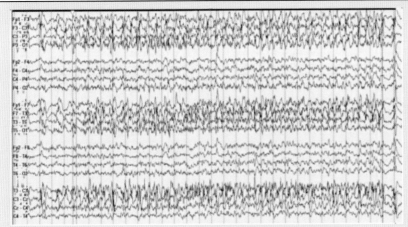

Electroencephalogram of a 67-y-old man with large left parietal intracerebral hemorrhage. This shows a 20-channel bipolar montage with a compressed time base of 15 mm/s.

Focal Seizure

This EEG shows an ictal onset in 1 region with spread in neighbor regions (shown as spread to nearby leads).

Shown are left hemisphere epileptiform discharges initially. Then, note at the left parietal (P3) region, the epileptiform abruptly changes in morphology (sharp and spike waves), and increases in frequency and amplitude. There is a clear abrupt end. This seizure lasts 25 s.

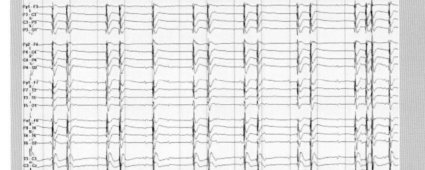

Electroencephalogram of a 64-y-old man status post PEA arrest who is comatose. This shows a 20-channel bipolar montage with a compressed time base of 30 mm/s.

Generalized Periodic Discharges (GPD)

This EEG shows spike and wave discharges that occur in regular intervals (here, every 1 second). Generalized periodic discharges are nonspecific and commonly encountered in metabolic encephalopathies and cerebral hypoxia. Prognostic and clinical significance of GPDs are unclear. It is controversial whether this pattern by itself is ictal and whether treatment would change outcome. However, this pattern is associated with occurrence of seizures.

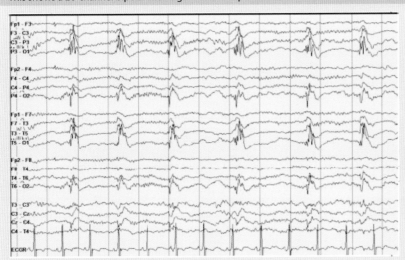

Electroencephalogram of a 40-y-old woman with status epilepticus with left parieto-occipital pachymeningitis. The patient is awake but Confused. This shows a 20-channel bipolar montage with a compressed time base of 30 mm/s.

Lateralized Periodic Discharges (LPD)

This EEG shows focal regional discharges that occur in regular intervals (here, sharp and wave discharges, predominantly left occipital with some right occipital spread occurring at about 1.5 Hz). This is a finding associated with structural (eg, stroke, hemorrhage, tumor), infectious, epileptic, and/or metabolic processes involving the cerebral hemisphere in which they occur. They are typically seen in the setting of an acute insult and are highly associated with seizures and status epilepticus.

(Continued)

TABLE 16-8 Commonly Encountered Electroencephalography Patterns (Continued)

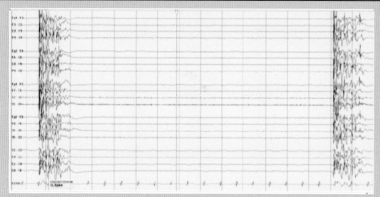

Electroencephalogram of a man of unknown age involved in a car accident with ROSC after cardiac arrest. This shows a 20-channel bipolar montage with a compressed time base of 30 mm/s.

Burst Suppression

This EEG has more than 50% of the record consisting of attenuation or suppression and intermixed with bursts of cerebral activity (here, a burst of generalized sharp discharges lasting 90 s on a suppressed background). Burst suppression is consistent with a process that has diffusely affected the cerebrum, including toxic, metabolic, and posthypoxic processes as well as diffuse structural abnormalities. The bursts of activity may be epileptiform, as in this case, or nonepileptiform.

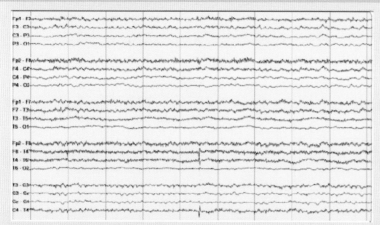

Encephalogram of a 26-y-old man who presented with self-hanging and PEA arrest and suffered hypoxic-ischemic encephaolopathy. This shows a 20-channel bipolar montage with a compressed time base of 30 mm/s.

Alpha or Theta Coma

This EEG shows a monotonous, frontally accentuated alpha and/or theta rhythm that lacks variability in a comatose patient. Etiologies include infection, toxic-metabolic encephalopathies, brainstem lesions, and hypoxic-ischemic encephalopathy. If not reactive, this sign predicts poor outcome.

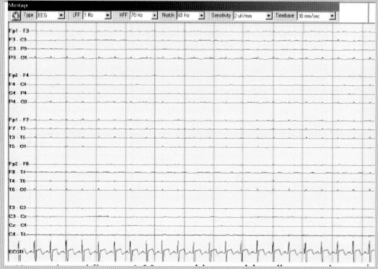

Electroencephalogram of a 29-y-old man with epilepsy and polysubstance abuse with 40 min of PEA arrest. This shows a 20-channel bipolar montage with a compressed time base of 30 mm/s.

Electro-cerebral Inactivity

This EEG shows no spontaneous cerebral activity at high sensitivity. Marked hypothermia, severe intoxication, hypoxic-ischemic encephalopathy can manifest as such. A specific EEG technique and criteria must be fulfilled to use as a sign of brain death. The EEG cannot be used alone to diagnose brain death, which is a clinical diagnosis.

Here, there is no EEG activity at 2 μV sensitivity except for ECG artifact (EEG spikes time-marked with ECG discharges).

EEG technical parameters for brain death:
- complete complement of electrodes
- electrode pairs at least 10 cm apart
- Interelectrode impedances < 10,000 Ohms but over 100 Ohms
- integrity of the entire recording system tested
- sensitivity 2 μV/mm for at least 30 min
- low-pass filter > 30 Hz, high-pass filter < 1 Hz
- no EEG reactivity
- only a qualified technologist can perform

ECG = electrocardiography; ECMO = extracorporeal membrane oxygenation; EEG = electroencephalogram; EMG = electromyography; GABA = γ-aminobutyric acid; NSTEMI = non-ST-elevation myocardial infarction; PEA = pulseless electrical activity

TABLE 16-9 Electroencephalographic Pattern Characterization and Descriptors

Location (Main Term 1)	Pattern Name (Main Term 2)	Seizure-like (Plus[a]) Features	Morphology	Temporal	Modulation	Response to Intervention
Generalized (G) Lateralized (L) Bilateral Independent (BI) Multifocal (Mf)	Periodic discharges (PD) Rhythmic delta activity (RDA) Spike-and-wave or sharp-and-wave (SW)	+F: superimposed fast (PD or RDA) +R: superimposed rhythmic delta (PD) +S: superimposed sharp or spikes	Sharpness Number of phases Amplitude Polarity	Prevalence Frequency Duration Onset: sudden vs gradual Dynamics: evolving, fluctuating, static	Stimulus-induced vs Spontaneous	Yes/No

[a]Plus features indicates a superimposed pattern suggestive to be more seizure-like; they apply to PD or RDA only. Refer to Hirsch et al[95] for further reading and examples.

For example, focal dysfunction is more concerning for an underlying structural etiology. Generalized dysfunction and certain patterns are usually consistent with a more global issue (such as from toxic, metabolic, or infectious etiologies).

Although the interpretation of raw cEEG is often regarded as subjective, the American Clinical Neurophysiology Society (ACNS) has produced a standard nomenclature aimed at defining terminology frequently encountered in hospital-based cEEG.[95] The standardization of cEEG terminology provides a framework for understanding patterns frequently encountered in the ICU and facilitates communication with reading electroencephalographers. Further, the use of quantitative EEG provides a method to review larger volumes of cEEG visually, with evidence to suggest that review time can be reduced substantially while preserving reasonable sensitivity for detecting seizures.[96,97] Educational materials are provided by the ACNS (available at https://www.acns.org/practice/guidelines#continuous_eeg_monitoring). Table 16-9 lists commonly used terminology.[1,95]

CONTROVERSIAL TOPICS

Management of Non-convulsive Status Epilepticus

The majority of seizures observed in the ICU setting are nonconvulsive. Often, there is uncertainty about the impact of NCSE on outcome, as much of the morbidity and mortality in these patients is associated with the underlying etiology.[98] Mortality overall is significantly higher in NCSE compared with CSE in 1 randomized, controlled trial of SE management (65% vs 27%).[47] The duration of NCSE contributes to mortality according to a retrospective study of 49 patients with NCSE that demonstrated that cases treated and resolved within 10 hours had 10% versus 85% mortality if seizures continued longer than 20 hours.[99] Moreover, NCSE is common in acute brain injury and is associated with secondary injury and adverse physiologic effects (Table 16-10). These findings argue for urgent treatment, but some have suggested that, in contrast to the prehospital data for generalized CSE, aggressive treatment with benzodiazepines specifically in elderly hospitalized patients with nonconvulsive seizures may not improve outcome and in fact may prolong hospital stay.[100]

Ultimately, treatment decisions may hinge on etiology. A decision analysis was performed and described a risk-benefit ratio in favor of nonaggressive treatment in cases of NCSE associated with a history of epilepsy and in favor of aggressive (eg, cIV anesthetic) treatment in cases of NCSE associated with intracerebral hemorrhage, where the risk of worsening the underlying brain injury outweighed the risks of therapeutic coma. In postanoxic SE, which exhibits an intrinsically high mortality, outcomes were poor regardless of the treatment chosen in this model.[114] Discussion between the patient's surrogate decision maker(s) and other members

TABLE 16-10 Effects of Nonconvulsive Status Epilepticus After Acute Brain Injury

Population and Incidence of NCSz/NCSE	Effects
Subarachnoid hemorrhage, 3–13%[101,102]	• NCSz associated with inflammation and poor outcome[103] • Depth EEG (cortical) seizures accompanied by elevated heart rate, blood pressure, and respiratory rates[104]
Traumatic brain injury, 22%[105]	• Increase in neuroexcitatory extracellular glutamate[105] • Increased episodic and mean intracranial pressure (22 mmHg vs 13 mmHg in episodic and 18 mmHg vs 12 mmHg overall, compared to without seizure)[106] • Metabolic crisis: increased lactate/pyruvate[106,107] • Hippocampal atrophy (21% vs 12% compared to without seizure)[108] • Elevations in glycerol, presumably because of cell membrane breakdown[109]
Intracerebral hemorrhage, 18–28%[110,111]	• Increased midline shift[111] • Expansion of hematoma[110]
Acute ischemic stroke, 3.6%[112]	• Three-fold increase in mortality associated with SE after stroke compared with isolated stroke or SE alone[113]

EEG = electroencephalography; NCSE, nonconvulsive status epilepticus; NCSz = nonconvulsive seizures; SE = status epilepticus.

of the treatment team are warranted before making decisions regarding aggressive care where there is equipoise regarding the need for third-line agents beyond conventional ASDs.

Management of the Ictal-Interictal Continuum

The ictal-interictal continuum (IIC) encompasses periodic or rhythmic EEG patterns described in Table 16-9 that do *not* fulfil Salzburg criteria for electrographic seizures and SE. These patterns are frequently associated with seizures, and in certain cases, represent seizure activity (ie, are "ictal") despite their appearance. When these patterns are encountered, further information is required. First, these patterns may be treated as seizures if evidence exists that they are creating neuronal injury. Diagnostic tests that can point to neuronal injury in patients with IIC patterns include fluorodeoxyglucose-positron emission tomography (FDG-PET),[115] magnetic resonance imaging (MRI) diffusion-weighted imaging, perfusion imaging (NM single-photon emission computed tomography),[116-118] or serum tests such as neuron-specific enolase.[119] Second, a potentially ictal pattern may be clarified by the use of a trial of antiseizure drug therapy (Trial of Org 10172 in Acute Stroke Treatment or TOAST; Fig. 16-2).[5] One retrospective case series applied this paradigm to patients with generalized periodic discharges with triphasic morphology, a pattern that is often difficult to interpret, and found that a TOAST resulted in a 42% response rate.[120] There is no unifying guideline that exists on the management of ictal-interictal patterns;

however, if there is evidence of neuronal injury or if a TOAST exhibits a positive response, consideration of the pattern as NCSE is reasonable.

SUMMARY

Status epilepticus is a medical emergency. Effective treatment of SE requires urgent, adequate measures to stop seizures while simultaneously evaluating for underlying causes. Benzodiazepines have Class IA evidence as first-line therapy for SE. There lacks strong evidence for any single second-line anti-seizure drug, and therefore, the choice will vary based on individual patient characteristics. Evidence-based guidelines and recommendations have been published (Table 16-11). These guidelines are based on rating of articles from Class I to Class IV. Class I consists of prospective, randomized controlled clinical trials with masked outcome assessment and requires less than 2 primary outcomes, concealed allocation, well defined exclusion/inclusion criteria, relevant baseline characteristics which are equivalent between treatment groups, or appropriate statistical adjustment for differences, adequate accounting for dropouts, and superiority in a superiority study design or demonstration of noninferiority using 10% margin in a noninferiority design.[46] Class II is a prospective, randomized controlled clinical trial with masked outcome but lacks at least one of additional requirements for Class I or a prospective matched group cohort study with masked outcome assessment.[46] Class III is all other controlled trials where outcome is independently assessed or independently derived by objective outcome measurements.[46]

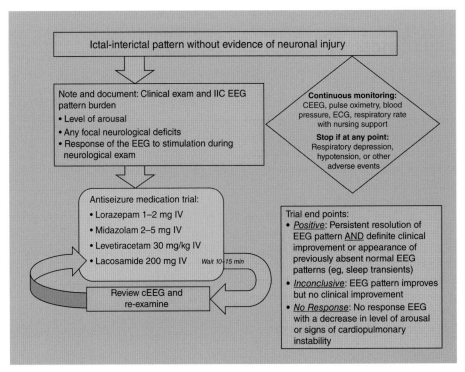

FIGURE 16-2 A stepwise approach to performing a trial of antiseizure drug therapy. cEEG = continuous EEG; ECG = electrocardiography; EEG = electroencephalography; IIC = ictal-interictal continuum; IV = intravenous.

TABLE 16-11 2016 Evidence-Based Guideline for Treatment of Convulsive Status Epilepticus by the American Epilepsy Society

Summary of Conclusions	Level of Recommendation
What are the best initial and subsequent therapies?	
In adults, IM midazolam, IV lorazepam, IV diazepam, and IV phenobarbital are efficacious at stopping seizures lasting at least 5 min.	A
IM midazolam has superior effectiveness compared with IV lorazepam in adults with convulsive status epilepticus without established IV access.	A
IV lorazepam is more effective than IV phenytoin in stopping seizures lasing at least 10 min.	A
There is no difference in efficacy between IV lorazepam followed by IV phenytoin, IV diazepam plus phenytoin followed by IV lorazepam, and IV phenobarbital followed by IV phenytoin.	A
IV valproic acid has similar efficacy to IV phenytoin or continuous IV diazepam as second therapy after failure of a benzodiazepine.	C
Insufficient data exist in adults about the efficacy of levetiracetam as either initial or second therapy.	U
What adverse events are associated with anticonvulsant administration?	
Respiratory and cardiac symptoms are the most common encountered treatment-emergent adverse events associated with IV anticonvulsant administration in adults with status epilepticus.	A
The rate of respiratory depression in patients with status epilepticus treated with benzodiazepines is lower than in patients with status epilepticus treated with placebo, indicating that respiratory problems are an important consequence of untreated status epilepticus.	A
No substantial difference exists between benzodiazepines and phenobarbital in the occurrence of cardiorespiratory adverse events in adults with status epilepticus.	A
Which is the most effective benzodiazepine?	
In adults with status epilepticus without established IV access, IM midazolam is established as more effective compared with IV lorazepam.	A
No significant difference in effectiveness has been demonstrated between lorazepam and diazepam in adults with status epilepticus.	A
Is IV fosphenytoin more effective than IV phenytoin?	
Insufficient data exist about the comparative efficacy of phenytoin and fosphenytoin.	U
Fosphenytoin is better tolerated compared with phenytoin.	B
When both are available, fosphenytoin is preferred based on tolerability, but phenytoin is an acceptable alternative.	B
When does anticonvulsant efficacy drop significantly?	
In adults, the second anticonvulsant administered is less effective than the first "standard" anticonvulsant, while the third anticonvulsant administered is substantially less effective than the first "standard" anticonvulsant.	A
Treatment Recommendations and Proposed Algorithm	
Stabilization phase (0–5 min)	
ABC, time of seizure onset, monitor vitals, ECG, pulse oximetry, fingerstick glucose and treat hypoglycemia, IV access with labs	
Initial therapy phase (5–20 min)	
A benzodiazepine (specifically IM midazolam, IV lorazepam, or IV diazepam) is recommended as the initial therapy of choice, given their demonstrated efficacy, safety, and tolerability.	A
• IM midazolam (10 mg for > 40 kg or 5 mg 13–40 kg) single dose	
• IV lorazepam (0.1 mg/kg/dose, max 4 mg/dose, may repeat once)	
• IV diazepam (0.15–0.2 mg/kg/dose, max 10 mg/dose, may repeat once)	
Although IV phenobarbital is established as efficacious and well tolerated as initial therapy (LOE A, 1 class I RCT), its slower rate of administration, compared with the 3 recommended benzodiazepines, positions it as an *alternative initial* therapy rather than a drug of first choice.	A
• IV phenobarbital (15 mg/kg/dose, single dose)	
For prehospital settings or where the *3 first-line benzodiazepine options are not available*, rectal diazepam, intranasal midazolam, and buccal midazolam are reasonable initial therapy alternatives.	B
• Rectal diazepam (0.2–0.5 mg/kg, max 20 mg/dose, single dose)	
• Intranasal midazolam (0.2 mg/kg max 10 mg/dose)	
• Buccal midazolam (10 mg/mL)	
Initial therapy should be administered as an adequate single full dose rather than broken into multiple smaller doses. Initial therapies should not be given twice except for IV lorazepam and diazepam, which can be repeated at full doses once.	A

(Continued)

TABLE 16-11 2016 Evidence-Based Guideline for Treatment of Convulsive Status Epilepticus by the American Epilepsy Society (Continued)

Summary of Conclusions	Level of Recommendation
Second therapy phase (20–40 min), failed initial therapy	
IV therapy: reasonable options include fosphenytoin, valproic acid, and levetiracetam. There is no clear evidence that any 1 of these options is better than the others.	U (fosphenytoin, levetiracetam), B (valproic acid)
IV phenobarbital is a reasonable second-therapy alternative (LOE B, 1 class II study) if none of the 3 recommended therapies is available.	B
Third therapy phase (> 40 min), failed second therapy	
There is no clear evidence to guide therapy in this phase. Choices included repeat second-line therapy or anesthetics (with cEEG).	U
Third therapy is substantially less effective than initial therapy.	A

ABC = airway, breathing, circulation; cEEG = continuous EEG; ECG = electrocardiogram; EEG = electroencephalogram; IM = intramuscular; IV = intravenous; LOE = Level of Evidence; RCT = randomized controlled trial.

Class IV is evidence from uncontrolled studies, case series, case reports, or expert opinion.[46] Recommendation Level A is based on more than or equal to 1 class I studies or more than or equal to 2 class II studies.[46] Recommendation Level B is more than or equal to class II studies or more than or equal to 3 class III studies.[46] Recommendation Level C is more than or equal to 2 class III studies.[46] Recommendation Level U is lack of studies meeting A, B, or C.[46] The use of continuous EEG to guide further treatment and monitor for ongoing seizures or SE cannot be understated. The use of continuous intravenous anesthetic agents to induce therapeutic coma depends largely on seizure semiology and underlying etiology. Decisions regarding the treatment of NCSE and patterns that lie along the ictal-interictal continuum may be challenging and deserve extra consideration.

QUESTIONS

1. An 80-year-old man with a past medical history of epilepsy on home carbamazepine and mild cognitive impairment is witnessed by his wife to have a generalized tonic-clonic seizure at home lasting 25 minutes. Emergency medical services (EMS) arrives on the scene while he is seizing and administers midazolam 10 mg intramuscularly which stops the seizure activity. He is somonolent but opens his eyes to voice, states his name and city, and follows simple commands. In the ED, an initial set of vital signs demonstrates a temperature of 37°C, heart rate (HR) of 108 beats/min, blood pressure (BP) of 130/89 mmHg, respiration rate (RR) of 12 breaths/min, pulse oximetry of 98% on room air, and a fingerstick glucose of 180 mg/dL. He has another GTC seizure lasting 6 minutes. He has IV access; therefore, lorazepam 4 mg IV is administered. This time, he is lethargic, disoriented, and no longer reliably following commands. How would you describe this patient's problem?

   A. An isolated seizure
   B. Early status epilepticus
   C. Established status epilepticus
   D. Refractory status epilepticus

2. A patient is noted to have status epilepticus. While the lorazepam is being administered, what do you order?

   A. Levetiracetam 60 mg/kg IV or 4500 mg max
   B. Fosphenytoin 20 mg/kg IV or 1500 mg max
   C. Valproic acid 40 mg/kg IV or 3000 mg max
   D. Any of the above

3. A 71-year-old woman with a medical history of prior non-convulsive status epilepticus on home lacosamide 100 mg twice daily (BID), end-stage renal disease on hemodialysis, hypertension, acute pulmonary embolism, chronic obstructive pulmonary disease, and colon cancer presents from her nursing facility for altered mental status. She is found to have a urinary tract infection and pneumonia, and you are treating her in your ICU with ampicillin, vancomycin, and cefepime. She becomes more unresponsive over the course of her stay, and eventually requires intubation. You initiate continuous EEG which shows the pattern in Figure 16-3.
   What should be the next step in management?

   A. Do not treat with an antiseizure drug. The pattern does not represent a potentially ictal pattern and instead reflects her sepsis and renal failure. Treat her infection by tailoring her antibiotics.
   B. Lorazepam 1 mg IV with continuous clinical and EEG monitoring.
   C. Treat by increasing her lacosamide to 150 mg BID.
   D. Treat by placing her on a propofol drip.

4. A patient is noted to have end-stage renal disease. What common antiepileptic medications should be renally dosed?

   A. Levetiracetam
   B. Valproic acid
   C. Phenytoin
   D. All of the above

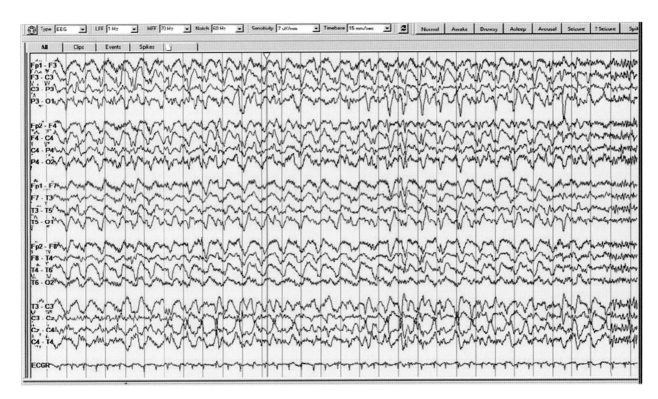

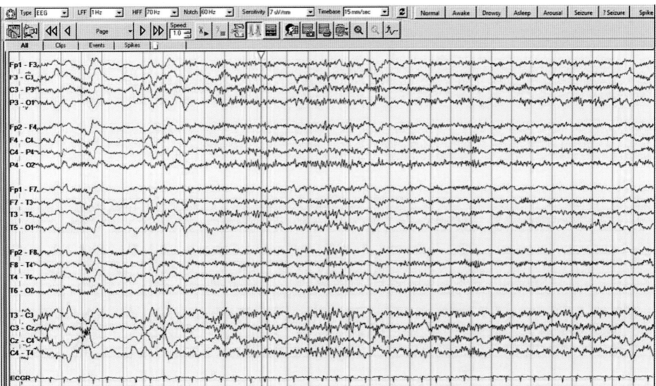

FIGURE 16-3 (A) A 20-channel continuous electroencephalography (EEG) recording in longitudinal bipolar montage, before a trial of antiseizure drug therapy. (B) A 20-channel continuous EEG recording in longitudinal bipolar montage, after a trial of antiseizure drug therapy.

5. An 18-year-old, 48-kg woman with a known history of juvenile myoclonic epilepsy (a primary generalized epilepsy syndrome), previously well-controlled on lamotrigine and successfully weaned off a year prior, presents to the hospital with 2 days of nausea, emesis, and anorexia. She is found to have acute appendicitis with complicated abscess. She is admitted to your surgical ICU after urgent laparoscopic appendectomy. On admission, she develops recurrent myoclonic and generalized tonic-clonic seizures without recovery to baseline. You immediately administer the first-line antiseizure drug lorazepam 4 mg intravenously which stops the seizure activity. If she seizes again (established status epilepticus), what medication might you quickly load as second-line therapy?

A. Phenytoin
B. Valproic acid
C. Carbemazepine
D. All of the above

6. What lab tests should you monitor for patients on valproic acid?

A. Hepatic panel
B. Lipase, amylase
C. Urine human chorionic gonadotropin (hCG)
D. All of the above

7. A 75-year-old man with a history of hypertension, alcohol-related dementia, and a 30-pack-year smoking history presents in the middle of the night from a nursing home with new-onset seizures. There, he was witnessed to have left-sided facial twitching, arm and leg shaking, and some episodes of apparently generalized shaking that lasted for 1 hour. He is given lorazepam 4 mg IV on arrival, which stops the seizure activity. In the ED, he is sleepy and afebrile but periodically desaturates on 5 Liters of oxygen via nasal cannula. His venous blood gas is pH 7.17/PCO_2 = 85 mmHg/PO_2 = 42 mmHg. He is given vancomycin, azithromycin, and cefepime after chest radiograph demonstrates a right lower lobe infiltrate. Head CT is negative for acute pathology. On arrival to your ICU, his mental status begins to decline and he is intubated with rocuronium and etomidate. He had no further apparent clinical seizures. You initiate continuous EEG. What does the cEEG (Fig. 16-4, red box) show?

A. A reactive background
B. A focal temporal onset seizure
C. Generalized spike-and-wave seizure
D. Lateralized periodic discharges

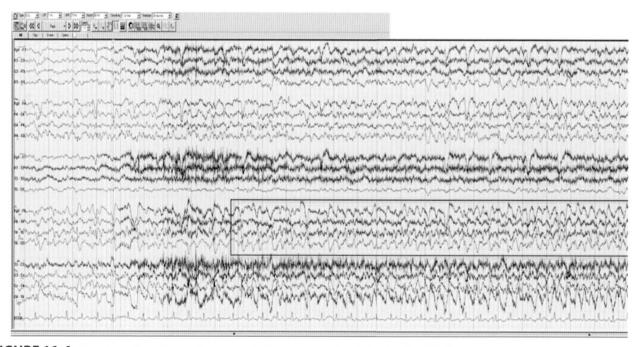

FIGURE 16-4 A 20-channel continuous electroencephalography recording in longitudinal bipolar montage.

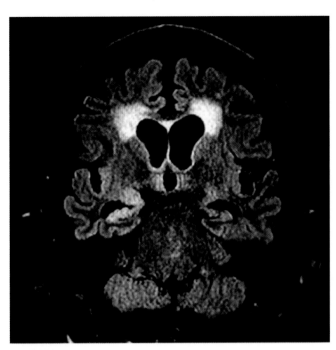

FIGURE 16-5 A T2-weighted fluid attenuated inversion recovery (FLAIR) magnetic resonance image (MRI) of the brain showing mesial temporal hyperintensity. A T1-weighted MRI with contrast image did not reveal definitive enhancement.

8. For the patient in question 7, you obtain an MRI of the brain with and without contrast in the morning shown in Figure 16-5. What should you be your next step in the workup?

    A. MR angiography of the head and neck
    B. CT chest with and without contrast
    C. Bronchoscopy
    D. Lumbar puncture

9. A 72-year-old woman with a history of non–small cell lung carcinoma and left frontal brain metastases status post recent gamma knife surgery currently on palliative chemotherapy presents with acute onset confusion and "babbling" while eating dinner. On arrival, the patient is noted to be nonverbal but quickly develops shaking of right extremity with lip smacking in the ED. She receives a total of 4 mg of IV lorazepam and 2 g of IV levetiracetam with resolution of clinical signs. Head CT shows a low attenuation in the left posterior frontal lobe with evidence of previous left posterior frontal craniotomy and a new left parietal lobe lesion. An urgent MRI is obtained (Fig. 16-6).

She was admitted to your neuroscience ICU for further management. On examination, she remains somnolent and verbal with some expressive aphasia and follows commands intermittently. She has a left gaze preference, right facial droop, and mild right hemiparesis. You start continuous EEG monitoring (Fig. 16-7).

The pattern lasts 2 minutes, then recurs 3 minutes later. During each event, the patient babbles. She regards you, but she continues to be aphasic and does not return to baseline. What is her diagnosis at this point?

    A. Convulsive status epilepticus
    B. Generalized nonconvulsive status epilepticus
    C. Focal nonconvulsive status epilepticus without impaired consciousness
    D. Lateralized periodic discharges

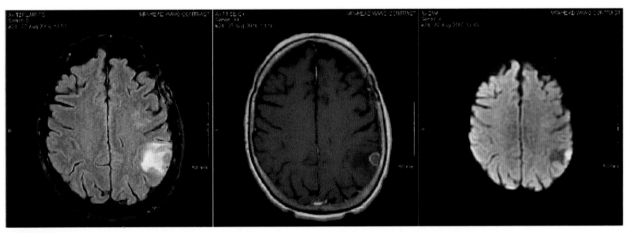

FIGURE 16-6 A T2-weighted fluid attenuated inversion recovery magnetic resonance image showing left parietal hyperintensity representing vasogenic edema surrounding a rim-enhancing lesion on contrast and diffusion restriction.

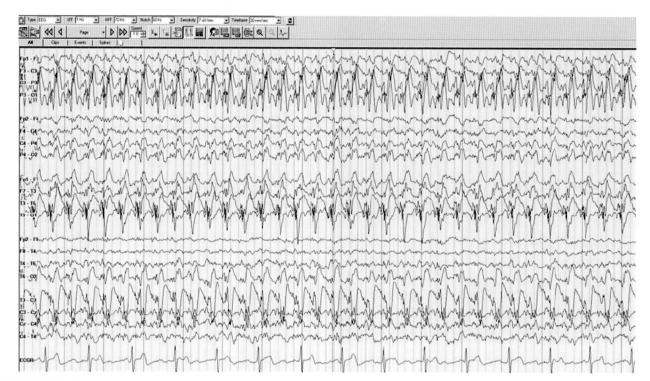

FIGURE 16-7 A 20-channel continuous electroencephalography recording in longitudinal bipolar montage during ongoing focal nonconvulsive seizures.

10. For the patient in question 9, she is appropriately treated, but her EEG continues to demonstrate the following (Fig. 16-8). How would you describe this pattern?

A. Generalized periodic discharges
B. Lateralized periodic discharges
C. Bilateral independent discharges
D. Multifocal rhythmic spike and wave

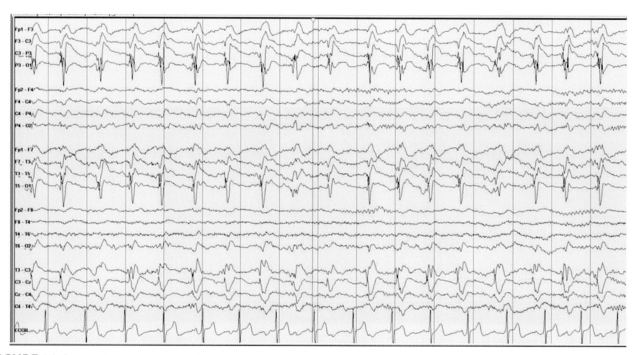

FIGURE 16-8 A 20-channel continuous electroencephalography recording in bipolar montage after treatment with an additional antiseizure drug.

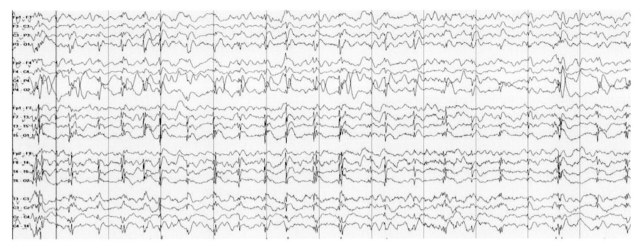

FIGURE 16-9 A 20-channel continuous electroencephalography recording in longitudinal bipolar montage.

11. A 20-year-old, 50-kg previously healthy man presents to your medical ICU after cardiac arrest secondary to electrocution while he was carrying a ladder that struck live wires. He was found down with pulseless ventricular fibrillation/tachycardia with return of spontaneous circulation (ROSC) achieved after 15 minutes. His initial Glasgow coma score was 4T, and he is intubated and postarrest hypothermic protocol at 33 degrees is initiated. Continuous EEG is started and showed severe generalized slowing and generalized suppression. Clinically, he has preserved brainstem reflexes but no motor responses. When stimulated, he has slight eye opening and blinking. During the initial rewarming, myoclonic movements of the upper extremities are observed for at least 40 minutes. You witness the EEG recording in Figure 16-9 and note that each discharge appears to correlate with the myoclonus. What is your diagnosis?

A. Generalized periodic discharges
B. Focal convulsive status epilepticus
C. Focal nonconvulsive status epilepticus
D. Myoclonic status epilepticus

ANSWERS

1. C. Established status epilepticus

He meets definition for generalized convulsive status epilepticus with seizure lasting longer than 5 minutes, so it is not early status epilepticus (choice B); in addition, he has had recurrent seizures without return to baseline. Specifically, this would be considered established status epilepticus because he failed first-line benzodiazepine. He meets criteria for status epilepticus, thus this is not an isolated seizure (choice A). He has not been given and failed a second-line agent, which defines refractory status epilepticus (choice D).

2. D. Any of the above

First-line therapy has failed, and an urgent second-line agent is needed. There is no strong evidence for use of one over another. Levetiracetam, fosphenytoin, and valproic acid are commonly used (choices A–C); lacosamide and perhaps brivatacetam are reasonable options as well. Because of his somnolence, valproic acid or levetiracetam might be better choices in this case. Neither is associated with significant cardiorespiratory depression.

3. B. Lorazepam I mg IV with continuous clinical and EEG monitoring.

This EEG pattern is described as 1-Hz generalized periodic discharges with triphasic morphology (sometimes called "triphasic waves").[95] Classically, triphasic waves were associated with toxic metabolic encephalopathies (eg, hepatic encephalopathy, renal failure, infections),[121,122] and therefore were not felt to be associated with seizures. However, more recent studies have shown that this pattern is highly associated with seizures[123,124] and in some cases may reflect an ictal pattern. A case series of 10 renal failure patients who received cephalosporin (similar to this patient) demonstrated that clonazepam administration resulted in clinical improvement in all patients (20% in less than 24 hours; the remainder within 7 days).[125]

Because the pattern is less than 2.5 Hz, this EEG cannot be considered ictal without further information. A trial of antiseizure drug therapy (see Fig. 16-2) at bedside with monitoring for EEG and clinical improvement is appropriate to determine if the patient is treatment responsive. In 1 retrospective case series, 34.4% of 64 patients with triphasic morphology positively responded to a benzodiazepine or nonsedating antiseizure drug, and an additional 10.9% possibly responded.[120] Figure 16-3B shows the improvement in EEG that this patient experienced, although clinically there was no improvement. This represents an inconclusive response and further monitoring is warranted;

lacosamide was continued at its current dose in this patient and a recommendation was made to transition to an alternative non-cephalosporin antibiotic.

The uncertainty of the response to antiseizure medication of improvement in EEG tracing but no clinical improvement should prompt further investigation with first tier antiepileptic medications (choice A). Increasing home medication that is renally cleared might not be appropriate (choice C), and propofol (choice D) might mask clinical improvement.

4. A. Levetiracetam

Levetiracetam and partially lacosamide are mainly (93–95%) renally metabolized and excreted while the other medications are highly hepatically metabolized. Therefore, it is important to dose-adjust for renal failure, and since both are dialyzed, an extra dose post-hemodialysis is required. Valproic acid and phenytoin (choices B and C) do not have to be dose-adjusted but may need post-dialysis dose supplementation in the setting of high-efficiency dialyzers. In these cases, drug levels should be monitored for dose adjustment. Therefore choice D, all of the above, is also incorrect.

5. B. Valproic acid

Valproic acid should be loaded at 40 mg/kg IV followed by a maintenance dose of 10 to 20 mg/kg every 6 hours. Valproic acid is the most efficacious in this primary generalized epilepsy syndrome, controlling seizures in 80% of patients.[126] In patients with primary generalized epilepsy, especially juvenile myoclonic epilepsy, selective sodium channel blockers such as phenytoin or carbemazipine should be avoided due to potential of aggravating seizure[127] (choices A, C, and D).

6. D. All of the above

You should monitor a liver panel due to hepatotoxicity risk, which is rare, but can be fatal.[128] If abdominal pain develops, lipase may be warranted; valproic acid has been associated with life-threatening cases of pancreatitis.[129,130] Alterations in mental status might similarly prompt testing for ammonia, which rises as a result of valproic acid toxicity. Finally, it is imperative to check hCG for any female of child-bearing age, since valproic acid is highly teratogenic (major malformations rate 9–11%, pregnancy category D).[131,132] If maintenance dosing is planned, a prescription for folate 1 mg twice a day is recommended. Not listed is complete blood count to assess baseline due to thrombocytopenia risk (17.7%).[133]

7. B. A focal temporal onset seizure

This is also a good example of convulsive SE transitioning into nonconvulsive seizures,[47,89] especially in setting of iatrogenic paralysis. The major etiology of this patient's respiratory failure is likely due to prolonged seizure rather than treating his seizures appropriately with lorazepam.[9,45] Given the prolonged duration of his status epilepticus and depressed level of consciousness, the utmost priority is seizure cessation. Note an abrupt onset of right temporal (corresponding to F8/T4) sharp-and-slow waves that evolve in frequency up to 3 Hz and spread posteriorly to O2. Similarly, abrupt offset was also observed (not shown) which is an attribute of seizures. These episodes lasted approximately 45 to 60 seconds. This is a seizure, since it has an abrupt start with evolution in time and space, not a reactive background or lateralized periodic discharge (choices A and D). It does not affect all leads, thus is not generalized (choice C).

8. D. Lumbar puncture

The MRI shows right mesial temporal hyperintensity on T2 FLAIR without enhancement. The next diagnostic step is to obtain a lumbar puncture to evaluate for infection, particularly herpes simplex encephalitis, which is classically associated with temporal periodic discharges. If herpes simplex encephalitis is considered, acyclovir should be started empirically until the results of the lumbar puncture return. Choices A through C are not appropriate at this time.

9. C. Focal nonconvulsive status epilepticus without impaired consciousness

This is focal nonconvulsive status epilepticus (NCSE) manifesting as episodic aphasia and behavioral change without return to baseline. This patient has new onset seizures (high amplitude polyspike and wave discharges arising from P3/O1 that evolve in amplitude, morphology, and frequency to 3 Hz). This area correlates with the new left parieto-occipital metastatic lesion seen on imaging. Although this is refractory status epilepticus, it is not generalized CSE, nor has the patient's level of consciousness become impaired. Therefore, the morbidity associated with third-line anesthetics would be very high in this patient with stage 4 lung cancer. In this case, it is reasonable to maximize second-line agents, ideally avoiding those that are hepatically metabolized through the same cytochrome P450 enzymes that metabolize her chemotherapy. In addition to typical IV second-line antiseizure drugs, oral agents such as gabapentin, oxcarbazepine, pregabalin, topiramate, or zonisamide could be trialed.[134] Ultimately, the treatment of the underlying etiology (ie, vasogenic edema and tumor burden) will improve her seizure burden.

She currently does not have convulsions, thus choice A is incorrect. This is focal, not generalized in distribution on EEG (choice B). This is a seizure on EEG, given its evolution; it is not lateralized periodic discharges (choice D) which do not evolve.

10. B. Lateralized periodic discharges

These are best described as lateralized periodic discharges (LPDs) at 1 Hz. Like many ictal-interictal patterns, it is controversial as to whether these discharges result in adverse neurologic consequences or simply represent metabolic and electrographic dysfunction within the brain. Nevertheless, it is an abnormal pattern representing cortical irritability that is highly associated with seizures.[135] In the absence of evidence of ongoing neurological injury, this pattern does not warrant additional treatment. However, because of the high prevalence of seizures associated with LPDs, the patient should be monitored closely with cEEG for at least 48 hours to ensure that seizures do not recur. Choices A, C, and D are not correct because the EEG clearly shows spike-wave discharges at a frequency of 1 per second, affecting the left side in a periodic regular manner.

11. D. Myoclonic status epilepticus

Clinically, myoclonic status epilepticus is a prolonged (lasting 30 minutes or longer) condition characterized by synchronous or asynchronous, generalized or multifocal, repetitive myoclonic jerks, which correlate with discharges on EEG. Observed on EEG is occurrence of generalized poly-spike/spike-and-wave at approximately 1 to 2 Hz. There is no evolution. However, each discharge is temporally associated with myoclonic jerking of the upper proximal extremity and thus is epileptic. In order to be sure that this EEG pattern does not represent muscle artifact, a trial of a paralytic would result in the same EEG pattern. Generalized periodic discharges (choice A) can appear similarly on EEG, but the discharges would not temporally correlate with myoclonus, as in this case. This is not focal (choices B and C).

REFERENCES

1. Trinka E, Cock H4, Hesdorffer D, et al. A definition and classification of status epilepticus—Report of the ILAE Task Force on Classification of Status Epilepticus. *Epilepsia.* 2015;56(10):1515-1523.
2. Theodore WH, Porter RJ, Albert P, et al. The secondarily generalized tonic-clonic seizure: a videotape analysis. *Neurology.* 1994;44(8):1403-1407.
3. Kramer R. Levisohn P.The duration of secondarily generalized tonic-clonic seizures. *Epilepsia.* 1992;33:68.
4. Brophy GM, Bell R, Claassen J, et al; Neurocritical Care Society Status Epilepticus Guideline Writing Committee. Guidelines for the evaluation and management of status epilepticus. *Neurocrit Care.* 2012;17(1):3-23.
5. Jirsch J, Hirsch LJ. Nonconvulsive seizures: developing a rational approach to the diagnosis and management in the critically ill population. *Clin Neurophysiol.* 2007;118(8): 1660-1670.
6. Beniczky S, Hirsch LJ, Kaplan PW, et al. Unified EEG terminology and criteria for nonconvulsive status epilepticus. *Epilepsia.* 2013;54(Suppl 6):28-29.
7. Leitinger M, Trinka E, Gardella E, et al. Diagnostic accuracy of the Salzburg EEG criteria for non-convulsive status epilepticus: a retrospective study. *Lancet Neurol.* 2016;15(10):1054-1062.
8. Chin RFM, Neville BGR, Scott RC. A systematic review of the epidemiology of status epilepticus. *Eur J Neurol.* 2004;11(12):800-810.
9. Alldredge BK, Gelb AM, Isaacs SM, et al. A comparison of lorazepam, diazepam, and placebo for the treatment of out-of-hospital status epilepticus. *N Engl J Med.* 2001;345(9):631-637.
10. Hesdorffer DC, Logroscino G, Cascino G, Annegers JF, Hauser WA. Incidence of status epilepticus in Rochester, Minnesota, 1965-1984. *Neurology.* 1998;50(3):735-741.
11. Knake S, Rosenow F, Vescovi M, *et al.* Incidence of status epilepticus in adults in Germany: a prospective, population-based study. *Epilepsia.* 2001;42(6):714-718.
12. Coeytaux A, Jallon P, Galobardes B, Morabia A. Incidence of status epilepticus in French-speaking Switzerland: (EPISTAR). *Neurology.* 2000;55(5):693-697.
13. DeLorenzo RJ, Hauser WA, Towne AR, et al. A prospective, population-based epidemiologic study of status epilepticus in Richmond, Virginia. *Neurology.* 1996;46(4):1029-1035.
14. Dham BS, Hunter K, Rincon F. The epidemiology of status epilepticus in the United States. *Neurocrit Care.* 2014;20(3):476-483.
15. Penberthy LT, Towne A, Garnett LK, Perlin JB, DeLorenzo RJ. Estimating the economic burden of status epilepticus to the health care system. *Seizure.* 2005;14(1):46-51.
16. Jallon P. Mortality in patients with epilepsy. *Curr Opin Neurol.* 2004;17(2):141-146.
17. Leitinger M, Höller Y, Kalss G, et al. Epidemiology-based mortality score in status epilepticus (EMSE). *Neurocrit Care.* 2015;22(2):273-282.
18. Kang BS, Kim DW, Kim KK, et al. Prediction of mortality and functional outcome from status epilepticus and independent external validation of STESS and EMSE scores. *Crit Care.* 2015;20:25.
19. Rossetti AO, Logroscino G, Milligan TA, et al. Status Epilepticus Severity Score (STESS): a tool to orient early treatment strategy. *J Neurol.* 2008;255(10):1561-1566.
20. Rossetti AO, Logroscino G, Bromfield EB. A clinical score for prognosis of status epilepticus in adults. *Neurology.* 2006;66(11):1736-1738.
21. Leitinger M, Kalss G, Rohracher A, et al. Predicting outcome of status epilepticus. *Epilepsy Behav.* 2015;49:126-130.
22. Sutter R, Kaplan PW, Rüegg S. Independent external validation of the status epilepticus severity score. *Crit Care Med.* 2013;41(12):e475-e479.
23. Rossetti AO, Hurwitz S, Logroscino G, Bromfield EB. Prognosis of status epilepticus: role of aetiology, age, and consciousness impairment at presentation. *J Neurol Neurosurg Psychiatry.* 2006;77(5):611-615.
24. Agarwal P, Kumar N, Chandra R, et al. Randomized study of intravenous valproate and phenytoin in status epilepticus. *Seizure.* 2007;16(6):527-532.
25. DeLorenzo RJ, Towne AR, Pellock JM, Ko D. Status epilepticus in children, adults, and the elderly. *Epilepsia.* 1992;33(Suppl 4): S15-S25.
26. Kowalski RG, Ziai WC, Rees RN, et al. Third-line antiepileptic therapy and outcome in status epilepticus: the impact of vasopressor use and prolonged mechanical ventilation. *Crit Care Med.* 2012;40(9):2677-2684.

27. Claassen J, Hirsch LJ, Emerson RG, Bates JE, Thompson TB, Mayer SA. Continuous EEG monitoring and midazolam infusion for refractory nonconvulsive status epilepticus. *Neurology*. 2001;57(6):1036-1042.

28. Cheng JY. Latency to treatment of status epilepticus is associated with mortality and functional status. *J Neurol Sci*. 2016;370:290-295.

29. DeLorenzo RJ, Garnett LK, Towne AR, et al. Comparison of status epilepticus with prolonged seizure episodes lasting from 10 to 29 minutes. *Epilepsia*. 1999;40(2):164-169.

30. Towne AR, Pellock JM, Ko D, DeLorenzo RJ. Determinants of mortality in status epilepticus. *Epilepsia*. 1994;35(1):27-34.

31. Walton NY. Systemic effects of generalized convulsive status epilepticus. *Epilepsia*. 1993;34 (Suppl 1):S54-S58.

32. Hocker S. Systemic complications of status epilepticus—an update. *Epilepsy Behav*. 2015;49:83-87.

33. Fujikawa DG. The temporal evolution of neuronal damage from pilocarpine-induced status epilepticus. *Brain Res*. 1996;725(1):11-22.

34. Mazarati AM, Wasterlain CG, Sankar R, Shin D. Self-sustaining status epilepticus after brief electrical stimulation of the perforant path. *Brain Res*. 1998;801(1-2):251-253.

35. Chen WB, Gao R, Su YY, et al. Valproate versus diazepam for generalized convulsive status epilepticus: a pilot study. *Eur J Neurol*. 2011;18(12):1391-1396.

36. Naylor DE, Liu H, Wasterlain CG. Trafficking of GABA(A) receptors, loss of inhibition, and a mechanism for pharmacoresistance in status epilepticus. *J Neurosci*. 2005;25(34):7724-7733.

37. Naylor DE, Liu H, Niquet J, Wasterlain CG. Rapid surface accumulation of NMDA receptors increases glutamatergic excitation during status epilepticus. *Neurobiol Dis*. 2013;54:225-238.

38. Fritsch B, Stott JJ, Joelle Donofrio J, Rogawski MA. Treatment of early and late kainic acid-induced status epilepticus with the noncompetitive AMPA receptor antagonist GYKI 52466. *Epilepsia*. 2010;51(1):108-117.

39. Chen JWY, Wasterlain CG. Status epilepticus: pathophysiology and management in adults. *Lancet Neurol*. 2006;5(3):246-256.

40. Jones DM, Esmaeil N, Maren S, Macdonald RL. Characterization of pharmacoresistance to benzodiazepines in the rat Li-pilocarpine model of status epilepticus. *Epilepsy Res*. 2002;50(3):301-312.

41. Mazarati AM, Wasterlain CG. N-methyl-D-asparate receptor antagonists abolish the maintenance phase of self-sustaining status epilepticus in rat. *Neurosci Lett*. 1999;265(3):187-190.

42. Kapur J, Macdonald RL. Rapid seizure-induced reduction of benzodiazepine and Zn^{2+} sensitivity of hippocampal dentate granule cell GABAA receptors. *J Neurosci Off J Soc Neurosci*. 1997;17(19):7532-7540.

43. Mazarati AM, Baldwin RA, Sankar R, Wasterlain CG. Time-dependent decrease in the effectiveness of antiepileptic drugs during the course of self-sustaining status epilepticus. *Brain Res*. 1998;814(1-2):179-185.

44. Cascino GD, Hesdorffer D, Logroscino G, Hauser WA. Treatment of nonfebrile status epilepticus in Rochester, Minn, from 1965 through 1984. *Mayo Clin Proc*. 2001;76(1):39-41.

45. Vignatelli L, Rinaldi R, Baldin E, et al. Impact of treatment on the short-term prognosis of status epilepticus in two population-based cohorts. *J Neurol*. 2008;255(2):197-204.

46. Glauser T, Shinnar S, Gloss D, et al. Evidence-based guideline: treatment of convulsive status epilepticus in children and adults: report of the Guideline Committee of the American Epilepsy Society. *Epilepsy Curr Am Epilepsy Soc*. 2016;16(1):48-61.

47. Treiman DM, Meyers PD, Walton NY, et al. A comparison of four treatments for generalized convulsive status epilepticus. Veterans Affairs Status Epilepticus Cooperative Study Group. *N Engl J Med*. 1998;339(12):792-798.

48. Silbergleit R, Durkalski V, Lowenstein D, et al; NETT Investigators. Intramuscular versus intravenous therapy for prehospital status epilepticus. *N Engl J Med*. 2012;366(7):591-600.

49. Prasad M, Krishnan PR, Sequeira R, Al-Roomi K. Anticonvulsant therapy for status epilepticus. *Cochrane Database Syst Rev*. 2014;(9):CD003723.

50. Claassen J, Riviello JJ, Silbergleit R. Emergency neurological life support: status epilepticus. *Neurocrit Care*. 2015;23 (Suppl 2):136-142.

51. Gaspard N, Foreman BP, Alvarez V, et al; Critical Care EEG Monitoring Research Consortium (CCEMRC). New-onset refractory status epilepticus: etiology, clinical features, and outcome. *Neurology*. 2015;85(18):1604-1613.

52. Mundlamuri RC, Sinha S, Subbakrishna DK, et al. Management of generalised convulsive status epilepticus (SE): A prospective randomised controlled study of combined treatment with intravenous lorazepam with either phenytoin, sodium valproate or levetiracetam—pilot study. *Epilepsy Res*. 2015;114:52-58.

53. Bleck T, Cock H, Chamberlain J, et al. The established status epilepticus trial 2013. *Epilepsia*. 2013;54 (Suppl 6):89-92.

54. Trinka E. What is the relative value of the standard anticonvulsants: Phenytoin and fosphenytoin, phenobarbital, valproate, and levetiracetam? *Epilepsia*. 2009;50 (Suppl 12):40-43.

55. Hodges BM, Mazur JE. Intravenous valproate in status epilepticus. *Ann Pharmacother*. 2001;35(11):1465-1470.

56. Zeller JA, Schlesinger S, Runge U, Kessler C. Influence of valproate monotherapy on platelet activation and hematologic values. *Epilepsia*. 1999;40(2):186-189.

57. Ramael S, Daoust A, Otoul C, et al. Levetiracetam intravenous infusion: a randomized, placebo-controlled safety and pharmacokinetic study. *Epilepsia*. 2006;47(7):1128-1135.

58. Carunchio I, Pieri M, Ciotti MT, Albo F, Zona C. Modulation of AMPA receptors in cultured cortical neurons induced by the antiepileptic drug levetiracetam. *Epilepsia*. 2007;48(4):654-662.

59. Alvarez V, Januel JM, Burnand B, Rossetti AO. Second-line status epilepticus treatment: comparison of phenytoin, valproate, and levetiracetam. *Epilepsia*. 2011;52(7):1292-1296.

60. Trinka E, Dobesberger J. New treatment options in status epilepticus: a critical review on intravenous levetiracetam. *Ther Adv Neurol Disord*. 2009;2(2):79-91.

61. Yasiry Z, Shorvon SD. The relative effectiveness of five antiepileptic drugs in treatment of benzodiazepine-resistant convulsive status epilepticus: a meta-analysis of published studies. *Seizure*. 2014;23(3):167-174.

62. Rogawski MA, Tofighy A, White HS, Matagne A, Wolff C. Current understanding of the mechanism of action of the antiepileptic drug lacosamide. *Epilepsy Res*. 2015;110:189-205.

63. Lang N, Lange M, Schmitt FC, et al. Intravenous lacosamide in clinical practice—results from an independent registry. *Seizure*. 2016;39:5-9.

64. Krauss G, Ben-Menachem E, Mameniskiene R, et al; SP757 Study Group. Intravenous lacosamide as short-term replacement for oral lacosamide in partial-onset seizures. *Epilepsia.* 2010;51(6):951-957.

65. Legros B, Depondt C, Levy-Nogueira M, et al. Intravenous lacosamide in refractory seizure clusters and status epilepticus: comparison of 200 and 400 mg loading doses. *Neurocrit Care.* 2014;20(3):484-488.

66. Goodwin H, Hinson HE, Shermock KM, Karanjia N, Lewin JJ. The use of lacosamide in refractory status epilepticus. *Neurocrit Care.* 2011;14(3):348-353.

67. Ryvlin P, Werhahn KJ, Blaszczyk B, Johnson ME, Lu S. Adjunctive brivaracetam in adults with uncontrolled focal epilepsy: results from a double-blind, randomized, placebo-controlled trial. *Epilepsia.* 2014;55(1):47-56.

68. Klein P, Schiemann J, Sperling MR, et al. A randomized, double-blind, placebo-controlled, multicenter, parallel-group study to evaluate the efficacy and safety of adjunctive brivaracetam in adult patients with uncontrolled partial-onset seizures. *Epilepsia.* 2015;56(12):1890-1898.

69. Klein P, Biton V, Dilley D, Barnes M, Schiemann J, Lu S. Safety and tolerability of adjunctive brivaracetam as intravenous infusion or bolus in patients with epilepsy. *Epilepsia.* 2016;57(7):1130-1138.

70. Wallis W, Kutt H, McDowell F. Intravenous diphenylhydantoin in treatment of acute repetitive seizures. *Neurology.* 1968;18(6):513-525.

71. Sinha S, Naritoku DK. Intravenous valproate is well tolerated in unstable patients with status epilepticus. *Neurology.* 2000;55(5):722-724.

72. Trinka E, Höfler J, Zerbs A, Brigo F. Efficacy and safety of intravenous valproate for status epilepticus: a systematic review. *CNS Drugs.* 2014;28(7):623-639.

73. Brigo F, Storti M, Del Felice A, Fiaschi A, Bongiovanni LG. IV valproate in generalized convulsive status epilepticus: a systematic review. *Eur J Neurol.* 2012;19(9):1180-1191.

74. Aiguabella M, Falip M, Villanueva V, et al. Efficacy of intravenous levetiracetam as an add-on treatment in status epilepticus: a multicentric observational study. *Seizure.* 2011;20(1):60-64.

75. Gillard M, Fuks B, Leclercq K, Matagne A. Binding characteristics of brivaracetam, a selective, high affinity SV2A ligand in rat, mouse and human brain: relationship to anti-convulsant properties. *Eur J Pharmacol.* 2011;664(1-3):36-44.

76. Klitgaard H, Matagne A, Nicolas JM, et al. Brivaracetam: rationale for discovery and preclinical profile of a selective SV2A ligand for epilepsy treatment. *Epilepsia.* 2016;57(4):538-548.

77. Ramsay RE, Sabharwal V, Khan F, et al. Safety and pK of IV loading dose of lacosamide in the ICU. *Epilepsy Behav.* 2015;49:340-342.

78. Garcés M, Villanueva V, Mauri JA, et al. Factors influencing response to intravenous lacosamide in emergency situations: LACO-IV study. *Epilepsy Behav.* 2014;36:144-152.

79. Rossetti AO, Milligan TA, Vulliémoz S, Michaelides C, Bertschi M, Lee JW. A randomized trial for the treatment of refractory status epilepticus. *Neurocrit Care.* 2011;14(1):4-10.

80. Claassen J, Hirsch LJ, Emerson RG, Mayer SA. Treatment of refractory status epilepticus with pentobarbital, propofol, or midazolam: a systematic review. *Epilepsia.* 2002;43(2):146-153.

81. Ferlisi M, Shorvon S. The outcome of therapies in refractory and super-refractory convulsive status epilepticus and recommendations for therapy. *Brain J Neurol.* 2012;135(Pt 8):2314-2328.

82. Fernandez A, Lantigua H, Lesch C, et al. High-dose midazolam infusion for refractory status epilepticus. *Neurology.* 2014;82(4):359-365.

83. Höfler J, Rohracher A, Kalss G, et al. (S)-Ketamine in refractory and super-refractory status epilepticus: a retrospective study. *CNS Drugs.* 2016;30(9):869-876.

84. Hocker SE, Britton JW, Mandrekar JN, Wijdicks EFM, Rabinstein AA. Predictors of outcome in refractory status epilepticus. *JAMA Neurol.* 2013;70(1):72-77.

85. Alvarez V, Lee JW, Westover MB, et al. Therapeutic coma for status epilepticus: Differing practices in a prospective multicenter study. *Neurology.* 2016;87(16):1650-1659.

86. Pandian JD, Cascino GD, So EL, Manno E, Fulgham JR. Digital video-electroencephalographic monitoring in the neurological-neurosurgical intensive care unit: clinical features and outcome. *Arch Neurol.* 2004;61(7):1090-1094.

87. Ney JP, van der Goes DN, Nuwer MR, Nelson L, Eccher MA. Continuous and routine EEG in intensive care: utilization and outcomes, United States 2005-2009. *Neurology.* 2013;81(23):2002-2008.

88. Kilbride RD, Costello DJ, Chiappa KH. How seizure detection by continuous electroencephalographic monitoring affects the prescribing of antiepileptic medications. *Arch Neurol.* 2009;66(6):723-728.

89. DeLorenzo RJ, Waterhouse EJ, Towne AR, et al. Persistent nonconvulsive status epilepticus after the control of convulsive status epilepticus. *Epilepsia.* 1998;39(8):833-840.

90. Claassen J, Mayer SA, Kowalski RG, Emerson RG, Hirsch LJ. Detection of electrographic seizures with continuous EEG monitoring in critically ill patients. *Neurology.* 2004;62(10):1743-1748.

91. Kamel H, Betjemann JP, Navi BB, et al. Diagnostic yield of electroencephalography in the medical and surgical intensive care unit. *Neurocrit Care.* 2013;19(3):336-341.

92. Towne AR, Waterhouse EJ, Boggs JG, et al. Prevalence of nonconvulsive status epilepticus in comatose patients. *Neurology.* 2000;54(2):340-345.

93. Jordan KG. Nonconvulsive seizure (NCS) and nonconvulsive status epilepticus (NCSE) detected by continuous EEG monitoring in the neuro ICU. *Neurology.* 1992;42(Suppl 3):194-195.

94. Westover MB, Shafi MM, Bianchi MT, et al. The probability of seizures during EEG monitoring in critically ill adults. *Clin Neurophysiol.* 2015;126(3):463-471.

95. Hirsch LJ, LaRoche SM, Gaspard N, et al. American Clinical Neurophysiology Society's standardized critical care EEG terminology: 2012 version. *J Clin Neurophysiol.* 2013;30(1):1-27.

96. Moura LM, Shafi MM, Ng M, et al. Spectrogram screening of adult EEGs is sensitive and efficient. *Neurology.* 2014;83(1):56-64.

97. Haider HA, Esteller R, Hahn CD, et al; Critical Care EEG Monitoring Research Consortium. Sensitivity of quantitative EEG for seizure identification in the intensive care unit. *Neurology.* 2016;87(9):935-944.

98. Shneker BF, Fountain NB. Assessment of acute morbidity and mortality in nonconvulsive status epilepticus. *Neurology.* 2003;61(8):1066-1073.

99. Young GB, Jordan KG, Doig GS. An assessment of nonconvulsive seizures in the intensive care unit using continuous EEG monitoring: an investigation of variables associated with mortality. *Neurology.* 1996;47(1):83-89.

100. Litt B, Wityk RJ, Hertz SH, et al. Nonconvulsive status epilepticus in the critically ill elderly. *Epilepsia.* 1998;39(11):1194-1202.

101. Dennis LJ, Claassen J, Hirsch LJ, Emerson RG, Connolly ES, Mayer SA. Nonconvulsive status epilepticus after subarachnoid hemorrhage. *Neurosurgery.* 2002;51(5):1136-1143; discussion 1144.

102. Kondziella D, Friberg CK, Wellwood I, Reiffurth C, Fabricius M, Dreier JP. Continuous EEG monitoring in aneurysmal subarachnoid hemorrhage: a systematic review. *Neurocrit Care.* 2015;22(3):450-461.

103. Claassen J, Albers D, Schmidt JM, et al. Nonconvulsive seizures in subarachnoid hemorrhage link inflammation and outcome. *Ann Neurol.* 2014;75(5):771-781.

104. Claassen J, Perotte A, Albers D, et al. Nonconvulsive seizures after subarachnoid hemorrhage: multimodal detection and outcomes. *Ann Neurol.* 2013;74(1):53-64.

105. Vespa PM, Nuwer MR, Nenov V, et al. Increased incidence and impact of nonconvulsive and convulsive seizures after traumatic brain injury as detected by continuous electroencephalographic monitoring. *J Neurosurg.* 1999;91(5):750-760.

106. Vespa PM, Miller C, McArthur D, et al. Nonconvulsive electrographic seizures after traumatic brain injury result in a delayed, prolonged increase in intracranial pressure and metabolic crisis. *Crit Care Med.* 2007;35(12):2830-2836.

107. Vespa P, Tubi M, Claassen J, et al. Metabolic crisis occurs with seizures and periodic discharges after brain trauma. *Ann Neurol.* 2016;79(4):579-590.

108. Vespa PM, McArthur DL, Xu Y, et al. Nonconvulsive seizures after traumatic brain injury are associated with hippocampal atrophy. *Neurology.* 2010;75(9):792-798.

109. Vespa P, Martin NA, Nenov V, et al. Delayed increase in extracellular glycerol with post-traumatic electrographic epileptic activity: support for the theory that seizures induce secondary injury. *Acta Neurochir Suppl.* 2002;81:355-357.

110. Claassen J, Jetté N, Chum F, et al. Electrographic seizures and periodic discharges after intracerebral hemorrhage. *Neurology.* 2007;69(13):1356-1365.

111. Vespa PM, O'Phelan K, Shah M, et al. Acute seizures after intracerebral hemorrhage: a factor in progressive midline shift and outcome. *Neurology.* 2003;60(9):1441-1446.

112. Belcastro V, Vidale S, Gorgone G, et al. Non-convulsive status epilepticus after ischemic stroke: a hospital-based stroke cohort study. *J Neurol.* 2014;261(11):2136-2142.

113. Waterhouse E, Vaughan JK, Barnes TY, et al. Synergistic effect of status epilepticus and ischemic brain injury on mortality. *Epilepsy Res.* 1998;29(3):175-183.

114. Ferguson M, Bianchi MT, Sutter R, et al. Calculating the risk benefit equation for aggressive treatment of non-convulsive status epilepticus. *Neurocrit Care.* 2013;18(2):216-227.

115. Struck AF, Westover MB, Hall LT, Deck GM, Cole AJ, Rosenthal ES. Metabolic correlates of the ictal-interictal continuum: FDG-PET during continuous EEG. *Neurocrit Care.* 2016;24(3):324-331.

116. Chu K, Kang DW, Kim JY, Chang KH, Lee SK. Diffusion-weighted magnetic resonance imaging in nonconvulsive status epilepticus. *Arch Neurol.* 2011;58(6):993-998.

117. Huang YC, Weng HH, Tsai YT, et al. Periictal magnetic resonance imaging in status epilepticus. *Epilepsy Res.* 2009;86(1):72-81.

118. Szabo K, Poepel A, Pohlmann-Eden B, et al. Diffusion-weighted and perfusion MRI demonstrates parenchymal changes in complex partial status epilepticus. *Brain.* 2005;128(Pt 6):1369-1376.

119. DeGiorgio CM, Heck CN, Rabinowicz AL, Gott PS, Smith T, Correale J. Serum neuron-specific enolase in the major subtypes of status epilepticus. *Neurology.* 1999;52(4):746-749.

120. O'Rourke D, Chen PM, Gaspard N, et al. Response rates to anticonvulsant trials in patients with triphasic-wave EEG patterns of uncertain significance. *Neurocrit Care.* 2016;24(2):233-239.

121. Sutter R, Stevens RD, Kaplan PW. Significance of triphasic waves in patients with acute encephalopathy: a nine-year cohort study. *Clin Neurophysiol.* 2013;124(10):1952-1958.

122. Karnaze DS, Bickford RG. Triphasic waves: a reassessment of their significance. *Electroencephalogr Clin Neurophysiol.* 1984;57(3):193-198.

123. Foreman B, Claassen J, Abou Khaled K, et al. Generalized periodic discharges in the critically ill: a case-control study of 200 patients. *Neurology.* 2012;79(19):1951-1960.

124. Foreman B, Mahulikar A, Tadi P, et al; Critical Care EEG Monitoring Research Consortium (CCEMRC). Generalized periodic discharges and "triphasic waves": a blinded evaluation of inter-rater agreement and clinical significance. *Clin Neurophysiol.* 2016;127(2):1073-1080.

125. Martínez-Rodríguez JE, Barriga FJ, Santamaria J, et al. Nonconvulsive status epilepticus associated with cephalosporins in patients with renal failure. *Am J Med.* 2001;111(2):115-119.

126. Marson AG, Al-Kharusi AM, Alwaidh M, et al; SANAD Study Group. The SANAD study of effectiveness of valproate, lamotrigine, or topiramate for generalised and unclassifiable epilepsy: an unblinded randomised controlled trial. *Lancet.* 2007;369(9566):1016-1026.

127. Chaves J, Sander JW. Seizure aggravation in idiopathic generalized epilepsies. *Epilepsia.* 2005;46 (Suppl 9):133-139.

128. Bryant AE 3rd, Dreifuss FE. Valproic acid hepatic fatalities. III. U.S. experience since 1986. *Neurology.* 1996;46(2):465-469.

129. Grosse P, Rüsch L, Schmitz B. Pancreatitis complicating treatment with intravenous valproic acid. *J Neurol.* 2002; 249(4):484-485.

130. Gerstner T, Büsing D, Bell N, et al. Valproic acid-induced pancreatitis: 16 new cases and a review of the literature. *J Gastroenterol.* 2007;42(1):39-48.

131. Harden CL, Pennell PB, Koppel BS, et al; American Academy of Neurology; American Epilepsy Society. Practice parameter update: management issues for women with epilepsy—focus on pregnancy (an evidence-based review): vitamin K, folic acid, blood levels, and breastfeeding: report of the Quality Standards Subcommittee and Therapeutics and Technology Assessment Subcommittee of the American Academy of Neurology and American Epilepsy Society. *Neurology.* 2009;73(2):142-149.

132. Wyszynski DF, Nambisan M, Surve T, Alsdorf RM, Smith CR, Holmes LB; Antiepileptic Drug Pregnancy Registry. Increased rate of major malformations in offspring exposed to valproate during pregnancy. *Neurology.* 2005;64(6):961-965.

133. Nasreddine W, Beydoun A. Valproate-induced thrombocytopenia: a prospective monotherapy study. *Epilepsia.* 2008;49(3):438-445.

134. Maschio M. Brain tumor-related epilepsy. *Curr Neuropharmacol.* 2012;10(2):124-133.

135. Sen-Gupta I, Schuele SU, Macken MP, Kwasny MJ, Gerard EE. "Ictal" lateralized periodic discharges. *Epilepsy Behav.* 2014;36:165-170.

Disorders of the Spinal Cord and Peripheral Nervous System in Critical Care

Edward W. Bahou, MD, Yaojie Wu, MD, and Shanna K. Patterson, MD

INTRODUCTION

This chapter will discuss the spinal cord, peripheral nerves, neuromuscular junction (NMJ), and their associated disorders. Focus will be placed on those disorders that potentially cause respiratory muscle weakness and hemodynamic instability. These are common findings in neurological disease that necessitate intensive care.

THE SPINAL CORD

The spinal cord is divided longitudinally into the cervical, thoracic, lumbar, and sacral cord. The cervical cord is made up of 8 segments, the thoracic cord is made up of 12 segments, the lumbar cord is made up of 5 segments, and the sacral cord is made up of 5 segments. There is also a single coccygeal segment, for a total of 31 spinal cord segments. Each segment of the cord gives off a ventral and dorsal spinal nerve root, which ultimately become the peripheral motor and sensory fibers, respectively. The cord is surrounded along its entire length by the bony vertebral column. Each vertebral body, except for C8, corresponds to its respective spinal cord segment. There is no C8 vertebral body. From C1 to C7, each root exits above its respective vertebral body. The C8 nerve root exits between the C7 and T1 vertebrae, and each root inferior to this level exits below its respective vertebrae. The spinal cord itself extends to approximately the lower margin of the first lumbar vertebral body (L1) in adults. Below this level, the spinal canal contains the lumbar, sacral, and coccygeal spinal roots that make up the cauda equina.

DISORDERS OF THE SPINAL CORD

Spinal cord injury (SCI) is a potential cause for neurogenic shock and respiratory compromise and is therefore an important reason for admission to the intensive care unit.

Traumatic Spinal Cord Injury

Most SCIs are traumatic. In the United States in 2014, the incidence of traumatic SCI is approximately 40 cases per million people.

The most common causes are motor vehicle accidents, falls, violent acts, and sports injuries.[1] Acute causes of SCI lead to fractures and dislocations of the vertebrae, resulting in displaced bony fragments and disc material. The direct mechanical injury to spinal cord axons caused by these events is known as primary injury, and also includes compression and laceration. Secondary injury may continue for hours to days after the initial injury, and includes ischemia, increased intracellular calcium, extracellular glutamate, free radicals, inflammation, and apoptosis.[2] In a cat model, as a result of these secondary phenomena, spinal cord edema develops within hours of injury, becomes maximal by day 3 to 6, and begins to recede by day 9.[3]

The severity is graded using the American Spinal Injury Association (ASIA) Impairment Scale (Fig. 17-1). Spinal cord injury is first determined to be complete or incomplete. A *complete* lesion is defined by the total absence of sensory and motor function in the lower sacral segments, S4 to S5. An *incomplete* injury will leave partial preservation of sensory and/or motor function, known as sacral sparing. Assessment for sacral sparing involves evaluation of sacral innervated muscle strength (anal sphincter tone) and regional reflexes, such as anal wink and bulbocavernosus reflex. The *neurological level* is then determined, which is the most caudal spinal segment with normal bilateral sensory and motor function.[4] The ASIA Impairment Scale grades a complete injury as A, with grades B-E representing varying degrees of injury (grade E is a normal exam).

Recovery after spinal cord injury mostly occurs during the first 6 to 9 months and relates to the severity of injury. A complete injury may convert to an incomplete injury in about 10% to 20% of patients, with the conversion from ASIA grade A to grade D occurring in only a minority of those patients.[4] Very few patients with complete injury regain the ability to ambulate, whereas 20% to 50% of those with an initial injury severity of ASIA grade B may ambulate by 1 year.[4]

Methylprednisolone is the only treatment in the acute setting of traumatic, nonpenetrating SCI that has been suggested by clinical trials to improve outcomes. The National Acute Spinal Cord Injury Study (NASCIS) II enrolled patients between 1985 and 1988 and compared methylprednisolone, naloxone, and placebo in acute traumatic SCI.

ASIA Impairment Scale (AIS)

A = Complete. No sensory or motor function is preserved in the sacral segments S4 to S5.

B = Sensory Incomplete. Sensory but not motor function is preserved below the neurological level and includes the sacral segments S4 to S5 (light touch or pin prick at S4 to S5 or deep anal pressure) AND no motor function is preserved more than 3 levels below the motor level on either side of the body.

C = Motor Incomplete. Motor function is preserved at the most caudal sacral segments for voluntary anal contraction (VAC) OR the patient meets the criteria for sensory incomplete status (sensory function preserved at the most caudal sacral segments [S4 to S5] by LT, PP, or DAP), and has some sparing of motor function more than 3 levels below the ipsilateral motor level on either side of the body.
(This includes key or non-key muscle functions to determine motor incomplete status.) For AIS C, less than half of key muscle functions below the single NLI have a muscle grade ≥ 3.

D = Motor Incomplete. Motor incomplete status as defined above, with at least half (half or more) of key muscle functions below the single NLI having a muscle grade ≥ 3.

E = Normal. If sensation and motor function as tested with the ISNCSCI are graded as normal in all segments, and the patient had prior deficits, then the AIS grade is E. Someone without an initial SCI does not receive an AIS grade.

Using ND: To document the sensory, motor, and NLI levels; the ASIA Impairment Scale grade; and/or the zone of partial preservation (ZPP) when they are unable to be determined based on the examination results.

FIGURE 17-1 American Spinal Injury Association: International Standards for Neurological Classification of Spinal Cord Injury. (Scale updated November 2015. © 2011 American Spinal Injury Association. Reprinted with permission. http://asia-spinalinjury.org/wp-content/uploads/2016/02/International_Stds_Diagram_Worksheet.pdf.)

At 1 year, no statistically significant differences in motor or sensory function were found between groups. However, in a subgroup analysis, those treated with methylprednisolone within 8 hours of injury demonstrated significantly improved motor recovery. Administration of methylprednisolone in acute SCI became standard of care in the years after NASCIS II.[2,5,6] This data has been heavily scrutinized in the past, with most critiques focusing on the post-hoc subgroup analysis, clinical significance of the reported motor improvement, and poor reproducibility. Others cite the risks associated with high-dose steroids, particularly wound infections, systemic infections, and gastrointestinal hemorrhage.[2] In 2013, the American Association of Neurological Surgeons and Congress of Neurological Surgeons stated that, based on the available evidence, the use of glucocorticoids in acute spinal cord injury is not recommended.[7] Some groups maintain the use of steroids as a treatment option (rather than a treatment standard) and to be considered in the clinical setting, arguing that the catastrophic results of SCI may lead to patient preference to receive treatment.[7]

Nontraumatic Causes of Spinal Cord Injury

Although trauma is the leading cause of acute SCI, a myriad of conditions can present similarly. Table 17-1 provides a differential diagnosis for nontraumatic acute SCI.[8] Figure 17-2 illustrates the vascular supply of the spinal cord and tracts. Figure 17-3 illustrates spinal cord syndromes. Table 17-3 further elaborates on spinal cord syndromes. Figure 17-4 illustrates the sympathetic and parasympathetic nervous system.

The symptomatology associated with each process listed in Table 17-1 depends on the spinal cord levels involved and the tracts of the spinal cord involved. For example, neuromyelitis optica (NMO) is an inflammatory disorder of the central nervous system characterized by severe demyelination and axonal damage that predominantly targets the optic nerves and spinal cord.[9] The brain parenchyma tends to be relatively spared in NMO. A common presentation of NMO is with transverse myelitis (TM), an inflammatory spinal cord dysfunction that may involve both gray and white matter. The transverse myelitis of NMO is typically longitudinally extensive (extending across 3 or more contiguous vertebral segments). If the lesion extends from the brainstem or high spinal cord downward, patients may present with quadriplegia and bladder dysfunction, and potentially

TABLE 17-1 Steps in Classifying Spinal Cord Injury, Grades and Definitions

Steps in Classifying Spinal Cord Injury	Grades and Definitions
1. Assess sensory level on both sides for pin prick and light touch.	Sensory Grading: • Absent = 0 • Altered = 1 • Normal = 2
2. Assess motor level on both sides.	Motor Grading: • Total Paralysis = 0 • Palapable or Visible Contractions = 1 • Full ROM with Gravity Eliminated = 2 • Full ROM against gravity = 3 • Full ROM against gravity with moderate resistance = 4 • Full ROM against gravity with full resistance = 5
3. Assess Neurologic Level of Injury (NLI)	• Most caudal segment with Motor Grade ≥ 3 and intact sensation
4. Complete or Incomplete	• Complete if no voluntary anal contraction, S4–S5 sensory grade is absent or 0, and no sensation to deep anal pressure
5. Determine ASIA Impairment Scale	• Grade A = Complete Impairment • Grade B = Sensory Incomplete • Grade C = Motor Incomplete with less than half of key motor functions below NLI have muscle grade ≥ 3 • Grade D = Motor Incomplete with at least half of key motor functions below NLI have grade ≥ 3 • Grade E = normal

ROM = Range of Motion.

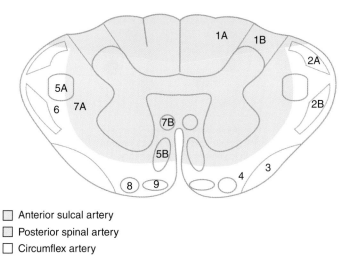

☐ Anterior sulcal artery
☐ Posterior spinal artery
☐ Circumflex artery

FIGURE 17-2 Spinal Cord Vascular Supply Distribution and Tracts. The anterior sulcus artery and the circumflex artery arise from the anterior spinal artery. The afferent or ascending tracts are: The Dorsal Column Medial Meniscus (1A = Gracile Fasciculus and 1B = Cuneatus Fasciculus); 2A = Posterior Spinocerebellar tract; 2B = Anterior Spinocerebellar Tract; 3 = Anterior and lateral spinothalamic tract; and 4 = spino-olivary fibers. The motor or descending tracts are: 5A = lateral corticospinal tract; 5B = anterior corticospinal tract; 6 = rubrospinal tract; 7A and 7B = reticulospinal–tracts; 8 = olivospinal tract; and 9 = vestibulospinal tract.

with respiratory distress because of involvement of the muscles of respiration innervated by the cervical roots.

Acute spinal cord infarction, on the other hand, most often occurs because of occlusion of the anterior spinal artery (ASA).[8] The ASA is fed along its length by radicular arteries, the largest of which is the artery of Adamkiewicz arising from the 9th to 12th intercostal arteries. The artery of Adamkiewicz is an important arterial supply of the ASA's distribution over the lower third of the spinal cord, including the conus medullaris, and is vulnerable to occlusion by aortic aneurysm and aortic repair procedures. Rostral to the artery of Adamkiewicz, there is relatively low collateral flow, making the midthoracic region of the cord particularly vulnerable to systemic hypoperfusion.[8] Other causes of spinal cord infarctions include cardiogenic embolism, aortic dissection, aortic thrombosis, vertebral artery dissection, spinal vascular malformations, or cocaine abuse.[10]

Because the ASA supplies the corticospinal and spinothalamic tracts, while the posterior spinal artery supplies the posterior columns, most patients with a spinal cord infarct will present with flaccidity and loss of reflexes below the level of infarction, and loss or reduction of sensation to pain and temperature, with relative sparing of vibratory and proprioceptive sense. Acute back pain is commonly associated and occurs near the level of infarction.[8]

Certain pathological processes preferentially involve the anterior horn cells of the spinal cord. West Nile virus, for example, can present in a similar way to polio virus, leading to progressive asymmetric weakness over as short a time as 48 hours. This typically occurs in the setting of meningitis or encephalitis. Facial weakness and bulbar symptoms, such as dysphagia or dysarthria, increase the risk for impending respiratory failure. In 1 study, respiratory failure requiring intubation was seen in 38% of patients with West Nile virus–associated paralysis.[11] Amyotrophic

lateral sclerosis (ALS) is a neurodegenerative process that also involves the anterior horn cells, although progression to respiratory failure tends to occur over the course of months to years.

Spinal Cord Injury: Considerations in the Critical Care Setting

Respiratory Compromise

Impairment of ventilatory musculature may lead to acute respiratory compromise and the need for mechanical ventilation. In a study of respiratory failure among patients with cervical SCI, 90% of cases that required mechanical ventilation occurred in the first 3 days after injury.[12]

The primary muscle of inspiration is the diaphragm, which is innervated by the phrenic nerve. The phrenic nerve is derived from the C3 to C5 nerve roots. Accessory muscles of inspiration include the scalenes, external intercostals, clavicular portion of the pectoralis major, and sternocleidomastoids. Muscles of expiration include the abdominal wall muscles and the internal intercostals. Although expiration is normally passive, these muscles are required for forced exhalation, such as is needed to effectively cough.

Injury to the spinal cord above the level of C3 will produce near-total paralysis of ventilation. Patients with injury to the high cervical cord will therefore require immediate mechanical ventilation. Injury from C3 to C5 will produce variable levels of weakness of both the diaphragm and the accessory muscles, and typically also will require intubation.[8,13] In patients with injury below C5, the diaphragm is spared and expiration will occur via passive recoil of the chest wall. However, these patients will still suffer from a weak cough mechanism and are at risk for respiratory fatigue in the setting other systemic

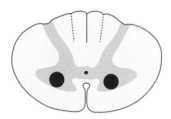

Poliomyelitis:
Lower motor neuron lesions in
anterior horn leading to flaccid paralysis

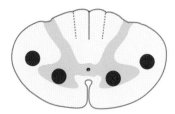

Amyotrophic Lateral Sclerosis:
upper and lower motor neuron
Involvement and no sensory deficit

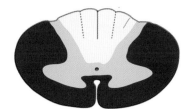

Complete occlusion of
anterior spinal artery

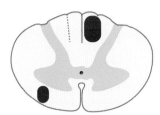

Multiple Sclerosis:
Random asymmetric lesions of the
white matter usually in cervical area
leading to scanning speech, tremor
and nystagmus

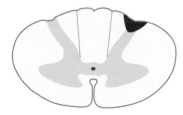

Tabes dorsalis:
Destruction of the fibers at the
posterior root, especially thoracic
and lumbosacral regions causing
stabbing pain, paraesthesias, loss
of pain sensation, and ataxia

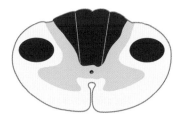

Vitamin B12 deficiency
and Friedreich's ataxia:
Demyelination of dorsal columns,
lateral corticospinal tracts and
spinocerebellar tracts, leading to ataxia,
hyperreflexia, and impaired position
and vibration sense

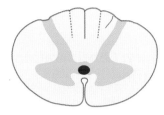

Syringomyelia:
Damage to crossing fibers of the
spinothalamic tract, causing bilateral
loss of pain and temperature sensation

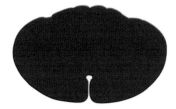

Complete Cord
Transection Syndrome:
Loss of sensation and muscle
movement below the lesion

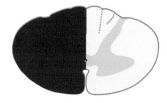

Brown-Sequard Syndrome:
Incomplete spinal cord lesion
resulting in upper motor neuron
paralysis, loss of proprioception,
and contralateral loss of pain
and temperature sensation

FIGURE 17-3 Spinal cord syndromes.[9] (Reprinted with permission from Crout TM, Parks LP, Majithia V. Neuromyelitis optica (Devic's syndrome): an appraisal. *Curr Rheumatol Rep.* 2016;18(8):54.)

TABLE 17-2 Innervation of Respiratory Musculature

Innervation	Muscles of Inspiration
Phrenic nerve (C3–C5)	Diaphragm
C4–C8	Scalenes
Thoracic nerve roots	External intercostals
Spinal accessory nerve	Sternocleidomastoid
Lateral pectoral nerve (C5–C7)	Pectoralis major, clavicular head
	Muscles of Expiration
Lower thoracic, lumbar nerve roots	Abdominal wall muscles
Thoracic nerve roots	Internal intercostals

pulmonary conditions such as pneumonia.[14] Table 17-2 lists the nerve and associated muscle of inspiration and expiration. Figure 17-3 illustrates the spinal cord syndromes, and Table 17-3 lists the spinal cord syndromes, associated tracts, causes, and symptoms.[8,13-15]

Disruption of the Autonomic Nervous System: Neurogenic Shock

The term *spinal shock* refers to sudden and transient suppression of all neural functions below the level of a spinal cord lesion. In this state, a flaccid paralysis of skeletal muscle occurs, and all tendon, cutaneous, and autonomic reflexes are abolished or greatly reduced.[16] *Neurogenic shock* refers to a state of hemodynamic instability following spinal cord injuries, or in some case, severe head trauma.

TABLE 17-3 Spinal Cord Syndromes

Spinal Cord Syndrome	Involved Tracts	Causes	Symptoms
Posterior cord syndrome	Bilateral dorsal columns, corticospinal tracts, descending central autonomic tracts	Multiple sclerosis, subacute combined degeneration, vascular malformations, atlantoaxial subluxation	Dorsal columns: loss of vibration and proprioception, gait ataxia, paresthesias Corticospinal: weakness Autonomic: urinary incontinence
Anterior cord syndrome	Bilateral corticospinal tracts, spinothalamic tracts, descending autonomic tracts	Anterior spinal artery stroke, intervertebral disc herniation	Corticospinal: weakness Spinothalamic: loss of pain and temperature Autonomic: urinary incontinence
Central cord syndrome	Decussating spinothalamic fibers at level of lesion	Syringomyelia, hyperextension injury with underlying cervical spondylosis, intramedullary tumor	Loss of pain and temperature along respective dermatomes Sensation normal above and below lesion
Brown-Sequard syndrome	Unilateral dorsal column, spinothalamic tract, corticospinal tract	Stab wounds, bullet wounds, demyelination	Dorsal columns: ipsilateral loss of vibration and proprioception Spinothalamic: contralateral loss of pain and temperature Corticospinal: ipsilateral weakness
Conus medullaris syndrome	Terminus of spinal cord	Lesions at L1–L2; intervertebral disc herniation, fracture, tumor	Flaccid paralysis of bladder and rectum, impotence, saddle anesthesia, bilateral leg weakness
Cauda equina syndrome	Lumbosacral nerve roots below the conus medullaris: L2–L5, S1–S5	Disc herniation, lumbar spondylosis, epidural abscess, acute or chronic inflammatory demyelinating polyradiculoneuropathy, carcinomatous meningitis, viral infection, Lyme disease, tuberculosis	Low back pain with radiation to legs, bilateral leg weakness and sensory loss to all modalities, bladder and sphincter paralysis

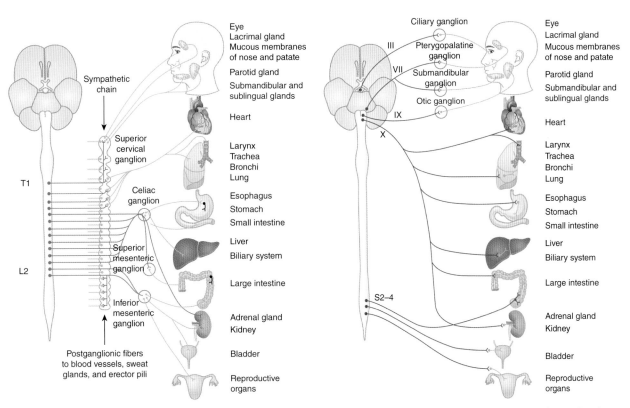

FIGURE 17-4 Sympathetic (left) and parasympathetic (right) nervous system. Sympathetic preganglionic neurons are located within the lateral horns of the T1–L2 spinal segments, and are under tonic excitatory input from descending pathways originating in the medulla. Preganglionic parasympathetic neurons are located in the brainstem and the S2–S4 spinal segments.[20] (Reprinted with permission from Neary D, Crossman AR. *Neuroanatomy: An Illustrated Colour Text*. 5th ed. Edinburgh: Churchill Livingstone; 2015. Internet resource.)

The sympathetic preganglionic neurons are located within the lateral horns of the spinal gray matter of the thoracic and upper lumbar spinal segments (T1–L2). These neurons are under tonic excitatory input from descending pathways originating in the medulla. High spinal cord lesions, especially at the level of the cervical cord or high thoracic cord, may disrupt these sympathoexcitatory fibers leading to alterations in sympathetic and parasympathetic control of cardiovascular dynamics.[17]

Initially after injury, sympathetic hypoactivity occurs. Over time, there is also alteration in morphology of the sympathetic preganglionic neurons, plastic changes within spinal circuits (including sprouting and the formation of inappropriate synaptic connections), and the development of peripheral α-adrenergic receptor hyperresponsiveness.[18]

During the period of sympathetic hypoactivity, there is uninhibited parasympathetic input via an intact vagus nerve. Profound hypotension and persistent bradycardia may occur, which are common features of neurogenic shock. The mainstay of treatment in neurogenic shock is pressor support as needed, as well as maintenance of appropriate blood volume. It is recommended that mean arterial pressure be maintained at a level of at least 85 to 90 mmHg for the first week after acute SCI in order to promote adequate spinal perfusion[19] (the extent and duration of the resulting hypotension is associated with the severity of spinal cord injury, with greater and more complete injuries requiring longer duration of pressor therapy.[17]

Disruption of the Autonomic Nervous System: Autonomic Dysreflexia

Autonomic dysreflexia (AD) refers to the loss of coordinated autonomic response to various cardiovascular demands. Whereas loss of supraspinal sympathoexcitatory pathways can lead to neurogenic shock and chronic low resting blood pressure, AD is a potentially life-threatening condition in which sudden, extreme rises in blood pressure result from uncontrolled surges in sympathetic tone in response to noxious stimuli.[20] Autonomic dysreflexia is typically seen in patients with spinal cord lesions above the level of T6. With a noxious impulse below the level of the lesion, an afferent signal stimulates the sympathetic neurons in the spinal cord in the intermediolateral gray matter. Normal descending inhibitory pathways are unable to pass the level of injury, resulting in widespread vasoconstriction below the level of injury, particularly in the splanchnic vasculature. Peripheral resistance increases, and blood volume that is normally congested is shunted into the systemic circulation. This combination of increased vascular tone and increased volume leads to sudden, potentially dangerous rises in blood pressure, to upwards of 300 mmHg systolic and 200 mmHg diastolic.[20,21] Potentially severe consequences of this rise in blood pressure include intracerebral hemorrhage, retinal detachment, or seizures.

In response to sympathetic drive, intact baroreceptors then activate the parasympathetic response. While there is vasoconstriction below the lesion, parasympathetic response activity results in peripheral vasodilation above the level of

the lesion, which can cause severe headache, sweating, facial flushing, and nasal congestion.[20] This may additionally be accompanied by bradycardia. Arrhythmias such as atrial fibrillation, premature ventricular contractions, and atrioventricular conduction abnormalities have been reported.[20,21]

Although it has been reported, AD is typically not seen in lesions below the level of T6, because intact splanchnic innervation allows for preserved vasodilation of the splanchnic vasculature. Autonomic dysreflexia is most commonly seen in the chronic stages after SCI; however, it has been proposed that early cases of AD are under-recognized. Krossioukov and colleagues reported cases of autonomic dysreflexia occurring as early as 4 days after SCI.[18]

Episodes of AD can be triggered by any noxious stimulus below the level of the spinal cord lesion. The most frequent causes include bladder distention secondary to retention or catheter blockage. Other common triggers include bowel distention, pressure ulcers, hemorrhoids, urinary tract infections, or procedures such as cystoscopy.[20]

DISORDERS OF THE PERIPHERAL NERVE AND MUSCLE

Fundamentals of Nerve Conduction Study and Needle Electromyography

A nerve conduction study (NCS) is divided into motor and sensory nerve responses. Motor responses are known as compound muscle action potentials (CMAP), which represent the summation of all underlying individual muscle fiber action potentials (see Fig. 17-5). The CMAP is a biphasic potential with an initial negativity (upward deflection from the baseline). For each stimulation site, the latency, amplitude, duration, and area of the CMAP are measured. A motor conduction velocity can be calculated after 2 sites, 1 distal and 1 proximal, have been stimulated.

Compound muscle action potential amplitude is measured from the baseline to the negative peak and reflects the number of muscle fibers that depolarize. The latency is

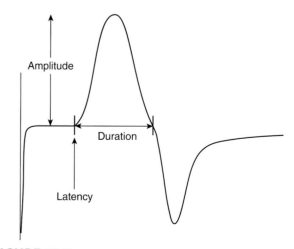

FIGURE 17-5 Compound muscle action potential (CMAP).

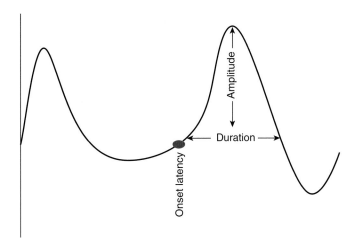

FIGURE 17-6 Sensory nerve action potential (SNAP).

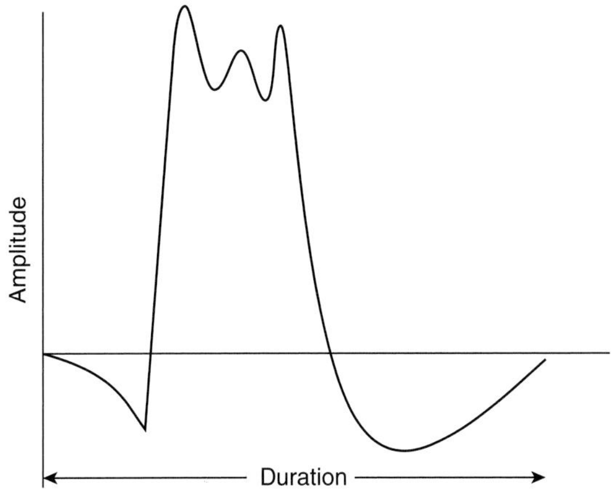

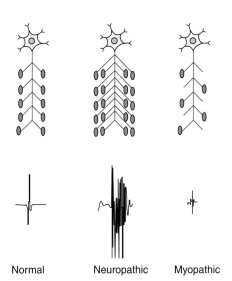

FIGURE 17-7 Motor unit action potential (MUAP).

the time from the stimulus to the initial CMAP deflection from baseline. Duration of CMAP is measured from the initial deflection from the baseline to the first baseline crossing (ie, negative peak duration). Motor conduction velocity is a measure of the speed of the fastest conducting motor axons in the nerve being studied, which is calculated by dividing the distance traveled by the nerve conduction time.

Sensory responses are known as sensory nerve action potentials (SNAP), which represent nerve fiber responses that are much smaller than CMAPs. (Notice in Fig. 17-6 that the scale is on the order of microvolts.) For SNAP, amplitude is measured from the baseline to the negative peak and reflects the sum of all of the individual sensory fibers that depolarize. Duration is measured from the onset of the potential to the first baseline crossing. Onset latency is the time from the stimulus to the initial negative deflection from baseline. Peak latency is measured at the midpoint of the first negative peak.

After a nerve conduction study is completed, then needle electromyography (EMG) proceeds to evaluate motor unit action potentials (MUAPs), which are assessed for morphology (duration, amplitude, phases), stability, and firing characteristics. The pattern of MUAP abnormalities will allow a determination of whether a disorder is primarily neuropathic or myopathic and often helps determine the time course (acute vs chronic) and severity of the lesion.

Motor unit action potential amplitude reflects those muscle fibers very close to the needle and is measured from peak to peak (see Fig. 17-7). Duration is measured as the time from initial deflection of the MUAP from baseline to its final return to baseline; it is the parameter that best reflects the number of muscle fibers in the motor unit. Phases can be counted by the number of baseline crossings and adding 1. The major spike is the largest positive-to-negative deflection; satellite potentials may occur after the main potential and usually represent early reinnervation of muscle fibers.

Normal MUAPs have 2 to 4 phases. In chronic neuropathic lesions after reinnervation, the number of muscle fibers per motor unit increases, resulting in long duration,

high-amplitude, and polyphasic MUAPs (see Figs. 17-7 and 17-8).

In myopathies or in neuromuscular junction disorders with block, the number of functional muscle fibers in the motor unit decreases, leading to short duration, small amplitude, and polyphasic MUAPs.

Phrenic Neuropathy

Phrenic neuropathy may occur in isolation secondary to surgery or tumor or may occur in diabetic generalized neuropathy.[22] Diagnosis of phrenic neuropathy can be made with a combination of clinical symptoms (eg, severe dyspnea and orthopnea), chest imaging findings, and respiratory electrodiagnostic results.[23] Criteria for diagnosis of phrenic neuropathy may include (1) amplitude of the phrenic nerve CMAP

Normal   Neuropathic   Myopathic

FIGURE 17-8 Motor unit action potential (MUAP) morphologies. (Reprinted with permission from Preston DC, Shapiro BE. *Electromyography and Neuromuscular Disorders: Clinical-Electrophysiological Correlations*, 4th edition. London: Elsevier Butterworth-Heinemann; 2013. Internet resource.)

of 0.2 mV or less (our lower reference limit: 0.46 mV); (2) denervation activity, severe reduction of MUP recruitment, or pronounced signs of diaphragm reinnervation on needle electromyography (EMG); (3) elevated position and reduced or paradoxical respiratory motility of the diaphragm on imaging studies; and (4) absent neuropathic changes in muscles innervated by similar spinal segments as the diaphragm.[23]

Acute Inflammatory Demyelinating Polyradiculoneuropathy

Acute inflammatory demyelinating polyradiculoneuropathy (AIDP), also known as Guillain-Barré syndrome, is an immune-mediated cause of flaccid paralysis with areflexia. The pathophysiology of AIDP results from an immune-mediated response to a preceding infection, which cross-reacts with neural tissue in the peripheral nervous system. Approximately two-thirds of patients provide a history of preceding upper respiratory or gastrointestinal illness.[24] The most commonly identified organism is *Campylobacter jejuni*. Acute inflammatory demyelinating polyradiculoneuropathy has also occurred in association with human immunodeficiency virus (HIV), Epstein-Barr virus (EBV), cytomegalovirus (CMV), West Nile virus, and most recently, the Zika virus. A small percentage of patients develop AIDP after immunization or surgery.

Classically, patients present with ascending, symmetric muscle weakness that begins in the legs, often accompanied by paresthesias and reduced or absent reflexes. Symptoms typically progress over 2 weeks, with maximal weakness occurring by 4 weeks in more than 90% of patients. Symptoms can start in the arms or the face in about 10% of patients.[25] Because AIDP involves the nerve roots, lumbar back pain and radiculopathic pain are also frequent early symptoms. Of note, early in the disease course, reflexes may be present, and the appearance of areflexia may only occur days into the illness.[26]

Cranial nerve deficits are present in nearly half of patients with AIDP. The most common cranial nerve finding is bilateral facial weakness, followed by oropharyngeal weakness and ophthalmoparesis. In severe cases, laryngeal weakness can be seen, resulting in vocal cord paralysis and a much higher risk of aspiration.[26]

The hallmark finding in cerebrospinal fluid (CSF) analysis in AIDP is *albuminocytologic dissociation*, in which high protein content is seen in the absence of pleocytosis. This finding is supportive of the diagnosis but is not required. Cerebrospinal fluid may be normal in the early stages of the disease, so repeat lumbar puncture should be considered if clinical suspicion is high. The finding of greater than 50 cells/mm^3 should suggest an alternative diagnosis, such as West Nile virus infection–related flaccid paralysis, Lyme infection, or CMV-related radiculitis.[26]

Electrodiagnostic studies such as electromyography and nerve conduction studies can also be useful in the diagnostic evaluation. Electrophysiologic changes are most pronounced around 2 weeks from symptom onset, so a normal study does not rule out AIDP if performed early.[27] Electromyography and NCS are nevertheless often performed soon after presentation, as they serve an important role in ruling out other causes of progressive weakness, such as spinal cord disease or myopathic disorders. Common early electrodiagnostic findings include prolonged or absent F-waves, prolonged or absent H-reflexes, sensory response abnormalities that spare the sural nerves, and reduced motor recruitment on needle EMG. Demyelinating features, such as conduction block or temporal dispersion, are more common weeks after presentation, and have much greater specificity for diagnosis.[28]

Several variants of the classic form of AIDP exist. Antibodies to gangliosides have been implicated in AIDP and its variants (Table 17-4).[28]

TABLE 17-4 Variants of Acute Inflammatory Demyelinating Polyradiculoneuropathy and Associated Antibodies[79]

Name	Symptoms and Findings	Antibodies
Acute motor axonal neuropathy (AMAN)	Pure motor weakness, distal > proximal; face and respiratory system less frequently involved EMG/NCS shows axonal involvement and sparing of sensory potentials	GM1, GM1b, GD1a, GalNac-GD1a
Acute motor and sensory axonal neuropathy (AMSAN)	More severe form of AMAN with greater sensory symptoms EMG/NCS shows motor and sensory axonal loss	GM1
Miller Fisher syndrome (MFS)	Classic triad: ophthalmoplegia, ataxia, areflexia May also see extremity weakness	GQ1b
Bickerstaff encephalitis	Brainstem encephalitis, cranial nerve involvement (ophthalmoplegia, facial diplegia, bulbar weakness), extremity weakness May resemble MFS, with encephalopathic features	GQ1b
Pharyngeal-cervical-brachial weakness	Oropharyngeal weakness, neck weakness, arm > leg weakness, bulbar weakness	GQ1b (common with MFS overlap), GT1a, GM1b

EMG = electromyography; NCS = nerve conduction study.

In patients with AIDP, immune therapy with IV immunoglobulin (IVIG) or plasma exchange show comparable efficacy in reducing the rate of mechanical ventilation at 2 weeks, decreasing the time to walking, and improving the level of disability at 4 weeks.[26] Both therapies are most effective when initiated within 2 weeks of symptom onset. In clinical practice, IVIG is typically utilized prior to plasma exchange because IVIG does not require invasive line treatment and is therefore expected to have fewer systemic side effects. The combination of plasma exchange and IVIG is no more effective than either treatment alone, which is likely related to the fact that if IVIG precedes plasma exchange and the process of plasma exchange will effectively filter out the active immunoglobulins in IVIG. There is no role for high-dose steroids in the treatment of AIDP.[26]

Respiratory failure occurs in approximately 25% of patients with AIDP.[29] Clinical aspects that are associated with a greater risk of respiratory failure include rapid symptom progression, greater severity of appendicular weakness, and presence of bulbar or facial weakness.[29] These features warrant ICU admission for close monitoring, as diaphragmatic failure can develop rapidly. Serial measurements of forced vital capacity (FVC) and negative inspiratory force (NIF) are helpful in monitoring patients who may progress to needing mechanical ventilation. An FVC of less than 20 mL/kg, an NIF of less than −30 cm H_2O, or a reduction by 30% or more on serial measurements is associated with progression to respiratory failure and should warrant consideration for intubation.[26,29] Of note, in patients with facial weakness, a weak labial seal during pulmonary function testing may give unreliable measurements, so these values should only be interpreted in conjunction with the clinical context.

Dysautonomia is a major feature of severe AIDP, often seen in those patients who develop respiratory failure or severe weakness. The most common manifestation of dysautonomia is sinus tachycardia, but also seen are paroxysmal changes in blood pressure, urinary retention, gastroparesis, and ileus.[26] Other arrhythmias such as atrioventricular block, ventricular tachycardia, and even asystole have been reported to occur in AIDP.[30]

Critical Illness Myopathy and Polyneuropathy

Acquired neuromuscular disorders in the ICU commonly manifest as either acute myopathy associated with intravenous corticosteroids and neuromuscular junction blocking agents (also known as critical illness myopathy [CIM] or axonal sensorimotor polyneuropathy (also known as critical illness polyneuropathy [CIP]).[31] Both can contribute to difficulty weaning off the ventilator. Critical illness myopathy manifests as flaccid weakness, proximal more than distal. It can be diffuse with limb muscles, neck flexors, facial muscles, and diaphragm, and tendon reflexes are normal or depressed.[31] Pathology shows selective myosin loss and, therefore, muscle atrophy.

Risk factors are IV glucocorticoids, neuromuscular blockers, renal failure, hyperglycemia, and systemic inflammatory response syndrome (SIRS).[31-35] Most of these patients are difficult to wean from the ventilator.[31] Nerve conduction studies show low-amplitude, sometimes broad or absent CMAPs with relatively preserved SNAPs. Patients exposed to neuromuscular blockers may show features of prolonged NMJ blockage via repetitive nerve stimulation (RNS), especially during the week of discontinuation of the paralytic agent.[31] Needle electromyography will demonstrate fibrillation potentials and positive sharp waves in limb muscles in some, but not all, patients.[34] Fifty percent of patients have elevated creatine kinase with peak 4 days after initiation of glucocorticoid therapy and can last for 2 weeks.

Muscle biopsy should be considered if an inflammatory myopathy is suspected or if the histologic findings may affect management; in addition, it may help differentiate critical illness myopathy from a neurogenic disorder, but often a definitive pathologic diagnosis cannot be made.[32]

Critical illness polyneuropathy manifests in the setting of SIRS and is often preceded by septic encephalopathy.[36] It is hypothesized that there is injury to microcirculation of nerves. Patients have flaccid weakness of extremities, decreased limb response to painful stimuli. In more alert patients, there may be evidence of distal loss sensation to light touch, temperature, vibration, and pain, and deep tendon reflexes are usually reduced or absent but may be normal.[35] Nerve conduction studies show reductions in CMAP and SNAP amplitudes.[36] The decline in CMAP amplitude usually occurring within 2 weeks of onset of SIRS and before other electrophysiologic signs and a decrease in SNAP amplitudes.[37]

Managing CIM and CIP risk factors helps to prevent ICU-associated weakness. Specifically, aggressive treatment of sepsis is considered to be a cornerstone in the prevention of ICU-associated weakness. Insulin treatment aimed at normalizing hyperglycemia significantly reduced the incidence of electrophysiological signs of CIP/CIM and the need for prolonged mechanical ventilation in long-stay medical and surgical ICU patients.[38]

Another important target is reducing the duration of immobilization. Early mobilization and occupational therapy within 72 hours of initiation of mechanical ventilation, in addition to daily sedation interruption, improved outcome, including functional status, although the incidence of ICU-associated weakness was not reduced.[39] Parenteral nutrition within 7 days of ICU stay is also thought to be a risk factor for CIP.[38,40]

Most patients recover from ICU-associated weakness within months, reaching a plateau at around 1 year, as supported by a prospective study of ARDS patients with longest follow-up at 2 years.[41] Several small prospective studies have shown evidence of worse prognosis of CIP than of CIM,[42-45] as patients with CIM might recover more quickly and completely, whereas coexistent CIP possibly impedes recovery.[38]

DISORDERS OF THE NEUROMUSCULAR JUNCTION

Myasthenia Gravis

Myasthenia gravis (MG) is an autoimmune disorder targeting postsynaptic acetylcholine receptors (AChR) of the neuromuscular junction.[46] Myasthenia gravis will commonly present with fluctuating skeletal muscle weakness, usually with normal muscle bulk. Weakness may present with ocular symptoms or facial, oropharyngeal, or respiratory muscle weakness at the onset of illness. Ocular symptoms may manifest as fluctuating blurred vision or frank diplopia, usually not present immediately upon awakening. Diplopia occurs initially during lateral or upward gaze, and it typically worsens in the evening and resolves if 1 eye is closed (binocular diplopia). Other ocular symptoms include gaze paresis due to eye muscle weakness and asymmetric painless ptosis. Facial muscle weakness usually occurs together with ocular involvement and commonly involves the orbicularis oculi and orbicularis oris muscles, presenting as weak eyelid closure and inability to suck up liquid through a straw, respectively. Oropharyngeal muscle weakness may manifest as slurred speech, difficulty with chewing, and dysphagia. Respiratory muscle weakness presents as difficulty breathing, and a patient with MG who cannot maintain a patent airway is thought to be in myasthenic crisis.[47] Myasthenia gravis is largely a clinical diagnosis; when suspected, immunological confirmation with AChR binding antibody test and/or muscle-specific tyrosine kinase (MuSK) antibodies (if AChR antibodies are negative) should be performed. When serum antibodies are positive for MG in the context of supportive clinical history and neurological physical examination, it is usually not necessary to confirm the diagnosis with EMG. However, if EMG is performed, the results will demonstrate decremental responses with repetitive nerve stimulation.

Myasthenic crisis is considered a true neurological emergency defined by severe weakness of the bulbar and/or respiratory muscles causing respiratory failure that necessitates intubation and ventilatory support.[46] Myasthenic crisis affects 20% to 30% of myasthenic patients, usually within the first year of illness[48] and may be the first presentation of MG.[49] Confirmation of a diagnosis of MG may be done with electrophysiological testing with repetitive nerve stimulation (single-fiber EMG being the most specific, although it is less commonly available) where a compound muscle action potential decrement of 10% or more is characteristically seen; however, in patients with the ocular form of MG, repetitive nerve stimulation studies are often normal. Other confirmatory tests include pharmacologic testing with edrophonium and serological testing. A majority of MG patients will have circulating antibodies to the AChR; amongst the AChR antibody subtypes—binding, blocking, and modulating—binding AChR antibodies are the most useful. The remaining MG patients will demonstrate antibodies against MuSK. Myasthenia gravis is

also associated with other antibodies that recognize skeletal muscle proteins, such as titin and ryanodine, but their role in disease pathogenesis is unclear. A chest computed tomography (CT) scan may be needed to confirm the presence of a thymoma.[49] Thymomas occur in about 15% of adult patients with MG.[50] All MG patients with a thymoma have elevated serum AChR antibodies; almost all have skeletal muscle antibodies in their sera, but up to one-third of MG patients with skeletal muscle antibodies do not have a thymoma.[51] The presence of non-AChR skeletal muscle antibodies is highly predictive of a thymoma in patients under the age of 45 to 50 years.[52]

Predisposing factors to MG crisis are respiratory infection (40%), emotional stresses, microaspirations (10%), changes in medication regimen (8%), surgery, or trauma.[49] Arterial blood gas analysis may show hypercarbia before hypoxia.[49] The 20/30/40 rule (FCV < 20 mL/kg or < 1 Liter; more positive than NIF −30 cm H_2O [or −20 cm H_2O]; and PEP < 40 cm H_2O) is probably the most helpful guide for a decision on intubation.[49] Immunotherapy is considered standard of care for patients with myasthenic crisis and may consist of plasma exchange (PLEX), human IVIG, and/or corticosteroids (Table 17-5). Initial administration of high-dose prednisone (typically greater than a 40 mg/d dose) may exacerbate symptoms.[53] This occurs because prednisone has a direct and initially adverse effect on the neuromuscular junction.[47] Myasthenic patients who are being initiated with prednisone treatment should be monitored closely.

TABLE 17-5 Treatment of Myasthenia Gravis

Type of Treatment	Characteristics
Plasmapharesis	• Rapid immunotherapy for acute exacerbation • 5-day course or every other day for 10 d
Intravenous immunoglobulins	• 400 mg/kg body weight for 5 d or 1 g/kg/d for 2 d
Prednisone	• 1–1.5 mg/kg body weight daily
Pyridostigmine	• 30 mg PO TID and titrated to effect (max 120 mg every 4 h) • Onset 15–30 min with peak at 2 h • SE cramping, increased bronchial secretions, salivation, bradycardia, weakness from cholinergic crisis usually if >120 mg every 4 h • Adjunct administration to relieve SE include: glycopyrrolate, propantheline, hyoscyamine
Thymectomy	• Especially in patients symptomatic after medical treatment • Avoid thymectomy if > 60 y of age unless thymoma present
Adjunct Immunomodulation	• Azathioprine, mycophenolate mofetil, cyclosporine, cyclophosphamide

TABLE 17-6 Drugs That Adversely Affect Myasthenia Gravis

Name of Drug or Toxin
Adrenocorticosteroids and ACTH
• Thyroid preparations
• Neuromuscular blocking agents (including botulinum toxin)
• Anesthetic agents (including alcohol)
• Magnesium salts
• Epsom salts,
• Quinidine, procainamide, phenytoin, gabapentin, verapamil, intravenous lidocaine, or procaine,
• Gentamicin, tobramycin, neomycin, paromomycin, amikacin, kanamycin, streptomycin,
• Polymyxin B, colistin,
• chlortetracycline, oxytetracycline, tetracycline, demeclocycline, metacycline, doxycycline, minocycline,
• Clindamycin, lincomycin, ciprofloxacin, high-dose ampicillin, intravenous erythromycin, cocaine, cimetidine, chloroquine, diazepam, lithium, quinine, beta-blockers, trihexyphenidyl hydrochloride, gemfibrozil

Certain medications also can induce or adversely affect myasthenia gravis, as seen in Table 17-6.[47]

Lambert-Eaton Myasthenic Syndrome

Lambert-Eaton myasthenic syndrome (LEMS) is another autoimmune disorder that targets the neuromuscular junction, resulting in antibodies against presynaptic voltage gated calcium channel (VGCC) receptors of the P/Q-type.[54] The VGCCs trigger the fusion of acetylcholine-containing vesicles with the plasma membrane; anti-VGCC antibodies thus inhibit this function and reduce the amount of acetylcholine released from the presynaptic terminal, resulting in reduced strength of the muscle contraction.[54] Measuring anti-VGCC antibodies can help confirm diagnosis with associated clinical and electrophysiologic characteristics but in isolation can be found in amyotrophic lateral sclerosis, myasthenia gravis, scleroderma, and malignancy.[54] Lambert-Eaton myasthenic syndrome can be a paraneoplastic process usually associated with small-cell lung carcinoma (SCLC); therefore, screening for underlying lung malignancy is of utmost importance.[55]

Clinical manifestations of LEMS include symmetric proximal limb weakness, loss of tendon reflexes, and autonomic dysfunction owing to its involvement in acetylcholine release at the level of the nicotinic synapse of the sympathetic nervous system.[54] Characteristic electrophysiological patterns seen in LEMS include normal CMAP at rest, a decremental response in fatigable muscles with 3-Hz repetitive stimulation (NCS) and partial repair of the decrement after the third or fourth stimulus, resulting in a U-shaped curve.[56] In addition, post-activation facilitation may be observed after 30 to 60 seconds following muscle contraction, usually in the range of 10% to 25% and occasionally greater than 50%.[57] Single-fiber EMG is a sensitive test, but it cannot distinguish between MG and LEMS, as both groups demonstrate increased jitter, and as mentioned above, single-fiber EMG is becoming less commonly available in clinical practice.

The first-line medication used for symptomatic treatment of LEMS is 3,4-diaminopyridine, a molecule that blocks presynaptic voltage-gated potassium channels and provides a prolonged action potential, which increases the amount of acetylcholine released.[58] If there is limited response to 3,4-diaminopyridine, immunosuppressive treatments such as prednisolone and azathioprine must be considered, although other less well-studied drugs such as mycophenolate mofetil, cyclosporine, and rituximab are also used in the treatment of LEMS.[59] It is important to note that 3,4-diaminopyridine may not be available at pharmacies, or at every medical institution; it is a drug only available through specific compassionate-use protocols at select centers.

Cholinergic Crisis

Cholinergic crisis may result from an excess intake/exposure to AChE inhibitors, such as oral pyridostigmine or organophosphate (OP) poisoning/toxin ingestion (from insecticide or rodenticide).[60] Cholinergic crisis in the setting of MG crisis is uncommon and typically acetylcholinesterase inhibitors are significantly lowered or discontinued in MG crisis to avoid excessive pulmonary secretions in the setting of respiratory distress.[61] Organophosphate compounds inhibit esterase enzymes, in particular, AChE and butyrylcholinesterase (BuChE). Inhibition results in excessive acetylcholine and cholinergic overstimulation within the peripheral, central, and autonomic (both parasympathetic and sympathetic) nervous systems and tissues.[62] People exposed to organophosphate insecticides often give off a strong chemical smell from their breath and their clothes.[63]

Symptoms include miosis, sweating, lacrimation, salivation, increased pulmonary secretions, bronchospasm, nausea, vomiting, increased urination, diarrhea, and bradycardia. Management begins with decontamination with activated charcoal, which works best when given within 1 hour of ingestion. Medication includes atropine, which is an acetylcholine antagonist in the muscarine receptors, and pralidoxime, a cholinesterase reacting agent that treats nicotine and muscarinic symptoms. Atropine is started at 2 to 5 mg IV and doubled every 3 to 5 minutes until respiratory secretions are cleared and bronchoconstriction improves. Pralidoxime is usually given concomitantly with atropine. In adults, there is an initial slow bolus of 30 mL/kg over 30 minutes followed by 8 mg/kg/h. Infusion can last for days.

With organophosphate poisoning, there are 2 other associated neurologic disorders: intermediate syndrome and organophosphorus agent–induced delayed neuropathy. The intermediate syndrome occurs 24 to 96 hours after OP insecticide exposure and consists of weakness or paralysis of the respiratory muscles, proximal limb muscles, neck flexors, and motor cranial nerves in the absence of cholinergic symptoms.[63] It is typically unresponsive to increases in atropine dose in the absence of muscarinic signs.[63] Supportive care is necessary and red blood cell acetylcholinesterase levels directly correlate to improvement. Organophosphorus agent–induced delayed neuropathy involves neuropathy target esterase inhibition resulting in stocking glove paresthesias followed by lower extremity weakness ascending to upper extremities.

Botulism

Botulism is a severe neuroparalytic disease caused by the action of the botulinum neurotoxins (BoNTs) produced by anaerobic spore-forming *Clostridium botulinum* and others. There are 4 forms of botulism (foodborne, infant, wound, and animal) that can cause acute weakness of muscles, resulting in difficulty speaking and swallowing, with diplopia and blurred vision in all 4 forms.[64] This is followed by progressive, descending symmetric flaccid paralysis starting from the head and throat that does not affect mental status.[64] Botulism is confirmed by detection of BoNT in a patient's serum or stool or in a sample of food consumed before onset of illness.[65] Infant botulism has been the most diagnosed form of botulism since 1979[66] with source of spores arising from honey or environmental exposure.[67,68] Treatment with antitoxin should be instituted early in the course of illness; available antitoxins are equine antitoxin from the Centers for Disease Control (neutralizing antibodies against BoNT types A, B, and E) and heptavalent (against types A, B, C, D, E, F, and G) antitoxin.[69] More than 80% of patients with adult botulism are treated with antitoxin, but approximately 9% of those patients develop hypersensitivity reactions. Use of equine-derived antitoxin for treatment of food-borne botulism produced a 36% decrease in mortality when given within 24 hours of symptom onset, and a 31% decrease in mortality when given after 24 hours of symptom onset, compared to patients not receiving antitoxin. A shorter median number of days of hospitalization was associated with antitoxin use (56 days if no antitoxin, 41 days if antitoxin infused > 24 hours after symptom onset, 10 days if antitoxin infused < 24 hours after symptom onset).[70]

BabyBIG, derived from the blood of human donors vaccinated with a pentavalent (against types A, B, C, D, and E) toxoid vaccine, is only available for infant botulism.[71] The prognosis for infantile botulism is excellent, largely in part to the availability of immunoglobulin; the fatality rate is less than 2% for all cases. Recovery is progressive as the motor end plates regenerate. Diaphragmatic function tends to recover before peripheral muscles fully recover, allowing discontinuation of mechanical ventilation earlier in the recovery process.[72,73] Neurologic sequelae are rarely seen in infantile botulism, although persistent hypotonia to some degree may still be present at time of discharge.[72]

QUESTIONS

1. A 34-year-old woman presents with progressive weakness in all 4 limbs that reaches a nadir after 8 hours. She is taken to the emergency room, where her husband reports she had complained of neck and back pain earlier in the day. She has flaccid paralysis of all 4 limbs. She is areflexic. She is dysarthric, is pooling secretions, and is intubated for airway protection. Her MRI demonstrates T2 hyperintensity spanning the rostral medulla to the level of T4, which diffusion restricts. Upon directed questioning, her husband also mentions that she has a history of recent vision impairment, of unclear etiology. What is the most likely diagnosis?

   A. Neuromyelitis optica
   B. Anterior spinal artery infarct
   C. Acute inflammatory demyelinating polyradiculoneuropathy
   D. West Nile virus–associated flaccid paralysis

2. After 6 days, the blood pressure (BP) of the patient in question 1 suddenly increases to 260/145 mmHg, with a heart rate of 46 beats/min. She is noted to have facial flushing and diaphoresis. What is the next best step in management?

   A. Anticoagulation for suspected new stroke
   B. Immediate nicardipine drip
   C. Assessment for urinary retention or constipation
   D. Lumbar puncture

3. A 29-year-old man presents to the emergency department (ED) with a 2-day history of progressive weakness in his legs, first noted by dragging his feet and later by having difficulty with climbing up stairs. He recalls having abrupt onset lower back pain prior to the weakness, but he denies trauma. He denies recent infection. Examination shows moderate bilateral facial weakness, dysarthric speech, and weakness of the ankles and hip flexors. Deep tendon reflexes are intact and normal. What is the most likely diagnosis?

   A. Radiculopathy secondary to herniated disk
   B. Transverse myelitis of the thoracic cord
   C. Acute inflammatory demyelinating polyradiculoneuropathy
   D. Amyotrophic lateral sclerosis

4. For the patient in question 3, what is the next step?

   A. Lumbar puncture
   B. MRI
   C. Electromyography and nerve conduction studies
   D. Measurement of forced vital capacity and negative inspiratory pressure

5. A 29-year-old man presents to the ED after a suicide attempt by ingesting a large amount of rat poison, which according to emergency medical services (EMS), occurred just prior to arrival. His friend is not sure what brand of rodenticide is ingested, but he states that he purchased the toxin at a small, independent neighborhood corner store. In the ED, he is diaphoretic and in moderate

respiratory distress. His vital signs are significant for a heart rate of 100 beats/min, a respiratory rate of 28 breaths/min, and oxygen saturation of 88% on room air. Initially, he is awake but appeared to be confused. He is moving all extremities with some muscle fasciculations. He has urinated on himself and his pupils are 2 mm and nonreactive to light. His toxicology screen is negative and his coagulation profile is normal. His electrocardiogram shows sinus tachycardia. Fifteen minutes later, he deteriorates rapidly with development of excessive salivation and subsequent respiratory failure. What is the next best action(s)?

A. Administration of IV lorazepam followed by intubation then placement of nasogastric tube for gastric lavage

B. Administration of IV lorazepam followed by intubation then administration of IV atropine and pralidoxime and then placement of nasogastric tube for gastric lavage

C. Decontamination with exposure of the body and washing with soap and water

D. None of the above

6. A 34-year-old woman presents to the ED after several weeks of progressive difficulty with speaking and swallowing. She tells you that in the last 2 days, she has trouble finishing her sentences, and when she eats, food spills out of her mouth. She has also noticed that her left eyelid is droopy and has also been experiencing fluctuating blurry vision. On exam, there is dysarthria with left-sided facial paresis (weak eyelid closure and asymmetric smile) and dysconjugate gaze. Pulmonary function tests are normal. An EMG is ordered. Upon completing urgent electrodiagnostic testing at the bedside, you review the data shown in Figure 17-9 from trapezius-accessory nerve (CN XI) system 3-Hz repetitive nerve stimulation portion of the patient's nerve conduction studies. What is the most significant diagnostic finding from the above 3-Hz repetitive nerve stimulation data?

A. The 3-Hz RNS demonstrates little or no decrement of the compound muscle action potential.

B. The 3-Hz RNS demonstrates a diagnostic decrement of 10% or more of the compound muscle action potential.

C. The 3-Hz RNS demonstrates postexercise exhaustion.

D. The 3-Hz RNS demonstrates postexercise increment.

7. Which of the following statements is true regarding myasthenia gravis and pregnancy?

A. Myasthenia gravis typically improves after delivery.

B. Myasthenic weakness does not affect progression of labor.

C. Standard drugs used to treat MG, such as anticholinesterase medications or prednisone, should be avoided during pregnancy.

D. Pregnancy does not worsen the long-term outcome of MG.

Baseline:

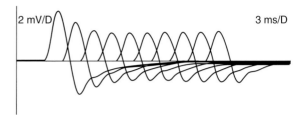

2 mV/D   3 ms/D

Immediately after 10 s of exercise:

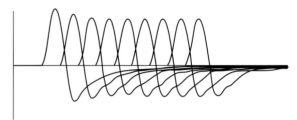

Three minutes after 60 s of exercise:

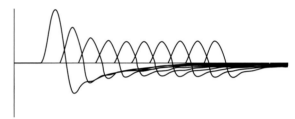

FIGURE 17-9 A 3-Hz repetitive nerve stimulation test in a woman with subacute onset dysphagia, dysarthria, and ptosis. (A) Baseline. (B) Immediately after 10 seconds of exercise. (C) Three minutes after 60 seconds of exercise. (Reprinted with permission from Preston DC, Shapiro BE. *Electromyography and Neuromuscular Disorders: Clinical-Electrophysiological Correlations*, 4th edition. London: Elsevier Butterworth-Heinemann; 2013. Internet resource.)

ANSWERS

1. A. Neuromyelitis optica

Neuromyelitis optica is an immune-mediated inflammatory disorder of the central nervous system characterized by severe demyelination and axonal damage that predominantly targets the optic nerves and spinal cord. A common presentation of NMO is with transverse myelitis. The transverse myelitis of NMO is typically longitudinally extensive (extending across 3 or more contiguous vertebral segments). Neuromyelitis optica typically affects women, and the median age of onset is in the fourth decade of life.[9] Acute spinal cord infarct (choice B) and transverse myelitis can present similarly. However, given the patient's age and lack of identified vascular risk factors, acute spinal cord infarct is less likely. In addition, the explicit mention of recent visual deficits raises a concern for pathology encompassing more than just the spinal cord (ie, NMO).

Like cerebral infarcts, spinal cord infarcts and the resulting spinal shock have an abrupt onset, but less commonly can occur rapidly over minutes to a few hours. Transverse myelitis typically progresses over hours to days. Patients may complain of local back or neck pain in both infarct and TM.[8,9] Although diffusion restriction is seen in strokes, it can also be seen in TM. Similar to cerebral infarcts, spinal cord infarcts tend to occur in older patients with cardiovascular risk factors. The temporal progression of the patient's symptoms, as well as her age and medical history, make NMO the most likely diagnosis. The lack of prodromal viral illness makes AIDP and West Nile virus less likely (choices C and D).

2. **C. Assessment for urinary retention or constipation**

Autonomic dysreflexia may occur from any spinal cord lesion above T6. Although it most commonly occurs in the chronic setting after spinal cord injury, it can also occur acutely.[18] Sudden elevation in blood pressure, with associated bradycardia, diaphoresis, headache, and facial flushing are common. It is caused by noxious stimuli below the level of the spinal cord lesion, which in the majority of cases is secondary to bladder distention, bowel distention, or pressure ulcers.[20] Episodes of AD can be prevented by adequate skin, bowel, and urinary care. Treatment is aimed first at removing the trigger. Treatment with antihypertensive agents (choice B) should be reserved for circumstances in which treating the underlying cause does not correct the blood pressure. Treatment should be conservative, as the autonomic dysfunction can lead to severe overcorrection. While hypertension can occur in the setting of a new stroke, there are no new focal findings to suspect an infarct (choice A). Lumbar puncture has no role in management in this case (choice D).

3. **C. Acute inflammatory demyelinating polyradiculoneuropathy**

Only two-thirds of patients with AIDP report antecedent viral prodrome, so the absence of this history does not rule out AIDP.[24] Additionally, deep tendon reflexes may be normal in the early phase of the disease.[26] While radiculopathy or transverse myelitis could potentially explain his lower extremity symptoms, these would not explain the described bulbar symptoms, including facial weakness (choices A and B). Acute inflammatory demyelinating polyradiculoneuropathy commonly affects the cranial nerves, with facial diplegia being the most frequent manifestation.[26] Amyotrophic lateral sclerosis (choice D) can produce dysarthric speech and bulbar weakness but tends to occur in older patients and progress over months to years. In addition, a strong clinical suspicion of ALS requires the presence of both upper and lower motor neuron findings on examination, and there is no mention of upper motor neuron findings in this case (eg, hyperreflexia, spasticity).

4. **D. Measurement of forced vital capacity and negative inspiratory pressure**

The patient's facial weakness and the presence of bulbar symptoms (dysarthria) are concerning for impending respiratory failure.[28] Serial monitoring of FVC and NIF will help guide the need for intubation. An FVC of less than 20 mL/kg, an NIF of less negative than –30 cm H_2O, or a reduction in either parameter by 30% or more on serial measurements are indications for intubation.[26] Note should be made if the patient is able to form a tight lip seal during pulmonary function testing, as facial diplegia may give falsely low results. While the finding of albuminocytologic dissociation by lumbar puncture is helpful in the diagnosis of AIDP (choice A), and MRI and EMG are often obtained to rule out other conditions such as transverse myelitis (choices B and C), the most important *next* step for this patient is to ensure stability of his respiratory status.

5. **B. Administration of IV lorazepam followed by intubation then administration of IV atropine and pralidoxime and then placement of nasogastric tube for gastric lavage**

The vignette refers to a case report in which an illegal rodenticide sold in the United States, called *Tres Pasitos* (Spanish for "three little steps," referring to the number of steps the mice take before dying), was used in a suicide attempt. The active ingredient in Tres Pasitos is aldicarb, which is a potent inhibitor of human cholinesterase, resulting in autonomic dysfunction and CNS toxicity. After stabilization of the airway, breathing, and circulation, and recognition of possible organophosphate exposure/toxin ingestion, treatment involves blockade of acetylcholine effects at both muscarinic and nicotinic receptors. Atropine provides inhibition of muscarinic receptors in both the central and peripheral systems; pralidoxime reverses both nicotinic and muscarinic toxicity and markedly increases the regeneration of acetylcholinesterase. In addition to treatment with reversal agents, the patient should be decontaminated, as aldicarb is rapidly absorbed through the skin; gastric lavage with airway protection should be utilized as well.[28,74] Choices A, C, and D are wrong.

6. **B. The 3-Hz RNS demonstrates a diagnostic decrement of 10% or more of the compound muscle action potential.**

In normal subjects, slow frequency RNS (3 Hz) results in little or no decrement in CMAP at baseline, whereas in myasthenia gravis, a CMAP decrement of 10% or more is characteristically seen at baseline. If a CMAP decrement is present at baseline, one should test for postexercise facilitation (seen in the second tracing), or repair of decrement following a 10-second maximum isometric contraction with slow RNS study. In addition, if a CMAP decrement is present at baseline, one should look for postexercise exhaustion (seen in the third tracing), in which a similarly significant decrement develops.[50] Postexercise increment is a finding seen in Lambert-Eaton

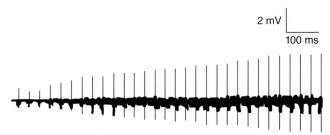

FIGURE 17-10 Characteristic increment with high frequency (50-Hz) repetitive nerve stimulation in Lambert-Eaton myasthenic syndrome. (Reprinted with permission from Preston DC, Shapiro BE. *Electromyography and Neuromuscular Disorders: Clinical-Electrophysiological Correlations,* 4th edition. London: Elsevier Butterworth-Heinemann; 2013. Internet resource.)

myasthenic syndrome, in which high frequency repetitive nerve stimulation (50 Hz) produces a marked increment (> 250%) in CMAP amplitude (Fig. 17-10).

7. D. Pregnancy does not worsen the long-term outcome of MG.

Myasthenia gravis symptoms typically do not worsen during pregnancy. In 1 study of 54 pregnant women with MG, 20% improved during pregnancy, 20% worsened during pregnancy, and 60% remained unchanged. After delivery, MG symptoms worsened in 28%[75] (choice A). Standard drugs used to treat MG, such as anticholinesterase medications or prednisone, are not associated with significant risk for congenital defects and are compatible with breastfeeding (choice C). Plasmapheresis and intravenous immunoglobulin treatments have been safely carried out during pregnancy. Obstetrical problems are uncommon as the uterus is composed of smooth muscle, but myasthenic weakness may be problematic when voluntary striated abdominal muscles are used to push during the second stage of labor[47] (choice B).

REFERENCES

1. Singh A, Tetreault L, Kalsi-Ryan S, Nouri A, Fehlings MG. Global prevalence and incidence of traumatic spinal cord injury. *Clin Epidemiol.* 2014;6:309-331.
2. Breslin K, Agrawal D. The use of methylprednisolone in acute spinal cord injury: a review of the evidence, controversies, and recommendations. *Pediatr Emerg Care.* 2012;28(11):1238-1245.
3. Lewin MG, Hansebout RR, Pappius HM. Chemical characteristics of traumatic spinal cord edema in cats. Effects of steroids on potassium depletion. *J Neurosurg.* 1974;40(1):65-75.
4. Burns AS, Marino RJ, Flanders AE, Flett H. Clinical diagnosis and prognosis following spinal cord injury. *Handb Clin Neurol.* 2012;109:47-62.
5. Bracken MB, Shepard MJ, Collins WF Jr, et al. Methylprednisolone or naloxone treatment after acute spinal cord injury: 1-year follow-up data. Results of the second National Acute Spinal Cord Injury Study. *J Neurosurg.* 1992;76(1):23-31.
6. Hulbert RJ, Hadley MN, Walters BC, et al. Pharmacological therapy for acute spinal cord injury. *Neurosurgery.* 2013;72 (Suppl 2);93-105.
7. Bowers CA, Kundu B, Hawryluk GW. Methylprednisolone for acute spinal cord injury: an increasingly philosophical debate. *Neural Regen Res.* 2016;11(6):882-885.
8. Weathred NR, Harel NY. Chapter 16: Acute spinal cord syndromes. In: Louis ED, Mayer SA, Rowland LP, eds. *Merritt's Neurology.* Philadelphia, PA: Lippincott Williams & Wilkins; 2016: 130-136.
9. Crout TM, Parks LP, Majithia V. Neuromyelitis optica (Devic's syndrome): an appraisal. *Curr Rheumatol Rep.* 2016;18(8):54.
10. Nardone R, Pikija S, Mutzenbach JS, et al. Current and emerging treatment options for spinal cord ischemia. *Drug Discov Today.* 2016;21(10):1632-1641.
11. Sejvar JJ, Bode AV, Marfin AA, et al. West Nile virus–associated flaccid paralysis. *Emerg Infect Dis.* 2005;11(7):1021-1027.
12. Mueller, G. Time-courses of lung function and respiratory muscle pressure generating capacity after spinal cord injury: a prospective cohort study. *J Rehabil Med.* 2008;40(4):269-276.
13. Stein DM, Pineda JA, Roddy V, Knight WA 4th. Emergency neurological life support: traumatic spine injury. *Neurocrit Care.* 2015;23 (Suppl 2):S155-S164.
14. De Troyer A, Estenne M, Heilporn A. Mechanism of active expiration in tetraplegic subjects. *N Engl J Med.* 1986;314(12):740-744.
15. Derenne JP, Macklem PT, Roussos C. The respiratory muscles: mechanics, control, and pathophysiology. *Am Rev Respir Dis.* 1978;118(1):119-133.
16. Nacimiento W, Noth J. What, if anything, is spinal shock? *Arch Neurol.* 1999;56(8):1033-1035.
17. Krassioukov A, Claydon VE. The clinical problems in cardiovascular control following spinal cord injury: an overview. *Prog Brain Res.* 2006;152:223-229.
18. Krassioukov AV, Furlan JC, Fehlings MG. Autonomic dysreflexia in acute spinal cord injury: an underrecognized clinical entity. *J Neurotrauma.* 2003;20(8):707-716.
19. Ryken TC, Hurlbert RJ, Hadley MN, et al. The acute cardiopulmonary management of patients with cervical spinal cord injuries. *Neurosurgery.* 2013;72 (Suppl 2):84-92.
20. Gunduz H, Binak DF. Autonomic dysreflexia: an important cardiovascular complication in spinal cord injury patients. *Cardiol J.* 2012;19(2):215-219.
21. Denton M, McKinlay J. Cervical cord injury and critical care. *Contin Educ Anaesth Crit Care Pain.* 2009;9(3):82-86.
22. Tang EW, Jardine DL, Rodins K, Evans J. Respiratory failure secondary to diabetic neuropathy affecting the phrenic nerve. *Diabet Med.* 2003;20(7):599-601.
23. Podnar S. Idiopathic phrenic neuropathies: a case series and review of the literature. *Muscle Nerve.* 2015;52(6):986-992.
24. Hahn AF. Guillain-Barré syndrome. *Lancet.* 1998;352(9128): 635-641.
25. Fokke C, van den Berg B, Drenthen J, Walgaard C, van Doorn PA, Jacobs BC. Diagnosis of Guillain-Barré syndrome and validation of Brighton criteria. *Brain.* 2014;137(Pt 1):33-43.
26. Rabinstein AA. Acute neuromuscular respiratory failure. *Continuum.* 2015;21(5):1324-1345.
27. Hadden RD, Cornblath DR, Hughes RA, et al. Electrophysiological classification of Guillain-Barré syndrome: clinical associations and outcome. Plasma Exchange/Sandoglobulin Guillain-Barré Syndrome Trial Group. *Ann Neurol.* 1998;44(5):780-788.

28. Washington University. Neuromuscular Disease Center website. http://neuromuscular.wustl.edu/antibody/pnimax.html. Accessed March 7, 2016.

29. Walgaard C, Lingsma HF, Ruts L, et al. Prediction of respiratory insufficiency in Guillain-Barré syndrome. *Ann Neurol.* 2010;67(6):781-787.

30. Mukerji S, Aloka F, Farooq MU, Kassab MY, Abela GS. Cardiovascular complications of the Guillain-Barré syndrome. *Am J Cardiol.* 2009;104(10):1452-1455.

31. Lacomis D. Electrophysiology of neuromuscular disorders in critical illness. *Muscle Nerve.* 2013;47(3):452-463.

32. Lacomis D, Zochodne D. Critical illness myopathy. *Muscle Nerve.* 2000;23(12):1785-1788.

33. Showalter CJ, Engel AG. Acute quadriplegic myopathy: analysis of myosin isoforms and evidence for calpain-mediated proteolysis. *Muscle Nerve.* 1997;20(3):316-322.

34. Campellone JV, Lacomis D, Kramer DJ, Van Cott AC, Giuliani MJ. Acute myopathy after liver transplantation. *Neurology.* 1998;50(1):46-53.

35. Bolton CF. Neuromuscular manifestations of critical illness. *Muscle Nerve.* 2005;32(2):140-163.

36. Bolton CF, Young GB, Zochodne DW. The neurological complications of sepsis. *Ann Neurol.* 1993;33(1):94-100.

37. Zifko UA, Zipko HT, Bolton CF. Clinical and electrophysiological findings in critical illness polyneuropathy. *J Neurol Sci.* 1998;159(2):86-193.

38. Hermans G, Van den Berghe G. Clinical review: intensive care unit acquired weakness. *Crit Care.* 2015;19:274.

39. Schweickert WD, Pohlman MC, Pohlman AS, et al. Early physical and occupational therapy in mechanically ventilated, critically ill patients: a randomised controlled trial. *Lancet.* 2009;373(9678):1874-1882.

40. Rossignol B, Gueret G, Pennec JP, et al. Effects of chronic sepsis on contractile properties of fast twitch muscle in an experimental model of critical illness neuromyopathy in the rat. *Crit Care Med.* 2008;36(6):1855-1863.

41. Fan E, Dowdy DW, Colantuoni E, et al. Physical complications in acute lung injury survivors: a 2-year longitudinal prospective study. *Crit Care Med.* 2013;42(4):849-859.

42. Intiso D, Amoruso L, Zarrelli M, et al. Long-term functional outcome and health status of patients with critical illness polyneuromyopathy. *Acta Neurol Scand.* 2011;123(3):211-219.

43. Koch S, Wollersheim T, Bierbrauer J, et al. Long-term recovery in critical illness myopathy is complete, contrary to polyneuropathy. *Muscle Nerve.* 2014;50(3):431-436.

44. Guarneri B, Bertolini G, Latronico N. Long-term outcome in patients with critical illness myopathy or neuropathy: the Italian multicentre CRIMYNE study. *J Neurol Neurosurg Psychiatry.* 2008;79(7):838-841.

45. Koch S, Spuler S, Deja M, et al. Critical illness myopathy is frequent: accompanying neuropathy protracts ICU discharge. *J Neurol Neurosurg Psychiatry.* 2011;82(3):287-293.

46. Phillips WD, Vincent A. Pathogenesis of myasthenia gravis: update on disease types, models, and mechanisms. *F1000Res.* 2016;27:5.

47. Keesey JC. Clinical evaluation and management of myasthenia gravis. *Muscle Nerve.* 2004;29(4):484-505.

48. Lee SJ, Hur J, Lee W, et al. Myasthenia gravis presenting initially as acute respiratory failure. *Respir Care.* 2015;60(1): e14-e16.

49. Godoy DA, Mello LJ, Masotti L, Di Napoli M. The myasthenic patient in crisis: an update of the management in neurointensive care unit. *Arq Neuropsiquiatr.* 2013;71(9A):627-639.

50. Rosai J, Levine GD. *Tumors of the Thymus.* Bethesda: Armed Forces Institute of Pathology; 1976;144:133-137. Atlas of Tumor Pathology, 2nd series, Fascicle 13.

51. Lanska DJ. Diagnosis of thymoma in myasthenics using antistriated muscle antibodies; predictive value and gain in diagnostic certainty. *Neurology.* 1991;41(4):520-524.

52. Cikes N, Momoi M, Williams CL, et al. Striational autoantibodies: quantitative detection by enzyme immunoassay in myasthenia gravis, thymoma, and recipients of D-penicillamine or allogeneic bone marrow. *Mayo Clin Proc.* 1988;63(5):474-481.

53. Pascuzzi RM, Coslett HB, Johns TR. Long-term corticosteroid treatment of myasthenia gravis: report of 116 patients. *Ann Neurol.* 1984;15(3):291-298.

54. Oger J, Frykman H. An update on laboratory diagnosis in myasthenia gravis. *Clin Chim Acta.* 2015;449:43-48.

55. Nicolle M, Stewart D, Remtulla H, Chen R, Bolton C. Lambert-Eaton myasthenic syndrome presenting with severe respiratory failure. *Muscle Nerve.* 1996;19(10):1328-1333.

56. Alboini PE, Damato V, Iorio R, Luigetti M, Evoli A. Myasthenia gravis with presynaptic neurophysiological signs: two case reports and literature review. *Neuromuscul Disord.* 2015;25(8):646-650.

57. Bekircan-Kurt CE, Derle Çiftçi E, Kurne AT, Anlar B. Voltage gated calcium channel antibody-related neurological diseases. *World J Clin Cases.* 2015;3(3):293-300.

58. Dhaked R, Singh M, Singh P, Gupta P. Botulinum toxin: bioweapon and magic drug. *Indian J Med Res.* 2010;132: 489-503.

59. Wendell L, Levine J. Myasthenic crisis. *Neurohospitalist.* 2011;1(1):16-22.

60. Cherington M. Botulism: update and review. *Semin Neurol.* 2004;24(2):155-163.

61. Hulse E, Davies J, Simpson A, Sciuto A, Eddleston M. Respiratory complications of organophosphorus nerve agent and insecticide poisoning. Implications for respiratory and critical care. *Am J Respir Crit Care Med.* 2014;190(12):1342-1354.

62. Eddleston M, Mohamed F, Davies JOJ, et al. Respiratory failure in acute organophosphorus pesticide self-poisoning. *QJM.* 2006;99(8):513-522.

63. Senanayake N, Karalliedde L. Neurotoxic effects of organophosphorus insecticides. An intermediate syndrome. *N Engl J Med.* 1987;316(13):761-763.

64. Hatheway CL. Botulism. In: Balows A, Hausler WH, Ohashi M, Turnano A, eds. *Laboratory Diagnosis of Infectious Diseases: Principles and Practice.* Vol. 1. New York, NY: Berlin Heidelberg Springer; 1988: 111-133.

65. Shapiro RL, Hatheway C, Swerdlow DL. Botulism in the United States: a clinical and epidemiologic review. *Ann Intern Med.* 1998;129(3):221-228.

66. Arnon SS, Midura TF, Damus K, Thompson B, Wood RM, Chin J. Honey and other environmental risk factors for infant botulism. *J Pediatr.* 1979;94(2):331-336.

67. Nevas M, Lindström M, Virtanen A, et al. Infant botulism acquired from household dust presenting as sudden infant death syndrome. *J Clin Microbiol.* 2005;43(1):511-513.

68. Tackett CO, Shandera WX, Mann JM, Hargrett NT, Blake PA. Equine antitoxin use and other factors that predict outcome in type A foodborne botulism. *Am J Med.* 1984;76:794-798.

69. Chalk CH, Benstead TJ, Keezer M. Medical treatment for botulism. *Cochrane Database Syst Rev.* 2014;(2):CD008123.

70. Francisco AM, Arnon SS. Clinical mimics of infant botulism. *Pediatrics.* 2007;119(4):826-828.

71. Brown N, Desai S. Infantile botulism: a case report and review. *J Emerg Med.* 2013;45(6):842-845.

72. Waseem M, Perry C, Bomann S, Pai M, Gernsheimer J. Cholinergic crisis after rodenticide poisoning. *West J Emerg Med.* 2010;11(5):524-527.

73. Tanenbaum, LN. Clinical applications of diffusion imaging in the spine. *Magn Reson Imaging Clin N Am.* 2013;21(2): 299-320.

74. Michael AP, Mostafa A, Cooper JM, Grice J, Roberts MS, Isbister GK. The pharmacokinetics and pharmacodynamics of severe aldicarb toxicity after overdose. Clin Toxicol (Phila). 2015;53(7):633-635.

75. Batocchi AP, Majolini L, Evoli A, Lino MM, Minisci C, Tonali P. Course and treatment of myasthenia gravis during pregnancy. *Neurology.* 1999;52(3):447-452.

Sepsis

Navitha Ramesh, MD, Matthew Frank, MD, Eric Bondarsky, MD, Lina Miyakawa, MD, and Ronaldo Collo Go, MD

INTRODUCTION

Sepsis is an important diagnosis in the critical care unit. This chapter will discuss its definition, pathogenesis, early goal directed therapy, and types of infection.

DEFINITION

Systemic inflammatory responses (SIRS) is defined as more than 2 of the following: temperature less than 36°C or greater than 38°C, heart rate (HR) greater than 90 beats/min, respiratory rate (RR) greater than 20 breaths/min, $Paco_2$ less than 32 mmHg, white blood cell (WBC) count less than 4000 per mm^3 or more than 12,000 per mm^3, or greater than 10% immature bands.[1] Systemic inflammatory responses associated with infection have been the definition of sepsis for 2 decades. Sepsis with organ dysfunction has been the definition of severe sepsis. Septic shock has been the definition of hypotension despite adequate fluid resuscitation requiring vasopressors and attributed to sepsis.

Improved understanding of this syndrome and the need for uniformity prompted a reevaluation of the criteria. From the Third International Surviving Sepsis Guidelines, the definition of sepsis is defined as life-threatening organ dysfunction by a dysregulated host response to infection.[2,3] Organ dysfunction is defined as an acute change of 2 points or more in total Sequential Organ Failure Assessment (SOFA) score secondary to infection.[2,3] Mortality is 10%. A bedside SOFA or quick SOFA (qSOFA) consists of RR of 22 or more per minute, altered mental status, and systolic blood pressure (SBP) of 100 mmHg or less. The full SOFA score is in Table 18-1.[4]

Septic shock is defined as persistent hypotension and lactic acid of 2 mmol/L (18 mg/dL) or greater despite adequate fluid resuscitation, and the need for vasopressors to maintain mean arterial pressure (MAP) of greater than 65 mmHg.[2,3,5] Mortality is 40%.

PATHOGENESIS

The pathogenesis of sepsis is complex, and this is a very brief summary. It is a response of the host to an infection with proinflammatory and anti-inflammatory components.[6]

The proinflammatory response attempts to kill the infective agent but consequently causes damage to the host tissue. The anti-inflammatory response attempts to mitigate the proinflammatory response but predisposes the host to secondary infections.

The paradoxical proinflammatory and inflammatory response of sepsis begins with identification of the infective agent through innate immunity. This is achieved via 4 groups of receptors (toll-like receptors, c-type lectin receptors, retinoic acid inducible gene 1–like receptors, and nucleotide-binding oligomerization domain–like receptors) that recognize pathogen-associated molecular patterns in infectious agents and damage-associated molecular patterns in injured cells.[7] There is an altered coagulation that leads to disseminated intravascular coagulation.[8] Organ dysfunction is partially secondary to impaired tissue oxygenation from hypotension, reduced red-cell deformability, and microvascular thrombosis. Humeral, cellular, and neurogenic mechanisms diminish the inflammatory response. This often leads to apoptosis of B cells, CD4 T cells, and follicular dendritic cells, which leads to further immunosuppression.[9,10]

EARLY GOAL-DIRECTED THERAPY

Early goal-directed therapy (EGDT) has been the gold standard for the management of sepsis.[11] However, current studies have challenged the benefits of EGDT. The Protocolized Management in Sepsis (PROMISE) trial showed that 184 out of 623 patients in EGDT and 181 out of 620 patients in the usual care group had died (relative risk in EGDT, 1.01; 95% confidence interval [CI], 0.85–1.20; $P = 0.90$) for absolute risk reduction (ARR) of −0.3 percentage points (95% CI, −5.4 to 4.7) and no significant differences in quality of life or rates of serious adverse effects.[12] Early goal-directed therapy increased costs, with cost-effectivity less than 20%.[12] The Australasian Resuscitation in Sepsis Evaluation (ARISE) and Australian and New Zealand Intensive Care Society (ANZICS) group showed that in 90 days after randomization, EGDT had 147 deaths and the usual care group had 150 deaths, with rates of 18.6% and 18.8%, respectively (absolute risk difference, −0.3 percentage points; 95% CI, 0.4 to 3.6; $P = 0.90$) and no difference in survival time, hospital mortality, duration of organ support, and

TABLE 18-1 Sequential (Sepsis-Related) Organ Failure Assessment Score[a]

System	Score				
	0	1	2	3	4
Respiration					
Pao$_2$/Fio$_2$, mm Hg (kPa)	≥ 400 (53.3)	< 400 (53.3)	< 300 (40)	< 200 (26.7) with respiratory support	<100 (13.3) with respiratory support
Coagulation					
Platelets, × 10^3/μL	≥ 150	< 150	< 100	< 50	< 20
Liver					
Bilirubin, mg/dL (μmol/L)	< 1.2 (20)	1.2–1.9 (20–32)	2.0–5.9 (33–101)	6.0–11.9 (102–204)	> 12.0 (204)
Cardiovascular	MAP ≥ 70 mmHg	MAP < 70 mmHg	Dopamine < 5 or dobutamine (any dose)[b]	Dopamine 5.1–15 or epinephrine ≤ 0.1 or norepinephrine ≤ 0.1[b]	Dopamine > 15 or epinephrine > 0.1 or norepinephrine > 0.1[b]
Central nervous system					
Glasgow Coma Scale score[c]	15	13–14	10–12	6–9	< 6
Renal					
Creatinine, mg/dL (μmol/L)	< 1.2 (110)	1.2–1.9 (110–170)	2.0–3.4 (171–299)	3.5–4.9 (300–440)	> 5.0 (440)
Urine output, mL/d				< 500	< 200

Fio$_2$ = fraction of inspired oxygen; MAP = mean arterial pressure; Pao$_2$ = partial pressure of oxygen.

[a]Adapted from Vincent et al.[4]

[b]Catecholamine doses are given as μg/kg/min for at least 1 hour.

[c]Glasgow Coma Scale scores range from 3–15; higher score indicates better neurological function.

Reprinted with permission from Vincent JL, Moreno R, Takala J, et al. Working Group on Sepsis-Related Problems of the European Society of Intensive Care Medicine. The SOFA (Sepsis-related Organ Failure Assessment) score to describe organ dysfunction/failure. *Intensive Care Med.* 1996;22(7):707-710.

length in hospital stay.[13] However, EGDT is still advocated, since there is no harm in the interventions, and clinicians need guidance in managing sepsis.

Resuscitation

Fluid resuscitation (30 mL/kg[11,12] or 2 Liters[13]) is recommended within the first 3 hours. Certain patients may require more fluid as determined by dynamic or functional hemodynamic monitoring, such as stroke volume variation (SVV), over static monitoring, such as central venous pressure (CVP). Central venous pressure is limited due to its inability to predict fluid responsiveness in patients with normal values (8–12 cm H$_2$O).[14,15] Crystalloids are preferred over colloids since crystalloids are cheaper and colloids have no clear benefit[2] (Strong Recommendation and Moderate Quality of Evidence). Well-balanced crystalloids are advocated, since hyperchloremia is thought to cause decreased glomerular filtration rate (GFR) due to constriction of afferent arteriole.[16] However, the 0.9% saline vs plasma-lyte 148 for icu fluid therapy (SPLIT) trial suggested that use of buffered crystalloid over normal saline did not reduce risk of acute kidney injury (AKI). Renal replacement

therapy (RRT) in the buffered crystalloid group is 38 of 1152 [3.3%] compared to 38 of 1110 [3.4%] in the saline group with absolute difference −0.1%; 95% CI, 01.6% to 1.4%).[17] However, a recent cluster-randomized, multiple-crossover trial in 5 intensive care units (ICUs) which compared balanced crystalloids such as lactated Ringer's solution or Plasma-lyte A versus normal saline showed 14.3% of balanced crystalloid group had major adverse kidney event compared to 15.4% in saline group (marginal odd's ratio 0.91; 95% confidence interval. 0.84–0.99; conditional odd's ratio 0.90; 95% CI 0.82–0.99; P=0.04).[18] In hospital mortality at 30 days was also less in the balanced crystalloid group (10.3%) compared to saline group (11.1%); incidence of new RRT was less in balanced crystalloid group (2.5%) compared to saline group (2.6%)(P=0.06).[18]

The use of albumin over crystalloid does not show consistent mortality benefit in multiple studies.[2,19-24] Hetastarches are associated with higher rates of RRT and their mortality benefit is variable[2,25] (Strong Recommendation and High Quality of Evidence). Gelatin, another colloid, did not increase mortality or AKI compared to albumin or crystalloid.[26]

The goal of fluid resuscitation is to maintain MAP above 65 mmHg and normalize lactate.[2] Mean arterial pressure is the driving force for tissue perfusion and at an MAP less than 65 mmHg, tissue perfusion becomes linearly dependent on arterial pressure.[2] Higher MAP goals have not been associated with improved mortality but have been associated with a higher risk of arrthymias.[2] Lactate is an indirect measure of perfusion, and early lactate clearance strategy has been shown to reduce mortality.[27-30]

Vasopressors can be utilized to meet these goals if fluid resuscitation is insufficient. Norepinephrine is the preferred first line vasopressor (Strong Recommendation and Moderate Quality of Evidence). Dopamine can be used in lieu of norepinephrine in patients who are bradycardic with a low incidence of tachyarrhythmias. If insufficient, vasopressin or epinephrine can be added (Weak Recommendation and Low Quality of Evidence). Dobutamine can be added if the patient has a persistent hypoperfused stated despite adequate fluid resuscitation and vasopressors (Weak Recommendation and Low Quality of Evidence).

Norepinephrine is preferred to dopamine because it has a more potent effect in increasing cardiac output, it is less protachyarrythmic, and it has no known association with immunosuppression.[31] A metanalysis of 11 randomized trials showed that norepinephrine had lower mortality (risk ratio, 0.89; 95% CI, 0.81–0.98) and lower arrhythmia risk (risk ratio, 0.48; 95% CI, 0.40–0.58).[32] It has been suggested that there is no difference in mortality with the use of epinephrine versus norepinephrine, but epinephrine may increase lactate production via β_2-adrenergic receptors in the skeletal muscle.[2] It also has been suggested that there is a relative vasopressin deficiency in septic shock, but most of the data regards vasopressin as a sparing effect to norepinephrine.[2] Dobutamine is considered a first-line inotropic agent to improve oxygen delivery. It has been shown to improve clinical outcomes, lactate, and central venous oxygen saturation ($Scvo_2$).[2] Phenylephrine causes splanchnic vasoconstriction and its effects on clinical outcomes have yet to be determined.[33] Low-dose dopamine does not improve urine output, RRT, intensive care unit stay, hospital stay, arrhythmias, and survival compared to placebo, and is generally not advocated.[2]

Antibiotics

Intravenous (IV) antibiotics should be administered within 1 hour of recognition of sepsis because each hour delay increases mortality, acute kidney injury, acute lung injury, and length of stay[34-37] (Strong Recommendation and Moderate Quality of Evidence). However, a recent meta-analysis suggested that there is no mortality benefit to administering antibiotics within 3 hours versus within 1 hour of sepsis or septic shock recognition.[38] Considerations for the choice of antibiotics include anatomic site of infection, prevalent pathogens in the community and resistance patterns, and presence of immunodeficiencies.[2] Duration of antibiotics is typically 7 to 10 days but can be longer if there is a slow response, undrainable foci, *Staphylococcus aureus* bacteremia, a fungal infection, a viral infection, or states of immunodeficiency[2] (Weak Recommendation and Low

Quality of Evidence). Daily assessment of antibiotic de-escalation should take place with clinical evaluation and culture results with or without utilization of biomarkers such as procalcitonin (PCT).

The patient should have cultures if there is no substantial delay to initiation of antibiotics (45 minutes).[2] Culture-negative sepsis is not uncommon. A prospective observation cohort suggested that culture-negative sepsis was associated with women, fewer comorbidities, lower Acute Physiology and Chronic Health Evaluation (APACHE) score, lower SOFA score, lower procalcitonin levels, less tachycardia, higher blood pressures, shorter duration of stay, and lower ICU mortality compared to culture-positive sepsis.[39]

Corticosteroids

Hydrocortisone 200 mg IV daily is suggested for septic shock despite adequate fluid resuscitation and vasopressor support[2] (Weak Recommendation and Low Quality of Evidence). The recommendation is weak due to the inconsistencies regarding whether it improves mortality.[40-47] Random cortisol levels are not useful, since they may underestimate or overestimate true values.[2]

TYPES OF INFECTIONS

Community-acquired pneumonia (CAP), nervous system infections such as meningitis, encephalitis, abscess, neuritis, infective endocarditis (IE), pericardial infections, skin and soft tissue infections, and infections during pregnancy are discussed in this chapter. Other types of infections are discussed in the following chapters: Chapter 19, "Healthcare-Acquired Infections"; Chapter 20, "The Immune System and Infection"; and Chapter 21, "Antimicrobials."

Community-Acquired Pneumonia

Clinical presentation of pneumonia can consist of fever, shortness of breath, cough, pleuritic chest pain, productive purulent or clear sputum, nausea, vomiting, diarrhea, or altered mental status, but the gold standard for confirmation is chest radiograph or chest computed tomography (CT). Typical pathogens associated with community acquired pneumonia are *Streptococcus pneumoniae*, *Haemophilus influenzae*, *S aureus*, group A streptococci, *Moraxella catarrhalis*, aerobic Gram-negative bacteria, atypical bacteria (*Mycoplasma pneumoniae*, *Chlamydia pneumoniae*, *C psittaci*, and *Legionella*), and viruses. In outpatient management of CAP, cultures are optional due to difficulty in obtaining good specimens, costs, and concerns for delay of treatment.[48] Cultures including sputum, blood, polymerase chain reaction (PCR), and urinary antigens for *S pneumoniae* and *Legionella* are advocated in hospitalized patients, especially for patients with severe pneumonia.

Site-of-care decision is based on risk of mortality, and from the observation that patients with less-severe CAP who are treated as outpatients generally recover faster, with less cost and less exposure to more resistant pathogens. Pneumonia severity index (PSI), CURB-65 (confusion, urea level, respiratory rate, blood pressure, and age less than 65 years), SMART-COP (systolic blood pressure, multilobar involvement, albumin level, respiratory rate, tachycardia, confusion, oxygenation, and arterial pH), and Severe Community-Acquired Pneumonia (SCAP) score are used to stratify risk and guide treatment[40] (Tables 18-2 and 18-3).

Nervous System Infections

In addition to neuroimaging, cerebrospinal fluid (CSF) analysis is crucial to identifying infectious and noninfectious pathologies of the CNS. There are 4 entities with normal CSF analysis: (1) early bacterial meningitis, (2) cryptococcal meningitis with HIV, (3) parimeningeal foci, and 4) herpes simplex encephalitis. Most common method to obtain CSF sample would be through a lumbar puncture. Prior to performing

TABLE 18-2 Stratification Tools for Pneumonia

CURB-65[49]	PSI[49,50]	SMART-COP[51,52]	SCAP Score[53,54]
• Confusion • Urea > 7 mmol/L (20 mg/dL) • Respiratory rate > 30 breaths/min • SBP < 90 mmHg or DBP ≤ 60 mmHg • Age ≥ 65 y	Sex • Male (0 points) • Female (−10 points) Demographics • Age (+1 point per year) • NH resident (+10 points) Comorbid illnesses • Neoplastic disease (+30 points) • Chronic liver disease (+20 points) • Heart failure (+10 points) • Cardiovascular (+10 points) • Chronic renal failure (+10 points) Physical examination • Altered mental status (20 points) • Respiratory rate ≥ 30 breaths/min (20 points) • SBP < 90 mmHg (+20 points) • Temperature < 35°C (95°F) or > 40°C (104°F) (+15 points) • Pulse ≥ 125/min (+10 points) Laboratory and radiographic findings • Arterial pH < 7.35 (+30 points) • BUN ≥ 30 mEq/L (+20 points) • Sodium < 130 mEq/L (+20 points) • Glucose > 250 mg/dL (14 mmol/L) (+10 points) • Hematocrit < 30% (+10 points) • Partial pressure or arterial oxygen < 60 mmHg or oxygen saturation < 90% (+10 points) • Pleural effusion (+10 points)	• SBP < 90 mmHg (2 points) • Multilobar (1 point) • Low albumin (1 point) • High respiratory rate (1 point) • Confusion (1 point) • Poor oxygenation (2 points) • Low arterial pH (2 points)	Major: • pH < 7.30 (13 points) • SBP < 90 mmHg (11 points) Minor: • Respiratory rate > 30 breaths/min (9 points) • Pao_2/Fio_2 < 250 mmHg (6 points) • BUN > 30 mg/dL (10.7 mmol/L) (5 points) • AMS (5 points) • Age ≥ 80 y (5 points) • Multilobar (5 points)
Score: • 0–1 point: outpatient • ≥ 2 points: inpatient • ≥ 3 points: ICU	Score: • Class I, 0.1% mortality • Class II, 0.6% mortality: 0–70 points (outpatient management) • Class III, 0.9% mortality: 71–90 points (outpatient vs observation admission) • Class IV, 9.3% mortality: 91–130 points (inpatient admission) • Class V, 27% mortality: 131–395 points (inpatient admission)	Score: • ≥ 3 points will require intensive respiratory and vasopressor support • Sensitivity increases for ages ≥ 50 • 0–2 points: low risk • 3–4 points: moderate risk • 5–6 points: high risk, consider ICU	Score: ≥ 10 points (1 major and 2 minor): predicts severe CAP

AMS = Altered mental status; BUN = blood urea nitrogen; DBP = diastolic blood pressure; Fio_2 = fraction of inspired oxygen; ICU = intensive care unit; SBP = systolic blood pressure.

TABLE 18-3 Recommended Empirical Antibiotics for Community-Acquired Pneumonia

Outpatient treatment

1. Previously healthy and no use of antimicrobials within the previous 3 months

   A macrolide (strong recommendation; level I evidence)

   Doxycycline (weak recommendation; level III evidence)

2. Presence of comorbidities such as chronic heart, lung, liver or renal disease; diabetes mellitus; alcoholism; malignancies; asplenia; immunosuppressing conditions or use of immunosuppressing drugs; or use of antimicrobials within the previous 3 months (in which case an alternative from a different class should be selected)

   A respiratory fluoroquinolone (moxifloxacin, gemifloxacin, or levofloxacin [750 mg]) (strong recommendation; level I evidence)

   A β-lactam **plus** a macrolide (strong recommendation; level I evidence)

3. In regions with a high rate (> 25%) of infection with high-level (MIC ≥ 16 μg/mL) macrolide-resistant *Streptococcus pneumoniae*, consider use of alternative agents listed above in (2) for patients without comorbidities (moderate recommendation; level III evidence)

Inpatients, non-ICU treatment

   A respiratory fluoroquinolone (strong recommendation; level I evidence)

   A β-lactam **plus** a macrolide (strong recommendation; level I evidence)

Inpatients, ICU treatment

   A β-lactam (cefotaxime, ceftriaxone, or ampicillin-sulbactam) **plus** either azithromycin (level II evidence) **or** a respiratory fluoroquinolone (level I evidence) (strong recommendation) (for penicillin-allergic patients, a respiratory fluoroquinolone and aztreonam are recommended)

Special concerns

   If *Pseudomonas* is a consideration

   An antipneumococcal, antipseudomonal β-lactam (piperacillin-tazobactam, cefepime, imipenem, or meropenem) plus either ciprofloxacin or levofloxacin (750 mg)

   or

   The above β-lactam plus an aminoglycoside and azithromycin

   or

   The above β-lactam plus an aminoglycoside and an antipneumococcal fluoroquinolone (for penicillin-allergic patients, substitute aztreonam for above β-lactam) (moderate recommendation; level III evidence)

   If CA-MRSA is a consideration, add vancomycin or linezolid (moderate recommendation; level III evidence)

CA-MRSA = community-acquired methicillin-resistant *Staphylococcus aureus*; ICU = intensive care unit; MIC = minimal inhibitory concentration.

Reprinted with permission from Mandell LA, Wunderink RG, Anzueto A, et al. Infectious Diseases Society of America/American Thoracic Society consensus guidelines on the management of community acquired pneumonia in adults. *Clin Infect Dis*. 2007;44 (Suppl 2):S27-S72.

this procedure, a computed tomography of the head must be obtained to rule out any space occupying lesion. Presence of seizures could also indicate transient increase in intracranial pressure; therefore, the lumbar puncture should be delayed by 30 minutes or more. Its presence could suggest the risk of herniation if the lumbar puncture is performed.

Cerebrospinal fluid is produced in the choroid plexus in the lateral, third, and fourth ventricles, circulated in the subarachnoid space, and reabsorbed in the arachnoid villi. The normal volume is 150 mL and produced at 20 mL/h. The normal CSF glucose–to–blood glucose ratio is 0.6 and glucose enters the CSF through choroid plexus and capillaries. The CSF glucose is decreased by consumption of white blood cells and organisms and/or decrease transfer from inflamed meninges. Protein generally is excluded in CSF but levels increase if there is a disruption of the blood–brain barrier. The normal levels along with the levels seen in several conditions are seen in Table 18-4.[55-57]

Encephalitis

Encephalitis is an inflammatory condition of the brain parenchyma secondary to an infectious or noninfectious cause. In infections, neural cells of gray matter are the target with associated perivascular inflammation, neuronal destruction, and tissue necrosis. It might be difficult to distinguish meningitis and encephalitis, and it is not uncommon that both processes can occur together and can have associated CSF pleocytosis called meningoencephalitis. In autoimmune or postinfectious causes, there is perivenular inflammation and demyelination of the white matter. Generally, patients with encephalitis will have abnormal brain function such as altered mental status, neurologic deficits, and personality changes, and may have abnormal radiographic findings.

Noninfectious causes include acute disseminated encephalomyelitis (ADEM), which is encephalitis triggered by an autoimmune response to prior antigen exposure. Prior antigen exposure can include immunization (1–14 days after vaccination) or febrile illness up to 1 week after the onset of a rash.[58] Although bacterial, protozoal, and parasitic infections can cause encephalitis, the most common infectious causes in the United States include herpes simplex, West Nile virus, enteroviruses, and herpesviruses.[58]

Investigation begins with an epidemiologic review of the patient's history, extraneurologic manifestations such as rash, and laboratories such as cultures, polymerase chain reaction, CSF analysis, and magnetic resonance imaging (MRI). Certain MRI patterns can suggest etiology. Herpes simplex encephalitis has temporal lobe involvement; flaviviruses and the Eastern equine encephalitis virus have mixed or hypodense lesions on T1 images of the thalamus, basal ganglia, and midbrain, and hyperintense lesions on T2 images; enterovirus 71 encephalitis has hyperintense lesions on T2 imaging and flair lesions in the midbrain, pons, and medulla; and ADEM has multifocal abnormalities usually in the subcortical white and sometimes even gray matter on T2 and fluid attenuation inversion recovery (FLAIR) sequences[58] (Table 18-5).[59-93]

Meningitis

Bacterial meningitis work-up should begin with CSF analysis, including a Gram stain, which identifies 60% to 90% of bacteria with a specificity of greater than 97%.[94,95] The likelihood that Gram stain can identify the bacteria is dependent on the concentration and the specific pathogen: *S pneumoniae* > *H influenza*

TABLE 18-4 Cerebrospinal Fluid Values and Associated Conditions

CSF Characteristics	Normal Values in Adults	Bacterial Meningitis	Aseptic Meningitis	Herpes Simplex	Fungal Meningitis	Tuberculosis
Color	Clear	Clear, cloudy, or purulent	Clear	Clear	Clear or cloudy	Clear or cloudy
Opening pressure	90–180 mm H_2O while lying lateral	> 250 mm H_2O	Normal or elevated	Normal	Variable; usually increased (Cryptococcus > 250 mm H_2O)	Variable; usually increased
Osmolarity	281 mOsm/L					
Specific gravity	1.006–1.008					
LDH	10% of serum value					
Lactic acid	1.1–2.8 mmol/L	> 3.9 mmol/L	Normal	Normal	> 2.8 mmol/L	> 2.8 mmol/L
Glucose	45–80 mg/dL or > 60% of serum glucose	< 40% of serum glucose	> 60% of serum glucose	> 60% of serum glucose	< 40% of serum glucose	Decreased, often falls progressively
Glutamine	8–18 mg/dL					
Proteins	20–40 mg/dL • Prealbumin 2–7% • Albumin 56–76% • $α_1$-globulin 2–7% • $α_2$-globulin 3.5–12% • γ-globulin: 7–12%	80–500 mg/dL	30–100 mg/dL	15–100 mg/dL	> 50 mg/dL	> 50 mg/dL
Immunoglobulins (Ig)	• IgG 10–40 mg/L • IgA 0–0.2 mg/L • IgM 0–0.6 mg/L					
Erythrocyte	0–10 cells/μL	Normal	Normal	Often increased	Normal	Normal
Leukocyte	0–5 cells/μL	> 100 cells/μL (> 90% PMN)	10–1000 cells/μL (lymph but PMN if early)	10–1000 cells/μL (lymph but PMN if early)	10–500 cells/μL (usually lymphocytic or mixed)	Variable; increased (usually lymphocytic or mixed)

CSF = cerebrospinal fluid; LDH = lactate dehydrogenase; PMN = polymorphonuclear leukocytes; TB = tuberculosis.

> *Neisseria meningitidis* > Gram-negative bacilli > *Listeria*.[96-98] Guidelines do not recommend routine use of latex agglutination tests although it can be used if the Gram stain is negative. Agglutination may be most useful for patients who have received empiric antibiotics and have negative Gram stain and culture. The limulus amoebocyte lysate assay has been suggested as a diagnostic tool to identify the presence of Gram negative infections; however, the assay rarely influences clinical practice and routine use is not suggested. Polymerase chain reaction testing may be useful in Gram stain and culture-negative cases in which suspicion for bacterial meningitis remains high.[94]

Meningitis is a neurologic emergency, and antibiotics should be started as soon as possible. Antibiotic regimen and duration are shown in Tables 18-6 and 18-7.[94-112] Adjunct dexamethasone therapy (0.15 mg/kg every 6 hours for 2–4 days with the dose administered 10–20 minutes before or concurrent with the first dose of the antimicrobial) in adults with suspected or proven pneumococcal meningitis is based on a study that showed unfavorable outcome and death was less in the dexamethasone group (26% vs 52%, $P = 0.006$ and 14% vs 34%, $P = 0.02$).[101] Adjunct dexamethasone may prevent hearing loss in patients with *H influenzae*. Ampicillin should be added to cover *Listeria* if there is advanced age, alcoholism, or immunocompromised states.

Patients with bacterial meningitis can be treated as outpatients if they have been treated with inpatient antimicrobials for 6 days or more, have been without fever for 24 hours or more prior to initiation of outpatient therapy, have no neurological deficits or seizure activity, are able to eat by mouth, have access to antimicrobial distribution, have reliable IV access,

TABLE 18-5 Causes of Encephalitis

Microorganism	Characteristics	Treatment
Eastern equine encephalitis	• Mortality rate of 30–70% with neurologic sequelae in 80% of patients	• Supportive
St Louis encephalitis (flavivirus)	• Inappropriate secretion of antidiuretic hormone and pyuria	• Supportive but Interferon-α-2 may decrease complications
Arboviral encephalitis from West Nile virus (flavivirus)	• Acute flaccid asymmetrical paralysis without pain or sensory loss in association with CSF pleocytosis from involvement of anterior horn cells of spinal cord and motor axons • Differential is GBS but does not have a symmetrical pattern with associated sensory changes, paresthesias, and CSF protein elevation without pleocytosis • Diagnosis was IgM antibody capture ELISA for IgM to WNV in serum or CSF • IgM does not cross BBB, and 90% of serum samples obtained within 8 days of symptom onset are + for IgM antibody.	• Supportive
HIV		• Supportive
Enterovirus (coxsackie A, B, and echoviruses)	• Diagnosis via pharyngeal, rectal, and urine viral cultures	• Supportive
Multifocal leukoencephalopathy secondary to DNA polyomavirus JC	• Demyelinating of white cerebral hemispheres • Patients present with confusion, disorientation, visual disturbances, which progress to cortical blindness and ataxia; CSF acellular and neuroimaging lack of mass effect • Neurologic improvement or stability at 2 mo after HAART in 26% compared to 3% who did not receive therapy • Decrease in JC virus DNA to undetectable levels predicted a longer survival • In context, PML may be fatal with 3–6 mo; a decrease in JC virus DNA predicted longer survival	• Supportive
Human rabies	• After inoculation, virus replicates in myocytes and travels in the nervous system via unmyelinated sensory and motor nerves until spinal cord is reached and paresthesias develop at wound site • Centrifugal spread along autonomic and somatic nerves to skin, intestine, salivary glands, and release in saliva • Early on, localizes in limbic structures and patient develops changes in personality • Ascending paralysis, hypertonicity, and hypersalivation with pain and/or weakness	• Rabies immunoglobulin at 20 IU/kg body weight dose infiltrated into and around the wound with remaining IM in deltoid or quadriceps • Rabies vaccine • Monoclonal antibodies • Ribavirin • Interferon-α • Ketamine • Prevention of exposure of family members or healthcare workers via vaccine
Powassan encephalitis	• Tick-borne encephalitis	• Supportive
HSV encephalitis	• HSV type 1 • Access to brain via olfactory nerve • Inflammation or necrosis localized to medial-temporal and orbital-frontal lobes • Acute, febrile, and focal with personality changes, headache, and focality • CSF maybe normal or shows increased ICP, CSF lymphocytosis, and presence of RBCs in CSF • CSF glucose is normal but patients may have hypoglycorrhachia • PCR analysis of CSF has 100% specificity and 75–98% sensitivity	• Acyclovir
Rickettsia, RMSF	• Late summer and early fall • Fever, petechiae on palms, soles, wrists, and ankles that start distally and progress to center	• Tetracycline • Alternative: chloramphenicol
Epidemic typhus secondary to *Rickettsia prowazekii*	• Winter • Central lesions moving distally	
Human mononuclear ehrlichiosis or human granulocytic ehrlichiosis	• Only 20% have rash • Symptoms include fever, leukopenia, thrombocytopenia, abnormal LFT, nervous system involvement, severe headache, confusion, lethargy, broad-based gait, hyperreflexia, clonus, photophobia, CN palsy, seizures, blurred vision, nuchal rigidity, and ataxia • CSF has lymphocytic pleocytosis with elevated protein level	• Tetracycline • Chloramphenicol

BBB = blood–brain barrier; CN = cranial nerve; CSF = cerebrospinal fluid; ELISA = enzyme-linked immunosorbent assay; GBS = Guillain-Barré syndrome; HAART = highly active antiretroviral therapy; HSV = herpes simplex virus; ICP = intracranial pressure; Ig = immunoglobulin; IM = intramuscular; IV = intravenous; JC = John Cunningham; LFT = liver function tests; PCR = polymerase chain reaction; PML = progressive multifocal leukoencephalopathy; RBC = red blood cell; RMSF = Rocky Mountain spotted fever; WNF = West Nile virus

TABLE 18-6 Empiric Antibiotics for Meningitis

Characteristics	Empiric Antibiotics
2–50 y of age	Vancomycin + third-generation cephalosporin
> 50 y of age	Vancomycin + ampicillin + third-generation cephalosporin
Penetrating head trauma, neurosurgery, or cerebrospinal fluid shunt	Vancomycin + ceftazidime OR vancomycin + cefepime OR vancomycin + meropenem
Immunocompromised	Vancomycin + ampicillin + cefepime OR vancomycin + ampicillin + meropenem

have daily availability of a physician or established health-care visits, are compliant, and live in a safe environment.[94] Repeat lumbar puncture may be indicated if the patient fails to improve clinically after 48 hours or more with treatment.[102,103]

Thrombophlebitis

Infection of thrombosis can occur as a complication of meningitis, paranasal sinusitis, middle ear or oropharynx infection, or infection of lungs and other distant organs. Most frequent pathogens are *S aureus*, coagulase-negative staphylococci, streptococci, Gram-negative bacilli, and anaerobes. Cavernous sinuses act as sleeves to microbes, and thromboses in this area can become infected. There are many important anatomical structures that pass through the cavernous sinus, including the internal carotid artery and sympathetic plexus and sixth cranial nerve (CN); the lateral walls have the third and fourth CN with ophthalmic and sometimes maxillary divisions of the trigeminal nerve.[113,114] Thrombosis and thrombophlebitis in this area can cause high fever, headaches, malaise, nausea, and vomiting. Patients progress to develop proptosis, chemosis, periorbital edema, and cyanosis of the ipsilateral forehead, eyelids, and root of the nose. Ophthalmoplegia may develop, with the sixth CN usually involved first. Trigeminal nerve involvement has decreased sensation about the eye, and ophthalmic nerve involvement causes photophobia and eye pain. Papilledema, diminished pupillary reactivity, and diminished corneal reflexes may develop. Treatment is antibiotics and surgical drainage. Other areas of thrombophlebitis include superior sagittal sinus thrombosis, which can result in bilateral leg weakness or communicating hydrocephalus; lateral sinus thrombosis with pain over the ear and mastoid and edema over the mastoid; superior petrosal sinus thrombosis with ipsilateral pain, sensory deficit, or temporary lobe seizures; and inferior petrosal sinus thrombosis producing ipsilateral facial pain and lateral rectus weakness, called Gradenigo syndrome.[115]

Brain Abscess

This results from hematogenous dissemination, extension from infected cranial structures along emissary veins from the sinuses or middle ear, or as a consequence of trauma or neurosurgery. Excision or aspiration of abscess may be performed if it is greater than 2.5 cm.[98,103,116-119] Others prefer to use empiric antibiotics without aspiration if the patient is neurologically stable and the abscess is less than 3 cm and not encroaching on the ventricular system; however, the patient must have serial imaging studies, and if the abscess is growing, it would warrant surgery.

Treatment includes metronidazole and penicillin or a third-generation cephalosporin such as ceftriaxone or cefotaxime. Alternative to metronidazole is chloramphenicol. If there is a penetrating trauma, neurosurgery, or endocarditis, staphylococcus coverage should be included. If it is otic or sinus in origin, coverage against *Enterobacteriaceae* and *H influenza* with a third-generation cephalosporin should be included.

Spinal epidural abscess is a neurosurgical emergency because delay in treatment can cause irreversible neurologic deficits, particularly when there is a delay in evacuating purulent material. The triad of findings that support the diagnosis includes fever, point tenderness over the spine, and focal neurologic deficits. Skin and soft tissue are probably the source of infection and abscesses may be a complication of lumbar puncture and epidural anesthesia. Usual pathogens include *S aureus*, streptococci, and Gram-negative bacilli.[120] Diagnosis of choice is gadolinium-enhanced MRI because it can also signal abnormalities consistent with acute transverse myelopathy and spinal cord ischemia.[121]

Subdural empyema occurs secondary to the spread of infection via emissary veins or extension of osteomyelitis of the skull. Half of cases are secondary to paranasal sinus infections, and the other half is caused by otitis. In young children, it is usually complication of meningitis. Clinical features include fever, headache, vomiting, meningeal irritation, AMS, and focal neurologic deficits that progress to focal seizures. Pathogens include streptococci, staphylococci, *H influenzae*, Gram-negative bacilli, and anaerobes including *Bacteroides fragilis*.

NEURITIS

While less common than vascular, inflammatory, or autoimmune causes, infectious agents can be a cause of peripheral nervous system (PNS) disease. These diseases can be a source of significant morbidity and even mortality manifesting as radiculopathies, peripheral neuropathies, and neuromuscular disorders. In this section, we will focus on a select group of the bacteria, viruses, and parasites responsible for these disorders. Table 18-8 highlights several of these pathogens.[104,122-133]

INFECTIVE ENDOCARDITIS

According to the Modified Duke Criteria, definitive diagnosis of infective endocarditis is made via pathologic criteria, which includes microorganisms of vegetation or intracardiac abscess

TABLE 18-7 Causes of Meningitis

Microorganism	Characteristics	Antibiotics
N meningitidis	• Reservoir nasopharynx • Causes bacteremia, meningococcemia (purpura fulminans and Waterhouse-Friderichsen syndrome), pneumonia, epiglottitis, otitis media, conjunctivitis, septic arthritis, urethritis, purulent pericarditis, and chronic meningococcemia • At risk includes children and young adults, military, cigarettes associated with closed settings, air travel for at least 8 h within 14 d • Meningococcal polysaccharide vaccine effective against serogroup C meningococcal disease with efficacy 85% for ages 2–29 y • Screen for late complement (C5–C8) deficiency via CH50, C5–C9	• Third-generation cephalosporin for 7 d • Alternatives: penicillin G, ampicillin, chloramphenicol, fluoroquinolone, aztreonam • Post-treatment with rifampin, ciprofloxacin, or ceftriaxone will help eradicate nasal carrier state; similar to chemoprophylaxis to close contacts, which should be administered within 24 h after contact; if >14 d since exposure, chemoprophylaxis has no value
H influenzae	• Nasopharynx or contiguous spread	• Third-generation cephalosporin for 7 d • Chloramphenicol, cefepime, ertapenem, fluoroquinolone
Streptococcus pneumoniae	• Most common • Steroids decrease vancomycin penetration • Rifampin if susceptible and delay with response	• Penicillin-susceptible (MIC ≤ 0.6): penicillin G or third-generation cephalosporin for 10–14 d • Penicillin-resistant (MIC ≥ 0.12) and cephalosporin-susceptible (MIC < 1.0): ceftriaxone or ceftazidime • Penicillin-resistant and cephalosporin-resistant (MIC ≥ 1): vancomycin + third-generation cephalosporin • Alternative: meropenem, fluoroquinolone
S agalactiae		• Ampicillin or penicillin G for 14–21 d • Alternative: third-generation cephalosporin
Listeria monocytogenes	• Patients with compromised cell-mediated immunity • After consumption of milk, cheese, and coleslaw • CSF PMN or lymphocytes with normal glucose • Predilection for meninges at base of brain causing hydrocephalus	• Ampicillin or penicillin G for ≥ 21 d • Alternative: trimethoprim-sulfamethoxazole, if penicillin allergy
Gram-negative	• Predisposing factors include urinary tract infections, *Strongyloides*, impaired cell-mediated immunity • Superinfection uncommon in CD4 ≥ 200 cells/mm³ with concomitant infection and organ transplantation with use of cyclosporine	• Aminoglycosides do not cross BBB after 28 d of life; therefore, intrathecal or intraventricular for 21 d • Chloramphenicol • Third-generation cephalosporin
Staphylococcus aureus	• Hospital-acquired has better prognosis than community-acquired • Due to DM, valvular disease, and alcohol	• Nafcillin for 14 d • Vancomycin
Anthrax	• Biphasic	• Penicillin • Chloramphenicol
Tuberculosis	• Needed repeated volumes of CSF (10–20 mL) to get improved yields of AFB • 4 positive smears 90% positive • CSF revealing increased adenosine deaminase or CSF chloride < 110 mEq/L in absence of bacterial infection supports TB meningitis	• RIPE for 6 mo • Steroids improve mortality
Cryptococcus neoformans	• Access through lungs • Lack of inflammation shows CSF WBC < 20 cells/μL and normal glucose • Mortality high from elevated ICP; therefore, daily lumbar puncture, acetazolamide, VP shunts for asymptomatic with ICP CSF > 320 mm H₂O or symptomatic with ICP CSF > 180 mm H₂O. • In absence of focal lesions, OP ≥ 250 mm H₂O should have large volumes of CSF drainage until CSF closing pressure is ≤ 200 mm H₂O or 50% of initial opening pressure • Diagnosis via latex agglutination test (cryptococcal antigen), India ink, silver stain, culture	• Amphotericin B (0.7 mg/kg/d) + flucytosine (100 mg/kg/d in persons with normal renal function) for 2 wk followed by fluconazole (400 mg/d oral) for 8–10 wk • Maintenance: fluconazole 200 mg PO daily

(Continued)

TABLE 18-7 Causes of Meningitis (Continued)

Microorganism	Characteristics	Antibiotics
Histoplasmosis	• Hydrocephalus because of preference for basal meninges	• Liposomal amphotericin B 5 mg/kg IV daily for 6 wk then itraconazole 200–300 BID–TID for > 1 y until resolution of symptoms and Histoplasma antigen
Coccidioides immitis	• Hydrocephalus because of preference for basal meninges • CSF: lymphocytes, low glucose, and occasional eosinophils • Complement fixing antibodies	• For meningitis, PO fluconazole for 3–6 mo • Alternative: itraconazole or intrathecal amphotericin B
Angiostrongylus cantonensis	• Asian and South Pacific • Caused by ingestion of mollusc hosts such as snails, slugs, and prawns or raw vegetables with larvae that penetrate gut wall and migrate to small vessels of meninges, causing fever, meningismus, and headache • CSF eosinophilia ("Eosinophilic meningitis") • Usually self-limited	• Supportive • Steroids for 2 wk • Avoidance of antihelminthic agents that can cause inflammatory response
Toxoplasma gondii	• HIV • Multiple, ≥ 3 nodular, contrast enhancing lesions with mass effect common in basal ganglia at gray-white matter junction • CSF pleocytosis usually a reactivation • IgG antibody is + in 95% of patients • Brain biopsy if atypical presentation or not responsive to antimicrobials	• Sulfadiazine, pyrimethamine, and leucovorin for 6 wk • Chemoprophylaxis with sulfadiazine + pyrimethamine + leucovorin after acute therapy is recommended to prevent recurrence but discontinued if CD4 ≥ 200 cells/mm³ for ≥ 6 mo • Alternatives include pyrimethamine, clindamycin, and leucovorin; leucovorin and atovaquone; or Aatovaquone, pyrimethamine, and leucovorin • Steroids considered if clinical deterioration or midline shift
Naegleria fowleri	• Free-living amoeba enters CNS via nasal mucosa at level of cribriform plate and can cause acute pyogenic meningitis after person swims in fresh water • CSF shows polymorphonuclear pleocytosis, many RBCs, and hypoglycorrhachia	• Amphotericin B 1.5 mg/kg/d in 2 doses for 3 d followed by 1 mg/kg/d for 11 d OR amphotericin B intrathecally 1.5 mg/d for 2 d followed by 1 mg/d for 8 d
Acanthamoeba	• Cell-mediated immunity, results in granulomatous amebic encephalitis • Concomitant pneumonitis • Preexisting skin lesions present for months before CNS and take form of ulcerative, nodular, or SQ abscess	• Uncertain: combination of miltefosine, fluconazole, and pentamidine with or without trimethoprim-sulfamethoxazole, metronidazole, and macrolide
Neurocysticercosis, caused by pork tapeworm Taenia solium	• Latin America, Asia, sub-Saharan Africa, and Oceania • Seizures, headache, hemiparesis, and ataxia; typically begin years after initial infection when host inflammation develops against T solium antigens released after death of parasite • Cystic or calcified but also chronic inflammation at the base of brain causing hydrocephalus • Serologies such as ELISA	• Albendazole or praziquantel; steroids should be given concomitantly to reduced edema • No treatment for inactive calcified lesions

BBB = blood–brain barrier; BID = twice daily; CD = cluster of differentiation 4; CNS = central nervous system; CSF = cerebrospinal fluid; DM = diabetes mellitus; ELISA = enzyme-linked immunosorbent assay; HIV = human immunodeficiency virus; ICP = intracranial pressure; Ig = immunoglobulin; MIC = minimum inhibitory concentration; PMN = polymorphonuclear leukocytes; PO = orally; RBCs = red blood cells; RIPE = rifampin, isoniazid, pyrazinamide, and ethambutol; SQ = subcutaneous; TB = tuberculosis; TID = 3 times daily; WBC = white blood cells.

demonstrated by culture or histology, or clinical criteria with 2 major criteria, 1 major criterion and 3 minor criteria, or 5 minor criteria.[134] Possible IE requires 1 major criterion and 1 minor criterion or 3 minor criteria (Table 18-9).[134]

Baddour et al. published guidelines with the diagnosis, treatment, and management of complications of infective endocarditis in adults.[135] Level of evidence (LOE) is defined as Level A if data is from multiple randomized clinical trials or meta-analyses, Level B if data from a single randomized trial or nonrandomized studies, and Level C if data is consensus opinion or case studies.[135] The class of recommendation is estimate of size of treatment effect and considered class I if benefits outweigh risks; Class IIa if benefits outweigh risks but additional studies with focused objectives needed; Class IIB if benefits may or may not outweigh risks and additional studies with broad objective needed; and Class III suggest that there is more harm than benefit.[135] Initial evaluation includes 3 sets of blood cultures and transthoracic echocardiogram (TTE) (Class I; LOE A). Transthoracic echocardiogram is preferred over transesophageal echocardiogram (TEE) as the

TABLE 18-8 Causes of Neuritis

	Characteristics	Treatment
Herpes simplex virus 2	• Virus lies dormant in sensory ganglia after primary infection • Reactivation can cause lumbosacral radiculomyelitis with radicular pain, paresthesia, genital discomfort, and lower extremity weakness • Involvement of the conus medullaris or cauda equina may result in associated urinary retention • Immunocompromised individuals are at risk for disseminated infection, which may result in fatal ascending myelitis	• IV acyclovir
Varicella-zoster virus	• Primary infection results in chicken pox • Reactivation results in shingles: itching, paresthesia, dysesthesia, allodynia, hyperesthesia, and severe neuropathic pain • Segmental zoster paresis can occur via spread to anterior horn, resulting in myotomal weakness as well	• Oral acyclovir, valacyclovir, or famciclovir shortens the duration of rash and sensory symptoms within 72 h of rash onset • IV acyclovir for disseminated herpes zoster or immunocompromised patients • Prevention with vaccine
HIV	• Distal, symmetric, sensory-predominant polyneuropathy	• Supportive
West Nile virus	• Meningoencephalitis picture is most common • Can rarely (5%) present as isolated motor paralysis without symptoms of meningoencephalitis; weakness can be profound and often involves respiratory muscles	• Supportive
Borrelia burgdorferi (Lyme)	• Ixodes scapularis • Early neurologic disease includes radiculopathy, cranial neuropathy, mononeuropathy multiplex, lymphocytic meningitis, and encephalomyelitis • Cranial nerve 7 palsy is the most common cranial neuropathy and is usually bilateral • Late Lyme disease is associated with stocking glove neuropathy which can include reduced vibratory sensation in the lower extremities and encephalopathy	• Early Lyme without neurologic manifestations: doxycycline, amoxicillin, or cefuroxime for 14–21 d. • Lyme meningitis: ceftriaxone, cefotaxime, penicillin G

Mycobacterium leprae	• Directly infects nerves
	• Long incubation period of 2 to 12 y
	• 2 forms:
	  • Tuberculoid leprosy: localized to the skin, sensory loss
	  • Lepromatous leprosy: widespread involvement of peripheral nerves; over time, there is spread to peripheral nerve trunks, most commonly causing ulnar neuropathy
		• Dapsone and rifampin for tuberculoid disease, with addition of clofazimine for lepromatous disease

Corynebacterium diphtheriae	• Produces toxins that injure peripheral nerves • Noninflammatory demyelination that initially produces local paralysis of the soft palate and posterior pharyngeal wall followed by CN involvement and peripheral nerves • Myocarditis in two-thirds but < 25% have clinical dysfunction	• Antitoxin + antibacterial with penicillin and erythromycin with slower fever clearance and higher GI side effects with erythromycin
Clostridium tetani	• Produces toxins that injure peripheral nerves • Toxin is transported up to axons and binds to presynaptic endings on motor neurons on anterior horn cells of spinal cord, blocks inhibitory signals, and results in uncontrolled motor input to skeletal muscle and tetanic spasm • Prevention is key and antibody levels decline over time	• Antitoxin not yet available but tetanus immune globulin and tetanus toxoid given
Clostridium botulinum	• Produces toxins that injure peripheral nerves • Toxin binds to presynaptic axon terminal of NM junction with inhibition of acetylcholine release, leading to symmetrical, descending, flaccid paralysis of motor and autonomic nerves, usually beginning with CN • Food-borne outbreaks with contaminated fish, commercial cheese sauce, baked potatoes held in aluminum for days at room temperature, drug users who inject Mexican black tar heroin • Neurologic and GI symptoms such as nausea, vomiting, diminished salivation, drying of mouth, difficulty focusing of eyes, progression to CN palsies, diplopia, dysarthria, dysphagia, then to symmetrical descending flaccid voluntary muscle weakness that may result in respiratory compromise • Diagnosis via (1) EMG showing > 50% in evoked train of compound muscle action potentials with rapid repetitive stimulation (20–50 Hz), (2) stool culture + for C botulinum, and (3) blurred vision, dysphagia, or dysarthria in person who did not have EMG findings indicating botulism and who did not have C botulinum in stool • High risk for death with decreased gag but no diarrhea • Intestinal botulism usually occurs in infants, which might be caused by colonization of GI tract by C botulinum or C baratii with role for botulism immune globulin IV, and does not respond to antitoxin	• Antitoxin is indicated for adult botulism and for wound botulism

(Continued)

TABLE 18-8 Causes of Neuritis (Continued)

	Characteristics	Treatment
Trypanosome	• Directly infects nerves • Autonomic neuropathy typically manifests as GI dysmotility	
Ciguatera fish poisoning	• Grouper, red snapper, and barracuda produced by microalgae known as dinoflagellates • GI, cardiovascular, and neurological symptoms, such as perioral paresthesias, and in distal extremities with debilitating hot-to-cold reversal dysesthesia • Toxins include ciguatoxin (which induces membrane depolarization by opening voltage-dependent sodium channels), maitotoxin (opens calcium channels), and palytoxin (muscle injury)	• Supportive
Paralytic shell fish poisoning	• Saxitoxin (a heat-stable alkaloid neurotoxin) or related compounds resulting in sensory, cerebellar, and motor dysfunction	• Supportive

CN = cranial nerve; EMG = electromyography; GI = gastrointestinal; HIV = human immunodeficiency virus; IV = intravenous; NM = neuromuscular.

initial diagnostic approach due to cost. However, TEE can be considered as the initial diagnostic test if patient has chronic obstructive pulmonary disease (COPD), is morbidly obese, or had prior cardiovascular surgery.[135] False negatives are secondary to small vegetations, vegetation that has already embolized, echocardiogram performed too early, or perivalvular abscess.[136,137] False positives include prior scarring or Lambl excrescenses.[135] Potential organisms include viridans group streptococci, *Streptococcus bovis*, HACEK (*Haemophilus species, Aggregatibacter, Cardiobacterium hominis, Eikenella corrodens*, and *Kingella*), *S aureus*, enterococci, *Brucella, Legionella, Tropheryma whipplei*, fungi, and *Mycobacterium* (Table 18-10).[135]

Transesophageal echocardiogram is performed if suspicion is high and initial TTE is negative (Class I; LOE B).[135] If the TEE is negative and suspicion is still high, it can be repeated in 3 to 5 days (Class I; LOE B).[135] Transesophageal echocardiogram can also be performed if there is a new intracardial complication (Class I; LOE B).[135]

Blood cultures are redrawn every 24 to 48 hours until they are negative. Duration of antibiotics is determined from the time of initial negative culture (Class IIa; LOE C). Type of IE and antimicrobial treatment is seen in Table 18-11.[135]

Surgery is considered for heart failure, 1 or more embolic events during first 2 weeks of antimicrobial therapy, fungal IE, highly resistant organisms, heart block, annular or aortic abscess, persistent bacteremia or fever lasting more than 5 days, recurrent emboli or persistent enlarging vegetations despite appropriate antibiotic treatment, severe valvular regurgitation, and mobile vegetation greater than 10 mm, particularly in the anterior mitral leaflet.[135] Surgery may be delayed for up to 4 weeks for intracranial hemorrhage or large ischemic cerebrovascular accident (CVA).[138]

Skin and Soft Tissue Infections

Cellulitis and *erysipelas* have been used interchangeably to mean a superficial diffuse skin infection that is not associated with collections of pus.[139] Distinction between the two have been suggested, such as erysipelas being most closely associated with the face and limited only to the upper dermis, including superficial lymphatics.[140] They are erythematous, swollen, warm, and tender, sometimes resembling an orange peel.[139] The most common cause is streptococci, particularly group A.[139] Blood cultures are often necessary, and aspirate or skin biopsies are only necessary for patients with cancer, sepsis, immersion injury, animal bites, neutropenia, and cell-mediated immunodeficiency.[141] Cellulitis that requires hospitalization might require a 5-day course of antibiotics, and steroids have been suggested to decrease inflammation.[139] Duration might be increased depending on the microbe isolated and if there is no improvement after 5 days.

Necrotizing fasciitis is an aggressive subcutaneous infection along the superficial fascia, usually in the lower extremities. Fournier gangrene is a type of necrotizing infection

TABLE 18-9 Modified Duke Criteria

Major Criteria	• 2 separate positive blood cultures > 12 h apart, or all 3 or a majority of ≥ 4 separate blood cultures with the first and last drawn at least 1 h apart • Single positive blood culture for *Coxiella burnetii* or anti-phase 1 IgG titer ≥ 1:800 • Evidence of endocardial involvement • Echocardiogram positive for IE: oscillating intracardiac mass on valve or other structures in absence of other explanation, abscess, new partial dehiscence of prosthetic valve, or new valvular regurgitation
Minor Criteria	• Predisposing heart condition or intravenous drug user (IDU) • Temperature > 38°C • Arterial emboli, pulmonary septic infarcts, mycotic aneurysms, intracranial hemorrhage, conjunctival hemorrhages, Janeway lesions • Glomerulonephritis, Osler nodes, Roth spots, and rheumatoid factor positive • Positive blood culture without meeting a major criterion

IDU = intravenous drug user; Ig = immunoglobulin.

TABLE 18-10 Epidemiologic Feature and Associated Microorganism in Endocarditis

Epidemiologic Feature	Common Microorganism	Epidemiologic Feature	Common Microorganism
IDU	S aureus, coagulase-negative staphylococci, β-hemolytic streptococcus, fungi, aerobic Gram-negative bacilli such as Pseudomonas, polymicrobial	Diabetes mellitus	S aureus, β-hemolytic streptococci, S pneumoniae
Indwelling cardiovascular medical device	S aureus, coagulase-negative staphylococci, fungi, aerobic Gram-negative bacilli, Corynebacterium spp	Early (≤ 1 y) prosthetic valve placement	Coagulase-negative staphylococci, S aureus, aerobic Gram-negative bacilli, fungi, Corynebacterium spp, Legionella spp
Genitourinary disorders, infection, and manipulation, including pregnancy, delivery, and abortion	Enterococcus spp, group B streptococci, Listeria monocytogenes, aerobic Gram-negative bacilli, Neisseria gonorrhea	Late (> 1 y) prosthetic valve placement	Coagulase-negative staphylococci, S aureus, viridans group streptococci, Enterococcus spp, fungi, Corynebacterium spp
Chronic skin disorders	S aureus, β-hemolytic streptococci	Dog or cat exposure	Bartonella spp, Pasteurella spp, Capnocytophaga spp
Poor dental health	Viridans group streptococci, nutritionally variant streptococci, Abiotrophia defectiva, Granulicatella spp, Gemella spp, HACEK	Contact with contaminated milk or infected farm animals	Brucella spp, Coxiella burnetii, Erysipelothrix spp
Alcoholism, cirrhosis	Bartonella spp, Aeromonas spp, Listeria spp, S pneumoniae, β-hemolytic streptococci	Homeless, body lice	Bartonella spp
Burn	S aureus, anaerobic Gram-negative bacilli such as Pseudomonas, fungi	AIDS	Salmonella spp, S pneumoniae, S aureus
Pneumonia, meningitis	S pneumoniae	Gastrointestinal lesions	S gallolyticus (S bovis), Enterococcus spp, Clostridium septicum
Solid organ transplantation	S aureus, Aspergillus fumigatus, Enterococcus spp, Candida spp		

involving the scrotum and penis or vulva. There may or may not be a visible initial lesion that rapidly progresses, leading to shock and multiorgan failure. There is severe pain, failure to respond to antibiotics, a wooden hard induration of the subcutaneous tissue on palpation, crepitus on palpation, edema, bullous lesions, and skin necrosis or ecchymosis.[139] It can be secondary to 1 organism such as S pyogenes, S aureus, Vibrio vulnificus, Aeromonas hydrophila, or Peptostreptococcus, or it could be polymicrobial, particularly in the setting of perianal abscesses, penetrating trauma, bowel surgery, decubitus ulcers, injections from drug use, or spread from genital sites.[139] Although CT or MRI may aid with the diagnosis by showing edema tending along the fascial plain, it should not delay initiation of treatment. Primary therapeutic modality is surgical debridement and antibiotics. Empirical antibiotics are usually penicillin and clindamycin, which suppress streptococcal toxin and cytokines.[142-146] Other empirical antibiotics include vancomycin or linezolid with piperacillin-tazobactam or carbapenem, or plus ceftriaxone and metronidazole.[139]

Myonecrosis or clostridial gas gangrene is caused by Clostridium perfringens, C novyi, C histolyticium, or C septicum.[139] C perfringens is most closely associated with trauma-associated gas gangrene, and C septicum is associated with neutropenia and malignancy.[147] It is characterized by increasing severe pain within 24 hours and skin color changes from pale to bronze to purplish-red.[139] Gas within the tissues is suggested by crepitus on palpation. There is a rapid development of shock and multiorgan failure. Treatment involves antibiotics such as penicillin and clindamycin and surgical debridement.

Pyomyositis is pus in the muscles and usually is caused by S aureus.[139] There is localized pain, tenderness, and fever. Serum creatine kinase is normal. Magnetic resonance imaging is used to visualize the muscle inflammation and/or abscess. Treatment is antibiotics with or without drainage if there is an abscess.

Pericardial Infectious Diseases

The pericardial sac consists of the visceral pericardium, which is a single layer of mesothelial cells and comes in contact with the myocardium, and the parietal pericardium, which is less than 2 mm thick and composed of collagen and elastin.[148-150] There is a space in between 2 layers of the pericardium that

TABLE 18-11 Type of Infective Endocarditis and Antimicrobial Treatment

Type of Infective Endocarditis	Treatment
Native valve IE with viridans group streptococci, *S gallolyticus* (MIC ≤ 0.12 µg/mL)	• Aqueous crystalline penicillin G 12–18 million U/24 h for 4 wk • Ceftriaxone 2 g IV/IM daily for 4 wk • Vancomycin 30 mg/kg per 24 h (trough 10–15 µg/mL) • Aqueous crystalline penicillin G or ceftriaxone with gentamicin (3 mg/kg per 24 h) for 2 wk
Native valve IE with viridans group streptococci, *S gallolyticus* (MIC >0.12–< 0.5 µg/mL)	• Aqueous crystalline penicillin G 12–18 million U/24 h for 4 wk and gentamicin (3 mg/kg per 24 h) for 2 wk • Vancomycin 30 mg/kg per 24 h (trough 10–15 µg/mL) • Ceftriaxone 2 g IV/IM daily for 4 wk and gentamicin (3 mg/kg per 24 h) for 2 wk if sensitive to ceftriaxone
Prosthetic valve IE with viridans group streptococci, *S gallolyticus*	• Aqueous crystalline penicillin G or ceftriaxone for 6 wk with or without gentamicin (3 mg/kg per 24 h) for first 2 wk • Aqueous crystalline penicillin G or ceftriaxone for 6 wk with or without gentamicin (3 mg/kg per 24 h) for 6 wk if MIC > 0.12 µg/mL
Native valve IE with staphylococci	• Nafcillin or oxacillin 12 g/24 h IV for 6 wk or 2 wk for uncomplicated right-sided IE • Cefazolin 6 g/24 h for 6 wk • Vancomycin 30 mg/kg 24 h for 6 wk (trough 10–20 µg/ml) for oxacillin-resistant strains • Daptomycin ≥ 8 mg/kg/dose for 6 wk for oxacillin-resistant strains
Prosthetic valve IE with staphylococci	• Nafcillin or oxacillin 12 g/24 h IV for 6 wk with rifampin 900 mg/24 h > 6 wk with gentamicin 3 mg/kg 24 h IV for 2 weeks • Vancomycin 30 mg/kg 24 h for 6 wk with rifampin 900 mg/24 h > 6 wk with gentamicin 3 mg/kg 24 h IV for 2 wk for oxacillin-resistant strains
IE with enterococcus	• Ampicillin 2 g IV every 4 h for 4 to 6 wk or aqueous crystalline penicillin G 12–18 million U/24 h for 4–6 wk plus gentamicin 3 mg/kg (> 3 mo for prosthetic valve IE) • Double β-lactam ampicillin 2 g IV every 4 h for 6 wk with ceftriaxone 2 g IV every 12 h for 6 wk • Ampicillin 2 g IV every 4 h for 4–6 wk or aqueous crystalline penicillin G 12–18 million U/24 h for 4–6 wk plus streptomycin 15 mg/kg/24 h IV for gentamicin-resistant strains • Linezolid 600 mg IV or PO every 12 h for > 6 wk if resistant to penicillin, aminoglycosides, and vancomycin • Daptomycin 10–12 mg/kg per dose > 6 wk if resistant to penicillin, aminoglycosides, and vancomycin
IE with HACEK	• Ceftriaxone 2 g/24 h IV for 4 wk • Ampicillin 2 g IV every 5 h • Ciprofloxacin 1000 mg/24 h PO or 800 mg/24 h IV for 4 wk

HACEK = *Haemophilus species, Aggregatibacter, Cardiobacterium hominis, Eikenella corrodens,* and *Kingella*; IE = infective endocarditis; IM = intramuscular; IV = intravenous; MIC = minimal inhibitory concentration; PO = orally.

contains 15 to 35 mL of serous fluid. It is relatively inelastic, therefore limiting cardiac dilation and enhancing interaction of the cardiac chambers.

Pericarditis can be acute, subacute, or chronic and can be with or without pericardial effusion. The most common infectious causes are viruses such as enteroviruses, herpesviruses, adenovirus, and parvovirus B19. Tuberculosis is the most common bacterial cause but other bacterial considerations includes *Coxiella burnetii, Borrelia burgdorferi,* pneumococcus, meningococcus, gonococcus, streptococcus, staphylococcus, *Haemophilus, Chlamydia, Mycoplasma, Legionella, Leptospira, Listeria,* and *Providencia stuartii.* Rare causes include *Histoplasma, Aspergillus, Blastomyces, Candida, Echinococcus,* and *Toxoplasma.*[150]

Diagnosis of acute pericarditis involves 2 of the following 4 criteria: (1) pericarditic chest pain, (2) pericardial rubs, (3) new widespread ST elevation or PR depression on electrocardiography (ECG), and (4) new or worsening pericardial effusions.[150] Supportive findings include elevated C-reactive protein (CRP), erythrocyte sedimentation rate (ESR), white blood cell count (WBC), and pericardial inflammation on CT and cardiac MRI.[150] Incessant pericarditis lasts more than 4 weeks but less than 3 months, and chronic pericarditis lasts for longer than 3 months. Recurrent is recurrence of pericarditis after more than a 4-week symptom-free interval. Predominant pericarditis with myocardial involvement, or *myopericarditis,* is defined as acute pericarditis with elevated markers of myocardial injury without focal or diffuse impairment of the left ventricle on echocardiography or cardiac MR. Predominant myocarditis with pericardial involvement, or *perimyocarditis,* has new focal or diffuse reduction of left ventricular function with elevated markers of myocardial injury. Myocarditis requires biopsy for confirmation of diagnosis; however, it is usually not necessary if there is no evidence of left ventricular dysfunction.[151,152]

Initial evaluation involves chest radiograph (which can show increased cardiothoracic ratio if >300 mL pericardial effusion), ECG, echocardiogram, and markers of inflammation.[150] Pericardial effusion is considered mild if it is less than 10 mm, moderate if it is 10 to 20 mm, and large if it is greater than 20 mm of diastolic echo-free space. Echographic evidence of tamponade includes swinging of the heart, early diastolic collapse of the right ventricle, late diastolic collapse of the right atrium, abnormal ventricular septal motion, exaggerated respiratory variability (> 25%) in mitral inflow velocity, inspiratory decrease and expiratory increase in pulmonary vein diastolic forward flow, respiratory variation in ventricular chamber size, aortic outflow velocity, and inferior vena cava plethora.[150]

Risk factors for poor prognosis include fever greater than 38°C, subacute course, large pericardial effusion (diastolic echo-free space > 20 mm), tamponade, and failure to respond to 7 days of nonsteroidal anti-inflammatory drugs (NSAIDs).[153,155]

Treatment for acute pericarditis includes aspirin (750–1000 mg every 8 hours for 1–2 weeks, decreased by 250–500 mg every 1–2 weeks) or NSAIDs (eg, ibuprofen 600 mg every 8 hours for 1–2 weeks, decreased by 200–400 mg every 1–2 weeks) with gastro protection. (LOE B) Colchicine (0.5 mg [< 70 kg] or 0.5 mg twice daily [≥ 70 kg]) for 3 to 6 months is given as adjunct to reduce recurrence in acute and recurrent pericarditis.[150](LOE A) C-reactive protein is used to gauge response to treatment. Corticosteroids (prednisone 0.2–0.5 mg/kg/d) is indicated if there is incomplete resolution with aspirin and NSAIDs. (LOE B) Patients who cannot tolerate colchicine can be given azathioprine, intravenous human immunoglobulins, and anakinra.[150] (LOE C) Pericardiocentesis or surgery is recommended for tamponade, symptomatic moderate or large pericardial effusions not responsive to medical therapy, and suspicion of unknown bacterial or neoplastic etiology.[150] Evaluation of the pericardial fluid is via Light criteria and will help determine the etiology.

Constrictive pericarditis has impaired diastolic filling due to pericardial disease with signs of heart failure but preserved right and left ventricular function.[150] Diagnosis may require chest radiograph, CT, and/or MRI and cardiac catheterization.[150] It is important to distinguish constrictive pericarditis from restrictive cardiomyopathy. They are compared in Table 18-12.[156]

Pleural Effusions

Aspiration is generally not required on bilateral effusions when the clinical setting suggests transudative effusions, unless it has atypical features or treatment fails.[157] Potential causes of transudative pleural effusions include congestive heart failure, liver cirrhosis, hypoalbuminemia, peritoneal dialysis, nephrotic syndrome, hypothyroidism, mitral stenosis, constrictive pericarditis, Meigs syndrome, and urinothorax.[157] The British Thoracic Society Pleural Disease Guideline defined their grades of recommendation as such: Grade A has more than or equal to 1 meta-analysis, systemic review or randomized trial; Grade B has high quality systemic review of case-control or cohort studies or meta-analysis and/or randomized control trials with high risk of bias; Grade C well conduced case-control or cohort studies with low risk of confounding, bias, or chance; and Grade D is case reports, case series, and expert opinion.[157] Definition of exudate versus transudate is based on Light criteria, which defines an exudate as 1 or more of the following: pleural fluid protein/serum protein greater than 0.5; pleural lactate dehydrogenase (LDH)/serum LDH greater than 0.6; and pleural fluid LDH greater than one-half the upper limit of the normal value for serum LDH[158] (Grade B).

TABLE 18-12 Comparison Between Constrictive Pericarditis and Restrictive Cardiomyopathy

Diagnostic Evaluation	Constrictive Pericarditis	Restrictive Cardiomyopathy
Physical findings	Kussmaul sign, pericardial knock	Regurgitant murmur, Kussmaul sign may be present, S3 (advanced)
EGG	Low voltages, nonspecific ST/T changes, atrial fibrillation	Low voltages, pseudoinfarction, possible widening of QRS, left-axis deviation, atrial fibrillation
Chest x-ray	Pericardial calcifications (one-third of cases)	No pericardial calcifications
Echocardiography	• Septal bounce • Pericardial thickening and calcifications • Respiratory variation of the mitral peak E velocity of > 25% and variation in the pulmonary venous, peak D flow velocity of > 20% • Color M-mode flow propagation velocity (V_p) > 45 cm/sec • Tissue Doppler: peak e' > 8.0 cm/s	• Small left ventricle with large atria, possible increased wall thickness • E/A ratio > 2, short DT • Significant respiratory variations of mitral inflow are absent • Color M-mode flow propagation velocity (V_p) < 45 cm/sec • Tissue Doppler: peak e' < 8.0 cm/s.
Cardiac catheterization	"Dip and plateau" or "square root" sign, right ventricular diastolic and left ventricular diastolic pressures usually equal, ventricular interdependence (ie, assessed by the systolic area index > 1.1)[a]	Marked right ventricular systolic hypertension (> 50 mmHg) and left ventricular diastolic pressure exceeds right ventricular diastolic pressure (LVEDP > RVEDP) at rest or during exercise by 5 mmHg or more (RVEDP < 1/3 RVSP).
CT/CMR	Pericardial thickness > 3–4 mm pericardial calcifications (CT), ventricular interdependence (real-time cine CMR)	Normal pericardial thickness (< 3.0 mm), myocardial involvement by morphology and functional study (CMR)

a = systolic area index is the ratio of the RV area (mmHg × s) to the LV area (mmHg × s) in inspiration versus expiration; CMR = cardiovascular magnetic resonance; CT = computed tomography; RVSP = right ventricular systolic pressure

Reprinted with permission from Imazio M, Brucato A, Mayosi BM, et al. Medical therapy of pericardial diseases: part II: noninfectious pericarditis, pericardial effusion and constrictive pericarditis. *J Cardiovasc Med (Hagerstown).* 2010;11(11):785-794.

Aspiration should be guided by ultrasound with a 21G needle and 50-mL syringe[157] (Grade B). The characteristic of the pleural fluid and the associated laboratory findings will help guide in the etiology of the effusion (Table 18-13).[157]

Drainage are indicated for pleural effusions that are loculated, or have greater than 50% hemithorax, positive pleural Gram stain or positive culture, and/or purulent pleural fluid with pleural pH less than 7.20, glucose less than 60 mg/dL, lactate dehydrogenase 3 times the upper normal limit of serum[157-159] (Grade B). The evolution of parapneumonic effusion to empyema comes in 3 stages. The first stage is exudate with rapid fluid flow secondary to increased capillary permeability and characterized by negative studies, glucose greater than 60 mg/dL, pleural pH greater than 7.20, and pleural LDH less than 3 times the upper normal limit of serum.[159,160] The second stage is the fibropurulent stage characterized by positive bacterial studies, glucose less than 60 mg/dL, pH less than 7.20, and pleural LDH more than 3 times the upper normal limit of serum.[159,160] The third stage is defined by growth of fibroblasts, producing a thick pleural peel.[159] Table 18-14 characterizes parapneumonic effusions and empyema based on anatomy, bacteriology, chemistry, risk of poor outcome, and drainage.[161]

Once the characteristic for drainage is met, it is important to drain it within 24 hours or the evolution of the effusion can progress and it will be difficult to drain.[162,163] Rahman et al found no significant difference in mortality or the need for surgery from varying sizes of chest tubes, although the bigger chest tubes were associated with more pain (size < 10F, number dying or needing surgery, 21/58 [36%]; size 10–14F, 75/208 [36%]; size 15–20F, 28/70 [40%]; size > 20F, 30/69 [44%]; chi^{2}trend, 1; and degrees of freedom [df] = 1.21; $P = 0.27$).[164] Rahman et al also showed that combination of intrapleural tissue plasminogen activator (t-PA) and DNAse improved drainage of pleural effusion and reduced surgical referral and duration of hospital stay compared to either agent alone.[165]

Maternal Infections

Pyelonephritis

This is the most common cause of septic shock during pregnancy and is related to relative obstruction of the urinary tract from the uterus, progesterone-induced dilation of the ureters, and lack of protective peristalsis.[166,167] The most common pathogen is *Escherichia coli* but other common pathogens include *Klebsiella*, *Proteus*, and *Enterobacter*.[168] Empiric treatment begins with clindamycin and ampicillin and failure to respond should prompt investigation for nephrolithiasis or abscess.

Chorioamnionitis

This is an infection of the chorion, amnion, and placenta in the setting of ruptured membranes, but it can occur with intact membranes.[166,167] Risk factors include young age, prolonged labor, nulliparity, prolonged rupture of membranes, multiple vaginal examinations, meconium-stained amniotic fluid, internal monitoring, group B streptococcus colonization, and bacterial vaginosis.[166] *Ureaplasma urealyticum* and *Mycoplasma hominis* are the most common causes but others include *Gardnerella vaginalis*, *Bacteroides*, group B streptococci, and Gram-negative rods such as *E coli*.[169,170] Empiric treatment is ampicillin with gentamicin with or without metronidazole, and clindamycin if cesarean delivery.[166]

Septic Abortion

This is fetal loss at less than 20 weeks' age of gestation and is associated with an infection, although associated more with induced abortion. The approach is to administer broad spectrum antibiotics and evacuate uterine contents.

TABLE 18-13 Differential Based on Pleural Fluid Characteristics

Characteristics	Disease
Odor and/or color	• Putrid odor: anaerobic empyema • Food particles: esophageal rupture • Bile: chylothorax • Milky: chylothorax/pseudochylothorax • Anchovy sauce: rupture of amoebic abscess
Cell count	• Lymphocytosis (> 50% are lymphocytes) seen predominantly in tuberculosis but other differential includes lymphoma, rheumatoid pleurisy, sarcoidosis, and late coronary artery bypass graft effusions • Neutrophils predominate in pulmonary embolism, acute tuberculosis, and benign asbestos pleural effusions • Eosinophilic (≥10%) from air or blood in pleural space, drug induced, benign asbestos pleural effusions, pulmonary infarction, parasitic disease, Churg-Strauss syndrome
pH	• pH < 7.30: malignant effusions, complicated parapneumonic effusions, empyema, connective tissue disease (particularly rheumatoid arthritis), tuberculous effusions, esophageal rupture
Glucose	• Glucose < 60 mg/dL: malignant effusions, complicated parapneumonic effusions, empyema, connective tissue disease (particularly rheumatoid arthritis), tuberculous effusions, esophageal rupture
Amylase	• Elevated if pleural > serum amylase or ratio > 1.0 • Elevated in acute pancreatitis, pancreatic pseudocysts, ectopic pregnancy, pleural malignancy, esophageal rupture
Triglycerides, cholesterol	• > 110 mg/dL if chylothorax, which is from disruption of the lymphatic duct and tributaries • > 200 mg/dL and/or presence of cholesterol crystals suggests pseudochylothorax
Hematocrit	• > 50% pleural hematocrit/serum hematocrit suggests hemothorax
Cytology	• Evaluation for malignancy

TABLE 18-14 **Characteristics of Parapneumonic Effusions and Empyema**

Pleural Space Anatomy		Pleural Fluid Bacteriology		Pleural Fluid Chemistry	Category	Risk of Poor Outcome	Drainage
A_0: Minimal, free-flowing effusion (< 10 mm on lateral decubitus)	and	B_x: culture and Gram stain results unknown	and	C_x: pH unknown	1	Very low	No
A_1: Small to moderate free-flowing effusion (> 10 mm and < one-half hemithorax)	and	B_0: negative culture and Gram stain	and	C_0: pH ≥ 7.20	2	Low	No
A_2: Large, free-flowing effusion (≥ one-half hemithorax) loculated effusion, or effusion with thickened parietal pleura	or	B_1: positive culture and Gram stain	or	C_1: pH < 7.20	3	Moderate	Yes
		B_2: pus			4	High	Yes

Endometritis

This is generally a polymicrobial infection that occurs post-partum and includes endometrial lining, myometrium, and parametrium.[166] Typical anaerobes include *Peptostreptococcus*, *Bacteroides*, and *Clostridium*, and aerobes include group B strep-tococci, enterococci, and *E coli*.[166] Empirical antibiotics include gentamycin, clindamycin, and ampicillin. Complications include uterus perforation, peritonitis, and septic thrombophlebitis.

QUESTIONS

1. A 40-year-old man with chronic lymphocytic leukemia was admitted for small bowel obstruction. He had an exploratory laparotomy and lysis of adhesions. Postop day 4, he is found nauseous and vomiting. He is awake and following com-mands. Vital signs are as follows: BP of 130/70 mmHg, HR of 70 beats/min, RR of 18 breaths/min; O_2 sat of 99% on 2 Liters via nasal cannula (NC), temp of 97.1°F. On ausculta-tion, he is noted to have rhonchi at the right base. His labs are obtained 6 hours later and include the following:

WBC	$14 \times 10^3/\mu L$
Hemoglobin	10 g/dL
Platelets	$100 \times 10^3/\mu L$
Sodium	135 mEq/L
Potassium	4 mEq/L
Chloride	108 mEq/L
Blood urea nitrogen	20 mg/dL
Creatinine	2 mg/dL
Glucose	100 mg/dL
Procalcitonin	0.20 mEq/L

On the chest radiograph, he is noted to have right lower lobe infiltrate. What is the next step?

A. Start piperacillin-tazobactam and vancomycin
B. Start ceftriaxone and azithromycin
C. Observation
D. Send to the ICU

2. A 24-year-old man with no past medical history was complaining of fevers, chills, cough, and shortness of breath. He claims he recently traveled to South America. His pulse oximetry was 85% on room air, and he was placed on 6 Liters of oxygen supplementation via nasal cannula, and his O_2 saturation increased to 95%. His vital signs include the following: BP of 102/60 mmHg, HR of 108 beats/min, RR of 34 breaths/min, O_2 sat of 95% on 6 Liters NC, and temp of 105°F. His physical examination is otherwise unremarkable except for bilateral rhonchi. His labs include the following:

WBC	$12 \times 10^3/\mu L$
Hemoglobin	14 g/dL
Hematocrit	38%
Platelets	$100 \times 10^3/\mu L$
Sodium	129 mEq/L
Chloride	111 mEq/L
Potassium	4.5 mEq/L
Blood urea nitrogen	35 mg/dL
Creatinine	0.76 mg/dL
Calcium	8 mEq/L
Glucose	100 mg/dL

His pH is 7.38, and his P_{O_2} 86. His chest radiograph shows bilateral infiltrates. What is the next step?

A. Outpatient management
B. Admit to observation
C. Admit to inpatient
D. Admit to ICU

3. A 55-year-old woman, weighing 65 kg, with past medical history of CVA with residual right-sided weakness, diabetes mellitus on insulin, obstructive sleep apnea on continuous positive airway pressure (CPAP) at night, coronary artery disease, systolic heart failure with an ejection fraction (EF) of 35%, and hypertension was found unresponsive in the nursing home. She had a BP of 90/60 mmHg, HR of 120 beats/min, RR of 8 breaths/min, O_2 saturation of 90% on room air and a temperature of 94.5°F. She was transferred to the emergency department (ED), where repeat vital signs were as follows: BP of 70/50 mmHg, HR of 150 beats/min, RR of 8 breaths/min, and O_2 saturation of 90% on room air. The patient was responsive to sternal rub. Physical examination showed decreased breath sounds bilaterally, and her abdomen was soft and nontender. Her labs include the following:

WBC	$27 \times 10^3/\mu L$
Hemoglobin	10 g/dL
Platelets	$250 \times 10^3/\mu L$
Sodium	151 mEq/L
Chloride	116 mEq/L
Potassium	4 mEq/L
Blood urea nitrogen	50 mg/dL
Creatinine	2.5 mg/dL
Calcium	9 mEq/L
Glucose	70 mg/dL
Lactic acid	5 mmol/L

Her chest radiograph was unremarkable. Her urinalysis showed WBC 62/HPF, positive leukocyte esterase, and positive nitrates. The patient was given a 2-L normal saline bolus and started on ceftriaxone. Her repeat blood pressure was noted to be SBP 85/50 mmHg. What is the next step?

A. Noninvasive cardiac output monitoring
B. Norepinephrine 5 µg/kg/h IV
C. Albumin
D. Normal saline 1000 mL IV bolus

4. A 28-year-old nurse presents to the ED with a fever that started yesterday right before lunch. She denies cough, chest pain, dysuria, chills, or sweats. There has been no recent weight loss. Around the same time as the fever began, she noticed myalgia and headache and lost her appetite. She has returned from volunteering at an Ebola clinic 12 days ago. She has no known allergies and no other chronic medical issues. On exam, she appears fatigued. Her vitals are as follows: BP of 102/62 mmHg, HR of 94 beats/min, RR of 14 breaths/min, temperature of 102.1°F, and O_2 saturation of 98% on room air. Her physical examination is remarkable for dry mucous membranes and diffuse abdominal tenderness. The patient has no rash. Her labs include the following:

WBC	2.6×10^3 µL
Hemoglobin	11.1 g/dL
Platelets	$102 \times 10^3/\mu L$
Sodium	144 mEq/L
Potassium	4.1 mEq/L
Chloride	107 mEq/L
CO_2	24 mEq/L
Blood urea nitrogen	24 mg/dL
Creatinine	1.1 mg/dL
Glucose	74 mg/dL
Rapid HIV	negative

The phlebotomy lab calls you and informs you that "headphone-like" inclusions are seen inside the erythrocytes on the blood smear. A urine pregnancy test is consistent with a first-trimester pregnancy. Which is the most appropriate course of treatment?

A. Antipyretics and fluid supplementation
B. Atovaquone and azithromycin
C. Chloramphenicol and a tetracycline
D. Quinine and clindamycin

5. A 42-year-old man presents to the ED with multiple episodes of vomiting. He was hiking in North Carolina 6 days ago when he noticed a tick over his medial malleolus. He cannot recall the appearance of the tick in order to identify the species. Last night, he has developed a severe headache, fevers, and chills. He has developed a rash that was initially on the wrists and ankles, and then it spread to the trunk; now, he has noted it on his palms. He has been vomiting for over 24 hours, which prompted a visit to the ED.

On physical exam, he has pink blanchable macules over his forearms and palms. Petechiae are seen on his upper and lower extremities. He has no meningeal signs, and the remainder of his physical exam, including vital signs, are normal. His labs include the following:

WBC	$2.6 \times 10^3/\mu L$
Hemoglobin	11.1 g/dL
Platelets	$90 \times 10^3/\mu L$
Sodium	135 mEq/L
Potassium	4.1 mEq/L
Chloride	107 mEq/L
CO_2	24 mEq/L
Blood urea nitrogen	24 mg/dL
Creatinine	1.1 mg/dL
Glucose	74 mg/dL

Which of the following is true?

A. Indirect fluorescent antibody is the gold standard for diagnosis.
B. Antibodies against *Proteus vulgaris* antigens OX2 and OX19 (Weil-Felix test) and latex agglutination are the gold standard for diagnosis.
C. Latex agglutination
D. Chloramphenicol is the treatment of choice.

6. Which of the following is a true statement?

   A. Doxycycline can treat Lyme disease, human granulocytic anaplasmosis, and babeiosis.
   B. Erythema migrans appears immediately after the *Ixodes* tick is removed.
   C. Stocking glove neuropathy is an early manifestation of Lyme disease.
   D. Cranial nerve VII palsy is the most common CN neuropathy associated with Lyme disease.

7. A 27-year-old woman with no significant past medical history went hiking at a nearby park. Forty-eight hours later, she noted an adult tick that was still attached to her skin. Lyme disease rate of infection in the area is 20%. She has no allergies to medications. What is the next step?

   A. Give doxycycline 200 mg PO × 1 day
   B. Give ceftriaxone 2 g IV daily × 14 days
   C. Rifampin 300 mg twice daily for 7 to 10 days as an alternative
   D. Atovaquone 750 mg PO 12 hours plus azithromycin 500 mg PO on day 1 and 250 mg on subsequent days

8. Which of the following is not an indication for CT scan before lumbar puncture for meningitis?

   A. Altered mental status
   B. HIV
   C. Seizure
   D. None of the above

9. A 32-year-old man with no past medical history presents with headache, fevers, and neck stiffness for the last 3 days. Vital signs are the following: HR of 92 beats/min, RR of 12 breaths/min, BP of 122/72 mmHg, temperature of 101.9°F, and SpO_2 of 98% on room air. Physical exam is remarkable for a positive Kernig sign. A lumbar puncture is performed.

   Which of the following findings from the lumbar puncture are consistent with bacterial meningitis?

   A. Opening pressure, 150 mm H_2O; WBC, 4000/μL; neutrophils, 85%; protein, 200 mg/dL; glucose, 60 mg/dL
   B. Opening pressure, 350 mm H_2O; WBC, 5000/μL; neutrophils, 90%; protein, 200 mg/dL; glucose, 30 mg/dL
   C. Opening pressure, 350 mm H_2O; WBC, 4500/μL; neutrophils, 20%; protein, 300 mg/dL; glucose, 10 mg/dL
   D. Opening pressure, 400 mm H_2O; WBC, 4500/μL; neutrophils, 90%; protein, 250 mg/dL; glucose, 65 mg/dL

10. A 24-year-old man was complaining of nonproductive cough, headache, and sore throat. This was followed by abdominal pain, left shoulder pain, fatigue, anorexia, nausea, and vomiting. On physical examination, his vitals were as follows: SBP of 88/50 mmHg, HR of 123 beats/min, RR of 24 breaths/min, temperature greater than 38°C, and O_2 saturation of 94% on room air. A small pinkish rash was noted on his trunk and lower extremities. His abdominal CT scan shows adrenal hemorrhage and his blood Gram stain shows Gram-negative diplococci. What is the pathogen?

    A. *N meningitides*
    B. *H influenzae*
    C. *Listeria*
    D. *S pneumoniae*

11. A 30-year-old man was complaining of intermittent episodes of stabbing pains on the face, back, and limbs. He also complained of abdominal pain, nausea, and vomiting. On physical examination, his left pupil was noted to be small, not responding to light or dilating to painful stimuli. There is normal accommodation and convergence. He is noted to have jerky movement when he walks. His head CT was negative. Lumbar puncture was performed and showed the following:

WBC	50/μL
Lymphocytes	90%
Protein	75 mg/dL
Glucose	80 mg/dL
Venereal Disease Research Laboratory test	reactive

    What is the treatment?

    A. Penicillin G benzathine 2.4 million units IM weekly for 3 weeks
    B. Penicillin G procaine 2.4 million units IM daily plus probenecid 500 mg orally 4 times daily for 10 to 14 days
    C. Doxycycline 100 mg PO twice daily for 4 weeks
    D. Penicillin G benzathine 2.4 million units IM × 1

12. An 80-year-old man from a nursing home in New York City presents, complaining of lower extremity weakness. The patient is noticed to have a fine tremor on his upper extremities and lower extremity weakness, with his right greater than the left. He has a maculopapular rash on his abdomen. His head CT and MRI head were unremarkable. EEG shows global slowing. Laboratory findings is remarkable for WBC 2.8×10^3/μL. A lumbar puncture is performed and shows the following:

Opening pressure	180 mmH$_2$0
WBC	100/μL
Protein	150 mg/dL
Glucose	60 mg/dL

    What is the most likely diagnosis?

    A. West Nile virus
    B. Listeriosis
    C. Guillain-Barré syndrome
    D. St Louis encephalitis

13. A 44-year old-woman with no significant past medical history was complaining of fever, malaise, nausea, vomiting, retro-orbital pain, hematemesis, and headaches. She has returned from a 3-week trip to Southeast Asia. On physical examination, her vital signs were as follows: BP of 80/60 mmHg, HR of 120 beats/min, RR of 18 breaths/min, temperature of 105°F, and O_2 saturation of 88% on room air. She was noted to have blanching rash on her anterior and posterior trunk, extending to her extremities. She had bleeding gums. She was also noted to have rales on auscultation. Her laboratory findings include the following:

WBC	$3 \times 10^3/\mu L$
Hemoglobin	15 g/dL
Platelets	$100 \times 10^3/\mu L$
Aspartate aminotransferase	1000 U/L
Alanine aminotransferase	1000 U/L

Her dengue immunoglobulin M (IgM) was 3 mg/dL and her IgG was less than 0.8 mg/dL; 6 days later, her IgM was 4 mg/dL and her IgG was 6 mg/dL.

What is your diagnosis?

A. Dengue fever
B. Dengue hemorrhagic fever
C. Dengue with warning signs
D. Severe dengue

14. What is the appropriate chemoprophylaxis for meningo-coccal exposure in a 30-year-old man?

A. Rifampin 10 mg/kg every 12 hours
B. Ceftriaxone 125 mg IM dose
C. Rifampin 20 mg/kg every 12 hours
D. Ceftriaxone 250 mg IM × 1

15. A 25-year-old man with no past medical history has returned from a trip to Africa complaining of fever, chills, nausea, vomiting, and abdominal pain. His physical examination was unremarkable except for icteric sclera and bleeding gums. His labs showed the following:

WBC	$3 \times 10^3/\mu L$
Platelets	$70 \times 10^3/\mu L$
Hemoglobin	15 g/dL

His tourniquet test was positive. Which of the following statements is *false*?

A. Yellow fever and dengue fever both have triphasic clinical presentation.
B. Chikungunya can be clinically distinguished from dengue with its predominant arthritic manifestations and fewer hemorrhagic complications.
C. Positive tourniquet test is suggested by more than 10 petechiae in 1 square inch underneath the cuff.
D. Infection with 1 serotype of dengue does not give you immunity to that serotype.

16. A 35-year-old man is complaining of headaches, dizziness, neck stiffness, and fevers for the last 4 days. He has no past medical history. He is a nonsmoker and socially drinks alcohol. He is a farmer. In the ED, his vital signs are the following: BP of 120/60 mmHg, HR of 101 beats/min, RR of 18 breaths/min, temperature of 100.4°F, and O_2 saturation of 96% on room air. His physical examination is unremarkable except for conjunctival suffusion and neck stiffness. His laboratory examination includes the following:

Hemoglobin	15 g/dL
Platelets	$300 \times 10^3/\mu L$
WBC	$16 \times 10^3/\mu L$ with 90% segmented neutrophils and 14.1% lymphocytes
Creatinine	0.9 mg/dL
Aspartate aminotransferase	34 IU/L
Alanine aminotransferase	12 IU/L
Glucose	109 mg/dL

He has a lumbar puncture, which shows an opening pressure of 240 mm H_2O, WBC of 254 cells/μL with 90% mononuclear cells and 9% segmented neutrophils, RBC of 2 cells/μL, glucose of 60 mg/dL, and protein of 90 mg/dL. He was started on ceftriaxone 2 g every 12 hours and acyclovir 500 mg IV every 8 hours, with some improvement. What is the most likely diagnosis?

A. Leptospirosis
B. Rocky Mountain spotted fever
C. Ehrlichiosis
D. Infective endocarditis

17. A 65-year-old Asian man, who is obese and has a history of DM, recently returned from Hong Kong complaining of shortness of breath, cough, fever, sore throat, and chills for 1 day. He arrived at the airport and his symptoms progressed, so he went to the ED. He was noted to have persistent tachypnea and hypoxia to 80% on nonrebreather, and he was subsequently intubated. Rapid testing for influenza was negative but the sputum PCR was positive for influenza B. Which of the following medications would you prescribe?

A. Amantadine
B. Ceftriaxone and azithromycin
C. Oseltamivir
D. Rimantadine

18. A 65-year-old man with history of coronary artery disease and hypertension had a recent mitral valve replacement 3 months ago. He presents with fever, chills, and shortness of breath. His chest radiograph was unremarkable, but his chest CT with contrast shows multiple nodular infiltrates. He was started on ceftriaxone and azithromycin. His blood cultures subsequently grew *S aureus*. His echocardiogram showed a 12-mm vegetation on the anterior leaflet of the mitral valve. What is the next step?

A. Refer to surgery
B. Finish course of antibiotics and then refer to surgery
C. Change antibiotics
D. Do not change treatment

19. A 59-year-old man with a history of atrial fibrillation on anti-coagulation, hypertension, COPD, and diabetes mellitus was admitted for fever, chills, and shortness of breath. Initially, he was treated for sepsis from multilobar pneumonia. He was started on ceftriaxone and azithromycin. Preliminary readings of initial blood cultures grew coagulase-negative streptococci. His transthoracic echocardiogram was essentially unremarkable. On day 3, the patient was noted to have collapsed after having a bowel movement. Initially, it was thought to be vasovagal, but a CT showed a large intracerebral hemorrhage. He was intubated. Neurosurgery and palliative consults were called. His intracerebral hemorrhage has stabilized after 3 days, but he continued to have fevers. Three additional sets of cultures have been performed, but all were negative. A transesophageal echocardiogram showed a vegetation in the aortic valve. What is the next step?

A. Surgery
B. Serologies for *Bartonella*, *C burnetii*, and *T whipplei*
C. Change antibiotics
D. Start antifungal

20. A 45-year-old man is complaining of low fever, chills, productive cough, and pleuritic chest pain for the last 3 days. He works at a horse farm, smokes 1 pack per day, and socially drinks. In the ED, he is noted to have oxygen saturation of 80% on room air, with a BP of 70/50 mmHg, HR 130 beats/min, and RR of 25 breaths/min. On physical examination, he has unilateral axillary adenopathy and pustule skin lesions on the right arm. His labs show the following:

Lactic acid	5 mmol/L
WBC	$20 \times 10^3/\mu L$
Platelets	$200 \times 10^3/\mu L$
Creatinine	1.5 mg/dL

His chest radiograph shows bilateral infiltrates. The patient was given crystalloid bolus and started on ceftriaxone and azithromycin. The axillary lymph node was aspirated for culture and histopathology. What is the most likely diagnosis?

A. *Yersinia pestis*
B. *Burkholderia mallei*
C. *Erysipelothrix rhusiopathiae*
D. *Bartonella* species

21. A 48-year-old man presents to the ED with fever and malaise for the last 4 days. This morning, he develop a cough and dyspnea. He denies headaches, neck pain, or stiffness. He has no past medical history and works in a wool mill. His vitals are as follows: BP of 124/72 mmHg, HR of 108 beats/min, RR of 22 breaths/min, temperature of 100.7°F, and O₂ saturation

of 89% on room air. The patient is alert and oriented but appears dyspneic. His chest x-ray demonstrates mediastinal widening and small bilateral pleural effusions. You are concerned about inhalation anthrax. Appropriate antibiotics for this condition would be which of the following?

A. Ciprofloxacin 500 mg every 12 hours for 5 days
B. Ciprofloxacin 400 mg every 8 hours and clindamycin 900 mg every 8 hours for 2 weeks or until clinically stable (whichever is longer)
C. Ciprofloxacin 400 mg every 8 hours and rifampin 600 mg every 12 hours
D. Ciprofloxacin 400 mg (IV) every 8 hours, meropenem 2 g every 8 hours, and linezolid 600 mg every 12 hours for 2 to 3 weeks (whichever is longer)

22. A 27-year-old female nurse comes to you in panic. She just discovered that a patient she triaged at a local clinic 6 days ago had developed symptoms of Ebola virus disease and was being quarantined in an isolated ICU for supportive care and management. The patient was asymptomatic at the time of encounter but noted that he had returned the day prior from an area with a recognized epidemic of Ebola hemorrhagic fever. She was not wearing personal protective equipment (PPE) when she took his vital signs and is concerned that she contracted the virus. She denies fever, chills, myalgia, headaches, diarrhea, or other complaints. Vital signs reveal the following: BP of 136/82 mmHg, HR of 82 beats/min, RR of 14 breaths/min, and temperature of 98.7°F. Her physical exam is unremarkable. Which of the following is the most appropriate next step in management?

A. Immediate isolation and admission to an ICU equipped for management of Ebola virus disease
B. Restrict the patient to her house for monitoring for 21 days without sending reverse transcription polymerase chain reaction for Ebola virus
C. Restrict the patient to her house for monitoring for 21 days and send reverse transcription polymerase chain reaction for Ebola virus
D. Reassure the patient without monitoring or sending of diagnostic studies

23. A 29-year-old woman (gravida 1 para 0) presents at 20 weeks of pregnancy with sudden onset fever, vomiting, and flank pain. Her pregnancy has been uncomplicated thus far. There is no abdominal pain, dysuria, or vaginal bleeding. Vitals reveal the following: BP of 105/60 mmHg, HR of 112 beats/min, RR of 15 breaths/min, and temperature of 101.0°F. Physical exam reveals an uncomfortable female. Her abdomen is gravid but not tender. She has left costovertebral angle tenderness. Fetal heart rate measures 145 beats/min. Laboratory examination demonstrates the following:

WBC	$16.2 \times 10^3/\mu L$
Hemoglobin	10.2 g/dL
Platelets	$210 \times 10^3/\mu L$

Her electrolytes, kidney function, and hepatic function panel are normal. Urinalysis reveals 3+ leukocyte esterase and more than 300 WBCs. Lactic acid is 2.8 mmol/L. You suspect pyelonephritis. Which of the following antimicrobials is most appropriate?

A. Cefepime
B. Fosfomycin
C. Levofloxacin
D. Trimethoprim-sulfamethoxazole

24. A 45-year-old man who recently immigrated from Africa and has a history of HIV was complaining of progressive shortness of breath, low-grade fever, chills, night sweats, and weight loss for the last 2 to 3 weeks. Today, he also noted chest pain and prompted him to see further evaluation. In the ED, his vital signs were BP of 70/50 mmHg, HR of 130 beats/min, RR of 22 breaths/min, temperature of 101°F, and O_2 saturation of 88% on room air. Physical examination is remarkable for a cardiac rub. His ECG shows diffuse ST elevations. His bedside echocardiogram shows a 20-mm pericardial effusion, no wall motion abnormalities, and preserved ejection fraction. Fluid resuscitation has taken place. What would be the next step?

A. Initiate rifampin, isoniazid, pyrazinamide, and ethambutol
B. Start prednisone
C. Perform pericardiocentesis
D. Start aspirin and colchicine

25. A 44-year-old man with history of alcohol abuse was complaining of fevers, chills, cough, and chest pain. Chest radiograph and CT of the chest revealed a right-sided loculated pleural effusion. Pleural aspiration was performed and the pleural studies showed pleural pH of 6.9 and glucose less than 10 mg/dL and was purulent in color and consistency. Therefore, a 14F tube thoracotomy was inserted. What is the appropriate next step?

A. Deoxyribonuclease 5 mg and tissue plasminogen activator 10 mg intrapleural for 1 hour every 12 hours for 3 days
B. Streptokinase 10 mg intrapleural for 1 hour every 12 hours for 3 days
C. Deoxyribonuclease 5 mg intrapleural for 2 hours every 12 hours for 3 days
D. Deoxyribonuclease 1 mg and tissue plasminogen activator 2 mg intrapleural for 15 minutes every 6 hours for 3 days

26. A 60-year-old woman who recently arrived from India is complaining of fever, night sweats, hemoptysis, and weight loss. Chest radiograph shows right-sided loculated pleural effusion. What would be helping in diagnosing tuberculous pleural effusion?

A. Pleural acid-fast bacilli
B. Pleural biopsy
C. Pleural lymphocytosis
D. Pleural adenosine deaminase

ANSWERS

1. C. Observation

Procalcitonin is a biomarker that has helped with antibiotic stewardship. It is normally secreted from the thyroid gland and lungs and is a precursor to calcitonin. In the setting of bacterial infection, it is also secreted from the spleen, kidneys, liver, adrenal glands, brain, spine, pancreas, stomach, small intestine, colon, heart, muscle, skin, fat, and testes.[10] It is more specific than leukocytosis or CRP for bacterial infection and rises within 3 to 6 hours, peaks at 6 to 12 hours, and has a half-life of 24 hours. It is not affected by immunosuppression.[171] In the setting of massive surgery, trauma, or burns, the initial levels would be falsely elevated, but subsequently, levels will trend down if there is no infection. If there is a concomitant infection, the levels will remain elevated.[172] For initial evaluation of bacterial infection, with a PCT of less than 0.1 ng/L or a PCT of 0.1 to 0.25 ng/L, antibiotics are discouraged[172,173] (choice C). However, antibiotics are still considered with these levels if (1) PCT is less than 0.1 ng/L with CAP with PSI class V, CURB-65 greater than 3, and/or COPD with Global Initiative for Obstructive Lung Disease (GOLD) IV; or (2) PCT less than 0.25 μg/L with CAP with PSI class IV or V, CURB-65 greater than 2, and COPD with GOLD III or IV.[172,173] If the PCT is between 0.25 and 0.5 ng/L or greater than 0.5 ng/L, antibiotics are encouraged.[172,173] If antibiotics are initiated, repeat PCT on day 3, 5, and 7 and stop if (1) PCT is 0.1 to 0.25 ng/L or (2) peak PCT is high but has decreased 80% to 90% from peak and repeat PCT is less than 0.5 μg/L.[172,173] Treatment failure occurs if PCT remains high.

The Effect of Procalcitonin-Based Guidelines vs Standard Guidelines on Antibiotic Use in Lower Respiratory Tract Infections (ProHOSP) trial suggested that the use of procalcitonin to guide antibiotic administration in lower respiratory tract infections lowered the rates of antibiotic exposure and antibiotic-associated diarrhea, and the rates of adverse effects were similar in PCT and control groups (15.4% [n = 103] vs 18.9% [n = 130]; difference, −3.5%; 95% CI, −7.6% to 0.4%).[173] Use of procalcitonin to reduce patients' exposure to antibiotics in intensive care units (PRORATA) also showed similar findings. Mortality of patients in the procalcitonin group seemed to be noninferior to those in the control group at day 28 (21.2% [65/307] vs 20.4% [64/314]; absolute difference, 0.8%; 90% CI, −4.6 to 6.2) and day 60 (30.0% [92/307] vs 26.1% [82/314]; absolute difference, 3.8%; 90% CI, −2.1 to 9.7). Patients in the procalcitonin group had significantly more days without antibiotics than did those in the control group (14.3 days [SD 9.1] vs 11.6 days [SD 8.2]; absolute difference, 2.7 days; 95% CI, 1.4–4.1; $P < 0.0001$).[174] The placebo controlled trial of sodium selenite and procalcitonin guided antimicrobial therapy in severe sepsis (SISPCT) multicenter randomized clinical trial did not show improved survival.[175] It has been suggested that PCT on the first day of ICU admission was associated with lower hospital and ICU length of stay.[176]

If the PCT was 0.25 ng/L or higher or the patient was hemodynamically unstable, antibiotics would be warranted. He would have required piperacillin-tazobactam with vancomycin since he would have had hospital-acquired pneumonia (choice A). Even if the patient met the criteria to use antibiotics, ceftriaxone and azithromycin would be the wrong choice of antibiotics (choice B). The patient is currently hemodynamically stable and would not need ICU right now (choice D).

2. **C. Admit to inpatient**

Based on CURB-65, his score is 2, warranting inpatient admission. Based on the Pneumonia Severity Index, his score is 109, also warranting inpatient admission. His SMART-COP score is 4, which also warrants inpatient admission. The patient is too sick to be treated as an outpatient, and he most likely will require hospitalization for greater than 24 hours (choices A and B). However, he currently does not have the criteria to be admitted to the ICU (choice D).

3. **A. Noninvasive cardiac output monitoring**

There was a partial response to initial fluid resuscitation and further fluid resuscitation might be limited due to her history of systolic heart failure. In this instance, dynamic or functional monitoring of fluid responsiveness is key. Starting norepinephrine may be premature (choice B). There is no benefit for albumin over crystalloid in fluid resuscitation (choice C). Further fluid resuscitation might cause an exacerbation of her congestive heart failure (choice D).

4. **D. Quinine and clindamycin**

"Headphone-like" rings are a typical appearance of *Plasmodium falciparum*. This parasite is transmitted through mosquitoes in endemic areas such as West Africa. Pregnant women are more likely to be infected than their nonpregnant counterparts, possibly due to the affinity of mosquitoes to pregnant women. Untreated malarial infection in pregnancy increases maternal mortality and leads to low neonatal birth weight. Quinine and clindamycin are the first-line agents for the treatment of *P falciparum* for pregnant women in the first trimester (choice D). Antipyretics and fluid supplementation would be appropriate management of infections that do not have proven antimicrobial therapy, such as dengue fever (choice A). Atovaquone and azithromycin are appropriate for first-line treatment of

babesiosis, which may present as "Maltese crosses" on a blood smear (choice B). Chloramphenicol or a tetracycline (tetracycline is a second-line treatment in pregnancy) would be appropriate treatment for a pregnant patient with Rocky Mountain spotted fever (RMSF), which is not endemic to West Africa (choice C).

5. **A. Indirect fluorescent antibody is the gold standard for diagnosis.**

The patient most likely has Rocky Mountain spotted fever. Due to various sensitivities and specificities, indirect fluorescent antibody (IFA) has emerged as the gold standard serologic test.[177] The Centers for Disease Control and Prevention (CDC) collected surveillance data in the 1980s and determined the sensitivities of the Weil-Felix (Choice B) and latex agglutination tests (Choice C) to be 47% to 70% and 71%, respectively[178] while the indirect fluorescent antibody test was 94% sensitive. The use of PCR as a diagnostic test for RMSF was also found to be lacking sensitivity[179] and therefore is not recommended to make the diagnosis (choice C). An alternative to make the diagnosis in this patient would be to perform a biopsy of the rash and check a PCR, a test which would have 73% sensitivity and 100% specificity.[180] Doxycycline is undoubtedly the treatment of choice in cases of suspected RMSF.[181] There is evidence[182] that initiation of treatment within 5 days of symptom onset reduced mortality from 22.9% to 6.5%, underscoring the importance of initiating treatment even without objective evidence of the organism. Chloramphenicol is the only other drug that has been studied in the treatment of RMSF and has been shown to be inferior to doxycycline[183] and therefore is used only in rare cases of doxycycline adverse reactions or in pregnant women (choice D).

6. **D. Cranial nerve VII palsy is the most common CN neuropathy associated with Lyme disease.**

The tick species *Ixodes scapularis* and *Ixodes pacificus* transmit the spirochete *B burgdorferi*, which causes Lyme disease. *I scapularis* also transmit *Anaplasma phagocytophilum*, which causes human granulocytic anaplasmosis (HGA), and *Babesia microti*, which causes babesiosis. Coinfection in patients with suspected Lyme disease should be considered when there is persistent fever for more than 48 hours after antibiotic treatment and unexplained anemia, thrombocytopenia, or leukopenia.[184]

An erythematous skin lesion, less than 5 cm, which appears within 48 hours of *Ixodes* attachment and disappears within 48 hours, is a hypersensitivity reaction and not infectious (choice B). Primary erythema migrans is a round, expanding lesion that appears 7 to 10 days after *Ixodes* has been removed.[185-194] It can be solitary or multiple secondary to hematogenous dissemination. Vesicles or pustules can be found in the center and generally are not associated with pruritus.[195] Diagnosis can be made based on this lesion but if still uncertain, serum samples during the acute and convalescent phases (2 weeks after) should be obtained.[184] Early neurologic disease includes radiculopathy, cranial neuropathy, mononeuropathy multiplex, lymphocytic meningitis, and encephalomyelitis. Cranial nerve VII palsy is the most common cranial neuropathy and is usually bilateral.[130,131] Late Lyme disease is associated with stocking glove neuropathy, which can include reduced vibratory sensation in the lower extremities and encephalopathy (choice C). Other late manifestations include arthritis and acrodermatitis chronica atrophicans.[184]

For early Lyme disease (erythema migrans) in the absence of neurologic manifestations or advanced heart block, treatment consist of doxycycline 100 mg twice daily (BID), amoxicillin 500 mg 3 times daily (TID), or cefuroxime 500 mg BID for 14 to 21 days. For Lyme meningitis, treatment is ceftriaxone 2 g IV daily for 10 to 28 days, or the alternatives are cefotaxime 2 g IV every 8 hours or penicillin G 18 to 24 million units daily every 4 hours for 10 to 28 days. Lyme carditis with atrioventricular heart block and/or myopericarditis can be treated with PO or parenteral antibiotics for 14 to 21 days. Pacemakers are recommended. Late Lyme disease, such as arthritis, is treated with doxycycline 100 mg BID, amoxicillin 500 mg TID, or cefuroxime axetil 500 mg BID for 28 days.

Human granulocytic anaplasmosis is associated with fever, chills, headache, thrombocytopenia, leukopenia, and increased liver enzymes within 3 weeks of exposure to *I scapularis* or *I pacificus*. It is a rickettsial infection of the neutrophils.[184] Diagnosis is based on identification of intragranulocytic inclusions on blood smear and antibodies to *A phagocytophilum*. Treatment is doxycycline 100 mg BID for 10 days. Rifampin 300 mg BID for 7 to 10 days is an alternative. Asymptomatic seropositive patients are not recommended to be treated.

Babesiosis is diagnosed with a viral-like infection and identification of parasites in blood smear or PCR. This viral-like infection consists of fever, nausea, vomiting, myalgia, fatigue, jaundice, hemolytic anemia, and hepatosplenomegaly. Asymptomatic babesiosis should not be treated but can be considered if there is persistent parasitemia for 3 months or more. Recommended treatment is atovaquone 750 mg PO 12 hours plus azithromycin 500 mg PO on day 1 and 250 mg on subsequent days, or clindamycin 300 to 600 mg every 6 hours IV plus quinine 650 mg PO every 6 to 8 hours for 7 to 10 days in severe babesiosis (choice A). Red blood cell exchange transfusions may be indicated if parasitemia is 10% or greater, if there is significant hemolysis, or if there is renal, hepatic, or pulmonary impairment.[184] Lyme carditis can occur concurrently, right after, or within 2 months of erythema migrans or neurologic Lyme disease. Presence of *B burgdorferi* antibodies in the acute or convalescent phase may be indicated when there is not a clear-cut correlation.

7. A. Give doxycycline 200 mg PO × 1 day

Antimicrobial prophylaxis and serologies for Lyme disease are not routinely recommended unless all of the following exist: (1) the tick is a nymph or adult *I scapularis* attached for 36 hours or more; (2) prophylaxis can be started within 72 hours from the time the tick is removed; (3) the local rate of infection is 20% or greater; and (4) doxycycline is not contraindicated.[184] Prophylaxis is a single dose of 200 mg of doxycycline (choice A).

Ceftriaxone 2 g IV daily for 10 to 21 days is the treatment for Lyme disease with early neurologic manifestations or Lyme carditis (choice B).

Rifampin 300 mg BID for 7 to 10 days is the alternative to doxycycline for HGA (choice C).

Atovaquone 750 mg PO 12 hours plus azithromycin 500 mg PO on day 1 and 250 mg on subsequent days is the treatment for babesiosis (choice D).

8. D. None of the above

Complications from lumbar punctures can be deadly. The incidence of brain herniation is unknown; however, some studies have quoted the risk to be less than 1.2%. A study involving 301 adult patients with bacterial meningitis described that CT scan has a negative predictive value of 97%. These findings led to the guidelines in Table 18-15 (Grade B-II).[94]

TABLE 18-15 Recommended Criteria for Adult Patients With Suspected Bacterial Meningitis Who Should Undergo CT Prior to Lumbar Puncture

Criterion	Comment
Immunocompromised state	HIV infection or AIDS, receiving immunosuppressive therapy, or after transplantation
History of CNS disease	Mass lesion, stroke, or focal infection
New onset seizure	Within 1 wk of presentation; some authorities would not perform a lumbar puncture on patients with prolonged seizures or would delay lumbar puncture for 30 min in patients with short, convulsive seizures
Papilledema	Presence of venous pulsations suggestions absence of increased intracranial pressure
Abnormal level of consciousness	—
Focal neurological defect	Including dilated nonreactive pupil, abnormalities of ocular motility, abnormal visual fields, gaze palsy, arm or leg drift

AIDS = acquired immunodeficiency syndrome; CNS = central nervous system; HIV = human immunodeficiency virus.

Reprinted with permission from Tunkel AR, Hartman BJ, Kaplan SL, et al. Practice guidelines for the management of bacterial meningitis. *Clin Infect Dis.* 2004;39(9):1267-1284.

9. **B. Opening pressure, 350 mm H$_2$O; WBC, 5000/μL; neutrophils, 90%; protein, 200 mg/dL; glucose, 30 mg/dL**

As indicated in Table 18-4, choice B is most consistent with bacterial meningitis.[55-59] Choice A may be seen in early viral meningitis, but the normal opening pressure makes bacterial meningitis less likely. Choice C is incorrect, as one would expect neutrophil predominance in bacterial meningitis. Choice D is less likely, as one would expect a lower CSF glucose in bacterial meningitis.

10. **A. *N meningitides***

N meningitides causes meningitis, meningitis and meningococcemia, or meningococcemia. It is the leading cause of meningitis in children and young adults and even with antibiotic treatment carries a 13% to 15% mortality.[196] The main toxin is the lipopolysaccharide that is located in the outer membrane and directly proportional to symptoms.[197] Meningococcemia can cause acute massive adrenal hemorrhage with Waterhouse-Friderichsen syndrome, disseminated intravascular coagulation, and purpura fulminans. Diagnosis is made through blood cultures, skin biopsies, and CSF analysis. Gram stain would show Gram-negative diplococci. Treatment is with third-generation cephalosporin such as ceftriaxone, penicillin, or chloramphenicol. Treatment with ceftriaxone, rifampin, or ciprofloxacin will eradicate nasal carriage.[198] Similarly, chemoprophylaxis in close contacts should be administered within 24 hours after contact and maintain droplet precautions for the first 24 hours. If it has been more than 14 days, chemoprophylaxis no value.

Small pleomorphic Gram-negative coccobacilli rare usually *H influenzae* (choice B). Gram-positive rods and coccobacilli are usually *Listeria* (choice C). Gram-positive diplococci are usually *S pneumoniae* (choice D).

11. **B. Penicillin G procaine 2.4 million units IM daily plus probenecid 500 mg orally 4 times daily for 10 to 14 days**

The patient has tabes dorsalis, which is a form of neurosyphilis. Tabes dorsalis can occur from 3 to 20 years after initial infection. The stages of syphilis with clinical manifestations and treatment are listed in Table 18-16.[199-203] Although the patient has lymphocytic meningitis with normal glucose and positive serologies, which is typical for neurosyphilis, the CSF and serum nontreponemal test may be normal in tabes dorsalis. Nontreponemal testing such as the Venereal Disease Research Laboratory (VDRL) test and rapid plasma regain (RPR) test also may be falsely positive in systemic lupus erythematosus, fungal infections, and tuberculosis. Treponemal tests such as the fluorescent treponemal antibody absorption test (FTA-ABS), the *Treponema pallidum* particle agglutination assay (TPPA), or syphilis enzyme immunoassay (EIA) should be performed because they remain reactive throughout life. The VDRL-CSF is highly specific. The FTA-ABS on CSF is less specific but has high sensitivity; therefore, a negative test excludes neurosyphilis. Reactive VDRL-CSF and CSF WBC of 10 cells/μL or more diagnoses neurosyphilis. The CSF-VDRL might not normalize after treatment, unlike CSF WBC or serum rapid plasma regain reactivity in HIV patients.[200-203]

Monitoring for treatment response in neurosyphilis is done via neurologic examination and lumber puncture at 3 to 6 months after treatment and then every 6 months afterward until WBC CSF is normal and VDRL is nonreactive. Retreatment is indicated if WBC CSF fails to

TABLE 18-16 Stages of Syphillis, Clinical Manifestations, and Treatment

Stages	Clinical Manifestations	Treatment
Early syphilis • Early latent • Primary • Secondary	• Asymptomatic but positive serologies within first year • Single painless chancre with adenopathy • Constitutional symptoms with rash and pharyngitis, arthritis, alopecia, and/or condyloma lata	• Penicillin G benzathine 2.4 million units IM × 1 • Alternative: doxycycline 100 mg PO BID for 2 wk, ceftriaxone 1–2 g daily IM/IV for 10–14 d, tetracycline 500 mg PO QID for 14 d, or amoxicillin 3 g plus probenecid 500 mg PO BID for 14 d
Late syphilis • Tertiary • Late latent	• Involving cardiovascular or gummatous disease • Asymptomatic but positive serologies > 1 y	• Penicillin G benzathine 2.4 million units IM weekly for 3 wk • Alternative: doxycycline 100 mg PO BID for 4 wk or ceftriaxone 2 g daily IM/IV for 10–14 d
Neurosyphilis • Early • Late	• Meningitis or meningovascular disease such as endarteritis of the middle cerebral artery • Dementia or tabes dorsalis	• Aqueous penicillin G 3–4 million units IV every 4 h (or 18–24 million units continuous IV infusion) for 10–14 d • Penicillin G procaine 2.4 million units IM daily plus probenecid 500 mg orally 4 times daily for 10–14 d • Alternative: ceftriaxone 2 g IV daily 10–14 d

BID = twice daily; IM = intramuscular; IV = intravenous; PO = orally; QID = 4 times daily.

Penicillin G benzathine 2.4 million units IM weekly for 3 weeks (choice A) and doxycycline 100 mg PO BID for 4 weeks (choice C) are treatments for late syphilis. One dose of penicillin G benzathine 2.4 million units IM (choice D) is treatment of early syphilis.

decrease after 6 months or VDRL fails to decline 4-fold or to become nonreactive after treatment.

12. A. West Nile virus

West Nile virus is a member of the genus *Flavivirus*, with a bird-mosquito-bird transmission cycle, and the vector is from the mosquito *Culex* genus.[204] The virus travels to infected dendritic cells or keratinocytes, the lymph nodes, and the central nervous system via (1) direct viral, crossing the blood-brain barrier via increased permeability; (2) infected macrophages; and (3) retrograde axonal transport from olfactory or peripheral nerves.[205] Transmission can also occur from blood product transfusions or transplantation.[204] The incubation period can last up to 21 days and symptoms include headache, malaise, low grade fever, chills, and a morbilliform, maculopapular, nonpruritic rash on the torso and extremities, sparing the palms and soles.[206,207] Neurologic symptoms include parkinsonism—coarse, postural, kinetic tremor particularly in the upper extremities—upper extremity clonus, ataxia, edema, seizures, and asymmetrical paralysis secondary to destruction of anterior horn cells of the spinal cord.[204] Other manifestations include choriditis, myocarditis, pancreatitis, hepatitis, stiff-person syndrome, and rhabdomyolysis.[204] WBC may be within normal range or low. Electroencephalogram show global slowing. Cerebrospinal fluid shows fewer than 500 WBC per µL, with neutrophils dominant early in disease, but later with lymphocytosis, normal glucose, and elevated protein less than 150 mg/dL.[208] Imaging studies are usually normal but may show lesions in the pons, basal ganglia, thalamus, anterior horns, and enhancement of leptomeninges.[204] A PCR might be helpful in immunocompromised patients, but IgM antibodies in the serum and CSF is gold standard for diagnosis. A plaque-reduction neutralization test may be helpful to distinguish false positives from yellow fever or Japanese encephalitis vaccinations or recent infection from St Louis encephalitis or dengue.[204] Full recovery is not unexpected, but fatigue and neuropsychiatric sequalae are common. Immunity may develop after initial infection, although its efficacy can dwindle over time.

St Louis encephalitis (choice D) also belongs to the genus *Flavivirus* and is similar to the West Nile virus' mode of infection, symptoms, and diagnosis.[209,210] St Louis encephalitis is characterized with an incubation period 4 to 21 days followed by high fevers, sore throat, cough, and malaise. In the acute phase, there is leukocytosis. There is less paralysis and seizures more common in children. Facial nerve weakness is common. Treatment is supportive.

Guillain-Barré syndrome (GBS; choice C) is secondary to an immune response against the myelin or axon of the peripheral nerves as a consequence of preconditioning based on molecular mimicry from prior infection. Cerebrospinal fluid analysis suggestive of GBS is albuminocytologic dissociation (protein > 0.55 g/L without elevation in WBC), which is 50% in the first week and more than

75% in the third week of infection; therefore, it is not always present. Serum autoantibodies are helpful in obtaining the diagnosis and variants (Table 18-17). Normal CSF protein may be encountered if the sample was obtained 1 week or less after onset of symptoms. Treatment includes supportive care for respiratory failure and dysautonomia. Disease-modifying treatments with equivalent efficacy are plasma exchange and IVIG.

13. D. Severe dengue

Dengue is a member of the genus *Flavivirus* transmitted by *Aedes aegypti* or *A albopictus* mosquitoes. There are 4 serotypes: DENV-1, DENV-2, DENV-3, and DENV-4. Incubation period is 3 to 14 days.[211] The 1997 World Health Organization (WHO) defined dengue fever (choice A) as a febrile illness with 2 or more of the following: headache, retro-orbital or ocular pain, myalgia or bone pain, arthralgia, rash, hemorrhagic manifestations, and leukopenia.[212] Hemorrhagic manifestations include positive tourniquet test, petechiae, purpura, ecchymosis, epistaxis, gum bleeding, hematemesis, hematuria, melena, or vaginal bleeding. Dengue hemorrhagic fever (DHF; choice B) is defined as fever for 2 to 7 days, hemorrhagic manifestations, thrombocytopenia of 100,000 cells/mm^3 or less, and plasma leakage (hematocrit rise $\geq$ 20%, drop in hematocrit with volume replacement, pleural effusions, ascites, or hypoproteinemia).[212] Dengue shock syndrome (DSS) is DHF with rapid and weak pulse, and/or narrow pulse pressure (20 mmHg), hypotension, or cold and clammy skin, and restlessness.[212] In 2009, this WHO criteria was revised. Dengue without warning signs is fever with 2 or more of the following: nausea and vomiting, rash, pain (headaches, eye pain, muscle or joint pain), leukopenia, and positive tourniquet test.[213] Dengue with warning signs (choice C) includes the criteria above with any of the following: abdominal pain, persistent vomiting, fluid accumulation such as ascites and pleural effusions, mucosal bleeding, lethargy or restlessness, hepatomegaly greater than 2 cm, and increase in hematocrit with concurrent decrease in platelets.[213] Severe dengue includes dengue with plasma leakage via shock or fluid accumulation, severe bleeding, and severe organ involvement such as aspartate aminotransferase (AST) or alanine aminotransferase (ALT) of 1000 units/L, altered mental status, and other organ failure.[213]

The fever is characterized as "saddleback" since initially it can rise to 102°F to 105°F, last for 2 to 7 days, defervesce for a few days, and rebound.[211] There are 2 types of rash: facial flushing or erythematous mottling before fever that disappears 2 days after symptoms and a scarlatiniform or maculopapular rash from the trunk that spreads outward and occurs on days 2 to 6 and lasts for up to 3 days.[211] After the febrile phase, petechiae may appear.

Dengue has 3 phases, which all occur in dengue with warning signs and severe dengue. The febrile phase is defined by high-grade biphasic fever, headache, vomiting, myalgias, arthralgias, hemorrhagic manifestations, leukopenia,

TABLE 18-17 Variants of Guillian Barre Syndrome

GBS Variant	Characteristics	Electrodiagnostic Study Findings
Acute inflammatory demyelinating polyneuropathy (AIDP)	• 85–90% of cases • Progressive, symmetrical muscle weakness with depressed or absent DTR	• Absent F waves and H reflexes followed by increased distal latencies and conduction slows with temporal dispersion of motor responses • Slowed nerve conduction velocities only on third to fourth week • Sural sparing
Miller Fisher syndrome	• More common in Japan • 5% in the United States • Associated with antibody to GQ1b • Ophthalmoplegia with ataxia and areflexia • One-quarter have extremity weakness	• Reduced or absent sensory responses without slowing of sensory conduction velocities, and motor nerve conduction abnormalities may be present if there is associated extremity weakness
Acute motor axonal neuropathy (AMAN)	• 5–10% of cases • *Campylobacter jejuni* • Similar to AIDP but sometime preserved DTR • Associated with antibodies to GM1, GD1a, GalNAC-GD1a, GD1b	• Selective involvement of motor nerves with distal motor amplitudes that are low and increase with recovery, reflecting reversible conduction failure at motor nerve terminal or node of Ranvier
Acute motor sensorimotor axonal neuropathy (AMSAN)	• 5–10% of cases • Severe form of AMAN due to both motor and sensory involvement	• Motor and sensory studies are reduced or absent
Bickerstaff brainstem encephalitis	• Hyperreflexia with ophthalmoplegia and ataxia • Clinically linked to Miller Fisher • Anti-GQ1b • Flaccid symmetrical tetraparesis • Disturbance of consciousness • Brainstem has perivascular lymphocytic infiltrate with edema and glial nodules	
Pharyngeal-cervical-brachial weakness	• Weakness of oropharyngeal neck and swallow dysfunction • Antibodies to GT1a, GQ1b, GD1a	
Acute pandysautonomia		
Pure sensory		
Facioplegia and distal limb paresthesia		
Acute bulbar palsy with areflexia, ophthalmoplegia, ataxia, and facial palsy		
Sixth nerve palsy and distal paresthesia		

Listeriosis (choice B) is a food-borne disease that causes febrile gastroenteritis, cellulitis, eye infections, lymphadenitis, septic arthritis, and meningoencephalitis, cerebritis, cerebral abscess, and rhombencephalitis. Symptoms include hemiplegia, ataxia, seizures, CN deficits, and deafness. The bacterium, *Listeria monocytogenes*, is aerobic, facultatively anaerobic, and Gram positive. Cerebrospinal fluid analysis would show pleocytosis with polymorphonuclear leukocytes, monocytes, or lymphocytes. Listeria is the only nontuberculous bacterial meningitis that can have lymphocytosis greater than 20%. Cerebrospinal fluid cultures are only 50% positive, even in the setting of cerebral abscess. Polymerase chain reaction is not readily available. Treatment for CNS infections is ampicillin with gentamicin for 3 to 6 weeks. Trimethoprim-sulfamethoxazole is an alternative.

thrombocytopenia, and transaminitis. The critical phase is a period of defervescence, usually lasting 24 to 48 hours, and patients may develop plasma leakage, bleeding, organ failure, and shock. The convalescence phase is when the patient improves. A pruritic rash for 1 to 5 days may occur.[211]

Diagnosis is clinical and laboratory with detection of viral nucleic acid via PCR or viral antigen nonstructural protein 1 (NS1) during the first week of the illness. Nonstructural protein 1 has a sensitivity of 90% during first infection and decreases to 60% to 80% during second infection. A 4-fold rise on IgM between the acute and convalescent phases can suggest acute infection. Primary infection is characterized by slow rise in IgG, whereas secondary infection is characterized by rapid rise in IgG.

Treatment is largely supportive. Primary infection may cause a lifelong immunity to that serotype and transient immunity to other dengue serotypes. Vaccine is available in Southeast Asia and Latin America but not in the United States.

14. D. Ceftriaxone 250 mg IM × 1

There are several available options for postexposure meningococcal chemoprophylaxis. It should be offered to close contacts of patients with meningococcal infection as early as possible after exposure (< 24 hours after contact). Recommended regimens include (1) rifampin, (2) ciprofloxacin, and (3) ceftriaxone. Rifampin is given for 2 days in the following dosing: for infants less than 1 month old, 5 mg/kg every 12 hours; for children older than 1 month, 10 mg/kg every 12 hours; and for adults, 600 mg every 12 hours. Ciprofloxacin 500 mg as a single dose may be administered to adults. Ceftriaxone dosing is 125 mg IM once for patients less than 15 years old (choice B) and 250 mg IM once for adults over 15 years old. Chemoprophylaxis has no role if the exposure occurred more than 14 days prior.

15. D. Infection with 1 serotype of dengue does not give you immunity to that serotype.

Infection with 1 serotype of dengue can give you immunity to that serotype and transient immunity to other serotypes.

The tourniquet test determines microvascular fragility. It is performed by inflating the blood pressure cuff on the arm midway between systolic and diastolic pressure for 5 minutes. Pressure is released and examination below the cuff is performed. It is positive if there are more than 10 petechiae in 1 square inch (choice C).

Chikungunya fever is often confused for dengue because it is transmitted via *Aedes* mosquito, and the clinical presentation is similar, with the high-grade biphasic fever, rash, headache, fatigue, nausea, and vomiting. Unlike dengue, there is predominant arthralgic manifestations, often symmetrical, in wrists, elbows, fingers, knees, and ankles, and they can result in a broad-based gait that can persist for months[214] (choice B). Diagnosis is via PCR and enzyme-linked immunosorbent assay (ELISA) for IgM and IgG. Treatment is supportive.

Yellow fever is a member of the genus *Flavivirus* that is transmitted by mosquitos from the genus *Haemagogus* in South America and *Aedes* in Africa.[215,216] Like dengue, it has a triphasic clinical presentation: phase 1 consists a viral exanthem with fever, myalgias, nausea, vomiting, dizziness, leukopenia, transaminitis, and jaundice; phase 2 has improvement of symptoms that may last for 2 days; and phase 3 involves return of symptoms with bleeding diathesis[204] (choice A). Neurologic involvement is rare. Diagnosis is dependent on cultures, PCR, and IgM. Treatment is largely supportive. The vaccine is effective in more than 90% patients and may confer immunity to other members of *Flavivirus*.[215,216]

16. A. Leptospirosis

Leptospirosis is the most common zoonosis. *Leptospira interrogans* enters the human host via abrasions on skin or through conjunctiva. It is linked to exposure of urine from rats or other rodents and infected dogs and has 2 syndromes. Anicteric leptospirosis is self-limited and has 2 stages: a septicemic 7 to 12 days incubation with fever, chills, nausea, vomiting, headache, and conjunctival suffusion, and with the organism isolated from blood or CSF, and after 1 to 3 days, an asymptomatic period with an immune stage that is characterized by aseptic meningitis. *Leptospira* are seen in urine during this stage and persist for up to 3 weeks. The second syndrome is icteric leptospirosis or Weil syndrome, which is potentially fatal and rare. It consists of jaundice, renal involvement, hypotension, and hemorrhage. The biphasic nature of the disease is obscured with persistence of jaundice and azotemia through the illness. *Leptospira* are isolated in blood, CSF, and urine. Diagnosis is demonstrated via rising antibody titers. Treatment is with IV penicillin 1.4 million units every 5 hours to shorten the duration of the fever, renal dysfunction, and hospital stay. Ceftriaxone and penicillin G are equally effective (choice A). The patient's response to ceftriaxone aides in the diagnosis since RMSF and Ehrlichiosis do not respond to ceftriaxone.

Rocky Mountain spotted fever, from *Rickettsia*, has normal CSF unless the patient is stuporous or in a coma and shows lymphocytic pleocytosis, elevated proteins, and normal glucose. It is characterized by a blanching erythematous rash that begins on the wrists and ankles and spreads to the trunk, and later to the palms and soles. The drug of choice is doxycycline. (choice B). Ehrlichiosis has lymphocytic pleocytosis with elevated protein and sometimes normal or low CSF glucose. In a minority of patients, there is also a rash. Patients have leukopenia, because of the intracellular location of organisms, and thrombocytopenia, both of which are not present in this patient. Treatment is doxycycline, chloramphenicol, or rifampin. (choice C). Infective endocarditis may cause lymphocytic pleocytosis with normal glucose that is the result of vasculitis, but there is no evidence of embolic phenomenon, cardiac murmur, or other systemic effects (choice D).

17. C. Oseltamivir

Influenza predisposes patients to secondary infections such as bacterial pneumonia. This can be seen by an exacerbation of constitutional and respiratory symptoms after a period of improvement. The most common bacterium is *S pneumoniae*. However, this is not the case for this patient, who did not have a period of improvement.

Treatment is recommended for residents of nursing homes or care facilities; for adults 65 years of age and older; women during pregnancy and for 2 weeks postpartum; individuals with chronic conditions such as pulmonary disease, cardiovascular disease, active malignancy, chronic kidney disease, chronic liver disease, hemoglobinopathies, immunocompromise, neurologic conditions that prevent clearance of secretions; Native Americans and Alaskan natives; patients with a body mass index (BMI) of 40 or greater; and patients with illnesses requiring hospitalization regardless of immunization status. Antiviral treatment should be initiated within 48 hours of symptoms for maximum benefit. Prevention and treatment of influenza includes neuraminidase inhibitors such as zanamivir, oseltamivir, and peramivir, which are active against influenza A and B, and amantadine and rimantadine, which are active against influenza A (choice A and D).

18. A. Refer to surgery

Early surgery (within 48 hours after diagnosis of IE) has been suggested to reduce embolisms without increasing the risk of mortality and recurrence of IE.[138,217] As stated earlier in the chapter, indications include heart failure, 1 or more embolic events during the first 2 weeks of antimicrobial therapy, fungal IE, highly resistant organisms, heart block, annular or aortic abscess, persistent bacteremia or fever for more than 5 days, recurrent emboli or persistent enlarging vegetations despite appropriate antibiotic treatment, severe valvular regurgitation, and a 10-mm or greater mobile vegetation, particularly in anterior mitral leaflet.[152] Intracerebral hemorrhage or large ischemic CVA are indications to postpone surgery. Continuing antibiotics and then surgery (choice B) or no change in treatment (choice D) will predispose the patient to further emboli complications. There is no need to change antibiotics (choice C) because the sensitivities are not back yet.

19. B. Serologies for *Bartonella*, *C burnetii*, and *T whipplei*

The patient continued to have fevers and has a vegetation that is seen on transesophageal echocardiogram, making culture-negative infective endocarditis likely. Culture-negative infective endocarditis requires 3 independent negative cultures after 5 days of incubation. The most common infectious causes are zoonotic agents, fungus, and *Streptococcus* spp in patients who have had prior antibiotic treatment. Other infectious causes includes HACEK, Q fever, *Bartonella*, *T whipplei*, *Legionella*, and *Mycobacterium tuberculosis*.[218-220] The noninfectious differential diagnoses of culture-negative endocarditis include antiphospholipid syndrome, acute rheumatic fever, atrial myxoma, nonbacterial thrombotic endocarditis, vasculitis, connective tissue disease, cholesterol emboli syndrome, shunts, and Lambl excrescences.

At this point, it is prudent to consider histopathological examination of the vegetation with special stains for *Bartonella*, *C burnetii*, and *T whipplei*. Other techniques include serologic assay such as *C burnetii* phase I antibody titers (positive if > 800) and *Bartonella* IgG greater than 800. The patient cannot have a histopathologic examination of the vegetation due to the recent intracerebral hemorrhage (choice A). Changing antibiotics or initiating antifungal would be premature (choices C and D).

20. B. *Burkholderia mallei*

Glanders is caused by *B mallei*, an aerobic Gram-negative rod that infects solipeds, but humans become hosts by inhalation or skin contact.[139] Clinically, it is associated with pustular skin lesions or ulcers and lymphadenopathy. It can metastasize from the skin or lung into the brain, spleen, liver, and kidneys. It can progress to septicemia and multiorgan failure from 2 to 14 days. It is difficult to diagnose. Exposure with solipeds such as horses and mules might help with diagnosis. Indirect hemagglutination assay (IHA) has been used in endemic areas.[221] Treatment is with imipenem, meropenem, ceftazidime, trimethoprim-sulfamethoxazole, doxycycline, or amoxicillin clavulanate[139,221]

Bubonic plague is caused by *Y pestis*, a Gram-negative coccobacillus that infects rodents and is transmitted to humans via fleas.[139] Clinically, patients develop fever, headaches, and tender erythematous lymphadenopathy, usually in groin, axilla, or neck, after a 6-day inoculation period. There can be an associated pneumonia. Septicemia can be associated with disseminated intravascular coagulopathy and characterized by acral cyanosis, ecchymosis, and digital gangrene. The patient is in septic shock yet do not have these manifestations. Diagnosis is aspiration from lymph node for stains and culture or PCR. Treatment is streptomycin, gentamicin, or ciprofloxacin for 10 to 14 days (choice A).

Erysipeloid is caused by the Gram-positive rod *E rhusiopathiae*, and a risk factor is handling marine life, swine, or poultry.[139] Within 7 days, maculopapular lesions appear, usually on the hands, and spread centrifugally with central clearing. Thirty percent of patients have associated lymphadenopathy.[139] Diagnosis is via culture of the lesions, and treatment includes cephalosporins, clindamycin, and fluoroquinolones[139](choice C).

The Gram-negative *Bartonella* species can cause cat scratch disease, which usually occurs in immunocompetent patients, and bacillary angiomatosis in immunocompromised patients. The disease begins with a papule that progress through erythematous, vesicular, papular, and crusted stages, with associated regional adenopathy. Bacillary angiomatosis carries a more fulminant course and often can mimic Kaposi sarcoma, epithelioid hemangioma, and pyogenic granuloma.[222] Cultures are difficult to obtain and serologies for *B henselae* antibodies are often used for diagnosis.[222] Positive Warthin-Starry silver stain can confirm the diagnosis but cannot differentiate between species.[139] Treatment for cat scratch disease is azithromycin, and treatment for bacillary angiomatosis is erythromycin or doxycycline[139] (choice D).

21. B. Ciprofloxacin 400 mg every 8 hours and clindamycin 900 mg every 8 hours for 2 weeks or until clinically stable (whichever is longer)

Anthrax is caused by *Bacillus anthracis*.[223] While the incidence of anthrax in the United States is low, anthrax epizootics still do occur, and its potential role as a bioterrorist agent make it an important pathogen to recognize.

Anthrax can take the form of 3 distinct clinical syndromes. Cutaneous anthrax is the most common and occurs when spores are introduced into the subcutaneous space from infected animals or products. It often manifests as a small, pruritic papule, which then develops a central bulla, followed by erosion, eventually leaving a painless necrotic eschar. Gastrointestinal tract anthrax develops after ingestion of undercooked meat infected by anthrax. It may cause erosion and hemorrhage of the intestine or painful swallowing from ulceration of the esophagus. Inhalation anthrax develops after inhalation of *B anthracis* spore-containing particles and has been described in individuals working with contaminated animal products (wool, hair, hides).[223]

The presentation of inhalation anthrax can be difficult to distinguish from other, more common respiratory conditions like influenza or bacterial pneumonia, and early recognition and treatment are necessary for survival. Patients will often present with a prodrome of fever, chills, malaise, headaches, and myalgias, followed by dyspnea, nausea, and chest pain. Hemoptysis and odynophagia have also been described. Chest x-ray will have widening of the mediastinum secondary to mediastinitis and may show pulmonary infiltrates and pleural effusions.[223] Diagnosis is via culture, PCR, and serologies, and may include pleural fluid and CSF sampling as well.[223]

First-line treatment of systemic anthrax without meningitis includes ciprofloxacin and clindamycin or ciprofloxacin and linezolid (choice B is correct). If clindamycin or linezolid are unavailable, acceptable alternatives include doxycycline or rifampin (choice C). Choice A would be appropriate treatment for cutaneous anthrax without systemic involvement. Choice D would be the correct treatment for systemic anthrax with possible or confirmed meningitis.[224] Antitoxins should also be administered for systemic anthrax.[225]

22. D. Reassure the patient without monitoring or sending of diagnostic studies

Ebola virus disease is caused by *Ebolavirus*, which belongs to the *Filoviridae* family of viruses.[226] Ebola has been responsible for several epidemics; however, it only made its way into the United States during the 2014 to 2016 epidemic in West Africa.

Transmission occurs via direct contact with body fluids from an infected human or animal. Patients present with symptoms 6 to 12 days after exposure. It should be noted that there is no evidence that transmission can occur before patients become symptomatic. Most cases present with sudden onset of fever and chills as well as myalgias, headaches, vomiting, and diarrhea. There may be a diffuse erythematous rash usually involving the face, neck, and trunk. Patients may develop hemorrhagic shock.[226-228]

Laboratory findings include leukopenia, thrombocytopenia, and hepatic dysfunction. Significant hemolysis may be present along with renal impairment.[226]

Ebola can present as severe hemorrhagic fever and is associated with high mortality. However, hemorrhage is seldom the cause of death as the disease causes hypovolemia through severe sepsis and may result in DIC and multiorgan failure.[226]

Currently, treatment remains supportive; however, early diagnosis is imperative to reduce the risk of transmission and implement supportive measures. Patients should be assessed for symptoms and screened for risks of exposure. Asymptomatic individuals without an identifiable risk factor do not need to be monitored or have diagnostic testing for Ebola.[227-229] This patient has no identifiable risk of exposure, as asymptomatic individuals do not transmit the virus, and she does not require monitoring. (Choice D is correct; choices A, B, and C are incorrect). Asymptomatic individuals with an identifiable risk should be monitored; however, the determination of where to monitor this individual is dependent on local regulations.[229] Symptomatic patients with any identifiable risk factor should trigger infection control precautions with standard, contact, and droplet precautions, as well personal protective equipment. Further information is available from the CDC (https://www.cdc.gov/vhf/ebola/healthcare-us/preparing/clinicians.html).

Diagnostic testing traditionally includes PCR for RNA sequences of the virus; however, they should be offered only to symptomatic patients with any exposure to Ebola (choice C is incorrect).[229]

23. A. Cefepime

Pyelonephritis is the most common cause of septic shock during pregnancy and is related to relative obstruction of the urinary tract from the uterus, progesterone-induced dilation of the ureters, and lack of protective peristalsis.[166,167] The most common pathogen is *E coli*, but the other common pathogens include *Klebsiella*, *Proteus*, and *Enterobacter*.[168] Risk factors for pyelonephritis include asymptomatic bacteriuria, advanced maternal age, nulliparity, sickle cell anemia, diabetes, nephrolithiasis, drug abuse, history of pyelonephritis, and urinary tract defects.[230] Given the potential severity of pyelonephritis, women with asymptomatic bacteriuria should be treated during pregnancy. Pyelonephritis should be suspected in pregnant women who present with symptoms of fever, chills, nausea, vomiting, and costovertebral tenderness. Dysuria is not always present. Urinalysis will show pyuria and there will be 10^5 or more colony-forming units (CFU)/mL in a midstream urine culture.[230] Treatment of mild or moderate pyelonephritis should be with ceftriaxone, cefepime (choice A), or aztreonam (if allergic to penicillin). Severe pyelonephritis should be treated with piperacillin-tazobactam or a carbapenem.[230] Fosfomycin does not achieve therapeutic levels in the kidneys and should be avoided in pyelonephritis (choice B). Levofloxacin is Food and Drug Administration category C in pregnancy and should be avoided (choice C). Trimethoprim-sulfamethoxazole may be considered if needed in the second and third trimesters and would be appropriate for asymptomatic bacteriuria or cystitis in pregnancy but is inadequate and not recommended for the treatment of pyelonephritis (choice D).

24. C. Perform pericardiocentesis

The most common bacterial cause of pericarditis and pericardial effusion in the developing world is tuberculosis. Definite tuberculous pericarditis is defined as tubercle bacilli in smear or culture of pericardial fluid and/or tubercle bacilli or caseating granulomas in histopathologic examination of pericardium.[231] Tuberculous pericarditis is considered if there is pericardial effusion in a patient with a history of extracardiac tuberculosis and/or lymphocytic pericardial exudate and elevated adenosine deaminase (ADA) and/or good response to antituberculosis chemotherapy.[231] The best approach for this patient is to perform pericardiocentesis of this moderate effusion to rule out pericardial tuberculosis.

Due to hemodynamic instability and the high likelihood of tuberculosis, aspirin and colchicine will not be able to treat this condition (choice D). Rifampin isoniazid, pyrazinamide, and ethambutol for 2 months and then rifampin and isoniazid for 4 months (for a total of 6 months) is the chemotherapy for tuberculosis pericarditis and would be prudent to initiate once diagnosis is confirmed (choice C). Prednisone has been advocated to prevent progression to constrictive pericaritidis.[149] However, for tuberculosis in patients with HIV, it is not recommended due to the increased risk of malignancy[232] (choice B).

25. A. Deoxyribonuclease 5 mg and tissue plasminogen activator 10 mg intrapleural for 1 hour every 12 hours for 3 days

Deoxyribonuclease (DNAse) was hypothesized to cleave uncoiled DNA, and the tissue plasminogen activator facilitated the drainage through disruption of the fibrinous septations. It his hypothesized that DNAse disruption of the uncoiled DNA or biofilm did not clear the infection since the bacterial or inflammatory components were systematically absorbed and not cleared from the body without tPA. Choices B, C, and D did not have the right dosage or lack the dual therapy.

26. D. Pleural adenosine deaminase

Adenosine deaminase (ADA) is excreted by lymphocytes, and a level over 45 has a sensitivity of 92% to 100% and a specificity of 90% to 97% for TB pleural disease.[233-237] It is not altered in patients who are immunocompromised. Pleural lymphocytosis is nonspecific (choice C). Pleural acid-fast bacilli are only positive in 20% to 30% of HIV-negative patients[238] (choice A). Pleural biopsy has a diagnostic yield of 60% to 90%[238-240] (choice B).

REFERENCES

1. Bone RC, Balk RA, Cerra FB, et al. American College of Chest Physicians/Society of Critical Care Medicine Consensus Conference: definitions for sepsis and organ failure and guidelines for the use of innovative therapies in sepsis. *Crit Care Med.* 1992;20(6):864-874.
2. Singer M, Deutschman CS, Seymour CW, et al. The Third International Consensus definitions for sepsis and septic shock (Sepsis-3). *JAMA.* 2016;315(8):801-810.
3. Rhodes A, Evans L, Alhazzani W, et al. Surviving Sepsis Campaign: International Guidelines for management of sepsis and septic shock. *Crit Care Med.* 2017.45(3):1-67.
4. Vincent JL, de Mendonca A, Cantraine F et al. Use of the SOFA score to assess the incidence of organ dysfunction/failure in intensive care units: results of a multicenter, prospective study. Working group on "sepsis-related problems" of the European Society of Intensive Care Medicine. *Crit Care Med.* 1998;26(11):1793-1800.
5. Angus DC, van der Poll T. Severe sepsis and septic shock. *New Engl J Med.* 2013;369(9):840-851.
6. Chan JK, Roth J, Oppenheim JJ, et al. Alarmins: awaiting a clinical response. *J Clin Invest.* 2012;122(8):2711-2719.
7. Levi M, van der Poll T. Inflammation and coagulation. *Crit Care Med.* 2010;38(2 Suppl):S26-S34.
8. Hotchkiss RS, Tinsley KW, Swanson PE, et al. Depletion of dendritic cells, but not macrophages, in patients with sepsis. *J Immunol.* 2002;168(5):2493-2500.
9. Hotchkiss RS, Tinsley KW, Swanson PE, et al. Sepsis-induced apoptosis causes progressive profound depletion of B and CD4+ T lymphocytes in humans. *J Immunol.* 2001;166(11): 6952-6963.
10. Muller B, White JC, Nylén ES, Snider RH, Becker KL, Habener JF. Ubiquitous expression of the calcitonin-I gene in multiple tissues in response to sepsis. *J Clin Endocrin Metab.* 2001;86(1): 394-404.
11. Rivers E, Nguyen B, Havstad S, et al; Early Goal-Directed Therapy Collaborative Group. Early goal-directed therapy in the treatment of severe sepsis and septic shock. *New Engl J Med.* 2001;345(19):1368-1377.
12. Mouncey PR, Osborn TM, Power S, et al; ProMISe Trial Investigators. Trial of early, goal-directed resuscitation for septic shock. *New Engl J Med.* 2015;372(14):1301-1311.
13. ARISE Investigators; ANZICS Clinical Group; Peake SL, Delaney A, Bailey M, et al. Goal-directed resuscitation for patients with early septic shock. *New Engl J Med.* 2014;371(16):1496-1506.
14. Cecconi M, DeBacker D, Antonelli M, et al. Consensus on circulatory shock and hemodynamic monitoring. Task Force of the European Society of Intensive Care Medicine. *Intensive Care Med.* 2014;40(12):1795-1815.
15. Eskesen TG, Wetterslev M, Perner A. Systemic review including re-analyses of 1148 individual data sets of central venous pressure as a predictor of fluid responsiveness. *Intensive Care Med.* 2016;42(3):324-332.
16. Yunos NM, Bellomo R, Hegarty C, et al. Association between a chloride-liberal vs chloride-restrictive intravenous fluid administration strategy and kidney injury in critically ill adults. *JAMA.* 2012;308(15):1566-1572.
17. Young P, Bailey M, Beasley R, et al. Effect of a buffered crystalloid solution vs saline on acute kidney injury among patients in the intensive care unit. *JAMA.* 2015;314(16):1701-1710.

18. Semler MW, Evans LE, Alhazzani W, et al. Balanced crystalloids versus saline in critical ill adults. *N Engl J Med.* 2018;378(9):829-839.

19. Finfer S, Norton R, Bellomo R, Boyce N, French J, Myburgh J. The SAFE study: saline vs albumin for fluid resuscitation in the critically ill. *Vox Sang.* 2004;87 (Supp 2):123-131.

20. Delany AP, Dan A, McCaffrey J, Finfer S. The role of albumin as a resuscitation fluid for patients with sepsis: a systemic review and metanalysis. *Crit Care Med.* 2011;39(2):386-391.

21. Rochwerg B, Alhazzani W, Gibson A, et al; FISSH Group (Fluids in Sepsis and Septic Shock). Fluid type and the use of renal replacement therapy in sepsis: a systemic review and network meta-analysis. *Intensive Care Med.* 2015;41(9):1561-1571.

22. Xu JY, Chen QH, Xie JF, et al. Comparison of the effects of albumin and crystalloid on mortality in adult patients with severe sepsis and septic shock: a meta-analysis of randomized clinical trials. *Crit Care.* 2014;18(6):702.

23. Uhlig C, Silva PL, Deckert S, Schmitt J, de Abreu MG. Albumin versus crystalloid solutions in patients with acute respiratory distress syndrome: a systematic review and meta-analysis. *Crit Care.* 2014;18(1):R10.

24. Patel A, Laffan MA, Waheed U, Brett SJ. Randomised trials of human albumin for adults with sepsis: a systemic review and meta-analysis with trial sequential analysis of all-cause mortality. *BMJ.* 2014;349:g4561.

25. Haase N, Perner A, Hennings LI, et al. Hydroxyethyl starch 130/0.38-0.45 versus crystalloid or albumin in patients with sepsis: systemic review with meta-analysis and trial sequential analysis. *BMJ.* 2013;346:f839.

26. Moeller C, Fleischmann C, Thomas-Rueddel D, et al. How safe is gelatin? A systematic review and meta-analysis of gelatin-containing plasma expanders vs crystalloids and albumin. *J Crit Care.* 2016;35:75-83.

27. Jansen TC, van Brommel J, Schoonderbeek FJ, et al; LACTATE Study Group. Early lactate-guided therapy in intensive care unit patients: a multicenter, open-label, randomized controlled trial. *Am J Respir Crit Care Med.* 2010;182(6):752-761.

28. Jones AE, Shapiro NI, Trzeciak S, et al; Emergency Medicine Shock Research Network (EMShockNET) Investigators. Lactate clearance vs central venous oxygen saturation as goals of early sepsis therapy: a randomized clinical trial. *JAMA.* 2010;303(8):739-746.

29. Lyu X, Xu Q, Cai G, Yan J, Yan M. [Efficacies of fluid resuscitation as guided by lactate clearance rate and central venous oxygen saturation in patients with septic shock.] *Zhonghua Yi Xue Za Zhi.* 2015;95(7):496-500.

30. Yu B, Tian HY, Hu ZJ, et al. [Comparison of the effect of fluid resuscitation as guided either by lactate clearance rate or by central venous oxygen saturation in patients with sepsis.] *Zhonghua Wei Zhong Bing Ji Jiu Yi Xue.* 2013;25(10):578-583.

31. Beck GCh, Brinkkoetter P, Hanusch C, et al. Clinical review: immunomodulatory effects of dopamine in general inflammation. *Crit Care.* 2004;8(6):485-491.

32. Avni T, Lador A, Lev S, Leibovici MP, Grossman A. Vasopressors for the treatment of septic shock: systemic review and meta-analysis. *PLoS One.* 2015;10(8):e0129305.

33. Zhou F, Mao Z, Zeng X, et al. Vasopressors in septic shock: a systematic review and network meta-analysis. *Ther Clin Risk Manag.* 2015;11:1047-1059.

34. Kumar A, Roberts D, Wood KE, et al. Duration of hypotension before initiation of effective antimicrobial therapy is the critical determinant of survival in human septic shock. *Crit Care Med.* 2006;34(6):1589-1596.

35. Ferrer R, Martin-Loeches I, Philips G, et al. Empiric antibiotic treatment reduces mortality in severe sepsis and septic shock from the first hour: results from a guideline-based performance improvement program. *Crit Care Med.* 2014;42(8):1749-1755.

36. Zhang D, Micek ST, Kollef MH. Time to appropriate antibiotic therapy is an independent determinant of postinfection ICU and hospital lengths of stay in patients with sepsis. *Crit Care Med.* 2015;43(10):2133-2140.

37. Bagshaw SM, Lapinsky S, Dial S, et al; Cooperative Antimicrobial Therapy of Septic Shock (CATSS) Database Research Group. Acute kidney injury in septic shock: clinical outcomes and impact of duration of hypotension prior to initiation of antimicrobial therapy. *Intensive Care Med.* 2009;35(5):871-881.

38. Sterling SA, Miller WR, Pryor J, Pusckarich MA, Jones AE. The impact of timing of antibiotics on outcomes in severe sepsis and septic shock: a systematic review and meta-analysis. *Crit Care Med.* 2015;43(9):1907-1915.

39. Phua J, Ngerng W, See K, et al. Characteristics and outcomes of culture negative versus culture positive severe sepsis. *Crit Care.* 12 2013;17(5):R202.

40. Annane D, Bellissant E, Bollaert PE, et al. Corticosteroids in the treatment of severe sepsis and septic shock in adults: a systematic review. *JAMA.* 2009;301(22):2362-2375.

41. Bollaert PE, Charpentier C, Levy B, Debouverie M, Audibert G, Larcan A. Reversal of late septic shock with supraphysiologic doses of hydrocortisone. *Crit Care Med.* 1998;26(4):645-650.

42. Briegel J, Forst H, Haller M, et al. Stress doses of hydrocortisone reverse hyperdynamic septic shock: a prospective randomized double-blind single-center study. *Crit Care Med.* 1999;27(4):723-732.

43. Sprung CL, Annane D, Keh D, et al; CORTICUS Study Group. Hydrocortisone therapy for patients with septic shock. *New Engl J Med.* 2008;358(2):111-124.

44. Sligl WL, Milner DA Jr, Sundar S, Mphatswe W, Majumdar SR. Safety and efficacy of corticosteroids for treatment of septic shock. *Clin Infect Dis.* 2009;49(1):93-101.

45. Annane D, Bellissant E, Bollaert PE, Briegel J, Keh D, Kupfer Y. Corticosteroids for treating sepsis. *Cochrane Database Syst Rev.* 2015;(12):CD002243.

46. Volbeda M, Wetterslev J, Gluud C, et al. Glucocorticosteroids for sepsis: systematic review with meta-analysis and trial sequential analysis. *Intensive Care Med.* 2015;41(7):1220-1234.

47. Annane D, Sébille V, Charpentier C, et al. Effect of treatment with low dose hydrocortisone and fludrocortisone on mortality in patients with septic shock. *JAMA.* 2002;288(7):862-871.

48. Mandell LA, Wunderink RG, Anzueto A, et al; Infectious Diseases Society of America; American Thoracic Society. Infectious Diseases Society of America/American Thoracic Society consensus guidelines on the management of community acquired pneumonia in adults. *Clin Infect Dis.* 2007;44 (Suppl 2):S27-S72.

49. Fine MJ, Auble TE, Yealy DM, et. al. A prediction rule to identify low-risk patients with community-acquired pneumonia. *N Engl J Med.* 1997;336(4):243-250.

50. Marras TK, Gutierrez C, Chan CK. Applying a prediction rule to identify low-risk patients with community acquired pneumonia. *Chest.* 2000;118(5):1339-1343.

51. Charles PG, Wolfe R, Whitby M, et al; Australian Community-Acquired Pneumonia Study Collaboration. SMART-COP: A

tool for predicting the need for intensive respiratory or vasopressor support in community acquired pneumonia. *Clin Infect Dis.* 2008;47(3):375.

52. Chalmers JD, Singanayagam A, Hill AT. Predicting the need for mechanical ventilation and/or inotropic support for young adults admitted to the hospital with community-acquired pneumonia. *Clin Infect Dis.* 2008;47(12):1571-1574.

53. España PP, Capelastegui A, Gorordo I, et al. Development and validation of a clinical prediction rule of severe community acquired pneumonia. *Am J Respir Crit Care Med.* 2006;174(11):1249-1256.

54. Yandiola PP, Capelastegui A, Quintana J, et al. Prospective comparison of severity scores for predicting clinically relevant outcomes for patients hospitalized with community-acquired pneumonia. *Chest.* 2009;135(6):1572-1579.

55. Privitera MD, Zakaria T, Khatri R. Nervous system. In: Kaplan LA, Pesce AJ, eds. *Clinical Chemistry: Theory Analysis, Correlation.* 5th ed. St Louis, MI: Elsevier Inc; 2010: 904-928.

56. King Strasinger S, Schaub DiLorenzo M. Cerebrospinal fluid. In: *Urinalysis and Body Fluids Testing.* 5th ed. Philadelphia, PA: F.A. Davis; 2008: 177-199.

57. Saraya AW, Wacharapluesadee S, Petcharat S, et al. Normocellular CSF in herpes simplex encephalitis. *BMC Res Notes.* 2016;9:95.

58. Tunkel AR, Glaser CA, Bloch KC, et al; Infectious Diseases Society of America. The management of encephalitis: clinical practice guidelines by the Infectious Diseases Society of America. *Clin Infect Dis.* 2008;47(3):303-327.

59. Whitley RJ, Lakeman F. Herpes simplex virus infections of the central nervous system: therapeutic and diagnostic considerations. *Clin Infect Dis.* 1995;20(2):414-420.

60. Tebas P, Nease RF, Storch GA. Use of the polymerase chain reaction in the diagnosis of herpes simplex encephalitis: a decision analysis model. *Am J Med.* 1998;105(4):287-295.

61. Centers for Disease Control and Prevention. Guidelines for the surveillance, prevention, and control of West Nile virus infection—United States. *MMWR Morb Mortal Wkly Rep.* 2000;49(2):25-28.

62. Petersen LR, Marfin AA. West Nile virus: a primer for the clinician. *Ann Intern Med.* 2002;137(3):173-179.

63. Watson NK, Bartt RE, Houff SA, et al. Focal neurological deficits and West Nile virus infection. *Clin Infect Dis.* 2005;40(7):e59-e62.

64. Centers for Disease Control and Prevention. Acute flaccid paralysis syndrome associated with West Nile virus infection—Mississippi and Louisiana. *MMWR Morb Mortal Wkly Rep.* 2002;51(37):825-828.

65. Gea-Banacloche J, Johnson RT, Bagic A, et al. West Nile virus: pathogenesis and therapeutic options. *Ann Intern Med.* 2004;140(7):545-553.

66. Centers for Disease Control and Prevention. Arboviral disease—United States, 1994. *MMWR Morb Mortal Wkly Rep.* 1995;44(35):641-644.

67. De Luca A, Giancola ML, Ammassari A, et al. The effect of potent antiretroviral therapy and JC virus load in cerebrospinal fluid on clinical outcome of patients with AIDS-associated progressive multifocal leukoencephalopathy. *J Infect Dis.* 2000;182(4):1077-1083.

68. Plotkin SA. Rabies. *Clin Infect Dis.* 2000;30(1):4-12.

69. Centers for Disease Control and Prevention. Human rabies—Montana and Washington, 1997. *MMWR Morb Mortal Wkly Rep.* 1997;46(33):770-774.

70. Srinivasin A, Burton EC, Kuehnert MJ, et al. Transmission for rabies virus from an organ donor to four transplant recipients. *New Engl J Med.* 2005;352(1):1103-1111.

71. Centers for Disease Control and Prevention. Human rabies—Texas and New Jersey, 1998. *MMWR Morb Mortal Wkly Rep.* 1998;47(1):1-5.

72. Jackson AC, Warrell MJ Ruppert CE, et al. Management of rabies in Humans. *Clin Infect Dis.* 2004;36(1):60-63.

73. Ruppercht CE, Gibbons RV. Prophylaxis against rabies. *New Engl J Med.* 2004;351(25):2626-2635.

74. Johnson RT. Acute encephalitis. *Clin Infect Dis.* 1996;23(2):219-226.

75. Farr RW. Leptospirosis. *Clin Infect Dis.* 1995;21(1):1-6.

76. Panaphut T, Domrongkitchaiporn S, Vibhagool A, et al. Ceftriaxone compared with sodium penicillin G for treatment of severe leptospirosis. *Clin Infect Dis.* 2003;36(12):1507-1513.

77. Ratnasamy N, Everett ED, Roland WE, et al. Central nervous system manifestations of human ehrlichiosis. *Clin Infect Dis.* 1996;23(2):314-319.

78. Salgado AV, Furlan AJ, Keys TF,- et al. Neurologic complications of endocarditis: a 12-year experience. *Neurology.* 1989;39(2 PT 1):173-178.

79. Verdon R, Chevret S, Laissy JP, et al. Tuberculous meningitis in adults: review of 48 cases. *Clin Infect Dis.* 1996;22(6):982-988.

80. Lopez-Cortes LF, Cruiz-Ruiz M, Gomez-Mateos J, et al. Adenosine deaminase in the CSF of patients with aseptic meningitis: utility in the diagnosis of tuberculous meningitis or neurobrucellosis. *Clin Infect Dis.* 1995;20(3):525-530.

81. American Thoracic Society/Centers for Disease Control and Prevention/Infectious Disease Society of America. Treatment of tuberculosis. *Am J Respir Crit Care Med.* 2003;167(4):603-662.

82. Thwaites GE, Bang ND, Dung NH, et al. Dexamethasone for the treatment of tuberculous meningitis in adolescents and adults. *New Engl J Med.* 2004;351(17):1741-1751.

83. Donald PR, Schoeman JF. Tuberculous meningitis. *New Engl J Med.* 2004;351(17):1719-1720.

84. van der Horst CM, Saag MS, Clud CA, et al. Treatment of cryptococcal meningitis associated with the acquired immunodeficiency syndrome. *New Engl J Med.* 1997;337(1):15-21.

85. Graybill JR, Sobel J, Saag M, et al. Diagnosis and management of increased intracranial pressure in patients with AIDS and cryptococcal meningitis. *Clin Infect Dis.* 2000;30(1):47-54.

86. Galgiani JN, Ampel NM, Ctanzaro A, et al. Practice guidelines for the treatment of coccidioidomycosis. *Clin Infect Dis.* 2000;30(4):71-718.

87. Wheat LJ, Musial CE, Jenny-Avital EJ. Diagnosis and management of central nervous system histoplasmosis. *Clin Infect Dis.* 2005;40(6):844-852.

88. Lo Re V III, Gluckman SJ. Eosinophilic meningitis. *Am J Med.* 2004;114(3):217-223.

89. Slom TJ, Cortese MM, Gerber SI, et al. An outbreak of eosinophilic meningitis caused by *Angiostrongylus cantonensis* in travelers returning from the Caribbean. *New Engl J Med.* 2002;346(9):668-675.

90. Centers for Disease Control and Prevention. Primary amebic meningoencephalitis—Georgia, 2002. *MMWR Morb Mortal Wkly Rep.* 2003;52(40):962-964.

91. Brooks TJ, Phillpotts RJ. Interferon-alpha protects mice against lethal infection with St Louis encephalitis virus delivered by the aerosol and subcutaneous routes. *Antiviral Res.* 1999;41(1):57-64.

92. Bookstaver PB, Mohorn, PL, Shah A, et al. Management of viral central nervous system infections: a primer for clinicians. *J Cent Nerv Syst Dis*. 2017;9;1179573517703342.

93. Hinten SR, Beckett GA, Gensheimer KF, et al. Increased recognition of Powassan encephalitis in the United States, 1999-2005. *Vector Borne Zoonotic Dis*. 2008;8(6):733-740.

94. Tunkel AR, Hartman BJ, Kaplan SL, et al. Practice guidelines for the management of bacterial meningitis. *Clin Infect Dis*. 2004;39(9):1267-1284.

95. Van de Beek D, Brouwer MC, Thwaites GE, Trunkel AR. Advances in treatment of bacterial meningitis. *Lancet*. 2012;380(9854):1693-1707.

96. Mylonakis E, Hohmann EL, Calderwood SB. Central nervous system infection with *Listeria monocytogenes*. 33 years' experience at a general hospital and review of 776 episodes from the literature. *Medicine (Baltimore)*. 1998;77(5):313-336.

97. Greenlee JE, Carroll KC. Cerobrospinal fluid in CNS infections. In: Scheld WM, Witley RJ, Durack DT, eds. *Infections of the Central Nervous System*. 2nd ed. Philadelphia: Lippincott-Raven; 1997: 899-922.

98. Gray LD, Fedorko DP. Laboratory diagnosis of bacterial meningitis. *Clin Microbiol Rev*. 1992;5(2):130-145.

99. Radetsky M. Duration of treatment in bacterial meningitis: a historical inquiry. *Pediatr Infect Dis J*. 1990;9(1):2-9.

100. O'Neill P. How long to treat bacterial meningitis. *Lancet*. 1993;341(8844):530.

101. deGans J, van de Beek D; European Dexamethasone in Adulthood Bacterial Meningitis Study Investigators. Dexamethasone in adults with bacterial meningitis. *New Engl J Med*. 2002;347(20):1549-1556.

102. Kaplan SL, Mason EO Jr. Management of infections due to antibiotic-resistant *Streptococcus pneumoniae*. *Clin Microbiol Rev*. 1998;11(4):628-644.

103. Kaplan SL. Management of pneumococcal infections. *Pediatr Infect Dis J*. 2002;21(6):589-591.

104. Krieger S. Neurologic infections. In: Frontera JA, ed. *Decision Making in Neurocritical Care*. New York: Thieme; 2009: 134-148.

105. Walker M, Zunt JR. Parasitic central nervous system infections in immunocompromised hosts. *Clin Infect Disc*. 2005;40(7):1005-1015.

106. Lorber B. Listeriosis. *Clin Infect Disc*. 1997;24(1):1-11.

107. Lerche A, Rasmussen N, Wandall JH, et al. *Staphylococcus aureus* meningitis: a review of 28 consecutive community-acquired cases. *Scand J Infect Dis*. 1995;27(6):569-573.

108. Busch LM, Abrams BH, Beall A, et al. Index case of fatal inhalational anthrax due to bioterrorism in the United States. *New Engl J Med*. 2001;345(22):1607-1610.

109. Mayer TA, Bersoff-Matcha S, Murphy C, et al. Clinical presentation of inhalation anthrax following bioterrorism exposure: report of 2 surviving patients. *JAMA*. 2001;286(2):2549-2553.

110. Durand ML, Calderwood SB, Weber DJ, et al. Acute bacterial meningitis in adults: a review of 493 episodes. *New Engl J Med*. 1993;328(1):21-28.

111. Galgiani JN, Ampel NM, Blair JE, et al. 2016 Infectious Diseases Society of America (IDSA) clinical practice guideline for the treatment of coccidioidomycosis. *Clin Infect Dis*. 2016;63(6):e112-e146.

112. Chotmongkol V, Kittimongkolma S, Niwattavakul K, et al. Comparison of prednisolone plus albendazole with prednisolone alone for treatment of patients with eosinophilic meningitis. *Am J Trop Med Hyg*. 2009;81(3):443-445.

113. Southwick FS, Richardson EP, Swartz MN. Septic thrombosis of the dural venous sinuses. *Medicine*. 1986;65(2):82-106.

114. Bleck TP, Greenlee JE. Suppurative intracranial phlebitis. In: Mandell GL, Bennett JE, Dolin R, eds. *Mandell, Douglas, and Bennett's Principles and Practice of Infectious Diseases*. 5th ed. Philadelphia, PA: Churchill Livingstone; 2000: 1034-1036.

115. Fragata I, Patel A. Cerebral sinus thrombosis. In: Frontera JA, ed. *Decision Making in Neurocritical Care*. New York: Thieme; 2009: 95-105.

116. Tattevin P, Bruneel F, Clair B, et al. Bacterial brain abscesses: a retrospective study of 94 patients admitted to an intensive care unit (1980-1999). *Am J Med*. 2003;115(2):143-146.

117. Tunkel AR, Wispelwey B, Scheld WM. Brain abscess. In: Mandell GL, Bennett JE, Delin R, eds. *Mandell, Douglas, and Bennett's Principles and Practice of Infectious Diseases*. 5th ed. Philadelphia, PA: Churchill Livingstone; 2000: 1016-1028.

118. Walot I, Miller BL, Chang L, Mehringer CM. Neuroimaging findings in patients with AIDS. *Clin Infect Dis*. 1996;22(6):906-919.

119. Kaplan JE, Masur H, Holmes KK; USPHS; Infectious Disease Society of America.. Guidelines for preventing opportunistic infections among HIV-infected persons—2002. Recommendations of U.S. Public Health Service and Infectious Diseases Society of America. *MMWR Recomm Rep*. 2002;51(RR-8):1-52.

120. Darouchie RO, Hamill RJ, Greenberg SB, et al. Bacterial spinal epidural abscess: review of 43 cases and literal survey. *Medicine*. 1992;71(6):369-385.

121. Stabler A, Reiser MF. Imaging of spinal infection. *Radiol Clin North Am*. 2001;39(1):115-135.

122. Kneen R, Pham NG, Solomon T, et al. Penicillin vs erythromycin in the treatment of diphtheria. *Clin Infect Dis*. 1998;27(4):845-850.

123. Gergen PJ, McQuillan GM, Kiely M, et al. A population-based serologic survey of immunity to tetanus in the United States. *New Engl J Med*. 1995;332(12):761-766.

124. Angulo FJ, Getz J, Taylor JP, et al. A large outbreak of botulism: the hazardous baked potato. *J Infect Disc*. 1998;178(1):172-177.

125. Centers for Disease Control and Prevention. Outbreak of botulism type E associated with eating a beached whale—Western Alaska, July 2002. *MMWR Morb Mortal Wkly Rep*. 2003;52(2):24-26.

126. Warma JK, Katsitadze G, Moiscrafishvili M, et al. Signs and symptoms predictive of death in patients with foodborne botulism—Republic of Georgia, 1980-2002. *Clin Infect Dis*. 2004;39(3):357-362.

127. Centers for Disease Control and Prevention. Infant botulism—New York City, 2001-2002. *MMWR Morb Mortal Wkly Rep*. 2003;52(2)21-24.

128. Shapiro RL, Hatheway C, Swerdlow DL. Botulism in the United States: a clinical and epidemiologic review. *Ann Intern Med*. 1998;129(3):221-228.

129. Arnon SS, Schecter R, Inglesby TV, et al. Botulism toxin as a biological weapon: medical and public health management. *JAMA*. 2001;285(8):1059-1070.

130. Clark JR, Carlson RD, Sasaki CT, Pachies AR, Steere AC. Facial paralysis in Lyme disease. Laryngoscope. 1985;95(11):13411345.

131. Shapiro ED, Gerber MA. Lyme disease and facial nerve palsy. *Arch Pediatr Adolesc Med*. 1997;151(12):1183-1184.

132. Hehir MK, Logigian EL. Infectious neuropathies. *Continuum (Minneap Minn)*. 2014;20(5):1274-1292.

133. Etheridge SM. Paralytic shellfish poisoning: seafood safety and human health perspectives. *Toxicon*. 2010;56(2):108-122

134. Li JS, Sexton DJ, Mick N, Proposed modifications to the Duke Criteria for the diagnosis of infective endocarditis. *Clin Infect Dis*. 2000;30(4):633-638.

135. Baddour LM, Wilson WR, Bayer AS, et al; American Heart Association Committee on Rheumatic Fever, Endocarditis, and Kawasaki Disease of the Council on Cardiovascular Disease in the Young, Council on Clinical Cardiology, Council on Cardiovascular Surgery and Anesthesia, and Stroke Council. Infective endocarditis in adults: diagnosis, antimicrobial therapy and management of complications: a scientific statement for healthcare professionals from the American Heart Association. *Circulation*. 2015;132(15):1-50.

136. Bayer AS. Infective endocarditis. *Clin Infect Dis*. 1993;17(3): 313-320; quiz 321-322.

137. Daniel WG, Mügge A, Martin RP, et al. Improvement in the diagnosis of abscesses associated with endocarditis by transesophageal echocardiography. *N Engl J Med*. 1991;324(12):795-800.

138. Kang DH. Timing of surgery in infective endocarditis. *Heart*. 2015;101(22):1786-1791.

139. Stevens DL, Bisno AL, Chambers HF, et al; Infectious Diseases Society of America. Practice guidelines for the diagnosis and management of skin and soft tissue infections: 2014 update by the Infectious Diseases Society of America. *Clin Infect Dis*. 2014;59(2):e10-e52.

140. Hirschman JV, Raugi GJ. Lower limb cellulitis and its mimics: part I. Lower limb cellulitis. *J Am Acad Dermatol*. 2012;67(2):163.e1-12; quiz 175-176.

141. Kielhofner MA, Brown B, Dall L. Influence of underlying disease process on the utility of cellulitis of needle aspirates. *Arch Intern Med*. 1988;148(11):2451-2452.

142. Zimbelman J, Palmer A, Todd J. Improved outcome of clindamycin compared with beta-lactam antibiotic treatment for invasive *Streptococcus pyogenes* infection. *Pediatric Infect Dis J*. 1999;18(12):1096-1100.

143. Mulla ZD, Leaverton PE, Wiersma ST. Invasive group A streptococcal infections in Florida. *South Med J*. 2003;96(10):968-973.

144. Tanz RR, Shulman ST, Shortridge VD, et al. Community-based surveillance in the United States of macrolide resistant pediatric pharyngeal group A streptococci during 3 respiratory disease seasons. *Clin Infect Dis*. 2004;39(12):1794-1801.

145. Jaggi P, Beall B, Rippe J, Tanz RR, Shulman ST. Macrolide resistance and emm type distribution of invasive pediatric group A streptococcal isolates: three-year prospective surveillance from a children's hospital. *Pediatr Infect Dis J*. 2007;26(3):253-255.

146. Stevens DL. Dilemmas in the treatment of invasive *Streptococcus pyogenes* infections. *Clin Infect Dis*. 2003;37(3):341-343.

147. Stevens DL, Aldape MJ, Bryant AE. Life-threatening clostridial infections. *Anaerobe*. 2012;18(2):254-259.

148. Little WC, Freeman GL. Pericardial disease. *Circulation*. 2006;113(12):1622-1632.

149. Adler Y, Charron P, Imazio M, et al; ESC Scientific Document Group. 2015 ESC guidelines for the diagnosis and management of pericardial diseases: The Task Force for the Diagnosis and Management of Pericardial Diseases of the European Society of Cardiology (ESC) Endorsed by: The European Association for Cardio-Thoracic Surgery (EACTS). *Eur Heart J*. 2015;36(42):2921-2964.

150. Imazio M, Gaita F, LeWinter M. Evaluation and treatment of percarditis. *JAMA*. 2015;314(14):1498-1506.

151. Imazio M, Brucato A, Barbieri A, et al. Good prognosis for pericarditis with and without myocardial involvement: results from a multicenter, prospective cohort study. *Circulation*. 2013;128(1):42-49.

152. Imazio M, Cooper LT. Management of myopericarditis. *Expert Rev Cardiovasc Ther*. 2013;11(2):193-201.

153. Lilly LS. Treatment of acute and recurrent idiopathic pericarditis. *Circulation*. 2013;127(16):1723-1726.

154. Imazio M, Cecchi E, Demichelis B, et al. Indicators of poor prognosis of acute pericarditis. *Circulation*. 2007;115(21):2739-2744.

155. Imazio M, Brucato A, Mayosi BM, et al. Medical therapy of pericardial diseases: part I: idiopathic and infectious pericarditis. *J Cardiovasc Med (Hagerstown)*. 2010;11(10):712-722.

156. Imazio M, Brucato A, Mayosi BM, et al. Medical therapy of pericardial diseases: part II: noninfectious pericarditis, pericardial effusion and constrictive pericarditis. *J Cardiovasc Med (Hagerstown)*. 2010;11(11):785-794.

157. Hooper C, Lee YCG, Maskell N. Investigation of a unilateral pleural effusion in adults: British Thoracic Society pleural disease guideline 2010. *Thorax*. 2010;65(Suppl 2):ii4-ii17.

158. Light RW, MacGregor MI, Luchsinger PC, et al. Pleural effusions: the diagnostic separation of transudates and exudates. *Ann Intern Med*. 1972;77(4):507-513.

159. Light RW. Parapneumonic effusions and empyema. *Proc Am Thorac Soc*. 2006;3(1):75-80.

160. Andrews NC, Parker EF, Shaw RR, Wilson NJ, Webb WR. Management of nontuberculous empyema. *Am Rev Respir Dis*. 1962;85:935-936.

161. Colice GL, Curtis A, Deslauriers J, et al. Medical and surgical treatment of parapneumonic effusions: an evidence-based guideline. *Chest*. 2000;118(4):1158-1171.

162. Bartlett JG, Finegold SM. Anaerobic infections of the lung and pleural space. *Am Rev Respir Dis*. 1974;110(1):56-77.

163. Cham CW, Haq SM, Rahamim J. Empyema thoracis: a problem with late referral? *Thorax*. 1993;48(9):925-927.

164. Rahman NM, Maskell NA, Davies CWH, et al. The relationship between chest tube size and clinical outcome in pleural infection. *Chest*. 2010;137(3):536-543.

165. Rahman NM, Maskell NA, West A, et al. Intrapleural use of tissue plasminogen activator and DNAse in pleural infection. *New Engl J Med*. 2011;365(6):518-526.

166. Chebbo A, Tan S, Kassis C, Tamura L, Carlson RW. Maternal sepsis and septic shock. *Crit Care Clin*. 2016;32(1):119-135.

167. Morgan J, Roberts S. Maternal sepsis. *Obstet Gynecol Clin N Am*. 2013;40(1):69-87.

168. Gilstrap LC, Cunningham FG, Whalley PJ. Acute pyelonephritis in pregnancy: an anterospective study. *Obstet Gynecol*. 1981;57(4):409-413.

169. Sperling RS, Newton E, Gibbs RS. Intraamniotic infection in low-birth-weight infants. *J Infect Dis*. 1988;157(1):113-117.

170. Waites KB, Katz B, Schelonka RL. Mycoplasmas and ureaplasmas as neonatal pathogens. *Clin Microbiol Rev*. 2005;18(4):757-789.

171. Glamerllos-Gourgoulis EJ, Grecka P, Poulakou G, Anargyrou K, Katsilambros N, Giamarellou H. Assessment of procalcitonin as a diagnostic marker of underlying infection in patients with febrile neutropenia. *Clin infect Dis*. 2001;32(12): 1718-1725.

172. Sager R, Kurtz A, Mueller B, Schuetz P. Procalcitonin-guided diagnosis and antibiotic stewardship revisited. *BMC Med.* 2017;15(1):15.

173. Schuetz P, Christ-Crain M, Thomann R, et al; ProHOSP Study Group. Effect of procalcitonin-based guidelines vs standard guidelines on antibiotic use in lower respiratory tract infections: the ProHOSP randomized controlled trial. *JAMA.* 2009;302(10):1059-1066.

174. Bouadma L, Luyt CE, Tubach F, et al; PRORATA trial group. Use of procalcitonin to reduce patients' exposure to antibiotics in the intensive care units (PRORATA trial): a multicenter randomized controlled trial. *Lancet.* 2010;375(9713):463-474.

175. Bloos F, Trips E, Nierhaus A, et al. Effect of sodium selenite administration and procalcitonin-guided therapy on mortality in patients with severe sepsis or septic shock: a randomized clinical trial. *JAMA Intern Med.* 2016;176(9):1266-1276.

176. Balk RA, Kadri SS, Cao Z, Robinson SB, Lipkin C. Effect of procalcitonin testing on health-care utilization and costs in critically ill patients in the United States. *Chest.* 2017;151(1):23-33.

177. Brezina R. Diagnosis and control of rickettsial diseases. *Acta Virol.* 1985;29(4):338-349.

178. Kaplan JE, Schonberger LB. The sensitivity of various serologic tests in the diagnosis of Rocky Mountain spotted fever. *Am J Trop Med Hyg.* 1986;35(4):840-844.

179. Sexton DJ, Kani SS, Wilson K, et al. The use of a polymerase chain reaction as a diagnostic test for Rocky Mountain spotted fever. *Am J Trop Med Hyg.* 1994;50(1):59-63.

180. Walker DH, Burday MS, Folds JD. Laboratory diagnosis of Rocky Mountain spotted fever. *South Med J.* 1980;73(11):1443-1446.

181. Chapman AS, Bakken JS, Folk SM, et al; Tickborne Rickettsial Diseases Working Group; CDC. Diagnosis and management of tickborne rickettsial diseases: Rocky Mountain spotted fever, ehrlichioses, and anaplasmosis—United States: a practical guide for physicians and other health-care and public health professionals. *MMWR Recomm Rep.* 2006;55(RR-4):1-27.

182. Kirkland KB, Wilkinson WE, Sexton DJ. Therapeutic delay and mortality in cases of Rocky Mountain spotted fever. *Clin Infect Dis.* 1995;20(5):1118-1121.

183. Biggs HM, Behravesh CB, Bradley KK, et al. Diagnosis and management of tickborne rickettsial diseases: Rocky Mountain spotted fever and other spotted fever group rickettsioses, ehrlichioses, and anaplasmosis—United States. *MMWR Recomm Rep.* 2016;65(2):1-44.

184. Wormser GP, Dattwyler RJ, Shapiro ED, et al. The clinical assessment, treatment, and prevention of Lyme disease, human granulocytic anaplasmosis, and babesiosis: clinical practice guidelines by the Infectious Diseases Society of America. *Clin Infect Dis.* 2006;43(9):1089-1134.

185. Nadelman RB, Wormser GP. Erythema migrans and early Lyme disease. *Am J Med.* 1995;98(Suppl 4A):15S-24S.

186. Steere AC. Lyme disease. *N Engl J Med.* 1989;321(9):586-596.

187. Nadelman RB, Wormser GP. Lyme borreliosis. *Lancet.* 1998;352(9127):557-565.

188. Stanek G, Strle F. Lyme borreliosis. *Lancet.* 2003;362(9814):1639-1647.

189. Smith RP, Schoen RT, Rahn DW, et al. Clinical characteristics and treatment outcome of early Lyme disease in patients with microbiologically confirmed erythema migrans. *Ann Intern Med.* 2002;136(6):421-428.

190. Steere AC. Lyme disease. *N Engl J Med.* 2001;345(2):115-125.

191. Centers for Disease Control and Prevention. Case definitions for infectious conditions under public health surveillance: Lyme disease (revised 9/96). *MMWR Morb Mortal Wkly Rep.* 1997;46(RR-10):1-51.

192. Wormser GP, McKenna D, Carlin J, et al. Brief communication: hematogenous dissemination in early Lyme disease. *Ann Intern Med.* 2005;142(9):751-755.

193. Wormser GP. Clinical practice: early Lyme disease. *N Engl J Med.* 2006;354(26):2794-2801.

194. Goldberg NS, Forseter G, Nadelman RB, et al. Vesicular erythema migrans. *Arch Dermatol.* 1992;128(11):1495-1498.

195. Nowakowski J, Schwartz I, Liveris D, et al. Laboratory diagnostic techniques for patients with early Lyme disease associated with erythema migrans: a comparison of different techniques. *Clin Infect Dis.* 2001;33(12):2023-2027.

196. Durand ML, Calderwood SB, Weber DJ, et al. Acute bacterial meningitis in adults. A review of 493 episodes. *N Engl J Med.* 1993;328(1):21-28.

197. Brandtzaeg P, Ovsteboo R, Kierulf P. Compartmentalization of the lipopolysaccharide production correlates with clinical presentation in meningococcal disease. *J Infect Dis.* 1992;166(3):650-652.

198. Control and prevention of meningococcal disease: recommendations of the Advisory Committee on Immunization Practices (ACIP). MMWR Recomm Rep. 1997;46(RR-5):1-51.

199. Benson CA, Kaplan JE, Masur H, et al. Treating opportunistic infections among HIV-infected adults and adolescents: recommendations from Centers for Disease Control and Prevention, National Institutes of Health, HIV Medicine Association/Infectious Diseases Society of America. HIV Infected adults and adolescents. *MMWR.* 2004;53(RR-15):1-112.

200. Marra CM, Maxwell CL, Tantalo K, et al. Normalization of cerebrospinal fluid abnormalities after neurosyphilis therapy: does HIV status matter? *Clin Infect Dis.* 2004;38(7):1001-1006.

201. Lukehart SA, Hook EW 3rd, Baker Zander SA, Collier AC, Critchlow CW, Handsfield HH. Invasion of the central nervous system by treponema pallidum: implications for diagnosis and treatment. *Ann Intern Med.* 1988;109(11):855-862.

202. Lee JW, Wilck M, Venna M. Dementia due to neurosyphilis with persistently negative CSF VDRL. *Neurology.* 2005;65(11):1838.

203. Marra CM, Maxwell CL, Tantalo LC, Sahi SK, Lukehart SA. Normalization of serum rapid plasma reagin titer predicts normalization of cerebrospinal fluid and clinical abnormalities after treatment of neurosyphilis. *Clin Infect Dis.* 2008;47(7):893-899.

204. Petersen LR, Brault AC, Nasci RS. West Nile virus: review of the literature. *JAMA.* 2013;310(3):308-315.

205. Cho H, Diamond MS. Immune responses to West Nile virus infection in the central nervous system. *Viruses.* 2012;4(12):3812-3830.

206. Rhee C, Eaton EF, Concepcion W, Blackburn BG. West Nile virus encephalitis acquired via liver transplantation and clinical response to intravenous immunoglobulin. *Transpl Infect Dis.* 2011;13(3):312-317.

207. Ferguson DD, Gershman K, LeBailly A, Petersen LR. Characteristics of the rash associated with West Nile virus fever. *Clin Infect Dis.* 2005;41(8):1204-1207.

208. Tyler KL, Pape J, Goody RJ, Corkill M, Kleinschmidt-DeMasters BK. CSF findings in 250 patients with serologically confirmed

West Nile virus meningitis and encephalitis. *Neurology.* 2006;66(3):361-336.

209. Brinker KR, Monath TP. The acute disease. In: Monath TP, ed. St Louis Encephalitis. Washington, DC: American Public Health Association; 1980: 503.

210. Powell KE, Blakely DL. St. Louis encephalitis: clinical and epidemiologic aspects, Mississippi, 1974. *South Med J.* 1976;69(9):1121-1125.

211. Gubler DJ. Dengue and dengue hemorrhagic fever. *Clin Microbiol Rev.* 1998;11(3):480-496.

212. World Health Organization. *Dengue Haemorrhagic Fever: Diagnosis, Treatment, Prevention and Control.* 2nd ed. Geneva: WHO; 1997.

213. World Health Organization. Dengue: *Guidelines for Diagnosis, Treatment, Prevention and Control.* New edition. Geneva: WHO; 2009.

214. Staples JE, Breiman RF, Powers AM. Chikungunya fever: an epidemiological review of a re-emerging infectious disease. *Clin Infect Dis.* 2009;49(6):942-948.

215. Barnett ED. Yellow fever: epidemiology and prevention. *Clin Infect Dis.* 2007;44(6):850-856.

216. Monath TP, Vasconcelos PFC. Yellow fever. *J Clin Virol.* 2015;64:160-173.

217. Delahaye F, Célard M, Roth O, de Givigney G. Indications and optimal timing for surgery in infective endocarditis. *Heart.* 2004;90(6):618-620.

218. Baron EJ, Scott JD, Tompkins LS. Prolonged incubation and extensive subculturing do not increase recovery of clinically significant microorganisms from standard automated blood cultures. *Clin Infect Dis.* 2005;41(11):1677-1680.

219. Petti CA, Bhally HS, Weinstein MP, et al. Utility of extended blood culture incubation for isolation of *Haemophilus, Actinobacillus, Cardiobacterium, Eikenella, Kingella* organisms: a retrospective multicenter evaluation. *J Clin Microbiol.* 2006;44(1):257-259.

220. Fournier PE, Thuny F, Richet H, et al. Comprehensive diagnostic strategy for blood culture-negative endocarditis: a prospective study of 819 new cases. *Clin Infect Dis.* 2010;51(2):131-140.

221. Van Zndt KE, Greer MT, Gelhaus HC. Glanders: an overview of infection in humans. Orphanet J Rare Dis. 2013;8:131.

222. Mazur-Melewska K, Mania A, Kemnitz P, Figlerowicz M, Służewski W. Cat-scratch disease: a wide spectrum of clinical pictures. *Postepy Derm Alergol.* 2015;32(3):216-220.

223. Swartz MN. Recognition and management of anthrax—an update. *N Engl J Med.* 2001;345(22):1621-1626

224. Hendricks KA, Wright ME, Shadomy SV, et al. Centers for Disease Control and Prevention expert panel meetings on prevention and treatment of anthrax in adults. *Emerg Infect Dis.* 2014;20(2).e130687.

225. Artenstein AW, Opal SM. Novel approaches to the treatment of systemic anthrax. *Clin Infect Dis.* 2012;54(8):1148-1161.

226. Kelvin KW, Jasper FW, Alan KL, et al. Ebola virus disease: a highly fatal infectious disease reemerging in West Africa. *Microbes Infect.* 2015;17(2):84-97.

227. Centers for Disease Control and Prevention. Epidemiologic risk factors to consider when evaluating a person for exposure to Ebola virus. Centers for Disease Control and Prevention Web site. http://www.cdc.gov/vhf/ebola/exposure/risk-factors-when-evaluating-person-for-exposure.html. Accessed February 2, 2015.

228. Centers for Disease Control and Prevention. Assessment of persons under investigation having low (but not zero) risk of exposure to Ebola. Centers for Disease Control and Prevention Web site. http://www.cdc.gov/vhf/ebola/healthcare-us/evaluating-patients/persons-under-investigation-low-exposure-ebola.html. Accessed July 1, 2015.

229. Centers for Disease Control and Prevention. Interim guidance for U.S. hospital preparedness for patients with possible or confirmed Ebola virus disease: a framework for a tiered approach. Centers for Disease Control and Prevention Web site. http://www.cdc.gov/vhf/ebola/hcp/us-hospital-preparedness.html. Accessed April 1, 2017.

230. Matuszkiewicz-Rowińska J, Małyszko J, Wieliczko W. Urinary tract infections in pregnancy: old and new unresolved diagnostic and therapeutic problems. *Arch Med Sci.* 2015;11(1):67-77.

231. Mayosi BM, Burgess LJ, Doubell AF. Tuberculous pericarditis. *Circulation.* 2005;112(23):3608-3616.

232. Mayosi BM, Ntsekhe M, Bosch J. Prednisolone and *Mycobacterium indicus pranii* in tuberculous pericarditis. *N Engl J Med.* 2014;371(12):1121-1130.

233. Liang QL, Shi HZ, Wang K, Qin SM, Qin XJ. Diagnostic accuracy of adenosine deaminase in tuberculous pleurisy: a meta-analysis. *Respir Med.* 2008;102(5):744-754.

234. Valdes L, Alvarez D, San José E, et al. Tuberculous pleurisy: a study of 254 patients. *Arch Intern Med.* 1998;158(18):2017-2021.

235. Riantawan P, Chaowalit P, Wongsangiem M, Rojanaraweewong P. Diagnostic value of pleural fluid adenosine deaminase in tuberculous pleuritis with reference to HIV coninfection and a Bayesian analysis. *Chest.* 1999;116(1):97-103.

236. Ocaña I, Martinez-Vazquez JM, Segura RM, Fernandez-De-Sevilla T, Capdevila JA. Adenosine deaminase in pleural fluids. Test for diagnosis of tuberculous pleural effusions. *Chest.* 1983;84(1):51-53.

237. Vales L, San José E, Alvarez D, et al. Diagnosis of tuberculous pleurisy using the biologic parameters adenosine deaminase, lysozyme, and interferon gamma. *Chest.* 1993;103(2):458-465.

238. Gopi A, Madhavan SM, Sharma SK, Sahn SA. Diagnosis and treatment of tuberculous pleural effusion in 2006. *Chest.* 2007;131(3):880-889.

239. Kirsch CM, Kroe DM, Azzi RL, Jensen WA, Kagawa FT, Wehner JH. The optimal number of pleural biopsy specimens for a diagnosis of tuberculous pleurisy. *Chest.* 1997;112(3):702-706.

240. Levine H, Metzger W, Lacera D, Kay L. Diagnosis of tuberculous pleurisy by culture of pleural biopsy specimen. *Arch Intern Med.* 1970;126(2):269-271.

Healthcare-Acquired Infections

Matthew Frank, MD, Navitha Ramesh, MD, and Ronaldo Collo Go, MD

INTRODUCTION

A healthcare-associated infection (HAI), or nosocomial infection, is defined as a localized or systemic condition resulting from the presence of an infectious agent(s) or its toxin(s) that develop in a hospital or other healthcare facility that were not present or incubating at the time of admission.[1] Healthcare-associated infections increase healthcare costs and contribute to extended intensive care unit (ICU) length of stay and increased morbidities. Mortality rates associated with healthcare-associated infections are significantly higher than those associated with community-acquired infections. While reports vary, recent data suggests that on a given day, 1 of every 25 inpatients at US acute care hospitals had at least 1 HAI.[2] Recent estimates suggest that the annual direct cost of HAIs to the healthcare system is approximately $6.65 billion.[3] Risk factors for development of an HAI include length of hospital stay, the presence of a central catheter, presence in a critical care unit, and mechanical ventilation. The leading causes of HAIs include pneumonias, surgical-site infections (SSIs), gastrointestinal infections (including those caused by *Clostridium difficile*), catheter-associated urinary tract infections, and bloodstream infections.[2]

INFECTION CONTROL

The mode of infection that develops in the hospital is thought to be due to either (1) autoinfection or an infection that was present with the patient on admission but without signs or symptoms of infection or (2) cross-contamination or the patient acquires an infective agent in the hospital and subsequently becomes infected. Controlling the infection also requires separating the source and cutting the modes of transmission. There are standard, droplet, airborne, contact, neutropenic, and bone marrow transplant precautions.

Standard precautions include the use of handwashing, gloves, mask, eye protection and/or face shield, gown, patient care equipment, environmental control, and occupational health to prevent injuries from needles, scalpels, and other sharp devices. Controlling the infection also requires separating the source and cutting the modes of transmission.

Droplet precautions prevent the transmission of respiratory particles larger than 5 microns in size, and can travel up to 3 feet away.[4] Transmission can occur when healthcare workers' (HCWs) mucosal membranes (eyes, nose, and mouth) come in contact with the patient's respiratory secretions. Patients should be in private rooms, although cohorting of patients with the same infection is appropriate. Surgical masks are advised for healthcare workers who come in direct contact with the patient. Because of the closed circuit and ventilator filters, transmission of organisms from patients who are intubated is unlikely. However, a surgical mask should still be worn, particularly when the patient is being transported, because the endotracheal tube can get disconnected.

Airborne precautions address respiratory particles smaller than 5 microns that can remain suspended in the air. Patients should be in private rooms with negative pressure and a minimum of 6 to 12 air changes per hour.[4] Healthcare workers must wear respirators with 95% filtering efficiency. In order to function reliably, these devices must not allow leakage. Therefore, HCWs must be fit-tested to ensure reliable protection. Transport of patients should be minimized; when necessary, the patient should be masked.

Patients on contact precautions warrant private rooms, and transmission occurs via direct contact or indirect contact with a contaminated object or person. Healthcare workers must perform hand hygiene and wear gloves, and if contact with the patient is anticipated or the patient has diarrhea, they should wear gowns. The gowns must be disposed of after leaving the room and healthcare workers must perform hand hygiene again.

Neutropenic precautions aim to prevent a neutropenic patient from acquiring an infection from the environment. The definition of neutropenia is institution dependent but generally includes an absolute neutrophil count (ANC) of less than 500 cells/μL. Neutropenic precautions include hand washing, nonspecific protective gear, avoiding plants or dried flowers, avoiding rectal temperatures, and avoiding suppositories.

Bone marrow transplant patients should be in a room with high-efficiency particulate arrestance (HEPA) filtration, which removes particles larger than 0.3 μ in diameter; directed, positive pressure airflow; and 12 air changes per hour to prevent invasive fungal infections.[4] Hematopoietic cell transplantation (HCT) recipients with multidermatomal varicella zoster virus (VZV) should be placed in contact and airborne precautions. The contact precautions should be enforced until all skin lesions are crusted. The airborne precautions should be enforced from 8 days after exposure to VZV until 21 days from last exposure, or 28 days postexposure if the patient receives VZV immune globulin (VZIG) because patients are infectious before rash appears.[4]

Appropriate precautions for specific pathogens are summarized in Table 19-1.[4,5]

DECOLONIZATION

Decolonization is used to prevent hospital acquired infections and target the nose, skin, and gastrointestinal tract. It is most effective for patients who are at risk of infection for a short period of time, such as surgical patients and ICU patients. Highest level of evidence is preventing surgical site infections.[6] There are two approaches: horizontal approach which targets a broad range of microbes and vertical approach which targets a specific microbe. There is also universal versus targeted decolonization.[6] Universal decolonization is for any high risk patient regardless of colonization status and targeted decolonization requires screening prior to decolonization. For 1 study, universal decolonization via intranasal mupirocin for 5 days and daily chlorhexidine impregnated cloths reduced MRSA clinical isolates and blood stream infections from any pathogens more effectively than targeted decolonization.[7] Mupirocin is produced by *Pseudomonas fluorescens* and is affective against staphylococci, streptococci, and Gram-negative organisms such as *N. gonorrhoeae*, *H. influenza*, and *M. catarrhalis*.[6] Chlorhexidine has good coverage against Gram-positive and Gram-negative bacteria and yeast.[6]

Nasal agents for decolonization include mupirocin, bacitracin, retapamulin, povidone-iodine, and investigational agents (tea tree oil, photodynamic therapy, omiganan pentahydrochloride, lysostaphin).[6] Topical agents include chlorhexidine gluconate, hexachlorophene, povidone-iodine, triclosan, and sodium hypochlorite.[6] Although currently not recommended, oral agents that have been used for decolonization include rifampin, quinolones, trimethoprim-sulfamethoxazole, novobiocin, clindamycin, doxycycline, and minocycline.[6]

HOSPITAL-ACQUIRED PNEUMONIA AND VENTILATOR-ASSOCIATED PNEUMONIA

Hospital-acquired pneumonia (HAP) is pneumonia that develops 48 hours or more after admission and did not appear to be incubating at the time of admission. It was previously thought that patients with healthcare associated pneumonia (HCAP)—defined as pneumonia in patients from nursing homes, hemodialysis centers, or clinics, or who were hospitalized in the

last 3 months—were also at high risk for multidrug-resistant organisms (MDRO). However, the Infectious Disease Society of America (IDSA) 2016 guidelines suggest that this risk has been overstated and that treating MDROs empirically as HAP does not improve outcomes.[8-10]

Multidrug resistance, particularly with Gram-negative bacilli, is resistance to 2 or more antibiotics. Extensive drug-resistant Gram-negative bacilli are resistant to all antibiotics except for colistin, tigecycline, and aminoglycosides. Panresistance is resistance to all systemic antibiotics. Table 19-2 lists the risk factors.[8-10]

In the 2016 IDSA guidelines, ventilator associated pneumonia (VAP) was noted to be a distinct entity from hospital-acquired pneumonia rather than a subset. Reported incidence varies, ranging from 10% to 25% with an all-cause mortality of 25% to 50%.[8,11] Ventilator-acquired pneumonia develops after more than 48 hours of mechanical ventilation, but diagnosis may be difficult. At present, the consensus is that VAP is suspected when there is clinical deterioration defined as an increase in positive end-expiratory pressure (PEEP) by 3 cm H_2O or an increase in the fraction of inspired oxygen (FIO_2) by 0.20 (a ventilator-associated condition) in association with aberration in temperature or white blood cell count. Possible VAP is present when these findings are found in concert with purulent secretions or isolation of a potential pathogen from respiratory cultures.[8,11]

Prevention should focus on avoiding intubation when possible, minimizing sedation and avoiding benzodiazepines, maintaining and improving physical conditioning with early mobilization and exercise, minimizing pooling of secretions above the endotracheal tube cuff by means of endotracheal tubes with subglottic secretion drainage ports, and elevating the head of the bed to 30 degree to 45 degree.[12] Endotracheal tubes are now available with subglottic secretion drainage ports. The use of subglottic drainage may reduce the incidence of VAP by 55% and may further reduce antibiotic utilization. Current evidence supports the use of oral care with chlorhexidine in intubated patients, particularly for preventing postoperative respiratory infections in cardiac surgery patients. At this time, data suggests that these oral antiseptics may lower VAP rates but insufficient data is available to determine the impact on duration of mechanical ventilation or mortality.[12]

Initiation of antibiotics should be dependent on clinical judgment and not on biomarkers such as procalcitonin, C-reactive protein (CRP), and soluble triggering receptor expressed on myeloid cells-1 (sTREM-1).[8] Typical pathogens include aerobic Gram-negative bacilli (eg, *Escherichia coli*, *Klebsiella pneumoniae*, *Enterobacter* species, *Pseudomonas aeruginosa*, *Acinetobacter* species) and Gram-positive cocci (eg, *Staphylococcus aureus*, including methicillin-resistant *S aureus* [MRSA], *Streptococcus* species). Nosocomial pneumonia due to viruses or fungi is significantly less common, except in the immunocompromised patient.[13]

Current guidelines recommend empiric therapy of HAP and VAP with antimicrobials providing coverage for *S aureus*, *P aeruginosa*, and other Gram-negative bacilli.

TABLE 19-1 Isolation Precautions

Precautions	Disease/Organism	Duration of Precautions
Droplet	Influenza	• Until patient is afebrile and symptom free for 24 hours OR 7 days since symptom onset
	Adenovirus[a]	• Duration of illness for pneumonia
	Parvovirus B19	• Duration of illness
	Diphtheria	• Until antibiotics are completed and chest x-ray is negative
	Bordetella	• 5 days
	Mycoplasma pneumoniae	• Duration of illness
	Haemophilus influenzae type B	• 24 h after therapy mostly for infants; adults warrant standard precautions
	Rubella	• 7 d after onset of rash
	Mumps	• 5-9 d
	Neisseria meningitides	• 24 h after therapy
	Ebola	• Duration of illness
	SARS	• Duration of illness + 7 d after resolution of fever
Airborne	SARS	• Duration of illness + 7 d after resolution of fever
	Small pox	• Duration of illness
	Measles	• 4 d after onset of rash
	Varicella[d]	• Until lesions dry and crusted
	Tuberculosis	• Precautions discontinued if clinically infectious TB is unlikely and any of the following is present: 3 consecutive acid-fast bacilli smears are negative, an alternate diagnosis is confirmed, or a sputum nucleic acid amplification test and a sputum acid-fast bacilli smear are both negative
Contact	Adenovirus[a]	• Contact precautions for duration of illness in gastroenteritis and conjunctivitis
	Cutaneous diphtheria[b]	• Until antibiotics are completed and chest x-ray is negative
	RSV	• Duration of illness
	Parainfluenza	• Duration of illness
	Enterovirus	• Only warrant contact precautions in children in diapers or in incontinent individuals to control institutional outbreaks.
	HSV	• Until lesions are dry and crusted
	MRSA	• Duration of illness
	VRE	• Duration of illness
	Drug-resistant organisms	• Duration of illness
	Clostridium difficile	• Duration of illness
	Escherichia coli O157:H7	• Duration of illness
	Anthrax if large amount of uncontained drainage (cutaneous)	• Duration of illness
	SARS	• Duration of illness + 7 d after resolution of fever
	Small pox	• Duration of illness

DI = duration of illness; HSV = herpes simplex virus; MRSA = methicillin-resistant *Staphylococcus aureus*; RSV = respiratory syncytial virus; SARS = severe acute respiratory syndrome; TB = tuberculosis; VRE = vancomycin-resistant enterococci.

[a] Droplet precautions should be used in pneumonia caused by adenovirus. For gastroenteritis, contact precautions should be used for diapered or incontinent individuals. For conjunctivitis, contact precautions should be used.

[b] Pharyngeal diphtheria warrants droplet precautions. Cutaneous diphtheria warrants contact precautions.

[c] Primary varicella infection warrants airborne precautions. Localized herpes zoster infections in immunocompetent adults requires standard precautions alone. Disseminated herpes zoster or localized herpes zoster in an immunocompromised individual warrants airborne and contact precautions.

TABLE 19-2 Multidrug Resistance Risk Factors

Type of MDR Infection	Risk Factors
MDR VAP	• IV antibiotics within 90 d • Septic shock at time of VAP • ARDS before VAP • ≥ 5 d prior to onset of VAP • Acute RRT prior to onset of VAP
MDR HAP	• IV antibiotics within 90 d
MRSA VAP/HAP	• IV antibiotics within 90 d
Pseudomonas VAP/HAP	• IV antibiotics within 90 d

ARDS = acute respiratory distress syndrome; HAP = hospital-acquired pneumonia; IV = intravenous; MDR = multidrug resistant; MRSA = methicillin-resistant *Staphylococcus aureus*; VAP = ventilator-acquired pneumonia.

MRSA should be covered with vancomycin or linezolid if MDR risk factors are present—particularly in patients who have received antibiotics within the last 90 days—or in hospital units with a high prevalence, greater than 10% to 20% of MRSA. Monotherapy for confirmed pseudomonal infections is recommended unless the patient is high risk for death, in septic shock, or has a structural lung disease such as bronchiectasis and cystic fibrosis. Dual therapy is then recommended. Aminoglycosides are generally avoided due to their high mortality risk, possibly greater than 25%.[8] Inhaled antibiotics are reserved for Gram-negative bacilli that are only susceptible to aminoglycosides or polymyxins as a last resort.

Tables 19-3 and 19-4 list the recommended empiric antibiotics for HAP and VAP.[8]

Treatment should be narrowed once culture results are available. Patients should be reassessed 72 hours after initiation of therapy for the possibility of narrowing the antibiotic regimen based on cultures and the clinical picture. The decision to de-escalate antibiotics can be particularly difficult in culture-negative HAP. However, current literature has found that patients with culture-negative HAP tend to have less severe disease. Serum procalcitonin may help support decisions to discontinue antibiotics but may have limited benefit since recent data suggests that treatment can be safely limited to 7 days regardless of pathogen.

Recent literature supports the use of respiratory cultures in guiding VAP therapy, particularly as a guide in the need for MDR coverage. The role of bronchoalveolar lavage (BAL) in collection of respiratory cultures is controversial. The use of bronchoscopic sampling does not improve mortality, duration of mechanical ventilation, or length of stay but may lead to more rapid de-escalation of antimicrobial therapy, potentially reducing antibiotic resistance. Current guidelines recommend noninvasive sampling (endotracheal aspiration [ETA]) rather than invasive sampling (eg, BAL); the yield of sputum culture via ETA is approximately 33% to 83%.[14,15] Bronchoalveolar lavage and ETA samples showing fewer than 10 epithelial cells and more than 25 polymorphonuclear leukocytes per low-power field are adequate for analysis. In the event of performing invasive methods, such as BAL or

TABLE 19-3 Empiric Antibiotics for Hospital-Acquired Pneumonia

Patients With HAP Who Do Not Require Ventilator Support and/or are Not in Septic Shock	Patients With HAP Who Not Require Ventilator Support and/or are Not in Septic Shock but Have an Increased Likelihood of MRSA, Such As Antibiotics Within 90 Days, MRSA Prevalence in Unit is Unknown, or > 20% MRSA Isolate In Unit	Patients With HAP Who are on Ventilator Support and/or in Septic Shock or Received Antibiotics Within 90 D
Piperacillin-tazobactam 4.5 g IV every 6 h or Cefepime 2 g IV every 8 h or Levofloxacin 750 mg IV daily or Imipenem 500 mg IV every 6 h Or Meropenem 1 g IV every 8 h	Piperacillin-tazobactam 4.5 g IV every 6 h or Cefepime 2 g IV every 8 h or Levofloxacin 750 mg IV daily or Ciprofloxacin 400 mg IV every 8 h or Imipenem 500 mg IV every 6 h Or Meropenem 1 g IV every 8 h or Aztreonam 2 g IV every 8 h PLUS Glycopeptides: Vancomycin 15 mg/kg IV every 8–12 h (loading dose 25–30 mg/kg × 1 in severe illness) *or* Oxazolidinones: Linezolid 600 mg IV every 12 h	Piperacillin-tazobactam 4.5 g IV every 6 h or Cefepime 2 g IV every 8 h or Levofloxacin 750 mg IV daily or Ciprofloxacin 400 mg IV every 8 h or Imipenem 500 mg IV every 6 h Or Meropenem 1 g IV every 8 h or Amikacin 15–20 mg/kg IV every 24 h or Gentamicin 5–7 mg/kg IV every 24 h or Tobramycin 5–7 mg/kg IV every 24 h or Aztreonam 2 g IV every 8 h PLUS Glycopeptides: Vancomycin 15 mg/kg IV every 8–12 h (loading dose 25–30 mg/kg × 1 in severe illness) *or* Oxazolidinones: Linezolid 600 mg IV every 12 h

IV = intravenous; HAP = hospital-acquired pneumonia; MRSA = methicillin-resistant *Staphylococcus aureus*

Data from Kalil AC, Metersky ML, Klompas M, et al. Management of adults with hospital-acquired and ventilator-associated pneumonia: 2016 clinical practice guidelines by the Infectious Diseases Society of America and the American Thoracic Society. *Clin Infect Dis*. 2016;63(5):e61-e111.

TABLE 19-4 Empiric Antibiotics for Ventilator-Acquired Pneumonia With Multidrug Resistance

Group A: Gram-Positive Antibiotics With MRSA Activity	Group B: Gram-Negative Antibiotics With Antipseudomonal Activity: β-Lactam–Based Agents	Group C: Gram-Negative Antibiotics With Antipseudomonal Activity: Non-β-Lactam–Based Agents
Glycopeptides: Vancomycin 15 mg/kg IV every 8–12 h (loading dose 25–30 mg/kg × 1 in severe illness) *or* Oxazolidinones: Linezolid 600 mg IV every 12 h	Piperacillin-tazobactam 4.5 g IV every 6 h or Cefepime 2 g IV every 8 h *or* Ceftazidime 2 g IV every 8 h or Imipenem 500 mg IV every 6 h or Meropenem 1 g IV every 8 h or Aztreonam 1 g IV every 8 h	Ciprofloxacin 400 mg IV every 8 h or Levofloxacin 750 mg IV every 24 h or Amikacin 15–20 mg/kg IV every 24 h or Gentamicin 5–7 mg/kg IV every 24 h or Tobramycin 5–7 mg/kg IV every 24 h or Colistin 5 mg/kg IV × 1 (loading dose) followed by 2.5 mg × (1.5 × CrCl + 30) IV every 12 h (maintenance) or Polymyxin B 2.5–3 mg/kg/d divided into 2 daily IV doses

Treatment for multidrug-resistant ventilator-acquired pneumonia requires 3 antibiotics, 1 from each group. CrCl = creatinine clearance; IV = intravenous; MRSA = methicillin-resistant *Staphylococcus aureus*

Data from Kalil AC, Metersky ML, Klompas M, et al. Management of adults with hospital-acquired and ventilator-associated pneumonia: 2016 clinical practice guidelines by the Infectious Diseases Society of America and the American Thoracic Society. *Clin Infect Dis.* 2016;63(5):e61-e111.

protected specimen brush (PSB), a BAL less than 10^4 colony-forming units (CFU)/mL and a PSB less than 10^3 CFU/mL are used as thresholds to withhold antibiotics to avoid unnecessary treatment, cost, and complications.[3] Respiratory secretions growing *Candida* often indicate colonization and rarely require antifungal therapy.[16] Currently, no evidence supports repeating sputum to ensure adequate treatment.

VENTILATOR-ASSOCIATED TRACHEITIS

Healthcare-associated tracheitis or ventilator-associated tracheobronchitis (VAT) is a localized disease that manifests with fever, increased or new sputum production, clinical signs (fever, leukocytosis, and purulent sputum), positive ETA culture (> 10^6 CFU/mL) yielding a new bacterium, and the absence of a new infiltrate on chest radiograph. Current guidelines do not recommend antibiotic treatment for VAT.[8,17]

CATHETER-RELATED INFECTIONS

Catheter-related infections are usually related to skin organisms at the insertion site but can occur due to direct contamination of the catheter or its hub, hematogenous seeding from another source, or infusate contamination.[18-22] A catheter-related bloodstream infection (CRBSI) should be suspected in patients with fever in the ICU. Localized signs of infection are often absent. The most common pathogens are coagulase-negative *Staphylococcus* (CoNS) followed by *S aureus* and enteric Gram-negative bacilli. *Candida* should be considered in patients receiving total parenteral nutrition (TPN) and in patients with femoral catheters.

Prevention of CRBSI and central line–associated bloodstream infection (CLABSI) is paramount. Prevention begins by selecting the most appropriate device. Peripheral catheters are preferred for short-term infusion of peripherally compatible solutions. Midline catheters are optimal for peripherally compatible solutions when duration of therapy is likely greater than 6 days and less than 14 days. Peripherally inserted central catheters (PICC) are appropriate in clinically stable patients who require prolonged (> 14-day) treatment, peripherally incompatible solutions, or frequent blood draws. Peripherally inserted central catheters are preferred to central venous access devices (CVAD) in critically ill patients in whom treatment for more than 15 days is anticipated or in those with bleeding disorders. Central venous access devices are the most appropriate choice for patients who are unstable and require hemodynamic monitoring, multiple medications, large fluid infusions, blood or blood products, or continuous parenteral nutrition, and for all patients requiring short-term critical access (< 14 days).[23,24] For central venous catheters (CVCs), femoral placement is avoided and subclavian site is preferred. Avoid the subclavian site in hemodialysis patients to prevent subclavian stenosis.[25] A chlorhexidine-impregnated sponge should be used for short-term catheters if the CLABSI rate is not decreasing despite adherence to basic preventive measures.[25] Chlorhexidine/silver sulfadiazine or minocycline/rifampin-impregnated catheters are recommended if catheters are expected to be in place for more than 5 days and the CLABSI rates are not decreasing.[25] Patients with recurrent or multiple CRBSI may benefit from prophylactic antimicrobial lock solution.[25]

Aseptic technique and hand hygiene are crucial during insertion, dressing changes, and removal of all catheters. Maximal barrier precautions should be employed when inserting midline and central catheters. Central catheters inserted emergently, where complete asepsis cannot be assured, should be removed and replaced within 48 hours.

Peripheral venous catheters are removed when there is warmth, erythema, tenderness, palpable venous cord, or malfunction, or when no longer clinically indicated.[25] Current guidelines do not support routinely changing catheters.

TABLE 19-5 Definitions of Catheter-Related Infections

Infection	Characteristics
Colonization	Growth ≥ 1 microorganism in quantitative culture of tip, subcutaneous segment, or hub
Phlebitis	Induration, erythema, warmth, and pain along tract of catheterized vein
Exit site infection, microbiological	Exudate at catheter exit site with microorganism ± bloodstream infection
Exit site infection, clinical	Exudate, induration, and/or tenderness within 2 cm of exit site and associated with other symptoms of infection ± bloodstream infection
Tunnel infection	Tenderness, erythema, and/or induration > 2 cm from exit site, along the subcutaneous tract of a tunnel catheter ± bloodstream infection
Pocket infection	Infected fluid in subcutaneous pocket of implanted device, with tenderness, erythema, and/or induration over pocket, along the subcutaneous tract of a tunnel catheter ± bloodstream infection
Bloodstream infection, infusate related	Concordance of microorganism from infusate and cultures of percutaneously obtained blood cultures
Bloodstream infection, catheter related	Bacteremia or fungemia in patients with intravascular device and > 1 positive blood culture (> 15 CFU per catheter segment via roll plate culture or > 10^2 CFU per catheter segment or sonication broth culture) from peripheral vein with a ratio of > 3:1 CFU/mL (catheter vs peripheral) and clinical signs of infection with no alternative source

Adapted from Mermel LA, Allon M, Bouza E, et al. Clinical practice guidelines for the diagnosis and management of intravascular catheter-related infection: 2009 update by the Infectious Diseases Society of America. *Clin Infect Dis.* 2009;49(1):1.

There are multiple kinds of catheter-related infections (Table 19-5). For suspected CRBSI, paired blood samples (1 from the catheter and 1 from a peripheral vein) should be obtained prior to initiation of antimicrobials. Catheter cultures should be performed when possible. For central venous catheters, the catheter tip, rather than the subcutaneous segment, should be sent for culture.[26]

Fever is sensitive but lacks specificity. Erythema, tenderness, and purulence at the catheter insertion site are specific but are not sensitive. According to the IDSA 2009 guidelines, the strength of recommendation is stratified as (A) if good evidence to support or go against a recommendation; (B) if moderate evidence to support or go against a recommendation; and (C) if poor evidence to support a recommendation. Quality of evidence is I if more than 1 properly randomized, controlled trial; II if evidence from more than 1 well designed clinical trial without randomization, from cohort or case-controlled analytic studies (preferably from > 1 center), from multiple time-series, or from dramatic results from uncontrolled experiments; and III if evidence is from opinions of authorities, clinical experiences, or descriptive studies.[26] A definitive diagnosis of CRSBI requires the same organism to grow from at least 1 percutaneous blood culture and from the catheter tip (Category AI) or that cultures from at least 2 blood samples meeting quantitative criteria for blood culture or differential time to positivity (growth detected from the catheter hub sample at least 2 hours before growth detected from the peripheral vein sample)[26] (Category AII).

Blood culture contamination is an issue and measures to prevent it include (1) having a dedicated phlebotomy team; (2) preparing skin with alcohol, alcohol chlorhexidine, or tincture of iodine; and (3) obtaining blood samples from peripheral veins over newly placed intravenous catheters.[26]

Use of antimicrobials should be based on clinical presentation and culture data. Initial empiric therapy should include MRSA coverage via vancomycin or alternatives such as daptomycin, where MRSA isolates have vancomycin minimum inhibitory concentration (MIC) greater than 2 μg/mL (Category A-II); an agent active against Gram-negative bacilli based on severity of illness and local resistance patterns (Category A-II); combination coverage, such as for *Pseudomonas* in neutropenic patients, sepsis, or patients with prior colonization of such pathogens (Category A-II); and empiric antifungal therapy for femoral catheters (Category A-II).[26] Empiric antifungal therapy should also be considered for patients on TPN, patients with prolonged use of broad-spectrum antibiotics, patients with hematologic malignancy, or transplant recipients (Category B-II).[26]

There is a low threshold to remove catheters, and suspicion of catheter-related blood stream infections should prompt its removal. To be specific, short-term catheters should be removed with infections from Gram-negative bacilli, *S aureus*, enterococci, fungus, and mycobacteria (Category A-II).[26] Long-term catheters should be removed in severe sepsis, thrombophlebitis, endocarditis, bacteremia despite more than 72 hours of antibiotics, and infections from *S aureus*, *P aeruginosa*, fungi, or mycobacteria (Category A-II).[26] In uncomplicated CRBSI of a long-term catheter due to species other than those mentioned above, antimicrobial therapy without catheter removal might be attempted. When attempting salvage therapy, treatment should include antimicrobial lock therapy (Category B-II) and/or systemic antibiotics through colonized catheter (Category C-III).[26]

Duration of treatment depends on the clinical situation but count starts with the first negative blood culture (Category C-III).[26] Treatment for uncomplicated CRBSI with

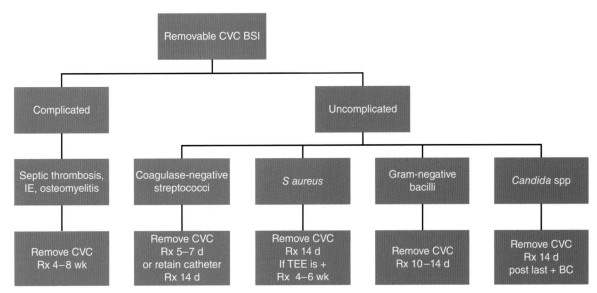

FIGURE 19-1 Approach to infected short-term central venous catheter. BC = blood culture; CVC = central venous catheter; BSI = bloodstream infection; CVC = central venous catheter; IE = infective endocarditis; Rx = Antibiotic Treatment; TEE = transesophageal echocardiogram. (Adapted from Mermel LA, Allon M, Bouza E, et al. Clinical practice guidelines for the diagnosis and management of intravascular catheter-related infection: 2009 update by the Infectious Diseases Society of America. *Clin Infect Dis.* 2009;49(1):1.)

catheter removal or exchange should typically continue for 10 to 14 days. For persistent bacteremia or fungemia (positive cultures > 72 hours after catheter removal), 4 to 6 weeks of antimicrobial therapy might be necessary (Category A-II).[26] Patients with infection due to *S aureus* require a minimum of 2 weeks of intravenous antibiotics. Certain situations such as endocarditis, venous thrombosis, or presence of implanted device may require longer duration of therapy.

Long-term catheters with evidence of abscess or tunnel infection but without associated bacteremia should have

the catheter removed followed by a 7- to 10-day course of antibiotics.[21] If there is an exit wound but no systemic evidence of infection, topical antibiotics might be sufficient.[25]

For hemodialysis catheters, immediate removal is indicated if cultures are positive for *Staphylococcus*, *Pseudomonas*, or *Candida*, but removal does not have to be immediate if cultures are positive for Gram-negative bacilli, as long as there is no evidence of metastatic infection.[26] If clinically warranted, a short-term dialysis can be placed until blood cultures are negative, at which point a long-term hemodialysis

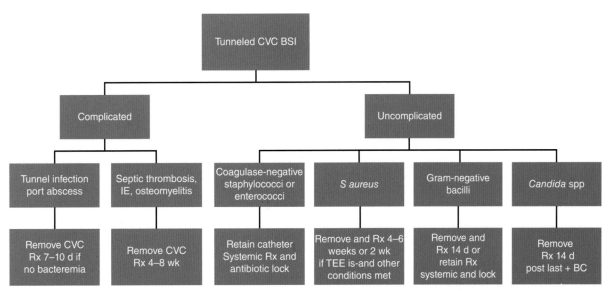

FIGURE 19-2 Approach to infected long-term catheter. BC = blood culture; BSI = bloodstream infection; CVC = central venous catheter; IE = infective endocarditis; Rx = antibiotic treatment; TEE = transesophageal echocardiogram. (Adapted from Mermel LA, Allon M, Bouza E, et al. Clinical practice guidelines for the diagnosis and management of intravascular catheter-related infection: 2009 update by the Infectious Diseases Society of America. *Clin Infect Dis.* 2009;49(1):1.)

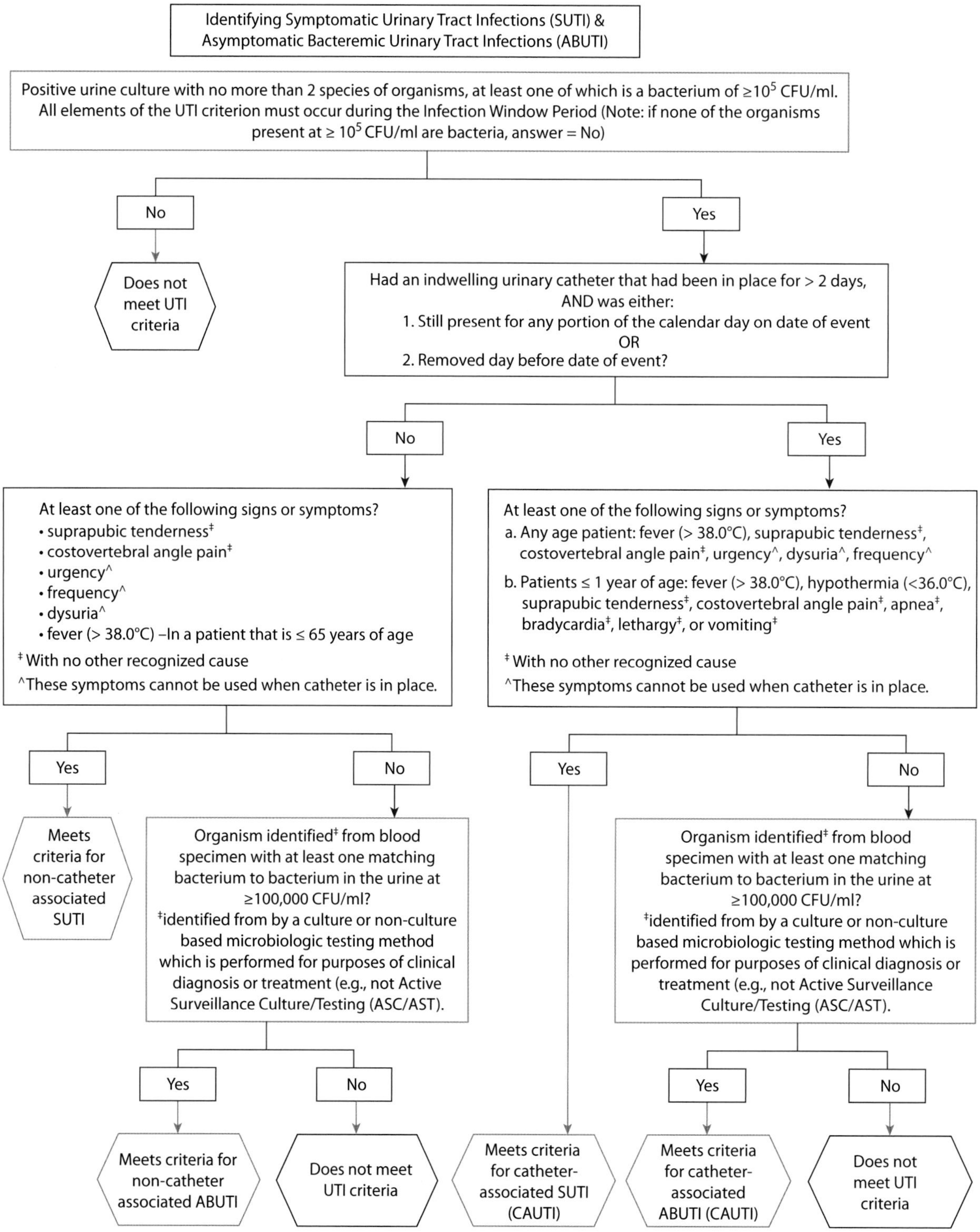

FIGURE 19-3 Center for Disease Control (CDC) Allgorithm for the Diagnosis of Catheter Associated Urinary Tract infection (CAUTI). (Reprinted from centers for disease control. Urinary Tract Infection (Catheter Associated Urinary Tract Infection) and Non-Catheter Associated Urinary Tract Infection and Other Urinary System Infection [USI] Events. (Jan 2018). www.cdc.gov/nhsn/pdfs/pscmanual/7psccauticurrent.pdf.)

catheter can be inserted. Antimicrobials should be continued for 4 to 6 weeks in cases where bacteremia or fungemia persists for more than 72 hours after catheter removal and 6 to 8 weeks if there is osteomyelitis.

Antibiotic lock therapy is an adjunct to systemic antibiotic therapy in infections in which there is no exit or tunnel infection and salvage therapy is the goal.[21,26-30] Antibiotic lock therapy is presumed to work by achieving the extremely high intraluminal antibiotic concentrations needed to eradicate organisms enmeshed in the catheter biofilm. However, this approach is less likely to be effective with infection due to *Staphylococcus* or *Candida*.[21,27-30] Catheters less than 2 weeks old usually have infection that is extraluminal and lock therapy might not work[21] (See Figs. 19-1 to 19-3).

CATHETER-ASSOCIATED URINARY TRACT INFECTIONS

In the ICU, indwelling urinary catheters remain the leading cause of urinary tract infections, and catheter-associated UTIs (CAUTIs) remain a leading cause of HAIs.[31] The key to CAUTI prevention is catheter avoidance. Therefore, the use of urinary catheters should be limited to patients with urinary retention, or those in whom accurate urine output is essential and who are unwilling or unable to collect urine.[31-33] When necessary, catheters should be inserted using sterile technique. Prompt removal of catheters should be performed when they are no longer needed.

In the catheterized patient, pyuria alone is not diagnostic and should not be used to distinguish colonization from infection. According to the IDSA 2009 guidelines, diagnosis of CAUTI in symptomatic patients with no other obvious source of infection requires a urinary culture growth of 10^3 CFU/mL or more of 1 or more bacterial species via single catheter specimen or midstream voided specimen, even if the urethral, suprapubic, or condom catheter was removed within the previous 48 hours (Category A-III).[31] Catheter-associated asymptomatic bacteriuria (CA-ASB) is defined a urinary catheter culture growth of 10^5 CFU/mL or more of 1 or more bacterial species without symptoms (Category A-II).[31] Signs and symptoms of CA-UTI include fever, rigors, altered mental status, malaise, flank or pelvic pain, and hematuria, although in patients with spinal cord injury, they may have increased spasticity, dysreflexia, and uneasiness (Category A-III). [31]

Prevention includes limiting unnecessary catheterization (Category A-III), prompt discontinuation as soon as it is no longer indicated (Category A-I), use of a close catheter drainage system (Category A-II), and use of antibiotic urinary catheters (Category B-II).[31]

In January 2018, The Centers for Disease Control (CDC) changed the definition of CAUTI (see Fig.19-3).[32] The following organisms are excluded from the diagnosis of UTI: Candida, yeast not otherwise specified, mold, dimorphic fungus, and parasites.[32] However, urinary system infection (USI) is considered when it meets at least one of the criteria: 1) organisms identified in fluid or tissue other than urine, 2) patient has an abscess or evidence of infection on anatomic examination or during invasive procedure; and/or 3) fever (> 38 C) with or without suprapubic tenderness and organisms identified in the blood or imaging study which if equivocal is supported by clinical correlation.[32]

Treatment of CAUTIs should be based on culture data when available. Duration of treatment should be 7 days in patients with prompt response; however, 10 to 14 days are recommended when there is a delayed response (Category A-III).[31] Patients who require chronic indwelling Foley catheters should have the catheters replaced at the initiation of antimicrobial therapy.[31]

SINUSITIS

Nosocomial sinusitis should be suspected in all intubated patients or if they have nasogastric tubes who have a fever without an obvious source, especially if there is purulent nasal drainage. The incidence of nosocomial sinusitis varies widely owing to differences in diagnostic criteria. Nasotracheal intubation should be avoided when possible and simultaneous nasotracheal and nasogastric intubation should be avoided.[34]

Diagnosis has traditionally relied on computed tomography (CT) imaging but endoscopically directed middle meatal culture has recently been shown to offer a simple, minimally invasive approach with comparable positive and negative predictive values. If encountered, nosocomial sinusitis should be treated with antimicrobials directed against pathogens found in sinus fluid culture and nasal tubes should be removed to allow drainage. If culture data is not available, empiric therapy should be similar to the antibiotic regimens suggested for VAP. Some may require surgical drainage.

DECUBITUS ULCERS

Decubitus ulcers result from extended elevations of arterial capillary pressure greater than 32 mmHg or venous capillary closing pressure greater than 12 mmHg[35,36] (see Table 19-6).

TABLE 19-6 Stages of Decubitus Ulcer

Stage 1: • Localized area of nonblanching erythema with intact skin • Treat with transparent film
Stage 2: • Partial-thickness skin loss with exposed dermis • Semiocclusive or occlusive dressings • Avoid wet to dry dressings
Stage 3: • Full-thickness loss with visible adipose and presence of granulation and wound edges • Debridement, dressing changes, and treatment of infection, if present
Stage 4: • Full-thickness skin and tissue loss with exposed fascia, muscle, tendon, ligament, cartilage, or bone • Debridement, dressing changes, and treatment of infection, if present
Unstageable: • Full-thickness, but the extent cannot be determined due to eschar or slough

Decubitus ulcers may lead to significant morbidity, including bacteremia with or without sepsis. Avoidance of pressure ulcers is predicated on nursing assessment of patient risk to inform optimal prevention strategies, which includes frequent positioning, minimization of head-of-bed elevation, having patients bend knees prior to elevating the head of the bed to decrease shear forces, and in high-risk patients, using pressure-reducing mattresses or specialized beds. Infection from a decubitus ulcer should be suspected if there is erythema extending from the ulcer site, induration, new or increasing pain or warmth, purulent discharge, increase in size, crepitus, discoloration, and systemic signs of infection such as fever, malaise, altered mental status, and lymph node enlargement.[37] Swab cultures will always be positive and have no diagnostic significance; postdebridement biopsy with qualitative culture may provide useful information. Localized infection may delay wound healing and should be addressed with silver-containing cream or antimicrobial-impregnated dressings. While relatively uncommon, sepsis from decubitus ulcers is associated with a high morbidity and mortality. Suspected wound sepsis should prompt blood cultures and empiric broad-spectrum antibiotics directed at the most common organisms: *P mirabilis*, group D streptococci, *E coli*, *S aureus*, *P aeruginosa*, and *Corynebacterium* species.[38]

CLOSTRIDIUM DIFFICILE

C difficile infection (CDI) is symptomatic illness due to the Gram-positive spore-forming bacterium *C difficile*, the severity of which varies from minimal to life-threatening toxic megacolon. *C difficile* infection should be suspected in any hospitalized patient with new-onset diarrhea, abdominal distension, or unexplained leukocytosis. The American College of Gastroenterology (ACG) published their guidelines in 2013 and the Infectious Diseases Society of America (IDSA) published their guidelines in 2017-2018. Methods for stratification of recommendation and quality of evidence are similar in both guidelines.

According to the 2013 guidelines published in the *American Journal of Gastroenterology*, only stools from patients with diarrhea should be sent for diagnosis of *C difficile* because the test cannot distinguish colonization from infection[39] (strong recommendation, high quality of evidence). The 2017 Update from the Infectious Diseases Society of America further elaborate that unexplained new-onset more than 3 unformed stools in 24 hours is the preferred population for testing. (weak recommendation, very low quality of evidence)[40] Although the *C difficile* cytotoxicity assay is the gold standard for diagnosis, it is impractical for widespread laboratory use. Nucleic acid amplification tests (NAATs) for *C difficile* toxin genes are superior to enzyme immunoassay (EIA) for toxins A and B for the diagnosis of CDI, but a stepped approach utilizing the glutamate dehydrogenase (GDH) antigen screening test with subsequent toxin A and

B EIAs may be a cost-effective strategy[37] (strong recommendation, moderate quality of evidence). Discordant results are then adjudicated with NAATs.[39] Repeat testing is discouraged (strong recommendation, moderate quality of evidence).[39]

Leukocytosis is a common but not universal feature of CDI and may precede gastrointestinal signs and symptoms. Marked leukocytosis, sometimes $50,000/\mu L$ or higher, and lactic acidosis may portend serious complications such as toxic megacolon.

The 2013 guidelines from the *American Journal of Gastroenterology* based treatment on disease severity. Mild disease is defined as CDI with diarrhea as the only symptom. Moderate disease is CDI with diarrhea and additional signs/symptoms not meeting the definition of severe or complicated CDI. Patients with severe CDI have hypoalbuminemia (serum albumin < 3g/dL) and either leukocytosis (white blood cell count [WBC] > 15,000 cells/μL) or abdominal tenderness. Complicated disease involves one of the following: (1) admission to ICU, (2) hypotension with or without vasopressor use, (3) fever of 38.5°C or higher, (4) ileus, (5) significant abdominal distention, (6) mental status change, (7) WBC greater than 35,000 cells/μL or less than 2,000 cells/μL, (8) lactate of greater than 2.2 mmol/L, or (9) evidence of end-organ failure.

However, the IDSA 2017 guidelines stratified treatment based on disease severity and sustained resolution for 1 month after treatment.[40] Between the two guidelines, treatment is similar except for a few exceptions such as the IDSA 2017 guidelines emphasis on fidaxomicin. Initial non-severe episode is associated with WBC less than 15,000 cells/μL and creatinine less than 1.5 mg/dL. Recommended treatment is vancomycin 125 mg PO every 6 hours for 10 days *OR* fidaxomicin 200 mg every 12 hours for 10 days. (strong recommendation, high quality of evidence).[40] Alternative is metronidazole 500 mg every 8 hours for 10 days (weak recommendation, high quality of evidence).[40] Initial severe episode is associated with WBC more than 15,000 cells/μL and creatinine more than 1.5 mg/dL. Recommended treatment is vancomycin 125 mg PO every 6 hours for 10 days *OR* fidaxomicin 200 mg every 12 hours for 10 days (strong recommendation, high quality of evidence).[40] Initial fulminant episode is associated with shock, ileus, and megacolon. Recommended treatment is vancomycin 500 mg every 6 hours by mouth (strong recommendation, high quality of evidence) *OR* 500 mg in 100 mL normal saline as retention enema per rectum every 6 hours (weak recommendation, low quality of evidence).[40]

Metronidazole 500 mg IV every 8 hours should be given as an adjunct (strong recommendation, moderate quality of evidence).[40]

ACG guidelines warrant surgical consultation in following cases: if complicated CDI with hypotension requiring pressors, lactic acid of greater than 5 mmol/L, WBC of greater than 50×10^3 cells/μL, mental status changes, sepsis and multiorgan failure, and/or failure to respond to medical management after 5 days.[39] IDSA guidelines elaborate on the type of surgery: subtotal colectomy with preservation of the rectum (strong recommendation, moderate quality of evidence) or diverting loop ileostomy with colonic lavage with antegrade vancomycin flushes (weak recommendation, low quality of evidence).[40]

According to the 2017 IDSA guidelines, treatment for the first recurrent include vancomycin 125 mg every 6 hours for 10 days if metronidazole was used for initial treatment OR pulse vancomycin regimen (eg, vancomycin 125 mg every 6 hours for 10–14 days, followed by 125 mg every 12 hours for 1 week, followed by vancomycin every 2–3 days for 2–8 weeks) (weak recommendation, low quality of evidence) OR fidaxomicin 200 mg every 12 hours for 10 days if vancomycin was used for initial episode (weak recommendation, moderate quality of evidence).[40]

Treatment for subsequent recurrence include vancomycin in tapered and pulsed regimen (weak recommendation, low quality) OR vancomycin 125 mg every 6 hours for 10 days followed by rifaximin 400 mg every 8 hours for 20 days (weak recommendation, low quality of evidence) OR fidaxomicin 200 mg every 12 hours for 10 day (weak recommendation, low quality of evidence) or fecal microbiota transplant (strong recommendation, moderate quality of evidence).[40]

Bezlotoxumab, a human monoclonal antibody that binds C difficile toxin B, has recently been shown to significantly lower the rate of recurrent CDI when added to standard treatment for primary or recurrent CDI. Cost is a significant factor and further data are needed to understand the relative cost effectiveness of this novel agent in comparison to other approaches and to define the patients likely to benefit most from this new drug.[41,42]

Strong evidence suggests that the use of probiotics (eg, Lactobacillus plantarum, Saccharomyces boulardii) may reduce antibiotic-associated diarrhea, but current data does not suggest that probiotics prevent CDI. The 2013 guidelines suggested that evidence supporting the role of probiotics in the treatment of CDI or the prevention of disease recurrence is lacking. (moderate recommendation, moderate quality of evidence)[39] Since then, further support for probiotics have surfaced. Shen et al's systemic review with meta-regression analysis showed that administration of probiotics given within 2 days of the first antibiotic administration reduced CDI risk by more than 50%.[43] Prevention of CDI requires judicious use of antibiotics and avoidance of gastric acid suppression (eg, proton pump inhibitors) when possible.[39,40,44]

Complications of CDI include dehydration, electrolyte disturbances, hypoalbuminemia, toxic megacolon, bowel perforation, hypotension, renal failure, systemic inflammatory response syndrome, sepsis, and death.

VENTRICULITIS AND MENINGITIS

Healthcare-associated ventriculitis and meningitis refer to the development of meningitis or ventriculitis in association with neurosurgical intervention or head trauma. While most patients become symptomatic during the acute hospital stay, symptoms may also develop after hospital discharge or, rarely, years later. As per the IDSA 2017 guidelines, signs and symptoms include (1) new headache, nausea, fatigue, or altered mental status; (2) erythema and tenderness over shunt tubing; (3) peritonitis or abdominal tenderness in patients with ventriculoperitoneal shunts; (4) pleuritis in ventriculopleural shunts; (5) bacteremia in ventriculoatrial shunt; (6) glomerulonephritis in ventriculoatrial shunt; and (7) fever in absence of another source (strong recommendation, moderate level of evidence).[45] These HAIs are distinguished from community-acquired meningitis and ventriculitis, as the causative agents tend be resistant Gram-negative bacilli and staphylococci.

Healthcare associated ventriculitis and/or meningitis is suggested by the presence of cerebrospinal fluid (CSF) pleocytosis, a positive culture, and associated symptoms.[43] Cerebrospinal fluid leukocytosis and hypoglycemia can often be associated with neurosurgical intervention and not necessarily an infection. However, WBC greater than 7500 cells/μL or CSF glucose less than 10 mg/dL might be more suggestive of an infection.[46] Cultures are imperative to the diagnosis, but a positive culture in a special media, light growth, or growth in minority of cultures, especially in an asymptomatic patient, may suggest contamination (strong recommendation, high level of evidence).[45] One of the most common bacterial contaminants is coagulase-negative staphylococci. Other CSF studies, such as CSF lactate, CSF procalcitonin, nucleic acid amplification tests, CSF β-D glucan, and CSF galactomannan, may be indicated to confirm the diagnosis.[45] If a CSF shunt or drain is present in a patient with a suspected infection, cultures should be held for at least 10 days to identify slow-growing organisms such as Propionibacterium acnes. (strong recommendation, high level of evidence).[45] Neuroimaging studies are recommended for all patients with suspected infections, and in patients with ventriculoperitoneal shunts and abdominal symptoms, abdominal ultrasonography or CT is recommended (strong recommendation, moderate level of evidence).[45]

Empiric treatment should consist of vancomycin and an antipseudomonal β-lactams and should be tailored to the culture and susceptibility results (strong recommendation, low level of evidence). Antimicrobial therapy should be continued for 10 to 14 days for most pathogens. Intraventricular antibiotics are given to patients who respond poorly to systemic antibiotics (strong recommendation, low level of evidence).[45] The agent is administered through a ventricular drain, which is clamped for 15 to 60 minutes. Additionally, current guidelines recommend removal of indwelling shunts and drains when possible.[45]

SURGICAL SITE INFECTIONS

Surgical site infections are divided into 3 classifications. They are all diagnosed by a surgeon or physician and are associated with at least one of the following: drainage, positive cultures, and signs of local inflammation. Superficial incisional SSI involves the subcutaneous space and occurs within 30 days of surgery.[47] Deep incisional SSI involves fascia and muscles and occurs within 3 days of surgery or within 1 year of receiving a prosthesis.[47] Organ/space SSI involves any part of the anatomy other than the original site and occurs within 3 days of surgery or within 1 year of receiving a prosthesis.[47] As per the IDSA 2014 guidelines, suture removal with incision and drainage is recommended for SSIs.[48] Surgical site infections should be considered with the presence of fever less than 4 days after the surgery, systemic illness, wound drainage or local signs of infection, and positive Gram stain for *Streptococcus* or *Clostridia* species.[48] Treatment would consist of debridement, penicillin, and clindamycin. Surgical site infections are also considered with the presence of fever more than 4 days after surgery, with erythema and/or induration noted on the surgical site, when the wound is open and associated with WBC of greater than 12,000 cells/μL, and with erythema more than 5 cm from the incision with induration or any necrosis.[48] For clean wounds following surgery of the trunk, head and neck, or extremities, systemic antibiotics with first-generation cephalosporin or antistaphylococcal penicillin for methicillin-sensitive *S aureus* (MSSA) is appropriate unless there are risk factors for MRSA (strong recommendation, low level of evidence).[48] For SSIs following surgeries on the axilla, gastrointestinal tract, perineum, or female genital tract, a cephalosporin or fluoroquinolone in combination with metronidazole are recommended.[48]

QUESTIONS

1. A 46-year-old man with a history of coronary artery disease, hypertension, and diabetes is transferred from the operating room to the ICU after undergoing 3-vessel coronary artery bypass graft. The procedure was complicated by vasodilatory shock requiring pressor support. Additionally, the patient required 2 units of packed red blood cells intraoperatively. He is afebrile and his blood pressure is 100/90 mmHg. His exam is significant for an intubated, sedated male status poststernotomy. All of the following are recommended to prevent the development of ventilator-associated pneumonia except:

   A. Utilization of silver-coated endotracheal tubes
   B. Elevating the head of the bed to 30° to 45°
   C. Interrupting sedation daily
   D. Changing the ventilator circuit if it is visibly soiled or malfunctioning

2. Regular use of oral care with chlorhexidine in mechanically ventilated patients has been associated with which of the following?

   A. Reduced rate of VAP
   B. Reduced duration of mechanical ventilation
   C. Reduced mortality benefit
   D. Lack of benefit in cardiac-surgery patients

3. A 26-year-old man with no significant medical history initially presented to the emergency department (ED) 3 days ago with altered mental status in the setting of opioid overdose. He was intubated in the ED and transferred to the ICU. This morning, his nurse reports that he is febrile to 101.4°F and increased respiratory secretions requiring frequent suctioning.

   His temperature is 101.4°F, his blood pressure (BP) is 110/68 mmHg, his heart rate (HR) is 108 beats/min, and respiratory rate (RR) of 14 breaths/min. On examination, he remains intubated and sedated. His lung exam reveals crackles in the right middle field.

   Blood work reveals leukocytosis with neutrophil predominance. His chest x-ray shows reticulonodular changes. Respiratory cultures are drawn. No prior respiratory cultures are available.

   The patient's girlfriend reports he has not seen a doctor in the last year. The ICU resistance rates show that less than 10% of Gram-negative bacilli are resistant to cefepime or levofloxacin. The ICU prevalence of MRSA is 5%.

   Which of the following is the most appropriate choice for empiric antibiotics?

   A. Ceftriaxone and azithromycin
   B. Cefepime
   C. Cefepime and levofloxacin
   D. Cefepime, levofloxacin, and vancomycin

4. For the patient in question 3, respiratory cultures grow *Candida albicans* along with *P aeruginosa*. Which of the following is the most appropriate treatment?

   A. Continue antibiotics only
   B. Continue antibiotics, start micafungin
   C. Continue antibiotics, start fluconazole
   D. Discontinue antibiotics, start amphotericin B

5. A 38-year-old man with a history of alcoholism presented to the hospital with severe acute pancreatitis. He developed acute respiratory distress syndrome (ARDS) and required mechanical ventilation and vasopressor use. Due to difficulty with liberation from the ventilator, the patient remained mechanically ventilated for 9 days prior to extubation yesterday. Since liberation, vasopressor use has dropped significantly and he has not required any vasopressors for the last 12 hours. Later that night, the patient develops chills and a subsequent temperature reading shows a fever of 101.9°F. He endorses no focal symptoms of infection and both chest x-ray and urinalysis do not reveal a source of infection. His abdominal exam is unremarkable, and his right subclavian triple lumen catheter and left forearm peripheral IV both appear clean, without visible drainage and without surrounding erythema. There are no murmurs, rubs, or gallops on his cardiac exam. There are no areas of skin breakdown. You suspect catheter-related bloodstream infection. Which of the following is the most appropriate method of diagnosis?

A. Draw blood cultures to check if the organism is a common bloodstream organism
B. Obtain qualitative broth culture of the catheter tip
C. Swab the area around the catheter entry point
D. Check quantitative blood cultures to ensure that blood obtained through the catheter hub is 3-fold greater than from a peripheral vein

6. For the patient in question 5, immediately after blood cultures are obtained, the Gram stain shows Gram-positive cocci in clusters. Your review of the hospital antibiogram shows a high prevalence of MRSA with vancomycin MIC values of 4 μg/mL. Which of the following would be the most appropriate empiric therapy?

A. Daptomycin
B. Linezolid
C. Vancomycin
D. Monitoring the patient until more definitive culture results return

7. A 52-year-old man with a history of alcohol abuse and cirrhosis has been evaluated for fever and malaise for the previous day. He has no other medical conditions. The patient was admitted to the hospital 5 days ago for massive upper gastrointestinal bleeding. A left internal jugular venous catheter was placed and the patient received isotonic fluids as well as 6 units of packed red blood cells. He has not required any transfusions in the last 24 hours.

On physical examination, his temperature is 100.9°F, his BP is 118/72 mmHg, and heart rate is 102 beats/min. The catheter site is mildly tender to palpation. There is minimal erythema and there is no drainage or fluctuance. The rest of the exam is unremarkable. Peripheral and central catheter blood cultures are drawn. Laboratory evaluation reveals WBC of 13.2 × 103/μL with a left shift and lactic acid of 1.8 mmol/L. Initial management should involve which of the following?

A. Catheter removal; IV vancomycin and IV cefepime
B. Catheter removal; IV vancomycin alone
C. Keep catheter in place; IV vancomycin and adjunct antibiotic lock therapy
D. Keep catheter in place; antibiotic lock therapy with vancomycin

8. For the patient in question 7, initial central and peripheral blood cultures grow MSSA. Repeat blood cultures are negative. A transthoracic echocardiogram (TTE) and transesophageal echocardiogram (TEE) do not reveal any vegetations. Which of the following is the most appropriate management?

A. Continue current therapy until 3 negative blood cultures are obtained
B. Discontinue current therapy, start IV nafcillin, perform repeat TEE at 2 weeks to determine duration of treatment

C. Discontinue current therapy, start IV nafcillin for a total of 2 weeks, with day 1 being the day of the first negative culture
D. Discontinue current therapy, start IV nafcillin for a total of 6 weeks, with day 1 being the day of the first negative culture

9. A 64-year-old woman with diabetes mellitus, multiple sclerosis with severe spasticity, and recurrent aspiration pneumonia presented 10 days ago with septic shock due to aspiration pneumonia. She required mechanical ventilation for 7 days and was transferred to a general medical floor yesterday. She complains today of suprapubic tenderness and fatigue, which are new compared to yesterday. She is not on any antibiotics.

Her temperature is 100.4°F, her BP is 104/58 mmHg, and her HR is 102 beats/min. On exam, she appears in mild distress, with mild suprapubic tenderness and a chronic indwelling bladder catheter.

Blood work shows leukocytosis with 84% neutrophils. Urine culture shows nitrites and leukocyte esterase as well as bacteria too numerous to count, without squamous epithelial cells.

Urine in her collection bag is not malodorous, nor is it cloudy. Review of prior urine cultures reveals *E coli*, *P aeruginosa*, and extended-spectrum β-lactamase (ESBL)–producing *Klebsiella*. Which of the following is the most appropriate choice for empiric antibiotics?

A. Ceftazidime
B. Imipenem
C. Ceftriaxone
D. Levofloxacin

10. For the patient in question 9, which of the following is the most appropriate foley catheter management in this patient?

A. The catheter should remain in place and antimicrobial management will not be affected.
B. The catheter should be removed and intermittent catheterization should be undertaken.
C. The catheter should be replaced at the completion of antimicrobial therapy.
D. The catheter should be replaced at the initiation of antimicrobial therapy.

11. A 62-year-old woman presents to the emergency department with 3 days of watery diarrhea, abdominal cramps, and fever. She was last seen by her primary care physician 2 weeks ago for right leg cellulitis and completed a course of clindamycin. One week after completing therapy, she developed abdominal cramps and 5 to 7 watery bowel movements a day.

Her temperature is 101.3°F, her HR is 110 beats/min, and her BP is 94/65 mmHg. Physical examination shows mild abdominal distention and tenderness but no guarding or rebound.

Her WBC is $18.4 \times 10^3/\mu L$, her serum albumin is 3.4 g/dL, her creatinine is 2.5 mg/dL, and her lactate is 4 mmol/L. Immunoassays for GDH antigen returns positive. Immunoassays for *C difficile* toxins A and B are sent and return negative. Which of the following is the most appropriate next step?

A. Repeat immunoassays for *C difficile* toxins A and B
B. Send stool cultures for ova and parasites
C. Send polymerase chain reaction of *C difficile* genes
D. Send *C difficile* cytotoxicity assay

12. For the patient in question 11, which of the following is the next best step in management?

A. Oral metronidazole alone
B. Oral vancomycin alone
C. Oral vancomycin and IV metronidazole
D. Oral rifaximin

13. A 65-year-old woman with diabetes, hyperlipidemia, and hypertension presents to the ED in late January with shortness of breath, fevers, and myalgias for 3 days. She works as a nurse in the hospital's ICU but has been unable to work since the onset of her symptoms. She has not received the flu shot this year but has been wearing a respiratory mask while caring for her patients. Her temperature is 103.1°F, her HR is 115 beats/min, her BP is 98/45 mmHg, her RR is 26 breaths/min, and her oxygen saturation is 91% on room air. Her physical exam is notable for diffuse rhonchi. Labs reveal WBC of $20 \times 10^3/\mu L$, creatinine of 1.3 mg/dL, and her lactate is 3.1 mmol/L. A flu swab returns positive. Her chest x-ray reveals bilateral infiltrates with small right pleural effusion. The patient's respiratory status rapidly decompensates and she requires intubation and medical ICU admission for ARDS. All of the following infection control measures are appropriate for preventing the transmission of influenzas *except*

A. promotion and administration of influenza vaccination to all hospital personnel annually.
B. postexposure prophylaxis with neuraminidase inhibitors or antiviral M2 protein inhibitors for unvaccinated hospital employees.
C. mandating hospital employees who decline vaccination to wear a face mask while at work.
D. isolating patients with influenza-like symptoms in airborne precautions.

14. For the patient in question 13, the appropriate precautions are used. In which of the following scenarios would it be appropriate to discontinue these precautions?

A. After 7 days of disease onset and finished treatment course of oseltamivir
B. After 24 hours if she remains afebrile and free of respiratory symptoms
C. Precautions should be continued throughout her hospital stay
D. After 5 days of treatment with oseltamivir

15. A 46-year-old man with uncontrolled diabetes mellitus presents to the ED with painful swelling of his right upper arm. Two weeks ago, the patient completed a 6-week course of nafcillin through a peripherally inserted central catheter inserted on his right arm but did follow up to have his PICC removed. On exam, he is febrile (101.2°F) and there is localized erythema, tenderness, and purulent drainage along the path of the PICC. Laboratory investigation revealed WBCs of $13.2 \times 10^3/\mu L$ and platelets of $516 \times 10^3/\mu L$. Cultures are sent from the blood and purulent drainage. Appropriate management of this patient includes which of the following?

A. Immediate surgical consultation for vein extraction
B. Removal of PICC; restarting nafcillin
C. Removal of PICC; vancomycin and ceftriaxone
D. Removal of PICC; vancomycin and piperacillin-tazobactam

16. A 47-year-old Colombian man with a history of recently diagnosed human immunodeficiency virus (HIV) infection presents to the ED with cough for the last 2 weeks. He also notes that he has had fevers, chills, and night sweats and admits to a 10-lb weight loss in the last 2 months. He denies hemoptysis. He emigrated from Columbia 2 months ago. He has never had a tuberculin skin test before and is unable to recall prior vaccinations. His physical examination has decreased breath sounds at the left apex, and his chest x-ray shows a cavity in the left upper lobe. You suspect pulmonary tuberculosis (TB) and appropriate precautions are used. Which of the following would be appropriate indications to discontinue these precautions?

A. Two sputum AFB smears 6 hours apart return negative
B. Tuberculosis is diagnosed; appropriate antituberculosis therapy is initiated and 3 subsequent AFB smears are negative
C. One sputum AFB smear is negative followed by a negative nucleic acid amplification test returns negative
D. Tuberculosis is diagnosed; appropriate antituberculosis therapy is initiated and 2 subsequent nucleic acid amplification tests return negative

17. A 57-year-old woman with recently diagnosed diffuse large B-cell lymphoma recently started on chemotherapy presents with fever for the last day. In the ED, she is febrile and hypotensive despite IV fluid resuscitation. She is started on broad-spectrum antibiotics. Norepinephrine infusion is initiated and she is admitted to the ICU. On the third day of admission, she is no longer febrile but her nurse notices she has a new rash. She is afebrile, her BP is 100/70 mmHg, and HR is 98 beats/min. There is a vesicular rash in a band-like distribution over the right hemithorax and a few erythematous papules. Her WBC count from the morning was $0.6 \times 10^3/\mu L$ (60% polymorphonuclear

leukocytes, 3% bands). The patient is placed under appropriate precautions. Precautions may be discontinued in which of the following scenarios?

A. Once antiviral therapy is initiated
B. After 7 days of antivirals
C. After all lesions have disappeared
D. After all lesions have dried and crusted over

18. A 64-year-old man with end-stage renal disease on hemodialysis secondary to long standing hypertension presents from his dialysis center for fevers and rigors after receiving 3 hours of dialysis. He notes fatigue for the last few days. His temperature is 100.3°F, his BP is 148/72 mmHg, his HR is 98 beats/min, his RR is 14 breaths/min, and his oxygen saturation is 98%. He has a right-sided hemodialysis port. Labs show a mild leukocytosis and creatinine of 3.2 mg/dL with normal electrolytes. Chest x-ray is unremarkable. Line infection is considered most likely. After discussion with his nephrologist, salvage therapy is attempted, and he is started on systemic antibiotics. Adjuvant antibiotic lock therapy (ALT) is most likely to be beneficial in which of the following scenarios?

A. The patient's dialysis catheter was placed 7 days ago.
B. There is erythema, tenderness, and fluctuance at the port insertion site.
C. The initial blood culture grows *Enterococcus*, and repeat blood cultures are negative at 72 hours.
D. Blood cultures grow *Candida* in 1 of 4 bottles, and repeat blood cultures are negative at 72 hours.

ANSWERS

1. A. Utilization of silver-coated endotracheal tubes

   Recommendations for the prevention of VAP include avoidance of intubation when possible; minimizing sedation and, particularly, avoiding benzodiazepines; avoiding daily sedation interruptions (choice C); maintaining and improving physical conditioning with early mobilization and exercise; and assessing readiness to extubate daily; minimizing pooling of secretions above the endotracheal tube cuff by means of endotracheal tubes with subglottic secretion drainage ports and elevating the head of the bed to 30° to 45°[49] (choice B). Current data does not support scheduled replacement of the ventilator circuit but does support changing the ventilator circuit if it is visibly soiled or malfunctioning (choice D). The use of silver-coated endotracheal tubes is generally not recommended. Although silver-coated endotracheal tubes may lower VAP rates, significant data suggests no impact on duration of mechanical ventilation, mortality, or length of stay[49] (choice A).

2. A. Reduced rate of VAP

   Current evidence suggests that regular oral care with chlorhexidine in intubated patients may lower VAP rates (choice A), but there is insufficient data to determine the impact on duration of mechanical ventilation or mortality[49] (choices B and C). The benefits of oral care with chlorhexidine are particularly pronounced in cardiac surgery patients[50-52] (choice D).

3. B. Cefepime

   Current guidelines recommend empiric therapy of VAP with antimicrobials providing coverage for *S aureus*, *P aeruginosa*, and other Gram-negative bacilli. MRSA should be covered with vancomycin or linezolid if MDR risk factors are present—particularly in patients who have received antibiotics within the last 90 days or in units with a high prevalence (> 10%) of MRSA. Similarly, empiric double coverage for *Pseudomonas* should be considered with MDR risk factors or in high-prevalence units, avoiding aminoglycosides when possible. Treatment should be narrowed once culture results are available. Recent data suggests that treatment can be safely limited to 7 days regardless of pathogen.

   This patient who has no MDR risk factors can be adequately treated with single-agent therapy with cefepime (choice B). Ceftriaxone and azithromycin would be the treatment for community-acquired pneumonia (choice A). Choices C and D are the treatment for VAP in patients with MDR risk factors or if the ICU resistance rates were higher.

4. A. Continue antibiotics only

   Respiratory secretions growing *Candida* often indicate colonization and rarely requires antifungal therapy (choice A). The *Candida* likely represents colonization and does not warrant therapy (choices B, C, and D are incorrect).

5. D. Check quantitative blood cultures to ensure that blood obtained through the catheter hub is 3-fold greater than from a peripheral vein

   The most sensitive finding for CRBSI is fever; however, this finding is not specific. Specific findings, such as inflammation or purulence around the insertion site, are not always present. Blood cultures that are positive for *S aureus*, coagulase-negative staphylococci, or *Candida* species should increase suspicion for CRBSI but are not pathognomonic (choice A). The IDSA guidelines from 2009 suggest against qualitative broth cultures of the catheter tip and only recommend swabbing catheter entry points if there is visible drainage[24] (choices B and C). These guidelines best define CRBSI as a colony count of microbes grown from blood obtained through the catheter hub that is at least 3-fold greater than the colony count from blood obtained from a peripheral vein[26] (choice D).

6. A. Daptomycin

   Vancomycin is recommended for empirical therapy in healthcare settings with an elevated prevalence of MRSA; for institutions in which the preponderance of MRSA isolates have vancomycin MIC values greater than 2 µg/mL, alternative agents, such as daptomycin, should be used (choice A and C). Linezolid should not be used for empirical therapy (ie, for patients suspected but not proven to have CRBSI) (choice B). Monitoring the patient until more definitive culture results return is not advised due to the high mortality rate of untreated bloodstream infections (choice D).

7. B. Catheter removal; IV vancomycin alone

   This patient fever is likely caused by a CRBSI. In general, there is a low threshold to remove short-term catheters. Absolute indications for catheter removal include septic shock; CRBSI due to *S. aureus*, *P aeruginosa*, *Candida* species, *Bacillus* species, or *Mycobacterium* species; or persistent bacteremia despite 3 days of antimicrobials.[26] Initial empiric therapy should include vancomycin; however, Gram-negative coverage (including *Pseudomonas*) is not necessary in this patient who is not septic or neutropenic (choices A and B). Leaving the central venous catheter in this patient would be inappropriate, particularly because this patient has been stable over the last 24 hours (choices C and D).

8. C. Discontinue current therapy, start IV nafcillin for a total of 2 weeks, with day 1 being the day of the first negative culture

   Patients with uncomplicated CRBSI due to *S. aureus* from a short-term catheter should have the CVC removed and should be started on vancomycin pending susceptibility data. Once identified, MSSA should be treated with nafcillin or oxacillin, and vancomycin should be discontinued (choice A). Patients with *S aureus* bacteremia warrant echocardiography to rule out infective endocarditis. A TTE should be obtained first. While it was previously suggested that all patients with *S. aureus* bacteremia and a negative TTE warrant TEE, some evidence suggests that a negative TTE alone in a select group of patients may be adequate. Uncomplicated cases without evidence of hematogenous complications (endocarditis, metastatic foci, venous thrombosis, presence of implanted device) can be treated with 2 weeks of antibiotics (choice C). A longer course of 4 to 6 weeks is appropriate in patients with known hematogenous complications (choice D). Repeating TEE is not required to determine duration of treatment (choice B). If required, a new catheter may be placed if additional blood cultures demonstrate no growth at 72 hours.

9. B. Imipenem

   In cases of CAUTI, previous culture results should be explored, if available. Usual treatment for urinary pathogens will not be adequate in this case where ESBL organisms have been cultured in the past. In these cases, a carbapenem should be the first line treatment, particularly in a case of a potentially or recently unstable patient (choice B). Cephalosporins and fluoroquinolones do not cover ESBL organisms (choices A, C, and D).

10. D. The catheter should be replaced at the initiation of antimicrobial therapy.

    Although antibiotics will be effective at sterilizing the urine in the bladder, there is evidence that the biofilm on the catheter itself will not be fully susceptible to the treatment.[31,53] Therefore, the catheter should be replaced at the initiation of antimicrobial therapy to allow the antibiotics to fully sterilize bladder contents (choice D). Maintaining the catheter or replacing the catheter after completed antimicrobial therapy is inappropriate (choices A and C). Although intermittent bladder catheterization may be an alternative to chronic bladder catheterization, the patient's severe spasticity will make self-catheterization difficult (choice B).

11. C. Send polymerase chain reaction of *C difficile* genes

    Several laboratory tests are available for *C difficile* testing. While the *C difficile* cytotoxicity assay is the gold standard for diagnosis, it is impractical for widespread laboratory use (choice D). Nucleic acid amplification tests for *C difficile* toxin genes are superior to EIA for toxins A and B for the diagnosis of CDI, but a stepped approach utilizing the GDH antigen screening test with subsequent toxin A and B EIAs may be a cost-effective strategy. Discordant results are then adjudicated with NAATs.

    Repeat testing of immunoassays is strongly discouraged (choice A). This patient's presentation is strongly suggestive of *C difficile* infection; therefore, sending stool cultures for ova and parasites is incorrect (choice B).

12. C. Oral vancomycin and IV metronidazole

    As per the IDSA guidelines, the patient has an initial severe episode of CDI based on the renal function and degree of leukocytosis. Treatment of CDI is dependent on disease severity. Patient should be treated with both oral vancomycin and IV metronidazole. Oral metronidazole is an alternative to oral vancomycin in initial nonsevere episode of CDI[40] (choice A). Oral vancomycin has a role for nonsevere initial episode of CDI (choice B). Rifaximin has a role for second or subsequent recurrence of CDI (choice D).

13. D. isolating patients with influenza-like symptoms in airborne precautions.

    Nosocomial influenza outbreaks can occur within the hospital and are associated with significant morbidity, mortality, and healthcare costs. A variety of infection control measures are available to prevent seasonal influenza in the healthcare setting. Patients with influenza-like symptoms which can include fevers, chills, myalgias, and generalized malaise should be placed on droplet precautions and rapid influenza swab should be sent.[54] Airborne precautions are not recommended for patients with suspected or confirmed influenza (choice D). Unvaccinated hospital employees should be offered prophylaxis during an outbreak within the institution (choice B). Nosocomial outbreaks can also be prevented by promoting and administrating influenza vaccination to hospital employees, and written declination of influenza vaccination with mandatory mask-wearing throughout influenza season (choices A and C). Despite the effectiveness of vaccination for influenza, it remains underused by healthcare providers.

14. A. After 7 days of disease onset and finished treatment course of oseltamivir

Hospitalized patients with suspected or confirmed influenza should be placed on droplet precautions. Precautions may be discontinued if influenza is ruled out. Those with confirmed influenza requiring hospitalization should be considered for treatment with a neuraminidase inhibitor (if resistance is not suspected). Droplet precautions should be maintained until the patient is afebrile and free of respiratory symptoms for at least 24 hours (choice B), or 7 days have elapsed since symptom onset, whichever is longer[4,54] (choice A). Treatment with oseltamivir alone does not affect the need for droplet precautions (choice D). Indefinite use of droplet precautions is unnecessary (choice C).

15. C. Removal of PICC; vancomycin and ceftriaxone

Suppurative thrombophlebitis is defined as venous thrombosis with inflammation in the setting of bacteremia. The diagnosis should be considered in individuals with persistent bacteremia after 72 hours of appropriate antimicrobial therapy, particularly in the setting of intravascular catheter. Management of suppurative thrombophlebitis involves removing the focus of infection (the PICC line, in this case) and administration of antibiotics. Antibiotics targeting staphylococci (such as vancomycin) and Enterobacteriaceae (such as ceftriaxone) should be promptly administered (choice C). Nafcillin would cover MSSA but would not cover MRSA and would also not provide Enterobacteriaceae coverage (choice B). *Pseudomonas* is not frequently associated with suppurative thrombophlebitis, and piperacillin-tazobactam is not necessary (choice D). While the management of suppurative thrombophlebitis may eventually include surgical intervention, antibiotics and source control with PICC removal are more appropriate in this patient (choice A).

16. B. Tuberculosis is diagnosed; appropriate antituberculosis therapy is initiated and 3 subsequent AFB smears are negative

Pulmonary mycobacterial tuberculosis should always be considered in patients presenting with prolonged cough and fevers, night sweats, and weight gain, particularly in the presence of risk factors such as HIV infection and recent emigration from an endemic country. Patients should be placed on airborne precautions and placed in an airborne infection isolation room when available. Healthcare workers should wear N95 masks when interacting with the patient.

These precautions may be discontinued if clinically infectious TB is deemed unlikely and one of the following criteria are met:

A. three consecutive sputum AFB smears at intervals of 8 to 24 hours apart are negative (choice A),
B. an alternative diagnosis is confirmed, and
C. demonstration of 2 negative-sputum nucleic acid amplification (NAA) tests (Note: a third sputum sample should still be sent for smear and culture; see below for further discussion).[55]

Isolation may also be discontinued in patients with confirmed infectious TB who have received antituberculosis therapy if there is clinical improvement and 3 subsequent sputum AFB smears are negative (choice B).

There have been several NAA tests developed to assist in the determination of the need for airborne infection isolation. In 2015, the Cepheid Xpert MTB/RIF (Xpert) assay was approved by the FDA.[56] It should not be used alone to rule out TB but should be taken in context of the clinical picture and sputum AFBs. The Xpert assay should not be used to release a confirmed TB patient from airborne isolation precautions (choice D). Choice C is incorrect because it is not enough specimen.

17. D. After all lesions have dried and crusted over

Infection by VZV causes 2 different clinical syndromes. Initial infection results in varicella (chicken pox). Herpes zoster (shingles) results from reactivation of latent VZV infection, which lies dormant in the dorsal root ganglia. Immunocompromised individuals are more prone to reactivation of VZV.

Immunocompetent patients with localized herpes zoster require only standard precautions. Rarely, immunocompetent patients can develop disseminated herpes zoster, which requires standard precautions as well as airborne and contact precautions. Immunocompromised patients require standard precautions as well as airborne and contact precautions, whether or not the disease is localized or disseminated. For these patients, airborne and contact precautions should only be discontinued when the lesions are dried and crusted (choice D).

Antiviral therapy should not influence the decision to continue precautions (choices A and B). It is not necessary to wait for all lesions to entirely disappear to discontinue airborne and contact precautions if the lesions are dried and crusted (choice C).

18. C. The initial blood culture grows *Enterococcus*, and repeat blood cultures are negative at 72 hours.

Bacteria and fungi may undergo profound alterations to form biofilms on catheter surfaces. These bacteria or fungi can be more difficult to eradicate with systemic antibiotics alone. Antibiotic lock therapy involves use of a highly concentrated antibiotic solution, often combined with an anticoagulant, suspended in the catheter lumen when the catheter is not in use. Antibiotic lock therapy is presumed to work by achieving extremely high intraluminal antibiotic concentrations needed to eradicate organisms enmeshed in the catheter biofilm.[24] Antibiotic lock therapy may be used as an adjunct to systemic antibiotic therapy in patients with infected long-term intravascular devices (> 14 days), including implanted ports and tunneled catheters. It is important to note that salvage therapy is not recommended in patients with hemodynamic instability; short-term catheters; recently placed catheters (choice A); infections due to *S aureus*, *P aeruginosa*, fungi, or mycobacteria (choice D); or tunnel infections, exit site infections, or port abscesses[26] (choice B). Antibiotic lock therapy is more likely to be effective in patients with infections caused by Gram-negative rods, vancomycin-sensitive enterococci, or coagulase-negative staphylococci (choice C).

REFERENCES

1. Horan TC, Andrus M, Dudeck MA. CDC/NHSN surveillance definition of health care-associated infection and criteria for specific types of infections in the acute care setting. *Am J Infect Control.* 2008;36(5):309-332.

2. Magill SS, Edwards JR, Bamberg W, et al. Multistate point-prevalence survey of health care–associated infections. *N Engl J Med.* 2014;370(13):1198-1208.

3. Scott RD. *The Direct Medical Costs of Healthcare-Associated Infections in U.S. Hospitals and the Benefits of Prevention.* Atlanta, GA: CDC; 2009: 13.

4. Siegel JD, Rhinehart E, Jackson M, Chiarello L; Health Care Infection Control Practices Advisory Committee. 2007 guideline for isolation precautions: preventing transmission of infectious agents in health care settings. *Am J Infect Control.* 2007; 35(10 Suppl 2):S65-S164.

5. Siegel JD, Rhinehart E, Cic RNMPH, Jackson M, Brennan PJ, Bell M. Management of organisms in healthcare settings, 2006. *Infect Control.* 2006:1-74.

6. Septimus EJ, Schweizer ML. Decolonization in prevention of healthcare associated infections. *Clin Microbiol Rev.* 2016;29(2):201-222.

7. Huang SS, Septimus E, Kleinman K, et al. Targeted versus universal decolonization to prevent ICU infection. *N Eng J Med.* 2013;368(24):2255-2265.

8. Kalil AC, Metersky ML, Klompas M, et al. Management of adults with hospital-acquired and ventilator-associated pneumonia: 2016 clinical practice guidelines by the Infectious Diseases Society of America and the American Thoracic Society. *Clin Infect Dis.* 2016;63(5):e61-e111.

9. Attridge RT, Frei CR. Health care-associated pneumonia: An evidence-based review. *Am J Med.* 2011;124(8):689-697.

10. Lopez A, Amaro R, Polverino E. Does health care associated pneumonia really exist? *Eur J Intern Med.* 2012;23(5):407-411.

11. Chastre J, Fagon J-Y. Ventilator-associated pneumonia. *Am J Respir Crit Care Med.* 2002;165(23):867-903.

12. Klompas M, Branson R, Eichenwald EC, et al. Strategies to prevent ventilator-associated pneumonia in acute care hospitals: 2014 update. *Infect Control Hosp Epidemiol.* 2014;3535(88): 915-936.

13. Joseph NM, Sistla S, Dutta TK, Badhe AS, Parija SC. Ventilator-associated pneumonia: a review. *Eur J Intern Med.* 2010;21(5): 360-368.

14. Luna CM, Bledel I, Raimondi A. The role of surveillance cultures in guiding ventilator-associated pneumonia therapy. *Curr Opin Infect Dis.* 2014;27(2):184-193.

15. Brusselaers N, Labeau S, Vogelaers D, Blot S. Value of lower respiratory tract surveillance cultures to predict bacterial pathogens in ventilator-associated pneumonia: systematic review and diagnostic test accuracy meta-analysis. *Intensive Care Med.* 2013;39(3):365-375.

16. Pappas PG, Kauffman CA, Andes DR, et al. Clinical practice guideline for the management of candidiasis: 2016 update by the Infectious Diseases Society of America. *Clin Infect Dis.* 2015;62(4):e1-e50.

17. Nseir S, Martin-Loeches I, Makris D, et al. Impact of appropriate antimicrobial treatment on transition from ventilator-associated tracheobronchitis to ventilator-associated pneumonia. *Crit Care.* 2014;18(3):R129.

18. Safdar N, Maki DG. The pathogenesis of catheter-related bloodstream infection with noncuffed short-term central venous catheters. *Intensive Care Med.* 2004;30(1):62-67.

19. O'Grady NP, Alexander M, Dellinger EP, et al. Guidelines for the prevention of intravascular catheter-related infections. *Am J Infect Control.* 2002;30(8):476-489.

20. Maki DG, Weise CE, Sarafin HW. A semiquantitative culture method for identifying intravenous-catheter-related infection. *N Engl J Med.* 1977;296(23):1305-1309.

21. Raad I, Costerton W, Sabharwal U, Sacilowski M, Anaissie E, Bodey GP. Ultrastructural analysis of indwelling vascular catheters: a quantitative relationship between luminal colonization and duration of placement. *J Infect Dis.* 1993;168(2): 400-407.

22. Dobbins BM, Kite P, Kindon A, McMahon MJ, Wilcox MH. DNA fingerprinting analysis of coagulase negative staphylococci implicated in catheter related bloodstream infections. *J Clin Pathol.* 2002;55(11):824-828.

23. Chopra V, Flanders SA, Saint S, et al. The Michigan appropriateness guide for intravenous catheters (MAGIC): results from a multispecialty panel using the RAND/UCLA Appropriateness Method. *Ann Intern Med.* 2015;163(6):S1-S39.

24. Moureau N, Chopra V. Indications for peripheral, midline, and central catheters: summary of the Michigan appropriateness guide for intravenous catheters recommendations. *J Assoc Vasc Access.* 2016;21(3):140-148.

25. O'Grady NP, Alexander M, Burns LA, et al. Guidelines for the prevention of intravascular catheter-related infections, 2011 Oklahoma Foundation for Medical Quality. *Healthc Infect Control Pract Advis Comm.* 2011;39(4):1-83.

26. Mermel LA, Allon M, Bouza E, et al. Clinical practice guidelines for the diagnosis and management of intravascular catheter-related infection: 2009 update by the Infectious Diseases Society of America. *Clin Infect Dis.* 2009;49(1):1-45.

27. Fernandez-Hidalgo N, Almirante B, Calleja R, et al. Antibiotic-lock therapy for long-term intravascular catheter-related bacteraemia: Results of an open, non-comparative study. *J Antimicrob Chemother.* 2006;57(6):1172-1180.

28. Benoit JL, Carandang G, Sitrin M, Arnow PM. Intraluminal antibiotic treatment of central venous catheter infections in patients receiving parenteral nutrition at home. *Clin Infect Dis.* 1995;21(5):1286-1288.

29. Arnow PM, Kushner R. Malassezia furfur catheter infection cured with antibiotic lock therapy. *Am J Med.* 1991;90(1):128-130.

30. Krzywda EA, Andris DA, Edmiston CE, Quebbeman EJ. Treatment of Hickman catheter sepsis using antibiotic lock technique. *Infect Control Hosp Epidemiol.* 1995;16(10):596-598.

31. Hooton TM, Bradley SF, Cardenas DD, et al. Diagnosis, prevention, and treatment of catheter-associated urinary tract infection in adults: 2009 International Clinical Practice Guidelines from the Infectious Diseases Society of America. *Clin Infect Dis.* 2010;50(5):625-663.

32. Centers for disease control. Urinary Tract Infection (Catheter Associated Urinary Tract Infection) and Non-Catheter Associated Urinary Tract Infection and Other Urinary System Infection [USI] Events. https://www.cdc.gov/nhsn/pdfs/pscmanual/7psccauticurrent.pdf. Accessed May 24, 2018.

33. Wong E. Guideline for prevention of catheter-associated urinary tract infections. *Am J Infect Control.* 1983;11(1):28-36.

34. Talmor M, Li P, Barie PS. Acute paranasal sinusitis in critically ill patients: guidelines for prevention, diagnosis, and treatment. *Clin Infect Dis.* 1997;25(6):1441-1446.

35. Gefen A. Reswick and Rogers pressure-time curve for pressure ulcer risk. Part 1. *Nurs Stand.* 2009;23(46):40-44.

36. Lindan O, Greenway R, Piazza J. Pressure distribution on the surface of the human body. *Arch Phys Med Rehabil.* 1965;46:378-385.

37. National Pressure Ulcer Advisory Panel, European Pressure Ulcer Advisory Panel, Pan Pacific Pressure Injury Alliance. *Prevention and Treatment of Pressure Ulcers: Quick Reference Guide.* Perth, Australia: Cambidge Media; 2014.

38. Gould L, Stuntz M, Giovannelli M, et al. Wound healing society 2015 update on guidelines for venous ulcers. *Wound Repair Regen.* 2016;24(1):136-144.

39. Surawicz CM, Brandt LJ, Binion DG, et al. Guidelines for diagnosis, treatment, and prevention of *Clostridium difficile* infections. *Am J Gastroenterol.* 2013;108(4):478-498.

40. McDonald LC, Gerding DN, Johnson S, et al. Clinical practice guidelines for clostridium difficile infection in adults and children: 2017 Update by the Infectious Disease (IDSA) and Society for Healthcare Epidemiology of America (SHEA). *Clin Infect Dis.* 2018;66(7):e1-e48.

41. Wilcox MH, Gerding DN, Poxton IR, et al. Bezlotoxumab for prevention of recurrent *Clostridium difficile* infection. *N Engl J Med.* 2017;376(4):305-317.

42. Bartlett JG. Bezlotoxumab—a new agent for *Clostridium difficile* infection. *N Engl J Med.* 2017;376(4):381-382.

43. Shen NT, Maw A, Tmanova LL, et al. Timely use of probiotics in hospitalized adults prevents Clostridium difficile infection: a systematic review with meta-regression analysis. *Gastroenterology.* 2017;152(8):1889-1900.

44. Howell MD, Novack V, Grgurich P, et al. Iatrogenic gastric acid suppression and the risk of nosocomial *Clostridium difficile* infection. *Arch Intern Med.* 2010;170(9):784-790.

45. Tunkel AR, Hasbun R, Bhimraj A, et al. 2017 Infectious Diseases Society of America's clinical practice guidelines for healthcare-associated ventriculitis and meningitis. *Clin Infect Dis.* 2017;64.

46. Forgacs P, Geyer CA, Freidberg SR. Characterization of chemical meningitis after neurological surgery. *Clin Infect Dis.* 2001;32(2):179-185.

47. Mangram AJ, Horan TC, Pearson ML, Silver LC, Jarvis WR. Guideline for prevention of surgical site infection, 1999. Hospital Infection Control Practices Advisory Committee. *Infect Control Hosp Epidemiol.* 1999;20(4):250-278.

48. Stevens DL, Bisno AL, Chambers HF, et al. Practice guidelines for the diagnosis and management of skin and soft tissue infections: 2014 update by the Infectious Disease Society of America. *Clin Infect Dis.* 2014;59(2):147-159.

49. Klompas M, Branson R, Eichenwald EC, et al; Society for Healthcare Epidemiology of America (SHEA). Strategies to prevent ventilator-associated pneumonia in acute care hospitals: 2014 update. *Infect Control Hosp Epidemiol.* 2014;35(8):915-936.

50. Klompas M, Speck K, Howell MD, Greene LR, Berenholtz SM. Reappraisal of routine oral care with chlorhexidine gluconate for patients receiving mechanical ventilation: systematic review and meta-analysis. *JAMA Intern Med.* 2014;174(5):751-761.

51. DeRiso AJ 2nd, Ladowski JS, Dillon TA, Justice JW, Peterson AC. Chlorhexidine gluconate 0.12% oral rinse reduces the incidence of total nosocomial respiratory infection and nonprophylactic systemic antibiotic use in patients undergoing heart surgery. *Chest.* 1996;109(6):1556-1561.

52. Segers P, Speekenbrink RG, Ubbink DT, van Ogtrop ML, de Mol BA. Prevention of nosocomial infection in cardiac surgery by decontamination of the nasopharynx and oropharynx with chlorhexidine gluconate: a randomized controlled trial. *JAMA.* 2006;296(20):2460-2466.

53. Trautner BW, Darouiche RO. Role of biofilm in catheter-associated urinary tract infection. *Am J Infect Control.* 2004;32(3):177-183.

54. Centers for Disease Control and Prevention. Prevention strategies for seasonal influenza in healthcare settings. CDC Website. https://www.cdc.gov/flu/professionals/infectioncontrol/healthcaresettings.htm. Accessed July 6, 2017.

55. Centers for Disease Control and Prevention. Report of an expert consultation on the uses of nucleic acid amplification tests for the diagnosis of tuberculosis. CDC Web site. https://www.cdc.gov/tb/publications/guidelines/amplification_tests/amplification_tests.pdf. Accessed July 5, 2017.

56. National TB Controllers Assotiation, Association of Public Health Laboratories. Consensus statement on the use of Cepheid Xpert MTB/RIF® assay in making decisions to discontinue airborne infection isolation in healthcare settings. April 2016. NTCA Web site. http://www.tbcontrollers.org/docs/resources/NTCA_APHL_GeneXpert_Consensus_Statement_Final.pdf.

The Immune System and Infection

Ronaldo Collo Go, MD, Navitha Ramesh, MD, Riffat Mannan, MD, Songyang Yuan, MD, and Mikyung Lee, MD

INTRODUCTION

The host defense consists of innate, or nonspecific, immunity and adaptive immunity. Innate immunity is present at birth and has 4 components: mechanical barriers such as skin and mucous membranes, secretion of chemicals and enzymes, phagocytosis, and inflammation. Adaptive immunity is acquired immunity that recognizes antigens after exposure and generates pathogen-specific response pathways. The immune response can also be categorized in terms of neutrophil defense, cell-mediated immunity (CMI), and humoral immunity. Abnormalities in the immune system predispose individuals to different types of infections depending on the site of the immune defect. This chapter will discuss the mechanisms of primary neutrophil defense, cell-mediated immunity, humoral immunity, strategies for infection prevention, and the types of commonly seen infections.

PRIMARY NEUTROPHIL DEFENSE

Polymorphonuclear neutrophils (PMNs) are major phagocytes for host immune response. They make up the majority of circulating white blood cells but migrate into tissue in response to a pathogen. Neutrophils kill microbes by engulfing the organism and using reactive oxygen metabolites and digestive enzymes. Neutrophil dysfunction can be qualitative or quantitative. Qualitative dysfunction is usually seen in children and includes abnormalities in (1) diapedesis, the mechanism by which PMNs leave the intravascular space via endothelial channels; (2) chemotaxis, which is the movement of the PMN to the site of infection; (3) ingestion; and (4) intracellular killing (via oxygen-dependent or oxygen-independent).[1,2]

Quantitative defects are categorized by the absolute neutrophil count (ANC), which is calculated by multiplying the percent of neutrophils by the total white blood cell (WBC) count. Neutropenia is defined as an ANC less than 1500 cells/μL,[3,4] while severe neutropenia is less than 500 cells/μL. Neutropenia may be due to benign ethnic neutropenia, which is rarely less than 1200 cells/μL, congenital neutropenias, and acquired neutropenia. Acquired neutropenia can be caused by hematologic conditions, including malignancy and myelodysplastic

syndromes, medications, infections, autoimmune, dietary deficiencies, such as vitamin B_{12}, folic acid, or copper, or paroxysmal nocturnal hematuria.[5] Neutropenic patients often present with fever, which is defined as single oral temperature greater than 38.3°C (101°F) or a temperature greater than 38°C (100.4°F) sustained over 1 hour.[3] Rectal temperatures are generally avoided in neutropenic patients to prevent bacterial translocation into tissues. Patients with neutropenia are at increased risk of bacterial and fungal infections.[3]

Patients with prolonged (> 7 days) and profound neutropenia (ANC ≤ 100 cells/μL) are at high risk of infection and should be admitted to the hospital for work-up and empiric intravenous (IV) antibiotics when they present with signs and symptoms suggestive of infection. Lower-risk patients with brief (≤ 7 days) neutropenia who are clinically stable may be eligible for outpatient management and oral therapy.[3] In cancer patients with neutropenic fever, risk stratification is determined via Multinational Association for Supportive Care in Cancer Risk-Index Score (MASCC score) using the patient's burden of illness (clinical symptoms), comorbidities, outpatient status at the time of onset of neutropenic fever, and age. A MASCC score less than 21 is considered high risk and should have inpatient treatment.[3] A MASCC score greater than 21 can be managed with outpatient treatment.[3]

The empirical antibiotics for neutropenic fever should include pseudomonal coverage and be bactericidal since patients do not have adequate neutrophils for host defense. High-risk patients who require hospitalization should receive monotherapy with an antipseudomonal β-lactam such as cefepime, carbapenem (imipenem or meropenem), or piperacillin-tazobactam. An additional agent such as an aminoglycoside can be considered in a patient who is unstable or for whom there is concern about resistant organisms.[3] Low-risk patients can receive the oral combination of ciprofloxacin and amoxicillin-clavulanate. Aerobic Gram-positive cocci coverage with vancomycin is not recommended as part of initial empiric therapy. Vancomycin might be started early if there is concern for methicillin-resistant *Staphylococcus aureus* (MRSA) infection, catheter-related infection, skin and soft tissue infection, pulmonary infection, or clinical instability.[3] Patients with mild penicillin allergies can be given cephalosporins, but patients with severe penicillin allergy, such as angioedema or anaphylaxis, should avoid β-lactams, including cephalosporins and carbapenems. Empirical antibiotics for neutropenic patients with unexplained fevers are often continued until ANC is greater than 500 cells/μL. The duration of antibiotics is determined by the duration for that specific infection as well as recovery of the marrow (ANC > 500 cells/μL). Antibiotic prophylaxis with an oral fluoroquinolone can be considered in patients whose signs and symptoms of infection have resolved but who have persistent neutropenia; fluoroquinolone prophylaxis is also considered in high-risk patients with prolonged and severe neutropenia (ANC ≤ 100 cells/μL for > 7 days).[6]

The addition of empirical antifungal therapy and evaluation for a possible invasive fungal infection (IFI) should be considered in patients with persistent or recurrent fever for more than 4 days who are anticipated to have neutropenia for more than 7 days.[6] These patients should be assessed clinically and radiographically, usually with computed tomography (CT) of the chest or sinuses, for evidence of IFI. Galactomannan and (1-3)-β-D-glucan are polysaccharides in fungal cell walls and can be measured in serum assays. These serum markers should be used in conjunction with the clinical setting and other diagnostic data when evaluating for IFI. Galactomannan is found in *Aspergillus* and *Penicillium* species with cross-reactivity to *Histoplasma capsulatum*. The test has a sensitivity of 58% to 65% and a specificity of 65% to 95%.[7] False positive results can occur with the use of β-lactam/β-lactamase inhibitor antibiotics, and false negatives may occur with the use of antifungals that have mold activity.[8] The (1, 3)-β-D-glucan test detects *Candida, Aspergillus, Pneumocystis,* and *Fusarium* with a sensitivity of 63% to 90% and a specificity of greater than 95%.[9-11] Lipid formulations of amphotericin B, such as liposomal amphotericin, are as effective as amphotericin B deoxycholate, which has been used as empiric antifungal therapy for decades; the lipid formulations have significantly fewer toxicities than amphotericin B desoxycholate. Voriconazole is an azole with mold activity that was found to be superior and better tolerated compared to amphotericin B deoxycholate for invasive aspergillosis.[12] Voriconazole is associated with more visual disturbances. Echinocandins such as caspofungin have excellent activity against *Candida,* including the azole-resistant species, with fewer side effects than amphotericin and are recommended for initial therapy for candidemia.[13] Antifungal prophylaxis is recommended for (1) high-risk for invasive candidiasis, such as allogeneic stem cell transplant recipients or patients with acute leukemia undergoing intensive remission-induction or salvage induction chemotherapy; (2) patients older than 13 years of age undergoing chemotherapy for acute myeloid leukemia (AML)/myelodysplastic syndrome (MDS); (3) prior invasive aspergillosis; or (4) neutropenia lasting more than 2 weeks in allogeneic or autologous transplant recipients.[6]

Antiviral therapy for herpes simplex virus (HSV) or varicella zoster virus (VZV) with acyclovir is indicated, if there is clinical or laboratory evidence of active viral disease.

Acyclovir prophylaxis is indicated for HSV seropositive patients undergoing allogeneic hematopoietic stem cell transplant (HSCT) or leukemia induction therapy.[6]

Colony stimulating factors (CSF) are not generally recommended in patients with established febrile neutropenia. Although some studies show decreased duration of fevers, time on antibiotics, and length of hospitalization with the use of myeloid CSFs, there is no evidence of overall clinical or survival benefit.[9] Myeloid CSF are more commonly used for prophylaxis in the following conditions: (1) during cycles of chemotherapy for which patients have a 20% or greater risk of febrile neutropenia based on patient-, disease-, and treatment-related factors; (2) for patients who have a prior neutropenic complication in which reduction dose or treatment delay of chemotherapy may compromise outcomes; (3) after autologous stem-cell transplantation; and (4) for diffuse aggressive lymphoma in patients 65 years and older treated with curative chemotherapy (cyclophosphamide, doxorubicin, vincristine, prednisone, and rituximab). Dosing regimen of CSF is seen in Table 20-1.[14] Colony stimulating factors should be avoided in patients with concomitant chemotherapy and radiation therapy particularly in the mediastinum.

CELL-MEDIATED AND HUMORAL IMMUNITY

Adaptive immunity has cell-mediated and humoral mechanisms. Cell-mediated immunity generally involves phagocytosis and cytotoxins rather than antibodies, which are key components of the humor response. T lymphocytes are divided into the subsets of helper T cells, which express CD4 surface proteins, and cytotoxic T cells, which express CD8 surface proteins. Although the distinctions are not exact, these immune responses have been categorized based on subpopulations of the T-helper lymphocytes into T helper type 1 (Th1) or type 1 immunity, which is primary cell mediated, and T helper type 2 (Th2) or type 2 immunity, which primarily stimulates the humoral response.[15] Naïve helper T cells are Th0 before being activated into either Th1 or Th2 cells. These subpopulations secrete distinct combinations of cytokines. Because of the overlap of secreted cytokines, the primary distinctions are between the secretion of interferon (IFN) γ, which is secreted by Th1 but not by Th2, and interleukin (IL)-4, which is secreted by Th2 but not by Th1. The Th1 cells secrete IFN-γ, IL-2, and lymphotoxin (LT)-α, which result in strong cell-mediated immunity and weak humoral immunity. The Th2 cells secrete IL-4, IL-5, IL-9, IL-10, and IL-13, which stimulate antibody production for a strong humoral response and suppress cell-mediated immunity.

Cell-Mediated Immunity

Cell-mediated immunity is driven by T lymphocytes in response to intracellular pathogens and abnormal cells such as

TABLE 20-1 Colony Stimulating Factors and Dosing Regimen

Agent	Dosing and Administration
Filgrastim	Filgrastim should be started 1–3 d after administration of myelotoxic chemotherapy; in setting of high-dose therapy and autologous stem cell rescue, filgrastim can be started 1–5 d after administration of high-dose therapy; filgrastim should be continued until reaching ANC ≥ 2 to 3 × 10⁹/L; for PBPC mobilization, filgrastim should be started ≥ 4 d before first leukapheresis procedure and continued until last leukapheresis In adults, recommended filgrastim dose is 5 µg/kg/d for all clinical settings other than PBPC mobilization; in setting of PBPC mobilization, dose of 10 µg/kg/d may be preferable; preferred route of filgrastim administration is subcutaneous
Filgrastim-sndz	Same as for filgrastim
Tbo-filgrastim	Tbo-filgrastim should be started 1–3 d after administration of myelotoxic chemotherapy; in adults, recommended tbo-filgrastim dose is 5 µg/kg/d; preferred route of tbo-filgrastim administration is subcutaneous
Pegfilgrastim	Pegfilgrastim 6 mg should be administered once 1–3 d after chemotherapy if possible; because some patients will not be able to return for dose of pegfilgrastim because of distance or immobility, for instance, alternatives to consider may include self-administered filgrastim or tbo-filgrastim or same-day pegfilgrastim, recognizing that although same-day pegfilgrastim is not as effective as later pegfilgrastim, it is better than no pegfilgrastim; pegfilgrastim is also available in a timed automated-inject device that delivers 6 mg of pegfilgrastim subcutaneously, 27 h after it is placed on skin and activated; pegfilgrastim is not currently indicated for stem cell mobilization; 6-mg formulation should not be used in infants, children, or small adolescents who weigh < 45 kg
Sargramostim	Because GM-CSFs have been licensed specifically for use in mobilization and after transplantation of autologous PBPCs, after autologous or allogeneic bone narrow transplantation, and for AML, manufacturer's instructions for administration are limited to those clinical settings; GM-CSFs should be initiated on day of bone marrow infusion and not < 24 h after last chemotherapy and 12 h after most recent radiotherapy; GM-CSFs should be continued until ANC > 1.5 × 10⁹/L for 3 consecutive days is achieved; drug should be discontinued early or dose reduced by 50% if ANC increases to > 20 × 10⁹/L; recommended dose for adults is 250 µg/m²/d

AML = acute myeloid leukemia; ANC = absolute neutrophil count; CSF = colony-stimulating factor; GM-CSF = granulocyte macrophage colony-stimulating factor; PBPC = peripheral-blood progenitor cell.

Data from Mhaskar R, Clark OA, Lyman G, et al. Colony-stimulating factors for chemotherapy-induced febrile neutropenia. *Cochrane Database Syst Rev.* 2014;10:CD003039.

cancer cells. T cells respond to antigen presenting cells (APCs) and signal an inflammatory cascade leading to activation of cytotoxic T cells and phagocytes and release of cytokines. Cell-mediated immunity plays an important role in fighting intracellular organisms such as viruses, mycobacteria, fungi, and certain other bacteria. It is also an important part of transplant immunology and autoimmune responses.

Aging and pregnancy both decrease the cellular immune response. Cell-mediated immunity deficiencies may also be caused by congenital deficiencies, thymic dysplasia, viral illnesses, medications, and T-cell malignancies. HIV infection leads to the destruction of T helper cells and ultimately leads to AIDS without antiretroviral (ART) therapy. Medications can lead to decreased CMI either by decreasing the number of T cells, as is the case with corticosteroids, or by decreasing lymphocyte function, in the case of cyclosporine.

Humoral Immunity

Humoral immunity is mediated by large extracellular molecules including immunoglobulins and complement proteins. The humoral response is driven by B lymphocytes, which secrete antibodies, but requires activation by T lymphocytes. B cells produce 5 immunoglobulin antibody subclasses with different functions (Table 20-2).[16] Antibodies are made up of 4 polypeptide chains, with 2 light and 2 heavy chains, which have variable and constant regions. The region

of the antibody that binds to the antigen is the Fab (antigen-binding) fragment, while the fragment of the antibody that interacts with cell surface receptors is the Fc (fragment crystallizable) region. Immunoglobulin M (IgM) and IgG form antigen-antibody complexes that activate the complement system and lead to opsonization, a process by which antigens are marked for phagocytosis.

The complement system assists with phagocytosis, pathogen lysis, and inflammation.[17,18] There are 3 pathways of the complement system: the classical, lectin, and alternative pathways. These pathways converge to assemble the membrane attack complex (MAC) for lysis and destruction of the pathogen (Fig. 20-1).[17] The classical pathway is triggered by antigen-antibody complexes, while the lectin pathway is activated by lectins, proteins that bind carbohydrates on the bacteria. Both lead to assembly of C4b2a, which causes proteolytic cleavage of C3 to C3b and leads to opsonization.

Defects of humoral immunity include (1) quantitative or qualitative disorders of immunoglobulins; (2) functional or actual asplenia; (3) complement deficiencies; and (4) impaired neutralization of toxins. Antibody deficiencies include IgA deficiency, x-linked or autosomal agammaglobulinemias, common variable immunodeficiency, specific antibody deficiency, IgG subclass deficiency, selective IgM deficiency, and selective IgE deficiency.[19-26] Medications such as anti-inflammatory agents, rheumatologic agents such as methotrexate, anticonvulsants, and rituximab can cause hypogammaglobulinemia.

TABLE 20-2 Immunoglobulin Antibody Subclasses and Function

Ig Antibody	Function
IgM	First immunoglobulin (Ig) expressed during B cell development (primary response; early antibody) • Opsonizing (coating) antigen for destruction • Complement fixation
IgG	Main Ig during secondary immune response • Only antibody capable of crossing the placental barrier • Neutralization of toxins and viruses • Opsonizing (coating) antigen for destruction • Complement fixation
IgD	Function unclear, appears to be involved in homeostasis
IgA	Mucosal response; protects mucosal surfaces from toxins, viruses, and bacteria through either direct neutralization or prevention of binding to mucosal surface
IgE	Associated with hypersensitivity and allergic reactions • Plays a role in immune response to parasites

Source: Warrington R, Watson W, Kim HL, Antonetti FR. An introduction to immunology and immunopathology. *Allergy Asthma Clin Immunol.* 2011;7 (Suppl 1):S1-S7.

Protein-losing conditions and severe malnutrition also increase risk of infection from hypogammaglobulinemia. Specific infectious complications depend on the specific disorder, but patients with humoral deficiencies often get recurrent respiratory infection from encapsulated bacteria, such as *Streptococcus pneumoniae* and *Haemophilus*, and respiratory and gastrointestinal (GI) viral infections.[19-26]

Complement disorders can be caused by different points in the classical or alternative pathways and may be acquired or hereditary.[18] The total hemolytic complement, or CH50, measures total complement activity and is the screening test for classical pathway deficiencies. Conditions associated with falsely low CH50 include laboratory error or cold activation via mixed cryoglobulin or cold-reacting complexes. C3 or C4 are usually normal. CH50, like C3 or C4, is an acute phase reactant and therefore would be increased in periods of stress. C3 (normal 80–160 mg/dL) and C4 (normal 16–48 mg/dL) can be low in autoimmune diseases such as systemic lupus erythematosus (SLE), antiphospholipid syndrome, cryoglobulinemia, Sjögren syndrome, and membranoproliferative glomerulonephritis. Low C4 can be seen in acquired C1 inhibitor deficiency and hereditary angioedema. AH50 measures for total activity of the alternative pathway. Complement disorders should be considered in people with recurrent bacterial infections, autoimmune processes,

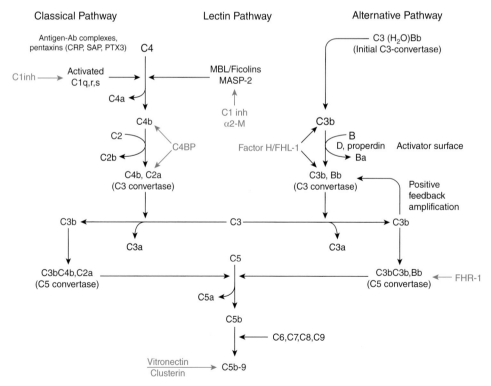

FIGURE 20-1 Schematic representing the activation of the complement cascade. The fragments released into solution are indicated in blue. The key fluid-phase regulators are indicated in green. α2-M = α2-macroglobulin; Ab = antibody; C1 inh = C1 inhibitor; C4BP = C4b binding protein; CRP = C-reactive protein; FHL-1 = factor H-like protein-1; FHR-1 = factor H-related molecule-1; MASP-2 = mannan-binding lectin serine peptidase 2; MBL = mannan-binding lectin; PTX3 = pentraxin 3; SAP = serum amyloid P component. (Reprinted from Ram S, Lewis LA, Rice PA. Infections of people with complement deficiencies and patients who have undergone splenectomy. *Clin Microbiol Rev.* 2010;23(4):740-780 with permission from American Society for Microbiology.)

and angioedema. The most common bacterial infections in patients with deficiencies in the classical pathway are recurrent *Neisseria meningitis* and bacteremia and recurrent infections with encapsulated bacteremia such as pneumococcus, *Haemophilus*, and *Neisseria*.[17]

The spleen is a hematopoietic organ that makes up 25% of the body's lymphoid tissue and has an active role in humoral and cellular immunity. Its functions include antibody production by B lymphocytes and removal of opsonin-coated organisms or damaged cells from circulation. Anatomic asplenia, functional asplenia, or hyposplenic states predispose patients to infection, particularly with encapsulated organisms.[20,21] Conditions that cause splenic infarction, such as sickle cell disease or splenic vein thrombosis, or splenic infiltration, such as autoimmune processes or hematologic disease, can cause hyposplenic states or functional asplenia. Pathogens associated with splenic dysfunction include encapsulated bacteria, such as *S pneumoniae*, *H influenzae* type b, and *N meningitidis*, and protozoa that infect red blood cells, such as malaria and *Babesia microti*.[22] Patients who have had splenectomies are also more susceptible to severe infection from *Capnocytophaga canimorsus*, a Gram-negative bacteria associated with dog bites.

INFECTIONS AFTER ORGAN TRANSPLANTATION

Infections in transplant recipients are common.[27] Development of immunosuppression after transplant has improved graft survival but has caused increased incidence of infections. Risk of infection after transplantation is dependent on exposure and overall immunosuppression of the patient.[28] Patients can be exposed to common community-acquired pathogens, such as influenza or *S pneumoniae*, or can have reactivation of latent infections, such as tuberculosis (TB), cytomegalovirus (CMV), or herpes zoster, either from the donor organ or from the recipient. The timing of these infections is divided into less than 1 month after transplant, 6 to 12 months after transplant, and greater than 12 months after transplant. The majority of infections occur within the first 6 months of organ transplant when immune suppression is higher.[29-32]

Infections within the first 30 days after solid organ transplantation can be due to hospital-acquired infection, technical complications from surgery, donor-derived infections, or recipient-derived infections. Opportunistic infections are uncommon early after transplant. Donor-acquired infections during this early period include active infections that were not diagnosed in the donor prior to transplant or activation of a latent infection. Bacterial and fungal infections are more common during this time. Organ transplant recipients do not always present with typical signs and symptoms of infection, as they are immune suppressed. Patients should be evaluated for infection when they present with altered mental status, hypotension, and evidence of graft dysfunction. Surgical site infections are also extremely common during the early post-transplant period.

In the intermediate period of 1 to 6 months after transplant, opportunistic pathogen and viral infections become more common. Transplant recipients are given prophylaxis for opportunistic infections such as pneumocystis, CMV, and toxoplasmosis during this period. Allograft rejection can also cause fevers during this intermediate post-transplant period. After 6 months, the risk and type of infections seen depend on the patient's net immunosuppression. Most patients are on lower stable doses of immunosuppression and are more likely to present with community-acquired infections rather than opportunistic infections. Transplant recipient who require higher levels of immunosuppression in the late transplant period are at risk for opportunistic pathogens as well as community-acquired infections.

INFECTION PREVENTION

Vaccines have played a crucial role in preventing communicable infections in the general population and are also important in immunocompromised hosts. Patients who anticipate immune suppression can be given live vaccines 4 months prior to immunosuppression and inactivated vaccines within 2 weeks of immunosuppression. Live vaccines such as measles-mumps-rubella (MMR), varicella, oral polio, rotavirus, and intranasal influenza vaccines should not be given to immunocompromised hosts. The intradermal influenza vaccine is inactivated and should be given to immunocompromised patients. Vaccines for tetanus and diphtheria, pneumococcus, meningococcus, human papilloma virus (HPV), hepatitis B (HBV), and hepatitis A are inactive vaccines and can be given to immunocompromised patients.[33-36]

The polysaccharide 23-valent pneumococcal vaccine (PPSV23 or Pneumovax) is recommended in smokers between ages 19 and 64 years, and adults of any age with chronic lung disease, chronic heart disease, chronic liver disease, diabetes mellitus, or alcoholism. Patients over 65 years of age or who are at higher risk of invasive pneumococcal disease should also receive the 13-valent pneumococcal conjugate vaccine (PCV13 or Prevnar); PCV13 should be given first, when possible, followed by PPSV23. Populations who should receive both pneumococcal vaccines include all individuals over 65 years of age, people with cochlear implants, persistent cerebrospinal fluid leaks, HIV infection, functional or anatomic asplenia, chronic renal disease, nephrotic syndrome, hematologic malignancies, organ transplant, or congenital or acquired immunodeficiencies. Revaccination with a single dose of PPSV23 is recommended for these high-risk groups or for people over 65 years of age who received their vaccine before the age of 65.

Patients who require splenectomy should receive pneumococcal, meningococcal, and *H influenzae* B vaccine at least 2 weeks before splenectomy. Meningococcal vaccine is also recommended for patients with terminal complement component deficiencies and functional asplenia.[37]

Prophylactic antimicrobials are given to immunocompromised patients such as those with HIV. CD4 T helper cell

TABLE 20-3 CD4 Indication and Prophylactic Regimen for Specific Microbes

	Indications for Prophylaxis	Prophylactic Regimens
Pneumocystis jirovecii pneumonia (PJP)	• CD4 less than 200 cells/mm³ • History of oral thrush • History of prior PCP • Prophylaxis can be discontinued when CD > 200 cells/mm³ for more than 3 months	• Trimethoprim-sulfamethoxazole DS daily • Trimethoprim-sulfamethoxazole single strength daily (may be better tolerated)
Mycobacterium avium complex	• CD4 less than 50 cells/mm³ • Prior to initiating prophylaxis, infection must be ruled out via AFB blood cultures • Prophylaxis can be discontinued if CD4 count remains above 100 for more than 3 months	• Azithromycin 1200 mg weekly • Clarithromycin 500 mg PO BID
Toxoplasmosis	• CD4 less than 100 cells/mm³ and seropositive to toxoplasma (positive toxoplasma IgG) • Prophylaxis can be discontinued if CD4 count remains above 200 for 3 months	• Trimethoprim-sulfamethoxazole DS daily
Histoplasmosis	• CD4 less than 150 cells/mm³ at high risk of exposure (time in endemic regions) • Prophylaxis can be stopped if CD4 > 150 cells/mm³ for more than 6 months	• Itraconazole 200 mg daily
Coccidioidomycosis	• Patients who have completed therapy for coccidioidomycosis should receive secondary prophylaxis • Primary prophylaxis is not recommended	• Fluconazole 400 mg daily

AFB = acid-fast bacilli; BID = twice daily; DS = double strength; IgG = immunoglobulin G; PO = orally.

levels are used to gauge which prophylactic antimicrobials are given (Table 20-3).[38,39]

TYPES OF MICROBE AND INFECTION

Streptococcus

This genus of bacteria is seen as Gram-positive cocci in pairs and chains on Gram stain and are facultative anaerobes. Streptococci, including nonpathogenic species, reside in the human nasopharynx, respiratory tract, intestines, and skin. Streptococci can be classified by their hemolytic properties on blood agar plates: α hemolysis is incomplete hemolysis leaving a green zone on the plate, β hemolysis is complete hemolysis with clearing of the red blood cells, and γ hemolysis is the absence of hemolysis. The most clinically important α hemolytic streptococci are *S pneumoniae* and viridans group streptococci. β hemolytic streptococci are further divided into their Lancefield groups and include group A strep (*S pyogenes*) and group B strep (*S agalactiae*).

S pneumoniae, or pneumococcus, is a common cause of otitis media, community-acquired bacterial pneumonia, and bacterial meningitis. It can cause serious invasive infections in patients with HIV and patients who have undergone splenectomy.[40] It contains several virulence factors. The polysaccharide capsule prevents iC3b and Fc of antibody from interacting with phagocytes, allowing pneumococcus to avoid phagocytosis.[41] Pneumococcus produces pneumolysin, a cytotoxin that binds to cholesterol, creating pores in cell membranes, and activates the classical complement pathway.

Pneumococcus has surface proteins such as hyaluronidase and neuraminidase, which cause inflammation and damage to the host. Diagnosis is by sputum and blood culture, although the yield is variable. Urinary pneumococcal antigen has a sensitivity of 70% to 90% and a specificity of 80% to 100% and can aid in the diagnosis.[42] Antibiotic options for pneumonia due to *S pneumoniae* include oral (PO) or IV penicillin, macrolides, quinolones, or third-generation cephalosporins such as ceftriaxone or cefotaxime. Because the incidence of penicillin resistance is increasing, third-generation cephalosporins are often used empirically while awaiting culture data. Treatment is usually for 5 days but is extended to 10 to 14 days if associated with bacteremia. For suspected pneumococcal meningitis, the empiric antibiotic treatment consists of vancomycin (15–20 mL/kg IV every 8–12 hours) with ceftriaxone 2 g IV every 12 hours or cefotaxime (2 g IV every 4–6 hours) for 14 days.[43] Penicillin G 4 million units IV every 4 hours can be used instead of a third-generation cephalosporin if the isolate is penicillin sensitive (minimum inhibitory concentration [MIC] < 0.06 µg/mL). Dexamethasone is often added at the beginning of treatment for bacterial meningitis to reduce incidence of hearing loss and other neurologic sequelae.

Group A streptococcus (GAS) resides in the nasopharynx and skin. It can cause pharyngitis and skin and soft tissue infections such as cellulitis, impetigo, myositis, necrotizing fasciitis, and streptococcal toxic shock syndrome. Complications of GAS infection include acute poststreptococcal glomerulonephritis (PSGN), acute rheumatic fever (ARF), and rheumatic heart disease (RHD).[44] Group A streptococcus contains 3 types of virulence factors: M proteins, cytolysins, and pyrogenic exotoxins.

M proteins, encoded by the *emm* gene, inhibit the binding of antibodies and opsonin and can protect the organism from phagocytosis by neutrophils. Group A streptococcus cytolysins include (1) streptolysin O, which creates cholesterol aggregates that facilitate cell lysis; (2) hyaluronidase, which hydrolyzes hyaluronic acid in deep tissues; (3) streptokinase, which converts plasminogen to plasmin and may contribute to the development of poststreptococcal glomerulonephritis; (4) nicotinamide-adenine dinucleotidase; and (5) deoxyribonucleases A, B, C, and D. Group A streptococcus exotoxins act as super antigens and can contribute to invasive disease and toxic shock syndrome.

Group A streptococcus is highly susceptible to penicillins and β-lactams. Acute pharyngitis can be treated with oral penicillin 2 to 4 times per day for 10 days; penicillin is the recommended first-line therapy, but other antibiotic options include a macrolide, such as azithromycin, or cephalosporin, such cefuroxime or cefpodoxime, for 5 days.[44] For impetigo, focal lesions can be managed with mupirocin or retapamulin ointments, but diffuse disease should be treated with oral or IV antibiotics with consideration for cross coverage for *Staphylococcus*, particularly MRSA.[44] In the event of necrotizing fasciitis, prompt surgical debridement is crucial. Antibiotics for necrotizing fasciitis due to GAS are penicillin G 3 to 4 million units IV every 4 hours and clindamycin 600 to 900 mg IV every 6 to 8 hours.[45,46] Clindamycin has antitoxin effects.[44]

Acute rheumatic fever is a nonsuppurative complication that can occur 1 to 5 weeks after streptococcal pharyngitis. Diagnosis is based on the Jones criteria. There are 5 major manifestations, which include carditis and valvulitis, arthritis, central nervous system (CNS) involvement known as Sydenham chorea, subcutaneous nodules, and erythema marginatum.[47] There are 4 minor manifestations, which include arthralgia, fever, elevated acute phase reactants, and prolonged PR interval on electrocardiogram (ECG).[47] Two major or 1 major and 2 minor manifestations in a patient with prior GAS infection are required for diagnosis. Late complications of ARF include rheumatic heart disease and Jaccoud arthropathy. Treatment consists of antibiotics to eradicate GAS carriage, symptomatic treatment of arthritis with nonsteroidal anti-inflammatory drugs (NSAIDs), and management of heart failure.[48] Secondary antibiotic prophylaxis to prevent rheumatic heart disease may be given with 1.2 million units of benzathine penicillin G intramuscularly (IM) every 4 weeks or oral penicillin twice daily.[49] The duration of antibiotics depends on the degree of cardiac involvement and the age of the patient.

Poststreptococcal glomerulonephritis is due to glomerular immune complex deposition and can occur 1 to 6 weeks after infection with nephritogenic strains of GAS. Clinical presentation can range from hematuria to acute nephritic syndrome (edema, hypertension, acute kidney injury with red to brown urine, and proteinuria).[50] Diagnosis is dependent on findings of nephritis with documented evidence of GAS infection by a positive culture or via serologic streptozyme test, such as antistreptolysin (ASO), antihyaluronidase (AHase), antistreptokinase

(ASKase), antinicotinamide-adenine dinucleotidase (anti-NAD), and anti-DNase B antibodies.[51,52] Treatment is largely supportive.

Haemophilus influenzae

This pleomorphic Gram-negative rod is a nonmotile facultative anaerobe that resides in the human respiratory tract.[53] It can cause otitis media, sinusitis, conjunctivitis, epiglottitis, pneumonia, and meningitis. It has 6 serotypes (A through F) that are associated with an outer capsule and a nontypeable serotype that is not associated with a capsule.[54] It has an outer membrane lipopolysaccharide that acts as an endotoxin and 3 types of IgA proteases. The currently available *H influenza* type B conjugate vaccine is active against the most common serotype B and induces bactericidal antibodies to capsular polysaccharides. The widespread use of the vaccine has reduced the incidence of invasive disease due to *H influenza* serotype B, but it has been suggested to have increased the incidence of infections due to nontypeable serotype.[53,54] *Haemophilus* is generally β-lactam susceptible. More serious infections such as meningitis should be treated with IV ceftriaxone or cefotaxime. Amoxicillin or an oral second- or third-generation cephalosporin can be used for pneumonia and less severe infections.[55]

Neisseria

The most common pathogens in this genus of Gram-negative diplococci are *N meningitides*, which causes meningitis and/or meningococcemia, and *N gonorrhoeae*, which primarily causes sexually transmitted genitourinary infections but can also present with pharyngitis, conjunctivitis, or proctitis. *N meningitides* presents with meningitis, meningitis with accompanying meningococcemia, or meningococcemia without meningitis. Patients may have a petechial rash that evolves into a purpuric rash, predominantly on the trunk and lower extremities. Diagnosis is via culture and cerebrospinal fluid analysis. Blood culture is positive 50% of the time. Antibiotics should be given promptly and should not be delayed while awaiting lumbar puncture (LP).[56] Cerebrospinal fluid cultures are less likely to be positive after antibiotics, but the Gram stain can be helpful. Cerebrospinal fluid studies for meningococcal meningitis typically show a high white blood cell count, a high protein level, and a low glucose level. Third-generation cephalosporins such as ceftriaxone or cefotaxime should be used for treatment.[57,58] Droplet precautions should be continued for 24 hours after initiation of appropriate antibiotics. Chemoprophylaxis should be given to close contacts, such as household contacts and healthcare workers exposed to oral secretions, within 24 hours of exposure. Options for prophylaxis are ciprofloxacin, rifampin, or ceftriaxone.[59,60]

Pseudomonas

This Gram-negative aerobic rod is found in the environment, particularly in water, and commonly causes infections in patients with decreased immune defenses and in the health-care system. It has virulence factors, including the formation of biofilm, which is in part secondary to a mucoid phenotype; exotoxins A, S, and U; endotoxin lipopolysaccharides; elastase; alkaline protease; and phenazines.[61-66] *Pseudomonas* is a common colonizer in the respiratory tract and skin, which is why it frequently causes hospital- or ventilator-associated pneumonia and infections in patients with burns. A colony count of 10^5 cells/µL or higher in the appropriate clinical setting can help distinguish colonization from true infection in burns.[65,67,68] Bacteremia is more common in immunocompromised hosts. Severe infections can be complicated by ecthyma gangrenosum, which are ulcerative lesions with violaceous margins, penetrating the dermis.[69] *Pseudomonas* is intrinsically resistant to many antibiotics and has several mechanisms of acquiring resistance. Although combination therapy with double coverage has previously been recommended, this is now reserved as empiric therapy for patients with serious infections and suspicion of *Pseudomonas* infections with possible drug resistance. Once susceptibility data is available, antibiotic therapy should be tailored appropriately. Antibiotics with good antipseudomonal activity include antipseudomonal β-lactams with β-lactamases (such as piperacillin/tazobactam and ticarcillin/clavulanate), antipseudomonal cephalosporins (ceftazidime and cefepime), aztreonam, fluoroquinolones, and carbapenems (with the exception of ertapenem, which does not cover *Pseudomonas*). Aminoglycosides have antipseudomonal activity but are not generally recommended for monotherapy.

Staphylococcus

This genus of Gram-positive cocci colonize the skin and upper respiratory tract and include the group known as coagulase-negative *Staphylococcus*, including *S epidermidis*, and *S aureus*, which is coagulase positive. They appear as clusters of Gram-positive cocci on Gram stain. Although coagulase-negative *Staphylococcus* is often a blood culture contaminant, it can cause bloodstream infections, particularly in the setting of catheters, endocarditis, and prosthetic joint infections. Virulence is associated with production of biofilm, protective exopolymer, and proinflammation properties of pathogen-associated molecular patterns (PAMPs). Coagulase-negative *Staphylococcus* has a higher resistance to methicillin compared to MRSA and appears to have acquired resistance to other antibiotics including rifamycin, fluoroquinolones, gentamicin, tetracycline, chloramphenicol, erythromycin, clindamycin, and sulfonamides.[70]

Staphylococcus aureus, which include methicillin-susceptible *S aureus* (MSSA) MRSA, is a very common cause of skin and soft structure infections (SSTIs), septic arthritis, prosthetic joint infections, necrotizing pneumonia, osteomyelitis, bloodstream infections, device-related infections, and endocarditis. Virulence factors for *S aureus* include the Panton-Valentine leukocidin (PVL), which lyses leukocytes and causes necrotizing infections; α-hemolysin; and phenol-soluble modulins.[71,72] The presence of the *mecA* gene encodes for methicillin resistance. Although MRSA was previously seen more in hospitalized patients, it has emerged as a common infection in the community. The USA300 strain of community-acquired MRSA (CA-MRSA) is the most common strain, and CA-MRSA is more closely associated with PVL compared to healthcare-associated MRSA.[73-75] *Staphylococcus aureus* skin and soft structure infections are generally purulent, with the development of pustules, furuncles, or abscesses, as opposed to the confluent cellulitis seen with *Streptococcal* cellulitis. Antistaphylococcal penicillins such as oxacillin or nafcillin, or cefazolin are the treatment of choice for MSSA infections. Vancomycin is generally the treatment for MRSA, although trimethoprim-sulfamethoxazole, tetracyclines, and clindamycin may be options for MRSA SSTIs. Bloodstream infections with *S aureus* require IV antibiotics, generally for at least 4 weeks. Endocarditis requires 6 weeks of treatment. Because *S aureus* forms biofilms on medical devices, removal of infected devices such as central lines and cardiac devices is crucial for clearance of infection.

Listeria

Listeria monocytogenes is an aerobic and facultatively anaerobic Gram-positive rod with "tumbling motility" that can cause febrile gastroenteritis, meningoencephalitis, cerebritis, rhombencephalitis, pneumonia, skin infections, eye infections, septic joints, biliary tract infections, and cholangitis. It can lead to stillbirth and abortion in pregnancy.[76,77] In addition to pregnant women, people at the extremes of age and immunocompromised hosts are more susceptible to listeriosis. It is diagnosed via culture. The bacteria are ingested and travel to the bloodstream and into the liver and spleen. They grow intracellularly in the cytosol of infected cells. First-line therapy is with ampicillin with gentamicin for synergy.[78-82] Duration is 14 days in bacteremia and 2 to 4 weeks in central nervous system infections.

Legionella

Legionella pneumophila is the most common species of this genus of aerobic Gram-negative bacilli. *Legionella* requires buffered charcoal yeast extract (BCYE) media to grow in cultures.[83] *Legionella* is found in fresh water and in water systems, such as cooling towers and plumbing systems, and infection occurs with inhalation of water droplets. Its virulence is related to its ability to inhibit phagosome-lysosome fusion via defective organelle trafficking (*dot*) genes and intracellular multiplication (*icm*) genes.[84] Suspicion for *Legionella* should be higher in patients with pneumonia and the following: GI symptoms, neurologic symptoms, fever greater than 39°C, hyponatremia, hepatitis, hematuria, and failure to respond to β-lactam therapy.[85] Although diagnosis can be made by culture on a BYCE plate, the *Legionella* urine antigen is more commonly used and has a sensitivity of 80% and specificity 97% to 100%. The urine antigen test is only for *Legionella* serogroup 1, but this serogroup causes the majority of infections.[86-90] Effective antibiotics must be able to reach high intracellular concentrations; options include macrolides, fluoroquinolones, and tetracyclines, with the newer macrolides and fluoroquinolones being the recommended treatment.[91-93] Levofloxacin was found to be superior than erythromycin or clarithromycin in terms of clinical response via defervescence, length of stay, and complications.[91] However, newer macrolides like azithromycin appear to have superior clinical response, with a 95% cure rate at 10 to 14 days and a 96% cure rate at 21 days.[92] For transplant patients, fluoroquinolones are preferred due to the interactions of macrolides and the immunosuppressant agents via the cytochrome P450 3A4 (CYP3A) enzyme.[94-97] The duration of antibiotics is dependent on the type of infection, although it is typically 14 to 21 days.

Nocardia

Nocardia is a genus of filamentous, branching Gram-positive rods that can partially stain acid fast.[98] The majority of infections are seen in immunocompromised hosts, particularly with defects in CMI, but a third of the infections are seen in immunocompetent hosts.[99] *Nocardia* is found in the environment and is inhaled, so infections are primarily pulmonary and radiographically appear as focal consolidation, pulmonary nodules, cavitary lesions, and pleural effusions. Extrapulmonary manifestations are secondary to hematogenous or contiguous spread. The CNS is the most common site of extra-pulmonary disease, so neuroimaging is recommended.[100] Cutaneous infections can occur with traumatic injury with direct inoculation. Diagnosis is via Gram stain and culture. Antibiotics with activity against *Nocardia* include amikacin, imipenem, meropenem, ceftriaxone, cefotaxime, minocycline, moxifloxacin, levofloxacin, linezolid, and tigecycline, but resistance to these agents is variable. Trimethoprim-sulfamethoxazole is the recommended first-line antibiotic.[98]

Actinomyces

Actinomyces is part of the flora in the oropharynx, GI tract, and urogenital tract; it is a filamentous, microaerophilic Gram-positive bacillus on Gram stain, often seen with sulfur granules.[101] Culturing the organism can be challenging, but the organism can be seen on Gram stain and pathology.[101,102] *Actinomyces* can appear as masses with abscesses and fistulae in the neck and face, lungs, and abdomen. Treatment includes surgical resection and prolonged course of antibiotics. *Actinomyces* is very susceptible to β-lactams. Recommended treatment is high dose IV penicillin G for 2 to 6 weeks followed by oral penicillin V or amoxicillin for 6 to 12 months.

Rhodococcus equi

This is an aerobic Gram-positive intracellular coccobacillus, previously known as *Corynebacterium equi*, and usually causes infection in immunocompromised patients, particularly those with HIV.[103] It is found in soil and in herbivores, such as horses. *Rhodococcus* most commonly causes cavitary pneumonia with or without pleural effusions in the immunocompromised,

making it difficult to distinguish from tuberculosis.[104] Its appearance on Gram stain with pleomorphic cocci and bacilli can make it difficult to distinguish from a contaminant, but *Rhodococcus* forms distinct salmon-colored colonies.[104] Recommended treatment is with 2 drugs, usually with a macrolide or fluoroquinolone in combination with rifampin; duration of antibiotics can be up to 6 months.

Corynebacterium

Corynebacterium is a genus of Gram-positive bacilli that are catalase positive, urease negative, cystinase positive, and pyrazinamidase negative.[105-107] *Corynebacterium diphtheria* is the most common species to cause infection by producing diphtheria toxin, leading to pseudomembrane formation and upper respiratory tract infection. Similar disease is less frequently caused by *C ulcerans* and *C pseudotuberculosis*. Symptoms of malaise, sore throat, lymphadenopathy, and low-grade fever usually starts 2 to 5 days after infection. Diagnosis is with culture, on Loeffler or Tinsdale medium, and toxin detection. Outbreaks of cutaneous infection have been seen. Dissemination of the diphtheria toxin can lead to systemic disease with involvement of the heart, nervous system, and kidneys. Antitoxin is effective if given before the toxin enters cells. Antibiotic treatment is with erythromycin or penicillin for 14 days.

Bartonella

This genus of Gram-negative intracellular bacteria include *Bartonella henselae*, which causes cat-scratch disease, and *B quintana*, which causes trench fever, bacillary angiomatosis, and culture-negative endocarditis.[108-110] Cat-scratch disease presents as cutaneous lesions with regional lymphadenopathy. Complications of *B henselae* infection include neuroretinitis, peliosis hepatis, Parinaud oculoglandular syndrome, osteomyelitis, encephalitis, or endocarditis.[110] In HIV patients, both *B henselae* and *B quintana* can cause bacillary angiomatosis, which are vascular lesions mostly involving the skin but can involve other organs, bacillary peliosis of the liver, and splenitis. *B quintana* is spread through lice and can cause trench fever with cyclical fevers that classically recur every 5 days, severe headache, bone pain, splenomegaly, and sometimes rash.[109] Both species can also cause culture-negative endocarditis. *Bartonella* is a fastidious organism and challenging to grow in culture, so diagnosis often includes serologies, histopathology and polymerase chain reaction (PCR) of tissue or blood. Treatment for cat-scratch disease is azithromycin 500 mg PO daily and 250 mg PO daily for 4 days.[111,112] Longer durations of combination therapy are used for more complicated *Bartonella* infections. For *Bartonella* endocarditis, treatment is doxycycline plus rifampin for 6 to 8 weeks.

Brucella

Brucella is a small, nonmotile, aerobic, intracellular Gram-negative coccobacilli that lacks a capsule, spores, and flagella.[113,114]

It is a zoonotic infection that occurs after contact with infected animals, such as sheep or cattle, or after ingestion of contaminated food from these animals, such as unpasteurized cheese or milk. The bacteria travel through the lymph nodes after being ingested by PMNs and macrophages, replicates intracellularly, and disseminates after cell lysis. *Brucella* has a smooth lipopolysaccharide and proteins that are involved in cell entry and likely help evade the immune response. Clinical manifestations are nonspecific and variable. Symptoms include fevers, night sweats, anorexia, weight loss, malaise, and arthralgias; complicated infections can lead to neurobrucellosis, endocarditis, and hepatic abscess. *Brucella* is associated with complications in pregnancy, including spontaneous abortion, premature delivery, and fetal death. Diagnosis is based on serologies and culture. Because of the risk of laboratory infection, the microbiology lab must be notified in advance if there is suspicion of brucellosis. Treatment is with the combination of either doxycycline and rifampin or doxycycline and streptomycin.[113]

Capnocytophaga canimorsus

Capnocytophaga is a facultative anaerobe and a long, slender Gram-negative rod found in the oral flora of dogs or cats. It can cause severe sepsis after a dog bite in immunocompromised patients, most often due to splenic abnormalities such as asplenia or splenectomy, cirrhosis, or alcohol abuse.[115-118] Diagnosis is via culture. Treatment is with β-lactams such as a β-lactam/β-lactamase combination, a cephalosporin, or a carbapenem, and duration is determined by clinical response.[115-118]

Enterococcus

Enterococcus is a genus of bacteria previously classified as group D *Streptococcus*. They appear as Gram-positive cocci in pairs and chains and are facultative anaerobes. The most common species that cause infection are *E faecalis* and *E faecium*, both of which reside in the human intestine.[119,120] Their virulence factors include surface adhesins such as the Enterococcal surface protein, which leads to bacterial adherence to the bladder, and gelatinase, which contributes to the development of endocarditis in animal models.[119] Enterococci are a common cause of nosocomial infections, including urinary tract infections, bloodstream infections, and endocarditis. Diagnosis is via culture. *Enterococcus faecalis* is usually susceptible to ampicillin, which is the antibiotic of choice, but *E faecium* is usually resistant to ampicillin and is often resistant to vancomycin. Antibiotic options for vancomycin-resistant *Enterococci* (VRE) include linezolid and daptomycin. Quinupristin-dalfopristin is the only active antibiotic against *E faecium* and is not active against *E faecalis*.

Escherichia coli

Escherichia coli is a Gram-negative rod that resides in the GI tract and a common cause of urinary tract infections and intestinal infections. *Escherichia coli* is a facultative anaerobe

and lactose fermenter. Enterohemorrhagic *E coli* (EHEC), particularly the strain O157:H7, expresses Shiga toxin, can cause hemorrhagic colitis, and is associated with hemolytic uremic syndrome (HUS; hemolytic anemia, acute renal failure, and thrombocytopenia).[120,121] Diagnosis is based on culture using sorbitol-MacConkey agar for O157:H7, O104:H4, and Shiga toxins in stool. Antibiotics are associated with development of HUS and are not recommended for EHEC.[122,123] Enterotoxigenic *E coli* (ETEC) expresses either a heat labile or heat stable cholera-like toxin that causes excretion of chloride and inhibits sodium chloride reabsorption in the intestinal tract, causing watery diarrhea. Enteropathogenic *E coli* (EPEC) adheres to enterocytes and alters electrolyte and water secretions.[124-128] Enteroaggregative *E coli* (EAEC) has mitogen-activated protein kinase, which releases IL-8, cytotoxin, and adherence fimbriae; it can cause an acute diarrheal illness. Diagnosis is via tissue culture adherence assay.[129-132]

Salmonella

This genus of enteric Gram-negative rods can further be classified into typhoidal *Salmonella*, which cause a systemic infection called typhoid fever with minimal diarrheal symptoms, and nontyphoidal *Salmonella*, which are common causes of diarrheal illnesses. *Salmonella typhi* and *S paratyphi* can cause typhoid fever. Symptoms of typhoid fever usually occur several days to weeks after ingestion of the bacteria and include high fevers, often with relative bradycardia, abdominal pain, and salmon-colored macules known as "rose spots."[133,134] Unlike infection with nontyphoidal *Salmonella*, typhoid fever can be associated with constipation. Diagnosis is by culture, with bone marrow cultures being the most sensitive; serologic tests such as the Widal test are of limited use in endemic areas as they may represent previous infection. Treatment includes fluoroquinolones, cephalosporins, and azithromycin. Patients can be chronic carriers of *S typhi*, shedding the bacteria in the urine and stool for more than 12 months after acute infection. Chronic carrier state also predisposes patients to biliary cancer.

Treponema pallidum

Treponema pallidum is the spirochete that causes syphilis. It cannot be grown in culture, so it is diagnosed with serology with non-treponemal tests, such as rapid plasmid regain (RPR), Venereal Disease Research Laboratory (VDRL) test, or treponemal antibodies, such as the fluorescent treponemal antibody absorption test (FTA-ABS).[135,136] The spirochete can also be seen with darkfield microscopy when a specimen is taken from a lesion. Clinically, syphilis can be divided into early infection (less than 1 year), which includes primary syphilis, secondary syphilis, and latent syphilis, or late infection. Primary syphilis presents as a painless genital ulcer. Secondary syphilis occurs weeks to months after the primary lesions with a diffuse maculopapular rash involving the soles and palms, constitutional symptoms, and lymphadenopathy. Secondary syphilis can also present with hepatitis, nephritis or nephrotic syndrome, and ocular disease.[137] Latent syphilis is asymptomatic. Early latent syphilis is when serologic tests are newly positive within the past 12 months, while late latent syphilis has positive testing either after 12 months or of unknown timing. Late syphilis can present up to 30 years from initial inoculation and consists of tertiary syphilis with gummatous syphilis, general paresis, tabes dorsalis, and cardiovascular syphilis.[137] Neurologic involvement can occur at any stage of infection and is diagnosed with a positive VDRL in the cerebrospinal fluid; cerebrospinal fluid VDRL is specific, though not sensitive.[135,136] Penicillin is the antibiotic of choice for all stages of syphilis. For early syphilis, treatment is 1 dose of penicillin G benzathine 2.4 million units IM. For late syphilis, treatment is penicillin G benzathine 2.4 million units IM weekly for 3 weeks.[137] Neurosyphilis treatment consists of penicillin G 3 to 4 million units IV every 4 hours for 10 to 14 days. Doxycycline or ceftriaxone can be used in patients who are allergic to penicillin, but there is limited data on efficacy and higher rates of failure in neurosyphilis.[137]

Mycobacterium tuberculosis

Mycobacterium is a genus of aerobic acid-fast bacteria. *Mycobacterium tuberculosis* is the most clinically significant species, as the cause of tuberculosis, which causes significant infectious mortality worldwide. Primary infection is pulmonary disease, but tuberculosis can cause latent and extrapulmonary infection. Infection is more complicated in immune-compromised hosts, such as patients with HIV. Patients who receive anti–tumor necrosis factor (TNF) therapy are also at increased risk of TB.[138] Primary tuberculosis occurs in patients not previously infected with tuberculosis and may be asymptomatic. Symptomatic patients can present with fevers and chest pain. Patients with intact immune systems can control further disease and will develop latent TB. The majority of TB cases seen are due to reactivated TB, which most often involve the upper lung lobes but can present as disseminated disease, particularly in patients with HIV. Symptoms of reactivated pulmonary TB include fever, night sweats, cough, dyspnea, hemoptysis, and weight loss. Miliary TB, which can be seen with primary or reactivated infection, is seen with hematogenous spread of TB and is more common in immunocompromised hosts. Extrapulmonary TB is distinguished as TB infection not involving the lungs and can involve the lymph nodes, GI tract, CNS, pericardium, and bones.

The diagnosis of latent TB infection (LTBI) is made by either the tuberculosis skin test (TST) or interferon gamma release assays (IGRAs) in patients with no clinical symptoms and no radiographic evidence of TB. A TST is read between 48 and 72 hours, and induration of 5 mm or more is positive in patients with direct TB exposure, patients with HIV, or patients on immunosuppressive therapy. A TST with induration of 10 mm or greater is positive in patients at increased risk of exposure, such as healthcare workers, immigrants from areas with high prevalence of TB, IV drug users, employees or residents of high-risk settings such as prisons

or nursing homes, and children younger than 4 years old. A TST with induration of 15 mm or greater is positive in all other populations.[139]

Radiographic findings in patients with tuberculosis include homogenous consolidation on any lobes, but particularly on the right middle or right lower lobe; unilateral adenopathy, particularly right paratracheal or right hilar; miliary disease; unilateral pleural effusion; or normal radiograph.[140-142] Ranke complex, the presence of Ghon complex and calcified hilar adenopathy suggests prior tuberculosis. If the lymph nodes are greater than 2 cm with or without areas of necrosis, it can suggest active disease.[140] Postprimary tuberculosis is a reactivation or reinfection and radiographically has upper lobe predilection, cavitation, and absence of lymphadenopathy. Coinfection with HIV tends to have atypical presentation of tuberculosis.

The diagnosis of active tuberculosis is based on clinical symptoms, risk factors, and isolation of *M tuberculosis* by culture. Patients with suspected active TB should be placed in airborne isolation. Sputum should be sent for acid-fast bacilli (AFB) smear and culture in patients with suspected TB; the sensitivity of sputum AFB smear increases with the number of specimens sent, so the recommendation is to send 3 specimens 8 hours apart. Molecular testing is also available for *M tuberculosis*, including nucleic acid amplification testing (NAAT); molecular diagnostics can lead to more rapid detection of TB, and depending on the specific test, can detect drug resistance.[139] Isolates of *M tuberculosis* are tested for antimicrobial susceptibility, and treatment is based on susceptibility results. All patients are started on empiric treatment with at least 4 agents.

Treatment of drug-susceptible pulmonary TB consists of a 2-month intensive phase with isoniazid (INH), rifampin (RIF), pyrazinamide (PZA), and ethambutol (EMB) followed by a 4-month continuation phase of isoniazid and rifampin.[143] If sensitivities show INH and RIF susceptibility, ethambutol is not necessary during the intensive phase.[143] Follow-up is via monthly AFB smear and culture until 2 consecutive specimens are negative. Cavitary disease and positive culture after 2 months of therapy are associated with relapse, and the continuation phase is extended for an additional 3 months.[143-145] Treatment is extended to 6 to 9 months if infection involves the bones and 9 to 12 months if there is CNS infection. Treatment should be continuous and without drug interruptions. If drug interruption is less than 14 days during the intensive phase, continue current regimen, but if the interruption is greater than 14 days during the intensive phase, all drugs would have to start from the beginning of the regimen.[143] If drug interruption occurs during the continuation phase after 80% or more of treatment has been given and AFB studies are negative, treatment can be discontinued.[143] If drug interruption occurs during the continuation phase when 80% or more of treatment has been given but AFB studies remain positive, treatment should be continued until all doses are completed.[143] If drug interruption occurs earlier in the continuation phase (< 80% of therapy given) and the lapses are less than 3 months total, continue treatment until all doses are completed.[143] If drug interruption occurs during the continuation phase when less than 80% of treatment is given and total lapses are greater than 3 months, treatment should be restarted from the beginning of the regimen.[143]

Multidrug resistant (MDR) tuberculosis is resistant to at least 2 drugs, including isoniazid and rifampin. Extensively drug-resistant (XDR) tuberculosis is resistant to isoniazid and rifampin plus any fluoroquinolone and at least 1 second-line agent such as amikacin, kanamycin, or capreomycin. Treatment for both MDR and XDR tuberculosis is prolonged and warrants consultation with an expert in resistant tuberculosis management

Patients with TB and HIV coinfection should be treated with both antiretroviral therapy and TB therapy, but special considerations include drug-drug interactions and the risk of immune reconstitution inflammatory syndrome (IRIS). Although the risk of IRIS is higher in patients with lower CD4, starting ARVs early is beneficial, particularly in patients with a CD4 of less than 50.[146] The exception is for TB meningitis in patients with HIV, in which more adverse events were seen with early ARV initiation.[147]

Nontuberculosis Mycobacteria

Nontuberculosis mycobacteria (NTM) such as *M avium* complex (MAC) and *M kansasii* are environmental organisms that can cause pulmonary disease in immunocompetent hosts with lung disease or disseminated infection in immunocompromised hosts such as patients with AIDS (CD4 < 50 cells/μL) and genetic disorders associated with IL-12 and interferon γ (IFN-γ).[148-150] Diagnosis of pulmonary NTM is dependent on the following criteria: clinical via pulmonary symptoms, nodular or cavitary opacities, or bronchiectasis with small nodules on chest radiograph and exclusion of other diagnosis; and microbial via (A) positive cultures from wash or lavage or 2 or more separated expectorated sputum samples, or (B) transbronchial or lung biopsy with mycobacterial histopathologic features and positive tissue culture for NTM, or (C) biopsy showing mycobacterial histopathologic features and 1 or more positive sputum or bronchial washing cultures.[151] Diagnosis of disseminated MAC in patients with AIDS is isolation of the organism in sterile sites such as the blood, bone marrow, or lymph nodes. Treatment of pulmonary MAC depends on the severity of the lung disease; treatment is with either clarithromycin or azithromycin plus ethambutol and rifampin. Treatment for pulmonary MAC is prolonged, with guidelines recommending 12 months of therapy from time of negative sputum cultures. Treatment of disseminated MAC in AIDS is usually combination therapy with clarithromycin and ethambutol with or without a rifamycin; patients should also be placed on ARV therapy. Prophylaxis for MAC in HIV patients with CD4 below 50 cells/μL was mentioned previously. For macrolide-sensitive MAC, initial treatment for nodular or bronchiectatic lung disease is clarithromycin 1000 mg or azithromycin 500 mg, ethambutol 25 mg/kg, and

rifampin 600 mg PO 3 times per week. For fibrocavitary or severe nodular bronchiectatic macrolide-sensitive MAC, treatment is clarithromycin 500 to 1000 mg/d or azithromycin 250 mg/d, ethambutol 15 mg/kg/d, and rifampin 10 mg/kg/d, with ethambutol removed after initial 2 months. The goal is 12 months of negative sputum cultures while on treatment. For macrolide-resistant NTM, treatment consists of ethambutol, rifampin or rifabutin, clofazimine, amikacin, and surgical resection. Treatment failure is considered if there is no clinical, radiographic, or microbiologic response after 6 months or there is a negative AFB sputum culture during 12 months of treatment.[151]

Acinetobacter

This Gram-negative coccobacillus is found in the environment and on animals. It colonizes our skin, respiratory tract, and GI tract. It is frequently seen with healthcare-associated infections and surgical site infections. Virulence factors include its ability to produce a biofilm, outer membrane protein A, K1 capsule, siderophore-mediated iron acquisition system, and fimbriae. *Acinetobacter* has multiple mechanisms of resistance including β-lactamase production. Antibiotic options for susceptible isolates include ampicillin-sulbactam, broad-spectrum cephalosporins such as cefepime, or carbapenems. Duration of antibiotics is dependent on the type of infection.

Aspergillus

Aspergillus is a genus of molds including *A fumigatus, A flavus*, and *A niger* that can cause a spectrum of pulmonary disease. These include aspergilloma, chronic pulmonary aspergillosis, allergic bronchopulmonary aspergillosis (ABPA), and invasive aspergillosis.[152]

A simple aspergilloma is a fungus ball that resides in preexisting cavitary lung disease. Diagnosis is radiographic with either a positive sputum culture or positive serum *Aspergillus* IgG.[153,154] This is often an incidental finding that does not require treatment. In patients who develop hemoptysis, treatment is with embolization or surgical resection. Antifungal therapy is not indicated.

Chronic pulmonary aspergillosis presents with systemic symptoms such as malaise, fevers, weight loss, elevated *Aspergillus*-specific IgG, and new or chronic cavities. This is primarily seen in immunocompetent hosts with chronic lung disease.[152] There may be intracavitary mycetoma, extensive parenchymal destruction, and fibrosis.[152,155] Cultures may be positive. For severe disease, treatment is with IV voriconazole or IV liposomal amphotericin.[152,156,157] Treatment for mild to moderate disease is with oral voriconazole or itraconazole.[152,156,157]

Allergic bronchopulmonary aspergillosis is a hypersensitivity reaction due to noninvasive colonization of *Aspergillus* in the setting of asthma or cystic fibrosis.[158-161] Symptoms are due to immune-mediated damage to airways and elevated *Aspergillus* IgE.[158-161] Diagnostic criteria include the following:

(1) a predisposing condition such as asthma or cystic fibrosis; (2) demonstration of fungal sensitization to *Aspergillus* via positive skin test or elevated IgE; (3) IgE IG greater than 1000 IU/mL, but it may be lower if the patient is on corticosteroids or during the less active phase of the disease; (4) elevated *Aspergillus* IgE and precipitins; and (5) mucous plugging and central bronchiectasis, although it may be absent in early disease.[162] Treatment is primarily with steroids. Antifungals such as itraconazole or voriconazole may be used as second-line treatment to improve lung function and decrease rates of exacerbation.

Invasive pulmonary aspergillosis (IPA) is an invasive disease seen in immunocompromised hosts, such as in patients with prolonged neutropenia, immunosuppression for stem cell transplant or organ transplant, inherited immunodeficiencies such as chronic granulomatous disease, or chronic pre-existing structural lung disease.[162,163] Patients typically have fevers, respiratory symptoms and chest pain, and focal radiographic findings such as pulmonary nodules with inflammation, consolidation, or cavitary lesions.[164] Proven diagnosis is based on histopathology showing invasive disease or isolation from a sterile site. Galactomannan is a cell wall component of *Aspergillus* that can be used as a serologic assay to support the diagnosis in the appropriate clinical setting. Preferred treatment is with voriconazole. Lipid formulations of amphotericin and posaconazole are alternative agents.[156,157,162] Echinocandins such as caspofungin have been used for salvage therapy.

Cryptococcus

Cryptococcus is an encapsulated yeast that can cause invasive disease in immunocompromised hosts. The most commonly seen pathogen is *C neoformans*. *Cryptococcus* is present in the soil and in bird droppings; it is inhaled and can spread hematogenously.[165] Immunocompromised hosts who are at risk of cryptococcal infection include patients with AIDS, liver disease, organ transplant, prolonged glucocorticoid therapy, and malignancies. Cryptococcal meningoencephalitis is most commonly seen in patients with AIDS with CD4 levels below 100 cells/μL; presentation is usually subacute with fever, headache, and malaise. Patients with cryptococcal infection can also present with cutaneous disease and pulmonary findings; pulmonary disease is worse in patients who are immunocompromised.[166] Diagnosis is based on cultures and cryptococcal antigen, which can be sent from the serum and cerebrospinal fluid. Serum cryptococcal antigen is a very sensitive test in AIDS patients with more subtle presentations; AIDS patients with a positive serum cryptococcal antigen should undergo a lumbar puncture after neuroimaging has excluded any mass lesions. Opening pressure should be measured, as cryptococcal meningoencephalitis causes increased intracranial pressure (ICP). Patients with a high opening pressure (> 20 cm H_2O) will require serial LPs to decrease their ICP. *Cryptococcus* can be seen on cerebrospinal fluid using the India ink stain. Unlike most CNS infections, WBC are often low in the cerebrospinal fluid with cryptococcal meningitis.

Fluconazole can be used to treat pulmonary and skin infections without CNS infection. Cryptococcal meningitis requires treatment with amphotericin IV and flucytosine for at least 2 weeks and followed by high-dose fluconazole.[167,168] Complications for amphotericin B include electrolyte disturbances and renal failure. Flucytosine causes hematologic toxicities, such as leukopenia and thrombocytopenia, and hepatic toxicity. Serum levels should be monitored, particularly in patients with renal insufficiency.

Histoplasma

Histoplasma is a dimorphic fungus found in soil and in bird and bat droppings; it is endemic to certain regions including the Ohio and Mississippi River valleys, eastern Asia, and part of Central and South America.[169-171] Clinical manifestations depend on the exposure and the patient's immune status and comorbidities; healthy patients exposed to a low inoculum may be asymptomatic, while immunocompromised hosts can present with severe pulmonary infection and disseminated disease. Clinical presentations can be similar to tuberculosis infection. Acute pulmonary histoplasmosis is often a self-limited infection in immunocompetent hosts with flu-like symptoms and patchy infiltrates and mediastinal lymphadenopathy; symptom duration is less than 1 month. Subacute pulmonary histoplasmosis presents with symptoms duration of more than 1 month, with pulmonary infiltrates and hilar and/or mediastinal adenopathy. Extrapulmonary manifestations such as pericarditis, erythema nodosum, pleuritis, or polyarthritis also can be seen. Chronic pulmonary histoplasmosis presents with more than 3 months of symptoms, including weight loss, dyspnea, cough, and hemoptysis; radiographic findings include apical cavitary lung lesions. Disseminated histoplasmosis is seen in the elderly or immunocompromised patients, such as those with AIDS, patients with hematologic malignancies, transplant recipients, and patients receiving anti-TNF therapy; disseminated disease can be either an acute or chronic infection with involvement of multiple organ systems, including the bone marrow, liver, spleen, adrenals, CNS, and skin. Diagnosis can be by histopathology, culture, and antigen testing. Pathology will show granulomas with possible narrow-based budding yeast in tissue; intracellular nonbudding yeast can also be seen in the WBCs on a buffy coat. Urine and serum can be sent for *Histoplasma* antigen testing, which is highly sensitive in disseminated disease. Severe or disseminated histoplasmosis is treated with liposomal amphotericin followed by itraconazole for several months and up to a year.[171] Itraconazole is the treatment of choice for mild to moderate disease.[171]

Candida

Candida is a genus of yeast that is part of the normal flora of the respiratory and GI tracts; *Candida* species, such as *C albicans*, are the most common cause of fungal infections. Local mucocutaneous infections such as oropharyngeal candidiasis (thrush) and intertriginous candidiasis can be seen in patients with normal immune systems. Pneumonia due to *Candida* is very rare.[172,173] *Candida* esophagitis is an AIDS-defining illness that presents with odynophagia and dysphagia. Immunocompromised patients at risk for candidemia and invasive *Candida* infections include patients with prolonged neutropenia due to hematologic malignancies or chemotherapy and patients who undergo stem cell or organ transplant. For this reason, those patient populations have guidelines for antifungal prophylaxis. Patients at risk for invasive candidiasis have conditions that compromise the skin or mucosal membranes, such as central venous catheters, total parenteral nutrition, antibiotics, high Acute Physiologic Assessment and Chronic Health Evaluation (APACHE) scores, acute kidney injury, recent surgery, particularly abdominal procedures, and GI tract perforations and leaks.[174,175] Although *C albicans* remains the most commonly encountered species, non-albicans *Candida*, such as *C krusei* and *C glabrata*, which often have decreased susceptibility or resistance to fluconazole have become increasingly common. For this reason, guidelines recommend empiric treatment with echinocandins, such as caspofungin for candidemia; antifungal susceptibility should be performed, and therapy can be directed once this data is known.[175]

Blastomyces

Blastomyces dermatitidis is a dimorphic fungus that is endemic to Midwestern US states and Canadian provinces that border the Great Lakes and the St Lawrence Seaway and the southeastern and south central United States near the Mississippi and Ohio Rivers.[176-183] *Blastomyces* resides in moist soil and organic debris and thrives in environments such as beaver dams; the conidia are inhaled and change into the yeast form in the lung. Acute infection can be asymptomatic or present as a self-limited respiratory infection. Symptoms often manifest 30 to 45 days after inoculation and include cough, night sweats, fever, chest pain, weight loss, and hemoptysis.[179,180] Radiographic findings include pneumonitis, nodules, or mass. Chronic pulmonary infection tends to have an upper lobe predominance of nodules and cavities. Blastomycosis can be disseminated to the skin as verrucous and crusting lesions with central abscess, to the CNS, and to the genitourinary tract. Culture of *Blastomyces* gives a definitive diagnosis, but direct visualization of *Blastomyces* on clinical specimens is usually faster and shows large, thick-walled, distinctive broad-based budding yeasts. Serologies for *Blastomyces* are of limited value due to cross-reactivity with other endemic fungi and due to low sensitivity.[184,185] Itraconazole can be used for mild to moderate disease, but lipid formulations of amphotericin should be used initially for moderate to severe infection before transitioning to itraconazole; treatment is continued to a total of 6 to 12 months.[176]

Coccidioides

Coccidioides is a dimorphic fungus endemic to the deserts in the southwest United States with the highest incidence in the San Joaquin Valley, Arizona, and northwestern Mexico. Infection occurs after inhalation of dust that contains the mold form. Presentation is variable and ranges from an acute or subacute self-limited pneumonia, referred to as valley fever, or disseminated disease in immunocompromised patients. Patients also can develop rash with erythema nodosum and may have residual fatigue and arthralgias that can last for weeks to months. Imaging shows mediastinal or hilar adenopathy; pulmonary nodules; cavitary lesions, which are usually solitary peripheral lesions; and pneumothorax.[186] Patients can develop chronic pulmonary infection with chronic fibrocavitary pneumonia. This presents with constitutional symptoms, chest pain, respiratory symptoms (such as cough, dyspnea and hemoptysis), and imaging showing extensive cavities, infiltrates, and hilar adenopathy. Extrapulmonary disease can cause a skin infection with granulomatous skin lesions or tissue abscess, joint infection, vertebral infection, and meningitis. Risk factors for disseminated coccidioidomycosis include AIDS, chronic corticosteroids, hematologic malignances, anti-TNF therapy, organ transplant, third trimester of pregnancy, male, African Americans, or Filipinos.[187] Diagnostic tests include serologic testing for *Coccidioides* species with IgM and IgG and *Coccidioides* antigens in blood and urine. The gold standard for diagnosis is culture or visualization of the *Coccidioides* spherules on histopathologic or cytopathologic specimens.[186] Primary pulmonary coccidioidomycosis with moderate to severe symptoms can be treated with fluconazole PO or itraconazole PO for 6 months or longer, if clinical and radiographic findings persist.[187] Patients at risk for disseminated coccidioidomycosis should be treated with the same regimen but for at least 12 to 18 months.

Pneumocystis

Pneumocystis jirovecii (previously *P carinii*) is a fungus that causes pulmonary infection in immunocompromised hosts. In HIV patients, *Pneumocystis* usually has a subacute presentation with several days to weeks of fever, dyspnea, and cough, and the majority of cases occur in AIDS patients with CD4 levels below 200 cells/μL. Patients are found with hypoxemia and an elevated lactate dehydrogenase (LDH). Imaging with chest x-rays can be unremarkable, but the most common finding is diffuse interstitial infiltrates. *Pneumocystis* can also affect HIV-uninfected immunocompromised populations, including organ transplant and stem cell transplant recipients; patients on long-term steroids, especially in combination with other immunosuppressive agents; and patients on other chemotherapy or immunosuppressive therapy. Clinical presentation in these populations is typically more acute and severe compared to HIV-infected patients. *Pneumocystis* cannot be grown in culture, so diagnosis is based on staining of the organism on microbiology of pathology specimens; direct fluorescent antibody (DFA) is most commonly used for respiratory specimens.[188-192] The DFA sensitivity of a bronchoalveolar lavage (BAL) specimen in HIV patients is 89% to 98%; sensitivity has historically been lower in HIV-uninfected immunocompromised patients.[188-192] The (1,3)β-D-glucan assay detects a fungal cell wall component and has a sensitivity of 92% and specificity of 86% for *Pneumocystis* when used in the appropriate patient with the appropriate clinical presentation.[193] Polymerase chain reaction testing of respiratory specimens can also be used in immunocompromised patients without HIV but is not readily available.[194] Trimethoprim-sulfamethoxazole is the most effective antibiotic for both treatment and prophylaxis. Alternative regimens for treatment include IV pentamidine or clindamycin plus primaquine; atovaquone can be used for treatment of mild infections.[195] Alternatives for prophylaxis are dapsone (if glucose-6-phosphate dehydrogenase screen is normal) or atovaquone. Steroids should be given with the initiation of antibiotics for patients with moderate to severe disease and hypoxemia as measured by a partial pressure of oxygen (Po_2) of less than 70 mmHg on room air and/or an alveolar-arterial oxygen gradient of 35 mmHg or greater. The use of steroids in these patients has been shown to decrease mortality and respiratory failure. [196-199]

Varicella-Zoster Virus

Varicella-zoster virus is a herpesvirus that can be transmitted via aerosolized droplets or direct contact with cutaneous vesicular fluid. Primary infection presents with fever, malaise, and pharyngitis, followed by the diffuse vesicular rash known as varicella or chickenpox. Varicella is usually an uncomplicated and self-limited disease that has become less common with the routine administration of the varicella vaccine during childhood. Varicella-zoster virus infects the sensory nerve endings to establish a latent infection that can be reactivated years later to cause zoster or shingles. Complications of primary varicella can include secondary bacterial skin and soft tissue infection, pneumonia, hepatitis, and neurologic complications such as cerebellar ataxia or diffuse encephalitis. The complication of varicella pneumonia is more common in adults than children, who mostly have the complication of group A streptococcal skin infections. Pregnancy, more than 100 skin lesions, prolonged fever, smoking, and pre-existing lung disease predispose patients to varicella pneumonia.[200-202] Reactivated infection or zoster is usually a dermatomal, painful vesicular rash; the most common complication of zoster is post-herpetic neuralgia. Reactivation in the trigeminal nerve is called herpes zoster ophthalmicus (HZO), which can lead to vision loss due to keratitis or iritis; vesicular lesions on the tip of the nose, known as Hutchison sign, is associated with HZO. Immunocompromised patients are more likely to have complicated primary infection or disseminated reactivated zoster. Diagnosis is primarily clinical but vesicular fluid can be sent for DFA, PCR, and viral culture. Treatment is largely supportive, but antiviral therapy with acyclovir and its related drugs can decrease duration of illness. Foscarnet also has activity and can be used for resistant herpesvirus infections.[203] Patients with HZO should be treated promptly with antivirals, usually IV acyclovir, and be evaluated by ophthalmology.

Herpes Simplex Virus

Infection from herpes simplex virus is due to either type 1 (HSV-1) or type 2 (HSV-2) virus. Herpes simplex virus also establishes dormant infection of the nerves which can lead to reactivation of infection. Primarily, HSV-1 causes herpes labialis involving oral lesions or "cold sores," and HSV-2 is associated with genital herpes involving multiple painful genital ulcers. Primary HSV infection may present with fevers and systemic symptoms but recurrent infections usually only present with focal vesicles.[204-206] Patients with decreased cellular immunity, such as patents with HIV or transplant recipients, can present with more extensive disease, such as esophagitis, pneumonitis, and eye infections, or more recurrences. Diagnosis of primary HSV infections is mostly clinical. Serologies for HSV are not helpful for recurrent infections because of the high prevalence of HSV in the community. Fluid from vesicular lesions can be sent for immunofluorescent staining, Tzanck smear, or viral culture. The detection of HSV in respiratory specimens is not diagnostic by itself, as asymptomatic viral shedding is common. The most severe form of HSV infection is herpes encephalitis, which can be caused by either virus but more commonly is caused by HSV-1. Herpes encephalitis presents acutely with fevers and neurologic deficits such as altered mental status with behavioral disturbances or decreased level of consciousness, cranial nerve palsies, or seizures; neuroimaging shows temporal lobe involvement. Herpes encephalitis has an extremely high mortality if not treated promptly with IV acyclovir. Even with prompt treatment, two-thirds of patients have significant neurologic sequelae.[207] This is very different from herpes meningitis, which is self-limited aseptic meningitis and often is caused by HSV-2. There is no clear role for acyclovir in herpes meningitis. Diagnosis of CNS herpes infection is with HSV PCR of the cerebrospinal fluid which is both highly sensitive and specific.[208] Treatment of HSV is with acyclovir or related antivirals. Herpes encephalitis should be treated with IV acyclovir. Foscarnet can be used for acyclovir-resistant HSV.

Cytomegalovirus

In immunocompetent patients, cytomegalovirus is another herpesvirus that causes a mild self-limited primary infection, often with mononucleosis, followed by latency within monocytes and dendritic cells.[209] Viral shedding occurs, but cell-mediated immunity often prevents overt disease.[210] Although organ involvement can occur with CMV infection in immunocompetent hosts, it is rarely severe. Organ systems include the GI tract, liver, CNS, and bone marrow.[209] Cytomegalovirus can cause serious organ-invasive disease in immunocompromised patients, such as transplant patients and patients with HIV. The most common presentation of CMV in AIDS is retinitis, while pneumonitis is more commonly seen in transplants rather than in AIDS.[211,212] In transplantation, donors and recipients are both screened for CMV, as CMV infection leads to increased risk of both graft rejection and other opportunistic infections.[213,214]

Available diagnostic tests include CMV serologies, qualitative and quantitative PCR, pp65 antigenemia, histopathologic examination, and culture. Serologies may indicate infection with the detection of CMV IgM or a more than 4-fold increase in CMV IgG titers at least 2 weeks apart,[215] but both CMV IgM and IgG may remain elevated for months after the infection.[216] Serum CMV PCR and CMV pp65 antigenemia testing are more sensitive than culture and have been used in transplant patients, but these tests are of limited use in HIV patients.[217,218] Organ-invasive disease may be present in AIDS patients, even in the absence of detectable viremia, and viremia does not always indicate invasive disease. Cytomegalovirus retinitis is diagnosed by dilated fundoscopic exam revealing yellow or white inflammation and hemorrhage.[219,220] If diagnosis is still uncertain, PCR of uveal fluid can be obtained. Histopathology can show viral inclusion bodies in the tissue and specific immunohistochemical staining can be performed.

There is no evidence to support antiviral therapy for primary infection in immunocompetent hosts. First-line therapy for CMV infection in immunocompromised patients is ganciclovir IV or oral valganciclovir, which is the prodrug of ganciclovir with improved bioavailability. Transplant recipients can receive either universal CMV prophylaxis or preemptive therapy based on weekly monitoring of CMV viremia. Cytomegalovirus immune globulin (Cytogam) is less commonly used in transplant for CMV prophylaxis.[221] Foscarnet is most commonly used for ganciclovir-resistant CMV; cidofovir is sometimes used for resistant infection. Cytomegalovirus infection in HIV is treated with ganciclovir or valganciclovir; CMV retinitis may also require intravitreal antivirals. Although initiation of ARV therapy may increase the risk of IRIS, ARVs should generally be started within 2 weeks of presentation.

Epstein-Barr Virus

Epstein-Barr virus (EBV) is a herpesvirus transmitted primarily from intimate contact with saliva. The B cells in the oropharynx become infected and resting memory B cells are sites of persistence of EBV. The number of latently infected cells can remain stable for years.[222,223] Humoral and cellular immunity both control EBV infection. Infectious mononucleosis (IM) due to primary EBV infection starts with nonspecific headache and fever followed by tonsillitis or pharyngitis, severe fatigue, painful cervical lymphadenopathy, and high fevers. A significant number of patients with infectious mononucleosis also develop splenomegaly, which puts them at risk of splenic rupture with trauma. Patients with mononucleosis from EBV have a lymphocytosis with atypical lymphocytes seen on peripheral smear. Other potential organ involvement can include pneumonia, myocarditis, pancreatitis, glomerulonephritis, nervous system involvement (such as meningoencephalitis, neuritis, aseptic meningitis, and Guillain-Barré syndrome) and hematologic abnormalities (such as hemolytic anemia, thrombocytopenia, and disseminated intravascular coagulation).[222-225] Diagnosis is primarily clinical but can be supported by heterophile antibody testing or EBV-specific antigens and antibodies.[222] Treatment for IM is largely supportive. Epstein-Barr virus can also cause several lymphoproliferative disorders and is associated with hematologic malignancies, particularly in HIV. Epstein-Bar virus is known to be 1 of the cause of hemophagocytic lymphohistiocytosis (HLH), which is a rapid and life-threatening condition caused by excessive immune activation with T-cell proliferation.[226] Diagnosis of HLH is based on molecular diagnosis of an HLH genetic mutation or 5 or more of the following criteria: (1) fever; (2) splenomegaly; (3) cytopenias affecting more than lineages such as hemoglobin less than 9 g/dL, platelets less than 100×10^9/L, and neutrophils less than 1×10^9/L; (4) hypertriglyceridemia ($\geq$ 265 mg/dL) and/or hypofibrinogenemia ($\leq$ 150 mg/dL); (5) hemophagocytosis in bone marrow, spleen, or lymph nodes; (6) low or absent natural killer (NK) cell activity; (7) ferritin of 500 µg/L or greater; and (8) soluble CD25 (ie, soluble IL2R) of 2400 µ/mL or greater.[227] Treatment includes etoposide, methotrexate, cyclophosphamide, dexamethasone, alemtuzumab, and/or stem cell transplant.[226] In transplant recipients, EBV causes a range of post-transplant lymphoproliferative disease (PTLD), such as mono-like syndromes, polyclonal B-cell proliferation, and even malignant B-cell lymphoma. Treatment is primary adjustment of immunosuppression.[222-225] Epstein-Barr virus is associated with a number of malignancies in HIV-infected patients, including non-Hodgkin lymphomas (NHL) and smooth muscle tumors. Patients with HIV can also have EBV-driven oral hairy leukoplakia. Other malignancies associated with EBV include Burkitt lymphoma, nasopharyngeal cancer, and certain forms of Hodgkin lymphoma.

Adenovirus

Adenoviruses are a group of respiratory viruses that mostly cause fever and upper respiratory infections (URI) in children. Adenovirus can persist in the lymphoreticular tissues such as the tonsils, adenoids, and intestines.[228-230] In immunocompetent hosts, adenovirus infection can cause pharyngitis, keratoconjunctivitis, pneumonia, hepatitis, colitis, and hemorrhagic cystitis.[228] Stem cell transplant recipients are at increased risk of viral infections due to depletion of T-cells in their graft, medications they receive, such as antithymocyte globulin (ATG) or alemtuzumab (anti-CD52+), and graft-versus-host disease.[231-240] Manifestations of infection include pneumonitis, encephalitis, hepatitis, colitis, nephritis, hemorrhagic cystitis, and disseminated infection. In organ transplants, adenovirus infection can be caused by reactivation or new infection and can range from asymptomatic viremia, organ invasive disease, or disseminated disease with multiple organ involvement; viral shedding is prolonged and can result in graft dysfunction.[230] Diagnosis can be confirmed with viral culture, direct viral antigen detection, histopathologic examination, and PCR. Treatment is primarily supportive with antiviral therapy being limited to severe infections in immunocompromised patients. Cidofovir is the antiviral that seems to have the best activity against adenovirus and has shown some clinical improvement, but the data is very limited. Pooled IV immunoglobulin has been used in some immunocompromised patients but the clinical data for this is also limited.

Measles

Measles is a highly contagious viral infection whose transmission and incidence has decreased significantly with vaccination, although recent outbreaks have occurred in people who have not received the vaccine. The incubation period is 6 to 21 days. Patients develop prodrome of fever, fatigue, and anorexia, followed by conjunctivitis, coryza, and cough. They then develop Koplik spots in the oral mucosa followed 48 hours later by the exanthem phase, characterized by a maculopapular, blanching rash that begins on the face and spreads cephalocaudally and centrifugally.[241,242] The most common complication is diarrhea, but other potential complications include pneumonia, bronchiolitis, gastroenteritis, hepatitis, and appendicitis.[243] Neurologic complications are rare but severe and can include acute encephalitis, acute disseminated encephalomyelitis (ADEM), and subacute sclerosing panencephalitis (SSPE).[243]

Acute disseminated encephalomyelitis is rare but generally seen in the postrecovery period, with demyelination of the central nervous system that is believed to be a postinfectious autoimmune response. Clinical manifestations occur 7 to 14 days after inoculation and consists of ataxia, altered mental status, brainstem symptoms, and motor and sensory deficits. Cerebrospinal fluid analysis is nonspecific, with lymphocytic pleocytosis, elevated albumin, and transient oligoclonal banding.[244,245] An MRI will show disseminated CNS demyelination with multifocal or extensive white matter lesions with or without deep gray matter lesions in the thalamus and basal ganglia.[246-250] A follow-up MRI 6 months later will show resolution or unchanged lesions, whereas new lesions would suggest multiple sclerosis.[245] Acute disseminated encephalomyelitis due to measles has a higher mortality rate than ADEM due to other causes.

Subacute sclerosing panencephalitis is a fatal, progressive degenerative disease of the CNS that occurs 7 to 10 years after measles infection. It has 4 stages: stage I involves personality changes; stage II involves repetitive myoclonic jerks, seizures, and dementia; stage III involves rigidity, extrapyramidal symptoms, and progressive unresponsiveness; and stage IV involves coma and autonomic failure.[251,252] Adult-onset SSPE typically occurs in males, with visual symptoms dominating over motor symptoms, and infrequent cerebellar and brainstem symptoms.[251] Diagnosis requires 2 major criteria and 1 minor criteria. Major criteria include (1) elevated cerebrospinal fluid measles antibody titers, and (2) typical history with acute, subacute, chronic, or relapsing-remitting history. Minor criteria include (1) periodic complexes on electroencephalogram; (2) increased cerebrospinal fluid IgG; (3) brain biopsy with measles antigen or measles genotype; and (4) identification of the genome with a molecular diagnostic test.[251] There is no curative treatment.[251] Ribavirin has in vitro activity against measles but no clinical data to support its use.

Vaccination with the measles, mumps, and rubella (MMR) vaccine and infection prevention with airborne precautions are important measures to prevent and control outbreaks.

Respiratory Syncytial Virus

Respiratory syncytial virus (RSV) is a seasonal paramyxovirus that is a common cause of lower respiratory infection, such as pneumonia and bronchiolitis in children; RSV mostly causes upper respiratory infections like a "common cold" in healthy adults but more complicated lower respiratory tract infections in the elderly, in patients with underlying cardiopulmonary disease, and in the immunocompromised.[253,254] Infection is usually self-limited but can be associated with airway reactivity. Diagnosis is via rapid antigen testing, PCR, or culture of respiratory secretions. Treatment is primarily supportive, though there are some limited data for the use of inhaled ribavirin and immunotherapy with IVIG or palivizumab in immunocompromised patients with severe infection.

Parainfluenza

This group of paramyxoviruses is also seasonal, with certain serotypes occurring throughout the year. Parainfluenza mostly causes self-limited URI in healthy adults but can cause complicated lower respiratory tract infections in immunocompromised patients, particularly patients with leukemia, stem cell transplant recipients, and organ transplant recipients.[255,256] Diagnosis is predominantly from viral culture or antigen detection, but PCR of respiratory secretions is the most sensitive test. Treatment is largely supportive and, if applicable, involves reduction of immunosuppression.

Influenza

Influenza viruses are orthomyxoviruses, with influenza A and B causing most infections. Influenza has hemagglutinin (H) and neuraminidase (N) surface proteins. Different strains of these proteins are used to categorize influenza A into further subtypes. Point mutations in these receptor proteins allow the virus to avoid neutralization by antibodies and cause "antigenic drift." Reassortment of genomic segments of influenza A viruses from mammalian hosts and avian reservoirs can lead to "antigenic shifts," which can lead to pandemic influenza. Influenza B can undergo antigenic drift but not antigenic shift, as it is almost exclusively found in humans. Uncomplicated influenza is a self-limited febrile illness with cough, URI symptoms, malaise, and myalgias. Influenza can be complicated by lower respiratory tract infection from influenza itself or a secondary bacterial infection, most commonly with pneumococcus or *S aureus*. Nonpulmonary complications of influenza include myositis, myocarditis, pericarditis, encephalitis, transverse myelitis, Guillain-Barré syndrome, toxic shock syndrome, and complications in pregnant women, such as fetal loss, preterm labor, and neural tube defects. Complications and mortality are higher in patients with cardiovascular disease, pulmonary disease, chronic renal disease, immunocompromised states, hemoglobinopathies, morbid obesity, neurologic conditions, and pregnancy.[257-261] Diagnostic tests include rapid antigen tests (DFA), real-time PCR, and viral culture.[257-259] Rapid antigen tests have a sensitivity of 62.3% and a specificity of 98.2%.[257] Polymerase chain reaction has a higher sensitivity and specificity and is the diagnostic test of choice. There are 2 classes of antiviral medications: neuraminidase inhibitors, such as oseltamivir, zanamivir, and peramivir, which are active against influenza A and B, and adamantanes, such as amantadine and rimantadine, which are active only against influenza A.[257-261] The benefits of treatment include decreased duration of symptoms, length of hospitalization, and mortality. Efficacy is better if antiviral treatment is given within 48 hours of onset of symptoms, but treatment with neuraminidase inhibitors in patients with complicated influenza can be beneficial if given within 5 days of symptom onset. The patients at risk of complications as previously noted, especially pregnant women, should be offered treatment even if they present more than 48 hours from symptom onset. Oseltamivir or zanamivir are the recommended antiviral for treatment.

Polyomaviruses

BK polyomavirus is asymptomatic during childhood and becomes latent in the kidney. Decreased cellular immunity leads to reactivation, causing nephropathy and ureteric stenosis in kidney transplant recipients or hemorrhagic cystitis in stem cell transplant recipients.[262-265] Treatment primarily involves decreasing immunosuppression. JC polyomavirus causes progressive multifocal leukoencephalopathy (PML), a demyelinating disease of the CNS white matter with neurologic deficits, depending on the area of demyelination. Progressive multifocal leukoencephalopathy has most often been associated with AIDS but is now being seen in patients who receive immunomodulatory therapies such as natalizumab. Treatment for PML in patients with HIV is antiretroviral therapy.[266]

Cystoisospora belli

Cystoisospora belli, formerly known as *Isospora belli*, is an opportunistic unicellular protozoan that attacks the intestinal epithelium. It causes a watery diarrheal illness sometimes associated with acalculous cholecystitis and, in HIV patients, reactive arthritis.[267-270] Infection in immunocompetent hosts is largely self-limited. Diagnosis involves detection of thin-walled, ellipsoidal oocysts in the stool. Treatment is trimethoprim-sulfamethoxazole.[271,272] The alternative treatment is ciprofloxacin, pyrimethamine, and nitazoxanide.[273-275] Patients with HIV should be promptly started on ARVs and should be kept on prophylactic trimethoprim-sulfamethoxazole.

Cryptosporidium parvum

Cryptosporidium is an intracellular protozoan that causes a gastrointestinal infection that is usually mild and self-limited in immunocompetent hosts but causes severe, prolonged diarrheal illness in patients with HIV. Other complications of cryptosporidiosis in HIV include cholecystitis, cholangitis, hepatitis, pancreatitis, and respiratory tract involvement.[276-278] Transmission is the fecal-oral route from contaminated water or food or person-to-person transmission. Diagnosis is by microscopic identification of oocysts, usually using modified acid-fast staining, although enzyme immunoassays and PCR are also available. Nitazoxanide and paromomycin have activity against *Cryptosporidium*, but prompt initiation of ARVs is crucial for patients with HIV.[279-281]

Microsporidia

Microsporidia are unicellular parasites previously classified as protozoa but now considered fungi. There are several species in this order. *Enterocytozoon bieneusi* is the most common and can lead to diarrhea, cholangitis, or calculous cholecystitis.[282] *Encephalitozoon Hellem or intestinalis*, *E cuniculi*, and *Trachipleistophora* causes keratoconjunctivitis, encephalitis, upper and lower respiratory tract disease, nephritis, cystitis, prostatitis, hepatitis, and peritonitis.[283,284] Infections are usually self-limited in immunocompetent hosts. Infection in HIV patients is less common with the introduction of ARVs. Diagnostic evaluation is via microscopic detection via modified trichrome stain, calcofluor white stain, or indirect immunofluorescent stain.[285] Treatment is albendazole except for *E bieneusi*, which is treated with systemic fumagillin.[286-289] Ocular involvement is treated with topical fumagillin, with or without concomitant albendazole, or topical voriconazole.

Amebic Central Nervous System Infections

The genera of free-living environmental ameba that cause human CNS infection are *Naegleria*, *Acanthamoeba*, *Balamuthia*, and *Sappinia*. *Acanthamoeba* and *B mandrillaris* have also been shown to cause skin infections and disseminated infection in patients with transplants or AIDS.[290-292] *Acanthamoeba* is also associated with keratitis in contact lens wearers.[291]

Granulomatous Amebic Encephalitis

Granulomatous amebic encephalitis (GAE) is a subacute to chronic infection caused by *Acanthamoeba*, *B mandrillaris*, and *S pedata*, with *Acanthamoeba* species being the most common pathogens. Granulomatous amebic encephalitis is mostly seen in patients with predisposing conditions such as alcoholism, cirrhosis, HIV, diabetes, chronic renal failure, systemic lupus, malignancy, and stem cell transplant. Symptoms include headache, fever, visual abnormalities, behavioral changes, and neurologic deficits. *Balamuthia* CNS infection may be preceded by a skin lesion. Cerebrospinal fluid will show pleocytosis with lymphocyte predominance, high protein, and low or normal glucose. Trophozoites may be seen in cerebrospinal fluid, but brain biopsy is needed for diagnosis. Treatment is unclear but is often with combination therapy and, if possible, surgical resection. *Acanthamoeba* is usually treated with a combination of antimicrobials that include fluconazole, pentamidine, and miltefosine with or without additional medications such as met-ronidazole, macrolide, or trimethoprim-sulfamethoxazole.[290-293] There is limited experience for treating *B mandrillaris*; the cases reported have used a combination of pentamidine, flucytosine, fluconazole, macrolide, and one of the of following: sulfadiazine, miltefosine, thioridazine, or liposomal amphotericin B.[290,293]

Primary Amebic Meningoencephalitis

Primary amebic meningoencephalitis (PAM) is caused by *N fowleri* after exposure to recreational fresh water. Presenta-tion is an acute meningoencephalitis, characterized by fever, headaches, photophobia, nausea, vomiting, behavioral distur-bances, and seizures. The infection progresses quickly, with altered mental status and increased cranial hypertension lead-ing to herniation and death. Imaging can show cerebral edema, meningeal enhancement, and brain lesions. The cerebrospinal fluid studies show significant pleocytosis with PMN predomi-nance, low glucose, elevated protein, and cerebrospinal fluid red blood cells; cerebrospinal fluid can become hemorrhagic with progression.[290] Mortality is very high. Diagnosis is estab-lished with visualization of trophozoites on cerebrospinal fluid or brain biopsy. Amphotericin B deoxycholate has the best in vitro activity but optimal treatment is unclear. Amphotericin B deoxycholate can be given in combination with rifampin, fluconazole, miltefosine, or azithromycin.[290,293]

Toxoplasma

Toxoplasma is a genus of intracellular parasites that can be acquired from ingestion of infected meat, exposure to oocysts in cat feces, or transmission by the maternal-fetal route.[294-297] Cats are the definitive host in which the parasite can complete its life cycle, but other animals ingest the oocysts and develop latent tissue infection. Consumption of undercooked meat is the most common form of transmission. Symptoms of acute infection in immunocompetent patients are usually mild, with fever, chills, lymphadenopathy, myalgias, pharyngitis, hepato-splenomegaly, and rash. Pneumonitis, pericarditis, polymyosi-tis, uveitis, and encephalitis are rare manifestations. Diagnosis of acute infection is usually with serologies. Central nervous system toxoplasmosis is a reactivated infection seen in HIV-infected patients with a CD4 count below 100 cells/μL. Patients usually present with fever, headache, and neurologic symptoms. Imaging reveals multiple ring-enhancing brain lesions. Diag-nosis is usually based on clinical presentation, imaging, and a positive serum *Toxoplasma* IgG. Patients are usually started on empiric treatment. Recommended first-line therapy is pyri-methamine with leucovorin (to prevent hematologic toxicity from pyrimethamine) and sulfadiazine; alternative regimens include trimethoprim-sulfamethoxazole or, in patients with sulfa allergies, clindamycin, pyrimethamine, and leucovorin.[298]

Leishmania

Leishmaniasis is a parasitic infection caused by *Leishmania* sand flies. Forms of infection include cutaneous leishmani-asis, presenting with skin sores, and visceral leishmaniasis

with internal organ involvement, most often the spleen, liver, and bone marrow. Cutaneous leishmaniasis is further catego-rized based on the number and severity of lesions, mucosal involvement, species causing infection, and whether or not the patient is immunosuppressed; uncomplicated cutane-ous disease can be treated locally, whereas more complicated infection warrants systemic therapy.[299] Diagnosis is usually by visualization of the parasite on tissue specimen, culture, or PCR.[300] Treatment for cutaneous leishmaniasis not at risk for mucocutaneous spread includes local therapy with cryo-therapy, thermotherapy, topical paromomycin, and photo-dynamic therapy.[299] Systemic oral therapy options include ketoconazole and fluconazole; parenteral therapy available in the United States is primarily formulations of amphotericin but pentavalent antimony is the traditional therapy.[299] Visceral leishmaniasis presents with fever, weight loss, malaise, mas-sive hepatosplenomegaly, and pancytopenia. Diagnosis can be made when the intracellular amastigotes are seen in the bone marrow or on splenic aspirates. Treatment for visceral leish-maniasis in the United States is with amphotericin B, but pen-tavalent antimony is the traditional treatment.[299]

Trypanosoma cruzi

Trypanosoma cruzi is a protozoan parasite spread via triato-mine or reduviid bugs that is the cause of Chagas disease.[301] *Trypanosoma cruzi* is mostly seen in Mexico and Central and South America. The acute phase of Chagas disease can last for weeks to months with parasitemia. Patients may be asymp-tomatic or have nonspecific symptoms of fever and malaise, but some patients will develop local inflammation and swell-ing at the site of inoculation, known as a chagoma.[302] The chronic phase of infection may be asymptomatic, but patients can develop cardiac and gastrointestinal complications years to decades later.[301] Cardiac disease can include conduction abnormalities and dilated cardiomyopathy. Gastrointestinal involvement is due to destruction of intramural neurons caus-ing achalasia, megaesophagus, constipation, and megacolon. These complications are almost exclusively seen in patients who acquire *T cruzi* in the southern cone of South America. In the chronic phase, serologic tests are used for diagnosis. Treat-ment is management of the complications. Benznidazole and nifurtimox are the effective antitrypanosomal therapy and can only be obtained through the Center for Disease Control.[301]

Strongyloides

Strongyloides stercoralis is a roundworm or nematode found in the soil, generally in rural areas of all continents, including the southeastern United States.[303-311] Infection occurs when skin is exposed to contaminated soil. Larvae migrate through the skin, spread through the bloodstream into the lungs, and are swal-lowed into the GI tract where they mature into adult worms. Patients can develop cutaneous reactions, usually in the feet, with larval penetration. Migration of the larvae through the lungs can cause cough, wheezing, and transient infiltrates that present as recurrent pneumonia. Worms in the GI tract can cause abdominal pain, nausea, vomiting, and diarrhea. *Strongyloides* hyperinfection syndrome (SHS) can occur due to autoinfection with high parasite burden. Hyperinfection syndrome is more common in immunocompromised hosts, such as patients on steroids or immunosuppression, human T-cell lymphotropic virus-1 (HTLV-1) infection, malignancies, or malnutrition. Common symptoms include fever, cough, wheezing, nausea, vomiting, abdominal pain, diarrhea, and anorexia. Other findings can include recurrent Gram-negative sepsis, pulmonary infiltrates, and eosinophilia. Because of the risk of *Strongyloides* hyperinfection in organ transplant, recipients and donors with appropriate exposure history should be screened with serum *Strongyloides* IgG. Recipients should receive prophylaxis with ivermectin at the time of transplant. Diagnosis is usually by examination of stool for ova and parasites; sensitivity is low for 1 stool specimen but diagnostic yield increases with multiple stool ova and parasites tests. *Strongyloides* serologies by enzyme-linked immunosorbent assay (ELISA) testing for IgG can be helpful in immunocompetent hosts. Evidence of strongyloidiasis is also sometimes found on endoscopic evaluation. Ivermectin is the treatment of choice; albendazole is an alternative agent.

QUESTIONS

1. A 50-year-old HIV-positive man presents to the emergency department (ED) with complaints of headache, fever (100.4–101.3°F) and confusion for the past 10 days. His physical examination is normal except for a decreased performance on mini–mental status examination. His chest radiograph and CT show right lower lobe consolidation and large pleural effusion. His labs show the following:

WBC	$14 \times 10^3/\mu L$
Hemoglobin	13 g/dL
Platelets	$300 \times 10^3/\mu L$
Sodium	145 mEq/L
Potassium	4 mEq/L
Chloride	110 mEq/L
CO$_2$	26 mEq/L
Blood urea nitrogen	30 mg/dL
Creatinine	1.6 mg/dL
Calcium	8 mg/dL
Glucose	100 mg/dL
Lactic acid	3 mmol/L

The patient proceeds to have a thoracentesis, which showed the following:

Protein	40 g/L
Glucose	20 mg/dL
LDH	188 IU/L
Cell count	470 /μL
Pleural adenosine deaminase	35 IU/L

Pleural fluid stained with India ink is positive for *Cryptococcus*. What is the next step?

A. Fluconazole
B. Lumbar puncture
C. Serial serum *Cryptococcus* antigen
D. CT head

2. A 65-year-old woman, a farmer from south Ohio, presents with low-grade fever, dry cough, and chest pain for 4 months. Physical examination reveals a temperature of 102.5°F. A chest radiograph reveals an apical consolidation with cavities in the right upper lobe. Her lung biopsy, shown below, depicted organisms within macrophages that stained positive with Gomori methenamine silver (GMS) (Fig. 20-2). What is the most likely diagnosis?

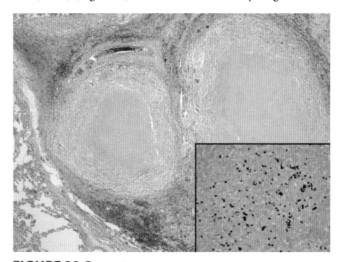

FIGURE 20-2 Lung biopsy.

A. Histoplasmosis
B. *Pneumocystis jirovecii* pneumonia
C. Blastomycosis
D. Toxoplasmosis

3. Which of the following laboratory test provides a rapid and accurate diagnosis for the patient in question 2?

A. Histopathology
B. Serology (complement fixation antibody tests)
C. Antigen detection in urine and serum
D. PCR assay

4. A 45-year-old homeless man was found unresponsive in a park and was brought to the emergency department by emergency medical services (EMS). His vital signs were stabilized after intravenous rehydration. HIV testing was positive for HIV-1. An MRI scan of the brain showed an ill-defined enhancing lesion in the left basal ganglia. There was extensive surrounding edema and a thick enhancing wall. The lesion was biopsied and a microscopic appearance of biopsy is shown in Figure 20-3. What is the most likely diagnosis?

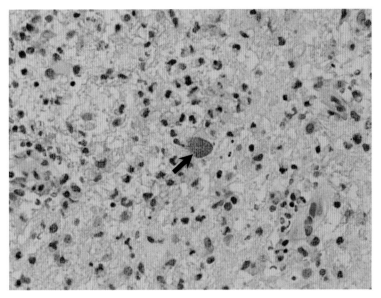

FIGURE 20-3 Brain biopsy.

A. Toxoplasmosis
B. Lymphoma
C. Brain abscess
D. Herpes simplex encephalitis

5. For the patient in question 4, which of following statement is true regarding his condition?

A. Immunocompetent individuals rarely get infected by this organism.
B. Humans are the definitive host of this organism.
C. Negative IgG serology to the organism definitively excludes this condition.
D. Empiric therapy should be started in HIV-infected patients with ring-enhancing lesions on MRI

6. A 45-year-old HIV-positive man presented to the ED with a 1-week history of shortness of breath. He also had a 2-month history of productive cough, night sweats, and fatigue. Physical examination revealed right cervical lymphadenopathy. His CD4 count was 43 cells/μL. A CT scan of his chest revealed moderate left pleural effusion with near-complete compressive atelectasis of the left lower lobe. Several solid nodules were seen scattered throughout both upper lobes; the largest measured 0.5 cm in greatest diameter. Microscopic appearance of the cervical lymph node biopsy is depicted in Figure 20-4.

Which of the following conditions does this patent have?

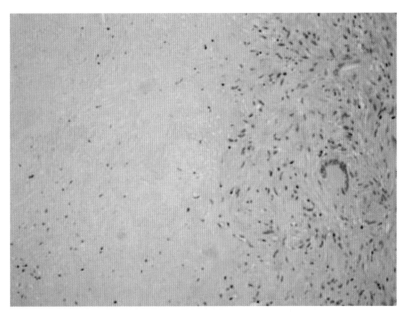

FIGURE 20-4 Cervical lymph node biopsy.

A. *Pneumocystis jirovecii* pneumonia
B. Tuberculous lymphadenitis
C. Acute suppurative lymphadenitis
D. Non-Hodgkin lymphoma

7. A 55-year-old man with recently diagnosed HIV was complaining of shortness of breath. Patient was found to have large right-sided pleural effusion. He had diagnostic and therapeutic thoracentesis. Pleural studies reveal show exudative characteristics and the pleural adenosine deaminase was elevated. Treatment was started. Two weeks later, he was readmitted to the ED 4 weeks later with recurrent fevers. His chest radiograph now reveals intrathoracic lymphadenopathy and worsening lung infiltrates. At this time, the cultures from the pleural fluid grew pan-sensitive tuberculous mycobacterium. CD4 count has increased from 50 cells/uL to 200 cells/uL. Which of the following is the most likely diagnosis?

A. Drug-resistant organism
B. Non-Hodgkin' lymphoma
C. Immune reconstitution inflammatory syndrome
D. Medication toxicity

8. A 62-year-old woman presented with fever, cough, and dyspnea. She has non-Hodgkin lymphoma for which she is receiving systemic chemotherapy. She was noted to be hypoxic to 80% on room air with diffuse crackles on auscultation. She was given supplemental oxygen via nasal cannula and her oxygen saturation improved to 95%. A chest radiograph revealed diffuse interstitial thickening with ground-glass opacities involving both lungs. A microscopic appearance of her transbronchial biopsy specimen is depicted below (Fig. 20-5).

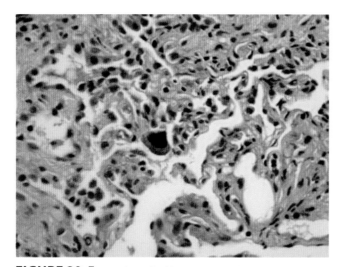

FIGURE 20-5 Transbronchial biopsy. (Reproduced with permission from Mannan A, Yuan S. Chapter 26: Pulmonary Pathology. In *Go R: Pulmonary Disease Examination and Board Review.* NY: McGraw-Hill, 2016.)

Which of the following is the most appropriate therapy for this patient?

A. Acyclovir
B. Amantadine
C. Ganciclovir
D. Lamivudine

9. A 28-year-old woman (gravida 1, para 0) at 32+4-weeks' gestation presented to the ED with 2 days' history of chill, fever, nausea, dysuria, and increased frequency of urination. She also complained of right-side back pain for 1 day. Her medical history was unremarkable. At presentation, her vital signs were as follows: BP of 110/80 mmHg, HR of 110 beats/min, RR of 28 breaths/min, and temperature of 101.8°F. Blood test results showed a leukocytosis of $21 \times 10^3/\mu L$. The urine sediment contained 25 leucocytes, 5 erythrocytes, and 4+ bacteria per high-power field. Which of the following is the most likely organism cultured from her urine or blood?

A. Group A *Streptococcus*
B. *Staphylococcus aureus*
C. *Pseudomonas aeruginosa*
D. *Escherichia coli*

10. A 65-year-old man with recently diagnosed leukemia is complaining of fever and sinus pain for the past 2 days. The patient is given a bolus of normal saline as well as vancomycin and cefepime. He is admitted to the hospital for febrile neutropenia after cultures are drawn. Twelve hours later, he becomes diaphoretic and hypotensive.

His vital signs are as follows: BP of 84/42 mmHg, HR of 122 beats/min, RR of 28 breaths/min, and O_2 sat of 94% on 4 L/min via nasal cannula. His physical examination is otherwise unremarkable except for sinus tenderness on palpation. His labs show the following:

WBC	$0.4 \times 10^3/\mu L$
Hemoglobin	7.1 g/dL
Platelets	$62 \times 10^3/\mu L$
Sodium	142 mEq/L
Potassium	4 mEq/L
Chloride	109 mEq/L
CO$_2$	18 mEq/L
Blood urea nitrogen	22 mg/dL
Creatinine	1.3 mg/dL (baseline creatinine 0.8 mg/dL)
Glucose	122 mg/dL
Lactic acid	4.2 mmol/L

The CT of his sinuses is seen below, and after he was stabilized, he proceeded to a biopsy (Fig. 20-6A and B). What is the initial treatment?

A. Posaconazole
B. Caspofungin
C. Amphotericin B
D. Voriconazole

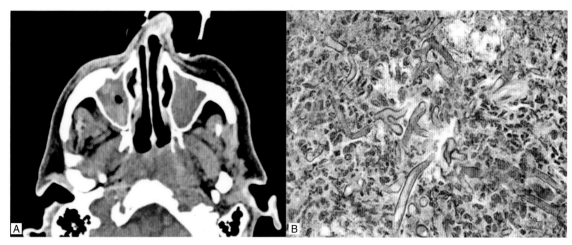

FIGURE 20-6 (A) CT of sinuses. (B) Sinus biopsy.

11. A 50-year-old man presents with cough and shortness of breath for 3 days. On admission, he is found to be febrile at 101.1°F and his oxygen saturation is 80% on room air. He is started on high-flow nasal cannula at 80% fraction of inspired oxygen Fio₂ and at 50 L/min and is currently being cared for in the intensive care unit. His past medical history includes kidney transplant 3 years ago and diabetes mellitus. His home medications include mycophenolate, tacrolimus, voriconazole, and prednisone. He is currently being treated with vancomycin and piperacillin-tazobactam. On examination, he appears lethargic and is oriented to person only. There are decreased breath sounds at the right upper lobe. He is intubated within a few hours for worsening hypoxia and altered mental status. His MRI brain shows multiple enhancing lesions. Bronchoscopy and BAL are performed. Transbronchial biopsies show weakly acid fast filamentous organism that branches in less than 90 degrees (Fig. 20-7).

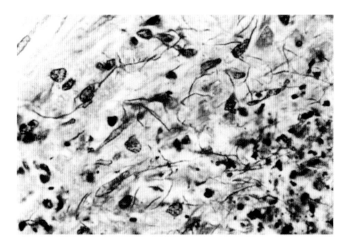

FIGURE 20-7 Sputum stain with modified weak acid fast method. (Reproduced with permission from Connor DH, Chandler FW, Schwartz DQ, et al. *Pathology of Infectious Diseases*. Stamford CT: Appleton & Lange, 1997.)

What is the next step?

A. Add a dose of aminoglycoside for double Gram-negative coverage
B. Discontinue current antibiotics and start the patient on trimethoprim-sulfamethoxazole
C. Discontinue current antibiotics and start the patient on amphotericin B
D. Continue current antibiotics, as they are sufficient to cover the organism

12. A 61-year-old woman with a history of asthma and recent admission for pneumonia now presents with 4 months of progressive dyspnea on exertion and weight loss. The patient complains of dysphagia and odynophagia. The exam reveals a chronically ill–appearing woman with notable findings of thrush in her oropharynx. She agreed to HIV testing; rapid HIV-1 test was positive with a CD4 count of 5 cells/μL. Her arterial blood gas reveals a Pao₂ of 65 mmHg. In addition to starting the patient on treatment for healthcare-associated pneumonia, what else would you like to start?

A. Trimethoprim-sulfamethoxazole
B. Trimethoprim-sulfamethoxazole plus prednisone
C. Atovaquone
D. Dapsone

13. A 22-year-old man with no past medical history presents to the ED with palpitations and presyncope in August. He had a recent febrile illness in early July after a hiking trip in Wisconsin in mid-June; he developed mild muscle aches and noted an erythematous rash with central clearing on his right thigh. His rash resolved, but the patient has been having some joint pain and headaches. He now presents after an episode of lightheadedness and diaphoresis during a concert. In the ED, vitals are remarkable for bradycardia. His ECG shows a first degree AV block. The patient is admitted to the telemetry unit and work up is sent. What is the most appropriate next step?

A. Echocardiogram
B. Emergent pacemaker placement
C. Initiation of doxycycline
D. Initiation of ceftriaxone

14. A 28-year-old woman with recent travel to Ghana is now presenting with several days of fevers, myalgias, dyspnea on exertion, and abdominal pain. She notes a mild headache but is alert and oriented. Temperature in the emergency room is 38.4°C, her HR is 140 beats/min, and her BP is 102/50 mmHg. She is pale and tired appearing, and her neurological exam is unremarkable. Her labs show a hemoglobin of 5 g/dL and creatinine of 1.5 mg/dL. A blood parasite smear shows *P falciparum* with 15% parasitemia. Blood films are seen below (Fig. 20-8).
The patient should be admitted and started on which of the following?

A. Atovaquone/proguanil
B. Artesunate IV
C. Chloroquine
D. Doxycycline

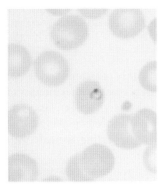

FIGURE 20-8 Blood films young and old trophozites of *P. falciparum.* (Reprinted from Bench. *Aids for the Diagnosis of Malaria Infections,* 2nd ed. © 2000 World Health Organization. http://www.who.int/malaria/publications/atoz/9241545240/en/)

15. A 56-year-old woman with prior deceased donor liver transplant for Hepatitis C Cirrhosis and hepatocellular carcinoma complains of abdominal pain and fever. She had received her liver from a 40-year-old donor from rural Ghana and was taking prophylactic trimethoprim-sulfamethoxazole and valganciclovir as well as tacrolimus, mycophenolate mofetil, and prednisone. Initial imaging including chest x-ray and abdominal x-ray were unremarkable. The patient developed Gram-negative bacteremia and initially improved with antibiotics, but she developed dyspnea and cough 6 days into her hospitalization. Her chest x-ray showed patchy infiltrates. The wet mount of the bronchoalveolar lavage is shown in Figure 20-9.

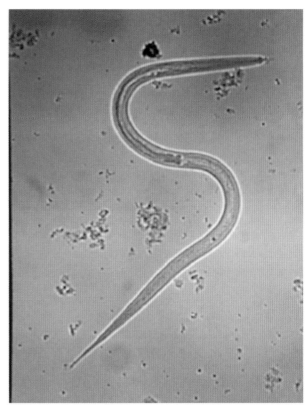

FIGURE 20-9 Wet mount of bronchoalveolar lavage. (Source: Public Health Image Library, Centers for Disease Control and Prevention.)

This organism is best treated with which of the following?

A. Thiabendazole
B. Praziquantel
C. Ivermectin
D. Nitazoxanide

16. A 36-year-old woman donated blood and was found to have positive serologies for *T cruzi.* She was originally born and raised in Mexico but has lived in New York State for 15 years. She is feeling well and has no complaints. She is afebrile with an unremarkable exam. What other study should be done to evaluate this patient?

A. *T cruzi* PCR to test for parasitemia
B. Electrocardiogram with a 30-second rhythm strip
C. Echocardiogram
D. Barium swallow study

17. A 43-year-old woman presented to the ED with cough with purulent sputum, wheeze, and dyspnea for 5 days' duration. She had rheumatoid arthritis for 8 years and was taking prednisone and azathioprine for last 2 months. On physical examination, her temperature was 99.8°F with no alterations on pulmonary auscultation. A chest CT image and a microscopic appearance of wedge biopsy with GMS stain are shown here (Fig. 20-10).

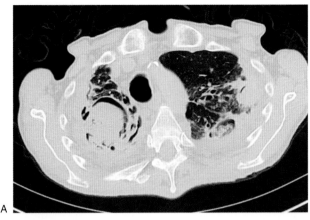

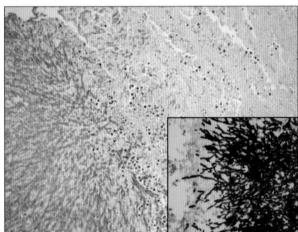

FIGURE 20-10 (A) CT chest. (B) Lung biopsy.

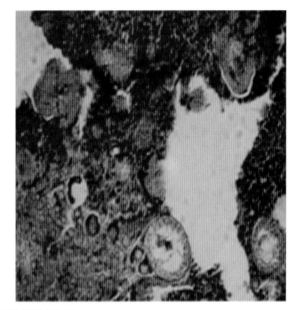

FIGURE 20-11 Lung biopsy of pulmonary nodules. (Reproduced with permission from Medical mycology. In: Carroll KC, Hobden JA, Miller S, et al., eds. *Jawetz, Melnick, & Adelberg's Medical Microbiology.* 27th ed. New York, NY: McGraw-Hill; 2016.)

Which condition is probably present in her lungs?

A. Acute invasive aspergillosis
B. *Candida* pneumonia
C. Pulmonary zygomycosis
D. Pulmonary histoplasmosis

18. A 35-year-old man presented with cough and fever for 5 days. Chest x-ray revealed multiple nodules in right lung. A biopsy specimen revealed changes as depicted in the image in Figure 20-11.

Which of the following statements is *not* true about the disease?

A. The disease is endemic in southwestern United States.
B. Disseminated disease is more prevalent in Filipinos.
C. The disease is caused by a protozoan.
D. Gomori methenamine silver stain can be used to demonstrate the organism.

19. A 20-year-old previously healthy man presented to the ED with a 2-day history of severe headache, stiff neck, and fever. He had just returned from Florida, where he had been swimming and wakeboarding at a local lake several days ago. A CT scan of the head without contrast was normal. A cerebrospinal fluid analysis indicated hypoglycorrhachia, elevated protein level, and neutrophilic pleocytosis. Gram-stain results were negative for bacteria, but wet preparation of cerebrospinal fluid showed motile parasites. Despite intensive treatment, the patient died after 4 days of admission. Which of the follow infections is this patient most likely to have?

A. *Trypanosoma brucei*
B. *Naegleria fowleri*
C. *Cryptococcus neoformans*
D. *Entamoeba histolytica*

20. A 43-year-old HIV-positive man presented to the ED with a 6-day history of crampy abdominal pain, watery diarrhea, and weakness. He had up to 10 watery bowel movements a day, without blood or mucus. On examination, he was afebrile with blood pressure of 80/50 mmHg. He was conservatively managed. An upper GI endoscopy was performed on his second day of admission. Stains of the patient's stool is seen in Figure 20-12.

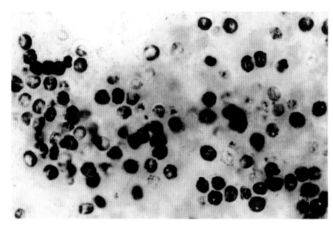

FIGURE 20-12 Acid fast stain of the patient's feces. (Reproduced with permission from Nester EW. *Microbiology: A Human Perspective*, 6th edition. NY:McGraw-Hill, 2009.)

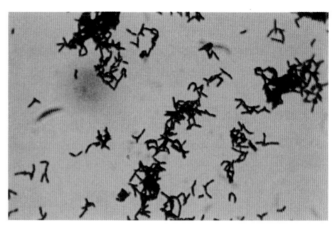

FIGURE 20-13 Sputum culture. Actinomyces and nocardia. (Reproduced with permission from Willey JM: *Prescott, Harley, & Klein's Microbiology*, 7th edition. McGraw-Hill, 2008.)

Which of the following infections is this patient most likely to have?

A. *Cystoisospora belli*
B. *Strongyloides stercoralis*
C. *Cryptosporidium parvum*
D. *Microsporidium*

21. A 63-year-old previously healthy man presented to the ED with a 5-day history of intermittent episodes of severe left flank and back burning pain accompanied by headache and malaise. Physical examination revealed an erythematous maculopapular rash with vesicles on the left side of the patient's back and chest wall. All vital signs were within normal limits. Which of the following would you consider relevant in his past history?

A. Rubella
B. Rubeola (measles)
C. Chickenpox
D. Infectious mononucleosis

22. A 60 year old man with history of alcohol abuse was intubated for acute respiratory failure secondary to pneumonia. He was noted to have poor dentition. Chest radiograph shows right middle and lower lobe consolidation. The sputum culture grows Gram-positive bacilli nonacid fast that branch in acute angels in microaerophillic conditions with sulfur granules (Fig. 20-13). What would be the appropriate antibiotic?

A. Penicillin G
B. Clindamycin
C. Erythromycin
D. Metronidazole

ANSWERS

1. D. CT head

   The patient has been diagnosed with pulmonary *Cryptococcus*. This fungus has a penchant for dissemination into the central nervous system, manifesting usually as meningoencephalitis and, in rare instances, as brain abscess. A CT head would be the appropriate initial step in patients who are immunocompromised and have CNS symptoms. This is followed by lumbar puncture (choice B) for evaluation of opening pressure as a surrogate to intracranial pressure and to obtain specimen for cerebrospinal fluid culture. Lumbar puncture may be repeated 2 weeks after induction therapy to determine whether pressures have improved and cerebrospinal fluid culture is cleared from *Cryptococcus*. Initial treatment is amphotericin B with flucytosine, due to its better penetration to the blood–brain barrier, for 2 weeks, followed by consolidation treatment with fluconazole (choice A) for 8 weeks. Serial *Cryptococcus* antigen (choice C) is only indicated when maintenance therapy is being discontinued. An initial serum or cerebrospinal fluid cryptococcal antigen might be useful if the diagnosis is not confirmed, since cultures can be falsely negative and/or take time to become positive.

2. A. Histoplasmosis

   Histoplasmosis (choice A) is caused by *Histoplasma capsulatum*, a dimorphic fungus that can be identified on hematoxylin-eosin sections as numerous intracellular yeasts within histiocytes measuring 2 to 4 µm. The biopsy confirmed the diagnosis of chronic pulmonary histoplasmosis. The natural habitat of *Histoplasma* is soil-containing feces of chickens, other birds, and bats.[312,313] Caves are frequently contaminated with *Histoplasma*. In the United States, highly endemic areas are the Ohio River and Mississippi River valleys. Primary infection is usually asymptomatic but remains dormant and reactivates as immune status declines. Clinically, 4 forms of histoplasmosis can be recognized: acute pulmonary histoplasmosis, subacute pulmonary histoplasmosis, chronic pulmonary histoplasmosis, and disseminated histoplasmosis. Disseminated histoplasmosis occurs in severely immunocompromised hosts, especially patients with AIDS, patients with hematologic malignancies, or transplant recipients. It can manifest as a mass lesion and be mistaken for a neoplasm. *Pneumocystis jirovecii* (choice B) does not stain with hematoxylin-eosin and is present mostly extracellularly. Blastomycosis (choice C) is characterized by large yeasts with broad-based budding. Toxoplasma (choice D) is a smaller obligate intracellular protozoan that can infect any parenchymal cell and is usually not seen in macrophages.

3. A. Histopathology

Demonstration of yeast on pathologic examination of tissue and isolation of the mold in culture of clinical specimens remain the gold standards for the laboratory diagnosis of histoplasmosis.[313,314] Histopathology of lung tissue can lead to rapid diagnosis of histoplasmosis. The typical histopathologic findings include caseating granulomas and characteristic budding yeast forms measuring 2 to 4 μm. However, histopathology requires obtaining tissue specimen by invasive procedures, which may not be feasible in critically ill patients or in those with coagulopathies. Serology testing is useful for chronic forms of histoplasmosis, in which circulating antibodies against *Histoplasma* are present. As with other serologic testing, a positive antibody test for *Histoplasma* indicates that the patient was exposed to the fungus at some point in the past (choice B). Serum and urine antigen tests are usually negative for chronic pulmonary histoplasmosis, due to low fungal burden (choice C). Polymerase chain reaction assays have been developed for histoplasmosis but are less sensitive than antigen detection or histopathology (choice D).

4. A. Toxoplasmosis

This patient has cerebral toxoplasmosis caused by *Toxoplasma gondii* (choice A). The histologic image shows large, encysted intracellular bradyzoites of toxoplasma. Central nervous lymphoma shows atypical lymphoid aggregates in a perivascular location (choice B). Brain abscess is characterized by collection of neutrophils (choice C). Herpes simplex encephalitis shows typical intranuclear viral inclusions (choice D).

5. D. Empiric therapy should be started in HIV-infected patients with ring-enhancing lesions on MRI

Toxoplasma gondii is known as one of the most common infectious protozoan parasites that have a worldwide distribution.[315]

Cats are recognized as the only definitive host (choice B). Humans can be infected by ingestion of raw or undercooked meat containing tissue cysts, unwashed vegetables, or contaminated water or soil. In immunocompetent individuals, most *T gondii* infections are subclinical, but severe infections can occur in immunocompromised individuals. An estimated 30% to 50% of HIV-seropositive individuals infected with *T gondii* develop cerebral toxoplasmosis. Toxoplasmosis is the most common cause of focal brain lesions in patients with AIDS and frequently localizes to the basal ganglia, although other sites in the brain and spinal cord may be affected. Multifocal lesions are frequently encountered. The most important differential diagnosis is CNS lymphoma. Brain biopsy showing tachyzoites or cysts provides a definitive diagnosis for cerebral toxoplasmosis. *Toxoplasma gondii* infection is commonly detected by performing serologic studies for anti-*Toxoplasma* antibodies. The serum IgG anti-*Toxoplasma* titer peaks between 1 and 2 months after primary infection and typically remains detectable for the rest of the patient's life. However, negative IgG serology does not definitively exclude toxoplasmosis (choice C), as patients with advanced HIV infection may become seronegative. A combination of pyrimethamine-sulfadiazine and folinic acid is considered the standard regimen for the treatment of toxoplasma encephalitis. Empirical treatment for *T gondii* should be started on patients with multiple ring-enhancing lesions on MRI, positive serology for *Toxoplasma* IgG, and absolute CD4 count less than 200 cells/mm. Immunocompetent individuals can be infected though the presentation is usually subclinical and not a CNS infection (choice A).

6. B. Tuberculous lymphadenitis

The image shows a necrotizing granuloma consisting of clusters of epithelioid macrophages, Langhans giant cells, and characteristic caseous necrosis in the center. An acid-fast stain (Ziehl-Neelsen acid-fast stain) revealed rare organisms as slender red rods. The HIV and TB co-epidemic is a major public health problem in many parts of the world.[316] In 2012, 1.1 million (13%) of the 8.7 million people who developed TB worldwide were HIV positive. HIV infection is estimated to increase the risk of TB 20-fold compared with HIV-seronegative individuals in high HIV prevalence countries.[316] Tuberculosis is a leading killer among people living with HIV. At least 1 in 4 deaths among people living with HIV can be attributed to TB. The increased incidence of TB in HIV-infected individuals can be attributed to 2 mechanisms: increased reactivation of latent TB and increased susceptibility to *M tuberculosis* infection. *Pneumocystis jirovecii* pneumonia (choice A) may be associated with pulmonary nodules but not granulomas. Acute lymphadenitis with abscess (choice C) usually shows neutrophilic infiltrate in the lymph node parenchyma to create abscesses. Non-Hodgkin lymphoma (choice D) is characterized by atypical lymphoid proliferations.

7. C. Immune reconstitution inflammatory syndrome

Immune reconstitution inflammatory syndrome (choice C) is the paradoxical worsening of symptoms and signs of TB after starting ART.[317] Although ART has positive effects through its suppression of the HIV-1 viral load and restoration of CD4+ T-cell numbers, this rapid restoration of the immune system can lead to this undesirable complication. Incidence of IRIS ranges from 8% to 43%. Following ART initiation, patients experience new, recurrent, or worsening features of TB, such as fever, lymph node swelling, serositis, and radiographic deterioration. It is important to note that IRIS is a diagnosis of exclusion. The onset of this syndrome is linked temporally to ART initiation and ART interruption followed by re-initiation. A strong suspicion of IRIS supplemented by the immunological tools of an increasing CD4 T-cell count and decreasing HIV viral load and ruling out other possible causes of clinical worsening will help clinch the diagnosis. The differential diagnosis is complex, including drug toxicity, drug resistance, and opportunistic infections (choices A and D). Non-Hodgkin lymphoma could occur or coexist with TB in HIV and may flare up after ART administration (choice B).

8. C. Ganciclovir

The photomicrograph shows characteristic intranuclear CMV inclusions, which were subsequently confirmed on immunohistochemistry as nuclear and cytoplasmic staining for the viral inclusion. Cytomegalovirus infection is a frequent complication in patients with immunosuppressive states such as in HIV/AIDS, organ transplants, or immunosuppressive therapy. The diagnosis of CMV pneumonia is based on viral culture and pathologic evaluation of lung biopsies or BAL specimens. Cytomegalovirus inclusions are characteristically observed in endothelial cells as nuclear and/or cytoplasmic inclusions. These can be appreciated on hematoxylin-eosin stains as acidophilic "owl-eye" inclusions in the nucleus, while in the cytoplasm, these can be seen as smaller, granular, basophilic inclusions. The first-line drug for therapy of CMV pneumonia is ganciclovir (choice C). Acyclovir is used more for HSV infections (choice A). Amantadine is effective for the treatment of influenza A virus (choice B). Lamivudine is used for the treatment of HIV/AIDS and chronic hepatitis B infection (choice D).

9. D. *Escherichia coli*

Urinary tract infections in pregnant women continue to pose a great challenge for physicians.[318] In about 80% of pregnant women, dilation of the urinary tract combined with mild hydronephrosis is observed. Simultaneously, the enlarged uterus compresses the urinary bladder. Urinary

stasis and impairment of the physiological antireflux mechanism may create favorable conditions for bacterial growth and ascending infection. There is a much higher risk (up to 40%) of progression to pyelonephritis in pregnant women. The pathogens responsible for infections during pregnancy are similar to those in the general population. Most infections are caused by *Escherichia coli* (choice D), which is responsible for 63% to 85% of cases. Other organisms listed in the choices (choices A, B, and C) are relatively infrequent causes of urinary tract infection in pregnant women.

10. C. Amphotericin B

Because of the rhino-orbital-cerebral area, surgical intervention should be sought while antimicrobials are broadened to include antifungal therapy. The patient has mucormycosis, which can appear as right-angle branching hyphae. Amphotericin B is the treatment for mucormycosis.[319] Voriconazole may be the better choice for invasive aspergillosis, which appears as narrow-branching hyphae (choice D). Posaconazole (choice A) is used for refractory or secondary mucormycosis prophylaxis.[319] Mucormycosis is resistant to caspofungin (choice B). Risk factors include hematologic malignancy, solid organ or stem cell transplantation, glucocorticoid treatment, iron overload, trauma, and deferoxamine use.

11. B. Discontinue current antibiotics and start the patient on trimethoprim- sulfamethoxazole

The organism isolated on the blood of this patient is *Nocardia*. It is a branching, weakly acid-fast organism. The branching typically occurs at an angle less than 90 degrees. *Nocardia* infects immunosuppressed patients. The treatment of choice is trimethoprim-sulfamethoxazole (choice B). Isolation of *Nocardia* always warrants treatment; it is not a colonizer organism. *Actinomyces* has characteristic sulfur-like clubs. This is not a fungus, so antifungals such as amphotericin B are not needed (choice C). There is no indication for adding Gram-negative coverage, as this is not a Gram-negative infection (and there is limited data to support double Gram-negative coverage [choice A]). The current antibiotics are not appropriate for this infection, so choice D is wrong.

12. B. Trimethoprim-sulfamethoxazole plus prednisone

This patient has AIDS and a presentation consistent with severe *Pneumocystis jirovecii* pneumonia (PJP). Trimethoprim-sulfamethoxazole is the most effective antibiotic for treating PJP. Atovaquone can be used for treatment of mild infections but not for severe PJP (choice C). Dapsone by itself is used for prophylaxis of PJP, but dapsone must be used in combination with trimethoprim when used to treat PJP and is not recommended for severe PCP (choice D). Steroids should be given with the initiation of antibiotics for patients with moderate to severe disease and hypoxemia as measured by partial pressure of oxygen less than 70 mmHg on room air and/or alveolar-arterial oxygen gradient of 35 mmHg or greater; the use of steroids in these patients have been shown to decrease mortality and respiratory failure.[196-198] Therefore, the correct answer is B, rather than A.

13. **D. Initiation of ceftriaxone**

This patient is presenting with Lyme carditis after a recent trip in the summer to an area where Lyme disease is endemic. His previous febrile illness with a rash is consistent with early Lyme disease causing erythema migrans (EM); early Lyme disease with EM is a clinical diagnosis. Lyme carditis can present several weeks to months later. Although doxycycline is the treatment of choice for Lyme disease, patients who present with neurologic symptoms or advanced heart block should be initiated on parenteral antibiotics with ceftriaxone (choice D).[320] Doxycycline is not an appropriate treatment for Lyme carditis (choice C). Heart block due to Lyme disease resolves with ceftriaxone; although temporary pacemakers may be needed in patients with severe heart block, these can be removed with response to antibiotics (choice B). Although obtaining an echocardiogram may be reasonable, prompt initiation of antibiotics is the most important step in treating symptomatic Lyme carditis (choice A).

14. **B. Artesunate IV**

The World Health Organization definition of severe *P falciparum* malaria is one or more of the following: neurologic involvement with seizures, prostration, impaired consciousness, acute renal failure (creatinine > 3 mg/dL) severe anemia (hemoglobin ≤ 5 g/dL), acute pulmonary edema, hypoglycemia, metabolic acidosis, bleeding, shock, or hyperparasitemia of greater than 10%.[321] This patient meets the definition based on her anemia and hyperparasitemia. The treatment of severe malaria is with IV artesunate; if intravenous artesunate is unavailable, intravenous quinidine in combination with doxycycline, tetracycline, or clindamycin is used for severe malaria. Uncomplicated malaria can be treated with atovaquone/proguanil (Malarone; choice A) or, in cases where there is no concern for chloroquine resistance, chloroquine (choice C), but they are not appropriate for severe malaria. Doxycycline is used in combination with quinidine for severe malaria, but monotherapy (choice D) is not appropriate.

15. **C. Ivermectin**

This patient is presenting with *Strongyloides* hyperinfection syndrome, which is more common in immunocompromised hosts, such as patients on steroids or immunosuppression after organ transplantation. Common symptoms include fever, cough, wheezing, nausea, vomiting, abdominal pain, diarrhea, and anorexia, and presentations can include recurrent Gram-negative sepsis, pulmonary infiltrates, and eosinophilia. Organ transplant recipients and donors with an exposure history should be screened with serum *Strongyloides* IgG. Both thiabendazole (choice A) and ivermectin (choice C) can be used to treat *Strongyloides*, but a randomized trial comparing ivermectin to thiabendazole showed that ivermectin had equal efficacy with much better tolerability and fewer side effects than thiabendazole.[322] Therefore C is the correct answer rather than choice A. Praziquantel (choice B) and nitazoxanide (choice D) will not eradicate this parasite.

16. **B. Electrocardiogram with a 30-second rhythm strip**

Trypanosoma cruzi, the parasite that causes Chagas disease, is endemic to Mexico, Central America, and South America. The acute phase of Chagas disease can last for weeks to months with parasitemia; patients may be asymptomatic or have nonspecific symptoms of fever and malaise, but some patients will develop local inflammation and swelling at the site of inoculation known as a chagoma.[323] The chronic phase of infection is usually asymptomatic but 20% to 30% of chronically infected people can develop cardiac manifestations and gastrointestinal complications years to decades later. In the chronic phase, serologic tests are used for diagnosis. Because parasitemia is low during the chronic phase, PCR testing is not recommended due to its variable sensitivity in the chronic phase (choice A). Cardiac complications of chronic Chagas disease are much more common than gastrointestinal complications; the gastrointestinal complications are almost exclusively seen in patients who acquire infection in the southern cone of South America. Ventricular conduction abnormalities precede onset of cardiac symptoms (choice B). Echocardiogram would be an appropriate step if the patient has symptoms or an abnormal ECG (choice C). This patient does not have any GI symptoms and acquired her infection from Mexico, so a barium swallow is not appropriate (choice D). Antitrypanosomal therapy, benznidazole and nifurtimox, can only be obtained through the Center for Disease Control and is generally considered in patients younger than 50 years of age without evidence of advanced Chagas cardiac disease.

17. **A. Acute invasive aspergillosis**

The computed tomography of the chest shows that the infection surpasses the right-sided mycetoma with involvement of both lung fields. The histologic image shows lung parenchyma with hemorrhagic necrosis. The GMS stain (inset) demonstrates hyphae with septa and branching at 45° angles, characteristic of *Aspergillus* species. Aspergillosis is a major cause of morbidity and mortality in immunocompromised patients.[324] *Aspergillus* species are widespread in the environment and are commonly isolated from soil, plant debris, and indoor environments, including hospitals. The most common portal entry is the respiratory system. *A fumigatus* is the pathogen that is isolated the most often from the lungs of immunocompromised patients and is responsible for fatal invasive aspergillosis. The risk factors for invasive aspergillosis include neutropenia, hematopoietic stem cell transplantation, solid organ transplantation, prolonged therapy with high-dose corticosteroids, advanced AIDS, and chronic granulomatous disease. Invasive aspergillosis is typically angiocentric and produces hemorrhagic infarcts. Voriconazole and amphotericin B remain the mainstays of therapy for patients with invasive aspergillosis. The mortality rate for invasive pulmonary aspergillosis can be 50% to 90%, with respiratory failure and massive hemoptysis as major complications. *Candida* species (choice B) are usually differentiated from other fungal forms by the presence of budding yeast forms and pseudohyphae. The hyphae of *Zygomycetes* and *Aspergillus* are different in tissue section. The hyphae of *Zygomycetes* (choice C) are broad, nonseptate, twisted, or folded, and have a branching pattern with 90° angles. *Histoplasma* (choice D) presents as yeasts and calcifications in the lung.

18. C. The disease is caused by a protozoan.

The image shows spherules characteristically observed in coccidioidomycosis. The disease, also known as San Joaquin Valley fever is endemic in the southwestern United States (choice A). It is caused by dimorphic fungus *Coccidioides immitis*, not a protozoan (choice C).[325] Most infected individuals develop a mild form of the disease. Disseminated coccidioidomycosis occurs in a small fraction of healthy individuals but more commonly in immunocompromised patients, pregnant women, and individuals of certain ethnicities such as Filipinos (choice B), African Americans, Hispanics, and Native Americans. Coccidioidomycosis can affect virtually any organ but is more frequently identified in the lungs. The diagnosis can be made by PCR, serologic studies, culture, or direct identification of the organisms. Histologically, the disease is characterized by granulomatous inflammation. Spherules are 40 to 70 μm in diameter and can be identified in tissue or body fluids. Spherules are filled with daughter cysts and eventually rupture to release endospores. Special stains such as GMS and periodic acid–Schiff are able to highlight the organism in tissue sections (choice D).

19. B. *Naegleria fowleri*

Naegleria fowleri is a free-living, thermophilic ameba that inhabits warm freshwater, such as ponds, lakes, rivers, and hot springs, and rarely infects humans. Infection with *Naegleria fowleri* causes a rapidly progressive, usually fatal primary amebic meningoencephalitis.[326] Primary amebic meningoencephalitis results when ameba-contaminated water incidentally enters the nose, followed by migration of amebae to the brain through the olfactory nerve. Symptoms are indistinguishable from fulminant bacterial meningitis and can include headache, fever, stiff neck, anorexia, vomiting, altered mental status, seizures, and coma. Death typically occurs several days to 2 weeks after the onset of

symptoms. Recognition of PAM depends on clinical suspicion, based on patient history. Only 27% of US cases were diagnosed before death. Cerebrospinal fluid findings mimic those of bacterial meningitis, with a predominantly polymorphonuclear leukocytosis and increased protein and decreased glucose concentration. In suspected PAM patients, a wet mount of CSF should be examined under a microscope immediately after collection for the presence of motile trophozoites. Only 3 survivors of PAM have been documented. Successful therapy appeared to be related to early diagnosis and administration of intravenous and intrathecal amphotericin B with intensive supportive care.

Trypanosoma brucei (choice A) is a unicellular protozoan parasite that causes African trypanosomiasis, the sleeping sickness in Sub-Saharan Africa. *Cryptococcus neoformans* (choice C) is an encapsulated yeast and causes cryptococcal meningitis. *Entamoeba histolytica* (choice D) is a protozoan parasite that may cause brain abscess.

20. C. *Cryptosporidium parvum*

Cryptosporidium species are protozoan parasites that infect a broad range of hosts, including humans, domestic animals, and wild animals.[327] *C parvum* undergoes both asexual (schizogony) and sexual (gametogony) stages of development, and multiplies in a single host (humans, cattle, cat, or dog). Humans acquire infection by ingestion of food and drinks contaminated with feces containing oocysts of the parasite. The sporozoites are released in the small intestine, invade the mucosal cells, and undergo asexual and sexual multiplication. The end product of the sexual multiplication is the formation of the oocysts, which are released in the lumen of the intestine and excreted in the feces. Human cryptosporidiosis is frequently accompanied by abdominal pain, fever, vomiting, malabsorption, and diarrhea that may sometimes be profuse and prolonged. Immunocompetent individuals typically experience self-limiting diarrhea and transient gastroenteritis lasting up to 2 weeks and recover without treatment. Immunocompromised individuals, including HIV/AIDS patients (not treated with antiretroviral therapy), often suffer from intractable diarrhea, which can be fatal. Detection of *Cryptosporidium* in clinical pathology laboratories still is based mainly on microscopic detection via stains and/or fluorescent antibodies (IFA) and other antigenic detection methods. On histology sections, *Cryptosporidium* appears as a spherical structure 2 to 4 μm in diameter attached to the luminal surface of crypts and surface epithelium. Modified acid-fast stain (modified Ziehl-Neelsen) staining is one of the most common differential staining techniques that highlights the organism. *Cystoisospora* (choice A) infection is not as common as infection with *C parvum*. *Cystoisospora belli* infection usually causes a mild and protracted illness in immunocompetent individuals, which may mimic inflammatory bowel disease and irritable bowel syndrome.[328]

Similar to *C parvum*, *C belli* infects the epithelial cells of the small intestine. However, the organism is much larger (up to 30 μm) and appears as ovoid structures with a parasitophorous vacuole in the perinuclear and subnuclear location within the host cells. In contrast, intracellular stages of *C parvum* reside within parasitophorous vacuoles in the microvillous region of the host cell. Microsporidia (choice D) causes intestinal infection in immunocompromised patients (specially AIDS patients) (Fig. 20-14). These appear as small (2- to 3-μm) spherules within the apical cytoplasm of enterocytes. *Strongyloides stercoralis* (choice B) is a parasitic nematode causing strongyloidiasis. Histopathological examination of the duodenal mucosa would show numerous cross sections of adult worms, eggs, and larvae developing in the crypts.

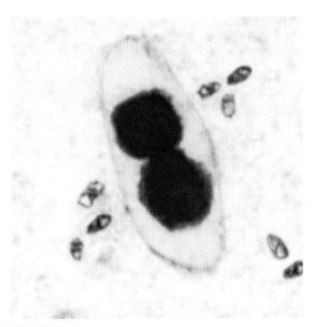

FIGURE 20-14 Large cell is isospora oocyst and small cells are microsporidian spores. (Reprinted with permission from Garcia LS: *J Clin Microbiol.* 2002;40:1892-1901.)

21. C. Chickenpox

Based on the history and physical examination, the patient is diagnosed with herpes zoster infection. Both chickenpox and shingles are caused by the same virus, the varicella-zoster virus.[329] After a person has had chickenpox, the virus rests in the dorsal root ganglia. The virus can remain latent for decades and reactivates following a decrease in virus-specific cell-mediated immunity. The lifetime risk of herpes zoster is estimated to be 10% to 20%. Rubella (choice A), also known as German measles, is an infection caused by the rubella virus. Rubeola (choice B), also known as measles, is a highly contagious infection caused by the measles virus in childhood. Infectious mononucleosis (choice D) is an infection caused by Epstein-Barr virus that predominantly affects adolescents.

22. A. Penicillin G

The patient has *Actinomyces*, Gram-positive rod that branches at acute angles and grows slowly under microaerophilic or strictly anerobic conditions. Characteristic form is the yellow-orange granules or sulfur granules, intertwined within the filaments. Even though clindamycin (choice B) and erythromycin (choice C) are effective, treatment of choice is Penicillin G. Metronidazole (choice D) is not effective.

REFERENCES

1. Mayadas TN, Cullere X, Lowell CA. The multifaceted functions of neutrophils. *Annu Rev Pathol.* 2014;9:181-218.
2. Urban CF, Lourido S, Zychlinsky A. How do microbes evade neutrophil killing? *Cell Microbiol.* 2006;8(11):1687-1696.
3. Freifeld AG, Bow EJ, Sepkowitz KA, et al; Infectious Diseases Society of America. Clinical practice guideline for the use of antimicrobial agents in neutropenic patients with cancer: 2010 update by the Infectious Diseases Society of America. *Clin Infect Dis.* 2011;52(4):e56-e93.
4. Valent P. Low blood counts: immune mediated, idiopathic, or myelodysplasia. *Hematology Am Soc Hematol Educ Program.* 2012;2012:485-491.
5. Shoenfeld Y, Alkan ML, Asaly A, Carmeli Y, Katz M. Benign familial leukopenia and neutropenia in different ethnic groups. *Eur J Haematol.* 1988;41(3):273-277.
6. Smith TJ, Bohlke K1, Lyman GH, et al; American Society of Clinical Oncology. Recommendations for the use of WBC growth factors: American Society of Clinical Oncology Clinical Practice Guideline Update. *J Clin Oncol.* 2005;33(28):3199-3212.
7. Pfeiffer CD, Fine JP, Safdar N. Diagnosis of invasive aspergillosis using a galactomannan assay: a meta-analysis. *Clin Infect Dis.* 2006;42(10):1417-727.
8. Asano-Mori Y, Kanda Y, Oshima K, et al. False-positive Aspergillus galactomannan antigenaemia after haematopoietic stem cell transplantation. *J Antimicrob Chemother.* 2008;61(2):411-416.
9. Odabasi Z, Mattiuzzi G, Estey E, et al. Beta-D-glucan as a diagnostic adjunct for invasive fungal infections: validation, cutoff development, and performance in patients with acute myelogenous leukemia and myelodysplastic syndrome. *Clin Infect Dis.* 2004;39(2):199-205.
10. Ostrosky-Zeichner L, Alexander BD, Kett DH, et al. Multicenter clinical evaluation of the (1–>3) beta-D-glucan assay as an aid to diagnosis of fungal infections in humans. *Clin Infect Dis.* 2005;41(5):654-659.
11. Senn L, Robinson JO, Schmidt S, et al. 1,3-Beta-D-glucan antigenemia for early diagnosis of invasive fungal infections in neutropenic patients with acute leukemia. *Clin Infect Dis.* 2008;46(6):878-885.
12. Herbrecht R, Denning DW, Patterson TF, et al; Invasive Fungal Infections Group of the European Organisation for Research and Treatment of Cancer and the Global Aspergillus Study Group. Voriconazole versus amphotericin b for primary therapy of invasive aspergillosis. *New Engl J Med.* 2002;347(6):408-415.
13. Pappas PG, Kauffman CA, Andes DR, et al. Clinical practice guideline for the management of candidiasis: 2016 update by the Infectious Disease Society of America. *Clin Infect Dis.* 2016;62(4):e1-e50.

14. Mhaskar R, Clark OA, Lyman G, et al. Colony-stimulating factors for chemotherapy-induced febrile neutropenia. *Cochrane Database Syst Rev.* 2014;10:CD003039.

15. Sellberg B, Edwards Jr JE. Type 1/type 2 immunity in infectious diseases. *Clin Infect Dis.* 2001;32(1):76-102.

16. Warrington R, Watson W, Kim HL, Antonetti FR. An introduction to immunology and immunopathology. *Allergy Asthma Clin Immunol.* 2011;7 (Suppl 1):S1-S7.

17. Ram S, Lewis LA, Rice PA. Infections of people with complement deficiencies and patients who have undergone splenectomy. *Clin Microbiol Rev.* 2010;23(4):740-780.

18. Nilsson B, Ekdahl KN. Complement diagnostics: concepts, indications, and practical guidelines. *Clin Dev Immunol.* 2012;2012:962702.

19. Cunningham-Rundles C. The many faces of common variable immunodeficiency. *Hematology Am Soc Hematol Educ Program.* 2012;2012:301-305.

20. Bonilla FA, Khan DA, Ballas ZK, et al. Practice parameter for the diagnosis and management of primary immunodeficiency. *J Allergy Clin Immunol.* 2015;136(5):1186-1205.

21. Notarangelo L, Casanova JL, Fischer A, et al. Primary immunodeficiency diseases: an update. *J Allergy Clin Immunol.* 2004;114:677.

22. Ballow M. Primary immunodeficiency disorders: antibody deficiency. *J Allergy Clin Immunol.* 2002;109(4):581-591.

23. Kainulainen L, Vuorinen T, Rantakokko-Jalava K, Osterback R, Ruuskanen O. Recurrent and persistent respiratory tract viral infections in patients with primary hypogammaglobulinemia. *J Allergy Clin Immunol.* 2010;126(1):120-126.

24. Wood P, Stanworth S, Burton J, et al; UK Primary Immunodeficiency Network. Recognition, clinical diagnosis and management of patients with primary antibody deficiencies: a systematic review. *Clin Exp Immunol.* 2007;149(3):410-423.

25. Agarwal S, Mayer L. Pathogenesis and treatment of gastrointestinal disease in antibody deficiency syndromes. *J Allergy Clin Immunol.* 2009;124(4):658-664.

26. Orange JS, Ballow M, Stiehm ER, et al. Use and interpretation of diagnostic vaccination in primary immunodeficiency: a working group report of the Basic and Clinical Immunology Interest Section of the American Academy of Allergy, Asthma & Immunology. *J Allergy Clin Immunol.* 2012;130(Suppl 3):S1-S24.

27. Green M. Introduction: infections in solid organ transplantation. *Am J Transplant.* 2013;13 (Suppl 4):3-8.

28. Fishman JA, Issa NC. Infection in organ transplantation: risk factors and evolving patterns of infection. *Infect Dis Clin North Am.* 2010;24(2):273-283.

29. Fishman JA, Greenwald MA, Grossi PA. Transmission of infection with human allografts: essential considerations in donor screening. *Clin Infect Dis.* 2012;55(5):720-727.

30. Chong PP, Razonable RR. Diagnostic and management strategies for donor-derived infections. *Infect Dis Clin North Am.* 2013;27(2):253-270.

31. Green M, Covington S, Trantano S. Donor-derived transmission events in 2013: a report of the organ procurement transplant network ad hoc disease transmission advisory committee. *Transplantation.* 2015;99(2):282-287.

32. Morris MI, Fischer SA, Ison MG. Infections transmitted by transplantation. *Infect Dis Clin North Am.* 2010;24(2):497-514.

33. Centers for Disease Control and Prevention (CDC). Use of 13-valent pneumococcal conjugate vaccine and 23-valent pneumococcal polysaccharide vaccine for adults with immunocompromising conditions: recommendations of the Advisory Committee on Immunization Practices (ACIP). *MMWR Morb Mortal Wkly Rep.* 2012;61(40):816-819.

34. McLean HQ, Fiebelkorn AP, Ternte JL, Wallace GS; Center for Disease Control and Prevention. Prevention of measles, rubella, congenital rubella syndrome, and mumps, 2013: summary recommendations of the Advisory Committee on Immunization Practices (ACIP). *MMWR Recomm Rep.* 2013;62(RR-04):1-34.

35. Rubin LG, Levin MJ, Ljungman P, et al; Infectious Diseases Society of America. 2013 IDSA clinical practice guideline for vaccination of the immunocompromised host. *Clin Infect Dis.* 2014;58(3):309-318.

36. van der Does-van den Berg A, Hermans J, Nagel J, van Steenis G. Immunity to diphtheria, pertussis, tetanus, and poliomyelitis in children with acute lymphocytic leukemia after cessation of chemotherapy. *Pediatrics.* 1981;67(2):222-229.

37. Centers for Disease Control and Prevention. Recommendations of the Advisory Committee on Immunization Practices (ACIP): use of vaccines and immune globulins for persons with altered immunocompetence. *MMWR Recomm Rep.* 1993;42(RR-7):1-20.

38. AIDS Education and Training Centers National Coordinating Resource Center (AETC NCRC). Opportunistic infection prophylaxis. 03 Jan. 2017.

39. U.S. Department of Health and Human Services. HIV/AIDS treatment guidelines. https://aidsinfo.nih.gov/contentfiles/lvguidelines/AdultandAdolescentGL.pdf. Accessed January 3, 2017.

40. Norris RP, Vergis EN, Yu VL. Overwhelming postsplenectomy infection: a critical review of etiologic pathogens and management. *Infect Med.* 1996;13(9):779-783.

41. Mitchell AM, Mitchell TJ. Streptococcus pneumoniae: virulence factors and variation. *Clin Microbiol Infect.* 2010;16(5):411-418.

42. Rosón B, Fernández-Sabé N, Carratalà J, et al. Contribution of a urinary antigen assay (Binax NOW) to the early diagnosis of pneumococcal pneumonia. *Clin Infect Dis.* 2004;38(2):222-226.

43. Tunkel AR, Hartman BJ, Kaplan SL, et al. Practice guidelines for the management of bacterial meningitis. *Clin Infect Dis.* 2004;39(9):1267-1284.

44. Walker MJ, Barnett TC, McArthur JD, et al. Disease manifestations and pathogenic mechanisms of group A Streptococcus. *Clin Microbiol Rev.* 2014;27(2):264-301.

45. Stevens DL, Bisno AL, Chambers HF, et al; Infectious Diseases Society of America. Practice guidelines for the diagnosis and management of skin and soft-tissue infections. *Clin Infect Dis.* 2005;41(8):1373-1406.

46. Allen U, Moore D. Invasive group A streptococcal disease: management and chemoprophylaxis. *Can J Infect Dis Med Microbiol.* 2010;21(3):115-118.

47. Gewitz MH, Baltimore RS, Tani LY, et al; American Heart Association Committee on Rheumatic Fever, Endocarditis, and Kawasaki Disease of the Council on Cardiovascular Disease in the Young. Revision of the Jones Criteria for the diagnosis of acute rheumatic fever in the era of Doppler echocardiography: a scientific statement from the American Heart Association. *Circulation.* 2015;131(20):1806-1818.

48. Walker KG, Wilmshurst JM. An update on the treatment of Sydenham's chorea: the evidence for established and evolving interventions. *Ther Adv Neurol Disord.* 2010;3(5):301-309.

49. Carapetis JR, McDonald M, Wilson NJ. Acute rheumatic fever. *Lancet*. 2005;366(9480):155-168.

50. Baldwin DS, Gluck MC, Schacht RG, Gallo G. The long-term course of poststreptococcal glomerulonephritis. *Ann Intern Med*. 1974;80(3):342-358.

51. Kaplan EL, Anthony BF, Chapman SS, Ayoub EM, Wannamaker LW. The influence of the site of infection on the immune response to group A streptococci. *J Clin Invest*. 1970;49(7):1405-1414.

52. Ayoub EM, Wannamaker LW. Streptococcal antibody titers in Sydenham's chorea. *Pediatrics*. 1966;38(6):946-956.

53. Agrawal A, Murphy TF. Haemophilus influenza infections in the *H. influenzae* type B conjugate vaccine era. *J Clin Microbiol*. 2011;49(11):3728-3732.

54. Langereis JD, de Jonge MI. Invasive disease caused by nontypeable *Haemophilus influenzae*. *Emerg Infect Dis*. 2015;21(10):1711-1718.

55. Nakamura S, Yanagihara K, Seki M, et al. Clinical characteristics of pneumonia caused by beta-lactamase negative ampicillin resistant *Haemophilus influenzae* (BLNAR). *Scand J Infect Dis*. 2007;39(6-7):521-524.

56. Mandell LA, Wunderink RG, Anzueto A, et al; Infectious Diseases Society of America; American Thoracic Society. Infectious Diseases Society of America/American Thoracic Society consensus guidelines on the management of community-acquired pneumonia in adults. *Clin Infect Dis*. 2007;44 (Suppl 2):S27-S72.

57. Apicella M. Diagnosis of meningococcal infection. In: Post TW, ed. UpToDate. Waltham, MA: UpToDate, Inc. http://www.uptodate.com. Accessed May 5, 2016.

58. Tunkel AR, Hartman BJ, Kaplan SL, et al. Practice guidelines for the management of bacterial meningitis. *Clin Infect Dis*. 2004;39(9):1267-1284.

59. Cohn AC, MacNeil JR, Clark TA, et al; Centers for Disease Control and Prevention (CDC). Prevention and control of meningococcal disease: recommendations of the Advisory Committee on Immunization Practices (ACIP). *MMWR Recomm Rep*. 2013;62(RR-2):1-28.

60. Schwartz B, Al-Tobaiqi A, Al-Ruwais A, et al. Comparative efficacy of ceftriaxone and rifampicin in eradicating pharyngeal carriage of group A *Neisseria meningitides*. *Lancet*. 1988;1(8597):1239-1242.

61. Pollack M, Taylor NS, Callahan LT 3rd. Exotoxin production by clinical isolates of pseudomonas aeruginosa. *Infect Immun*. 1977;15(3):776-780.

62. Somerville G, Mikoryak CA, Reitzer L. Physiological characterization of *Pseudomonas aeruginosa* during exotoxin A synthesis: glutamate, iron limitation, and aconitase activity. *J Bacteriol*. 1999;181(4):1072-1078.

63. Mayer-Hamblett N, Ramsey BW, Kulasekara HD, et al. *Pseudomonas aeruginosa* phenotypes associated with eradication failure in children with cystic fibrosis. *Clin Infect Dis*. 2014;59(5):624-631.

64. Hoffman LR, D'Argenio DA, MacCoss MJ, Zhang Z, Jones RA, Miller SI. Aminoglycoside antibiotics induce bacterial biofilm formation. *Nature*. 2005;436(7054):1171-1175.

65. Song Z, Wu H, Ciofu O, et al. *Pseudomonas aeruginosa* alginate is refractory to Th1 immune response and impedes host immune clearance in a mouse model of acute lung infection. *J Med Microbiol*. 2003;52(Pt 9):731-740.

66. Meluleni GJ, Grout M, Evans DJ, Pier GB. Mucoid *Pseudomonas aeruginosa* growing in a biofilm in vitro are killed by opsonic antibodies to the mucoid exopolysaccharide capsule but not by antibodies produced during chronic lung infection in cystic fibrosis patients. *J Immunol*. 1995;155(4):2029-2038.

67. Fujitani S, Sun HY, Yu VL, Weingarten JA. Pneumonia due to *Pseudomonas aeruginosa*: part I: epidemiology, clinical diagnosis, and source. *Chest*. 2011;139(4):909-919.

68. Sun HY, Fujitani S, Quintiliani R, Yu VL. Pneumonia due to *Pseudomonas aeruginosa*: part II: antibiotic resistance, pharmacodynamic concepts, and antibiotic therapy. *Chest*. 2011;139(5):1172-1185.

69. Vaiman M, Lazarovitch T, Heller L, Lotan G. Ecthyma gangrenosum and ecthyma-like lesions: review article. *Eur J Clin Microbiol Infect Disc*. 2015;34(4):633-639.

70. Rogers KL, Fey PD, Rupp ME. Coagulase-negative staphylococcal infections. *Infect Dis Clin North Am*. 2009;23(1):73-98.

71. Bubeck Wardenburg J, Bae T, Otto M, Deleo FR, Schneewind O. Poring over pores: alpha-hemolysin and Panton-Valentine leukocidin in *Staphylococcus aureus* pneumonia. *Nat Med*. 2007;13(12):1405-1406.

72. Tong SYC, Davis JS, Eichenberger E, Holland TL, Fowler Jr VG. *Staphylococcus aureus* infections: epidemiology, pathophysiology, clinical manifestations, and management. *Clin Microbiol Rev*. 2015;28(3):605-661.

73. Wang R, Braughton KR, Kretschmer D, et al. Identification of novel cytolytic peptides as key virulence determinants for community-associated MRSA. *Nat Med*. 2007;13(12):1510-1514.

74. Hsin H, Flynn NM, King JH, Monchaud C, Morita M, Cohen SH. Comparisons of community-acquired methicillin-resistant *Staphylococcus aureus* (MRSA) and hospital-associated MRSA infections in Sacramento, California. *J Clin Microbiol*. 2006;44(7):2423-2427.

75. Amin A, Batts D. In touch with the experts: community-acquired and healthcare-associated MRSA: improving patient outcomes. Medscape Web site. http://www.medscape.org/viewarticle/544583. Accessed August 8, 2017.

76. Freitag NE, Port GC, Miner MD. *Listeria monocytogenes*—from saprophyte to intracellular pathogen. *Nat Rev Microbiol*. 2009;7(9):1-15.

77. Liu D. Identification, subtyping and virulence determination of *Listeria monocytogenes*, an important foodborne pathogen. *J Med Microbiol*. 2006;55(Pt 6):645-659.

78. Lorber B. Listeriosis. *Clin Infect Dis*. 1997;24(1):1-9.

79. Lorber B. *Listeria monocytogenes*. In: Mandell GL, Bennett JE, Dolin R, eds. *Principles and Practice of Infectious Diseases*, 7th ed. Philadelphia: Churchill Livingstone; 2010: 2707-2714.

80. Mylonakis E, Hohmann EL, Calderwood SB. Central nervous system infection *with Listeria monocytogenes*. 33 years' experience at a general hospital and review of 776 episodes from the literature. *Medicine (Baltimore)*. 1998;77(5):313-336.

81. Hof H, Nichterlein T, Kretschmar M. Management of listeriosis. *Clin Microbiol Rev*. 1997;10(2):345-357.

82. Drevets DA, Canono BP, Leenen PJ, Campbell PA. Gentamicin kills intracellular *Listeria monocytogenes*. *Infect Immun*. 1994;62(6):2222-2228.

83. Phin N, Parry-Ford F, Harrison T, et al. Epidemiology and clinical management of Legionnaires' disease. *Lancet Infect Dis*. 2014; 14(10):1011-1021.

84. Roy CR, Berger KH, Isberg RR. Legionella pneumophila DotA protein is required for early phagosome trafficking decisions that occur within minutes of bacterial update. *Mol Microbiol*. 1998;28(3):663-674.

85. Mulazimoglu L, Yu VL. Can Legionnaires disease be diagnosed by clinical criteria? A critical review. *Chest.* 2001;120(4):1049-1053.

86. Yu VL, Plouffe JF, Pastoris MC, et al. Distribution of *Legionella* species and serogroups isolated by culture in patients with sporadic community-acquired legionellosis: an international collaborative survey. *J Infect Dis.* 2002;186(1):127-128.

87. Helbig JH, Uldum SA, Bernander S, et al. Clinical utility of urinary antigen detection for diagnosis of community-acquired, travel-associated, and nosocomial legionnaires' disease. *J Clin Microbiol.* 2003;41(2):838-840.

88. von Baum H, Ewig S, Marre R, et al; Competence Network for Community Acquired Pneumonia Study Group. Community-acquired *Legionella pneumonia*: new insights from the German competence network for community acquired pneumonia. *Clin Infect Dis.* 2008;46(9):1356-1364.

89. Domínguez J, Galí N, Matas L, et al. Evaluation of a rapid immunochromatographic assay for the detection of Legionella antigen in urine samples. *Eur J Clin Microbiol Infect Dis.* 1999;18(12):896-898.

90. Stout JE. Laboratory diagnosis of Legionnaires' disease: the expanding role of the Legionella urinary antigen test. *Clin Microbiol Newsletter.* 2000;22(8):62-64.

91. Pedro-Botet L, Yu VL. Legionella: macrolides or quinolones? *Clin Microbiol Infect.* 2006;12(3):25-30.

92. Marston BJ, Plouffe JF, File TM Jr, et al. Azithromycin in the treatment of Legionella pneumonia requiring hospitalization. *Clin Infect Dis.* 2003;37(11):1475-1480.

93. Pedro-Botet ML, Yu VL. Legionnaire's disease in solid organ transplants. Antimicrobe Web site. http://www.antimicrobe.org/t41.asp. Accessed May 1, 2017.

94. Amsden GW. Macrolides versus azalides: a drug interaction update. *Ann Pharmacother.* 1995;29(9):906-124.

95. Periti P, Mazzei T, Mini E, Novelli A. Pharmacokinetic drug interactions of macrolides. *Clin Pharmacokinet.* 1992;23(2):106-131.

96. Page RL 2nd, Ruscin JM, Fish D, Lapointe M. Possible interaction between intravenous azithromycin and oral cyclosporine. *Pharmacotherapy.* 2001;21(11):1436-1443.

97. Qaqish R, Polk RE. Drug-drug interactions. In: Hooper DC, Wolfson JS, eds. *Quinolones Antimicrobial Agents.* Washington, DC; ASM Press; 2003: 133-146.

98. Wilson JW. Nocardiosis: updates and clinical overview. *Mayo Clin Proc.* 2012;87(4):403-407.

99. Beaman BL, Burnside J, Edwards B, Causey W. Nocardial infections in the United States. 1972-1974. *J Infect Dis.* 1976;134(3):286-289.

100. Beaman BL, Beaman L. *Nocardia* species: host-parasite relationships. *Clin Microbiol Rev.* 1994;7(2):213-264.

101. Valour F, Sénéchal A, Dupieux C, et al. Actinomycosis: etiology, clinical features, diagnosis, treatment, and management. *Infect Drug Resist.* 2014;7:183-197.

102. Smego RA, Foglia G. Actinomycosis. *Clin Infect Dis.* 1998;26(6):1255-1263.

103. Weinstock DM, Brown AE. *Rhodococcus equi*: an emerging pathogen. *Clin Infect Dis.* 2002;34(10):1379-1385.

104. Le T, Cash-Goldwasser, Tho PV, et al. Diagnosis *Rhodococcus equi* infections in a setting where tuberculosis is highly endemic: a double challenge. *J Clin Microbiol.* 2015;53(4):1431-1433.

105. Clarridge JE, Popovic T, Inzana TJ. Diphtheria and other corynebacterial and coryneform infections. In: Hausler WJ, Sussman M, eds. *Topley and Wilson's Microbiology and Microbial Infections.* Vol 3. New York: Oxford University Press; 1998; 347.

106. Efstratiou A, Engler KH, Mazurova IK, Glushkevich T, Vuopio-Varkila J, Popovic T. Current approaches to the laboratory diagnosis of diphtheria. *J Infect Dis.* 2000;181 (Suppl 1):S138-S145.

107. Colman G, Weaver E, Efstratiou A. Screening tests for pathogenic corynebacteria. *J Clin Pathol.* 1992;45(1):46-48.

108. Weiss S, Efsfratiou A, Chiou CC. *Corynebacterium diphtheriae* (Diphtheria). Antimicrobe Web site. http://www.antimicrobe.org/b99.asp. Accessed. January 10, 2017.

109. Harms A, Dehio C. Intruders below the radar: molecular pathogenesis of *Bartonella* spp. *Clin Microbiol Rev.* 2012;25(1):42-78.

110. Prutsky G, Domecq JP, Mori L et al. Treatment outcomes of human bartonellosis: a systematic review and meta-analysis. *Int J Infect Dis.* 2013;17(10):e811-e819.

111. Nelson CA. Cat-scratch disease in the United States, 2005-2013. *Emerg Infect Dis.* 2016;22(10):1741-1746.

112. Spach DH, Kaplan SL. Treatment of cat scratch disease. In: Post TW, ed. UpToDate. Waltham, MA: UpToDate, Inc. http://www.uptodate.com. Accessed April 26, 2017.

113. Franco MP, Mulder M, Gilman RH, Smits HL. Human brucellosis. *Lancet Infect Dis.* 2007;7(12):775-786.

114. Figueirdo P, Ficht TA, Rice-Ficht A, Rossetti CA, Adams LG. Pathogenesis and immunobiology of brucellosis. *Am J Pathol.* 2015;185(6):1505-1517.

115. Janda JM, Graves MH, Lindquist D, Probert WS. Diagnosing *Capnocytophaga canimorsus* infections. *Emerg Infect Dis.* 2006;12(2):340-342.

116. Chiang-Mei Low S, Greenwood JE. *Capnocytophaga canimorsus*: infection, septicaemia, recovery, and reconstruction. *J Med Microbiol.* 2008;57(Pt 7):901-903.

117. Pers C, Gahrn-Hansen B, Frederiksen W. *Capnocytophaga canimorsus* septicemia in Denmark, 1982-1995: review of 39 cases. *Clin Infect Dis.* 1996;23(1):71-75.

118. Kullberg BJ, Westendorp RG, van 't Wout JW, Meinders AE. Purpura fulminans and symmetrical peripheral gangrene caused by *Capnocytophaga canimorsus* (formerly DF-2) septicemia--a complication of dog bite. *Medicine (Baltimore).* 1991;70(5):287-292.

119. Vu J, Carvalho J. Enterococcus: review of its physiology, pathogenesis, diseases, and the challenges it poses for clinical microbiology. *Front Biol.* 2011;6(5):357-366.

120. Arias CA, Murray BE. The rise of the *Enterococcus*: beyond vancomycin resistance. *Nat Rev Microbiol.* 2012;10(4):266-278.

121. Tarr PI, Gordon CA, Chandler WL. Shiga-toxin-producing *Escherichia coli* and haemolytic uraemic syndrome. *Lancet.* 2005;365(9464):1073-1086.

122. Slutsker L, Ries AA, Greene KD, Wells JG, Hutwagner L, Griffin PM. *Escherichia coli* O157:H7 diarrhea in the United States: clinical and epidemiologic features. *Ann Intern Med.* 1997;126(7):505-513.

123. Freedman SB, Xie J, Neufeld MS, Hamilton WL, Hartling L, Tarr PI; Alberta Provincial Pediatric Enteric Infection Team (APPETITE). Shiga toxin-producing *Escherichia coli* infection, antibiotics, and risk of developing hemolytic uremic syndrome: a meta-analysis. *Clin Infect Dis.* 2016;62(10):1251-1258.

124. Donnenberg MS, Tzipori S, McKee ML, O'Brien AD, Alroy J, Kaper JB. The role of the eae gene of enterohemorrhagic *Escherichia coli* in intimate attachment in vitro and in a porcine model. *J Clin Invest.* 1993;92(3):1418-1424.

125. Donnenberg MS, Calderwood SB, Donohue-Rolfe A, Keusch GT, Kaper JB. Construction and analysis of TnphoA mutants of enteropathogenic Escherichia coli unable to invade HEp-2 cells. *Infect Immun*. 1990;58(6):1565-1571.

126. Dytoc M, Fedorko L, Sherman PM. Signal transduction in human epithelial cells infected with attaching and effacing *Escherichia coli* in vitro. *Gastroenterology*. 1994;106(5):1150-1161.

127. Finlay BB, Rosenshine I, Donnenberg MS, Kaper JB. Cytoskeletal composition of attaching and effacing lesions associated with enteropathogenic *Escherichia coli* adherence to HeLa cells. *Infect Immun*. 1992;60(6):2541-2543.

128. Steiner TS, Nataro JP, Poteet-Smith CE, Smith JA, Guerrant RL. Enteroaggregative *Escherichia coli* expresses a novel flagellin that causes IL-8 release from intestinal epithelial cells. *J Clin Invest*. 2000;105(12):1769-1777.

129. Nataro JP, Deng Y, Cookson S, et al. Heterogeneity of enteroaggregative *Escherichia coli* virulence demonstrated in volunteers. *J Infect Di*s. 1995;171(2):465-468.

130. Benjamin P, Federman M, Wanke CA. Characterization of an invasive phenotype associated with enteroaggregative *Escherichia coli*. *Infect Immun*. 1995;63(9):3417-3421.

131. Khan K, Konar M, Goyal A, Ghosh S. Enteroaggregative *Escherichia coli* infection induces IL-8 production via activation of mitogen-activated protein kinases and the transcription factors NF-kappaB and AP-1 in INT-407 cells. *Mol Cell Biochem*. 2010;337(1-2):17-24.

132. Coburn B, Grassl GA, Finlay BB. Salmonella, the host and disease: a brief review. *Immunol Cell Biol*. 2007;85(2):112-118.

133. Andino A, Hanning I. *Salmonella enterica*: survival, colonization, and virulence differences among serovars. *ScientificWorld Journal*. 2015:2015;1-16.

134. Connor BA, Schwartz E. Typhoid and paratyphoid fever in travellers. *Lancet Infect Dis*. 2005;5(10):623-628.

135. Hart G. Syphilis tests in diagnostic and therapeutic decision making. *Ann Intern Med*. 1986;104(3):368-376.

136. Seña AC, White BL, Sparling PF. Novel *Treponema pallidum* serologic tests: a paradigm shift in syphilis screening for the 21st century. *Clin Infect Dis*. 2010;51(6):700-708.

137. Workowski KA, Bolan GA; Centers for Disease Control and Prevention. Sexually transmitted diseases treatment guidelines, 2015. *MMWR Recomm Rep*. 2015;64(RR-03):1-137.

138. Brassar P, Kezouh A, Suissa S. Antirheumatic drugs and the risk of tuberculosis. *Clin Infect Dis*. 2006;43(6):717-722.

139. Lewinsohn DM, Leonard MK, LoBue PA, et al. Official American Thoracic Society/Infectious Diseases Society of America/Centers for Disease Control and Prevention clinical practice guidelines: diagnosis of tuberculosis in adults and children. *Clin Infect Dis*. 2017;64(2):111-115.

140. Burrill J, Williams CJ, Bain G, Conder G, Hine AL, Misra RR. Tuberculosis: a radiologic review. *Radiographics*. 2007;27(5):1255-1273.

141. Nachiappan AC, Rahbar K, Shi X, et al. Pulmonary tuberculosis: role of radiology in diagnosis and management. *Radiographics*. 2017;37(1):52-72

142. Woodring JH, Vandiviere HM, Fried AM, Dillon ML, Williams TD, Melvin IG. Update: the radiographic features of pulmonary tuberculosis. *AJR Am J Roentgenol*. 1986;146(3):497-506.

143. Nahid P, Dorman SE, Alipanah N, et al. Official American Thoracic Society/Centers for Disease Control and Prevention/Infectious Diseases Society of America clinical practice guidelines: treatment of drug susceptible tuberculosis. *Clin Infect Dis*. 2016;63(7):853-867.

144. Jo KW, Yoo JW, Hong Y, et al. Risk factors for 1-year relapse of pulmonary tuberculosis treated with a 6-month daily regimen. *Respir Med*. 2014;108(4):654-659.

145. Benator D, Bhattacharya M, Bozeman L, et al. Rifapentine and isoniazid once a week versus rifampicin and isoniazid twice a week for treatment of drug-susceptible pulmonary tuberculosis in HIV-negative patients: a randomised clinical trial. *Lancet*. 2002;360(9332):528-534.

146. Havlir DV, Kendall MA, Ive P, et al; AIDS Clinical Trials Group Study A5221. Timing of antiretroviral therapy for HIV-1 infection and tuberculosis. *New Engl J Med*. 2011;365(16):1482-1491.

147. Török ME, Yen NT, Chau TT, et al. Timing of initiation of antiretroviral therapy in human immunodeficiency virus (HIV)—associated tuberculous meningitis. *Clin Infect Dis*. 2011;52(11):1374-1383.

148. American Thoracic Society. Mycobacterioses and the acquired immunodeficiency syndrome. Joint Position Paper of the American Thoracic Society and the Centers for Disease Control. *Am Rev Respir Dis*. 1987;136(2):492-496.

149. Dorman SE, Holland SM. Interferon-gamma and interleukin-12 pathway defects and human disease. *Cytokine Growth Factor Rev*. 2000;11(4):321-333.

150. Casanova JL, Abel L. Genetic dissection of immunity to mycobacteria: the human model. *Annu Rev Immunol*. 2002;20:581-620.

151. Griffith DE, Adsamit T, Brown-Elliott BA, et al; ATS Mycobacterial Diseases Subcommittee; American Thoracic Society; Infectious Disease Society of America. An official ATS/IDSA statement: diagnosis, treatment and prevention of nontuberculous mycobacterial diseases. *Am J Respir Crit Care Med*. 2007;175(4):367-416.

151a. Patterson KC, Strek ME. Diagnosis and treatment of pulmonary aspergillosis syndromes. *Chest*. 2014;145(5):1358-1368.

152. Riscili BP, Wood KL. Noninvasive pulmonary *Aspergillus* infections. *Clin Chest Med*. 2009;30(2):315-335.

153. Kravitz JN, Berry MW, Schabel SI, Judson MA. A modern series of percutaneous intracavitary instillation of amphotericin B for the treatment of severe hemoptysis from pulmonary aspergilloma. *Chest*. 2013;143(5):1414-1421.

154. Nam HS, Jeon K, Um SW, et al. Clinical characteristics and treatment outcomes of chronic necrotizing pulmonary aspergillosis: a review of 43 cases. *Int J Infect Dis*. 2010;14(6):e479-e482.

155. Schweer KE, Bangard C, Hekmat K, Cornely OA. Chronic pulmonary aspergillosis. *Mycoses*. 2014;57(5):257-270.

156. Limper AH. Clinical approach and management for selected fungal infections in pulmonary and critical care patients. *Chest*. 2014;146(6):1658-1666.

157. Walsh TJ, Anaissie EJ, Denning DW, et al; Infectious Diseases Society of America. Treatment of aspergillosis: clinical practice guidelines of the Infectious Diseases Society of America. *Clin Infect Dis*. 2008:46(3):327-360.

158. Agarwal R, Gupta D, Aggarwal AN, Saxena AK, Chakrabarti A, Jindal SK. Clinical significance of hyperattenuating mucoid impaction in allergic bronchopulmonary aspergillosis: an analysis of 155 patients. *Chest*. 2007;132(4):1183-1190.

159. Greenberger PA. When to suspect and work up allergic bronchopulmonary aspergillosis. *Ann Allergy Asthma Immunol.* 2013;111(1):1-4.

160. Agarwal R, Maskey D, Aggarwal AN, et al. Diagnostic performance of various tests and criteria employed in allergic bronchopulmonary aspergillosis: a latent class analysis. *PLoS ONE.* 2013;8(4):e61105.

161. Agarwal R, Chakrabarti A, Shah A, et al; ABPA Complicating Asthma ISHAM Working Group. Allergic bronchopulmonary aspergillosis: review of literature and proposal of new diagnostic and classification criteria. *Clin Exp Allergy.* 2013;43(8):850-873.

162. Patterson KC, Strek ME. Diagnosis and treatment of pulmonary aspergillosis syndromes. *Chest.* 2014;145(5):1358-1368.

163. Kousha M, Tadi R, Soubani AO. Pulmonary aspergillosis: a clinical review. *Eur Respir Rev.* 2011;20(121):156-174.

164. Greene RE, Schlamm HT, Oestmann JW, et al. Imaging findings in acute invasive pulmonary aspergillosis: clinical significance of the halo sign. *Clin Infect Dis.* 2007;44(3):373-379.

165. Li SS, Mody CH. Cryptococcus. *Proc Am Thorac Soc.* 2010;7(3):186-196.

166. Chang WC, Tzao C, Hsu HH, et al. Pulmonary cryptococcosis: comparison of clinical and radiographic characteristics in immunocompetent and immunocompromised patients. *Chest.* 2006;129(2):333-340.

167. Saag MS, Graybill RJ, Larsen RA, et al. Practice guidelines for the management of cryptococcal disease. Infectious Diseases Society of America. *Clin Infect Dis.* 2000;30(4):710-718.

168. van der Horst CM, Saag MS, Cloud GA, et al. Treatment of cryptococcal meningitis associated with the acquired immunodeficiency syndrome. National Institute of Allergy and Infectious Diseases Mycoses Study and AIDS Clinical Trials Group. *N Engl J Med.* 1997;337(1):15-21.

169. Kauffman CA. Histoplasmosis: a clinical and laboratory update. *Clin Microbiol Rev.* 2007;20(1):115-132.

170. Wheat LJ. Nonculture diagnostic methods for invasive fungal infections. *Curr Infect Dis Rep.* 2007;9(6):465-471.

171. McKinsey DS, McKinsey JP. Pulmonary histoplasmosis. *Semin Respir Crit Care Med.* 2011;32(6):735-744.

172. el-Ebiary M, Torres A, Fàbregas N, et al. Significance of the isolation of *Candida* species from respiratory samples in critically ill, non-neutropenic patients. *Am J Respir Crit Care Med.* 1997;156(2 Pt 1):583-590.

173. Ibrahim M, Staros EB. Sputum culture. Medscape Web site.http://emedicine.medscape.com/article/2119232.Accessed May, 2017.

174. Chow JK, Golan Y, Ruthazer R, et al. Risk factors for albicans and non-albicans candidemia in the intensive care unit. *Crit Care Med.* 2008;36(7):1993-1998.

175. Pappas PG, Kauffman CA, Andes DR, et al. Clinical practice guideline for the management of candidiasis: 2016 update by the Infectious Diseases Society of America. *Clin Infect Dis.* 2016;62(4):409-417.

176. Vaaler AK, Bradsher RW, Davies SF. Evidence of subclinical blastomycosis in forestry workers in northern Minnesota and northern Wisconsin. *Am J Med.* 1990;89(4):470-476.

177. Sarosi GA, Davies SF, Phillips JR. Self-limited blastomycosis: a report of 39 cases. *Semin Respir Infect.* 1986;1(1):40-44.

178. Light RB, Kralt D, Embil JM. Seasonal variations in the clinical presentation of pulmonary and extrapulmonary blastomycosis. *Med Mycol.* 2008;46(8):835-841.

179. Baumgardner DJ, Halsmer SE, Egan G. Symptoms of pulmonary blastomycosis: Northern Wisconsin, United States. *Wilderness Environ Med.* 2004;15(4):250-256.

180. Brown LR, Swensen SJ, Van Scoy RE, Prakash UBS, Coles DT, Colby TV. Roentgenologic features of pulmonary blastomycosis. *Mayo Clin Proc.* 1991;66(1):29-38.

181. Smith JA and Kauffman CA. Blastomycosis. *Proc Am Thorac Soc.* 2010;7(3):173-180.

182. Sheflin JR, Campbell JA, Thompson GP. Pulmonary blastomycosis: findings on chest radiographs in 63 patients. *AJR Am J Roentgenol.* 1990;154(6):1177-1180.

183. Winer-Muram HT, Beals DH, Cole FH Jr. Blastomycosis of the lung: CT features. *Radiology.* 1992;182(3):829-832.

184. Durkin M, Witt J, LeMonte A, Wheat B, Connolly P. Antigen assay with the potential to aid in diagnosis of blastomycosis. *J Clin Microbiol.* 2004;42(10):4873-4875.

185. Mongkolrattanothai K, Peev M, Wheat L, Marcinak J. Urine antigen detection of blastomycosis in pediatric patients. *Pediatr Infect Dis J.* 2006;25(11):1076-1078.

186. Malo J, Luraschi-Monjagatta C, Wlk DM, Thompson R, Hage CA, Knox KS. Update on the diagnosis of pulmonary coccidioidomycosis. *Ann Am Thorac Soc.* 2014;11(2):243-253.

187. Limper AH. Clinical approach and management for selected fungal infections in pulmonary and critical care patients. *Chest.* 2014;146(6):1658-1666.

188. Pagano L, Fianchi L, Mele L, et al. *Pneumocystis carinii* pneumonia in patients with malignant haematological diseases: 10 years' experience of infection in GIMEMA centres. *Br J Haematol.* 2002;117(2):379-386.

189. Jacobs JA, Dieleman MM, Cornelissen EI, Groen EA, Wagenaar SS, Drent M. Bronchoalveolar lavage fluid cytology in patients with *Pneumocystis carinii* pneumonia. *Acta Cytol.* 2001;45(3):317-326.

190. Thomas CF Jr, Limper AH. Pneumocystis pneumonia: clinical presentation and diagnosis in patients with and without acquired immune deficiency syndrome. *Semin Respir Infect.* 1998;13(4):289-295.

191. Shelhamer JH, Gill VJ, Quinn TC, et al. The laboratory evaluation of opportunistic pulmonary infections. *Ann Intern Med.* 1996;124(6):585-599.

192. Limper AH, Offord KP, Smith TF, Martin WJ 2nd. *Pneumocystis carinii* pneumonia. Differences in lung parasite number and inflammation in patients with and without AIDS. *Am Rev Respir Dis.* 1989;140(5):1204-1209.

193. Tasaka S, Hasegawa N, Kobayashi S, et al. Serum indicators for the diagnosis of pneumocystis pneumonia. *Chest.* 2007;131(4):1173-1180.

194. Azoulay E, Bergeron A, Chevret S, Bele N, Schlemmer B, Menotti J. Polymerase chain reaction for diagnosing pneumocystis pneumonia in non-HIV immunocompromised patients with pulmonary infiltrates. *Chest.* 2009;135(3):655-661.

195. Huang L, Morris A, Limper AH, Beck JM; ATS Pneumocystis Workshop Participants. An official ATS workshop summary: recent advances and future directions in pneumocystis pneumonia (PCP). *Proc Am Thorac Soc.* 2006;3(8):655-664.

196. Ewald H, Raatz H, Boscacci R, Furrer H, Bucher HC, Briel M. Adjunctive corticosteroids for *Pneumocystis jirovecii* pneumonia in patients with HIV infection. *Cochrane Database Syst Rev.* 2015;(4):CD006150.

197. Montaner JS, Lawson LM, Levitt N, Belzberg A, Schechter MT, Ruedy J. Corticosteroids prevent early deterioration in

patients with moderately severe *Pneumocystis carinii* pneumonia and the acquired immunodeficiency syndrome (AIDS). *Ann Intern Med.* 1990;113(1):14-20.

198. Bozzette SA, Sattler FR, Chiu J, et al. A controlled trial of early adjunctive treatment with corticosteroids for *Pneumocystis carinii* pneumonia in the acquired immunodeficiency syndrome. California Collaborative Treatment Group. *N Engl J Med.* 1990;323(21):1451-1457.

199. Gagnon S, Boota AM, Fischl MA, Baier H, Kirksey OW, La Voie L. Corticosteroids as adjunctive therapy for severe *Pneumocystis carinii* pneumonia in the acquired immunodeficiency syndrome. A double-blind, placebo-controlled trial. *N Engl J Med.* 1990;323(21):1444-1450.

200. Masih I, Boyle R, Donnelly A, Soye A, Kidney J. Varicella pneumonitis in an immunocompetent patient. *BMJ Case Reports.* 2011;2011:1-5.

201. Mohsen AH, Peck RJ, Mason Z, Mattock L, McKendrick MW. Lung function tests and risk factors for pneumonia in adults with chickenpox. *Thorax.* 2001;56(10):796-799.

202. Potgieter PD, Hammond JMJ. Intensive care management of varicella pneumonia. *Respir Med.* 1997;91(4):207-212.

203. Dworkin RH, Johnson RW, Breuer J et al. Recommendations for the management of herpes zoster. *Clin Infect Dis* 2007;44:(Suppl 1):S1-S26.

204. World Health Organization. Herpes simplex virus. World Health Organization Web site. http://www.who.int/mediacentre/factsheets/fs400/en/ Updated January 3, 2017.

205. Simoons-Smit AM, Kraan EM, Beishuizen A, Strack van Schijndel RJ, Vandenbroucke-Grauls CM. Herpes simplex virus type 1 and respiratory disease in critically-ill patients: real pathogen or innocent bystander? *Clin Microbiol Infect.* 2006;12(11):1050-1059.

206. Schuller D. Lower respiratory tract reactivation of herpes simplex virus. *Chest.* 1994;106(1):3S-7S.

207. Whitley RJ, Kimberly DW. Herpes simplex encephalitis: children and adolescents. *Semin Ped Infect Dis.* 2005;16(1):17-23.

208. Whitley RJ, Lakeman F. Herpes simplex virus infections of the central nervous system: therapeutic and diagnostic considerations. *Clin Infect Dis.* 1995;20(2):414-420.

209. Al-Omari A, Aljamaan F, Alhazzani W, Salih S, Arabi Y. Cytomegalovirus infection in immunocompetent critically ill adults: literature review. *Ann Intensive Care.* 2016;6(110):1-14.

210. Sinclair J. Human cytomegalovirus: latency and reactivation in the myeloid lineage. *J Clin Virol.* 2008;41(3):180-185.

211. Osawa R, Singh N. Cytomegalovirus infection in critically ill patients: a systematic review. *Crit Care.* 2009;13(3):1-10.

212. Tamm M, Traenkle P, Grilli B, Soler M, Bolliger CT, Dalquen P, Cathomas G. Pulmonary cytomegalovirus infection in immunocompromised patients. *Chest.* 2001;119(3):838-843.

213. Nichols WG, Corey L, Gooley T, Davis C, Boeckh M. High risk of death due to bacterial and fungal infection among cytomegalovirus (CMV) seronegative recipients of stem cell transplants from seropositive recipients of stem cell transplants from seropositive donors: evidence for indirect effects of primary CMV infection. *J Infect Dis.* 2002;185(3):273-282.

214. Ljungman P, Hakki M, Boeckh M. Cytomegalovirus in hematopoietic stem cell transplant recipients. *Hematol Oncol Clin North Am.* 2011;25(1):151-169.

215. Chou S. Newer methods for diagnosis of cytomegalovirus infection. *Rev Infect Dis.* 1990;12 (Suppl 7):S727-S736.

216. Razonable RR, Hayden RT. Clinical utility of viral load in management of cytomegalovirus infection after solid organ transplantation. *Clin Microbiol Rev.* 2013;26(4):703-727.

217. Bek B, Boeckh M, Lepenies J, et al. High-level sensitivity of quantitative pp65 cytomegalovirus (CMV) antigenemia assay for diagnosis of CMV disease in AIDS patients and follow-up. *J Clin Microbiol.* 1996;34(2):457-459.

218. van den Berg AP, Klompmaker IJ, Haagsma EB, et al. Antigenemia in the diagnosis and monitoring of active cytomegalovirus infection after liver transplantation. *J Infect Dis.* 1991;164(2):265-270.

219. Port AD, Orlin A, Kiss S, Patel S, D'Amico DJ, Gupta MP. Cytomegalovirus Retinitis: A review. *J Ocul Pharmacol Ther.* 2017;33(4):224-234.

220. Goldberg DE, Smithen LM, Angelilli A, Freeman WR. HIV-associated retinopathy in the HAART era. *Retina.* 2005;25(5):633-649.

221. Kotton CN, Kumar D, Caliendo AM, et al; Transplantation Society International CMV Consensus Group. Updated international consensus guidelines on the management of cytomegalovirus in solid-organ transplantation. *Transplantation.* 2013;96(4):333-360.

222. Geng L, Wang X. Epstein-Barr virus-associated lymphoproliferative disorders: experimental and clinical developments. *Int J Clin Exp Med.* 2015;8(9):14656-14671.

223. Odumade OA, Hogquist KA, Balfour Jr HH. Progress and problems in understanding and managing primary Epstein-Barr virus infections. *Clin Microbiol Rev.* 2011;24(1):193-209.

224. Dunmire SK, Hogquist KA, Balfour HH. Infectious mononucleosis. *Curr Top Microbiol Immunol.* 2015;390(Pt 1):211-240.

225. Hudson LB, Perlman SE. Necrotizing genital ulcerations in a premenarcheal female with mononucleosis. *Obstet Gynecol.* 1998;92(4 Pt 2):642-644.

226. Schram AM, Berliner N. How I treat hemaphagocytic lymphohistiocytosis in the adult patient. *Blood.* 2015;125(19):2908-2914.

227. Henter JI, Horne A, Aricó M, et al. HLH-2004: diagnostic and therapeutic guidelines for hemophagocytic lymphohistiocytosis. *Pediatr Blood Cancer.* 2007;48(2):124-131.

228. Lindemans CA, Leen AM, Boelens JJ. How I treat adenovirus in hematopoietic stem cell transplant recipients. *Blood.* 2010:116(25):5476-5485.

229. Mims CA. General features of persistent virus infections. *Postgrad Med J.* 1978;54(635):581-586.

230. Echavarria M. Adenovirus in immunocompromised hosts. *Clin Microbiol Rev.* 2008;21(4):704-715.

231. Feuchtinger T, Lang P, Handgretinger R. Adenovirus infection after allogeneic stem cell transplantation. *Leuk Lymphoma.* 2007;48(2):244-255.

232. Myers GD, Bollard CM, Wu MF, et al. Reconstitution of adenovirus-specific cell-mediated immunity in pediatric patients after hematopoietic stem cell transplantation. *Bone Marrow Transplant.* 2007;39(11):677-686.

233. Chakrabarti S, Mautner V, Osman H, et al. Adenovirus infections following allogeneic stem cell transplantation: incidence and outcome in relation to graft manipulation, immunosuppression, and immune recovery. *Blood.* 2002;100(5):1619-1627.

234. Heemskerk B, Lankester AC, van VT, et al. Immune reconstitution and clearance of human adenovirus viremia in pediatric stem-cell recipients. *J Infect Dis.* 2005;191(4):520-530.

235. Annels NE, Kalpoe JS, Bredius RG, et al. Management of Epstein-Barr virus (EBV) reactivation after allogeneic stem cell transplantation by simultaneous analysis of EBV DNA load and EBV-specific T cell reconstitution. *Clin Infect Dis.* 2006;42(12):1743-1748.

236. La Rosa AM, Champlin RE, Mirza N, et al. Adenovirus infections in adult recipients of blood and marrow transplants. *Clin Infect Dis.* 2001;32(6):871-876.

237. Versluys AB, Rossen JW, van Ewijk B, Schuurman R, Bierings MB, Boelens JJ. A strong association between respiratory viral infection early after HSCT and the development of life-threatening acute and chronic alloimmune lung syndromes. *Biol Blood Marrow Transplant.* 2010;16(6):782-791.

238. Myers GD, Krance RA, Weiss H, et al. Adenovirus infection rates in pediatric recipients of alternate donor allogeneic bone marrow transplants receiving either antithymocyte globulin (ATG) or alemtuzumab (Campath). *Bone Marrow Transplant.* 2005;36(11):1001-1008.

239. Robin M, Marque-Juillet S, Scieux C, et al. Disseminated adenovirus infections after allogeneic hematopoietic stem cell transplantation: incidence, risk factors and outcome. *Haematologica.* 2007;92(9):1254-1257.

240. Kampmann B, Cubitt D, Walls T, et al. Improved outcome for children with disseminated adenoviral infection following allogeneic stem cell transplantation. *Br J Haematol.* 2005;130(4):595-603.

241. Moss WJ, Griffin DE. Measles. *Lancet.* 2012;379(9811):153-164.

242. Perry RT, Halsey NA. The clinical significance of measles: a review. *J Infect Dis.* 2004;189 (Suppl 1):S4-S16.

243. Atkinson W, Wolfe C, Hamborsky J, eds. *Epidemiology and Prevention of Vaccine-Preventable Diseases (The Pink Book).* 12th ed. Washington, DC: The Public Health Foundation; 2011.

244. Menge T, Hemmer B, Nessler S, et al. Acute disseminated encephalomyelitis: an update. *Arch Neurol.* 2005;62(11):1673-1680.

245. Marchioni E, Tavazzi E, Minoli L, et al. Acute disseminated encephalomyelitis. *Curr Infect Dis Rep.* 2008;10(4):307-314.

246. Leake JA, Albani S, Kao AS, et al. Acute disseminated encephalomyelitis in childhood: epidemiologic, clinical and laboratory features. *Pediatr Infect Dis J.* 2004;23(8):756-764.

247. Murthy SN, Faden HS, Cohen ME, Bakshi R. Acute disseminated encephalomyelitis in children. *Pediatrics.* 2002;110(2 Pt 1):e21.

248. Dale RC, de Sousa C, Chong WK, Cox TC, Harding B, Neville BG. Acute disseminated encephalomyelitis, multiphasic disseminated encephalomyelitis and multiple sclerosis in children. *Brain.* 2000;123 (Pt 12):2407-2422.

249. Hynson JL, Kornberg AJ, Coleman LT, Shield L, Harvey AS, Kean MJ. Clinical and neuroradiologic features of acute disseminated encephalomyelitis in children. *Neurology.* 2001;56(10):1308-1312.

250. Prashanth LK, Taly AB, Ravi V, Sinha S, Arunodaya GR. Adult onset subacute sclerosing panencephalitis: clinical profile of 39 patients from a tertiary care centre. *J Neurol Neurosurg Psychiatry.* 2006;77(5):630-633.

251. Gutierrez J, Issacson RS, Koppel BS. Subacute sclerosing panencephalitis: an update. *Dev Med Child Neurol.* 2010;52(10):901-907.

252. Anlar B. Subacute sclerosing panencephalitis and chronic viral encephalitis. *Handb Clin Neurol.* 2013;112:1183-1189.

253. Falsey AR, Hennessey PA, Formica MA, Cox C, Walsh EE. Respiratory syncytial virus infection in elderly and high-risk adults. *New Engl J Med.* 2005;352(7):1749-1759.

254. Shah JN, Chemaly RF. Management of RSV Infections in adult recipients of hematopoietic stem cell transplantation. *Blood.* 2011;117(10):2755-2763.

255. Falsey AR. Current management of parainfluenza pneumonitis in immunocompromised patients: a review. *Infect Drug Resist.* 2012;5:121-127.

256. Henrickson KJ. Parainfluenza viruses. *Clin Microbiol Rev.* 2003;16(2):242-264.

257. Harper SA, Bradley JS, Englund JA, et al. Seasonal influenza in adults and children--diagnosis, treatment, chemoprophylaxis and institutional outbreak management: clinical practice guidelines of the Infectious Diseases Society of America for Seasonal Influenza in Adults and Children. *Clin Infect Dis.* 2009;48(8):1003-1032.

258. Centers for Disease Control and Prevention. Rapid influenza diagnostic tests. CDC Web site. Available at: www.cdc.gov/flu/professionals/diagnosis/clinician_guidance_ridt.htm#Table1. Accessed September 8, 2016.

259. Chartrand C, Leeflang MM, Minion J, Brewer T, Pai M. Accuracy of rapid influenza diagnostic tests: a meta-analysis. *Ann Intern Med.* 2012;156(7):500-511.

260. Glezen WP. Clinical practice. Prevention and treatment of seasonal influenza. *N Engl J Med.* 2008;359(24):2579-2585.

261. Fiore AE, Fry A, Shay D, Gubareva L, Bresee JS, Uyeki TM; Centers for Disease Control and Prevention (CDC). Antiviral agents for the treatment and chemoprophylaxis of influenza—recommendations of the Advisory Committee on Immunization Practices (ACIP). *MMWR Recomm Rep.* 2011;60(1):1-24.

262. Egli A, Helmersen DS, Taub K, Hirsch HH, Johnson A. Renal failure five years after lung transplantation due to polyomavirus BK-associated nephropathy. *Am J Transplant.* 2010;10(10):2324-2330.

263. Hirsch HH, Randhawa P; AST Infectious Diseases Community of Practice. BK polyomavirus in solid organ transplantation. *Am J Transplant.* 2013;13 (Suppl 4):179-188.

264. Hirsch HH. Polyoma and papilloma virus infections after hematopoietic stem cell or solid organ transplantation. In: Bowden P, Ljungman P, Snydman DR, eds. *Transplant Infections.* Philadelphia, PA: Lippincott Williams & Wilkins; 2010:465-482.

265. Arthur RR, Shah KV, Baust SJ, Santos GW, Saral R. Association of BK viruria with hemorrhagic cystitis in recipients of bone marrow transplants. *N Engl J Med.* 1986;315(4):230-234.

266. Drachenberg CB, Hirsch HH, Papadimitriou JC, et al. Polyomavirus BK versus JC replication and nephropathy in renal transplant recipients: a prospective evaluation. *Transplantation.* 2007;84(3):323-330.

267. DeHovitz JA, Pape JW, Boncy M, Johnson WD Jr. Clinical manifestations and therapy of Isospora belli infection in patients with the acquired immunodeficiency syndrome. *N Engl J Med.* 1986;315(2):87-90.

268. Benator DA, French AL, Beaudet LM, Levy CS, Orenstein JM. *Isospora belli* infection associated with acalculous cholecystitis in a patient with AIDS. *Ann Intern Med.* 1994;121(9):663-664.

269. Takahashi H, Falk GA, Cruise M, Morris-Stiff G. Chronic cholecystitis with *Cystoisospora belli* in an immunocompetent patient. *BMJ Case Rep.* 2015;2015.

270. González-Dominguez J, Roldán R, Villanueva JL, Kindelán JM, Jurado R, Torre-Cisneros J. *Isospora belli* reactive arthritis in a patient with AIDS. *Ann Rheum Dis.* 1994;53(9):618-619.

271. Panel on Opportunistic Infections in HIV-Infected Adults and Adolescents. Guidelines for the prevention and treatment of opportunistic infections in HIV-infected adults and adolescents: Recommendations from the Centers for Disease Control and Prevention, the National Institutes of Health, and the HIV Medicine Association of the Infectious Diseases Society of America. http://aidsinfo.nih.gov/contentfiles/lvguidelines/adult_oi.pdf. Accessed July 22, 2013.

272. DeHovitz JA, Pape JW, Boncy M, Johnson WD Jr. Clinical manifestations and therapy of Isospora belli infection in patients with the acquired immunodeficiency syndrome. *N Engl J Med.* 1986;315(2):87-90.

273. Verdier RI, Fitzgerald DW, Johnson WD Jr, Pape JW. Trimethoprim-sulfamethoxazole compared with ciprofloxacin for treatment and prophylaxis of *Isospora belli* and *Cyclospora cayetanensis* infection in HIV-infected patients. A randomized, controlled trial. *Ann Intern Med.* 2000;132(11):885-888.

274. Weiss LM, Perlman DC, Sherman J, Tanowitz H, Wittner M. *Isospora belli* infection: treatment with pyrimethamine. *Ann Intern Med.* 1988;109(6):474-475.

275. Nitazoxanide (Alinia)--a new anti-protozoal agent. *Med Lett Drugs Ther.* 2003;45(1154):29-31.

276. Soave R, Johnson WD Jr. *Cryptosporidium* and *Isospora belli* infections. *J Infect Dis.* 1988;157(2):225-229.

277. Cama VA, Ross JM, Crawford S et al. Differences in clinical manifestations among *Cryptosporidium* species and subtypes in HIV-infected persons. *J Infect Dis.* 2007;196(5):684-691.

278. Amadi B, Mwiya M, Musuku J, et al. Effect of nitazoxanide on morbidity and mortality in Zambian children with cryptosporidiosis: a randomised controlled trial. *Lancet.* 2002;360(9343):1375-1380.

279. Fox LM, Saravolatz LD. Nitazoxanide: a new thiazolide antiparasitic agent. *Clin Infect Dis.* 2005;40(8):1173-1180.

280. Rossignol JF, Ayoub A, Ayers MS. Treatment of diarrhea caused by *Cryptosporidium parvum*: a prospective randomized, double-blind, placebo-controlled study of Nitazoxanide. *J Infect Dis.* 2001;184(1):103-106.

281. Hussien SM, Abdella OH, Abu-Hashim AH, et al. Comparative study between the effect of nitazoxanide and paromomycin in treatment of cryptosporidiosis in hospitalized children. *J Egypt Soc Parasitol.* 2013;43(2):463-470.

282. Pol S, Romana CA, Richard S, et al. Microsporidia infection in patients with the human immunodeficiency virus and unexplained cholangitis. *N Engl J Med.* 1993;328(2):95-99.

283. Schwartz DA, Visvesvara GS, Leitch GJ, et al. Pathology of symptomatic microsporidial (*Encephalitozoon hellem*) bronchiolitis in the acquired immunodeficiency syndrome: a new respiratory pathogen diagnosed from lung biopsy, bronchoalveolar lavage, sputum, and tissue culture. *Hum Pathol.* 1993;24(9):937-943.

284. Scaglia M, Gatti S, Sacchi L, et al. Asymptomatic respiratory tract microsporidiosis due to *Encephalitozoon hellem* in three patients with AIDS. *Clin Infect Dis.* 1998;26(1):174-176.

285. Didier ES, Orenstein JM, Aldras A, Bertucci D, Rogers LB, Janney FA. Comparison of three staining methods for detecting microsporidia in fluids. *J Clin Microbiol.* 1995;33(12):3138-3145.

286. Molina JM, Chastang C, Goguel J, et al. Albendazole for treatment and prophylaxis of microsporidiosis due to Encephalitozoon intestinalis in patients with AIDS: a randomized double-blind controlled trial. *J Infect Dis.* 1998;177(5):1373-1377.

287. Dionisio D, Manneschi LI, Di Lollo S, et al. Persistent damage to *Enterocytozoon bieneusi*, with persistent symptomatic relief, after combined furazolidone and albendazole in AIDS patients. *J Clin Pathol.* 1998;51(10):731-736.

288. Gross U. Treatment of microsporidiosis including albendazole. *Parasitol Res.* 2003;90 (Supp 1):S14-S18.

289. Molina JM, Goguel J, Sarfati C, et al. Potential efficacy of fumagillin in intestinal microsporidiosis due to *Enterocytozoon bieneusi* in patients with HIV infection: results of a drug screening study. The French Microsporidiosis Study Group. *AIDS.* 1997;11(13):1603-1610.

290. Visvesvara GS, Martinez AJ, Klassen-Fischer MK, Neafie RC. Amebic meningoencephalitides and keratitis: challenges in diagnosis and treatment. *Curr Opin Infect Dis.* 2010;23(6):590-594.

291. Visvesvara GS. Infections with free-living amebae. *Handb Clin Neurol.* 2013;114:153-168.

292. Salameh A, Belle N, Becker J, Zangeneh T. Fatah granulomatous amoebic encephalitis caused by acanthamoeba in a patient with kidney transplant: a case report. *Open Forum Infect Dis.* 2015;2(3):1-4

293. Centers for Disease Control and Prevention. https://www.cdc.gov/parasites/acanthamoeba/index.html. Accessed February 2, 2017.

294. Jones JL, Parise ME, Fiore AE. Neglected parasitic infections in the United States: toxoplasmosis. *Am J Trop Med Hyg.* 2014;90(5):794-799.

295. Montoya JG, Remington JS. Management of *Toxoplasma gondii* infection during pregnancy. *Clin Infect Dis.* 2008;47(4):554-566.

296. Porter SB, Sande MA. Toxoplasmosis of the central nervous system in the acquired immunodeficiency syndrome. *N Engl J Med.* 1992;327(23):1643-1648.

297. Derouin F, Pelloux H. Prevention of toxoplasmosis in transplant patients. *Clin Microbiol Infect.* 2008;14(12):1089-1101.

298. Centers for Disease Control and Prevention. Parasites—toxoplasmosis (Toxoplasma infection): resources for health professionals. CDC Web site. https://www.cdc.gov/parasites/toxoplasmosis/health_professionals/. Accessed May 7, 2017.

299. Aronson N, Herwaldt BL, Libman M, et al. Diagnosis and treatment of leishmaniasis: clinical practice guidelines by the Infectious Diseases Society and the American Society of Tropical Medicine and Hygiene. *Clin Infect Dis.* 2016;63(12): e202-e264.

300. Shaw JJ, Lainson R. Leishmaniasis in Brazil: X. Some observations of intradermal reactions to different trypanosomatid antigens of patients suffering from cutaneous and mucocutaneous leishmaniasis. *Trans R Soc Trop Med Hyg.* 1975;69(3):323-335.

301. Montgomery SP, Starr MC, Cantey PT, Edwards MS, Meymandi SK. Neglected parasitic infections in the United States. Chagas disease. *Am J Trop Med Hyg.* 2015;90(5):814-818.

302. Bern C, Montgomery SP, Herwaldt BL, et al. Evaluation and treatment of Chagas disease in the United States: a systematic review. *JAMA.* 2007;298(18):2171-2181.

303. Williams SJ, Nunley D, Dralle W, Berk SL, Verghese A. Diagnosis of pulmonary strongyloidiasis by bronchoalveolar lavage. *Chest.* 1988;94(3):643-644.

304. Woodring JH, Halfhill H, Reed JC. Pulmonary strongyloidiasis: clinical and imaging features. *AJR Am J Roentgenol.* 1994;162(3):537-542.

305. Siddique AA, Berk SL. Diagnosis of *Strongyloides stercoralis* infection. *Clin Infect Dis.* 2001;33(7):1040-1047.

306. Keiser PB, Nutman TB. *Strongyloides stercoralis* in the immunocompromised population. *Clin Microbiol Rev.* 2004;17(1):208-217.

307. Newberry AM, Williams DN, Strauffer WM, Boulware DR, Hendel-Paterson BR, Walker PF. Strongyloides hyperinfection presenting as acute respiratory failure and Gram-negative sepsis. *Chest.* 2005;128(5):3681-3684.

308. Vadlamudi RJ, Chi DS, Krishnaswamy G. Intestinal strongyloidiasis and hyperinfection syndrome. *Clin Mol Allergy.* 2006;4:1-13.

309. Patel G, Arvelakis A, Sauter BV, Gondolesi GE, Caplivski D, Huprikar S. Strongyloides hyperinfection syndrome after intestinal transplantation. *Transplant Infect Dis.* 2008;10(2):137-141.

310. Vilela EG, Clemente WG, Mira RRL, et al. *Strongyloides stercoralis* hyperinfection syndrome after liver transplantation: case report and literature review. *Transplant Infect Dis.* 2009;11(2):132-136.

311. Roxby AC, Gottlieb GS, Limaye AP. Strongyloidiasis in transplant patients. *Clin Infect Dis.* 2009;49(9):1411-1423.

312. Knox KS, Hage CA. Histoplasmosis. *Proc Am Thorac Soc.* 2010;7(3):169-172.

313. Hage CA, Azar MM, Bahr N, Loyd J, Wheat J. Histoplasmosis: up-to date evidence-based approach to diagnosis and management. *Semin Respir Crit Care Med.* 2015;36(5):729-745.

314. Azar MM, Hage CA. Laboratory diagnostics for histoplasmosis. *J Clin Microbiol.* 2017;55(6):1612-1620.

315. Bowen LN, Smith B, Reich D, Quezado M, Nath A. HIV-associated opportunistic CNS infections: pathophysiology, diagnosis and treatment. *Nat Rev Neurol.* 2016;12(11):662-674.

316. Bruchfeld J, Correia-Neves M, Kallenius G. Tuberculosis and HIV coinfection. *Cold Spring Harb Perspect Med.* 2015;5(7):a017871.

317. Lai RPJ, Meintjes G, Wilkinson RJ. HIV-1 tuberculosis-associated immune reconstitution inflammatory syndrome. *Semin Immunopathol.* 2016;38(2):185-198.

318. Matuszkiewicz-Rowińska J, Małyszko J, Wieliczko M. Urinary tract infections in pregnancy: old and new unresolved diagnostic and therapeutic problems. *Arch Med Sci.* 2015;11(1):67-77.

319. Kontoyiannis DP, Lewis RE. How I treat mucormycosis. *Blood.* 2011;118(5):1216-1224.

320. Wormser GP, Dattwyler RJ, Shapiro ED, et al. The clinical assessment, treatment and prevention of Lyme disease, human granulocytic anaplasmosis, and babesiosis: clinical practice guidelines by the Infectious Diseases Society of America. *Clin Infect Dis.* 2006;43(9):1089-1134.

321. World Health Organization. *Guidelines for the Treatment of Malaria.* 3rd Ed. Geneva: World Health Organization; 2015.

322. Gann PH, Neva FA, Gam AA. A randomized trial of single- and two-dose ivermectin versus thiabendazole in the treatment of strongyloidiasis. *J Infect Dis.* 1994;169(5):1076-1079.

323. Bern C, Montgomery SP, Herwaldt BL, et al. Evaluation and treatment of Chagas disease in the United States: a systemic review. *JAMA.* 2007;298(18):2171-2181.

324. Kousha M, Tadi R, Soubani AO. Pulmonary aspergillosis: a clinical review. *Eur Respir Rev.* 2011;20(121):156-174.

325. DiCaudo DJ. Coccidioidomycosis: a review and update. *J Am Acad Dermatol.* 2006;55(6):929-942.

326. Cope JR, Ali IK. Primary amebic meningoencephalitis: what have we learned in the last 5 years? *Curr Infect Dis Rep.* 2016;18(10):31.

327. Tzipori S, Ward H. Cryptosporidiosis: biology, pathogenesis and disease. *Microbes Infect.* 2002;4(10):1047-1058.

328. Wiwanitkit V. Intestinal parasite infestation in HIV infected patients. *Curr HIV Res.* 2006;4(1):87-96.

329. Sauerbrei A. Diagnosis, antiviral therapy, and prophylaxis of varicella-zoster virus infections. *Eur J Clin Microbiol Infect Dis.* 2016;35(5):723-734.

Antimicrobials

Diana Gritsenko, PharmD, Marianna Fedorenko, PharmD, BCPS,
Navitha Ramesh, MD, and Anousheh Ghezel-Ayagh, MD

INTRODUCTION

It has been reported that for every 1-hour delay of effective antimicrobial therapy in patients with septic shock, there is a 7.6% decrease in survival.[1,2] Inadequate empiric therapy has also been associated with increased length of hospital stay.[3,4] In addition to timing and choice of antimicrobials, understanding the pharmacokinetics is vital to providing adequate coverage while minimizing resistance.[5]

PHARMACOKINETICS

Antibiotics can interfere with protein synthesis or common metabolic pathways of the target cells and/or compromise the integrity of the cell wall. They can be classified as either bacteriostatic—ie, inhibiting the growth and replication of bacteria—or bactericidal. Bacteriostatic antibiotics rely on the host's immune system in order to effectively clear the bacteria, whereas agents that are bactericidal are able to kill bacteria independent of the immune response.[6,7] These terms, however, are general categories and may not always apply for a given agent. For example, ampicillin and daptomycin, which are both regarded as bactericidal agents, are bacteriostatic against *Enterococcus*.[8] Azithromycin, a member of the traditionally bacteriostatic macrolide class, is bactericidal against *Legionella*.[9]

The minimum inhibitory concentration (MIC) is conventionally used to describe the susceptibility of the microorganism to an antimicrobial agent and is set by the Clinical and Laboratory Standard Institute (CLSI) using microbiologic, pharmacodynamic/kinetic, and clinical data.[10] It should be noted that MIC values are unique to the antibiotic with respect to an organism and cannot be compared across different agents. For example, levofloxacin with an MIC of less than 2 µg/mL is not less effective against *Pseudomonas aeruginosa* than piperacillin/tazobactam with an MIC of 4 µg/mL. In fact, in this scenario, levofloxacin would actually be categorized as "resistant," since the MIC breakpoint for *P aeruginosa* is 1 µg/mL or less.[11] Although MICs are useful in identifying potentially effective antibiotics, these values must be interpreted cautiously, as they do not reflect variable in vivo processes such as penetration of the antibiotic into the site of infection.[10,12]

Understanding the pharmacokinetic (PK) and pharmacodynamic (PD) properties of antibiotics can potentially optimize drug therapy and increase clinical effectiveness. By combining relative MICs with the PK/PD parameters of the drugs, antibiotics can be categorized as time-dependent or concentration-dependent. Figure 21-1 and Table 21-1 illustrate the pharmacokinetic and pharmacodynamics indices and associated antibiotics. Antibiotics that are considered to be concentration-dependent, such as fluoroquinolones or aminoglycosides, require a high concentration above the MIC in order to ensure maximal bactericidal activity. For time-dependent antibiotics, activity against microorganisms correlates best with the duration of time the concentration remains above the MIC (T > MIC).[12] In order to reach optimal bactericidal activity against Gram-negative bacteria, the free drug concentration needs to exceed the MIC for 60% to 70% of the dosing interval for penicillins, 70% to 80% for cephalosporins, and 40% to 50% for carbapenems.[13,14] Therefore, to optimize dosage for time-dependent antibiotics, one may consider giving doses more frequently rather than increasing the administered dose.

Alternatively, continuous infusion or an extended duration (3–4 hours) of infusion may be an appropriate method of administration in select circumstances. Studies utilizing Monte Carlo simulations to predict clinical response have supported the use of prolonged infusion strategies for infections caused by Gram-negative organisms with higher MICs. As demonstrated by Lodise et al, the probability of obtaining adequate bactericidal activity for treating *P aeruginosa* with an MIC of 16 mg/L (the susceptibility breakpoint) utilizing a 30-minute standard infusion of piperacillin/tazobactam 3.375 g intravenously (IV) every 6 hours was less than 25%, while a 4-hour infusion of 3.375 g every 8 hours had a probability of target attainment of 100%.[15]

SPECTRUM OF ACTIVITY AND SAFETY

The β-lactam ring is a core component of many antibiotic classes, such as the penicillins, cephalosporins, carbapenems, and monobactams. Penicillins are among the first antibiotics that were developed and initially maintained excellent

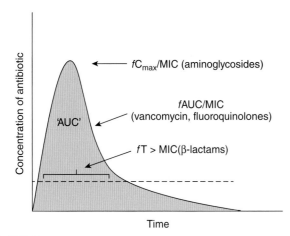

FIGURE 21-1 Pharmacokinetics-pharmacodynamics (PK-PD) Indices. Graphical representation of three commonly used PK-PD indices. fC_{max}/MIC: ratio of peak drug concentration to the organism minimum inhibitory concentration (MIC); commonly employed index for the aminoglycosides. $fAUC$/MIC: ratio of the area under the 24 hour concentration curve to the organism MIC; commonly employed index for vancomycin and the fluoroquinolones. $fT > MIC$: percent time of the dosing interval the drug concentration remains above the organism MIC; commonly employed index for the β-lactams. (Reprinted with permission from Labreche MJ, Graber CJ, Nguyen HM. Recent updates on the role of pharmacokinetics-pharmacodynamics in antimicrobial susceptibility testing as applied to clinical practice. *Clin Infect Dis*. 2015;61(9):1446-1452.)

TABLE 21-1 Pharmacokinetic and Pharmacodynamics Properties of Antibiotics

Antimicrobial Agent	Bactericidal Pattern of in Vitro Activity	PK/PD Measure(s)
Aminoglycosides	Concentration dependent	AUC_{0-24}:MIC, C_{max}:MIC
B-Lactams		
Penicillins	Time dependent	T > MIC
Cephalosporins	Time dependent	T > MIC
Carbapenems	Time dependent	T > MIC
Monobactams	Time dependent	T > MIC
Clindamycin	Time dependent	AUC_{0-24}:MIC
Glycopeptides/ lipopeptides		
Daptomycin	Concentration dependent	AUC_{0-24}:MIC, C_{max}:MIC
Oritavancin	Concentration dependent	T > MIC, C_{max}:MIC
Vancomycin	Time dependent	AUC_{0-24}:MIC
Macrolides and clindamycin		
Azithromycin	Time dependent	AUC_{0-24}:MIC
Clarithromycin	Time dependent	AUC_{0-24}:MIC
Metronidazole	Concentration dependent	AUC_{0-24}:MIC, C_{max}:MIC
Oxazolidinones		
Linezolid	Time dependent	AUC_{0-24}:MIC
Quinolones	Concentration dependent	AUC_{0-24}:MIC, C_{max}:MIC
Tetracyclines		
Doxycycline	Time dependent	AUC_{0-24}:MIC
Tigecycline	Time dependent	AUC_{0-24}:MIC

AUC_{0-24}:MIC = ratio of the area under the concentration-time curve at 24 h to the minimum inhibitory concentration; C_{max}:MIC = the ratio of the maximal drug concentration to the MIC; T > MIC = duration of time a drug concentration remains above the MIC.

Reprinted with permission from Ambrose PG, et al. Pharmacokinetics-Pharmacodynamics of Antimicrobial Therapy: It's Not Just for Mice Anymore. *Clin Infect Dis*. 2007;44(1):79-86.

activity against staphylococci, but due to the development of resistance, most staphylococci now are resistant to natural penicillins. However, the class still has excellent activity against most streptococci, including *Streptococcus pneumoniae*, and *Treponema pallidum*, while maintaining moderate activity against enterococci. The antistaphylococcal penicillins (ie, nafcillin, oxacillin, and methicillin) were developed with modifications that provided this class with activity against methicillin-sensitive *Staphylococcus aureus* (MSSA). The aminopenicillins, such as ampicillin or amoxicillin, have increased activity against some enteric Gram-negative organisms and *Haemophilus* species; however, this class does not have adequate antistaphylococcal activity because staphylococci usually produce penicillinases. Piperacillin is currently the only penicillin antibiotic that possesses activity against the *Pseudomonas* species, but it must be combined with a β-lactamase inhibitor like tazobactam to have antistaphylococcal activity.[16] The addition of β-lactamase inhibitors like tazobactam, sulbactam, or clavulanate not only enables activity against *Staphylococcus* species to the penicillins but also provides activity against anaerobes and β-lactamase–producing enteric Gram-negative organisms.[16,17]

The cephalosporin class is categorized into 5 "generations" that correspond to their spectrum of activity. The Gram-negative activity of the cephalosporins increases with each increase in generation, but only cefepime and ceftazidime possess antipseudomonal activity. Alternatively, the Gram-positive activity of the cephalosporins declines as the generations increase, with the exception of the fifth-generation antibiotics ceftaroline and ceftobiprole, which have activity against MRSA.[16-18]

Carbapenems, which represent the most broad-spectrum class, have activity against most Gram-negative, Gram-positive, and anaerobic organisms. The exception is ertapenem which is inactive against *Pseudomonas* species, *Enterococcus* species, and *Acinetobacter* species.[18] The last member of the β-lactam antibiotics is aztreonam—the only monobactam, which has activity against Gram-negative organisms only, including *Pseudomonas*, and does not cover anaerobes.[19] In general, the β-lactam antibiotics are very well tolerated, with nausea, vomiting, and diarrhea being the most reported side effects. All β-lactams, however, can cause hypersensitivity reactions ranging from mild rash to acute interstitial nephritis or anaphylaxis. Some β-lactams can have increased incidence of neurotoxicity (eg, seizures from carbapenems), which can occur when toxic levels of the antibiotic accumulate due to renal dysfunction.[17,18]

Glycopeptide antibiotics (eg, vancomycin), linezolid, and daptomycin only possess activity against Gram-positive organisms including MRSA. The latter agents are also effective against vancomycin-resistant Gram-positive organisms (eg, vancomycin-resistant *Enterococcus* spp, or VRE). These anti-MRSA agents are associated with adverse effects, such as nephrotoxicity and ototoxicity with vancomycin, thrombocytopenia and serotonin toxicity with linezolid, and increased creatinine phosphokinase and rhabdomyolysis with daptomycin.[20] Metronidazole, a nitroimidazole, is active against anaerobes, *Clostridium* species, and protozoa.[21] Clindamycin has activity against MRSA, streptococci, anaerobes, and certain protozoa.[22] Trimethoprim/sulfamethoxazole (TMX/SMP) has adequate MRSA coverage as well as activity against *Stenotrophomonas maltophilia* and *Pneumocystis jirovecii* but possesses no pseudomonal or enterococcal coverage. In addition to causing hyperkalemia, TMX/SMP can also cause an increase in serum creatinine without affecting the glomerular filtration rate by inhibiting a cationic transport in the convoluted tubules of the kidney, which is responsible for creatinine secretion.[23]

Fluoroquinolones have excellent oral bioavailability and a favorable side effect profile. Due to widespread use, Gram-negative resistance to these agents has increased and can vary by geographic region. These antibiotics can be categorized as "respiratory" (ie, levofloxacin and moxifloxacin) or "nonrespiratory" (ie, ciprofloxacin). It is important to note that these categories do not refer to the penetration of the fluoroquinolones into the lungs, since these drugs are able to concentrate in tissues (such as the lungs, kidneys, and prostate) at levels that exceed serum concentrations. Respiratory fluoroquinolones are thus named because they have activity against *S pneumoniae* (including penicillin-resistant strains) and can be initiated empirically for community-acquired pneumonia.[24,25] Fluoroquinolones have otherwise poor Gram-positive coverage (with the exception of levofloxacin and moxifloxacin's activity against *S pneumoniae*) but have great activity against atypical and Gram-negative organisms, including *Pseudomonas* species. Moxifloxacin, a newer generation fluoroquinolone, has activity against anaerobes but lacks anti-pseudomonal activity. Although moxifloxacin previously had excellent activity against *Bacteroides* species, resistance has become prevalent.[26] The most notable adverse effects with the fluoroquinolone class are QT prolongation, central nervous system (CNS) side effects (confusion, dizziness, somnolence), neuropathy, and arthralgias.[24]

Macrolide antibiotics are commonly used in both the inpatient and the outpatient setting. Although they have broad antimicrobial coverage, including excellent atypical coverage, there is increasing resistance to these agents, especially to *S pneumoniae*. This class is generally well tolerated, with gastrointestinal (GI) side effects being the most prevalent. Of the available agents, erythromycin has the most GI side effects as well as the most frequent dosing, which is why it is currently limited to use as a promotility agent.[25] Tetracyclines, such as minocycline and doxycycline, are also broad-spectrum antibiotics with excellent atypical coverage and have activity against community-acquired MRSA. These agents have poor anaerobe and Gram-negative coverage. Tigecycline, a tetracycline-derivative, can evade many of the tetracycline resistance mechanisms and has a similar spectrum of activity to the aforementioned class. In addition, tigecycline possesses activity against enterococci (including VRE), Gram-negatives organisms (with exception of *Pseudomonas* spp, *Proteus* spp, and *Providencia* spp), and anaerobes. Common side effects of these agents include nausea, vomiting, and diarrhea, as well as increased photosensitivity.[27,28] The aminoglycoside and the polymyxin classes (ie, colistin and polymyxin B) are used less frequently and are generally reserved for use in patients with multidrug-resistant Gram-negative infections due to an effort to preserve their activity and limit their use, due to the potential for systemic toxicity (eg, neurotoxicity and nephrotoxicity).[29,30]

RESISTANCE MECHANISMS

Antimicrobial resistance has continued to trend steadily upward over the past few decades and has given rise to multidrug-resistant organisms, or organisms that are nonsusceptible to at least 1 agent in 3 or more antibacterial classes.[31,32] There are 4 fundamental mechanisms by which antimicrobial resistance can develop: (1) alteration in the bacterial membrane permeability to antibiotics, (2) enzymatic degradation, (3) active efflux out of the bacterial cell, and (4) alteration of bacterial proteins that act as antimicrobial targets (Table 21-2).[33]

For β-lactam antibiotics, the most common mechanism of resistance is through hydrolysis by enzymes such as β-lactamases, acylases, and esterases. β-Lactamases, encoded on bacterial chromosomes or plasmids, are the most important mechanisms of resistance. This enzyme, predominantly secreted by Gram-negative bacteria, catalyzes the β-lactam ring into an open position, which thereby removes the drug's antibacterial properties. Extended spectrum β-lactamases (ESBLs) confer resistance to not only all penicillins and first- and second-generation cephalosporins (as seen with type I β-lactamases), but also to third-generation cephalosporins and aztreonam. Carbapenems and cephamycins (cefotetan and cefoxitin), however, are generally more resistant to degradation by most β-lactamases. In order to overcome β-lactamase–mediated resistance, certain antibiotics are coadministered with a β-lactamase inhibitor (ie, clavulanic acid, sulbactam, tazobactam)—that is, an agent that is capable of inhibiting β-lactamase activity.[34] Since the early 2000s, there has been a rise in the number of *Klebsiella pneumoniae*

TABLE 21-2 Resistance Mechanisms in Select Bacterial Pathogens

Pathogen	Antibiotic	Fundamental Mechanism of Resistance	Example of Specific Resistance Mechanism
Staphylococcus aureus	β-Lactams	Enzymatic degradation	Production of penicillinases
		Alteration in target site	Alteration of PBP2a via *mecA* gene
	Vancomycin	Alteration in membrane permeability	VISA: thickening of cell wall, which prevents adequate antibiotic penetration
		Alteration in target site	VRSA: transfer of *vanA* genes from VRE, resulting in D-ala-D-lac peptidoglycan layer
	Daptomycin	Alteration in membrane permeability	*mprF* mutation resulting in a charge-repulsive milieu for calcium-complexed daptomycin
			Increase in *dlt* operon expression leading to enhanced d-alanylation of cell wall teichoic acids
	Fluoroquinolones	Efflux pumps	MepA and NorA, NorB, and NorC efflux pumps
Streptococcus pneumoniae	β-Lactams	Alteration in target site	Alteration of PBP2X
	Fluoroquinolones	Alteration of target enzymes	Mutation of QRDRs of DNA gyrase via *gyrA* mutations and topoisomerase IV via *parC*
	Macrolides	Alteration of ribosomal target site	Methylation of adenine residue of the 23S subunit of rRNA encoded via the *ermB* gene
		Efflux pumps	Encoded via the *mef* genes; *mefA* encodes for a macrolide-specific efflux pump
Enterococcus spp	β-Lactams	Alteration of target enzymes	Alteration of PBP5 in *E faecium*
		Enzymatic degradation	Production of penicillinases in *E faecalis*
	Vancomycin	Alteration in target site	Production of *Van* genes (eg, *VanA* and *VanB*) resulting in D-ala-D-lac peptidoglycan layer
	Daptomycin	Alteration in membrane permeability	Reduced diffusion into bacteria through thickened cell walls of vancomycin-resistant strains
	Linezolid	Alteration of ribosomal target site	G2576U mutation in the peptidyl-transferase region of the 23S rRNA
Enterobacteriaceae spp	β-Lactams	Enzymatic degradation	Production of penicillinases, extended-spectrum β-lactamases, AmpC cephalosporinases, and carbapenemases
		Alteration in target site	Alterations in various PBPs
	Fluoroquinolones	Alteration of target enzymes	Mutation of QRDRs of DNA gyrase via *gyrA* mutations and topoisomerase IV via *parC*
	Aminoglycosides	Alteration of ribosomal target site	High-level resistance via 16S rRNA methyltransferases (*ArmA* and *RmtB*)
		Enzymatic degradation	Bacterial expression of drug-metabolizing enzymes such as AAC(6')-Ib
	Tetracyclines	Efflux pumps	Plasmid-mediated *Tet*(A) to *Tet*(E) determinants that code for the presence of efflux pump
		Alteration of ribosomal target site	Presence of ribosome protection proteins [eg, *Tet*(M) and *Tet*(O)] that bind to the 70S ribosome
Pseudomonas aeruginosa	β-Lactams	Efflux pumps	Presence of MexC-MexD-OprM pumps
		Alteration in membrane permeability	Carbapenem resistance via *OprD*
		Enzymatic degradation	Production of penicillinases, extended-spectrum β-lactamases, AmpC cephalosporinases, and carbapenemases
	Fluoroquinolones	Alteration of target enzymes	Mutation of QRDRs of DNA gyrase via *gyrA* mutations and topoisomerase IV via *parC*
		Efflux pumps	Presence of MexC-MexD-OprM pumps
	Aminoglycosides	Efflux pumps	Presence of multidrug efflux system (eg, MexXY)
		Alteration of ribosomal target site	High-level resistance via 16S rRNA methyltransferases (*ArmA* and *RmtB*)
		Enzymatic degradation	Bacterial expression of drug-metabolizing enzymes such as acetyltransferases [eg, AAC(6')-Ib]

PBP = penicillin-binding proteins; QRDR = quinolone resistance-determining region; VISA = vancomycin-intermediate *S aureus*; VRE = vancomycin-resistant enterococci; VRSA = vancomycin-resistant *S aureus*.

carbapenemase (KPC) producing bacteria, or more accurately, since other Gram-negative bacteria are capable of producing the same resistance mechanism, an increase in carbapenem-resistant Enterobacteriaceae (CRE). This resistance pattern renders all carbapenems ineffective.[35]

β-Lactam antibiotics such as methicillin, nafcillin, and oxacillin have increased stability to Gram-positive β-lactamases; however, resistance to these agents can be mediated through alteration of the penicillin-binding proteins (PBPs). Production of an altered PBP2—such as PBP2a in *Staphylococcus* species or PBP2X in *S pneumoniae*, confers a much lower affinity for methicillin as well as most other β-lactams.[35,36] In addition to β-lactams, fluoroquinolones, macrolides, and lincosamides are other examples of antibiotics in which resistance is mediated via alteration of the target enzyme. In fluoroquinolones, the A subunit of DNA gyrase is altered so that it no longer binds to the antibiotic, while resistance to macrolides and lincosamides is due to methylation of adenine in the 23S ribosomal RNA.[33] Resistance to fluoroquinolones, as well as β-lactams and tetracyclines, can also develop via mutations in porins, which provide a path through the outer membrane of Gram-negative bacteria. Gram-negative resistance can also be mediated via production of genes that code for efflux pumps; efflux pumps can expel a wide array of molecules from both the cytoplasm and the periplasm of the bacterial cell and therefore can render an organism resistant to antibiotics.[37]

In the 1980s, resistance to vancomycin was first identified within the *Enterococcus* species followed by the identification of vancomycin resistance in the *Staphylococcus* species. Vancomycin inhibits bacterial cell-wall formation by binding to the D-ala-D-ala portion of the cell wall precursor and therefore inhibits the synthesis of the peptidoglycan layer. Resistance to vancomycin, which is plasmid mediated and inducible, is believed to be due a transposon which alters the D-ala-D-ala to a dipeptide with a lower affinity for vancomycin, D-ala-D-lac.[38-40]

INHALED ANTIBIOTICS

Effective treatment of pneumonia requires the concentration of the antibiotic in the lung to be well above the MIC of the respective bacteria. Some systemically administered antibiotics, such as the β-lactams, polymyxins, and aminoglycosides, can have poor penetration into the lung parenchyma. An effective concentration can potentially be obtained by utilizing higher doses of the antibiotic, but this may increase the risk of systemic adverse effects. The rationale behind inhaled antibiotics is to maximize the drug delivery to the target site (ie, the lower airways) while minimizing the potential for systemic side effects.[41] Clinical studies have successfully demonstrated that nebulized antibiotics are able to achieve a concentration in the epithelial lining fluid (ELF) far above the MICs for even multidrug-resistant pathogens. For example, in Badia et al, tobramycin was administered via nebulization to

6 critically ill patients who were mechanically ventilated for greater than 48 hours. The antibiotic concentration found in the patients' bronchial specimens 1 hour after nebulization ranged from 68 mg/L to 855.7 mg/L, while serum drug concentrations were undetectable in 4 patients and were 0.4 mg/L and 0.6 mg/L in 2 of the patients.[42]

One concern involving the use of nebulized antibiotics is the potential for development of systemic resistance. In traditional medical teaching, concentrations below the effective MIC of the invading pathogen is thought to encourage the selection of resistant mutants. However, it appears that the low systemic concentrations seen with nebulized antibiotics fall outside the mutant selection window and therefore reduce the risk of resistance.[43,44] Furthermore, studies involving both critically ill patients and patients with cystic fibrosis have not reported an increase in the emergence of resistance.[45-47]

As few antibiotics have been formulated specifically for nebulized administration, intravenous preparations are usually administered utilizing a nebulizer. Ideal solutions for inhalation have a particle size in the range of 1 to 5 μm to effectively deposit in the alveoli. Although intravenous formulations are not designed to consistently deliver this ideal particle size, the use of a vibrating mesh nebulizer (which can produce particle sizes of 3 μm) can improve antibiotic delivery.[48] In addition, these formulations contain preservatives (eg, phenols) and may have suboptimal osmolarity, which can increase the risk of bronchospasm and coughing.[49] Antibiotics—such as colistin, tobramycin, and aztreonam—specifically formulated for nebulized administration have appeared on the market but are only approved by the US Food and Drug Administration (FDA) for patients with cystic fibrosis only.[41]

In the 2016 Clinical Practice Guidelines provided by the Infectious Diseases Society of America and the American Thoracic Society, the role of inhaled antibiotics was better elucidated to include patients with ventilator-associated pneumonia secondary to Gram-negative bacilli susceptible only to aminoglycosides or polymyxins. In this patient population, the concomitant use of inhaled and intravenous antibiotics was suggested, rather than the use of intravenous antibiotics alone.[50]

ANTIFUNGALS

Polyenes

The polyene agents include amphotericin B and nystatin. These agents bind to ergosterol in the fungal cell membrane, which disrupts cell permeability and results in rapid cell death. Nystatin is usually administered locally and for topical treatment due to its prohibitive toxicity when administered systemically.[51] Amphotericin B's broad spectrum of activity includes *Aspergillus* species (except for *A terreus*), *Candida* species (except *C lusitaniae*), *Cryptococcus*, *Coccidioides* species, *Blastomyces*, *Histoplasma*, and some activity against

Mucorales and *Fusarium* species. In addition to the conventional formulation of amphotericin B deoxycholate (AmBd), newer lipid formulations have been developed, aiming to minimize amphotericin B's nephrotoxicity. The lipid formulations include liposomal amphotericin B (AmBisome; L-AmB), amphotericin B lipid complex (Abelcet; ABLC), and amphotericin B colloidal dispersion (Amphotec; ABCD). Care should be taken when dosing amphotericin B, as weight-based dosing recommendations for lipid formulations (3–5 mg/kg/d) are 5 to 7 times that of the conventional amphotericin B deoxycholate (0.5–1.0 mg/kg/d). The most common adverse effects include nephrotoxicity, infusion-related reactions, and electrolyte imbalances (ie, hyperkalemia, hypokalemia, hypomagnesemia). To minimize nephrotoxicity, administering a saline load and maintaining adequate hydration has been recommended (eg, administering 500 mL of normal saline before and after each dose).[51-54] Resistance to amphotericin is infrequent; mechanisms include defects in the *ERG3* gene leading to disruption in ergosterol biosynthesis and decreased ergosterol levels in the fungal membrane or increased catalase activity, which leads to decreased susceptibility to oxidative damage.[55]

Azoles

Azoles exert their antifungal activity by inhibiting 14α-demethylase, a fungal cytochrome P450 (CYP)-dependent enzyme, which impedes ergosterol synthesis and results in accumulation of methylsterols, growth arrest, and eventual fungal cell death. Agents in the azole class differ in spectrum of activity, tissue distribution, toxicities, and pharmacokinetic properties (Tables 21-3 and 21-4). Monitoring for drug-drug interactions is warranted due to collateral inhibition of human CYP enzymes. Concomitant use of medications that are CYP substrates (ie, fentanyl, methylprednisolone) and azoles may result in increased concentrations of the substrates, which may potentiate or prolong adverse effects.[51-53] As a class, azoles have been associated with QTc-interval prolongation (except for isavuconazole) and hepatotoxicity. Fluconazole is well tolerated. Itraconazole may cause gastrointestinal effects, hypokalemia, hypertension, and edema, and has negative inotropic properties. Voriconazole has been associated with rash with retinoid-like phototoxic reactions, photopsia, and visual disturbances.[51-53] Posaconazole and isavuconazole are well tolerated with reports of gastrointestinal side effects.[51-53,56] Resistance to azoles may be due to efflux pumps and/or mutations in *ERG11*, which encodes the target enzyme 14α-demethylase, among others.[55]

Echinocandins

Echinocandins inhibit the synthesis of β-(1,3)-D-glucan, a key structural component of fungal cell walls, which leads to a loss of cell integrity and increased susceptibility to cell lysis. Agents in this class include caspofungin, anidulafungin, and micafungin, which are used interchangeably. Echinocandins are active against *Candida* species (including *C glabrata*) and *Aspergillus* species, with fungicidal and fungistatic activity, respectively.[51-53] Higher MIC values have been associated with *C parapsilosis*, but the clinical significance is controversial. Observational studies suggest that the echinocandins may be effective for treatment of *C parapsilosis*.[57-59] This class is generally well tolerated, with rare adverse effects, including liver function test abnormalities and infusion-related reactions.[51-53] Resistance to echinocandins may be due to mutations in the *FKS1* or *FKS2* genes that encode the β-(1,3)-D-glucan synthase complex or via efflux pumps.[55]

Flucytosine

As a pyrimidine analogue, flucytosine inhibits DNA and protein synthesis in the fungal cell. The spectrum of activity includes *Candida* and *Cryptococcus* species. Due to the high rate of hematologic toxicities (leukopenia, thrombocytopenia, and/or pancytopenia), its use is typically reserved for treatment of cryptococcal meningitis. Other adverse effects include hepatotoxicity and gastrointestinal effects.[53,60] Ideal body weight is recommended for dosing, and therapeutic drug monitoring is typically performed (target trough and peak of 25–50 and 50–100 mg/L, respectively).[60,61]

ANTIVIRALS

Below is a selected group of antivirals.

Herpes Simplex Virus and Varicella Zoster Virus

Acyclovir is a nucleoside analogue; once converted to its active form acyclovir triphosphate by viral thymidine kinase and cellular enzymes, it competes with deoxyguanosine for viral DNA polymerase and subsequently inhibits DNA synthesis and viral replication. Its antiviral activity includes the herpes simplex virus-1 (HSV-1) and HSV-2, varicella zoster virus (VZV), and Epstein-Barr virus. Acyclovir is available in both oral and parenteral formulations.[62] Due to acyclovir's poor oral absorption and bioavailability, valacyclovir was developed. As a prodrug, it is converted to acyclovir after oral administration and yields better bioavailability.[63] Intravenous formulation of acyclovir is typically initiated in severe infections to attain adequate concentrations, with potential transition to oral antivirals upon hospital discharge.[64] Acyclovir penetrates cerebrospinal fluid CSF with concentrations approximately 50% of corresponding plasma concentrations. It is primarily renally eliminated, and dosing modification for renal dysfunction is suggested. Though generally well tolerated, neurological toxicities and acute renal dysfunction secondary to crystalopathy and tubular obstruction have been reported with acyclovir, especially when administered intravenously. Maintaining adequate hydration with high urinary flow rates (100–150 mL/h) prior to acyclovir administration, prolonging the infusion rate, and

TABLE 21-3 Comparative Pharmacokinetic and Pharmacodynamic Parameters of Antifungal Agents

Drug	Typical Adult Dosing	Oral Bioavailability	C_{max} (µg/mL)	AUC (mg × b/L)	Protein (%)	CSF (%)	Vitreous (%)	Urine (%)	Metabolism	Elimination	$T_{1/2}$ (h)	PK:PD (total drug unless indicated)
AMB	0.6–1.0 mg/kg/d	< 5	0.5–2.0	17.0	> 95.0	0–4	0–38[a,b]	3–20	Minimal	Feces	50	C_{max}:MIC 4–10 or AUC:MIC > 100
ABCD	4 mg/kg/d	< 5	4.0	43.0	> 95.0	< 5	0–38[a,b]	< 5	Minimal	ND	30	ND
ABLC	5 mg/kg/d	< 5	1.7	14.0	> 95.0	< 5	0–38[a,b]	< 5	Minimal	ND	173	C_{max}:MIC > 40 or AUC:MIC > 100
LAMB	3–5 mg/kg/d	< 5	83	555	> 95.0	< 5	0–38[a,b]	5	Minimal urine; feces	Minor	100–153	C_{max}:MIC > 40 or AUC:MIC > 100
FLU	6–12 mg/kg/d	> 90	6–20	400–800	10.0	> 60	28–75[a,b]	90	Minor hepatic	Renal	31	AUC:MIC > 25
ITRA[c]	200 mg twice daily	50	0.5–2.3	29.2	99.8	< 10	10[a]	1–10	Hepatic	Hepatic	24	AUC:MIC > 25
VOR	6 mg/kg every 12 h for 2 doses, then 4 mg/kg every 12 h	> 90	3.0–4.6	20.3	59.0	60	38[a,b]	< 2	Hepatic	Renal	6	AUC:MIC > 25
POS	600–800 mg/d in divided doses	ND	1.5–2.2	8.9	99.0	ND	26[a,b]	< 2	Modest hepatic	Feces	25	AUC:MIC > 25 (8–25 free drug)
ANI[d]	200 mg × 1 loading dose, then 100 mg/d	< 5	6–7	99	84.0	< 5	0[b]	< 2	None	Feces	26	C_{max}:MIC > 10 or serum (unbound) AUC:MIC > 20
CAS	70-mg loading dose, then 50 mg/d	< 5	8–10	119	97.0	< 5	0[a]	< 2	Hepatic	Urine	30	C_{max}:MIC > 10 or serum (unbound) AUC:MIC > 20
MICA[a]	100–150 mg/d; 50 mg/d (prophylaxis)	< 5	10–16	158	99.0	< 5	< 1[b]	< 2	Hepatic	Feces	15	C_{max}:MIC > 10 or serum (unbound) AUC:MIC > 20
5-FC	100 mg/kg/d in divided doses	80	30–40	30–62	4.0	60–100	49[b]	90	Minor intestinal	Renal	3–6	Time > MIC 20–40%

ABCD = amphotericin B colloidal dispersion; ABLC = amphotericin lipid complex; AMB = amphotericin B; ANI = anidulafungin; AUC = area under the curve; CAS = caspofungin; C_{max} = maximum concentration; CSF = cerebrospinal fluid; 5-FC = flucytosine; FLU = fluconazole; ITRA = itraconazole; LAMB = liposomal AMB; MIC = minimum inhibitory concentration; MICA = micafungin; ND = not determined; PK-PD = pharmacokinetics-pharmacodynamics; POS = posaconazole; VOR = voriconazole; $T_{1/2}$ = half-life.

[a] Data derived from human studies.

[b] Data derived from animal studies.

[c] Oral solution formulation.

[d] Data are for the 100-mg dose.

Reprinted with permission from Lewis RE. Current concepts in antifungal pharmacology. *Mayo Clin Proc.* 2011;86(8):805-817.

TABLE 21-4 Cytochrome P450 Inhibition Profile of Triazole Antifungal Agents

Mechanism	Fluconazole	Itraconazole	Posaconazole	Voriconazole
Inhibitor				
CYP2C19	+	−	−	+++
CYP2C9	++	+	−	++
CYP3A4	++	+++	+++	++
Substrate				
CYP2C19	−	−	−	+++
CYP2C9	−	−	−	+
CYP3A4	+	+++	−	+

− = no activity; + = minimal activity; ++ = moderate activity; +++ = strong activity.

Data from Fernando-Ruiz M, Aguado JM, Almirante B, et al. Initial use of echinocandins does not negatively influence outcome in *Candida parapsilosis* blood stream infection: a propensity score analysis. *Clin Infect Dis*. 2014;58(10):1413-1421.

reducing the dose in patients with renal impairment re rec-ommended to minimize the risk of nephrotoxicity.[65] Valacy-clovir has been associated with mild adverse effects such as nausea, headache, and diarrhea. Resistance to acyclovir and valacyclovir can be conferred by alterations to viral thymidine kinase and viral DNA polymerase.[66,67] Penciclovir and its pro-drug, famciclovir, are other oral treatment options. Penciclovir shares a similar mechanism of action, chemical structure, and spectrum of activity as acyclovir.[68]

Influenza

Two antiviral classes are currently available for treatment and prophylaxis of influenza: neuraminidase inhibitors (NAI) and adamantanes. Neuraminidase inhibitors interfere with the enzyme that releases progeny virions from the infected host cell, which reduces viral replication and halts spread of infection. As a class, these agents—which include oseltamivir, zanamivir, and peramivir—are effective against all influenza strains.[69] Oselta-mivir is only available in an oral formulation and is generally well tolerated; the most frequent side effects include nausea, vomiting, and abdominal pain and rare reports of neuropsy-chiatric events.[69,70] As it is primarily renally excreted, dosing must be decreased in patients with renal dysfunction.[69] Zana-mivir is available as a dry powder for inhalation and should not be nebulized.[71] Its use is not recommended in patients with underlying pulmonary dysfunction (eg, asthma, chronic obstructive pulmonary disease [COPD]) as it has been asso-ciated with cough, bronchospasm, and reversible decreases in pulmonary function.[69] The only FDA-approved agent that can be administered parenterally is peramivir, but its effectiveness for critically ill patients is uncertain. A large multicenter trial of patients hospitalized with influenza comparing peramivir plus standard of care to placebo plus standard of care did not dem-onstrate clinical benefit. However, receipt of other NAIs was allowable as part of standard of care, which confounded study design.[72] Resistance to NAI can develop as a result of mutations in the neuraminidase target site.[73] Adamantanes (ie, amanta-dine and rimantadine) are not currently recommended for treatment in the United States, as they are inactive against the majority of circulating influenza strains.[74]

ANTIPARASITICS

Antimalarials

Severe malaria is typically caused by 1 of 4 possible *Plasmo-dium* species: *P falciparum*, *P vivax*, *P ovale*, and *P malariae*. Patients with severe malaria are those who present with par-asitemia and one or more of the following clinical or labora-tory features: impaired consciousness, jaundice, respiratory distress, severe anemia, hemoglobinuria, and pulmonary edema. Critically ill patients with severe malaria should be loaded with parenteral antimalarial drugs as quickly as possible, as most deaths from severe malaria occur within the first 24 to 48 hours.[75] In the United States, only 1 drug, quinidine, is FDA approved for intravenous administra-tion. Quinidine is a member of the quinoline class, along with chloroquine, mefloquine, quinine, and primaquine. Chloroquine, quinine, and quinidine work by interfering in the ability of the malaria parasite to detoxify hemoglobin metabolites, which results in toxic accumulation and even-tual parasitic death.[76,77] The quinoline class of antiparasit-ics is associated with various and unique side effects. As a class, the quinolines can cause dose-dependent cardiovas-cular toxicity including hypotension, QT prolongation, and ventricular arrhythmias. These cardiovascular effects are more common with intravenous quinidine, a class IA anti-arrhythmic agent, than with the other agents. Both quini-dine and quinine can stimulate the release of insulin, which can result in profound hypoglycemia if unmonitored, and quinine can cause cinchonism (headache, nausea, tinnitus, and visual disturbances) even at therapeutic doses. Meflo-quine should be avoided in patients with neuropsychiatric conditions, as it is associated with a wide range of psychi-atric disturbances, such as vivid dreams, mood swings, depression, and even psychosis. Neurotoxicity induced by mefloquine can be difficult to distinguish from postmalarial neurologic syndrome, which can typically last between 1 and days and is more common among patients with severe malaria.[78-80] Primaquine, on the other hand, has a different mechanism of action, whereby it affects parasite pyrimidine synthesis and disrupts the mitochondrial electron transport chain. A major adverse effect of primaquine is its ability to induce significant hemolysis especially in patients with glucose-6-phosphate dehydrogenase (G6PD) deficiency. It is important to test for the deficiency in patients before initiation of the drug. The metabolites of primaquine induce the oxidation of hemoglobin into methemoglobin; this occurs both in normal and in G6PD erythrocytes.[76,78] More frequently, physicians will utilize this drug as an alternative for the treatment of *Pneumocystis jirovecii* pneumonia (PJP) in conjunction with clindamycin.[81]

In patients with severe malaria who have contraindications to or cannot tolerate intravenous quinidine, artesunate is a potential new option. Currently available from the Centers of Disease Control and Prevention under an investigational new drug protocol, artesunate is available in intravenous form and is recommended by the World Health Organization in preference to intravenous quinidine for the treatment of severe malaria.[82] This derivative of the *Artemisia annua* plant is thought to work by creating an endoperoxide dioxygen bridge that accumulates in various parasite compartments and causes critical damage to parasite organelles.[83] Artesunate demonstrates excellent efficacy against all human malaria parasites, including those with multidrug resistance, and other parasites such as *Schistosoma*, *Leishmania*, and *Fasciola*.[84,85] Because artesunate is rapidly eliminated, it must always be partnered with a drug with a longer half-life (artemisinin combination therapy) such as atovaquone-proguanil (Malarone), mefloquine, or doxycycline.[86]

Anthelmintics

Helminths, or parasitic worms, can be categorized into roundworms (nematodes) or 1 of 2 types of flatworms: flukes (trematodes) or tapeworms (cestodes). With few exceptions, such as *Strongyloides stercoralis* and *Echinococcus*, helminths do not replicate within the human host. As a result, the number of parasites infecting the host (ie, infection intensity or "worm burden") is dictated by the extent of the exposure and is a determinant of morbidity.[87] Although initially developed for veterinary use, safe and effective anthelmintic drugs have been developed for human use with antihelminthic chemotherapy dominated by 3 drugs: albendazole, praziquantel, and ivermectin.[87,88] These drugs have specific efficacy against different classes of helminths. In general, albendazole or ivermectin can be utilized for infections due to nematodes, while praziquantel is generally used for trematodes. For infections due to cestodes, praziquantel is generally used for intestinal infections, while tissue infections outside of the GI tract can be treated with albendazole.[89]

Albendazole, a member of the benzimidazole class, exerts its action by disrupting cell division and various energy pathways through selective binding to the nematode tubulin, which prevents polymerization into microtubules. This results in a decrease of ATP production, which in turn leads to immobilization and eventual worm death.[88,90,91] The absorption of albendazole is pH dependent, so it should be taken with food. When albendazole was administered with food, the plasma concentration of its metabolite, albendazole sulfoxide, increased 5-fold.[92] Albendazole displays a higher affinity for the parasitic β-tubulin rather than the same β-tubulin target in other eukaryotic organisms, which accounts for its excellent safety profile. In mass treatment programs, the most frequent side effect (occurring in ~1% of the population) was mild gastrointestinal symptoms.[93] The development of resistance to albendazole is the result of amino acid substitutions on the worm's β-tubulin. Resistance is uncommon but is developing in parasites like *Trichuris trichiura* and *Wuchereria bancrofti*.[94,95]

Ivermectin, an antiparasitic agent derived from *Streptomyces avermitilis*, is active against a wide range of helminths and ectoparasites but is the drug of choice for onchocerciasis and strongyloidiasis and a second-line agent for scabies.[96] It exerts its mechanism of action by activating ligand-gated chloride channels and inducing hyperpolarization and muscle paralysis.[97] Ivermectin has a higher binding affinity for the nematode ligand, thereby causing paralysis of nematode pharynx and halting ingestion of nutrients, than for mammalian ligands, which explains its particular selectivity and its safety profile.[97,98] The most notable side effects of ivermectin include mild GI symptoms and a Mazzotti-like reaction to dying microfilariae in filarial infections.[99] Ivermectin also interacts with the gamma-aminobutyric acid (GABA) receptors, however with relatively low affinity in mammalian brains compared to invertebrate receptors (~100-fold higher affinity).[100] A theoretical concern exists for ivermectin use in patients with an impaired blood–brain barrier (eg, meningitis) in whom it is believed that continued use can lead to a benzodiazepine-like encephalopathy; however, independent of a Mazzotti-like reaction, this effect is rarely seen.[101]

Praziquantel, which is active against most cestodes and trematodes, is the drug of choice for the treatment of schistosomiasis and a component of therapy with albendazole for neurocysticercosis.[102] In order to achieve clinical efficacy with praziquantel, an intact immune system is believed to be required. At low concentrations, praziquantel is believed to cause increased muscular activity leading to contraction and spastic paralysis. At higher effective concentrations, praziquantel is believed to disrupt the parasite tegument, which causes loss of adherence to host tissue, which ultimately leads to parasite expulsion. It is also believed to interfere with the parasite's metabolism and to expose tegumental antigens.[103] For this reason, indirect effects such as fever, pruritus, arthralgias, and myalgias may occur as a result of parasite death. Eosinophilia may also occur as a result of the parasite burden and release of antigens. In patients with neurocysticercosis, inflammatory reactions as a result of praziquantel therapy may produce seizures, meningismus, and mental status changes. Praziquantel is also contraindicated in patients with ocular cysticercosis because the inflammatory host response can cause irreversible eye damage.[104-106]

ANTIMICROBIAL STEWARDSHIP

Antimicrobial resistance is rising, while the number of new agents in the drug development pipeline has declined.[107-110] Infections with multidrug-resistant (MDR) organisms are associated with increased mortality, prolonged lengths of hospital and intensive care unit (ICU) stays, and cost.[111,112] Recognizing that antimicrobials provide selective pressure for the emergence of resistant bacteria, minimizing unnecessary or inappropriate use by engaging in antimicrobial stewardship is vital. Antimicrobial stewardship generally refers to diverse interventions designed to improve appropriate use of antimicrobials by optimizing agent selection, dosing, duration of therapy, and route of administration.[113] These interventions are especially relevant in intensive care units, which are associated with high antibiotic use and resistance rates and includes critically ill patients for whom selection of optimal antibiotic regimens is complex.[114,115] Notably, implementation of antimicrobial stewardship interventions in the intensive care unit has been associated with improved antimicrobial utilization, antimicrobial susceptibility rates, and decreased adverse effects without compromising clinical outcomes.[116]

Antibiotic Selection

As timely and adequate antimicrobial therapy has been associated with improved mortality in patients with septic shock, initial therapy is often empiric, with selection of antimicrobials based on the presence of risk factors for MDR organisms (eg, recent antimicrobial use, prolonged hospital stay, prior infection with MDR organisms), local antimicrobial susceptibility patterns, and likely sources of infection.[117,118] Subsequently, de-escalation—the selection of antimicrobials with a narrower spectrum of activity or a reduction in the number of antimicrobials—may be made after identification of the organism and susceptibilities.[118,119]

Duration of Therapy

Prolonged duration of antimicrobial therapy provides selective pressure for antimicrobial resistance and increases patients' risk for side effects, including *Clostridium difficile* infections.[114,115] Consequently, recent studies demonstrate that short-duration regimens are effective for serious infections, such as pneumonia, urinary tract infections, intra-abdominal infections, and cellulitis, especially if adequate source control is obtained.[118,120-122] Furthermore, biomarkers may be used to assist with decisions to discontinue antimicrobial therapy. In a large randomized controlled trial of intensive care unit patients (PRORATA trial), procalcitonin-guided therapy was associated with reduced antibiotic exposure without affecting mortality rates.[123] Of note, longer durations are indicated for certain indications such as *S aureus* bacteremia, endocarditis, osteomyelitis, fungemia, febrile neutropenia, and/or cases with poor source control.[59,124-128]

QUESTIONS

1. An 85-year-old man with a past medical history of COPD and type 2 diabetes presents from a nursing home with acute cholangitis and septic shock. No recent travel history was described. The patient is now on day 3 of empiric treatment with cefepime. Blood cultures are growing *Enterobacter cloacae*, which is susceptible to gentamicin, ceftriaxone, ceftazidime, cefepime, piperacillin/tazobactam, meropenem, and ciprofloxacin, and is resistant to cefazolin and cefoxitin. What β-lactamase is most likely produced by the *E cloacae* isolated in this case?

   A. AmpC
   B. *Klebsiella pneumoniae* carbapenemase
   C. New Delhi metallo-β-lactamase
   D. CTX-M

2. For the patient in question 1, what is the most appropriate antimicrobial selection?

   A. De-escalate to ceftriaxone
   B. Change to piperacillin/tazobactam
   C. Continue cefepime
   D. Add gentamicin

3. Which of the following antibiotics is correctly paired with its likely resistance mechanism?

   A. Macrolide: reduced ribosome binding affinity via Tet(M) protein
   B. Penicillin: removed via efflux pump encoded by *mef*(A) gene
   C. Macrolide: modification of target site via *erm* gene
   D. Penicillin: increased levels of dihydrofolate reductase enzyme

4. A 22-year-old woman with a past medical history of cystic fibrosis (3120+1G>A and R1162X CFTR mutation), asthma, diabetes, pancreatic insufficiency, gastroparesis, depression, percutaneous endoscopic gastrostomy (PEG) tube, and history of MDR pseudomonas presented to the hospital with 3 days of shortness of breath and dyspnea on exertion. She developed a productive cough with yellow/green sputum associated with chest tightness.

   The patient was admitted to the floor and started on empiric coverage with ceftazidime 2 g IV every 8 hours (q8h) and ciprofloxacin 400 mg IV every 12 hours (q12h). Her vital signs are as follows: blood pressure (BP) of 103/79 mmHg, heart rate (HR) of 101 beats/min, respiratory rate (RR) of 22 breaths/min, temperature of 100.6°F, and O$_2$ saturation of 94% on 2 Liters via nasal cannula. Her labs are as follows:

Sodium	149 mEq/L
Potassium	4.3 mEq/L
Chloride	106 mEq/L
CO_2	24 mEq/L
Blood urea nitrogen	25 mEq/L
Creatinine	0.73 mg/dL
White blood cells	23×10^3 cell/μL
Hemoglobin	13.8 g/dL
Hematocrit	40.9 g/dL
Platelets	213×10^3 μ/L

Her chest x-ray showed bilateral patchy opacities on the right more than the left. Her blood culture showed no growth to date, and her sputum showed moderate (3+) mucoid *P aeruginosa*.

Organism	Kirby Bauer
Amikacin	Susceptible
Aztreonam	Intermediate
Cefepime	Intermediate
Ceftazidime	Intermediate
Ciprofloxacin	Resistant
Gentamicin	Susceptible
Imipenem	Resistant
Levofloxacin	Resistant
Piperacillin	Resistant
Tobramycin	Susceptible
Meropenem	Resistant
Organism	**Etest (μg/mL)**
Polymyxin B	0.38 (Susceptible)

According to the susceptibilities reported above, which of the following regimens would likely be the most effective while minimizing toxicity?

A. Ceftazidime 2 g IV q8h and gentamicin 3 mg/kg IV q8h
B. Polymyxin B 25,000 units/kg/d divided every 12 hours
C. Ceftazidime 2 g IV q8h and tobramycin 300 mg inhalation q12h
D. Amikacin 15–20 mg/kg/d IV once daily

5. The team wants to replace ceftazidime with an agent that is susceptible. Which additional susceptibilities should the team call the microbiology lab and ask for?

A. Ceftaroline
B. Ceftolozane/tazobactam
C. Ertapenem
D. Tigecycline

6. A 52-year-old man was admitted to the inpatient unit with a chief complaint of fever, wheezing, and cough with sputum production. He does not have any relevant past medical history and no recent antibiotic use or previous hospitalizations. A chest x-ray is performed and demonstrates the presence of bilateral infiltrates. Since the patient reports a childhood penicillin allergy (anaphylaxis), the medical resident decides to use a fluoroquinolone antibiotic. Which fluoroquinolone is not recommended for this indication due to a higher likelihood of resistance?

A. Moxifloxacin
B. Levofloxacin
C. Gemifloxacin
D. Ciprofloxacin

7. A 65-year-old woman presents with pneumonia complicated by septic shock and acute respiratory failure requiring intubation. Vancomycin 1.25 g IV q12h, cefepime 1 g IV q8h, and gentamicin 490 mg IV × 1 are initiated. Her past medical history includes hypertension, coronary artery disease, COPD, type 2 diabetes mellitus, hospitalization 3 weeks prior to admission for pneumonia requiring intubation, and a 5-day ICU stay. She has no known allergies. She lives in nursing home. Her vital signs are as follows: BP of 100/70 mmHg, HR of 110 beats/min, fraction of inspired oxygen (Fio_2) of 60%, positive end-expiratory pressure (PEEP) of 10 mmHg, and a maximum temperature of 100.8°F. Her weight is 85 kg and her height is 167 cm. Her labs are as follows:

White blood cells	20×10^3 cells/μL (15% bands)
Hemoglobin	11 g/dL
Platelets	180×10^3 μL
Sodium	135 mEq/L
Potassium	4.1 mEq/L
Chloride	107 mEq/L
CO_2	24 mEq/L
Blood urea nitrogen	18 mg/dL
Creatinine	0.8 mg/dL (baseline creatinine, 0.7 mg/dL)
Lactic acid	3.0 mmol/L

What are the therapeutic level goals for vancomycin?

A. 5–10 mg/L
B. 10–15 mg/L
C. 15–20 mg/L
D. 20–25 mg/L

8. For the patient in question 7, what is the next step for managing gentamicin?

   A. Order a dose to be administered 24 hours after the first dose
   B. Order a dose to be administered 8 hours after the first dose
   C. Order a peak to be drawn 1 hour after the first administered dose
   D. Order a random level 8 to 10 hours after the first administered dose

9. A 60-year-old woman with a past medical history of hypertension, diabetes mellitus, end-stage renal disease on hemodialysis (Monday, Wednesday, and Friday), and atrial fibrillation (not on anticoagulation) was brought in by emergency medical services for altered mental status. Per the patient's family, she was admitted to another hospital 1 week prior for severe community-acquired pneumonia. Her family reports that the patient has been having fevers (maximum temperature, 102°F), chills, nausea, and vomiting for the past day and skipped her dialysis session because she was feeling too weak. In the ED, the patient's vital signs are as follows: BP of 97/65 mmHg, HR of 123 beats/min, RR of 35 breaths/min, O_2 saturation of 89% on nonrebreather, and temperature of 101°F. She weighs 80 kg. The patient received a total of 3 liters of normal saline. Her chest x-ray revealed bilateral patchy infiltrates (R > L) and a small pleural effusion. Her labs are as follows:

Sodium	151 mEq/L
Potassium	6.5 mEq/L
Chloride	111 mEq/L
CO$_2$	29 mEq/L
Blood urea nitrogen	135 mEq/L
Creatinine	9.19 mg/dL
Albumin	1.9 g/L
Aspartate aminotransferase/alanine transaminase	546/491 IU/L
International normalized ratio	1.7
White blood cells	35 u/L
Hemoglobin	8.9 g/dL
Hematocrit	26.7 g/dL
Platelets	110×10^3 u/L

In the ED, the patient has already received meropenem 1000 mg IV × 1 and azithromycin 500 mg IV × 1. What loading dose of vancomycin would be the most optimal in this situation?

   A. Vancomycin 1000 mg IV (12.5 mg/kg)
   B. Vancomycin 1500 mg IV (18.75 mg/kg)
   C. Vancomycin 2000 mg IV (25 mg/kg)
   D. Vancomycin 1250 mg IV (15.6 mg/kg)

10. The patient in question 9 has been admitted to the medical ICU and was seen by nephrology who recommended initiating the patient on sustained low-efficiency daily diafiltration (SLEDD). What dose of meropenem would be most appropriate for the patient at this time?

   A. Meropenem 1000 mg IV q6h daily
   B. Meropenem 1000 mg IV q6h daily while on SLEDD
   C. Meropenem 500 mg IV q8h daily while on SLEDD
   D. Meropenem is not recommended with this modality due to its complete removal during SLEDD

11. A 46-year-old woman with a past medical history of hypertension and diabetes recently immigrated from Peru. She presents to the ED with new-onset seizures. Family members present at her bedside report that the patient has also been experiencing frequent headaches and nausea and vomiting for the past 2 weeks. An MRI of the brain revealed 2.3-mm and 4.3-mm cystic lesions adjacent to the occipital horn of the ventricular system and multiple 2- to 3-mm cysts within the subarachnoid space. The MRI shows the obstruction of cerebrospinal fluid flow with dilatation of the fourth ventricle. The team requested a cysticercus-specific IgG antibody level and an enzyme-linked immunosorbent assay of the CSF, which both returned positive. What treatment would you recommend?

   A. Praziquantel 50–100 mg/kg/d in 3 divided doses
   B. Albendazole 15 mg/kg/d in 2 divided doses taken on an empty stomach
   C. Albendazole 15 mg/kg/d in 2 divided doses taken with food PLUS praziquantel 50–100 mg/kg/d in 3 divided doses
   D. Ivermectin 200 µg/kg as a single dose

12. Which medication is conventionally given in conjunction with the treatment described in question 11?

   A. Diphenhydramine 25 mg IV q8h
   B. 0.9% sodium chloride at 50–100 mL/h
   C. Prednisone 1 mg/kg/d for 5–10 days
   D. Methotrexate 7.5 mg once a week

ANSWERS

1. A. AmpC

   Organisms that possess chromosomally encoded inducible AmpC β-lactamase are sometimes referred to as SPACE organisms (*Serratia, Providencia, Pseudomonas, Acinetobacter, Citrobacter, Enterobacter*). However, other organisms such as *Morganella morganii, Proteus vulgaris*, and *P penneri* may be included as well.[128,129] Since the *E cloacae* in this case was susceptible to meropenem, possession of a KPC (choice B) or New Delhi metallo-β-lactamase

(NDM1; choice C) is unlikely. In addition, the patient does not report recent travel, and NDM1 is associated with healthcare contact in India and Bangladesh.[130] As activity to ceftriaxone and ceftazidime was maintained, then the presence of a CTX-M (choice D), which is a type of extended spectrum β-lactamase, is also less likely.

2. **C. Continue cefepime**

Bacteria express 1 of 3 types of AmpC production: (1) low-level constitutive, which refers to a low basal level of production; (2) high-level constitutive, also known as "depressed," which refers to constant production of high concentrations of AmpC regardless of the presence or absence of an inducer; and (3) inducible production, which refers to low levels of AmpC production initially, but the presence of an inducer causes a surge in production. When the inducer is removed, production returns to basal levels. B-Lactams differ in their inducing ability and stability against AmpC hydrolysis. Strong inducers that are labile to AmpC include benzylpenicillin, ampicillin, amoxicillin, cefazolin, and cephalothin. Strong inducers stable to AmpC include cefoxitin and imipenem. Second- and third-generation cephalosporins, piperacillin, and aztreonam are weak inducers, which are also labile. Treatment with this last category of β-lactams (weak and labile inducers) can select for derepressed mutants, increasing the risk for clinical failure.[128-129] Therefore, answer choices A and B are not the best option. Cefepime (choice C) retains stability against AmpC and studies report favorable clinical outcomes, although this remains controversial.[128,131,132] There is no need to add gentamicin (choice D) because current treatment is active against the isolate.

3. **C. Macrolide: modification of target site via *erm* gene**

TetM (choice A) is a ribosome protection protein (RPR) that confers resistance to the tetracycline class of antibiotics by binding to their ribosomal target, the 70S ribosome.[133,134] Increased levels of dihydrofolate reductase enzyme (choice D), is mediated by a modification in the target enzyme, which is encoded in *dfr* genes. This modification confers resistance to trimethoprim, 1 of the 2 drug components of Bactrim.[135] Choices B and D both describe mechanisms of resistance to macrolide antibiotics. The *ermB* gene methylates an adenine residue within the 23S ribosomal RNA of the bacteria, which creates cross-resistance to macrolides and lacosamide (ie, clindamycin) antibiotics. The *mef* genes encode for the presence of the efflux pump. The *mefA* gene, for example, encodes for a macrolide-specific efflux pump.[136] Resistance to the penicillin class of antibiotics is generally mediated through amino acid substitutions in the penicillin-binding proteins, which creates a conformational change inhibiting the binding of the antibiotic. In *S pneumoniae*, PBP2X is responsible for resistance to β-lactam antibiotics.[137]

4. **C. Ceftazidime 2 g IV q8h and tobramycin 300 mg inhalation q12h**

Although the *Pseudomonas* is susceptible to all of the aminoglycosides and to polymyxin B, monotherapy with these agents (choices B and D) is not recommended due to the increased likelihood of developing resistance during treatment. Combining an aminoglycoside or polymyxin B with another antibiotic, even if the second antibiotic is resistant, can prevent the development of resistance. Combination therapy for *Pseudomonas* is also indicated in the setting of sepsis. Since the *Pseudomonas* has intermediate susceptibilities to ceftazidime, it is an acceptable second agent. Choice A is not ideal due to the poor penetration of aminoglycosides into the lung. The concentration of aminoglycoside in the epithelial lining fluid of the lung is approximately 30% of that of plasma.[138,139] The C_{max}:MIC ratio is an important predictor of efficacy in aminoglycosides. It has been shown that aminoglycosides eradicate bacteria more effectively when C_{max}:MIC is at least 8 to 10. Assuming the MIC of the *Pseudomonas* to gentamicin was 1 μg/mL, a peak plasma concentration of 8 to 10 μg/mL would only give us a theoretical ELF concentration of 2.4 to 3 μg/mL, which is ineffective. To achieve an ELF concentration of 8 to 10 μg/mL, we would need to target a plasma concentration of 26.7 to 33.3 μg/mL, which is well above the range where ototoxicity and nephrotoxicity can be expected to occur (12–14 μg/mL). Therefore, administration of the aminoglycoside directly into the site of infection via inhalation (choice C) is an effective option, since it can achieve exponentially higher concentrations well over the MIC of the organism and minimize systemic toxicity.

5. **B. Ceftolozane/tazobactam**

Unlike the other carbapenems in its class, ertapenem does not have anti-pseudomonal activity (choice C).[140] In general, tetracycline antibiotics do not have activity against *Pseudomonas*. Tigecycline, a glycylcycline antibiotic structurally related to the tetracyclines, also lacks activity to *Pseudomonas* due to the presence of efflux pumps (choice D).[141] Ceftaroline is a newer cephalosporin, which has excellent activity against MRSA but does not exhibit reliable activity against *Pseudomonas* (choice A).[142] Ceftolozane/tazobactam (Zerbaxa) is another broad-spectrum β-lactam and β-lactamase inhibitor combination drug that was approved by the FDA and that may retain activity against *Pseudomonas*.[143] To confirm susceptibilities, an E-test can be requested from the microbiology laboratory.

6. **D. Ciprofloxacin**

Moxifloxacin, levofloxacin, and gemifloxacin are all respiratory fluoroquinolones and are recommended by the 2007 IDSA/ATS Consensus Guidelines for the Management of Community-Acquired Pneumonia in Adults (choices A, B, and C).[144] Ciprofloxacin, although it possesses excellent penetration into the site of infection, is not considered to be a respiratory fluoroquinolone due to the rapid emergence of resistance in *S pneumoniae*. Fluoroquinolones target DNA gyrase and topoisomerase IV, which are essential for DNA replication in bacteria. Resistance to these agents is mediated through a mutation in the quinolone resistance–determining regions (QRDR) of various genes—in particular, the *parC* of topoisomerase IV and the *gyrA* of DNA gyrase.[145] Several studies have demonstrated that fluoroquinolone resistance occurs in a stepwise fashion, with point mutations in topoisomerase IV conferring low-level resistance, while the addition of gyrase mutations confers high-level resistance.[145-147] With ciprofloxacin, *parC* is the primary target, whereas with other fluoroquinolones *gyrA* is the primary target.[148] Therefore, resistance to the newer fluoroquinolones is less likely to be present.

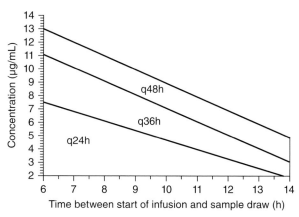

FIGURE 21-2 Hartford nomogram. ODA nomogram for gentamicin and tobramycin at 7 mg/kg. (Reprinted with permission from Nicolau DP, Freedman CD, Belliveu PP, et al. Experience with a once-daily aminoglycoside program to 2,184 patients. *Antimicrob Agents Chemother.* 1995;39(3):650-655.)

7. C. 15–20 mg/L

For treatment of severe infections or of those in which vancomycin penetration is suboptimal (eg, MRSA pneumonia, bacteremia, endocarditis, meningitis, osteomyelitis), consensus guidelines recommend aiming for vancomycin trough goals of 15 to 20 mg/L (choice C). Trough serum concentrations in that range are more likely to achieve the targeted vancomycin AUC:MIC ratio of greater than 400 for organisms with an MIC less than 1 mg/L. Lower trough goals are recommended for less complicated infections such as cellulitis (choices A and B). Obtaining troughs is indicated in select patients, including those in whom the target is 15 to 20 mg/L, those at high risk for nephrotoxicity (eg, with concurrent nephrotoxins), those with unstable renal function, and those requiring prolonged courses (> 3–5 days). It is recommended to obtain troughs at steady state, which is typically prior to the fourth dose in a patient with normal renal function.[149] Higher vancomycin trough levels have been associated with an increased risk of nephrotoxicity (choice D).[150] Of note, recent studies indicate that higher trough goals (15–20 mg/L) are not associated with improved outcomes, suggesting that troughs are a poor surrogate marker for the targeted PK/PD goal of an AUC:MIC of greater than 400.[151-153]

8. D. Order a random level 8 to 10 hours after the first administered dose

There are 2 types of dosage regimens for aminoglycosides: traditional dosing and extended-interval dosing. Extended-interval dosing differs from its predecessor in that the total daily dose is administered at one time (eg, 5 mg/kg or 7 mg/kg) with the frequency extended to either once per day or longer, depending on underlying renal function. Extended-interval dosing optimizes aminoglycoside PK/PD parameters (ie, C_{max}:MIC) by enabling higher concentrations and is associated with

decreased rates of nephrotoxicity as compared to traditional dosing. It is recommended to obtain aminoglycoside levels prior to administering subsequent doses in order to determine the appropriate dosage interval (choices A and B). As the patient received 7 mg/kg of gentamicin, the Hartford Nomogram can be used to determine when the next dose should be administered (Fig. 21-2). To use it, a random level is obtained 8 to 10 hours after dose administration (choice D). The resultant concentration is plotted on the nomogram according to the time the level was taken. The recommended dosing interval is chosen based on where the point lies. If the serum level is above the 48-hour interval, then traditional dosing should be used instead.[154]

Alternatively, the dosing interval can be determined by obtaining a level 24 hours after dose administration and redosing the aminoglycoside if the level is 1 µg/mL or lower for gentamicin or tobramycin or 4 µg/mL or lower for amikacin. If serum concentrations are above these thresholds, then random levels are repeated until the level falls below the thresholds.

Peak concentrations are generally not recommended, as extended-interval dosing achieves high concentrations, but they may be indicated in certain cases of organisms with high MICs and/or patients with altered pharmacokinetics, which is not reflective in this case (choice C).

9. C. Vancomycin 2000 mg IV (25 mg/kg)

In most institutions, initiating vancomycin at a dose of 1000 mg for all patients has become a knee-jerk reaction. But this dose is not appropriate for all patients. In this 80-kg patient, vancomycin 1000 mg IV (choice A) is approximately 12.5 mg/kg, which is below the recommended 15- to 20-mg/kg dose.[155] Vancomycin 1500 mg IV (choice B) and vancomycin 1250 mg IV (choice D) fall within this range and can be appropriate options, but given the severity of the patient's illness, these options may not be the most optimal. In patients presenting with septic shock, delaying appropriate treatment can increase the mortality risk by 7.6%.[156] Although this statistic pertains to patients who have received no antibiotic therapy, multiple studies have demonstrated that subtherapeutic doses of antibiotics can lead to worse clinical outcomes.[157,158] In critically ill patients, it is reasonable to administer a 25- to 30-mg/kg loading dose in order to attain target trough serum concentrations earlier in the course of disease.[155] Critically ill patients often have an increased volume of distribution (Vd) compared to their noncritically-ill counterparts for a myriad of reasons, including administration of resuscitative fluids, hypoalbuminemia, and compartmental fluid accumulation (Fig. 21-3). Therefore, these patients would require larger initial doses in order to reach a therapeutic drug concentration.[159] Furthermore, it is necessary also to take into account the suspected source of infection, which in this patient, appears to be the lungs. Vancomycin does not penetrate the lungs well; concentration in the epithelial lining fluid ranging between 5% and 41% of the serum levels have been reported in healthy patients.[159,160] In critically ill patients, vancomycin lung penetration is highly variable and a blood-to–epithelial lining fluid ratio of 6:1

has been reported.[161] One small study found that administering a loading dose of 25 mg/kg, infused at a rate of 500 mg/h, does not produce toxic peak levels and accelerates the accumulation of trough serum vancomycin concentrations above 8 ug/mL throughout the first 24 to 48 hours.[162]

10. C. Meropenem 500 mg IV q8h daily while on SLEDD
Sustained low-efficiency daily diafiltration is utilized as an alternate modality to continuous venovenous hemofiltration (CVVH) and uses conventional dialysis machines but programed at a lower efficiency. Typically, a session of SLEDD will last between 6 and 12 hours. The variation in the flow rates and treatment times that can be prescribed, combined with the limited pharmacokinetic data available with this modality, presents a challenge in terms of dosing antibiotics. During SLEDD, only 51% of meropenem is removed over the course of an 8-hour session (choice D). A good rule of thumb in patients undergoing SLEDD is to adjust the antibiotics that are renally cleared as they would be for continuous renal replacement therapy (creatinine clearance, 10–50 mL/min); therefore, the dosing provided by choices A and B may be too high. It is important to note that the patient's antibiotic regimen should be adjusted to his or her intrinsic renal function when he or she is not receiving SLEDD, in order to avoid overdosing.[163,164]

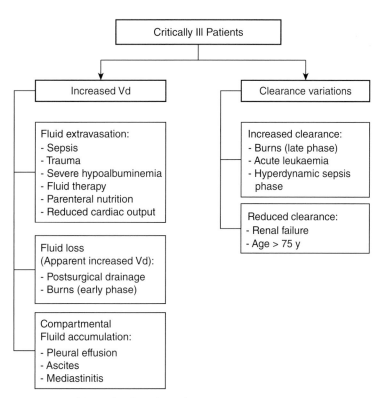

FIGURE 21-3 Schematic representation of the pathophysiological or iatrogenic conditions in critically ill patients affecting drug distribution and elimination. Vd = volume of distribution. (Reprinted with permission from Scaglione F, Paraboni L. Pharmacokinetics/pharmacodynamics of antibacterials in the intensive care unit: setting appropriate dosing regimens. *Int J Antimicrob Agents.* 2008;32(4):294-301.)

11. C. Albendazole 15 mg/kg/d in 2 divided doses taken with food PLUS praziquantel 50–100 mg/kg/d in 3 divided doses

Neurocysticercosis is a CNS infection caused by the larval form of the tapeworm *T solium*. Previously regarded as an "exotic" disease, neurocysticercosis is one of the leading causes of acquired epilepsy in the developing world and, as a result of immigration, is becoming more prevalent in industrialized nations.[165] There is controversy regarding the treatment of neurocysticercosis, as it is largely dependent on the type of disease, the number of cysts, and potential sequelae.[166] Although praziquantel alone (choice A) has been studied for the treatment of neurocysticercosis and has been generally efficacious, albendazole has better penetration into the cerebrospinal fluid and its concentrations are not affected when administered concomitantly with steroids.[167,168] Albendazole also appears to be the cheaper agent for treatment. Although albendazole can be used as monotherapy for this disease, its bioavailability is affected by the presence of food.[169-171] Only 5% to 10% of albendazole is absorbed after oral administration; however, the plasma concentration of its metabolite increases up to 5-fold when coadministered with a fatty meal (~40 g of fat).[171] Ivermectin (choice D) is active against a wide range of helminths and ectoparasites and is the drug of choice for strongyloidiasis. In neurocysticercosis, ivermectin is not a first-line agent and has only been studied as a therapeutic alternative in patients who are resistant to conventional treatment with albendazole and praziquantel.[172] The combination of albendazole and praziquantel is preferred in patients who have multiple cysts and intraparenchymal involvement.[173-175]

12. C. Prednisone 1 mg/kg/d for 5–10 days

Clinical manifestations of neurocysticercosis, such as seizures or focal neurologic deficits, are frequently a consequence of cerebral inflammation that occurs as a result of degenerating or dead cysts rupturing and releasing antigenic material. This can occur during the natural course of the disease or as a result of anthelmintic therapy.[176,177] Corticosteroids have been used in the treatment of neurocysticercosis for decades.[178] In a 1982 study, investigators noted that patients developed acute clinical symptoms and neurologic sequelae within the first week of initiating therapy with praziquantel.[179] Years later, multiple studies evaluating the role of corticosteroids found that the concurrent administration of prednisone decreased the incidence of seizures (typically around the 6- to 9-month mark) as well as significantly decreased the appearance of cysts on computed tomography scan.[180-182] Methotrexate (choice D) can be used in patients with neurocysticercosis; however, its role is limited to use as a corticosteroid-sparing agent in patients with chronic or recurrent cerebral inflammation who could no longer tolerate long-term corticosteroids.[183] Diphenhydramine (choice A) and 0.9% sodium chloride (choice B) are not necessary for the administration of the medication in question 11.

REFERENCES

1. Vincent JL, Rello J, Marshall J, et al. International study of the prevalence and outcomes of infections in intensive care units. *JAMA.* 2009;302(21):2323-2329.
2. Kumar A, Roberts D, Wood KE, et al. Duration of hypotension before initiation of effective antimicrobial therapy is the critical determinant of survival in human septic shock. *Crit Care Med.* 2006;34(6):1589-1596.
3. Garnacho-Montero J, Garcia-Garmendia JL, Barrero-Almodovar A, Jimenez-Jimenez FJ, Perez-Paredes C, Ortiz-Leyba C. Impact of adequate empirical therapy on the outcome of patients admitted to the intensive care unit with sepsis. *Crit Care Med.* 2033;31(12):2742-2751.
4. Shorr AF, Micek ST, Welch EC, Doherty JA, Reichley RM, Kollef MH. Inappropriate antibiotic therapy in gram-negative sepsis increases hospital length of stay. *Crit Care Med.* 2011;39(1):46-51.
5. Roberts JA, Lipman J. Pharmacokinetic issues for antibiotics in the critically ill patient. *Crit Care Med.* 2009;37(3):840-851.
6. Finberg RW, Moellering RC, Tally FP, et al. The importance of bactericidal drugs: future directions in infectious disease. *Clin Infect Dis.* 2004;39(9):1314-1320.
7. Mulligan MJ, Cobbs CG. Bacteriostatic versus bactericidal activity. *Infect Dis Clin North Am.* 1989;3(3):389-398.
8. Landman D, Quale JM. Management of infections due to resistant enterococci: a review of therapeutic options. *J Antimicrob Chemother.* 1997;40(2):161-170.
9. Edelstein PH, Edelstein MA. In vitro activity of azithromycin against clinical isolates of *Legionella* species. *Antimicrob Agents Chemother.* 1991;35(1):180-181.
10. Jorgensen JH, Ferraro MJ. Antimicrobial susceptibility testing: a review of general principles and contemporary practices. *Clin Infect Dis.* 2009;49(11):1749-1755.
11. Clinical and Laboratory Standards Institute. *M100 Performance Standards for Antimicrobial Susceptibility Testing.* 27th ed. Wayne, PA: Clinical and Laboratory Standards Institute; 2016.
12. Levison, ME, Levison JH. Pharmacokinetics and pharmacodynamics of antibacterial agents. *Infect Dis Clin North Am.* 2009;23(4):791-815, vii.
13. Craig WA. Basic pharmacodynamics of antibacterials with clinical applications to the use of beta-lactams, glycopeptides, and linezolid. *Infect Dis Clin North Am.* 2003;17(3):479-501.
14. Lodise TP, Lomaestro BM, Drusano GL; Society of Infectious Diseases Pharmacists. Application of antimicrobial pharmacodynamics concepts into clinical practice: focus on beta-lactam antibiotics: insights from the Society of Infectious Diseases Pharmacists. *Pharmacotherapy.* 2006;26(9):1320-1332.
15. Lodise TP, Lomaestro B, Drusano GL. Piperacillin-tazobactam for *Pseudomonas aeruginosa* infection: clinical implications of an extended infusion dosing strategy. *Clin Infect Dis.* 2007;44(3):357-363.
16. Kong KF, Schneper L, Mathee K. Beta-lactam antibiotics: from antibiosis to resistance to bacteriology. *APMIS.* 2010;118(1):1-36.

17. Bush K, Macielag MJ. New β-lactam antibiotics and β-lactamase inhibitors. *Expert Opin Ther Pat.* 2010;20(10):1277-1293.

18. Zhanel GG, WIebe R, Dilay L, et al. Comparative review of the carbapenems. *Drugs.* 2007;67(7):1027-1052.

19. Westley-Horton E, Koestner JA. Aztreonam: a review of the first monobactam. *Am J Med Sci.* 1991;302(1):46-49.

20. Tverdek FP, Crank CW, Segreti J. Antibiotic therapy of methicillin-resistant *Staphylococcus aureus* in critical care. *Crit Care Clin.* 2008;24(2):249-260.

21. Freeman CD, Klutman NE, Lamp KC. Metronidazole. A therapeutic review and update. *Drugs.* 1997;54(5):679-708.

22. Smieja M. Current indications for the use of clindamycin: a critical review. *Can J Infect Dis.* 1998;9:(1)22-28.

23. Samra M, Abcar AC. False estimates of elevated creatinine. *Perm J.* 2012;16(2):51-52.

24. King, DE, Malone R, Lilley SH. New classification and updated on the quinolone antibiotics. *Am Fam Physician.* 2000;61(9):2741-2748.

25. Blondeau JM. Update on the use of macrolides for community acquired respiratory tract infections. *Therapy.* 2006;3:619-650.

26. Stein GE, Goldstein EJ. Fluoroquinolones and anaerobes. *Clin Infect Dis.* 2006;42(11):1598-1607.

27. Chopra I, Roberts M. Tetracycline antibiotics: mode of action, applications, molecular biology, and epidemiology of bacterial resistance. *Microbiol Mol Biol Rev.* 2001;65(2):232-260.

28. Sum PE, Lee VJ, Testa RT, et al. Glycylcyclines. A new generation of potent antibacterial agents through modification of 9-aminotetracyclines. *J Med Chem.* 1994;37(1):184-188.

29. Andriole VT. The quinolones: past, present, and future. *Clin Infect Dis.* 2005:41(Suppl 2);S113-S119.

30. Izadpanah M, Khalili H. Antibiotic regimens for treatment of infections due to multidrug-resistant Gram-negative pathogens: an evidence-based literature review. *J Res Pharm Pract.* 2015;4(3):105-114.

31. McDonald LC. Trends in antimicrobial resistance in health care-associated pathogens and effect on treatment. *Clin Infect Dis.* 2006;42(Suppl 2):S65-S71.

32. Magiorakos AP, Srinivasan A, Carey RB, et al. Multidrug-resistant, extensively drug-resistant, and pandrug-resistant bacteria: an international expert proposal for interim standard definitions for acquired resistance. *Clin Microbiol Infect.* 2012;18(3):268-281.

33. Dever LA, Dermody TS. Mechanisms of bacterial resistance to antibiotics. *Arch Intern Med.* 1991;151(1):886-895.

34. Shaikh S, Fatima J, Shakil S, Rizvi SM, Kamal MA. Antibiotic resistance and extended spectrum beta-lactamases: types, epidemiology, and treatment. *Saudi J Biol Sci.* 2015;22(1):90-101.

35. Arnold RS, Thom KA, Sharma S, Phillips M, Kristie Johnson J, Morgan DJ. Emergence of *Klebsiella pneumoniae* carbapenemase (KPC)-producing bacteria. *South Med J.* 2011; 104(1):40-45.

36. Grebe T, Hakenbeck R. Penicillin-binding proteins 2b and 2x of streptococcus pneumonia are primary resistance determinants for different classes of beta-lactam antibiotics. *Antimicrob Agents Chemother.* 1996;40(4):829-834.

37. Delcour AH. Outer membrane permeability and antibiotic resistance. *Biochim Biophys Acta.* 2009;1794(5):808-816.

38. Arthur M, Courvalin P. Genetics and mechanisms of glycopeptide resistance in enterococci. *Antimicrob Agents Chemother.* 1993;37(8):1563-1571.

39. Gardete S, Tomasz A. Mechanisms of vancomycin resistance in *Staphylococcus aureus. J Clin Invest.* 2014;124(7):2836-2840.

40. Cetinkaya Y, Falk P, Mayhall CG. Vancomycin-resistant enterococci. *Clin Microbiol Rev.* 2000;13(4):686-707.

41. Bassetti M, Luyt CE, Nicolau DP, Pugin J. Characteristics of an ideal nebulized antibiotic for the treatment of pneumonia in the intubated patient. *Ann Intensive Care.* 2016;6(1):35.

42. Badia JR, Soy D, Adrover M, et al. Disposition of instilled versus nebulized tobramycin and imipenem in ventilated intensive care unit (ICU) patients. *J Antimicrob Chemother.* 2004;54(2):508-514.

43. Drlica K. The mutant selection window and antimicrobial resistance. *J Antimicrob Chemother.* 2003;52(1):11-17.

44. Drlica K, Zhao X. Mutant selection window hypothesis updated. *Clin Infect Dis.* 2007;44(5):681-688.

45. Ramsey BW, Dorkin HL, Eisenberg JD, et al. Efficacy of aerosolized tobramycin in patients with cystic fibrosis. *N Engl J Med.* 1993;328(24):1740-1746.

46. Burns JL, Van Dalfsen JM, Shawar RM, et al. Effect of chronic intermittent administration of inhaled tobramycin on respiratory microbial flora in patients with cystic fibrosis. *J Infect Dis.* 1999;179(5):1190-1196.

47. Palmer LB, Smaldone GB. Reduction of bacterial resistance with inhaled antibiotics in the intensive care unit. *Am J Respir Crit Care Med.* 2014;189(10):1225-1233.

48. Dhand R. The role of aerosolized antimicrobials in the treatment of ventilator-associated pneumonia. *Respir Care.* 2007;52(7):866-884.

49. Le J, Ashley ED, Neuhauser MM, et al. Consensus summary of aerosolized antimicrobial agents: application of guideline criteria. Insights from the Society of Infectious Disease Pharmacists. *Pharmacotherapy.* 2010;30(6):562-584.

50. Kalil AC, Metersky ML, Klompas M, et al. Management of adults with hospital-acquired and ventilator-associated pneumonia: 2016 clinical practice guidelines by the Infectious Diseases Society of America and the American Thoracic Society. *Clin Infect Dis.* 2016;63(5):e61-e111.

51. Ashley ESD, Lewis R, Lewis JS, Martin C, Andes D. Pharmacology of systemic antifungal agents. *Clin Infect Dis.* 2006;43(Suppl 1):S28-S39.

52. Mohr J, Johnson M, Cooper T, Lewis JS, Ostrosky-Zeichner L. Current options in antifungal pharmacotherapy. *Pharmacotherapy.* 2008;28(5):614-645.

53. Lewis RE. Current concepts in antifungal pharmacology. *Mayo Clin Proc.* 2011;86(8):805-817.

54. Gallis H, Drew RH, Pickard WW. Amphotericin B: 30 years of clinical experience. *Rev Infect Dis.* 1990;12(2):308-329.

55. Kanafani Za, Perfect JR. Resistance to antifungal agents: mechanisms and clinical impact. *Clin Infect Dis.* 2008;46(1):120-128.

56. Miceli MH, Kauffman CA. Isavuconazole: a new broad-spectrum triazole antifungal agent. *Clin Infect Dis.* 2015; 61(10):1558-1565.

57. Fernando-Ruiz M, Aguado JM, Almirante B, et al. Initial use of echinocandins does not negatively influence outcome in *Candida parapsilosis* blood stream infection: a propensity score analysis. *Clin Infect Dis.* 2014;58(10):1413-1421.

58. Andes DR, Safdar N, Baddley JW, et al. Impact of treatment strategy on outcomes in patients with candidemia and other forms of invasive candidiasis: a patient level quantitative review of randomized trials. *Clin Infect Dis.* 2012;54(8):1110-1122.

59. Pappas PG, Kauffman CA, Andes DR, et al. Clinical practice guidelines for the management of candidiasis: 2016 update by the Infectious Diseases Society of America. *Clin Infect Dis.* 2016;62(4):e1-50.

60. Vermes A, Guchelaar HJ, Dankert J. Flucytosine: A review of its pharmacology, clinical indications, pharmacokinetics, toxicity and drug interaction. *J Antimicrob Chemother.* 2000;46(2):171-179.

61. Gillum JG, Johnson M, Lavoie S, Venitz J. Flucytosine dosing in an obese patient with extrameningeal cryptococcal infection. *Pharmacotherapy.* 1995;15(2):251-253.

62. O'Brien JJ, Campoli-Richards DM. Acyclovir. An updated review of its antiviral activity, pharmacokinetic properties and therapeutic efficacy. *Drugs.* 1989;37(3):233-309.

63. Perry CM, Faulds D. Valacyclovir. A review of its antiviral activity, pharmacokinetic properties and therapeutic efficacy in herpesvirus infections. *Drugs.* 1996;52(5):754-772.

64. Dworkin RH, Johnson RW, Breuer J, et al. Recommendations for the management of herpes zoster. *Clin Infect Dis.* 2007;44 (Suppl 1):S1-S26.

65. Izzedine H, Launay-Vacher V, Deray G. Antiviral drug-induced nephrotoxicity. *Am J Kidney Dis.* 2005;45(5):804-817.

66. Piret J, Boivin G. Resistance to herpes simplex viruses to nucleoside analogues: mechanisms, prevalence, and management. *Antimicrob Agents Chemother.* 2011;55(2)459-472.

67. Sauerbrei A, Taut J, Zell R, Wutzler P. Resistance testing of clinical varicella-zoster virus strains. *Antiviral Research.* 2011;90(3):242-247.

68. Simpson D, Lyseng-Williamson KA. Famciclovir: a review of its use is herpes zoster and genital and orolabial herpes. *Drugs.* 2006;66(18):2397-2416.

69. Moscana A. Neuraminidase inhibitors for influenza. *N Engl J Med.* 2005;353(13):1363-1373.

70. Nakamura K, Schwartz BS, Lindegardh N, Keh C, Guglielmo BJ. Possible neuropsychiatric reaction to high-dose oseltamivir during acute 2009 H1N1 influenza A infection. *Clin Infect Dis.* 2010;50(7):e47-e49.

71. Steel HM, Peppercorn AF. Fatal respiratory events caused by zanamivir nebulization. *Clin Infect Dis.* 2010;51(1):121.

72. De Jong MD, Ison MG, Monto AS, et al. Evaluation of intravenous peramivir for treatment of influenza in hospitalized patients. *Clin Infect Dis.* 2014;59(12):e172-e185.

73. Samson M, Pizzorno A, Abed Y, Boivin G. Influenza virus resistance to neuraminidase inhibitors. *Antiviral Res.* 2013; 98(2):174-185.

74. Fiore AE, Fry A, Shay D, Gubareva L, Bresee JS, Uyeki TM; Centers for Disease Control and Prevention. Antiviral agents for the treatment and chemoprophylaxis of influenza—recommendations of the Advisory Committee on Immunization Practices (ACIP). *MMWR Recomm Rep.* 2011;60(1):1-24.

75. World Health Organization. *Guidelines for the Treatment of Malaria.* Geneva, Switzerland: WHO; 2006.

76. Egan TJ. Chloroquine and primaquine: combining old drugs as a new weapon against falciparum malaria? *Trends Parasitol.* 2006;22(6):235-237.

77. Minker E, Ivan J. Experimental and clinicopharmacological study of rectal absorption of chloroquine. *Acta Physiol Hung.* 1991;77(3-4):237-248.

78. Fernando D, Rodrigo C, Rajapakse S. Primaquine in vivax malaria: an update and review on management issues. *Malar J.* 2011;10:351.

79. Barrett PJ, Emmins PD, Clarke PD, Bradley DJ. Comparison of adverse events associated with use of mefloquine and combination of chloroquine and proguanil as antimalarial prophylaxis: postal and telephone survey of travelers. *Br Med J.* 1996;313(4056):525-528.

80. Foley M, Tilley L. Quinoline antimalarials: mechanisms of action and resistance and prospects for new agents. *Pharmacol Ther.* 1998;79(1):55-87.

81. Benfield T, Atzori C, Miller RF, et al. Second-line salvage treatment of AIDS-associated *Pneumocystis jirovecii* pneumonia: a case series and systematic review. *J Acquir Immune Defic Syndr.* 2008;48(1):63-67.

82. Centers for Disease Control and Prevention. Artesunate is available to treat severe malaria in the United States. Centers for Disease Control and Prevention Web site. https://www.cdc.gov/malaria/diagnosis_treatment/artesunate.html. Updated July 14, 2017. Accessed August 6, 2017.

83. Meshnick SR. Artemisinin: mechanisms of action, resistance, and toxicity. *Int J Parasitol.* 2002;32(13):1655-1660.

84. Marfurt J, Chalfein F, Prayoga P, et al. Comparative ex vivo activity of novel endoperoxides in multidrug-resistant *Plasmodium falciparum* and *P vivax. Antimicrob Agent Chemother.* 2012;56(10):5258-5263.

85. Brockman A, Price RN, van Vugt M, et al. *Plasmodium falciparum* antimalarial drug susceptibility on the northwestern border of Thailand during five years of extensive use of artesunate-mefloquine. *Trans R Soc Trop Med Hyg.* 2000;91(5):537-544.

86. Price R, Luxemburger C, van Vugt M, et al. Artesunate and mefloquine in the treatment of uncomplicated multidrug-resistant hyperparasitaemic falciparum malaria. *Trans R Soc Trop Med Hyg.* 1998;92(2):207-211.

87. Hotez PJ, Bindley PJ, Bethony JM, et al. Helminth infections: the great neglected tropical diseases. *J Clin Invest.* 2008;118(4):1311-1321.

88. Edwards G, Breckenridge AM. Clinical pharmacokinetics of anthelmintic drugs. *Clin Pharmacokinet.* 1988;15(2):67-93.

89. McCarthy JS, Moore TA. Drugs for helminths. In: Bennett JE, Dolin R, Blaser MD, eds. *Mandell, Douglas, and Bennett's Principles and Practice of Infectious Diseases.* 8th ed. New York. (NY): Elsevier; 2015: 519-527.

90. Horton J. Albendazole: a review of anthelmintic efficacy and safety in humans. *Parasitology.* 2000;121(Suppl):S113-S132.

91. Sheth UK. Mechanisms of anthelmintic action. *Prog Drug Res.* 1975;19:147-157.

92. Nagy J, Schipper HG, Koopmans RP, et al. Effect of grapefruit juice or cimetidine coadministration on albendazole bioavailability. *Am J Trop Med Hyg.* 2002;66(3):260-263.

93. Urbani C, Albonico M. Antihelminthic drug safety and drug administration in the control of soil-transmitted helminthiasis in community campaigns. *Acta Trop.* 2003;86(2-3):215-223.

94. Diawara A, Drake IJ, Suswillo RR, et al. Assays to detect beta-tubulin codon 200 polymorphism in *Trichuris trichiura* and *Ascaris luinbricoides. PLoS Negl Trop Dis.* 2009;3(3):e397.

95. Schwab AE, Boakye DA, Kyelem D, Prichard RK. Detection of benzimidazole resistance-associated mutations in the filarial nematode *Wucheria bancrofti* and evidence for selection by albendazole and ivermectin combination treatment. *Am J Trop Med Hyg.* 2005;73(2):234-238.

96. Campbell WC. Ivermectin, an antiparasitic agent. *Med Res Rev.* 1993;13(1):61-79.

97. Canga Gonzalez A, Sahagun Pedro AM, Jose Diez Liebana M, et al. The pharmacokinetics and interactions of ivermectin in humans—a mini-review. *AAPS J.* 2008;10(1):42-46.

98. Sangster NC, Gill J. Pharmacology of anthelmintic resistance. *Parasitol Today.* 1999;15(4):141-146.

99. Njoo FL, Beek WM, Keukens HJ, et al. Ivermectin detection in serum of onchocerciasis patients: relationship to adverse reactions. *Am J Trop Med Hyg.* 1995;52(1):94-97.

100. Schaeffer JM, Haines HW. Avermectin binding in *Caenorhabditis elegans*. A two-state model for the avermectin binding site. *Biochem Pharmacol.* 1989;38(14):2329-2338.

101. Gustafsson LL, Beerman B, Aden Abdi Y. *Handbook of Drugs for Tropical Parasitic Infections.* New York, (NY): Taylor & Francis; 1987.

102. Watt G, White NJ, Padre L, et al. Praziquantel pharmacokinetics and side effects in Schistosoma japonicum-infected patients with liver disease. *J Infect Dis.* 1988;157(3):530-535.

103. Xiao SH, Friedman PA, Catto BA, et al. Praziquantel-induced vesicle formation in the tegument of male *Schistosoma mansomi* is calcium dependent. *J Parasitol.* 1984;70(1):177-179.

104. Mandour ME, el Turabi H, Homeida MM, et al. Pharmacokinetics of praziquantel in healthy volunteers and patients with schistosomiasis. *Trans R Soc Trop Med Hyg.* 1990;84(3):389-393.

105. Polderman AM, Gryseels B, Gerold JL, Mpamila K, Manshande JP. Side effects of praziquantel in the treatment of *Schistosoma mansoni* in Maniema, Zaire. *Trans R Soc Trop Med Hyg.* 1984;78(6):752-754.

106. Matsumoto J. Adverse effects of praziquantel treatment of *Schistosoma japonicum* infections: involvement of host anaphylactic reactions induced by parasite antigen release. *Int J Parasitol.* 2002;32(4):461-471.

107. Center for Disease Control and Prevention. Antibiotic resistance threats in the Unites States, 2013. Centers for Disease Control and Prevention Web site. https://www.cdc.gov/drugresistance/pdf/ar-threats-2013-508.pdf. Accessed March 6, 2017.

108. Flournoy DJ, Reinert RL, Bell-Dixon C, Gentry CA. Increasing antimicrobial resistance in Gram-negative bacilli isolated from patients in intensive care units. *Am J Infect Control.* 2000;28(3):244-250.

109. Pop-Vicas AE, D'Agata EM. The rising influx of multi-drug resistant Gram-negative bacilli in a tertiary care hospital. *Clin Infect Dis.* 2005;40(12):1792-1798.

110. Boucher HW, Talbot GH, Benjamin DK, et al; Infectious Diseases Society of America. 10 x '20 progress-development of new drugs active against gram-negative bacilli: An update from the Infectious Diseases Society of America. *Clin Infect Dis.* 2013;56(12):1685-1694.

111. Slama TG. Gram-negative antibiotic resistance: there is a price to pay. *Crit Care.* 2008;12(Suppl 4):S4

112. Cosgrove SE. The relationship between antimicrobial resistance and patient outcomes: mortality, length of hospital stay, and healthcare costs. *Clin Infect Dis.* 2006;42(Suppl 2):S82-S89.

113. Barlam TF, Cosgrove SE, Abbo LM, et al. Implementing an antibiotic stewardship program: guidelines by the Infectious Diseases Society of America and the Society for Healthcare Epidemiology of America. *Clin Infect Dis.* 2016;62(10):e51-77.

114. Luyt C, Brechot N, Trouillet J, Chastre J. Antibiotic stewardship in the intensive care unit. *Critical Care.* 2014;18:480.

115. Vincent J, Basseti M, Francois B, et al. Advances in antibiotic therapy in critically ill. *Critical Care.* 2016;20:133.

116. Kaki R, Elligsen M, Walker S, Simor A, Palmay L, Daneman N. Impact of antimicrobial stewardship in critical care: s systematic review. *J Antimicrob Chemother.* 2011;66(6):1223-1230.

117. Kumar A, Roberts D, Wood KE, et al. Duration of hypotension before initiation of effective antimicrobial therapy is the critical determinant of survival in human septic shock. *Crit Care Med.* 2006;34(6):1589-1596.

118. Rhodes A, Evans LE, Alhazzani W, et al. Surviving Sepsis Campaign: international guidelines for management of sepsis and septic shock: 2016. *Crit Care Med.* 2017;45(3):486-552.

119. Tabah A, Cotta MO, Garnacho-Montero J, et al. A systematic review of the definitions, determinants, and clinical outcomes of antimicrobial de-escalation in the intensive care unit. *Clin Infect Dis.* 2016;62(8):1009-1017.

120. Eliakim-Raz N, Yahav D, Paul M, Leibovici L. Duration of antibiotic treatment for acute pyelonephritis and septic urinary tract infection—7 days or less versus longer treatment: systematic review and meta-analysis of randomized controlled trials. *J Antimicrob Chemother.* 2013;68(10):2183-2191.

121. Hepburn MG, Dooley DP, Skidmore PJ, Ellis MW, Starnes WF, Hasewinkle WC. Comparison of short-course (5 days) and standard (10 days) treatment for uncomplicated cellulitis. *Arch Intern Med.* 2004;164(15):1669-1674.

122. Sawyer RG, Claridge JA, Nathens AB, et al. Trial of short-course antimicrobial therapy for intraabdominal infection; STOP-IT Trial Investigators. *N Engl J Med.* 2015;372(21):1996-2005.

123. Bouadma L, Luyt C, Tubach F, et al; PRORATA Trial Group. Use of procalcitonin to reduce patients' exposure to antibiotics in intensive care units (PRORATA trial): a multicenter randomised controlled trial. *Lancet.* 2010;375(9713):463-474.

124. Liu C, Bayer A, Cosgrove SE, et al. Clinical practice guidelines by the Infectious Diseases Society of America for the treatment of methicillin-resistant *Staphylococcus aureus* infections in adults and children. *Clin Infect Dis.* 2011;52(3):e18-e55.

125. Holland TL, Arnold D, Fowler VG. Clinical management of *Staphylococcus aureus* bacteremia. *JAMA.* 2014; 312(13): 1330-1341.

126. Baddour LM, Wilson WR, Bayer AS, et al. Infective endocarditis in adults: diagnosis, antimicrobial therapy, and management of complications: a scientific statement for healthcare professionals from the American Heart Association. *Circulation.* 2015;132(15):1435-1486.

127. Freifeld AG, Bow EJ, Sepkowitz KA, et al. Clinical practice guidelines for the use of antimicrobial agents in neutropenic patients with cancer: 2010 update by the Infectious Diseases Society of America. *Clin Infect Dis.* 2011;52(4):e56-e93.

128. Fierer J. Vertebral osteomyelitis guidelines. *Clin Infect Dis.* 2016;62(7):953-954.

129. Jacoby GA. AmpC β-Lactamase. *Clin Microb Rev.* 2009;22(1):161-182.

130. Harris PNA, Ferguson JK. Antibiotic therapy for inducible AmpC β-lactamase-producing Gram-negative bacilli: what are the alternatives to carbapenems, quinolones and aminoglycosides? *Int J Antimicrob Agents.* 2012;40(4):297-305.

131. Rogers BA, Aminzadeh Z, Hayashi Y, Paterson DL. Country-to-country transfer of patients and the risk of multi-resistant bacterial infection. *Clin Infect Dis.* 2011;53(1):49-56.

132. Blanchette LM, Kuti J, Nicolau DP, Nailor M. Clinical comparison of ertapenem and cefepime for treatment of infections caused by AmpC beta-lactamase-producing Enterobacteriacae. *Scand J Infect Dis.* 2014;46(11):803-808.

133. Tamma PD, Girdwood SY, Gopaul R, et al. The use of cefepime for treating Amp-C β-lactamase-producing enterobacteriacae. *Clin Infect Dis.* 2013;57(6):781-788.

134. Burdett V. Tet(M)-promoted release of tetracycline from ribosomes is GTP dependent. *J Bacteriol.* 1996;178(11):3246-3251.

135. Donhofer A, Franckenberg S, Wickles S, et al. Structural bases for TetM-mediated tetracycline resistance. *Proc Natl Acad Sci U S A.* 2012;109(42):16900-16905.

136. Bergmann R, van der Linden M, Chhatwal GS, et al. Factors that cause trimethoprim resistance in streptococcus pyogenes. *Antimicrob Agents Chemother.* 2014;58(4):2281-2288.

137. Bean DC, Klena JD. Prevalence of *erm(A)* and *mef(B)* erythromycin resistance determinants in isolates of streptococcus pneumoniae from New Zealand. *J Antimicrob Chemother.* 2002;50(4):597-599.

138. Carapito R, Chesnel L, Vernet T, et al. Pneumococcal beta-lactam resistance due to a conformational change in penicillin-binding protein 2x. *J Biol Chem.* 2006;281(3):1771-1777.

139. Gatmaitan BG, Carruthers MM, Lerner AM. Gentamicin in treatment of primary Gram-negative pneumonias. *Am J Med Sci.* 1970;260(2):90-94.

140. Pines A, Raafat H, Plucinski K. 1967. Gentamicin and colistin in chronic purulent bronchial infections. *Br Med J.* 1967;2(5551):543-545.

141. Zhanel GG, WIebe R, Dilay L, et al. Comparative review of the carbapenems. *Drugs.* 2007;67(7):1027-1052.

142. Dean CR, Visalli MA, Projan SJ, et al. Efflux-mediated resistance to tigecycline (GAR-936) in pseudomonas aeruginosa PAO1. *Antimicrob Agents Chemother.* 2003;47(3):972-978.

143. Duplessis C, Crum-Cianflone NF. Ceftaroline: a new cephalosporin with activity against methicillin-resistant staphylococcus aureus (MRSA). *Clin Med Rev Ther.* 2011;3 pii:a2466.

144. Liscio JL, Mahoney MV, Hirsch EB. Ceftolozane/tazobactam and ceftazidime/avibactam: two novel β-lactam/β-lactamase inhibitor combination agents for the treatment of resistant Gram-negative bacterial infections. *Int J Antimicrob Agents.* 2015;46(3):266-271.

145. Mandell LA, Wunderink RG, Anzueto A, et al. Infectious disease society of America/American thoracic society consensus guidelines on the management of community-acquired pneumonia in adults. *Clin Infect Dis.* 2007;44(Suppl 2):S27-S72.

146. De la Campa AG, Balsalobre L, Ardanuy C, et al. Fluoroquinolone resistance in penicillin-resistant *Streptococcus pneumoniae* clones, Spain. *Emerg Infect Dis.* 2004;10(10):1751-1759.

147. Adams DE, Shekhtman EM, Zechiedrich EL, et al. The role of topoisomerase IV in partitioning bacterial replicons and the structure of catenated intermediates in DNA replication. *Cell.* 1992;71(2):277-288.

148. Kato J, Nishimura Y, Imamura H, et al. New topoisomerase essential for chromosome segregation in *E coli. Cell.* 1990;63(2):393-404.

149. Fukuda H, Hiramatsu K. Primary targets of fluoroquinolones in *Streptococcus pneumoniae. Antimicrob Agents Chemother.* 1999;43(2):410-412.

150. Rybak M, Lomaestro B, Rotschafer JC, et al. Therapeutic monitoring of vancomycin in adult patients: a consensus review of the American Society of Health-System Pharmacists, the Infectious Diseases Society of America, and the Society of Infectious Diseases Pharmacists. *Am J Health-System Pharm.* 2009;66(10):887.

151. Carreno JJ, Kenney RM, Lomaestro B. Vancomycin-associated renal dysfunction: where are we now? *Pharmacotherapy.* 2014;34(12):1259-1268.

152. Neely MN, Youn G, Jones B, et al. Are vancomycin trough concentrations adequate for optimal dosing? *Antimicrob Agents Chemother.* 2013;58(1):309-316.

153. Prybylski JP. Vancomycin trough concentrations as a predictor of clinical outcomes in patients with *Staphylococcus aureus* bacteremia: a meta-analysis of observational studies. *Pharmacotherapy.* 2015;35(10):889-898.

154. Nicolau DP, Freedman CD, Belliveu PP, Nightingale CH, Ross JW, Quintiliani R. Experience with a once-daily aminoglycoside program to 2,184 patients. *Antimicrob Agents Chemother.* 1995;39(3):650-655.

155. Rybak MJ, Lomaestro BM, Rotschafer JC, et al. Vancomycin therapeutic guidelines: a summary of consensus recommendations from the Infectious Diseases Society of America, the American Society of Health-system Pharmacists, and the Society of Infectious Disease Pharmacists. *Clin Infect Dis.* 2009;49(3):325-327.

156. Kumar A, Roberts D, Wood KE, et al. Duration of hypotension prior to initiation of effective antimicrobial therapy is the critical determinant of survival in human septic shock. *Crit Care Med.* 2006;34(6):1589-1596.

157. Roe JL, Fuentes JM, Mullins ME. Underdosing of common antibiotics for obese patients in the ED. *Am J Emer Med.* 2012;30(7):1212-1214.

158. Falagas ME, Thanasoulia AP, Peppas G, et al. Effect of body mass index on the outcome of infections: a systematic review. *Obes Rev.* 2009;10(3):180-189.

159. Wang JT, Fang CT, Chen YC, et al. Necessity of a loading dose when using vancomycin in critically ill patients. *J Antimicrob Chemother.* 2001;47(2):246.

160. Rybak MJ. The pharmacokinetic and pharmacodynamics properties of vancomycin. *Clin Infect Dis.* 2006;42(Suppl 1):S35-S39.

161. Cruciani M, Gatti G, Lazzarini L, et al. Penetration of vancomycin into human lung tissue. *J Antimicrob Chemother.* 1996;38(5):865-869.

162. Georges H, Leroy O, Alfandari S, et al. Pulmonary disposition of vancomycin in critically ill patients. *Eur J Clin Microbiol Infect Dis.* 1997;16(5):385-388.

163. Mushatt DM, Mihm LB, Dreisbach AW, Simon EE. Antibiotic dosing in slow extended daily dialysis. *Clin Infect Dis.* 2009;49(3):433-437.

164. Bogard KN, Peterson NT, Plumb TJ, et al. Antibiotic dosing during sustained low-efficiency dialysis: special considerations in adult critically ill patients. *Crit Care Med.* 2011;39(3):560-570.

165. Kimura-Hayama ET, Higuera JA, Corona-Cedillo R, et al. Neurocysticercosis: radiologic-pathologic correlation. *Radiographics.* 2010;30(6):1705-1719.

166. Garcia HH, Evans CAW, Nash TE, et al. Current consensus guidelines for treatment of neurocysticercosis. *Clin Microbiol Rev.* 2002;15(4):747-756.

167. Jung H, Hurtado M, Sanchez M, Medina MT, Sotelo J. Plasma and cerebrospinal fluid levels of albendazole and praziquantel in patients with neurocysticercosis. *Clin Neuropharmacol.* 1990;13(6):559-564.

168. Jung H, Hurtado M, Medina MT, Sanchez M, Sotelo J. Dexamethasone increases plasma levels of albendazole. *J Neurol.* 1990;237(5):279-280.

169. Göngora-Rivera F, Soto-Hernández JL, González Esquivel D, et al. Albendazole trial at 15 or 30 mg/kg/day for subarachnoid and intraventricular cysticercosis. *Neurology.* 2006;66(3):436-438.

170. Jagota SC. Albendazole, a broad-spectrum anthelmintic, in the treatment of intestinal nematode and cestode infection: a multicenter study in 480 patients. *Clin Ther.* 1986;8(2):226-231.

171. Lange H, Eggers R, Bircher J. Increased systemic availability of albendazole when taken with a fatty meal. *Eur J Clin Pharmacol.* 1988;34(3):315-317.

172. Diazgranados-Sanchez JA, Barrios-Arrazola G, Costa JL, et al. [Ivermectin as a therapeutic alternative in neurocysticercosis that is resistant to conventional pharmacologic treatment]. *Rev Neurol.* 2008;46(11):671-674.

173. Garcia HH, Pretell EJ, Gilman RH, et al; Cysticercosis Working Group in Peru. A trial of antiparasitic treatment to reduce the rate of seizures due to cerebral cysticercosis. *N Engl J Med.* 2004;350(3):249-258.

174. Garcia HH, Gonzales I, Lescano AG, et al; Cysticercosis Working Group in Peru. Efficacy of combined antiparasitic therapy with praziquantel and albendazole for neurocysticercosis: a double blind randomized controlled trial. *Lancet Infect Dis.* 2014;14(8):687-695.

175. Del Brutto OH, Sotelo J. Neurocysticercosis: an update. *Rev Infect Dis.* 1998;10(6):1075-1087.

176. Garg RK, Potluri N, Kar AM, et al. Short course of prednisolone in patients with solitary cysticercus granuloma: a double blind placebo controlled study. *J Infect.* 2006;53(1):65-69.

177. Garcia HH, Del Brutto OH, Nash Te, et al. New concepts in the diagnosis and management of neurocysticercosis (*Taenia solium*). *Am J Trop Med Hyg.* 2005;72(1):3-9.

178. Nash TE, Mahanty S, Garcia HH, et al. Corticosteroid use in neurocysticercosis. *Expert Rev Neurother.* 2011;11(8):1175-1183.

179. Spina-França A, Nobrega JP, Livramento JA, Machado LR. Administration of praziquantel in neurocysticercosis. *Tropenmed Parasitol.* 1982;33(1):1-4.

180. Mall RK, Agarwal A, Garg RK, Kar AM, Shukla R. Short course of prednisolone in Indian patients with solitary cysticercus granuloma and new-onset seizures. *Epilepsia.* 2003;44(11):1397–1401.

181. Kishore D, Misra S. Short course of oral prednisolone on disappearance of lesion and seizure recurrence in patients of solitary cysticercal granuloma with single small enhancing CT lesion: an open label randomized prospective study. *J Assoc Physicians India.* 2007:55:419-424.

182. Prakash S, Garg RK, Kar AM, et al. Intravenous methyl prednisolone in patients with solitary cysticercus granuloma: a random evaluation. *Seizure.* 2006;15(5):328-332.

183. Mitre E, Talaat KR, Sperling MR, et al. Methotrexate as a corticosteroid-sparing agent in complicated neurocysticercosis. *Clin Infect Dis.* 2007;44(4):549-553.

Endocrinology

Allison Ann Froehlich, MD

INTRODUCTION

In the setting of critical illness, the production and function of many hormones can be interrupted. As a result, new endocrine disorders may arise or preexisting endocrine disorders can become exacerbated.

DISORDERS OF THE PITUITARY GLAND

The pituitary gland, or "master gland," is a small, pea-shaped gland at the base of the brain. The anterior pituitary gland produces the majority of the hormones and is the portion of the gland that is most likely to become dysfunctional. It produces adrenocorticotrophic hormone (ACTH), luteinizing hormone (LH), follicle-stimulating hormone (FSH), prolactin, growth hormone (GH), and thyroid-stimulating hormone (TSH).[1] The posterior gland is responsible for producing vasopressin, also called antidiuretic hormone (ADH). A lack of vasopressin can lead to diabetes insipidus, or an inability to properly concentrate urine. The posterior gland also produces oxytocin, which helps with uterine contractions.

Most cases of hypopituitarism arise from surgery or radiation, and the rest are associated with tumors of the pituitary itself or extrapituitary tumors. Important considerations of pituitary dysfunction include pituitary dysfunction after transsphenoidal hypophysectomy or craniopharyngioma, apoplexy, and Sheehan syndrome.

In 1.1% of patients with transsphenoidal hypophysectomy or craniopharyngioma resection, a triphasic response of central diabetes insipidus, syndrome of inappropriate ADH secretion (SIADH), and chronic central diabetes insipidus may occur.[2] Table 22-1 shows the triphasic phase after transsphenoidal hypophysectomy or craniopharyngioma resection.

Apoplexy, or pituitary hemorrhage, may present with a sudden intense headache and visual changes and/or diplopia related to optic nerve compression.[3,4] There is often loss of hormones that are secreted from the anterior pituitary gland, including ACTH, resulting in central adrenal insufficiency,

with an immediate need for stress-dose steroids, in addition to neurosurgical intervention to decompress the hemorrhagic region.[5]

Sheehan syndrome is an infarction of the pituitary gland that occurs in pregnancy, typically in the setting of delivery complications (eg, excessive blood loss or severe hypotension).[6] Sometimes it can have a subtle presentation and the diagnosis is not made until the mother fails to lactate and/or menstruate postpartum.[7] As with pituitary apoplexy, central adrenal insufficiency is the most pressing concern, with a risk for mortality if unrecognized.

DISORDERS OF THE THYROID GLAND

Euthyroid Sick Syndrome

Euthyroid sick syndrome refers to abnormalities of thyroid function tests secondary to critical illness and is nonindicative of an actual thyroid problem. Often, during the initial phase of illness, the TSH level becomes slightly depressed (but not undetectable), related to pituitary thyrotropin cells in the pituitary gland going into a relative state of conservation, or reduced TSH secretion.[8] The T4 and T3 levels are also often low in the setting of critical illness, whereas the reverse T3 will be elevated.[9] Eighty percent of T3 is produced by peripheral deiodination of T4 to T3 via 5′-monodeiodinases in muscle, the liver, and the kidneys, and this process is diminished with low calorie intake.[10] T4 is low due to low levels of thyroid hormone–binding proteins or thyroxine-binding globulin (TBG) that adheres poorly to T4.[11] Reverse T3 is high due to inhibition of 5′-monodeiodinase acivity.[10]

The degree of thyroid dysfunction can often correlate with the severity of critical illness. Then, as the illness progresses and the pituitary gland recovers, the TSH may rise above the upper limit of the normal range (but typically remains below 10 mIU/L). Ultimately, the TSH will normalize within a span of several weeks. Thyroid medication is not indicated for this condition.[12,13] Table 22-2 summarizes the progressive changes seen in nonthyroidal illness.

TABLE 22-1 The Three Phases of the Triphasic Response

Phase	Timeframe	Presentation and Etiology	Classic Labs
First	Initial 4–5 d	Central diabetes insipidus due to initial ischemia or trauma to vasopressin-secreting cells of pituitary	High serum osmolality, low urine osmolality, and potential hypernatremia
Second	Next 1–2 d	SIADH due to vasopressin leak from damaged cells of posterior pituitary gland	Low serum osmolality, high urine osmolality, and hyponatremia
Third	Potentially persistent vs resolution after next 5–6 d	Chronic central diabetes insipidus, provided that 80–90% of the vasopressin-secreting cells have been destroyed	High serum osmolality, low urine osmolality, and hypernatremia (vs normal labs)

Unless there is a strong suspicion of an actual thyroid condition, thyroid function tests should not be routinely ordered in the setting of a critical illness.

Drug-Induced Thyroiditis

Drug-induced thyroid dysfunction is secondary to interferon-α, interleukin-2 (IL-2), lithium, and amiodarone. Amiodarone, a cardiac drug used to treat arrhythmias, has been clinically associated with development of both hypothyroidism and hyperthyroidism.[14] One of the reasons that amiodarone has a tendency to affect thyroid function is that it contains a large amount of iodine (roughly 35–40%),[15] which is the molecule that the thyroid gland uses for its production of thyroid hormone. Given this fact, sometimes the gland uses the excess iodine to overproduce thyroid hormone, particularly if the patient has a predisposing condition, such as Graves disease. On the other hand, amiodarone has a directly destructive effect on thyroid cells. Thyroid dysfunction can occur unpredictably, even after an extended duration of amiodarone use, so routine monitoring of thyroid function tests at baseline (before starting amiodarone), as well as periodic monitoring (while on amiodarone), can be helpful.

Amiodarone-induced hypothyroidism is thought to be due to the excess iodine causing a global inhibition of all thyroid hormone production, a phenomenon known as the Wolff-Chaikoff effect. Normally, the body is able to re-equilibrate to the excess iodine load. However, in the case of amiodarone-induced hypothyroidism, the body fails to adjust or escape from the Wolff-Chaikoff effect.[16] This condition is treated

with levothyroxine, generally without a need to discontinue amiodarone.

Amiodarone-induced thyrotoxicosis (AIT) is typically divided into 2 subtypes (1 and 2). Type 1 is typically associated with iodine-fueled overproduction of thyroid hormone. Conversely, type 2 is typically associated with an acute destruction of thyroid tissue.[17] Table 22-3 summarizes some of the diagnostic studies that are helpful in differentiating the 2 subtypes of AIT.[18] Also, Figure 22-1 illustrates the radioactive iodine uptake scan features that can be seen in the 2 subtypes.

In terms of treatment, type 1 AIT is initially treated with antithyroid medications (methimazole or propylthiouracil), potentially combined with potassium perchlorate. On the other hand, type 2 AIT generally responds best to steroid treatment. In cases of unclear etiology, antithyroid medication with steroid treatment is sometimes initiated. However, in patients who remain refractory to medication, sometimes a thyroidectomy is necessary, especially in severe cases of thyrotoxicosis.[19] Discontinuation of amiodarone is generally not helpful in the immediate context, as the amiodarone has a long half-life, so its effects can linger after its discontinuation.

Thyroid Storm

Severe thyrotoxicosis can have mortality rates estimated at roughly 20% to 30%.[20] This situation often occurs when

TABLE 22-2 Progressive Changes in Thyroid Function Tests During Nonthyroidal Illness

Initial Phase	Mid-Phase	Recovery Phase
↓ or Normal TSH	Normal or ↑ TSH	Normal TSH
↓ or Normal T4	↓ or Normal T4	Normal T4
↓ or Normal T3	↓ or Normal T4	Normal T3

TABLE 22-3 Studies Helpful for Differentiating Type 1 From Type 2 Amiodarone-Induced Thyrotoxicosis

	Type 1 Amiodarone-Induced Thyrotoxicosis	Type 2 Amiodarone-Induced Thyrotoxicosis
Thyroid radioiodine uptake	Typically normal	Decreased
Doppler ultrasound flow	Increased	Decreased
Interleukin-6	Normal or slightly increased	Increased

include elevated T4 and/or T3 levels and suppressed TSH. There may be associated hyperglycemia, hypercalcemia, leukopenia or leukocytosis, and elevated liver function tests.

The grading system is called the Burch-Wartofsky score and ranges from a total score of 0 to 45, with a score of 25 to 44 being suggestive of a diagnosis of thyroid storm, and a score greater than 45 as highly suggestive of a diagnosis of thyroid storm.[22] Details of this scoring system are listed in Table 22-4.

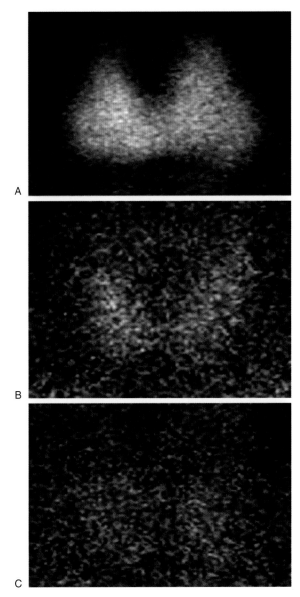

FIGURE 22-1 Radioactive iodine uptake in (A) amiodarone-induced thyrotoxicosis (AIT) type 1, (B) indeterminate AIT, and (C) AIT type 2.[18] (Reprinted with permission from Piga M, Cocco MC, Serra A, et al. The usefulness of ^{99m}Tc-sestaMIBI thyroid scan in the differential diagnosis and management of amiodarone-induced thyrotoxicosis. *Eur J Endocrinol.* 2008;159(4):423-429.)

TABLE 22-4 Burch-Wartofsky Scoring System for Thyroid Storm Diagnosis

Diagnostic Criterion	Points
Temperature (°F)	
99–99.9	5
100–100.9	10
101–101.9	15
102–102.9	20
103–103.9	25
> 104	30
Tachycardia (beats/min)	
90–109	5
110–119	10
120–129	15
130–139	20
> 140	25
Central nervous system impairment	
None/absent	0
Mild (agitation)	10
Moderate (psychosis)	20
Severe (coma)	30
Congestive heart failure	
None/absent	0
Mild (pedal edema)	5
Moderate (bi-basilar rales)	10
Severe (pulmonary edema)	15
Atrial fibrillation	
Absent	0
Present	10
Gastrointestinal/hepatic dysfunction	
Absent	0
Moderate (diarrhea/nausea/vomiting)	10
Severed (jaundice)	20
Precipitant history	
Negative	0
Positive	10
Total score	
< 25	Thyroid storm unlikely
25–44	Suggestive of thyroid storm
> 45	Highly suggestive of thyroid storm

Source: Burch HB, Wartofsky L. Life-threatening thyrotoxicosis. Thyroid storm. *Endocrinol Metab Clin North Am.* 1993;22(2):263-277.

a patient has preexisting hyperthyroidism that is exacerbated by another critical condition, such as major surgery, trauma, pregnancy, myocardial infarction, or infection. Although hyperthyroidism must be present for this diagnosis, certain clinical features also must be present to officially make this diagnosis.[21] In addition to fever, other clinical features include (1) gastrointestinal symptoms such as nausea, vomiting, diarrhea, and jaundice; (2) neurologic symptoms such as altered mental status or coma; and (3) cardiac symptoms such as tachycardia and cardiogenic pulmonary edema. Laboratory findings

Treatment includes thionamides such as methimazole or propylthiouracil to block the synthesis of thyroid hormones, iodine solution started 1 to 2 hours after initiation of the antithyroid medication to block the release of the thyroid hormones and induce Wolff-Chaikoff phenomenon, beta-blockers to block adrenergic effects, corticosteroids to reduce conversion of T3 to T4 and to treat adrenal insufficiency, and aggressive intravenous fluid hydration for hemodynamic support.[23]

Hashimoto Encephalopathy

Hashimoto encephalopathy (HE) is a form of relapsing encephalopathy that was first described by Sir Walter Russell Brain in 1966.[24] It is sometimes also referred to as steroid-responsive encephalopathy associated with autoimmune thyroiditis (SREAT), which alludes to the presence of high titers of classic Hashimoto antibodies (thyroid peroxidase [TPO] and antithyroglobulin [TgAb]), along with the clinical utility of steroids for treatment of this condition. However, the exact pathophysiology behind this condition is still not well understood.[25]

The typical clinical presentation of this condition occurs over a span of about 1 to 7 days, during which an individual might experience a relapsing course of encephalopathy. Some of the neurological symptoms include personality changes and/or altered mental status, mood changes, headaches, seizures, partial paralysis, tremors, ataxia, aphasia, and sleep disturbances. Although it is a very rare diagnosis, it should be considered in the differential for a patient with unexplained symptoms of encephalopathy, especially as failure to properly make this diagnosis could result in coma or death.

Myxedema Coma

Myxedema coma is a severe case of hypothyroidism that can arise in the setting of illness or another major stressor, such as trauma, myocardial infarction, pulmonary embolus, or even exposure to cold weather, particularly when an individual has preexisting untreated hypothyroidism for a prolonged interval of time.[26] It can have a high mortality risk of up to 40%.[27] It is typically characterized by a decompensated clinical state, with notable bradycardia, hypotension, hypothermia (temp < 94°F), hypoventilation, urinary retention, changes in mental status, seizures, and coma.[28] Electrocardiography (ECG) findings include bradycardia, low QRS voltage, T-wave inversions, QT prolongation, and first-degree atrioventricular block. Incidentally, the skin of an individual with myxedema coma may have an edematous appearance, which is due to the accumulation of intradermal proteins, rather than being true edema.[29] Although there is some debate over the official criteria required for a diagnosis of myxedema coma, largely due to the overall rarity of this condition, it is generally agreed that some degree of neurological impairment (ie, altered mental status) needs to be present to make this clinical diagnosis.

Patients have hyponatremia and hypoglycemia. The hyponatremia is thought to be related to decreased free water clearance from increased vasopressin excretion or decreased renal clearance. The hypoglycemia can be due to changes in metabolism from hypothyroid and/or concurrent adrenal insufficiency.

Given that it has a high mortality risk, it is imperative to initiate treatment as soon as a diagnosis is suspected, sometimes even before lab results are available. Treatment begins with empiric stress-dose steroid treatment (eg, hydrocortisone 100 mg every 8 hours), as an adrenal crisis could be precipitated if a patient has underlying adrenal insufficiency and is suddenly administered high-dose levothyroxine.[30,31] Then, a loading dose of intravenous T3 and T4 is initiated.[30] T4 at 200 to 400 μg intravenously (IV) is given as the initial dose, followed by 50 to 100 μg IV. T3 is given simultaneously at 5 to 20 μg, followed by 2.5 to 10 μg every 8 hours until there is clinical improvement. Serum T3 and T4 should be monitored daily. Additionally, if an individual is known to have underlying cardiovascular disease, the loading and maintenance doses of levothyroxine would be lowered.[30] It is also important to directly address any clinical symptoms associated with myxedema coma, such as using a warming blanket for hypothermia, administering aggressive intravenous fluids for hypotension, intubating for respiratory support, and treating any potential precipitating conditions.[26]

HYPOGLYCEMIA

Hypoglycemia is a condition in which the blood sugar drops below 55 mg/dL.[32] Normally, the body has counter-regulatory mechanisms to help restore euglycemia, including reduced production of insulin, along with increased secretion of glucagon, epinephrine, growth hormone, and cortisol.[33] When there is a process that interferes with the balance of glucose and counter-regulatory hormones, then prolonged hypoglycemia may occur. Symptoms associated with hypoglycemia include autonomic symptoms such as anxiety, sweating, palpitations, tremors, and headaches, and neurologic symptoms such as fatigue, confusion, and changes in mental status including coma and seizures. Common causes are listed in Table 22-5.

The workup consists of glucose, insulin, connecting peptide (C-peptide), β-hydroxybutyrate, proinsulin, and sulfonylurea and meglitinide screen. Plasma insulin levels greater than 3 μU/mL, proinsulin levels greater than 5 pmol/L, and C-peptide levels greater than 200 pmol/L occur in insulinoma, oral hypoglycemic-induced hyperinsulinemia, insulin autoimmune hypoglycemia, and noninsulinoma pancreatogenous hypoglycemia syndrome (NIPHS). Insulinoma also has a β-hydroxybutyrate level of less than 2.7 mmol/L. Hypoglycemia from insulinoma occurs during fasting, and hypoglycemia from NIPHS occurs 2 hours after a meal. Antibodies to insulin or insulin receptors can help distinguish autoimmune hypoglycemia from insulinoma.[34] Hypoglycemia from insulin autoimmune hypoglycemia

TABLE 22-5 Potential Causes of Fasting Hypoglycemia

Causes	Specific Types
Medication/drug side effects	Sulfonylurea, insulin, salicylates, antihistamines, angiotensin-converting enzyme inhibitors, alcohol
Systemic	Sepsis, malignancy, malnutrition/starvation, pregnancy, renal/hepatic disease, glycogen storage diseases
Hormone deficiencies	Adrenal insufficiency, glucagon deficiency, growth hormone deficiency
Excess insulin	Endogenous (eg, insulinoma) or exogenous (eg, accidental/intentional excess insulin administration)

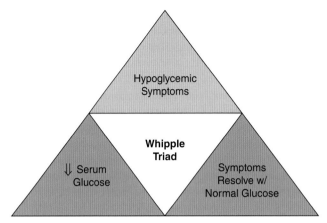

FIGURE 22-2 Components of the Whipple triad.

occurs after a meal, during fasting, or during both.[34] Imaging studies such as abdominal ultrasound, spiral computed tomography (CT), magnetic resonance imaging (MRI), 111In-pentetreotide imaging, and positron emission tomography (PET) are used to localize insulinoma.

Treatment of sulfonylurea-induced hypoglycemia consists of dextrose and octreotide 50-150 µg intramuscularly (IM) or subcutaneously (SQ) every 6 hours. Treatment for NIPHS involves nutritional modification and/or pancreatectomy. The treatment of choice for insulinoma is surgery, but patients who are not candidates can have medical therapy such as diazoxide, octreotide, and lanreotide.

Reactive hypoglycemia is an oversecretion of endogenous insulin in response to a consumed glucose load. The classic presentation of this particular diagnosis occurs in an individual who has had bariatric surgery and is now experiencing episodes of hypoglycemia less than 5 hours after consumption of a meal. This type of hypoglycemia is partly related to the increased rate of gastric emptying that occurs in bariatric surgery.[35] Reactive hypoglycemia can also sometimes be seen as the earliest manifestation of type 2 diabetes. In order to make the diagnosis of true hypoglycemia, a patient must fulfill the 3 components of the Whipple Triad,[36] which are illustrated in Figure 22-2.

Glucose Goal

In the critical care setting, causes of hypoglycemia include medication, sepsis, and renal dysfunction. Historically, there was often a push to achieve tight glycemic control in the critical care setting, especially after the breakthrough study published by Van den Berghe et al in 2001,[37] which indicated that there could be a clinical benefit to tight glycemic control (ie, intensive insulin therapy) in the surgical critical care setting. In that study, patients who were kept at glucose levels below 110 mg/dL were found to have substantially reduced mortality, both within the intensive care unit (ICU) and in the hospital, as well as overall reduced morbidity. However,

a subsequent large randomized critical care study called the Normoglycemia in Intensive Care Evaluation and Surviving Using Glucose Algorithm Regulation (NICE-SUGAR) trial that was published in 2009 looked at a population of patients in the medical ICU and found that use of intensive glucose control was actually associated with a 2.6% increased absolute risk of death at 90 days, with a number needed to harm of 38. Ultimately, this study concluded that a target blood glucose below 180 mg/dL would result in less mortality than a tighter glycemic target of 81 to 108 mg/dL.[38]

Treatment of hypoglycemia must focus on taking a good history, along with ordering appropriate laboratory tests. In particular, it is important to clarify preexisting medical conditions, weight changes, current medications, and family history. For fasting hypoglycemia, usually defined as less than 50 mg/dL, initial lab tests should involve fasting insulin, glucose, and c-peptide levels. High serum insulin levels and high C-peptide levels can be secondary to insulinoma or secretagogues such as sulfonylureas.[39] High serum insulin levels and low C-peptide levels can be secondary to exogenous insulin administration.[39] For reactive hypoglycemia, a prolonged glucose tolerance test should be performed, with confirmation of diagnosis if there is documentation of concordant hypoglycemia and there are symptoms several hours after receipt of an oral glucose load.

Hyperglycemic Emergencies

Diabetic Ketoacidosis

Diabetic ketoacidosis (DKA) refers to a state of insulin deficiency, which results in hyperglycemia. This condition generally involves individuals with type 1, or fully insulin-dependent, diabetes. There is reduced effective insulin concentration with increased catecholamines, cortisol, glucagon, and growth hormone.[40] The hyperglycemia is the result of increased gluconeogenesis, accelerated glycogenolysis, and impaired peripheral utilization.[41] Because of this impaired glucose utilization, lipolysis becomes a source of fuel. Free fatty acids are produced, which in turn become ketones via fatty acid oxidation. This leads to development of acidosis and ketonemia.[40,41] Dehydration is a key feature associated with this condition because the kidneys must eliminate the excess glucose, leading to concurrent water loss via osmotic diuresis.[42] In an insulin-dependent diabetic, this condition is generally provoked by a failure to take insulin or a defect in an insulin delivery device.[40,41] However, it can also be precipitated by a significant stressor, such as an acute infection, gastrointestinal bleed, myocardial infarction, stroke, or trauma.[41,43]

Hyperosmolar nonketotic coma (HONK) or hyperosmolar hyperglycemic state (HHS) generally occurs in individuals with type 2 diabetes with partial reserve of endogenous insulin. Therefore, lipolysis does not occur. It is defined as remarked hyperglycemia (glucose > 600 mg/dL) and hyperosmolarity (serum osmolarity > 320 mOsm/L), in the absence of acidosis (arterial pH > 7.30) and ketosis.[44] The osmolarity is calculated with the following equation: 2 (Na^+) + Glucose/18 + BUN/2.8, where BUN is the blood urea nitrogen level.

Risk factors for both DKA and HHS include inadequate insulin therapy, pancreatitis, myocardial infarction, cerebrovascular accident, thiazide, corticosteroids, sympathomimetics, pentamidine, antipsychotics, and new-onset type 1 diabetes. Table 22-6 lists the biochemical and clinical presentation of DKA. Table 22-7 lists the differences between DKA and HONK.[45,46]

Although a glucose level greater than 250 mg/dL is key in the diagnosis of either hyperglycemic emergencies, euglycemic (≤ 250 mg/dL) DKA does exist.[40] This can be attributed to pregnancy, food restriction, or inhibited gluconeogenesis.[41] Leukocytosis of 10,000 to 15,000/uL is secondary to elevated levels of norepinephrine and cortisol but a level greater than 25,000/uL is atypical in DKA.[47] This should prompt investigation for an infectious cause. The ketones (acetone, acetoacetate, and β-hydroxybutyrate) are the remaining byproducts of lipolysis that are not converted to acetyl coenzyme A, which subsequently enters the Krebs cycle. Urine and serum ketone values may not always agree. It is possible that the urine has been in the bladder for several hours preceding the development of the acute DKA presentation, so serum ketones levels may be a more accurate assessment of whether an individual is producing ketones. Additionally, the urine

TABLE 22-7 Differences Between Diabetic Ketoacidosis and Hyperosmolar Nonketotic Coma[41]

	Diabetic Ketoacidosis	Hyperosmolar Nonketotic Coma
Plasma glucose	> 250 mg/dL	> 600 mg/dL
Bicarbonate (HCO_3^-)	< 18 mEq/L	>18 mEq/L
Anion gap	Typically > 12 mEq/L	Typically < 12 mEq/L
Arterial pH	< 7.3	> 7.3
Urine ketones	Present	Absent
Fluid deficit	4–6 L	9–12 L
Typical patient	Younger	Older and/or disabled

ketone assay mostly detects acetoacetate, whereas the predominant ketone in DKA is β-hydroxybutyrate. Whether urine or serum ketones are measured, it is important to keep in mind that they can both be subject to confounding factors or false positive results. Some confounding conditions that produce positive ketones include starvation, alcoholism, hypoglycemia, hyperthyroidism, and certain medications (eg, salicylates). False positive results can be obtained in the setting of dehydration, as well as with the use of certain medications (eg, captopril, valproic acid, levodopa, acetylcysteine, and vitamin C).[48,49] Patients with HONK have enough endogenous insulin to prevent ketosis, so the condition will generally have a slow onset of polydipsia and polyuria over several weeks,[50] contributing to weight loss and an insidious onset of fatigue, neurologic deficits, and even coma.

Incidentally, lactic acidosis may also be seen in DKA, which is thought to be related to a combination of hypoperfusion from dehydration, along with alterations in metabolism from the diabetic ketoacidosis itself. It has not been shown to alter the ICU length of stay or patient mortality risk.[51] Sodium levels may be a reflection of hydration status, with hypernatremia suggesting severe dehydration. True sodium level is obtained by adding 1.6 mg/dL for every glucose level more than 100 mg/dL above 100 mg/dL.[40] Potassium may be normal (or even elevated initially) in DKA, but the potassium must still be monitored closely. As the hyperglycemia is addressed, there is an intracellular shift of potassium, resulting in a significant drop in serum potassium.[52] If the potassium is documented as below 5 mEq/L at the time of insulin initiation, it would be important to initiate potassium supplementation. If the potassium is ever documented as below 3.3 mEq/L, insulin should be held until the potassium is adequately addressed.

Triglycerides can become elevated during hyperglycemic states. In DKA, the excess free fatty acids that are produced from lipolysis are taken up by the liver, resulting in increased production of very low-density lipoprotein (VLDL), which are partly compromised of triglycerides and serve to transport triglycerides throughout the body. In both DKA and HONK,

TABLE 22-6 The Biochemical and Clinical Spectrum of Diabetic Ketoacidosis

	Mild	Moderate	Severe
Bicarbonate	15–18 mEq/L	10–15 mEq/L	< 10 mEq/L
Anion gap	> 10 mEq/L	> 12 mEq/L	> 12 mEq/L
Arterial pH	7.25–7.3	7.0–7.24	< 7.0
Clinical alertness	Alert	Drowsy	Stuporous/comatose

Data from Laffel L. Improving outcomes with POCT for HbA1c and blood ketone testing. *J Diabetes Sci Technol.* 2007;1(1):133-136; Kitabchi AE, Umpierrez GE, Murphy MB, et al. Hyperglycemic crises in diabetes. *Diabetes Care.* 2004;27(Suppl 1):S94-S102.

hyperglycemia inhibits lipoprotein lipase activity peripherally, thereby exacerbating hypertriglyceridemia. If the triglycerides exceed 1000 mg/dL, it is possible for acute or spontaneous pancreatitis to arise. In fact, hypertriglyceridemia is the third most common cause of acute pancreatitis and has been reported to account for 1% to 4% of cases in hospitalized patients.[53] Diagnosis of pancreatitis during DKA must rely mostly upon abdominal symptoms and CT findings, as lipase can become elevated in DKA in the absence of pancreatic inflammation. In fact, amylase and lipase are increased up to 25% of the time in DKA.[54] In any case, it is very important to ensure that these triglycerides are adequately addressed or lowered. Fortunately, use of insulin and restoration of euglycemia generally help to significantly lower the triglycerides. When attainment of euglycemia does not adequately lower triglycerides, intravenous heparin and plasmapheresis are other modalities that can be used for further lowering.

Treatment of hyperglycemic emergencies involves aggressive fluid hydration, intense insulin treatment, and close monitoring of the electrolytes. Bicarbonate therapy is not included as a standard component of the treatment algorithm, as it typically does not improve treatment outcomes.[55] It has been suggested that sodium bicarbonate can be given if the pH is less than 6.9.[40] In terms of the bodily water deficit in DKA, it can be in the order of 4 to 6 Liters.[56] Hydration typically is addressed with crystalloids, such as isotonic saline at 15 to 20 mL/kg/h or 1 to 1-5 L/h. Normal 0.9% saline may be used for subsequent replacement, or 0.45% saline at 250 to 500 mL/h if sodium is normal or elevated. Electrolytes are routinely monitored every 4 hours.

In uncomplicated cases of DKA, insulin can be administered via an intravenous or subcutaneous route, with injections dosed at overlapping 1- to 2-hour intervals; a study published by the American Diabetes Association in 2004 indicated that both approaches have relatively equivalent outcomes.[57] Nevertheless, the current standard of care has favored intravenous insulin administration, with insulin typically given in an initial bolus of 0.1 U/kg, followed by a continuous infusion that may be adjusted via a hospital-specific protocol. Plasma glucose is expected to decrease by 50 to 75 mg/dL/h. It has been suggested that more rapid decreases can precipitate cerebral edema. If the glucose does not decrease at the desired rate, the insulin drip may be increased. It is prudent to consider adding potassium to the intravenous fluids when there is a documented serum potassium below 5 mEq/L.[42]

Glucose monitoring is performed every hour. However, a point-of-care (POC) glucose level can be inaccurate in critical illness. In particular, if a patient has hypotensive shock, there will typically be associated decreased capillary blood, so the surrounding tissue tries to extract an increased amount of glucose from capillaries, resulting in falsely lower capillary blood glucose measurement.[58] Venous blood can be a much more accurate measurement in this scenario, but the slow turnaround time does not make it as practical as POC glucose.

Some hospitals have advocated the use of an arterial blood gas (ABG) analyzer as an alternative method of glucose measurement, especially when there is a strong clinical suspicion that the POC glucose may be inaccurate.[59]

In the management of DKA, the standard is to keep the patient from eating or drinking (nothing by mouth [NPO]). When the glucose drops below 250 mg/dL, the intravenous fluids can be switched to 5% dextrose in 0.9% sodium chloride (D5NS).[41] It is very important to avoid hypoglycemia in the treatment of DKA, as it can cause a rebound ketosis, thereby lengthening the duration of treatment.

Once the acidosis resolves (generally defined as a closure of the anion-gap of < 12 mEq/L, a serum bicarbonate level > 18 mEq/L, and an arterial blood gas pH > 7.3), the patient can be transitioned to an oral diet, and subcutaneous insulin can be started, making sure to overlap the initial insulin injection at least 1 to 2 hours with the continuous insulin infusion.[41,58] Several studies have supported using 80% of the total 24-h intravenous insulin requirements.

The importance of treating HONK as aggressively as DKA is best reflected by the fact that DKA has typically been associated with a mortality risk less than 5%, whereas HONK can have a mortality risk estimated above 15%.[50]

DISORDERS OF THE ADRENAL GLAND

The adrenal glands are above the kidneys and respond to regulatory signals from the pituitary gland. Specifically, the pituitary gland secretes adrenocorticotrophic hormone in response to corticotropin-releasing hormone (CRH) from the hypothalamus, which subsequently stimulates secretion of the glucocorticoid cortisol from the cortex of the adrenal gland. When there is a breakdown in this cascade of communication, adrenal insufficiency can arise. The cortex contains the glomerulosa, which secretes the mineralocorticoids aldosterone and corticosterone; the fasciculata, which secretes the glucocorticoids cortisol and cortisone; and the reticularis, which secretes estrogen and testosterone. The medulla secretes epinephrine, norepinephrine, somatostatin, and substance P.

An adrenal crisis can occur from an exacerbation of preexisting adrenal insufficiency, in the setting of an acute stressor, such as illness, pregnancy, trauma, or a major surgery.[60] Causes of adrenal insufficiency are typically subdivided into primary (involving the adrenal gland itself) and secondary (related to insufficient ACTH production from the pituitary gland). Table 22-8 outlines some causes of adrenal insufficiency.[61,62] Additionally, an adrenal crisis related to an adrenal infarction or hemorrhage can arise unexpectedly.

Autoimmune polyglandular deficiency syndromes are a rare cause of adrenal insufficiency, but it is important to have an awareness of these syndromes in the critical care setting. The 2 subtypes of this unique condition causing adrenal insufficiency are summarized in Table 22-9.[63,64]

TABLE 22-8 Primary and Secondary Causes of Adrenal Insufficiency

Primary Causes	Secondary Causes
Infection of adrenal gland (eg, tuberculosis, HIV-related opportunistic infections, and sepsis)	Infection of pituitary gland (eg, tuberculosis)
Metastatic adrenal carcinoma (pulmonary and breast) or other structural disease	Metastatic pituitary disease, pituitary adenoma, stalk lesion
Medications (eg, ketoconazole, rifampin, and phenytoin)	Exogenous steroids for prolonged duration
Familial/autoimmune/congenital (eg, Addison disease)	Familial/autoimmune/infiltrative (eg, neurosarcoidosis; lymphocytic hypophysitis
Adrenal hemorrhage/infarction	Pituitary apoplexy or infarction, trauma
Idiopathic	Idiopathic or isolated adrenocorticotrophic hormone deficiency

TABLE 22-9 Subtypes of Polyglandular Deficiency Syndromes

	Type 1	Type 2
Associated endocrine disorders	**Common:** Adrenal insufficiency Hypoparathyroidism Hypogonadism **Less common:** Type 1 diabetes Autoimmune thyroid disease (eg, Graves or Hashimoto)	**Common** Adrenal insufficiency Autoimmune thyroid disease (eg, Graves or Hashimoto) Type 1 diabetes Hypogonadism
Other conditions	Mucocutaneous candidiasis Celiac disease Pernicious anemia Autoimmune hepatitis Vitiligo Nail/tooth dystrophy	~5% of patients Vitiligo Pernicious anemia Alopecia Myasthenia gravis Celiac disease Sjögren syndrome Rheumatoid arthritis
Genetics	Idiopathic or autosomal recessive mutation of autoimmune regulator gene (*AIRE*) on chromosome 21	50% sporadic 50% familial (up to 90% have circulating antibodies to 21-hydroxylase)
Typical age of onset	6 mo to 20 y	20 to 30 y

If an individual has preexisting adrenal insufficiency and is on steroid replacement, the steroid dose is typically increased in the setting of a significant stressor to help prevent a potential adrenal crisis. However, there has been debate as to the full utility of this practice in the surgical setting.[65,66] Generally, perioperative steroid doses vary based on surgical risk, but hydrocortisone doses under 200 mg are often advised.[67]

Classic symptoms of an adrenal crisis from primary adrenal insufficiency include severe hypotension, nausea, vomiting, occasionally fever, and abdominal pain.[68] Additionally, a patient may develop hypoglycemia, along with hyponatremia, hyperkalemia, and metabolic acidosis. If there is no prior history of adrenal insufficiency in a patient in the critical care setting, a low serum cortisol, (below 15 μg/dL) may raise suspicion of this diagnosis,[69] and further assessment of the adrenal axis could be attained with a Cortrosyn (ACTH) stimulation test. For this test, 250 μg of Cortrosyn is administered either intramuscularly or intravenously and then serum cortisol is measured at intervals of 0 minutes (prior to injection), 30 minutes, and 60 minutes, with a "normal" response considered to be a final serum cortisol of over 18 μg/dL. However, one must keep in mind that 90% of the circulating cortisol in humans is bound to proteins (either cortisol-binding globulin [CBG] or albumin) and hypoproteinemia, manifested as low serum albumin, is not uncommon in the critical care setting. Some studies have proposed using free cortisol levels as an alternative means of assessing the adrenal function, but this is not currently considered a standard practice.[70]

Beyond the Cortrosyn stimulation test, there are certain tests that can be helpful for differentiating primary from secondary (or tertiary) adrenal insufficiency. Specifically, a serum ACTH level typically will be low in both secondary and tertiary adrenal insufficiency, whereas it would be elevated in primary adrenal insufficiency. If the baseline serum ACTH level is low, a CRH stimulation test can be helpful for differentiating secondary from tertiary adrenal insufficiency. In the case of secondary adrenal insufficiency, the ACTH level would not rise appreciably with CRH stimulation, whereas with tertiary adrenal insufficiency, there would be a normal or increased response of ACTH to CRH stimulation. A serum aldosterone level (which is under the regulation of angiotensin) typically is preserved in secondary and tertiary adrenal insufficiency. Therefore, electrolyte disturbances and hypotension are less common with secondary and tertiary adrenal insufficiency (compared with primary adrenal insufficiency). Also, clinically, the patient will not have hyperpigmentation of the skin or mucous membranes in secondary and tertiary adrenal insufficiency because the hyperpigmentation seen in primary adrenal insufficiency is due to melanocyte stimulation from excessive ACTH production. Table 22-10 summarizes key laboratory and

TABLE 22-10 Diagnostic Findings in Primary, Secondary, and Tertiary Adrenal Insufficiency

Adrenal Insufficiency Type	Baseline (8:00 AM) fasting serum Cortisol	Final Cortisol After Cortrosyn Stim Test	Baseline ACTH Level	ACTH After CRH Stim Test	Serum Aldosterone	K+ Level	Low Blood Pressure	Skin Darkening
Primary	Low	Low	High	N/A	Low	High	Common	Often Present
Secondary	Low	Normal or Subnormal	Low	No change	Normal	Normal	Uncommon	Absent
Tertiary	Low	Normal or Subnormal	Low	Increased	Normal	Normal	Uncommon	Absent

clinical findings in primary, secondary, and tertiary adrenal insufficiency.

Given that an adrenal crisis can be potentially fatal, if it is suspected, it must be treated aggressively, even prior to obtaining definitive lab results. Treatment for an adrenal crisis involves aggressive intravenous fluids, along with immediate intravenous stress-dose steroids. If there is a plan for adrenal axis testing, then dexamethasone would be the steroid of choice, as it does not interfere with the cortisol assay. Otherwise, in patients with preexisting adrenal insufficiency, hydrocortisone is appropriate. The key point in management is that initiation of steroids takes precedence over any additional testing of the adrenal axis. Table 22-11 summarizes treatment guidelines advocated by the Endocrine Society.[62,71] In unexplained causes of adrenal insufficiency, a subsequent CT of the adrenal glands could potentially reveal the presence of an adrenal hemorrhage. If there is concern for secondary adrenal insufficiency, a pituitary MRI could be performed.

TABLE 22-11 Treatment of Perioperative Adrenal Insufficiency and Adrenal Crisis in an Adult

Condition	Treatment
Minor/moderate surgery	25–75 mg hydrocortisone/d for 1–2 d
Major surgery (eg, general anesthesia, trauma, delivery)	100 mg intravenous hydrocortisone, followed by 50 mg every 6 h (total of 200 mg/d); steroid taper contingent on clinical status Continuous intravenous fluids- either D5 + 1/4 NS or D5 + 1/2 NS).
Acute adrenal crisis	Dexamethasone 4 mg intravenous bolus **OR** 100 mg intravenous hydrocortisone, followed by continuous infusion of hydrocortisone (200 mg/d), reduced by half the following day 1 L of NS or D5NS over 1 h, continuous dextrose infusion for hypoglycemia

Pheochromocytoma

A pheochromocytoma is a very rare catecholamine-secreting tumor of the adrenal gland that contributes to hypertension in over 90% of affected patients.[72] Medications such as beta-blockers, metoclopramide, opiates, and atropine can provoke a hypertensive crisis in patients with pheochromocytoma.[73]

In a classic presentation of a pheochromocytoma, an individual could have paroxysmal episodes of hypertension, lasting roughly 30 minutes, during which he or she may experience a classic triad of headache, sweating, and palpitations. These episodes can occur in the absence of any clear provoking factors, and other times, they may arise in the setting of abdominal palpation or simply vigorously shifting a patient in a bed.

Initial testing for this condition would involve a fasting serum metanephrine level. However, it is not uncommon for this test to be falsely positive, especially in the stressful setting of the critical care unit. An alternative method of testing involves a 24-hour urine collection of metanephrines and catecholamines.

A pheochromocytoma is usually best localized on an abdominal CT or MRI. In rare situations, an individual might have an extra-adrenal pheochromocytoma (or paraganglioma), which would be best visualized with an iodine-123-meta-iodobenzylguanidine (MIBG) scan, or sometimes a positron-emission tomography scan, if metastatic disease is involved.[74]

Ultimately, the treatment for a pheochromocytoma would entail surgery if the source can be identified. However, it is important to have the patient adequately alpha-blocked prior to surgery, typically using phenoxybenzamine, which is gradually titrated until adequate blood pressure control is achieved. Although a patient with a pheochromocytoma may have notable tachycardia, it is important to avoid beta-blockade until there is adequate alpha-blockade, in order to prevent provocation of a potential hypertensive crisis. In fact, the tachycardia is often predominantly caused by volume depression and responds best to aggressive intravenous fluid hydration, along with oral salt supplements. Inadequate fluid resuscitation prior to surgery can result in dramatic postoperative drops in blood pressure.

QUESTIONS

1. A 32-year-old man with a history of human immunodeficiency virus (HIV) is being treated in the ICU for cryptococcal meningitis. Due to severe alterations in his mental status, he has been intubated and has been placed on amphotericin B as part of his therapeutic regimen. During the course of his treatment, the nursing staff alerts you that this patient's urine output has increased dramatically, amounting to 500 mL of urine output per hour. A serum sodium comes back elevated at 147 mEq/L, a urine osmolality is 150 mOsm/kg, and a plasma osmolality is 300 mOsm/kg.

   The nurse administers a stat 2 µg IV push of desmopressin. If the amphotericin B is, in fact, the etiologic factor in his diabetes insipidus, which of the following responses would you NOT anticipate on a subsequent recheck of urine osmolality?

   A. Urine osmolality 100 mOsm/Kg
   B. Urine osmolality 250 mOsm/kg
   C. Urine osmolality 150 mOsm/kg
   D. Urine osmolality 160 mOsm/kg

2. A patient has diabetes insipidus from amphotericin B. Which of the following would be the best treatment strategy for this patient?

   A. Administering desmopressin intravenously at intervals of every 12 hours
   B. Administration of the intravenous vasopressin receptor antagonist conivaptan
   C. Aggressive IV fluid hydration, along with administration of salt tablets
   D. Aggressive IV fluid hydration and switching to liposomal amphotericin B

3. Which of the following disorders may become a chronic condition in Sheehan syndrome?

   A. Hypothyroidism
   B. Diabetes insipidus
   C. Osteoporosis
   D. Nephropathy

4. A 53-year-old man with history of hyperthyroidism is admitted for sepsis secondary to community-acquired pneumonia. He is started on levofloxacin. His labs are as follows:

Na	135 mEq/L
Cl	102 mEq/L
CO_2	22 mEq/L
K	4.2 mEq/L
BUN	22 mg/dL
Creatinine	1.2 mg/dL
TSH	0.2 mIU/L
Free T4	0.6 ng/dL
BNP	250 pg/mL

What is the next step?

A. Stat total T3 and reverse T3 levels
B. IV levothyroxine 25 µg
C. Repeat TSH and free T4 levels in the morning
D. No further thyroid labs and/or thyroid-related medications are necessary

5. A 57-year-old man with a history of atrial fibrillation, which has previously been stable on a combination of amiodarone and beta-blocker treatment, now presents to the emergency department (ED) with acute shortness of breath, anxiety, and a pulse of 160. His lower extremities are edematous, and there is evidence of jugular venous distension, along with decreased breath sounds at his lung bases.

   His O_2 saturation is low at 85%. His blood pressure is 115/76 mm Hg. A stat ECG indicates an irregularly irregular rhythm consistent with recurrent atrial fibrillation. His chest x-ray shows bilateral pleural effusions. He is placed on IV diltiazem, along with diuretic treatment, and 1 Liter of oxygen via nasal cannula. Stat lab work is ordered. The results of these labs are as follows:

Na	135 mEq/L
K	4.2 mEq/L
Cl	102 mEq/L
CO_2	20 mEq/L
BUN	18 mg/dL
Creatinine	1.3 mg/dL
Glucose	89 mg/dL
TSH	< 0.01 mIU/L
Free T4	2.2 ng/dL
Troponin I	< 0.01 ng/mL
Hemoglobin	11.8 g/dL
BNP	350 pg/mL

The patient reports that he has no prior known history of thyroid disease. On exam, you are unable to palpate any thyroid nodules. Which of the following studies would be most helpful in guiding your initial treatment of his thyroid condition?

A. Serum total T3 level
B. Thyroid Doppler ultrasound study
C. Serum IL-9 level
D. Thyroid antibody levels

6. For the patient in question 5, if the etiology of the hyperthyroidism is not clear based on additional studies, what would be the best approach to addressing his hyperthyroidism acutely?

A. Radioiodine treatment
B. Urgent surgical consult for thyroidectomy
C. Methimazole alone
D. Methimazole and prednisone

7. A 60-year-old homeless man is brought into the ED by ambulance after being observed by pedestrians to have tonic-clonic seizures on a busy city sidewalk. He is no longer seizing at the time of presentation but appears to be shivering, and his breath sounds are slow or widely spaced. Rectal temperature is 92°F. Of note, he is hypoxic with O_2 saturation of 85% on room air. A stat arterial blood gas reveals significant CO_2 retention, so the patient is emergently intubated. An ECG reveals sinus bradycardia in the 40s with some flattening of the T waves. His blood pressure is 125/87 mmHg. You notice on physical exam that he has what appears to be a well-healed thyroidectomy scar. What is the next best step in managing this patient?

A. Check a stat panel of thyroid function tests (TSH, free T4, and total T3 levels)
B. Administer stat IV steroids
C. Give stat loading dose of IV levothyroxine
D. Give stat dose of liothyronine (T3)

8. All of the following ancillary treatments would be potentially indicated to help stabilize a patient with myxedema coma, except for which one?

A. Inotrope treatment for his bradycardia
B. Warming blanket for his hypothermia
C. Antiseizure medication
D. Glucose administration

9. In a patient with accidental sulfonylurea ingestion, what insulin–C-peptide pattern will you see?

A. Low Insulin, high C-peptide
B. High Insulin, high C-peptide
C. Low Insulin, low C-peptide
D. High Insulin, low C-peptide

10. A 60-year-old woman with dementia and diabetes mellitus who had been prescribed glipizide 5 mg orally (PO) daily has had decreased appetite, nausea, and vomiting for the last 2 to 3 days. She was found unresponsive and hypoglycemic with levels in the 40s. Her sulfonylurea screen was negative and the CT of her abdomen shows an insulinoma.

The patient is not initially agreeable to getting a surgical consultation for a potential resection of this suspected insulinoma. You urge her to reconsider her decision and educate her about the potential risks of hypoglycemia. She states that she now "feels fine" and is demanding to be discharged home. However, she is agreeable to following up with an endocrinologist in the outpatient setting next week and is agreeable to following your outpatient instructions in the meantime. From the following treatment options, which would be the least effective in temporarily managing her hypoglycemic symptoms?

A. Small, frequent 30-g carbohydrate meals at intervals of roughly every 4 hours
B. Glucagon 1 mg to be administered daily in the evening and as needed for blood sugar below 50 mg/dL
C. Diazoxide orally 3 times per day
D. Metformin orally 3 times per day

11. An elderly woman is brought to the ED, having been found unconscious in a nearby public park, with a documented fingerstick glucose of 35 mg/dL by emergency medical services (EMS), which had been treated with 1 mg of glucagon on transit to the ED. Her labs were as follows:

Na	136 mEq/L
K	3.7 mEq/L
Creatinine	1.9 mg/dL
Glucose	45 mg/dL
Cortisol	15.8 µg/dL

You immediately administer an ampule of D50. As you are not clear on the identity of this woman or her current medications, you decide to run several additional tests, including a sulfonylurea drug screen. What treatment would be indicated to further address this woman's hypoglycemia in the meantime?

A. Immediate initiation of stress-dose steroids
B. IV hydration with D10 with hourly glucose checks
C. IV glucagon drip
D. IV fluids to address suspected dehydration, with ampules of dextrose as needed for glucose below 60 mg/dL

12. A 36-year-old insulin-dependent diabetic, on an insulin pump, reports that he began to experience a severe sore throat prior to admission, with accompanying fatigue, myalgias, and a dry cough. He has been eating very little, so he decided to reduce all his pump settings by 50%. This morning, his blood glucose is 350 mg/dL. He took his standard coverage bolus, but a repeat blood sugar about 1 hour later came back at 390 mg/dL. He performed a home urine ketone test and it came back positive, so he advised his wife to drive him to the ED for further evaluation. His vitals on admission are as follows: BP of 120/76 mmHg, HR of 115 beats/min, RR of 25 breaths/min, and temperature of 100.6°F. On exam, he appears quite dehydrated with poor skin turgor. Also, his breath has a fruity odor. Stat lab work is sent in the ED and comes back as follows:

Glucose	460 mg/dL
Na	128 mEq/L
K	4.9 mEq/L
Cl	95 mEq/L
HCO$_3$	14 mEq/L
Creatinine	2.0 mg/dL
AST	45 U/L
ALT	38 U/L
Urine ketones	positive

ABG:

pH	7.1
PO_2	100 mmHg
HCO_3	16 mmol/L
Pco_2	32 mmHg
Sao_2	98% (room air)
HbA1c	7.6%
WBC	$13.5 \times 10^3/\mu L$
Hemoglobin	13 g/dL

His ECG is notable for sinus tachycardia in the 110 range. A chest x-ray shows a few increased interstitial markings but is otherwise unremarkable. Which of the following options would be the best initial treatment for his condition?

A. Normal saline, bicarbonate, and insulin
B. 5% albumin and insulin
C. Normal saline and insulin
D. Normal saline, insulin, and potassium

13. Which of the following patterns of lab tests would be the best indication that his DKA has resolved?

A. Na, 140 mEq/L; K, 3.8 mEq/L; chloride, 105 mEq/L; bicarb, 21 mEq/L; ABG pH, 7.3
B. Na, 138 mEq/L; K, 3.8 mEq/L; chloride, 108 mEq/L; bicarb, 16 mEq/L; ABG pH, 7.25
C. Na, 136 mEq/L; K, 3.7 mEq/L; chloride, 107 mEq/L; bicarb, 20 mEq/L; ABG pH, 7.32
D. Na, 135 mEq/L; K, 4.0 mEq/L; chloride, 97 mEq/L; bicarb, 19 mEq/L; ABG pH, 7.35

14. A 23-year-old girl with type 1 diabetes is brought to the ED with complaints of feeling nauseous and very fatigued. She has been unable to eat or drink very much over the past 48 hours. Her glucose was 295 mg/dL, and her home urine ketone test was moderately positive. In the ED, she is found to be afebrile, with blood pressure of 100/65 mmHg, pulse of 105 beats/min, and oxygen saturation of 99%. Her labs are as follows:

Na	133 mEq/L
Cl	103 mEq/L
K	3.5 mEq/L
HCO_3	17 mEq/L
Calcium	8.8 mg/dL
Magnesium	2.0 mEq/L
Glucose	235 mg/dL
Lactic acid	4 mmol/L
WBC	$18 \times 10^3/\mu L$
ABG pH	7.3

Which of the following treatments would you initiate first?

A. IV fluid hydration with NS
B. A weight-based insulin bolus
C. Empiric antibiotics
D. Insulin drip

15. Which of the following electrolytes has the greatest risk of dropping dramatically in patients on insulin drip for DKA?

A. Sodium
B. Potassium
C. Magnesium
D. Calcium

16. An 18-year-old cachectic-appearing boy presents to the ED with severe dizziness, weakness, and spontaneous twitching of several muscle. His hands feel cool to the touch, and there are macular areas of hypopigmentation on the dorsum of his hands and forearms. His blood pressure on exam is 85/45 mmHg with a pulse of 95 beats/min. The patient is placed on IV fluid hydration and then stat lab work is drawn. Some of the initial lab results are as follows:

Na	127 mEq/L
Cl	108 mEq/L
K	5.8 mEq/L
Ca	6.5 mg/dL
Albumin	2.9 g/dL
Glucose	72 mg/dL
CO_2	22 mEq/L
Creatinine	0.9 mg/dL
Hemoglobin	11.2 g/dL
TSH	24 mIU/L
Cortisol (drawn 8:59 AM)	5 μg/dL

You suspect that this patient may have a new diagnosis of autoimmune polyglandular disease. For the immediate stabilization of this patient, which would be the next best step in management?

A. Intravenous levothyroxine
B. Intravenous steroids
C. Intravenous glucose
D. Intravenous calcium

17. Which of the following associated conditions would help you to classify the patient in question 16 as potentially having type 1 (instead of type 2) autoimmune polyglandular disease?

A. Hypoparathyroidism
B. Thyroiditis
C. Adrenal insufficiency
D. Vitiligo

18. Which test would be the most sensitive for determining if the patient has acquired adrenal insufficiency from past oral corticosteroid use?

A. An adrenal CT to look for adrenal atrophy
B. A pituitary MRI to look for pituitary hypoplasia
C. A midnight salivary cortisol collection
D. None of the above

ANSWERS

1. B. Urine osmolality 250 mOsm/kg

   If the patient has nephrogenic diabetes insipidus, the vasopressin receptors have significantly lost their ability to respond to DDAVP. Therefore, when exogenous desmopressin is administered, you would anticipate seeing less than a 50% rise in the urine osmolality (choice A, C, and D). In choice B, the urine osmolality has risen by 66%, so this answer would be more suggestive of central diabetes insipidus.

2. D. Aggressive IV fluid hydration and switching to liposomal amphotericin B

   The liposomal formulation of amphotericin B has been clinically shown to have a reduced incidence of nephrogenic side effects, so this formulation would be preferable, especially if it is determined that amphotericin is still a necessary component of this patient's medical treatment. Given that this patient has been temporarily unable to concentrate his urine, he likely has a significant free water deficit and it will be important to aggressively hydrate him until it appears that the nephrogenic diabetes insipidus is sufficiently resolved. Choice A is not appropriate, as you have already presumably determined that the patient does NOT have central diabetes insipidus. Choice B is not correct because he already has inhibition of his vasopressin receptors from the amphotericin B. The use of the vasopressin receptor antagonists is typically indicated in certain cases of hyponatremia from SIADH. Lastly, salt tablets (choice C) are not indicated in nephrogenic insipidus, as these patients typically have hypernatremia. Addressing the large fluid losses associated with nephrogenic diabetes insipidus is the priority in the clinical management of this specific condition.

3. A. Hypothyroidism

   Patients with Sheehan syndrome often develop anterior pituitary insufficiency. Other hormones (aside from ACTH) made by the anterior pituitary gland include TSH, LH/FSH, GH, and prolactin. Women with Sheehan syndrome often fail to lactate following delivery and may develop persistent amenorrhea. Central hypothyroidism (choice A) is the best answer. Diabetes insipidus (choice B) is not as relevant (as ADH is made by the posterior pituitary gland). It is possible that osteoporosis (choice C) may develop over time from hypopituitarism and potential chronic steroid replacement, but this should not occur in the near future. Lastly, nephropathy (choice D) would not be anticipated in the absence of a documented chronic contributing condition such as diabetes.

4. D. No further thyroid labs and/or thyroid-related medications are necessary

   There is no need to check additional thyroid function tests in this scenario, as the initial tests are already consistent with euthyroid sick syndrome or nonthyroidal illness. Checking total T3 and reverse T3 (choice A) would not significantly alter management. Also, choice B is not indicated, and in fact, IV levothyroxine may even prove harmful in this patient who has recently presented with a myocardial infarction. Euthyroid sick syndrome or nonthyroidal illness typically takes several weeks to fully resolve, so repeat TSH and free T4 levels in morning (choice C) would not change management.

5. B. Thyroid Doppler ultrasound study

   The patient has been on amiodarone for an unspecified period of time, and it is likely that he has developed AIT. The Doppler ultrasound (choice B) can be quite helpful in differentiating type 1 from type 2 AIT, as the former will typically have increased vascularity and the latter will have decreased vascularity on the ultrasound imaging. The serum T3 (choice A) would likely come back elevated but would not acutely impact the choice of treatment. Choice C is incorrect because it is IL-6 (not IL-9) that becomes acutely elevated in type 2 AIT. Lastly, thyroid antibodies (choice D) may indeed point to an underlying predisposing condition, such as Graves or Hashimoto disease, but these tests will likely not come back immediately, and the Doppler ultrasound still provides the most direct evidence of the specific subtype of AIT.

6. D. Methimazole and prednisone

   In cases of indeterminate AIT, it is generally best to use an approach that addresses both type 1 and type 2. Specifically, choice D is the best answer here, as it entails a combination of antithyroid medication and steroid treatment. Choice A is not the best answer in the acute setting because the patient's current use of amiodarone (which is high in iodine content) would greatly lessen the effectiveness of radioiodine treatment. This patient may ultimately require a thyroidectomy (choice B), if he does not respond effectively to a combination of antithyroid medication and steroid treatment. However, keep in mind that any surgery has inherent risks, so it would not be the next best choice, at least not before consideration of a trial of medication. Lastly, choice C would only be the best selection if it was clear that the patient had type 1 AIT. However, in this case, the cause of his hyperthyroidism remains undetermined, so combination treatment with methimazole and steroids is preferable.

7. B. Administer stat IV steroids

   The patient has evidence of a past thyroidectomy on physical exam, and it appears that he has several symptoms consistent with potential myxedema coma (eg, bradycardia, hypothermia, respiratory decompensation, and a recently observed tonic-clonic seizure). Your first priority should be immediate stabilization of this patient. If myxedema coma is suspected, IV steroids (choice B) would be indicated, before initiation of levothyroxine (choice C). Thyroid function tests (choice A) should be sent on this patient. However, if there is a very strong clinical suspicion of myxedema coma, treatment should be initiated, even before the test results are back. Lastly, liothyronine (choice D) is considered to have a debatable impact in the treatment of myxedema coma, and it would certainly not take precedence over initiation of corticosteroids.

8. **A. Inotrope treatment for his bradycardia**

This patient still has a reasonable blood pressure, so inotrope treatment (choice A) is not critically indicated for cardiovascular support. Additionally, in this patient with suspected myxedema coma, using an inotrope could provoke an arrhythmia, especially when levothyroxine is initiated. In general, inotropes should be avoided in individuals with suspected myxedema coma. The remaining choices (choices B, C and D) all appropriately address different critical aspects in the stabilization of this patient.

9. **B. High Insulin, high C-peptide**

Secretagogues help the beta cells of the pancreas to secrete additional insulin. C-peptide is a metabolite of insulin, so it will become acutely elevated while on treatment with a sulfonylurea. In other words, both insulin and C-peptide levels will become elevated in this scenario, so choice B is the correct answer, and choices A, C, and D are incorrect.

10. **D. Metformin orally 3 times per day**

In the case of an insulinoma, there is a major risk for recurrent hypoglycemia. All measures possible should be taken to help keep the glucose elevated until surgery can be performed. Ingesting glucose at regular intervals (choice A) is a way to help keep the serum glucose at a steadier state. Also, the glucagon at night (choice B) can be used as a preventative measure to help raise her overnight glucose level, as it will likely drop significantly throughout the evening. Also, diazoxide (choice C) is a powerful inhibitor of insulin secretion from the pancreas, provided that this patient can tolerate the potential side effect of edema. Metformin (choice D) would be the least helpful, as it is an insulin sensitizer that is best utilized in individuals with insulin resistance. It may have a small impact on decreasing the insulin secretion, but its impact would likely be trivial compared with the other answer selections.

11. **B. IV hydration with D10 with hourly glucose checks**

Given that this patient is demonstrating recurrent or refractory hypoglycemia, it will be important to select a modality of treatment that will be more proactive in achieving euglycemia. In this case, a continuous infusion of dextrose-containing fluids would be the best choice. A continuous glucagon infusion (choice C) would be a much less cost-effective choice. Additionally, continuous glucagon could be associated with undesirable side effects of nausea, vomiting, and tachycardia. Steroids alone (choice A) are not an appropriate choice, as the serum cortisol has already been documented as normal. Also, intravenous fluids with dextrose ampules as needed (choice D) would not serve to preventatively treat the hypoglycemia.

12. **D. Normal saline, insulin, and potassium**

The patient fulfills criteria for diagnosis of DKA with an ABG pH of less than 7.3, anion-gap metabolic acidosis, and presence of ketones in the urine. Generally, with DKA, you can anticipate that there will be a fluid deficit on the order of 4 to 6 Liters. It is appropriate to start with normal saline (rather than 5% albumin; choice B), as the patient simply needs hydration and does not have any evidence of hypotension or impending shock. Additionally, keep in mind that the cost of 5% albumin is significantly higher than normal saline, so you would need a strong indication to justify its use.

Diabetic ketoacidosis occurs when there is a deficiency of insulin, so insulin would be a core component of the selected treatment regimen. Bicarbonate treatment is not necessary (choice A) and, in fact, can pose a risk for cerebral edema, along with risk for hypokalemia with rapid administration. Only in rare cases, when the pH is 6.9, can the use of bicarbonate be arguably justified. However, even with that situation, great caution must be taken to ensure that the bicarbonate is slowly administered in free water, as a nearly isotonic solution.

Choice D is the best answer because, aside from normal saline and insulin (choice C), it addresses the need for potassium replacement. Even though the potassium in the case is technically normal at 4.9 mEq/L, initiation of insulin treatment can provoke a precipitous drop in potassium, related to intracellular shifts of potassium. Aggressive replacement of potassium (starting when potassium is < 5.0 mEq/L) is indicated.

13. **C. Na, 136 mEq/L; K, 3.7 mEq/L; chloride 107 mEq/L; bicarb, 20 mEq/L; ABG pH, 7.32**

In the case of resolution of DKA, you would need to have closure of the anion-gap acidosis. Choice C is the only answer that has full closure of the anion-gap acidosis, with a rise in ABG pH to more than 7.3.

14. **A. IV fluid hydration with NS**

This patient only has mild acidosis, but her lactic acid level and white blood cell count are both elevated, in the setting of having had very little oral fluid intake over the past 48 hours. Also, she has borderline low blood pressure and mild tachycardia. All these findings would be consistent with dehydration. Treating dehydration is the priority because the acidosis is from starvation ketosis and lactic acidosis from hypoperfusion. It is possible that the acidosis may actually improve or resolve with rehydration alone.

Antibiotics (choice C) may or may not be indicated; but dehydration should be addressed first. Insulin (choice B and D) can be initiated after hydration.

15. B. Potassium

Insulin quickly drives the potassium from the blood into the cells via activation of the sodium-potassium pump. If the potassium level becomes too low, it can predispose a patient to critical cardiac arrhythmias. In an individual with DKA, it is important to proactively initiate potassium replacement whenever the potassium is below 5.3 mEq/L to help prevent development of hypokalemia. Also, insulin treatment should be temporarily held whenever the potassium is documented below 3.3 mEq/L. Sodium (choice A) would typically rise as hyperglycemia improves via insulin treatment. Magnesium and calcium (choice C and D) would not be expected to change significantly with insulin treatment.

16. B. Intravenous steroids

This patient appears to have several classic features that are associated with a diagnosis of type 1 autoimmune polyglandular disease, also known as APECED (Autoimmune polyendocrinopathy-candidiasis-ectodermal dystrophy) and (APS-1). Specifically, he appears to have adrenal insufficiency, with a documented morning serum cortisol of less than 15 mEq in a state of being critically ill, with an associated low blood pressure. Also, when his serum calcium is corrected for the low albumin, using the formula below, the calcium only corrects to 7.38 mg/dL, which is considered low.

Corrected Calcium = Serum Calcium (mg/dL) + ([4.0 − Serum Albumin (g/dL)] × 0.8)

A parathyroid hormone has not yet been checked, but it is quite likely that this young man has hypoparathyroidism. In type 2 autoimmune polyglandular disease, you would not typically expect to see hypoparathyroidism as one of the presenting endocrinopathies. Furthermore, this patient has thyroid dysfunction, with a notably elevated TSH level. Although thyroid disease is more commonly seen in type 1 autoimmune polyglandular disease, it can also be seen in type 2. Also, he appears to have vitiligo, which can be a clinical feature of both type 1 and type 2 autoimmune polyglandular disease. Glucose (choice C) and calcium (choice D) are low and patient does have thyroid dysfunction (choice A) but these measures will not immediately stabilize the patient and improve blood pressure. Therefore, they are wrong.

17. A. Hypoparathyroidism

As mentioned in the answer to question 16, it is the presence of hypocalcemia, likely due to hypoparathyroidism, that would be more consistent with a diagnosis of type 1 (as opposed to type 2) autoimmune polyglandular disease.

Adrenal insufficiency (choice C), vitiligo (choice D), and thyroiditis (choice B) can be seen in type 1 and type 2 autoimmune polyglandular disease.

18. D. None of the above

In the case of adrenal insufficiency secondary to steroids, it is unusual to see notable structural anomalies on pituitary (choice B) or adrenal (choice A) imaging. Midnight salivary cortisol (choice C) is incorrect because that test is best utilized for the diagnosis of excess cortisol production or Cushing disease. In other words, a low or undetectable midnight salivary cortisol does not secure a diagnosis of adrenal insufficiency. Therefore, choice D is the best answer.

REFERENCES

1. Higham CE, Johannsson G, Shalet SM. Hypopituitarism. *Lancet*. 2016;388(10058):2403-2415.
2. Hensen J, Henig A, Fahlbusch R, et al. Prevalence, predictors and patterns of postoperative polyuria and hyponatremia in the immediate course after transsphenoidal surgery for pituitary adenomas. *Clin Endocrinol (Oxf)*. 1999;50(4):431-449.
3. Schneider HJ, Aimaretti G, Kreitschmann-Andermahr I, Stalla GK, Ghigo E. Hypopituitarism. *Lancet*. 2007; 369(9571): 1461-1470.
4. Nawar RN, AbdelMannan D, Selman WR, Arafah BM. Pituitary tumor apoplexy: a review. *J Intensive Care Med*. 2008; 23(2): 75-90.
5. Capatina C, Inder W, Karavitaki N, Wass JA. Management of endocrine disease: pituitary tumour apoplexy. *Eur J Endocrinol*. 2015;172(5):R179-R190.
6. Molitch ME. Chapter 41: Pituitary and adrenal disorders in pregnancy. In: Gabbe SG, Niebyl JR, Simpson JL, Landon MB, Galan HL, Jauniaux ERM, Driscoll DA, eds. *Obstetrics: Normal and Problem Pregnancies*. 6th ed. Philadelphia, PA: Elsevier Mosby; 2012: 953-961.
7. Kelestimur F. Sheehan's syndrome. *Pituitary*. 2003;6(4):181-188.
8. Chopra IJ. Clinical review 86: Euthyroid sick syndrome: is it a misnomer? *J Clin Endocrinol Metab*. 1997;82(2):329-334.
9. Langouche L, Van den Berghe G. Thyroidal changes during critical illness. In: Preiser JC, ed. *The Stress Response of Critical Illness: Metabolic and Hormonal Aspects*. Brussels, Belgium: Springer Cham; 2016: 125-136.
10. Davidson MB, Chopa IJ. Effect of carbohydrate and noncarbohydrate sources of calories on plasma 3,5,3'-triiodothyronine concentrations in man. *J Clin Endocrinol Metab*. 1979;48(4): 577-581.
11. Jirasakuldech B, Schussler GC, Yap MG, Drew H, Josephson A, Michl J. A characteristic serpin cleavage product of thyroxine-binding globulin appears in sepsis sera. *J Clin Endocrinol Metab*. 2000;85(11):3996-3999.
12. Utiger RD. Altered thyroid function in nonthyroidal illness and surgery. To treat or not to treat? *N Engl J Med*. 1995;333(23): 1562-1563.
13. Brent GA, Hershman JM. Thyroxine therapy in patients with severe nonthyroidal illnesses and low serum thyroxine concentration. *J Clin Endocrinol Metab*. 1986;63(1):1-8.
14. Danzi S, Klein I. Amiodarone-induced thyroid dysfunction. *J Intensive Care Med*. 2015;30(4):179-185.

15. Ursella S, Testa A, Mazzone M, Gentiloni SN. Amiodarone-induced thyroid dysfunction in clinical practice. *Eur Rev Med Pharmacol Sci.* 2006;10(5):269-278.

16. Leung AM, Braverman LE. Consequences of excess iodine. *Nat Rev Endocrinol.* 2014;10(3):136-142.

17. Brogioni S, Dell'Unto E, Cosci C, et al. Amiodarone-induced thyrotoxicosis. *Int J Endocrinol Metabol.* 2006;4(1):52-62.

18. Piga M, Cocco MC, Serra A, Boi F, Loy M, Mariotti S. The usefulness of 99mTc-sestaMIBI thyroid scan in the differential diagnosis and management of amiodarone-induced thyrotoxicosis. *Eur J Endocrinol.* 2008;159(4):423-429.

19. Bogazzi F, Bartalena L, Martino E. Approach to the patient with amiodarone-induced thyrotoxicosis. *J Clin Endocrinol Metab.* 2010;95(6):2529-2535.

20. Tietgens ST, Leinung MC. Thyroid storm. *Med Clin North Am.* 1995;79(1):169-184.

21. Roth RN, McAuliffe MJ. Hyperthyroidism and thyroid storm. *Emerg Med Clin North Am.* 1989;7(4):873-983.

22. Burch HB, Wartofsky L. Life-threatening thyrotoxicosis. Thyroid storm. *Endocrinol Metab Clin North Am.* 1993;22(2):263-277.

23. Nayak B, Burman K. Thyrotoxicosis and thyroid storm. *Endocrinol Metab Clin North Am.* 2006;35(4):663-686.

24. Brain L, Jellinek EH, Ball K. Hashimoto's disease and encephalopathy. *Lancet.* 1966;2(7462):512-514.

25. Mocellin R, Walterfang M, Velakoulis D. Hashimoto's encephalopathy: epidemiology, pathogenesis and management. *CNS Drugs.* 2007;21(10):799-811.

26. Wartofsky L. Myxedema coma. *Endocrinol Metab Clin North Am.* 2006;35(4):687-698, vii-viii.

27. Beynon J, Akhtar S, Kearney T. Predictors of outcome in myxoedema coma. *Crit Care.* 2008;12(1):111.

28. Fliers E, Wiersinga WM. Myxedema coma. *Rev Endocr Metab Disord.* 2003;4(2):137-141.

29. Myers L, Hays J. Myxedema coma. *Crit Care Clin.* 1991;7(1):43-56.

30. Jonklaas J, Bianco AC, Bauer AJ, et al. Guidelines for the treatment of hypothyroidism: prepared by the American Thyroid Association Task Force on thyroid hormone replacement. *Thyroid.* 2014;24(12):1670-1751.

31. Klubo-Gwiezdzinska J, Wartofsky L. Thyroid emergencies. *Med Clin North Am.* 2012.96(2):385-403.

32. Field JB. Hypoglycemia. Definition, clinical presentations, classification, and laboratory tests. *Endocrinol Metabol Clin North Am.* 1989;18(1):27-43.

33. Mitrakou A, Ryan C, Veneman T, et al. Hierarchy of glycemic thresholds for counter regulatory hormone secretion, symptoms, and cerebral dysfunction. *Am J Physiol.* 1991;260(1):E67-E74.

34. Lupsa BC, Chong AY, Cochran EK, Soos MA, Semple RK, Gorden P. Autoimmune forms of hypoglycemia. *Medicine (Baltimore).* 2009;88(3):141-153.

35. Patti ME, Goldfine, AB. The rollercoaster of post-bariatric hypoglycaemia. *Lancet Diabetes Endocrinol.* 2016;4(2):94-96.

36. Cryer PE, Axelrod L, Grossman AB, et al. Evaluation and management of adult hypoglycemic disorders: an Endocrine Society clinical practice guideline. *J Clin Endocrinol Metab.* 2009;94(3):709-728.

37. Van den Berghe G, Wouters P, Weekers F, et al. Intensive insulin therapy in critically ill patients. *N Engl J Med.* 2001;345(19):1359-1367.

38. NICE-SUGAR Study Investigators; Finfer S, Chittock DR, Su SY. Intensive versus conventional glucose control in critically ill patients. *N Engl J Med.* 2009;360(13):1283-1297.

39. Cryer PE. Chapter 34: Hypoglycemia. In: Melmed S, Polonsky KS, Larsen PR, Kronenberg HM, eds. *Williams Textbook of Endocrinology.* 13th ed. Philadelphia, (PA): Elsevier; 1582-1607.

40. Kitabchi AE, Umpierrez GE, Miles JM, Fisher JN. Hyperglycemic crises in adult patients with diabetes. *Diabetes Care.* 2009; 32(7):1335-1343.

41. Gosmanov AR, Gosmanova EO, Dillard-Cannon E. Management of adult diabetic ketoacidosis. *Diabetes Metab Syndr Obes.* 2014;7:255-264.

42. Chiasson JL, Aris-Jilwan N, Bélanger R. Diagnosis and treatment of diabetic ketoacidosis and the hyperglycemic hyperosmolar state. *CMAJ.* 2003;168(7):859-866.

43. Kitabchi AE, Nyenwe EA. Hyperglycemic crises in diabetes mellitus: diabetic ketoacidosis and hyperglycemic hyperosmolar state. *Endocrinol Metab Clin N Am.* 2006;35(4):725-751.

44. Pasquel FJ, Umpierrez GE. Hyperosmolar hyperglycemic state: a historic review of the clinical presentation, diagnosis, and treatment. *Diabetes Care.* 2014;37(11):3124-3131.

45. Kitabchi AE, Umpierrez GE, Murphy MB, et al. Hyperglycemic crises in diabetes. *Diabetes Care.* 2004;27(Suppl 1):S94-S102.

46. Trachenbarg DE. Diabetic ketoacidosis. *Am Fam Physician.* 2005;71(9):1705-1714.

47. Slovis CM, Mork VG, Slovis RJ, Bain RP. Diabetic ketoacidosis and infection: leukocyte count and differential as early predictors of serious infection. *Am J Emerg Med.* 1987;5(1):1-5.

48. Schwab TM, Hendey GW, Soliz TC. Screening for ketonemia in patients with diabetes. *Ann Emerg Med.* 1999;34:342-346.

49. Laffel L. Improving outcomes with POCT for HbA1c and blood ketone testing. *J Diabetes Sci Technol.* 2007;1(1):133-136.

50. Umpierrez GE, Murphy MB, Kitabchi AE. Diabetic ketoacidosis and hyperglycemic hyperosmolar syndrome. *Diabetes Spectr.* 2002:15(1);28-36.

51. Cox K, Cocchi MN, Salciccioli JD, Carney E, Howell M, Donnino MW. Prevalence and significance of lactic acidosis in diabetic ketoacidosis. *J Crit Care.* 2012:27(2);132-137.

52. Arora S, Cheng D, Wyler B, Menchine M. Prevalence of hypokalemia in ED patients with diabetic ketoacidosis. *Am J Emerg Med.* 2012;30(3):481-484.

53. Fortson MR, Freedman SN, Webster PD 3rd. Clinical assessment of hyperlipidemic pancreatitis. *Am J Gastroenterol.* 1995; 90(12):2134-2139.

54. Yadav D, Nair S, Norkus EP, Pitchumoni CS. Nonspecific hyperamylasemia and hyperlipasemia in diabetic ketoacidosis: incidence and correlation with biochemical abnormalities. *Am J Gastroenterol.* 2000;95:3123-3128.

55. Morris LR, Murphy MB, Kitabchi AE. Bicarbonate therapy in severe diabetic ketoacidosis. *Ann Intern Med.* 1986;105(6): 836-840.

56. Kitabchi AE, Umpierrez GE, Murphy MB, et al. Management of hyperglycemic crises in patients with diabetes. *Diabetes Care.* 2001;24(1):131-153.

57. Umpierrez GE, Cuervo R, Karabell A, Latif K, Freire AX, Kitabchi AE. Treatment of diabetic ketoacidosis with subcutaneous insulin aspart. *Diabetes Care.* 2004;27(8):1873-1878.

58. Juneia D, Pandey R, Singh O. Comparison between arterial and capillary blood glucose monitoring in patients with shock. *Eur J Intern Med.* 2011;22(3):241-244.

59. Shigeaki I, Moritoki E, Joji K, Kiyoshi M. Accuracy of blood-glucose measurements using glucose meters and arterial blood

gas analyzers in critically ill adult patients: systemic review. *Crit Care*. 2013;17(2):R48.

60. Hahner S, Spinnler C, Fassnacht M, et al. High incidence of adrenal crisis in educated patients with chronic adrenal insufficiency: a prospective study. *J Clin Endocrinol Metab*. 2015; 100(2):407-416.

61. Weibke A, Allolio B. Adrenal insufficiency. *Lancet*. 2003; 361(9372):1881-1893.

62. Bornstein SR, Allolio B, Arlt W, et al. Diagnosis and treatment of primary adrenal insufficiency: an Endocrine Society clinical practice guideline. *J Clin Endocrinol Metab*. 2016;101(2):364-389.

63. Kahaly GJ. Polyglandular autoimmune syndromes. *Eur J Endocrinol*. 2009;161(1):11-20.

64. Eisenbarth GS, Gottlieb PA. Autoimmune polyendocrine syndromes. *N Engl J Med*. 2004;350(20):2068-2079.

65. Salem M, Tainsh RE Jr, Bromberg J, Loriaux DL, Chernow B. Perioperative glucocorticoid coverage: a reassessment 42 years after emergence of a problem. *Ann Surg*. 1994;219(4):416-425.

66. Yong SL, Coulthard P, Wrzosek A. Supplemental perioperative steroids for surgical patients with adrenal insufficiency. *Cochrane Database Syst Rev*. 2012;12:CD005367.

67. Jung C, Inder WJ. Management of adrenal insufficiency during the stress of medical illness and surgery. *Med J Aust*. 2008; 188(7):409-413.

68. Puar TH, Stikkelbroeck NM, Smans LC, Zelissen PM, Hermus AR. Adrenal crisis: still a deadly event in the 21st century. *Am J Med*. 2016;129(3):339.e1-9.

69. Cooper MS, Stewart PM. Corticosteroid insufficiency in acutely ill patients. *N Engl J Med*. 2003;348(8):727-734.

70. Hamrahian AH, Oseni TS, Arafeh BM. Measurement of serum free cortisol in critically ill patients. *N Engl J Med*. 2004;350(16):1629-1638.

71. Allolio B. Extensive expertise in endocrinology: adrenal crisis. *Eur J Endocrinol*. 2015;172(3):R115-R124.

72. Fitzgerald PA. Endocrinology. In: Tierney LM, McPhee SJ, Papadakis MA, eds. *Current Medical Diagnosis Treatment*. 45th ed. New York, (NY): McGraw-Hill; 2006: 1098-1193.

73. Eisenhofer G, Rivers G, Rosas AL, Quezado Z, Manger WM, Pacak K. Adverse drug reactions in patients with phaeochromocytoma: incidence, prevention and management. *Drug-Saf*. 2007;30(11):1031-1062.

74. Lenders JW, Duh QY, Eisenhofer G, et al. Pheochromocytoma and paraganglioma: an endocrine society clinical practice guideline. *J Clin Endocrinol Metab*. 2014;99(6):1915-1942.

Hematology and Oncology

Ronaldo Collo Go, MD, and Michael H. Kroll, MD

INTRODUCTION

This chapter will discuss anemia, thrombocytopenia, coagulation disorders, and oncologic emergencies that are seen in the critical care setting.

ANEMIA

Two-thirds of patients admitted to the intensive care unit (ICU) will have a hemoglobin level less than 12 g/dL, and 97% will have anemia by day 8.[1-4] The lifespan of a red blood cell (RBC) is 120 days, and normal aging leads to increased oxygen hemoglobin affinity, decreased repair of oxidant injury, and decreased ability to membrane deformability during transit.[1,5] Red blood cell formation begins at 20 mL/d and can increase to 200 mL/d in hemolysis and heavy blood loss in a healthy patient.[6] Increasing levels of erythropoietin stimulate red cell production, inhibit erythroid precursor apoptosis, and enhance the removal of senescent RBCS. In addition to erythropoietin, healthy RBC production requires iron, zinc, folate, vitamin B_{12}, thyroxine, androgens, cortisol, and catecholamines.[1]

Anemia in the ICU is due to blood loss and decreased production.[1] Insensible blood loss occurs from phlebotomy, especially for patients with arterial catheters; stress gastritis exacerbated by mechanical ventilation, nutritional deficiencies, antithrombotic medication, and renal failure; and invasive procedures and surgical interventions.[1,7-12] Decreased production may be secondary to nutritional deficiencies, anemia of inflammation (AI), and medications. In AI, cytokines such as interleukin-1 (IL-1), tumor necrosis factor-α (TNF-α), and IL-6 increase hepatic hepcidin synthesis, which inhibits iron absorption and delivery to the bone marrow compartment and blocks iron release from bone marrow macrophages to the erythron.[1,13-16] Medications such as norepinephrine and phenylephrine inhibit hematopoietic maturation and angiotensin-converting enzyme inhibitors (ACEI), calcium channel blockers, theophylline, and β-adrenergic blockers suppress the secretion of erythropoietin by the kidney in response to anemia-induced hypoxemia.[17-20]

Anemia has been shown to be associated with adverse effects and poor outcomes in patients with normal renal function, chronic renal failure, chronic obstructive pulmonary disease (COPD), congestive heart failure, and acute myocardial infarction.[21-31] Anemia can persist up to 6 months after ICU stay.[32]

Evaluation

Anemias are classified based on the mean corpuscular volume (MCV) and the reticulocyte count (Table 23-1). The next step in the diagnosis of anemia is examining the leukocyte count and differential, the platelet count, and the blood smear (Table 23-2). Anemias are normocytic, microcytic, and macrocytic, and within each category, they are subdivided into normoproliferative, hypoproliferative, and hyperproliferative, if the reticulocyte count is normal, decreased, or increased, respectively. Healthy reticulocyte production should increase 1.5-fold for a hematocrit (Hct) of 30% to 40%, should double with Hct of 20% to 30%, and should triple with Hct of 15% or less; these increases are designated maturation factors. The reticulocyte production index (RPI) is used to determine proliferation status:

$$RPI = (Reticulocyte\ Count \times Hct\ of\ Patient/45)/Maturation\ Factor$$

For example, the RPI for a patient with a Hct of 20% and a reticulocyte count of 10% can be calculated as $(10 \times 20/45)/2 = 2.2$, which is normal. An RPI less than 2 suggests a hypoproliferative anemia and an RPI of greater than 4 suggests a hyperproliferative anemia.

Hemolytic Anemia

Hemolytic anemia is the premature destruction of red blood cells. It can occur intravascularly or extravascularly within the spleen.[33,34] Extravascular hemolysis is usually due to an immunoglobulin G (IgG)-mediated process, designated as warm antibody autoimmune hemolytic anemia (AIHA). Investigation begins with careful history and physical examination that includes review of any infectious process and medications. Laboratory findings that indicate hemolysis include an elevated or rising mean corpuscular volume, increased reticulocytes, increased lactate dehydrogenase (LDH), increased indirect bilirubin, low haptoglobin, and the presence of microspherocytes

TABLE 23-1 Classification of Anemia

Normocytic Anemia (MCV 80–100 fL)	Microcytic Anemia (MCV < 80 fL)	Macrocytic Anemia (MCV > 100 fL)
Hypoproliferative • Anemia of inflammation or chronic disease • Chronic or end-stage renal failure • Hypothyroidism • Copper deficiency • Myelophthisis • Chemotherapy • Myelodysplasia **Normohyperproliferative** • Sickle cell disease • Mild hemolysis or hemorrhage	**Hypoproliferative** • Iron deficiency (low MCHC) • Anemia of inflammation or chronic disease **Hyperproliferative** • Thalassemia (normal MCHC with small target cells)	**Hypoproliferative** • Ethanol • Folate deficiency • Vitamin B_{12} deficiency • Myelodysplastic syndrome • Drug-induced megaloblastic anemias • Hypothyroidism • Liver disease **Hyperproliferative** • Reticulocytosis associated with moderate to severe hemolysis or hemorrhage

MCHC = mean corpuscular hemoglobin concentration; MCV = mean corpuscular volume.

(small red cells without any central pallor) on blood smear. The diagnosis is confirmed by indirect and direct antiglobulin test (DAT) also referred to as Coombs testing. The indirect Coombs test looks for an autoantibody in the patient's serum. The direct Coombs test looks for an autoantibody on the patient's red cells. Table 23-3 lists the pattern of Coombs testing

TABLE 23-2 Peripheral Smear Examination

Peripheral Smear Findings	Causes
Elliptocytes	Hereditary elliptocytosis
Spherocytes	Hereditary spherocytosis, autoimmune hemolytic anemia, alloimmune hemolytic anemia
Schistocytes	Burns, microangiopathic hemolytic anemia
Bite cells, blister cells, and irregular contracted cells	Oxidant-induced hemolysis such as in G6PD deficiency, pentose shunt defect, glutathione synthesis defect, dapsone use, Wilson disease
Macrocytes, hypersegmented neutrophils	Vitamin B_{12} deficiency
Round macrocytes, target cells, stomatocytes	Liver disease, alcohol abuse
Macrocytosis with polychromasia	Hemolysis or recent blood loss
Hypogranular or hypolobulated neutrophils, blast cells, giant or hypogranular platelets, Pappenheimer bodies	Myelodysplastic syndromes
Microcytes with Pappenheimer bodies and red cell dimorphism	Sideroblastic anemia
Basophilic stippling	Lead poisoning
Boat-shaped cells, contracted cells, sickle cells, target cells	Sickle cell anemia if hemoglobin S and C present
Platelet clumping	Pseudothrombocytopenia

G6PD = glucose-6-phosphate-dehydrogenase.

for IgG-mediated AIHA (antibodies that bind to red cells at body temperature), IgM-mediated AIHA (antibodies that bind to red cells only at lower temperatures, the so-called cold agglutinins) and hapten-mediated AIHA (an antibody that binds to the red cell modified by the presence of a membrane-bound substance such as penicillin).

Treatment of AIHA begins with identifying and treating the underlying disease. For idiopathic warm AIHA, corticosteroid treatment is first-line therapy. Second-line treatment for patients with refractory AIHA from corticosteroids includes splenectomy or rituximab.[34] Patients with AIHA after splenectomy are high risk for venous thromboembolism. Although transfusion therapy of patients with AIHA is complicated by difficulties with patient blood typing and cross-matching, it is imperative that life-threatening anemia be treated with transfusion, often using the least incompatible blood, such as O negative.

Transfusion Therapy

It has been hypothesized that euvolemic resting patients with an acute drop of hemoglobin of 5 g/dL can have elevated cardiac index and oxygen extractions with no tissue hypoxia.[35] Chronicity allows the body to tolerate even lower values.[36] The 2016 American Association of Blood Bank (AABB) Guidelines recommend a restrictive transfusion threshold of 7 g/dL over a liberal transfusion threshold of 10 g/dL because the 30-day critical care outcome has 3 fewer deaths per 1000

TABLE 23-3 Coomb's Testing Pattern for IgG Mediated AIHA

Syndrome	Indirect Coombs (Antibody in Serum)	Direct Coombs (Antibody on Red Cell)
IgG (warm)	+ IgG	+ IgG; ± C3
IgM (cold)	+ IgM	− IgM; ++ C3
Hapten	− Ig	+ Ig; ± C3

C3 = complement C3; Ig = immunoglobulin. (+) = presence; (−) = absence.

with the restrictive transfusion threshold, shows no evidence of harm, and does not affect length of stay, functional status, and fatigue.[37] A transfusion threshold of 8 g/dL is sometimes recommended for orthopedic surgery, cardiac surgery, or known cardiovascular disease because that was the threshold used for the randomized control trials.[37] The restrictive threshold has not been advocated for patients with acute coronary syndrome because the liberal threshold was associated with a trend toward decreased mortality.[38,39] According to AABB, it also has not been advocated for patients with hematologic and oncologic disorders, severe thrombocytopenia at risk for bleeding, and transfusion-dependent anemia.[37] The Society of Critical Care Medicine (SCCM) and the Eastern Association for the Surgery of Trauma (EAST) still recommend an individualized approach to transfusion threshold.[40] It takes 15 minutes for the blood to equilibrate after blood transfusion.[41,42] However, in certain scenarios, such as trauma or active bleed, a follow-up complete blood count (CBC) should not be used to direct further transfusion. Worsening hemodynamic instability or ongoing bleeding should prompt further transfusion.

One unit of packed red blood cells is 450 to 500 mL and can increase the hemoglobin by 1 g/dL or hematocrit by 3% to 4%.[43] Donor blood must be serologically compatible with the recipient's blood prior to administration, except in cases of life-threatening hemorrhage or anemia. Blood type O negative is the universal donor. Blood type AB can receive blood from any other blood type. Although rare, transfusions are associated with infections. These include human immunodeficiency virus (HIV) (1 in 1,467,000), hepatitis C (1 in 1,149,000), hepatitis B (1 in 282,000), West Nile virus, cytomegalovirus (CMV), bacteria (1 in 2000–3000), and parasites such as *Trypanosoma cruzi*, which causes Chagas disease.[43] There are also noninfectious adverse effects such as those listed in Table 23-4.

Transfusion is the most important cause of clinically significant immunization against blood group antigens. In addition, there are naturally occurring antibodies to A, B, P, and other antigens in children and nontransfused adults due to their production by gut microbes. The antigens responsible for major hemolytic transfusion reactions are in descending order: ABO system > anti-D (part of the Rh system) > anti-K (Kell system) > anti-E (Rh system). Blood typing and screening will establish the patient's ABO and Rh type and examine for any antibodies against minor antigens, such as the Kell antigens or other systems that could cause minor or delayed hemolytic transfusion reactions (eg, the Lutheran, Lewis, Duffy, and Kidd systems). Crossmatching will provide red blood cells that are ABO and Rh compatible and that lack any antigens identified as targets in the antibody screen (the purpose of which is to identify alloantibodies).

Blood products are also modified to decrease the risk of adverse effects. These modifications include leukocyte reduction, washing, irradiation, and volume reduction. Leukocyte reduction is achieved by differential centrifugation or filtration where 99.9% of leukocytes are removed to reduce the incidence of nonfebrile hemolytic transfusion reactions (NFTR);

CMV transmission, particularly in neonates, pregnancy patients, patients with HIV, organ transplant recipients and other immunocompromised patients, and fetuses receiving intrauterine transfusions; human leukocyte antigen (HLA) alloimmunization; and transfusion-related immunomodulation (TRIM).[49,50] Washing consists of instilling normal saline with or without dextrose to remove residual plasma. This will decrease the risk of anaphylaxis from an IgA-deficient recipient with anti-IgA antibodies, severe allergies, sensitivity to hyperkalemia, and paroxysmal nocturnal hemoglobinuria. Twenty percent of the RBC may be lost.[43] Shelf-life of the washed product is 24 hours if stored at 1°C to 6°C, and 4 hours if stored at 20°C to 24°C.[43] Irradiation is used to prevent transfusion-associated graft-versus-host disease (GVHD), which is almost always fatal in the following circumstances: (1) the donor is family member, an HLA-selected donor, or a donor with a relationship that has not been established; (2) the patient has acute leukemia with HLA-matched or family-donated products; (3) the patient is an allogenic hematopoietic progenitor cell (HPC) transplant recipient; (4) the patient was an allogenic HPC donor 7 days prior to or during harvest; (5) the patient is an autologous HPC recipient; (6) the patient has Hodgkin disease; (7) the patient has a history of purine analogs and related drugs such as fludarabine; (6) the patient has a history of alemtuzumab use; and (7) the patient had aplastic anemia treated with cyclosporine A and antithymocyte globulin.[43]

Packed RBC transfusion alternatives such as erythropoietin, blood substitutes, and iron supplementation have been investigated. Administration of high-dose erythropoietin can produce the equivalent of 1 unit of packed RBCs after 7 days, but its use in the critically ill has been controversial since it has not been shown to improve survival and can increase thrombotic events in patients.[51,52] Blood substitutes such as hemoglobin-based oxygen carriers and perfluorocarbons are not available. Iron absorption may be limited due to the effect of critical illness on hepcidin secretion, and IV administration is preferred.[1] These alternatives may be contemplated in severely anemic symptomatic patients who refuse blood transfusions.

POLYCYTHEMIA

Polycythemia is defined as increased red blood cells with increased hemoglobin or hematocrit (hemoglobin [Hgb] > 16.5 g/dL or Hematocrit(Hct) ≥ 49% in men and Hgb >16 g/dL or ≥ Hct 48% in women). Relative polycythemia has elevated hemoglobin, hematocrit, and RBC count but no increase in red cell mass. This can be from Gaisbock disease or stress erythrocytosis, or it can be spurious. If there is an associated increase with red cell mass, this is called absolute polycythemia, which comes in primary and secondary forms. Symptoms due to increased blood viscosity include headaches, chest pain, abdominal pain, and shortness of breath. Treatment should include treatment of the underlying cause.

TABLE 23-4 Adverse Effects From Transfusion, Mechanisms, Presentation, and Treatment

Adverse Effects From Transfusions	Mechanism	Clinical Presentation and Diagnosis	Treatment
Acute hemolytic transfusion reaction	• Preformed antibodies[43] • ABO incompatibility[43]	• Chills, fever, shock, DIC, hemoglobinuria[43]	• IV hydration, treat DIC
Delayed hemolytic transfusion reaction	• Amnestic response to incompatible red cell antigen[43]	• 1–2 wk after transfusion with fever, dropping hemoglobin from hemolysis, jaundice[43]	
Febrile nonhemolytic transfusion reaction	• Anti-WBC antibodies in recipient[43]	• Fever	• Leukoreduction[43] • Premedication with acetominophen[43]
Urticarial reactions	• Antibody to donor plasma protein[43]	• Itching, rash, flushing, and mild wheezing	• Pause transfusion and give diphenhydramine and may resume transfusion[43]
Anaphylaxis	• Antibody to donor plasma protein (IgA, C4, haptoglobin)[43]	• Similar to urticarial reactions but more severe and associated with shock and angioedema	• Hemolysis work-up[43] • Epinephrine, antihistamines, steriods[43]
Transfusion-related acute lung injury (TRALI)	• Two-hit mechanism, with the first hit being priming of neutrophils to pulmonary endothelium and the second hit being activation of neutrophils, releasing reactive oxygen species[44-46] • Transfusion of antileukocyte antibodies or bioreactive substances, such as lipids like lysophosphatidylcholine, into recipients[45]	• Noncardiogenic pulmonary edema associated with fever, shortness of breath, hypoxia, and diffuse bilateral infiltrates on radiographs ≥ 6 h of ≥ 1 transfusion	• Cessation of transfusion • Supportive care
Transfusion-related circulatory overload (TACO)	• Hydrostatic pulmonary edema[47]	• Pulmonary edema secondary to right atrial hypertension or volume overload and characterized by shortness of breath, hypoxia, and diffuse bilateral infiltrates on radiographs ± hypertension ≥ 6 h of ≥ 1 transfusion[44,47]	• Supportive care
Transfusion-related immunomodulation (TRIM)	• Immunosuppression with decreased T cells, decreased response to mitogens, decreased NK cell function, reduced in delayed-type hypersensitivity, defective antigen presentation, decreased cytokine production, increased production of anti-idiotypic and anticlonotypic antibodies[48]		
Transfusion-associated graft-versus-host disease	• Immunocompetent donor T cells proliferate in recipient; risk eliminated by irradiating blood product	• Skin, liver and GI toxicity in severely immunosuppressed patients (solid organ and stem cell transplant recipients, patients with hematological malignancies; not AIDS)	• Corticosteroids and calcineurin inhibitors

AIDS = acquired immunodeficiency syndrome; DIC = disseminated intravascular coagulation; GI = gastrointestinal; IgA = immunoglobulin A; IV = intravenous; NK = natural killer; WBC = white blood cells.

Primary polycythemia (polycythemia vera) is treated immediately with phlebotomy, aiming to achieve a hematocrit less than 45%. Patients with secondary polycythemia from hypoxia often do not require phlebotomy, but if phlebotomy is done, the target hematocrit is 55%.[53,54]

THROMBOCYTOPENIA

Thrombocytopenia is defined as a platelet count of less than $150 \times 10^3/\mu L$ (150,000/μL), although less than $100 \times 10^3/\mu L$ (100,000/μL) is considered the threshold for bleeding risk.[55-57] Thrombocytopenia has been used as a prognostic marker, and its magnitude is correlated with length of ICU stay and mortality.[57-66] About 150 billion platelets are produced daily, and they circulate for 10 days.[58] A decrease in platelet count causes increased soluble thrombopoietin, which stimulates megakaryocytopoiesis. The timeframe of thrombocytopenia onset offers clues to its etiology. Rapidly developing thrombocytopenia can be the result of bacteremia, disseminated intravascular coagulation (DIC), or immune clearance by platelet autoantibodies or alloantibodies. Slowly progressive thrombocytopenia suggests medication- or chemotherapy-induced thrombocytopenia, or a primary or secondary bone marrow disorder affecting thrombopoiesis.[58] Heparin-induced thrombocytopenia (HIT) almost never occurs before day 4 of heparin therapy in patients not exposed during the previous 3 months and will not develop among patients who have been treated continuously for 2 weeks or longer (Table 23-5).

In thrombocytopenic patients, it is important to identify associated coagulation defects that contribute to bleeding risk. The current AABB guidelines recommend the following platelet transfusion thresholds: (1) 10,000/μL for asymptomatic hospitalized patients; (2) 20,000 to 30,000/μL for minor procedures such as central catheter placement, thoracentesis, or paracentesis; (3) 50,000/μL for lumbar puncture, major elective non-neuraxial surgery, and endoscopic and percutaneous needle biopsies; and (4) 100,000/μL for spinal cord or neurosurgery.[67] The AABB guidelines do not recommend for or against transfusion for intracranial hemorrhage on antiplatelet therapy.[67] Platelet units are derived from the whole blood of multiple donors and pooled, or they are collected by plateletpheresis. There are approximately 5.5×10^{10} platelets in 45 to 65 mL of plasma per unit of whole blood and approximately 3×10^{11} platelets in 200 mL of plasma collected per donor plateletpheresis, equivalent to about 4 to 6 units of pooled random donor platelets. Each unit of transfused platelets will raise the blood platelet count by 5,000 to 10,000/μL; when the platelet increment is less than 3,000/μL, the transfusion recipient is designated as platelet transfusion refractory. Platelet transfusion refractoriness is due to platelet antibodies (allo- and autoantibodies), fever, medications (especially heparin and amphotericin), hypersplenism, and DIC.

TABLE 23-5 Mechanisms of Thrombocytopenia and Causes

Mechanisms of Thrombocytopenia	Causes
Pseudothrombocytopenia	• Hemodilution • Clotting in sample • EDTA-induced clumping • Platelet satellite • Macrothrombocytes
Platelet consumption	• Bleeding • Infection • DIC • Intravascular devices (aortic balloon pump, cardiac assist devices) • Thrombotic microangiopathy
Platelet destruction	• Drug induced • Autoimmune • Passive and active posttransfusion purpura • Infection
Decreased production	• Myelosuppression • Liver disease • Alcohol abuse • Malignancy • Bacterial toxins/infection • Radiation • Delayed engraftment after bone marrow transplantation[57]
Increased sequestration	• Hypersplenism[57] • Hypothermia[57]

DIC = disseminated intravascular coagulation; EDTA = ethylenediaminetetraacetic acid.

COAGULATION DISORDERS

Extrinsic Pathway

The prothrombin time (PT) is initiated by tissue factor binding to factor VII. This causes the calcium- and phospholipid-dependent cleavage and activation of factor X, which subsequently cleaves prothrombin to thrombin, a reaction requiring the essential cofactor factor V. Thrombin cleaves fibrinogen to fibrin monomers, which polymerize linearly and are then covalently cross-linked by factor XIII.[68] A mild deficiency in factor VII due to liver disease, warfarin, or vitamin K deficiency usually will result in prolonged PT with a normal activated partial thromboplastin time (aPTT).

Intrinsic Pathway

The aPTT begins when kaolin (or clay) is added to citrate-anticoagulated plasma followed by recalcification. This sequentially activates factor XII, factor XI, and factor IX. Activated factor IX plus its essential cofactor factor VII plus calcium and phospholipid then cleaves and activates factor X, which cleaves prothrombin to thrombin, which cleaves fibrinogen as above. Deficiencies or inhibitors of any of these coagulation factors prolong the aPTT.[68]

Other Tests

The activated clotting time (ACT) is used routinely to measure heparin anticoagulation during extracorporeal blood flow. The thrombin time measures the conversion of fibrinogen to fibrin and will be prolonged with qualitative and quantitative abnormalities of fibrinogen. The dilute Russell viper venom test is used to identify a lupus anticoagulant. Fibrin degradation products (FDP) and d-dimers reflect plasmin degradation of monomeric and cross-linked fibrin, respectively.[68] The first step in evaluating an elevated coagulation time is to perform and 1:1 mix with normal plasma. If the elevated time corrects, the patient has a coagulation factor deficiency; if it fails to correct, the patient has a coagulation factor inhibitor.

Disseminated intravascular coagulation is a complication of many diseases such as sepsis, trauma, pancreatitis, malignancy, liver failure, ABO incompatibility, transplant rejection, aneurysms, amniotic fluid embolism, snake bites, and recreational drugs. Its pathogenesis involves inflammation; tissue factor–activated thrombin generation; dysfunction of the natural anticoagulant system (including antithrombin, protein C, and tissue factor pathway inhibitor); and both hyper- and hypofibrinolysis. It is a dynamic process that is often clinically silent, but it can be associated with bleeding and, less frequently, microvascular thrombosis.

Diagnosis is based on clinical presentation and a combination of laboratory abnormalities. Ninety-eight percent of patients with DIC have thrombocytopenia.[69] The rate of platelet consumption can be considered when diagnosing DIC. The Japanese Association for Acute Medicine criteria gives 1 point to a platelet reduction of more than 30% in 24 hours and 3 points to a platelet reduction of more than 50% in 24 hours.[70] Fibrin degradation products and d-dimers reflect the degree of fibrinolysis.[71] Consumption of coagulation factors is suggested by prolonged PT and aPTT, which are found in 95% DIC.[72] Fibrinogen is an acute phase reactant and, therefore, can be elevated despite ongoing consumption.[71] Low levels of fibrinogen are detected in the severe form of DIC.[69] Yu et al have suggested a combination of d-dimer and FDP has a diagnostic accuracy of 95% with a sensitivity of 91% and a specificity of 95%.[73] There are multiple scoring criteria; the International Society on Thrombosis and Haemostasis criteria is shown in Table 23-6.

Treatment begins with treating the underlying cause. Control of hemorrhage with blood product transfusions and fibrinolysis inhibitors such as tranexamic acid or aminocaproic acid can be started. Fresh frozen plasma at 250 mL is given at a dose of 15 mL/kg (4–6 units) and will increase factor levels by 20% to 30%.[74] Cryoprecipitate is given when the fibrinogen level falls below 100 mg/dL. Microvascular

TABLE 23-6 ISTH DIC Score

Criteria	Points
Platelet count	• > 100 × 10³ /uL (0 point) • 50–100 × 10³ /uL (1 point) • < 50 × 10³ / uL (2 points)
Increase in fibrin markers	• No change (0 point) • Moderate rise (2 points) • Strong rise (3 points)
Prothrombin time prolongation	• 3 sec or less (0 point) • 3–6 sec (1 point) • > 6 sec (2 points)
Fibrinogen	• > 1 g/L (0 point) • <1 g/L (1 point)
Interpretation	• < 5 points DIC not over, repeat • > 5 points DIC probable, repeat daily

Data from Levi M, Toh CH, Thachil J, Watson HG. Guidelines for the diagnosis and management of disseminated intravascular coagulation. *Br J Haematol.* 2009 Apr;145(1):24-33.

thrombosis associated with DIC is treated with low-dose unfractionated heparin (UFH).

ONCOLOGY

The survival rates of critically ill cancer patients are lower than those of critically ill patients with no comorbidities.[75] However, their in-hospital mortality rates are no higher than patients with other comorbidities.[76] Azoulay et al have suggested that (1) short-term survival after critical illness has improved due to improved identification of etiology of critical illness, implementation of noninvasive approaches to diagnoses, more intensive chemotherapy regimen, and improved available targeted treatment; (2) classic predictors of mortality are not relevant, and age or early phase of advanced-stage malignancy should not be used to discriminate ICU admission; (3) there is improved understanding of organ dysfunction; (4) bedridden patients, patients receiving a bone marrow transplant who have severe GVHD, patients with multiple organ failure from delayed ICU admission, patients with carcinomatosis lymphangitis with respiratory failure, patients with carcinomatosis meningitis with coma, and patients with extrahematopoietic cancer cells with medullary insufficiency generally have high mortality; (5) the current triage ICU criteria is unreliable in oncology patients; (6) a trial of critical care for 3 days may benefit certain cancer patients; (7) early admission to ICU may improve outcomes; (8) doing everything early may improve outcomes; and (9) broadening ICU admission and clarification of code status needs to occur on admission.[75]

Tumor lysis syndrome is a laboratory or clinical diagnosis of metabolic derangements secondary to release of massive cellular components after initiation of chemotherapy, or it

TABLE 23-7 Risk Stratification for Tumor Lysis Syndrome

Risk Factors
- NHL, ALL, AML, CLL, CML, MM, Solid Tumors
- High cell proliferation rate
- Chemosensitivity
- Large tumor burden suggested by > 10 cm diameter of disease and / or WBC > 50 × 10³ uL),
  serum lactate dehydrogenase ≥ 2 times normal, organ or bone marrow involvement
- Pretreatment serum uric acid > 7.5 mg/dL or hyperphosphoatemia
- Preexisting nephropathy or dehydration

Highest Risk
- Burkitt, Lymphoblasitc, B-ALL
- ALL with WBC ≥ 100 x 10³ uL
- AML with WBC ≥ 50 x 10³ uL and monoblastic

Lowest Risk
- Indolent NHL
- ALL and WBC ≤ 50 x 10³ uL
- AML and WBC ≤ 10 x 10³ uL
- CLL and WBC ≤ 10 x 10³ uL

ALL = acute lymphoblastic leukemia; AML = acute myeloid leukemia; B-ALL = Burkitt acute lymphoblastic leukemia; CLL = chronic lymphocytic leukemia; CML = chronic myeloid leukemia; DLBCL = diffuse large B-cell lymphoma; NHL = non-Hodgkin lymphoma; Tx = treatment; WBC = white blood cell.

can appear spontaneously in hematologic malignancies such as acute lymphocytic leukemia (ALL) and Burkitt lymphoma. These derangements include hyperuricemia, hyperkalemia, hyperphosphatemia, and hypocalcemia. Symptoms are usually secondary to these derangements and include nausea, vomiting, diarrhea, edema, hematuria, congestive heart failure, seizures, arrhythmia, tetany, cramps, and death.[77-79] The laboratory Cairo-Bishop definition of tumor lysis syndrome is 2 or more laboratory changes 3 days before or 7 days after chemotherapy, including: uric acid of 476 µmol/L or higher, or an 8-mg/dL or 25% increase from baseline; potassium of 6 meq/L or more, or 25% increase from baseline; phosphorus of 1.45 mmol/L or more or a 25% increase from baseline; or calcium of 1.75 mmol/L or less or a 25% decrease from baseline.[77]

The best approach is to prevent the development of complications from tumor lysis syndrome by identifying low- to high-risk patients, as shown in Table 23-7.[77] Low-risk patients can be monitored; intermediate risk patients can be treated with hydration and allopurinol, but rasburicase can be started if hyperuricemia develops; and high-risk patients can be treated with hydration and rasburicase.[77]

Leukostasis (hyperleukocytosis), in which there are 100 × 10³ or more immature white blood cells per µL, is typically associated with blast crisis chronic myeloid leukemia, acute myeloid leukemia, or acute lymphocytic leukemia.[80-82] The pathophysiology is secondary to increased viscosity from less deformity of blasts, localized hypoxia from high metabolic drive of blasts, and release of cytokines.[83-86] Most causes of death are related to neurologic and/or pulmonary complications. Treatment involves hydration, induction chemotherapy, and prophylaxis for tumor lysis syndrome.[87-90] In patients who cannot tolerate induction chemotherapy, hydroxyurea (50–100 mg/kg daily) may be used until the WBC count is less than 50,000/µL. Leukapheresis in addition to hydroxyurea may be used if induction chemotherapy is delayed.

Superior vena cava syndrome secondary to malignancy causes intrinsic or extrinsic compression of the superior vena cava, leading to collateral formation, and head and neck interstitial edema. This is a chronic process, and emergent intervention is necessary if the patient develops stridor. A tracheal stent and radiotherapy are warranted to secure the airway. A caveat to radiotherapy is that it might obscure biopsy results.

QUESTIONS

1. A 60-year-old man was complaining of fatigue and shortness of breath. His vital signs and physical examination were otherwise unremarkable. He was noted to have a WBC count of 15 × 10³/µL with 20% blasts, a hemoglobin of 10 g/dL, and platelets of 90 × 10³/µL. Auer rods were noted on the peripheral smear and flow cytometry was positive for CD7, CD19, and CD2. He was started on induction chemotherapy with cytarabine 200 mg/m² for 7 days, daunorubicin 60 mg/m² for 3 days, normal saline at 150 mL/h, and rasburicase. On subsequent serologies, he was noted to have a drop in hemoglobin from 10 g/dL to 6 g/dL. His haptoglobin was 10 mg/dL, his LDH was 1000 U/L, his total bilirubin was 4 mg/dL, and his direct bilirubin was 1 mg/dL. He was ordered for 1 unit of packed red blood cells and then developed a fever. Transfusion was stopped and the patient was given acetaminophen. His urinalysis was unremarkable. What type of anemia does the patient have?

   A. Febrile nonhemolytic transfusion reaction
   B. G6PD deficiency
   C. Acute blood loss anemia
   D. Thrombotic thrombocytopenic purpura

2. A 26-year-old Greek man is admitted to the leukemia service for treatment of acute lymphoblastic leukemia. He has diffuse palpable lymphadenopathy and an enlarged spleen extending 10 cm below the left costal margin. His WBC count is 237 × 10³/μL with 90% lymphoblasts, his hemoglobin was 10 g/dL, and his platelet count was 26 × 10³/μL. His serum creatinine is 1.6 mg/dL. He is given allopurinol 100 mg/d, and hyper-CVAD (cyclophosphamide, vincristine, doxorubicin [Adriamycin], and dexamethasone) therapy is begun. On day 2 of therapy, the patient's chemistry panel reveals a serum uric acid of 14 mg/dL and uricase is administered. The next morning, he complains of shortness of breath on going to the restroom.

His laboratory data reveals serum uric acid of 6 mg/dL, hemoglobin of 6 g/dL, elevated lactic dehydrogenase levels, and indirect bilirubin of 4.6 mg/dL with a total bilirubin of 6 mg/dL. His corrected reticulocyte count is 1%. The blood smear is shown below:

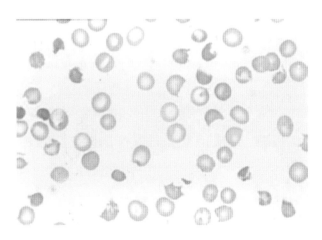

The red blood cell morphology shown above is the result of the spleen removing which of the following from the red blood cells?

A. Uric acid crystals
B. Denatured hemoglobin
C. Malaria parasite
D. All of the above

3. A patient receiving 1 unit of red blood cells develops a fever. The patient has no other symptoms. What is the next step?

A. Stop transfusion
B. Give acetaminophen and continue transfusion
C. Give corticosteroids
D. Order urinalysis

4. A 70-year-old man with a past medical history of hypertension, diabetes, and systolic heart failure was complaining of abdominal pain. His computed tomography angiogram (CTA) showed a ruptured abdominal aortic aneurysm. He had an endovascular repair and subsequently was sent to inpatient rehabilitation for 1 week. He then complained of shortness of breath and was found to be hypoxic and with new-onset atrial fibrillation. He was readmitted to your hospital. He had a CTA, which showed bilateral pulmonary embolism. A lower extremity ultrasound showed no deep venous thrombosis. His vital signs were as follows: blood pressure (BP) of 100/60 mmHg, heart rate (HR) of 80 beats/min, respiratory rate (RR) of 18 breaths/minute, and O_2 saturation of 99% on nasal cannula. His physical examination was unremarkable. What is your next step?

A. No additional treatment
B. Tissue plasminogen activator
C. Heparin drip
D. Inferior vena cava filter

5. For the patient in question 4, his platelets decreased from 220 × 10³/μL to 80 × 10³/μL on the fifth day of heparin therapy. While waiting for diagnostic serologies, he was pre-emptively started on argatroban, and his current dose is 2 μg/kg/h. After the second day, his international normalized ratio (INR) was greater than 3. What is your next step?

A. Continue current treatment
B. Administer coumadin with no heparin bridge
C. Stop anticoagulation
D. Start direct oral anticoagulant

6. A 50-year-old man with a history of thalassemia was involved in a motor vehicle accident. He was found to have hypovolemic shock and required massive blood transfusion protocol. There was concern for iron overload. His labs revealed the following:

Hgb	10 g/dL
Ferritin	500 μg/L
TSAT	> 50%
AST	10 U/L
ALT	12 U/L
T bili	8 Mg/dL

What would be the next step?

A. Do nothing
B. Perform phlebotomy
C. Administer deferoxamine
D. Administer deferoxamine and deferiprone

7. A 55-year-old woman with history of hypertension and diabetes is recently diagnosed with limited small cell lung carcinoma. Her physical examination shows BP of 130/80 mmHg, HR of 86 beats/min, and temperature of 97.8°F. She is started on cisplatin 80 mg/m^2 IV, etoposide 100 mg/m^2 IV, IV fluids, and metoclopramide 10 mg IV every 6 hours. She develops lightheadedness, nausea, and vomiting despite antiemetics. Her labs are as follows:

Glucose	98 mg/dL
BUN	198 mg/dL
Serum creatinine	2.5 mg/dL
Uric acid	27.4 mg/dL
Total protein	4.8 g/dL
Serum albumin	3.0 g/dL
Calcium	6.5 mg/dL
Phosphate	8.7 mg/dL
Potassium	6.1 meq/L
LDH	856 IU/L
WBC	$10 \times 10^3/\mu L$
Hgb	10 g/dL
Hct	17%
Platelets	$200 \times 10^3/\mu L$

Arterial blood gas analysis was evaluated as metabolic acidosis (pH, 7.22; HCO_3^-, 13 mEq/L; Pco_2, 27 mmHg; and Po_2, 96 mmHg). What is the next step?

A. Allopurinol
B. Rasburicase
C. IV fluids and diuretics
D. Alkalinization of urine

8. A 28-year-old man with sickle cell disease is complaining of progressive shortness of breath on exertion and associated with productive cough for the last 2 days. His chest radiograph shows lower lobe infiltrates. Antibiotics are started. His labs are as follows:

WBC	$12 \times 10^3/\mu L$
Hgb	6 g/L
Platelets	$200 \times 10^3/\mu L$
BUN	24 mg/dL
Creatinine	3 mg/dL

What is the next step?

A. A. Washed packed red blood cell transfusion
B. Exchange transfusion
C. Hydroxyurea
D. Corticosteroids

9. For the patient in question 8, what is the next step to prevent these crises?

A. Hydroxyurea
B. Plasmapheresis
C. Corticosteroids
D. Simple blood transfusion

10. A 50-year-old woman with a history of pulmonary embolism was recently started on unfractionated heparin and subsequently developed thrombocytopenia. How can you make a diagnosis of HIT type II?

A. Onset of thrombocytopenia
B. Platelet factor 4 IgG enzyme immunoassay
C. Magnitude of thrombocytopenia
D. Serotonin release assay

11. Which of the following is true regarding HIT?

A. Platelets should be monitored every 2 to 3 days from day 4 until day 14.
B. Platelets should be given to improve thrombocytopenia prior to an emergent cardiac catheterrization.
C. Once vitamin K antagonists and thrombin inhibitor overlap therapy are initiated, the thrombin inhibitor can be discontinued once the INR is therapeutic.
D. Anticoagulation is continued for 3 months.

12. A 50-year-old woman with a history of hypertension and diabetes was admitted for hospital-acquired pneumonia. The sputum was positive for methicillin-resistant *Staphylococcus aureus* (MRSA) and the patient was started on linezolid. On hospital day 3, the platelet count was 66,000/μL and the hemoglobin was 12 g/dL. On hospital day 5, the platelet count was 39,000/μL and the hemoglobin was 7.8 g/dL. Her neurological examination was unremarkable. Hematology consultation was obtained because of the thrombocytopenia. Laboratory examination revealed a decreased haptoglobin, elevated d-dimer, elevated LDH, normal PT/PTT, elevated thrombin time, and increased C-reactive protein and reticulocyte count. Schistocytes were observed on the peripheral smear. What is your diagnosis?

A. Sepsis-induced thrombocytopenia
B. Drug-induced thrombocytopenia
C. Thrombotic thrombocytopenic purpura
D. Idiopathic thrombocytopenic purpura

13. For the patient in question 12, what is your first-line treatment?

A. Plasma exchange
B. Corticosteroids
C. Eculizumab
D. Rituximab

14. A 32-year-old man with acute myeloid leukemia has finished induction chemotherapy. Now, he has persistent thrombocytopenia. He was previously transfused with red blood cells and platelets prior to induction chemotherapy. Now, his platelet count is $2 \times 10^3/\mu L$. One hour after transfusion of 6 units of single-donor platelets, his platelet count is $6 \times 10^3/\mu L$. A platelet antibody screening shows

the presence of HLA antibodies. An HLA-matched platelet transfusion is planned. Which of the following processing step is most appropriate prior to his next transfusion?

A. Washing
B. Leukoreduction
C. Irradiation
D. Deglycerolization

15. Which of the following statements is correct regarding the risk of thrombosis and bleeding in patients with myeloproliferative neoplasms (MPN)?

A. The risk of bleeding is higher than in thrombosis.
B. Normal hematocrit and platelet counts eliminate the risk of thrombosis in MPN patients.
C. Myocardial infarction and stroke are the most common thrombotic complications in a patient with MPN.
D. Anagrelide therapy is associated with a lower rate of arterial thrombosis than is hydroxyurea in essential thrombocythemia (ET) patients.

16. A 32-year-old woman (gravida 2, para 2) is referred for evaluation for spontaneous, severe subcutaneous bleeding 1 week after giving birth to her second child. Past history is negative for excessive bruising, epistaxis, menorrhagia, or bleeding issues with a prior pregnancy. Her medical history is negative for autoimmune disorders, use of medications other than prenatal vitamins, and malignant disorders. The patient reports that her lochia is excessive as compared with her first pregnancy and is requiring pad changes every hour. She reports development of painful bruises on her arms and legs beginning 2 days postpartum without identified antecedent injury. Her aPTT is 65 seconds and does not correct with a 1:1 mix. Her PT is 13 seconds. What is the diagnostic entity that is most likely the cause of this patient's bleeding?

A. Immune thrombocytopenic purpura
B. Factor XI deficiency
C. Acquired von Willebrand syndrome
D. Acquired factor VIII deficiency due to an inhibitor

ANSWERS

1   B. G6PD deficiency

The patient does not have concomitant schistocytes and thrombocytopenia, so he does not have thrombotic thrombocytopenic purpura (TTP) (choice D). The patient does not have a febrile nonhemolytic transfusion reaction because there is no evidence of hemolysis (choice A). The patient does not have iron deficiency anemia, which would

be strange due to the rapid blood drop (choice C). The patient has G6PD deficiency, a genetic defect of G6PD that generates nicotinamide adenine dinucleotide phosphate (NADPH), which protects RBCs from oxidative stress. Triggers includes food, illness, henna, fava beans, and medications such as dapsone, nitrofurantoin, primaquine, dimercaprol, methylene blue, phenazopyridine, toluidine blue, uricase, aniline dyes, and naphthalene. Diagnosis via G6PD activity assays can produce false negatives in a patient in an acute hemolytic episode.

2   B. Denatured hemoglobin

The lack of the G6PD enzyme in the red blood cells causes a decrease in glutathione production. This results in a decrease in the ability of hemoglobin to withstand exposure to unopposed oxidative agents. The presence of unopposed oxidizing agents leads to oxidation of the sulfhydryl bridges between parts of the hemoglobin molecule. This decreases the solubility of hemoglobin, leading to precipitations called Heinz bodies. The laboratory investigation of G6PD deficiency is commonly done by a quantitative spectrophotometric analysis or by a rapid fluorescent spot test detecting the generation of NADPH from NADP. Genetic tests based on polymerase chain reaction detect specific mutations and may be used for population screening, family studies, or prenatal diagnosis. Removal of the denatured hemoglobin, Heinz bodies, by the spleen results in formation of "bite cells" and "blister cells." Note: the reticulocyte count is not high, as the patient is being treated for acute lymphoblastic leukemia. Malarial parasites (choice C) will have various presentations depending of stage such as immature or mature trophozites and ring stage which are not present here. There are no crystals to suggest uric acid. (choice A). Therefore choice D is wrong as well.

3   A. Stop transfusion

This patient is having a febrile nonhemolytic transfusion reaction (FNHTR), as suggested by the fever and the lack of other systemic manifestations, such as flank pain, chills, hypotension, and dark urine. FNHTR is a diagnosis of exclusion. Therefore, initial approach would be to stop the transfusion (choice A) and obtain urinalysis to help determine if there is hemolysis through the presence of hemoglobinuria (choice D). If the urine maintains a red color after it is centrifuged, it is a hemoglobinuria but if sediment settles at the bottom, it is hematuria. If negative, patient can resume transfusion but would need to be premeditated with acetaminophen (choice B) and/or be given leukocyte-reduced blood products. For bacterial contamination that can lead to sepsis, transfusion is stopped and cultures are obtained. Corticosteroids would be indicated if there is clinical and laboratory evidence of anaphylaxis (choice C).

4. **C. Heparin drip**

Qureshi et al's retrospective cohort suggested it is safe to restart anticoagulation for atrial fibrillation after 7 days post-gastrointestinal (GI) bleeding to decrease the risk of thromboembolism without increased risk of GI bleeding (hazard ratio, 0.67; 95% confidence interval [CI], 0.56–0.81; P < 0.0001 and hazard ratio, 1.18; 95% CI, 0.94–1.10, P = 0.47, respectively).[91] According to the European Stroke Initiative, anticoagulation is restarted 10 to 14 days after intracerebral hemorrhage in patients with high risk for thromboembolism, such as atrial fibrillation.[92] For mechanical valves with recent GI bleeding, it is recommended to initiate anticoagulation after 48 to 72 hours for an extracerebral bleed, and after 7 to 10 days for an intracerebral bleed.[92,93] If the acute primary intracerebral hemorrhage is stable, pharmacologic deep vein thrombosis prophylaxis such as unfractionated heparin or low molecular weight heparin is started between days 2 and 4.[94]

The recent GI bleed is a contraindication for thrombolytics (choice B). An inferior vena cava filter might prevent another bout of pulmonary embolism, but the patient's history of atrial fibrillation places him at risk for another type of thromboembolic event, such as cerebrovascular accident (choice D). Doing nothing will not benefit the patient (choice A).

5. **A. Continue current treatment**

Patients with HIT can develop arterial and venous thrombosis up to 30 days after the cessation of heparin and are at risk for limb gangrene and skin necrosis during initiation of warfarin. Therefore, anticoagulation is still necessary, and nonheparin forms of anticoagulation include argatroban danaparoid, bivalirudin, and fondaparinux, as seen in Table 23-8[95] (choice C). Novel oral anticoagulants have not been fully evaluated for HIT (choice D). Warfarin can be initiated while on bridging anticoagulation with a platelet count greater than 150 × 10³/uL (choice B). Argatroban is preferred for patients with renal insufficiency since it is hepatically metabolized. Like the other direct thrombin inhibitors such as bivalirudin and lepirudin, it influences the INR. Argatroban infusion usually is continued until the INR is greater than 4 on both argatroban and warfarin (choice A).

TABLE 23-8 Alternative Anticoagulants, Dosing and Monitoring in Heparin Induced Thrombocytopenia

Anticoagulant	Dosing	Monitoring
Argatroban	• 2 µg/kg/min • 0.5–1.2 µg/kg/min in liver dysfunction (total bilirubin >1.5 mg/dL), heart failure, postcardiac surgery	• APTT 1.5-3 times patient baseline

Danaparoid	• Bolus depends on weight:
	  • < 60 kg →1500 U
	  • 60-75 kg → 2250 U
	  • 75-90 kg → 3000 U
	  • >90 kg → 3750 U
	• Accelerated initial infusion:
	  • 400 U/h × 4 h then 300 U/h × 4 h
	• Maintenance infusion:
	  • Creatinine < 2.5 mg/dL → 200 U/h
	  • Creatinine ≥ 2.5 mg/dL → 150 U/h
		• Anti Xa 0.5-0.8 U/mL

Bivalirudin	• 0.15 mg/kg/h • Dose reduced in renal or hepatic impairment	• APTT 1.5-2.5 times patient baseline
Fondaparinux	• < 50 kg → 5 mg SQ daily • 50-100 kg → 7.5 mg SQ daily • >100 kg → 10 mg SQ daily • Creatinine clearance < 30 ml/min contraindicated	• Peak Anti-Xa activity of 1.5 fondaparinux-specific U/mL
Rivaroxaban	• 15 mg PO twice a day	• Currently not FDA approved for HIT
Apixaban	• 5 mg PO twice a day	• Currently not FDA approved for HIT
Dabigatran	• 150 mg PO twice a day • 75 mg PO twice a day for creatinine clearance 15-30 ml/min	• Currently not FDA approved for HIT

aPTT = activated partial thromboplastin time; FDA = US Food and Drug Administration; HIT = heparin-induced thrombocytopenia; NOAC = novel oral anticoagulant; SQ = subcutaneously.

Data from Cuker A, Crowther MA. *2013 Clinical Guidelines on the Evaluation and Management of Adults with Suspected Heparin Induced Thrombocytopenia.* Washington DC: American Society of Hematology; 2013; Warkentin TE, Pain M, Linkins LA, Direct oral anticoagulants for treatment of HIT: update of Hamilton experience and literature review. *Blood* 2017;130(9):1104-1113.

6. A. Do nothing

The patient does have iron overload but treatment via phlebotomy and chelation is not indicated at this time. There is no active mechanism to remove iron from the body, and patients requiring multiple units of blood transfusions may develop iron overload. Mechanisms of iron overload include (1) decrease in hepcidin such as in hemochromatosis; (2) high erythropoietic drive causing relative hepcidin deficiency such as in thalassemias; and (3) oversaturated transferrin leading to large amounts of nontransferrin-bound iron (NTBI) that is taken up in the tissues due to hepcidin or a portion of NTBI, the chelating labile plasma iron, causing oxidative damage.[96] Symptoms have cardiac, hepatic and endocrinologic manifestations. Diagnosis is based on (1) serum ferritin >200 ug/L and >150 ug/L; (2) transferrin saturation >45% in >2 measurements; (3) liver and/or cardiac magnetic resonance imaging (MRI) with liver iron concentration greater than 3 to 7 mg/g dry weight and cardiac T2 <20 milliseconds respectively; (4) biopsy and/or; (5) response to phlebotomy. Phlebotomy removes 200 to 250 mg of iron in 500 mL of blood. The goal of phlebotomy is to obtain hemoglobin less than 12 g/dL, MCV of less than 75 to 80 fL, transferrin saturation less than 15%, and ferritin less than 20 μg/L (choice B). The goal of chelation therapy is to achieve ferritin levels less than 1000 μg/L, liver iron concentration less than 7 mg/g, and/or T2-weighted MRI greater than 20 milliseconds.[97-100] For this patient, chelation is not indicated (choices C and D). Chelation medications include deferoxamine, deferiprone, and deferasirox. There is evidence to suggest that combination therapy is helpful if iron overload is refractory (choice D).

7. B. Rasburicase

Although usually seen after chemotherapy of non-Hodgkin lymphoma and acute lymphocytic leukemia, tumor lysis syndrome can also be seen after chemotherapy of breast cancer, small cell lung cancer, neuroblastoma, medulloblastoma, germ cell tumors, gastrointestinal malignancies, urothelial cancer, and squamous cell carcinoma of the vulva, and spontaneous tumor lysis syndrome can occur in patients with non-Hodgkin lymphoma and acute leukemia without associated hypophosphatemia. Hydration is important in treatment and prevention. Crystalloid infusions (avoid crystalloids with potassium) should be given to maintain a urine output of 80 to 100 mL/m²/h. Diuretics can also be given in patients who are hypervolemic, but this patient is hypovolemic, as suggested by the respiratory variation and diameter of the inferior vena cava (choice C). Allopurinol (a 100-mg/m² dose every 8 hours for an oral dose with a maximum of 800 mg/d or a 200–400-mg/m² dose in 1–3 IV doses, with a maximum of 600 mg/d) is given 12 to 24 hours before chemotherapy and continued until uric acid, WBC, and other laboratory parameters return to low-risk levels. If the patient has preexisting elevated uric acid levels such as in this patient, allopurinol is not advocated (choice A). Allopurinol is believed to increase xanthine and hypoxanthine, which can precipitate and cause obstructive uropathy.[79,101] Alkalinization can increase uric acid solubility but decreases calcium phosphate solubility and decreases the solubility of xanthine and hypoxanthine. These can cause obstructive uropathies (choice D). Cortes et al showed that rasburicase only was the fastest and most effective way to decrease the level of uric acid compared to rasburicase with allopurinol, and allopurinol.[102] Plasma uric acid response was 87% with rasburicase in 4 hours, 78% with rasburicase and allopurinol in 4 hours, and 66% with allopurinol in 27 hours.[102] Rasburicase 0.15 to 2 mg/kg IV for 5 days to remove uric acid is contraindicated in G6PD deficiency since it can precipitate methemoglobinemia. Serial uric acid levels should be used to monitor response and duration of treatment.

8 B. Exchange transfusion

Sickle cells can last 10 to 20 days due to premature clearing by reticuloendothelial cells and release of proinflammatory heme and cell free hemoglobin. These patients generally suffer from a chronic inflammatory vasculopathy with acute vaso-occlusive crisis described as adhesions of platelets, red blood cells, and leukocytes on postcapillary venules and triggered by certain stressors such as infection. Sickle cell patients decompensate as a response to these stressors due to the chronic effects on their organs. There is an immune dysfunction due to functional asplenia predisposing patients to sepsis from encapsulated bacteria. The cardiopulmonary modification for anemia leads to biventricular dilatation, diastolic dysfunction, and pulmonary hypertension. There is a discrete progressive renal dysfunction that often is masked by normal levels of creatinine with an elevated glomerular filtration rate.

Acute chest syndrome (ACS) has one or more of the following signs and symptoms: fever (≥ 38.5°C), cough, chest pain, wheezes, rales, tachypnea, use of accessory respiratory muscles, Pao_2 less than 60 mmHg, and hypoxia (> 2% decrease in Spo_2 on room air) with new infiltrates on radiograph. It can overlap pneumonia and radiographically has a predilection to be multilobar in the lower lobes. Potential triggers can be hemolysis, as suggested by dropping hemoglobin and increasing LDH; fat embolization from bone marrow necrosis at the diaphysis of long bones, as suggested by lipid-laden alveolar macrophages via Oil Red O stain on bronchoalveolar lavage; hypoventilation and atelectasis from pain medication and infarcted ribs; and pulmonary thrombosis.

Treatment should include antibiotics for *Streptococcus pneumoniae* and atypical bacteria, volume expansion with or without a diuretic and exchange transfusion. The use of corticosteroids is controversial since withdrawal can lead to vaso-occlusive crisis (choice D). Hydroxyurea prevents the development of ACS but has no role in treating ACS (choice C). It is started at 10 mg/kg daily with a maximum dose of 25 to 35 mg/kg daily while monitoring for complications such as neutropenia (< 2500/μL), thrombocytopenia (< 80,000/μL), hydroxyurea levels, and fetal hemoglobin A levels.

Red blood cell transfusion is indicated for acute chest syndrome with increasing respiratory distress with or without hypoxemia, acute cerebrovascular accident (CVA), retinal artery occlusion, acute splenic sequestration with drop in hemoglobin, acute hepatic sequestration, aplastic crisis, persistent priapism, multiorgan failure (MOF), and acute life-threatening infections.[103] Besides the acute setting, transfusions have been indicated prior to high-risk surgical procedures or procedures with anesthesia in patients with end-organ damage; cardiac, pulmonary, renal, and liver disease; exacerbations during pregnancy; CVA prevention; and hemoglobin levels of 6 g/dL or less.[103] The blood produced must be leukocyte reduced; antigen matched for Cc, Ee, K, and hemoglobin greater than 10 g/dL or hematocrit of 30% to prevent alloimmunization and increased viscosity (choice A). The goal of exchange transfusion is a hemoglobin A of greater than 70% with a hemoglobin S of less than 30%.

9. **A. Hydroxyurea**

Hydroxyurea has been shown to reduce the incidence of vaso-occlusive crisis through 5 mechanisms: (1) fetal hemoglobin production, due to activation of guanylyl cyclase and change in erythroid dynamics; (2) ribonucleotide reductase inhibition, which leads to transient cytotoxicity and depressed neutrophils and reticulocytes; (3) decreasing adhesion receptors; (4) hemolysis reduction, due to improved hydration and decreased sickling; and (5) nitric oxide (NO) release and vasodilatation.[104] The presence of fetal hemoglobin (HgbF; a2y2) is variable among sickle cell patients but generally appears to reduce the symptoms of the disease. It has been associated with reduced incidences of painful episodes, leg ulcers, acute chest syndrome, and osteonecrosis, although there appears to be weaker correlation with reduction of incidence in vasculopathy, CVA, priapism, and urine albumin.[105,106] Hydroxyurea is started at 20 mg/kg/d with a target absolute neutrophil count (ANC) of 2 to 4 × 10³/μL and an absolute reticulocyte count (ARC) of 100 to 200 × 10³/μL. Other complications include headache, gastrointestinal symptoms, and dermatologic changes. Patients with multiorgan failure or ACS may develop secondary thrombotic thrombocytopenic purpura, at which time, plasma exchange maybe

helpful (Table 23-9).[107] Transfusions (choice D), plasmapheresis (choice B), and corticosteroids (choice C) do not prevent reoccurrence.

10. **D. Serotonin release assay**

There are 2 types of HIT. Type I is a nonimmune process in which heparin binds to platelet factor 4 (PF4) and causes platelet aggregation. Thrombocytopenia occurs 1 to 4 days after heparin administration and the platelet count usually does not fall below $100 × 10^3/μL$ and is self-limiting. Type II is an immunologic reaction in which IgG antibodies bind to platelet factor 4/HIT complexes on platelets, which results in a coagulative state with arterial and venous thrombosis.[108-110] Risk factors include use of unfractionated heparin, being a woman, and having cardiac or orthopedic surgery.[110] The 4Ts help identify HIT type II, as seen below (Table 23-10). Crystals to suggest uric acid are not present here.[108]

The magnitude of thrombocytopenia is generally nonspecific, and 25% of patients will develop thrombosis before thrombocytopenia (choice C).[108,110] Timing appears to have more of a diagnostic relevance (choice A). The typical HIT type II will have thrombocytopenia 5 to 10 days from exposure to heparin. Still, thrombocytopenia can manifest less than 24 hours after re-exposure to heparin if the patient has been exposed to heparin within the previous 100 days. Delayed-onset HIT manifests symptoms or worsens after heparin is discontinued. There is also a spontaneous HIT that occurs without heparin exposure. This occurs after orthopedic surgery or infection. Platelet factor 4 immunization's template appears to be either bacterial wall or cartilage origin.[111-113] The median time for thrombosis is day 10, with venous thrombosis over arterial thrombosis, and the most common sites are the lower extremities. Still, HIT has a penchant for developing thrombosis in the most unusual places, such as in the adrenal vein, the mesenteric veins, and the cerebral veins.[108]

Platelet factor 4–dependent immunoassays are not specific for HIT and frequently detect nonpathologic antibodies (choice B). The platelet serotonin release assay (SRA) is the gold standard. Serotonin is released when platelets are activated, such as in HIT. An SRA is performed under the following conditions: (1) buffer; (2) UFH, 0.1 IU/mL; (3) UFH, 0.3 IU/mL; (4) UFH 0.3 IU/mL with Fc receptor inhibiting antibody; and (5) UFH, 100 IU/mL.[114] The cut-off for serotonin release in positive assay is 20%. Heparin-induced thrombocytopenia usually has 80% serotonin release in UFH 0.1 IU/mL and UFH 0.3 IU/mL, but platelet activation is inhibited with high doses of heparin (UFH 100 IU/mL) and platelet activating inhibited by Fc receptor blocking antibody.[114] Platelet factor 4/IgG enzyme immunoassay has been used a quality control to reduce risk of reporting false-positive SRA.

TABLE 23-9 Acute Crises in Sickle Cell Disease and Recommended Interventions

Acute Crisis	Intervention[a]	Strength of Recommendation	Quality of Evidence
Acute chest syndrome	Antibiotic therapy with cephalosporin and macrolide[b]	Strong	Low
	Exchange transfusion If ↓ O_2 saturation on O_2 therapy, ↑ Respiratory distress, ↑ Pulmonary infiltrates, ↓ Hemoglobin despite transfusions	Strong	Low
	Simple transfusion[c] If hemoglobin > 1 g/dL below baseline, especially if baseline < 9 g/dL	Weak	Low
Multisystem organ failure syndrome	Simple or exchange transfusion[d]	Consensus	Panel expertise
Aplastic crisis	Simple transfusion Droplet isolation of patients	Consensus	Panel expertise
Splenic sequestration	Simple transfusion	Strong	Low
Hyperhemolysis crisis	Reserve transfusion for hemodynamic compromise; consider corticosteroids, immunoglobulins, erythropoietin	Not available	Not available
Thrombotic thrombocytopenic purpura–like syndrome	Consider plasma exchange in addition to exchange transfusion	Not available	Not available
Acute stroke	Exchange transfusion	Consensus	Panel expertise
Hepatic sequestration or acute intrahepatic cholestasis	Simple or exchange transfusion[e]	Consensus	Panel expertise

[a]It is critical that all packed RBC units administered for single or exchange transfusions be HbS negative; leukoreduced; and fully matched for C, E, and K antigens.

[b]Fluoroquinolones represent an alternative antibiotic regimen for patients with penicillin or cephalosporin allergies.

[c]The authors of this review favor an aggressive approach to transfuse all patients with SCD, with exchange transfusions reserved for patients with the most severe symptoms (see text).

[d]The authors of this review favor exchange transfusion if it is available without delay.

[e]The authors of this review favor exchange transfusion because of the risk of "reverse sequestration" (see text).

Data from Novelli EM, Gladwin M. Crises in sickle cell disease. *Chest*. 2016;149(4):1082-1093.

TABLE 23-10 4 "Ts" Scoring System

	Points (0, 1, or 2 for each of 4 categories; maximum possible score = 8)		
	2	1	0
Thrombocytopenia	> 50% platelet fall to nadir ≥ 20	30–50% platelet count fall (or > 50% directly resulting from surgery) or nadir of 10–19	< 30% platelet fall, or nadir < 10
Timing[a] of platelet count fall, thrombosis, or other sequelae (first day of putative immunizing exposure to heparin = day 0)	D 5–10: onset[a] (typical/delayed-onset HIT), or ≤ 1 d (with recent heparin exposure within past 30 d (rapid-onset HIT)	Consistent with fall on d 5–10, but not clear (eg, missing platelet counts), or ≤ 1 d (heparin exposure within past 31–100 d) (rapid-onset HIT), or platelet fall after d 10	Platelet count fall < 4 d (unless picture of rapid-onset HIT)
Thrombosis or other sequelae (eg, skin lesions, anaphylactoid reactions)	Proven new thrombosis, or skin necrosis (at injection site), or postintravenous heparin bolus anaphylactoid reaction	Progressive or recurrent thrombosis, or erythematous skin lesions (at injection site), or suspected thrombosis (not proven); hemofilter thrombosis	None
Other cause for thrombocytopenia	No explanation for platelet count fall is evident	Possible other cause is evident	Definite other cause is present
Pretest probability score: 6–8 = high; 4–5 = intermediate; 0–3 = low			

[a]First day of immunizing heparin exposure considered day 0; the day the platelet count begins to fall is considered the day of onset of thrombocytopenia (it generally takes 1–3 more days until an arbitrary threshold that defines thrombocytopenia is passed). Usually, heparin administered at or near surgery is the most immunizing situation (ie, day 0).

Reprinted with permission from Warkentin TE. Heparin-induced thrombocytopenia in critically ill patients. *Semin Thromb Hemost*. 2015;41(1):49-60.

11. A. Platelets should be monitored every 2 to 3 days from day 4 until day 14.

The latest *Chest* guidelines on HIT risk stratification are based on patient population and heparin preparation, as seen in Table 23-11.[110] If the risk is more than 1%, platelets should be monitored every 2 to 3 days starting at day 4 of heparin administration and up to day 14 (or until heparin is stopped)[110] (Grade C). Baseline platelets should probably be obtained prior to the initiation of heparin, particularly if there is concern for other types of thrombocytopenia or if there is exposure to heparin within 100 days.

If the suspicion for HIT or heparin induced thrombocytopenia complicated with thrombosis (HITT) is high or the diagnosis is confirmed, heparin products should be discontinued and anticoagulation should be started with one of the following products.[110]

Vitamin K antagonists (VKA) such as warfarin should not be started in lieu of another thrombin inhibitor in HIT, due to the risk of limb gangrene. Initiation of warfarin is heralded by a prothrombotic state due to depletion of anticoagulation protein C. Factor VII can serve as an indirect measure of the degree of depletion of protein C. Depletion of factor VII prolongs PTT. Limb gangrene is also associated with thrombocytopenia of less than $150 \times 10^3/\mu L$.[132] Vitamin K

TABLE 23-11 Incidence of Heparin-Induced Thrombocytopenia According to Patient Population and Type of Heparin Exposure

Patient Population (Minimum of 4-Day Exposure)	Incidence of HIT, %
Postoperative patients	
Heparin, prophylactic dose[115-118]	1–5
Heparin, therapeutic dose[118]	1–5
Heparin, flushes[a]	0.1–1
LMWH, prophylactic or therapeutic dose[117,118]	0.1–1
Cardiac surgery patients[117,119-121]	1–3
Medical	
Patients with cancer[122-124]	1
Heparin, prophylactic, or therapeutic dose[122]	0.1–1
LMWH, prophylactic, or therapeutic dose[123,125]	0.6
Intensive care patients[126]	0.4
Heparin, flushes[127]	< 0.1
Obstetrics patients[128-131]	< 0.1

HIT = heparin-induced thrombocytopenia; LMWH = low-molecular-weight heparin.

Characteristic	Lepirudin	Argatroban	Danaparoid	Bivalirudin	Fondaparinux
Target	Thrombin	Thrombin	Factor Xa (predominantly)	Thrombin	Factor Xa
Half-life	80 min	40–50 min	24 h	25 min	17–20 h
Elimination	Renal	Hepatobiliary	Renal	Enzymatic (80%)	Renal
Approved for patients with HIT[a]	Treatment	Treatment/PCI	Treatment	PCI/cardiac surgery	No
Method of administration	IV, SQ	IV	IV, SQ	IV	SQ
Monitoring	aPTT	aPTT	Anti-Xa level	aPTT	Anti-Xa level
	ECT (high doses)	ACT		ACT or ECT (high doses)	
Effect on INR	+	+ + +	0	+ +	0
Immunologic features	40–60% lepirudin Ab[b]	None	5% cross-reactivity with HIT Ab[c]	Potentially cross-reactive with anti-lepirudin Ab	May cause HIT[d]
Antidote available	No	No	No	No	No
Crosses placenta	Unclear[c]	Unclear[c]	No[c]	Unclear[c]	Yes[c]
Dialyzable	High-flux dialyzers	20%	Yes	25%	20%

Ab = antibodies; ACT = activated clotting time; aPTT = activated partial thromboplastin time; ECT = ecarin clotting time; FDA = US Food and Drug Administration; HIT = heparin-induced thrombocytopenia; INR = international normalized ratio; IV = intravenous; PCI = Percutaneous Coronary Intervention; SQ = subcutaneous.

[a]In some countries (check with local health regulatory authorities).

[b]Fatal anaphylaxis has been reported; therefore, patients should only be treated once with this agent.

[c]Clinical significance is uncertain and routine testing for cross-reactivity is not recommended.

[d]Case reports only.

antagonists should be continued with the thrombin inhibitor for at least 5 days prior to discontinuation of the thrombin inhibitor due to adverse complications seen when thrombin inhibitors are stopped after less than 5 days of bridge therapy.[133] The current *Chest* guidelines recommend to start VKA at a low dose (5 mg), once thrombocytopenia recovers (> $150 \times 10^3/\mu L$), and thrombin inhibitors should be stopped after 5 days of overlap therapy (Grade 2C)[110] (choice C). For HIT, anticoagulation is continued for 4 weeks, and for HITT, anticoagulation is continued for 3 months (choice D).

Platelet transfusion is indicated in HIT only if there is concern for bleeding. For emergent catheterrization, alternative thrombin inhibitors can be used, but if nonemergent, heparin should be used only if HIT resolves and HIT antibodies are negative (Grade 2C)[110] (choice A).

12. C. Thrombotic thrombocytopenic purpura

There appears to be an indirect correlation with sepsis-induced thrombocytopenia and increasing morbidity and mortality. Sepsis causes thrombocytopenia by myelosuppression, decreased platelet receptors, immune mediation, sequestration, and consumptive coagulopathy.[134] In addition to its role with homeostasis, a recent study suggested that thrombocytopenia in sepsis is associated with a disturbed host response with exaggerated cytokine activation and vascular endothelium, increased loss of vascular integrity, and decreased leukocyte adhesion, diapedesis, and signaling.[135] Sepsis-induced thrombocytopenia is a diagnosis of exclusion (choice A).

Diagnosis of idiopathic thrombocytopenic purpura is a diagnosis of exclusion with an isolated thrombocytopenia with no significant abnormalities on peripheral smear (choice D). If there are clumps of platelets causing pseudothrombocytopenia, it probably is related to ethylenediaminetetraacetic acid (EDTA). Samples should be repeated with tubes that are heparin anticoagulated or citrate anticoagulated. Bone marrow biopsy to evaluate for hypoplasia or fibrosis prior to splenectomy might be obtained. Secondary causes of idiopathic thrombocytopenic purpura include Evans syndrome, antiphospholipid syndrome, common variable immune deficiency, drug reaction, CMV, *Helicobacter pylori*, hepatitis C, HIV, varicella zoster, lymphoproliferative disorders, bone marrow transplantation, vaccination, and systemic lupus erythematosus.[136]

There are several mechanisms for drug-induced thrombocytopenia (DIT). It can be caused by myelosuppression, such as from linezolid or chemotherapy, or accelerated destruction from platelet antibodies, such as from quinidine, quinine, or heparin. Diagnosis begins with thrombocytopenia with a nadir less than $20 \times 10^3/\mu L$ and the onset is 5 to 10 days or within hours after initiation of the drug. Exclusion of other causes of thrombocytopenia is key and laboratory evidence of immunologic binding may confirm diagnosis[137,138] (choice B).

Thrombotic thrombocytopenic purpura and hemolytic uremic syndrome (HUS) are 2 diseases that present with thrombocytopenia and hemolytic anemia. Hemolytic anemia can be a consequence of vascular devices such as heart valves, ventricular assist devices, or extracorporeal oxygenation, or from arteriolar stenosis.[139] Arteriolar stenosis is secondary to von Willebrand platelet thrombosis from ADAMTS13 protein deficiency in TTP, platelet fibrin thrombosis in DIC, tumor cells in metastatic disease, vasculitis in autoimmune or infectious diseases, or thrombotic microangiopathy as seen in HUS.[139] ADAMTS13 prevents the formation of von Willebrand factor–platelet aggregates. Its deficiency, stress, and shear stress profile (> 50–90 dyne/cm²) predisposes the patient to TTP. Hemolytic uremic syndrome is a result of: (1) complement system defects such as in activation of factor H, membrane cofactor protein, factor I, or thrombomodulin; (2) gain of function mutations of factor B or C3; or (3) complement factor H autoantibodies.[139]

Thrombotic thrombocytopenic purpura does not necessarily have to fulfill the classic pentad of thrombocytopenia (70–100%), microangiopathic hemolytic anemia with schistocytes (70–100%), neurologic symptoms (50–90%), renal abnormalities (50%), and fever (25%).[140] Confirmation of diagnosis does not preclude treatment and presence of thrombocytopenia, and microangiopathic hemolytic anemia is sufficient to initiate treatment. Confirmation of TTP diagnosis is dependent on an ADAMTS13 level of 10% or less, with or without the presence of neutralizing or non-neutralizing antibodies to ADAMTS13 activity.[139]

13. A. Plasma exchange

The patient has thrombotic thrombocytopenic purpura. Treatment of TTP begins with daily plasma exchange to remove von Willebrand factor/platelet aggregates and autoantibodies, and restore ADAMTS13 until platelets, LDH, hemolysis, and organ dysfunction improve.[139-142] (choice A). With plasma exchange, survival improves by up to 90%.[141] Corticosteroids can be added or given after plasma exchange until remission begins. Remission is defined by resolution of symptoms and laboratory abnormalities, although the presence of ADAMTS13 and ADAMTS13-binding antibodies can persist for years.[141] Rituximab and splenectomy are for refractory TTP (choice D).

Treatment for idiopathic thrombocytopenic purpura is indicated if the patient is symptomatic or if the platelet count is less than $30 \times 10^3/\mu L$ (Grade 2C). First-line treatment includes (1) prednisone 1 mg/kg orally for 21 days, then tapering (Grade 2B); (2) intravenous immunoglobulin at 1g/kg (grade 2C); or (3) anti-D for Rh-positive nonsplenectomized patients (Grade 2C).[136] Prednisone and intravenous immunoglobulin can be given together if a rapid increase of platelets is desired (choice B). A response occurs if the platelet count is $30 \times 10^3/\mu L$ or more and there is a 2-fold increase in baseline on 2 occasions at least 7 days apart with no bleeding. A complete response occurs if the platelets count is $100 \times 10^3/\mu L$ or higher. In refractory idiopathic thrombocytopenic purpura, splenectomy or thrombopoietin receptor agonists are options. If all else fails, administer rituximab (Grade 2C).[136]

Treatment of hemolytic uremic syndrome also begins with plasma exchange, although appears to be not as effective. Mortality is higher and a substantial number of patients progress to renal failure.[141] Eculizumab, a monoclonal antibody to C5, is given intravenously at 900 mg weekly for 4 doses followed by 1200 mg intravenously on the subsequent weeks (choice C).[143]

14. C. Irradiation

All HLA-matched blood products require irradiation to prevent transfusion-associated graft-versus-host disease. Irradiation kills lymphocytes so that they cannot proliferate in the recipient. Transfusion-associated graft-versus-host disease also occurs with any type of transfusion in immunosuppressed recipients, such as patients who are post-transplant (solid-organ and stem cell) and those who have leukemia, lymphoma (Hodgkin and non-Hodgkin), and congenital immunodeficiencies (but not AIDS). Washing decreases the risk of anaphylaxis from IgA-deficient recipients with anti-IgA antibodies, severe allergies, sensitivity to hyperkalemia, and paroxysmal nocturnal hemoglobinuria (choice A). Leukocyte reduction reduces the incidence of nonfebrile hemolytic transfusion reactions; cytomegalovirus transmission, particularly in neonates, pregnancy, HIV, organ transplant recipients and other immunocompromised patients, and fetuses receiving intrauterine transfusions; HLA alloimmunization; and transfusion-related immunomodulation (choice B). Deglycerolization is the removal of glycerol, which is used as cryoprotection in freezing blood products (choice D).

15. C. Myocardial infarction and stroke are the most common thrombotic complications in a patient with MPN.

In patients with myeloproliferative neoplasms, the risk of thrombosis is higher than bleeding and the risk of arterial thrombosis is higher than venous thrombosis (choice A). However, one should consider the possibility of MPN in patients with venous thrombosis in unusual sites, such as Budd-Chiari syndrome, portal vein thrombosis, or cerebral venous thrombosis. Age and history of thrombosis are the main risk factors for arterial thrombosis in patients with myeloproliferative neoplasms and most arterial thromboses are in the form of myocardial infarction and stroke. Normal hematocrit and platelet counts do not eliminate risk of thrombosis in myeloproliferative neoplasms (choice B). Hydroxyurea provides better protection against arterial thrombosis in essential thrombocythemia patients than does anagrelide (choice D).

16. D. Acquired factor VIII deficiency due to an inhibitor

Acquired factor VIII deficiency due to a factor VIII inhibitor commonly presents either during pregnancy or in the postpartum period. Although acquired hemophilia is a rare disorder, occurring at a frequency of approximately 1 case per million population per year, the presentation in this case is classic for this disorder and requires primary consideration for appropriate diagnosis and management. Approximately 7% of cases of acquired hemophilia present in the postpartum period. Acquired hemophilia is associated with significant morbidity and risk of mortality; early and accurate diagnosis is critical to prevent poor outcomes. Immune thrombocytopenic purpura more commonly presents before or during pregnancy rather than in the postpartum period and is often associated with mild to moderate subcutaneous bleeding (choice A). Factor XI deficiency usually presents with bleeding associated with trauma or surgery and is not associated with spontaneous significant cutaneous hemorrhage (choice B). Acquired von Willebrand syndrome does not classically present in the postpartum period and is often associated with mild or moderate mucocutaneous bleeding (choice C).

REFERENCES

1. Hayden SJ, Albert TJ, Watkins TR, Swenson ER. Anemia in critical illness: insights into etiology, consequences, and management. *Am J Respir Crit Care Med.* 2012;185(10):1049-1057.
2. Vincent JL, Baron JF, Reinhart K, et al; ABC (Anemia and Blood Transfusion in Critical Care) Investigators. Anemia and blood transfusion in critically ill patients. *JAMA.* 2002; 288(12):1499-1507.
3. Corwin HL, Gettinger A, Pearl RG, et al. The CRIT Study: anemia and blood transfusion in the critically ill—current clinical practice in the United States. *Crit Care Med.* 2004; 32(1):39-52.
4. Thomas J, Jensen L, Nahirniak S, Gibney RT. Anemia and blood transfusion practices in the critically ill: a prospective cohort review. *Heart Lung.* 2010;39(3):217-225.
5. Stäubli M, Ott P, Waber U. Erythrocyte adenosine triphosphate depletion during voluntary hyperventilation. *J Appl Physiol.* 1985;59(4):1196-1200.
6. Hillman RS, Henderson PA. Control of marrow production by the level of iron supply. *J Clin Invest.* 1969;48(3):454-460.
7. Corwin HL, Parsonnet KC, Gettinger A. RBC transfusion in the ICU: is there a reason? *Chest.* 1995;108(3):767-771.
8. Barie PS. Phlebotomy in the intensive care unit: strategies for blood conservation. *Crit Care.* 2004;8(Suppl 2):S34-S36.
9. Hadfield RJ, Sinclair DG, Houldsworth PE, Evans TW. Effects of enteral and parenteral nutrition on gut mucosal permeability in the critically ill. *Am J Respir Crit Care Med.* 1995;152(5 Pt 1): 1545-1548.
10. Cook D, Heyland D, Griffith L, Cook R, Marshall J, Pagliarello J; Canadian Critical Care Trials Group. Risk factors for clinically important upper gastrointestinal bleeding in patients requiring mechanical ventilation. *Crit Care Med.* 1999;27(12):2812-2817.

11. Rodriguez RM, Corwin HL, Gettinger A, Corwin MJ, Gubler D, Pearl RG. Nutritional deficiencies and blunted erythropoietin response as causes of the anemia of critical illness. *J Crit Care*. 2001;16(1):36-41.

12. Prakash D. Anemia in the ICU: anemia of chronic disease versus anemia of acute illness. *Crit Care Clin*. 2012;28(3):333-343.

13. Fleming RE, Bacon BR. Orchestration of iron homeostasis. *N Engl J Med*. 2005;352(17):1741-1744.

14. Weiss G, Goodnough LT. Anemia of chronic disease. *N Engl J Med*. 2005;352(10):1011-1023.

15. Nemeth E, Rivera S, Gabayan V, et al. IL-6 mediates hypoferremia of inflammation by inducing the synthesis of the iron regulatory hormone hepcidin. *J Clin Invest*. 2004;113(9):1271-1276.

16. Corwin HL, Krantz SB. Anemia of the critically ill: "acute" anemia of chronic disease. *Crit Care Med*. 2000;28(8):3098-3099.

17. Fonseca RB, Mohr AM, Wang L, Sifri ZC, Rameshwar P, Livingston DH. The impact of a hypercatecholamine state on erythropoiesis following severe injury and the role of IL-6. *J Trauma*. 2005;59(4):884-889.

18. Bakris GL, Sauter ER, Hussey JL, Fisher JW, Gaber AO, Winsett R. Effects of theophylline on erythropoietin production in normal subjects and in patients with erythrocytosis after renal transplantation. *N Engl J Med*. 1990;323(2):86-90.

19. Linde T, Sandhagen B, Hägg A, Mörlin C, Danielson BG. Decreased blood viscosity and serum levels of erythropoietin after antihypertensive treatment with amlodipine or metoprolol: results of a cross-over study. *J Hum Hypertens*. 1996;10(3):199-205.

20. Vlahakos DV, Marathias KP, Madias NE. The role of the renin–angiotensin system in the regulation of erythropoiesis. *Am J Kidney Dis*. 2010;56(3):558-565.

21. Culleton BF, Manns BJ, Zhang J, Tonelli M, Klarenbach S, Hemmelgarn BR. Impact of anemia on hospitalization and mortality in older adults. *Blood*. 2006;107(10):3841-3846.

22. Martinez FJ, Foster G, Curtis JL, et al; NETT Research Group. Predictors of mortality in patients with emphysema and severe airflow obstruction. *Am J Respir Crit Care Med*. 2006;173(12):1326-1334.

23. Chambellan A, Chailleux T, Similowski T. Prognostic value of the hematocrit in patients with severe COPD receiving long term oxygen therapy. *Chest*. 2005;128(3):1201-1208.

24. Similowski T, Agustí A, MacNee W, Schönhofer B. The potential impact of anaemia of chronic disease in COPD. *Eur Respir J*. 2006;27(2):390-396.

25. Go AS, Yang J, Ackerson LM, et al. Hemoglobin level, chronic kidney disease, and the risks of death and hospitalization in adults with chronic heart failure: the Anemia in Chronic Heart Failure: Outcomes and Resource Utilization (ANCHOR) Study. *Circulation*. 2006;113(23):2713-2723.

26. Salisbury AC, Alexander KP, Reid KJ. Incidence, correlates, and outcomes of acute, hospital-acquired anemia in patients with acute myocardial infarction. *Circ Cardiovasc Qual Outcomes*. 2010;3(4):337-346.

27. Mehdi U, Toto R. Anemia, diabetes, and chronic kidney disease. *Diabetes Care*. 2009;32(7):1320-1326.

28. Khamiees M, Raju P, DeGirolamo A, Amoateng-Adjepong Y, Manthous CA. Predictors of extubation outcome in patients who have successfully completed a spontaneous breathing trial. *Chest*. 2001;120(4):1262-1270.

29. Thygesen K, Alpert JS, White HD; Joint ESC/ACCF/AHA/WHF Task Force for the Redefinition of Myocardial Infarction. Universal definition of myocardial infarction. *Eur Heart J*. 2007;28(20):2525-2538.

30. Rasmussen L, Christensen S, Lenler-Petersen P, Johnsen SP. Anemia and 90-day mortality in COPD patients requiring invasive mechanical ventilation. *Clin Epidemiol*. 2010;3:1-5.

31. Carson JL, Noveck H, Berlin JA, Gould SA. Mortality and morbidity in patients with very low postoperative Hb levels who decline blood transfusion. *Transfusion*. 2002;42(7):812-818.

32. Bateman AP, McArdle F, Walsh TS. Time course of anemia during six months follow up following intensive care discharge and factors associated with impaired recovery of erythropoiesis. *Crit Care Med*. 2009;37(6):1906-1912.

33. Dhaliwal G, Cornett PA, Tierney LM. Hemolytic anemia. *Am Fam Physician*. 2004;69(11):2599-2606.

34. Leschner K, Jager U. How I treat autoimmune hemolytic anemias in adults. *Blood*. 2010;116(11):1831-1838.

35. Weiskopf RB, Viele MK, Feiner J, et al. Human cardiovascular and metabolic response to acute, severe isovolemic anemia. *JAMA*. 1998;279(3):217-221.

36. Semenza GL. Regulation of oxygen homeostasis by hypoxia-inducible factor 1. *Physiology (Bethesda)*. 2009;24:97-106.

37. Carson JL, Guyatt G, Heddle NM, et al. Clinical practice guidelines from the AABB: red blood cell transfusion thresholds and storage. *JAMA*. 2016;316(10):2025-2035.

38. Carson JL, Brooks MM, Abbott JD, et al. Liberal versus restrictive transfusion thresholds for patients with symptomatic coronary artery disease. *Am Heart J*. 2013;165(6):964-971.e1.

39. Cooper HA, Rao SV, Greenberg MD, et al. Conservative versus liberal red cell transfusion in acute myocardial infarction (the CRIT Randomized Pilot Study). *Am J Cardiol*. 2011;108(8):1108-1111.

40. Napolitano LM, Kurek S, Luchette FA, et al; American College of Critical Care Medicine of the Society of Critical Care Medicine; Eastern Association for the Surgery of Trauma Practice Management Workgroup. Clinical practice guideline: red blood cell transfusion in adult trauma and critical care. *Crit Care Med*. 2009;37(12):3124-3157.

41. Wiesen AR, Hospenthal DR, Byrd JC, Glass KL, Howard RS, Diehl LF. Equilibration of hemoglobin concentration after transfusion in medical inpatients not actively bleeding. *Ann Intern Med*. 1994;121(4):278-280.

42. Elizalde JI, Clemente J, Marin JL, et al. Early changes in hemoglobin and hematocrit levels after packed red cell transfusion in patients with acute anemia. *Transfusion*. 1997;37(6):573-576.

43. Carson JL, Grossman BJ, Kleinman S, et al. Red blood cell transfusion: a clinical practice guideline from the AABB. *Ann Intern Med*. 2012;157(1):49-58.

44. Sayah DM, Looney MR, Toy R. Transfusion reactions: newer concepts on the pathophysiology, incidence, treatment and prevention of transfusion related acute lung injury (TRALI). *Crit Care Clin*. 2012;28(3):363-372.

45. Gajic O, Gropper MA, Hubmayr RD. Pulmonary edema after transfusion: how to differentiate transfusion-associated circulatory overload from transfusion-related acute lung injury. *Crit Care Med*. 2006;34(Suppl 5):S109-S113.

46. Looney MR, Gropper MA, Matthay MA. Transfusion-related acute lung injury: a review. *Chest*. 2004;126(1):249-258.

47. Roubinian NH, Murphy EL. Transfusion-associated circulatory overload (TACO): prevention, management, and patient outcomes. *Int J Clin Transfus Med*. 2015;3:17-28.

48. Vamvakas EC, Blajchman MA. Transfusion-related immunomodulation (TRIM): update. *Blood Rev*. 2007;21(6):327-348.

49. Blajchman MA. The clinical benefits of the leukoreduction of blood products. *J Trauma*. 2006;60(Suppl 6):S83-90.

50. Nichols WG, Price TH, Gooley T, Corey L, Boeckh M. Transfusion-transmitted cytomegalovirus infection after receipt of leukoreduced blood products. *Blood*. 2003;101(10):4195-4200.

51. Corwin HL, Gettinger A, Fabian TC, et al; EPO Critical Care Trials Group. Efficacy and safety of epoetin alfa in critically ill patients. *N Engl J Med*. 2007;357(10):965-976.

52. Milligan LJ, Bellamy MC. Anaesthesia and critical care of Jehovah's Witnesses. *Contin Educ Anaesth Crit Care Pain*. 2004;4(2):35-39.

53. McMullin MF, Bareford D, Campbell P, et al; General Haematology Task Force of the British Committee for Standards in Haematology. Guidelines for the diagnosis, investigation and management of polycythaemia/erythrocytosis. *Br J Haematol*. 2005;130(2):174-195.

54. Keohane C, McMullin MF, Harrison C. The diagnosis and management of erythrocytosis. *BMJ*. 2013;347:f6667

55. Rice TW, Wheeler AP. Coagulopathy in critically ill patients. Part 1: platelet disorders. *Chest*. 2009;136(6):1622-1630.

56. Mercer KW, Macik B, Williams ME. Hematologic disorders in critically ill patients. *Semin Respir Crit Care Med*. 2006; 27:286-296.

57. Drews RE, Weinberger SE. Thrombocytopenic disorders in critically ill patients. *Am J Respir Crit Care Med*. 2000; 162(2 Pt 1):347-351.

58. Greinacher A, Selleng K. Thrombocytopenia in the intensive care unit patient. *Hematology*. 2010;2010:135-143.

59. Drews RE. Critical issues in hematology: anemia, thrombocytopenia, coagulopathy, and blood product transfusions in critically ill patients. *Clin Chest Med*. 2003;24(4):607-622.

60. Vanderschueren S, De Weerdt A, Malbrain M, et al. Thrombocytopenia and prognosis in intensive care. *Crit Care Med*. 2000;28(6):1871-1876.

61. Strauss R, Wehler M, Mehler K, et al. Thrombocytopenia in patients in the medical intensive care unit: bleeding prevalence, transfusion requirements, and outcome. *Crit Care Med*. 2002;30(8):1765-1771.

62. Akca S, Haji-Michael P, de Mendonca A, et al. Time course of platelet counts in critically ill patients. *Crit Care Med*. 2002;30(4):753-756.

63. Stephan F, Hollande J, Richard O, et al. Thrombocytopenia in a surgical ICU. *Chest*. 1999;115(5):1363-1370.

64. Brogly N, Devos P, Boussekey N, et al. Impact of thrombocytopenia on outcome of patients admitted to ICU for severe community-acquired pneumonia. *J Infect*. 2007; 55(2):136-140.

65. Baughman RP, Lower EE, Flessa HC, Tollerud DJ. Thrombocytopenia in the intensive care unit. *Chest*. 1993; 104(4): 1243-1247.

66. Vandijck DM, Blot SI, De Waele JJ, et al. Thrombocytopenia and outcome in critically ill patients with bloodstream infection. *Heart Lung*. 2010;39(1):21-26.

67. Kaufman RM, Djulbergovic B, Gernsheimer T, et al. Platelet transfusion: a clinical practice guideline from AABB. *Ann Intern Med*. 2015;162(3):205-213.

68. Wheeler AP, Rice TW. Coagulopathy in critically ill patients. Part 2: soluble clotting factors and hemostatic testing. *Chest*. 2010;137(1):185-194.

69. Spero JA, Lewis JH, Hasiba U. Disseminated intravascular coagulation. Findings in 346 patients. *Thromb Haemost*. 1980;43(1):28-33.

70. Asakura H, Takahashi H, Uchiyama T, et al; DIC subcommittee of the Japanese Society on Thrombosis and Hemostasis. Proposal for new diagnostic criteria for DIC from the Japanese Society on Thrombosis and Hemostasis. *Thromb J*. 2016;14:42.

71. Levi M, Toh CH, Thachil J, Watson HG. Guidelines for the diagnosis and management of disseminated intravascular coagulation. *Brit J Haematol*. 2009;145(1):24-33.

72. Levi M, Van der Poll T. Disseminated intravascular coagulation: a review for the internist. *Intern Emerg Med*. 2013;8(1):23-32.

73. Yu M, Nardella A, Pecet L. Screening tests of disseminated intravascular coagulation: guidelines for rapid and specific laboratory diagnosis. *Crit Care Med*. 2000;28(6):1777-1780.

74. Holland LL, Brooks JP. Toward rational fresh frozen plasma transfusion: the effect of plasma transfusion on coagulation test results. *Am J Clin Pathol*. 2006;126(1):133-139.

75. Azoulay E, Soares M, Darmon M, Benoit D, Pastores S, Afessa B. Intensive care of the cancer patient: recent achievements and remaining challenges. *Ann Intensive Care*. 2011;1(1):5.

76. Tanvetyanon T, Leighton JC. Life-sustaining treatments in patients who died of chronic congestive heart failure compared with metastatic cancer. *Crit Care Med*. 2003;31(1):60-64.

77. Coiffier B, Altman A, Pui CH, Younes A, Cairo MS. Guidelines for the management of pediatric and adult tumor lysis syndrome: an evidence-based review. *J Clin Oncol*. 2008;26(16):2767-2778.

78. Howard SC, Jones DP, Pui CH. The tumor lysis syndrome. *New Engl J Med*. 2011;364(19):1844-1854.

79. Band PR, Silverberg DS, Henderson JF, et al. Xanthine nephropathy in a patient with lymphosarcoma treated with allopurinol. *N Engl J Med*. 1970;283(7):354-357.

80. Daver N, Kantarjian H, Marcucci G, et al. Clinical characteristics and outcomes in patients with acute promyelocytic leukaemia and hyperleucocytosis. *Br J Haematol*. 2015;168(5):646-653.

81. Cuttner J, Conjalka MS, Reilly M, et al. Association of monocytic leukemia in patients with extreme leukocytosis. *Am J Med*. 1980;69(4):555-558.

82. Hehlmann R. How I treat CML blast crisis. *Blood*. 2012; 120(4):737-747.

83. Lichtman MA, Weed RI. Peripheral cytoplasmic characteristics of leukocytes in monocytic leukemia: relationship to clinical manifestations. *Blood*. 1972;40(1):52-61.

84. Lichtman MA, Rowe JM. Hyperleukocytic leukemias: rheological, clinical, and therapeutic considerations. *Blood*. 1982; 60(2):279-283.

85. Stucki A, Rivier AS, Gikic M, Monai N, Schapira M, Spertini O. Endothelial cell activation by myeloblasts: molecular mechanisms of leukostasis and leukemic cell dissemination. *Blood*. 2001;97(7):2121-2129.

86. Azoulay E, Fieux F, Moreau D, et al. Acute monocytic leukemia presenting as acute respiratory failure. *Am J Respir Crit Care Med*. 2003;167(10):1329-1333.

87. Dutcher JP, Schiffer CA, Wiernik PH. Hyperleukocytosis in adult acute nonlymphocytic leukemia: impact on remission rate and duration, and survival. *J Clin Oncol*. 1987;5(9): 1364-1372.

88. van Buchem MA, te Velde J, Willemze R, Spaander PJ. Leucostasis, an underestimated cause of death in leukaemia. *Blut.* 1988;56(1):39-44.

89. Porcu P, Farag S, Marcucci G, Cataland SR, Kennedy MS, Bissell M. Leukocytoreduction for acute leukemia. *Ther Apher.* 2002;6(1):15-23.

90. Grund FM, Armitage JO, Burns P. Hydroxyurea in the prevention of the effects of leukostasis in acute leukemia. *Arch Intern Med.* 1977;137(9):1246-1247.

91. Qureshi W, Mittal C, Patsias I, et al. Restarting anticoagulation and outcomes after major gastrointestinal bleeding in atrial fibrillation. *Am J Cardiol.* 2014;113(1):662-668.

92. Steiner T, Kaste M, Forsting M, et al. Recommendations for the management of intracranial haemorrhage—part I: spontaneous intracerebral haemorrhage. The European Stroke Initiative Writing Committee and the Writing Committee for the EUSI Executive Committee. *Cerebrovasc Dis.* 2006; 22(4):294-316.

93. Panduranga P, Al-Mukhaini M, Al-Mushlai M, Haque MA, Shehab A. Management dilemmas in patients with mechanical heart valves and warfarin-induced major bleeding. *World J Cardiol.* 2012;4(3):54-59.

94. Lansberg MG, et al. Antithrombotic and thrombolytic therapy for ischemic stroke. *Chest.* 2012;141(2):e601s-e636s.

95. Cuker A, Crowther MA. *2013 Clinical Guidelines on the Evaluation and Management of Adults with Suspected Heparin Induced Thrombocytopenia.* Washington, DC: American Society of Hematology; 2013.

96. Mir MA, Logue GL. Transfusion-induced iron overload. Medscape Web site. http://emedicine.medscape.com/article/1389732-overview#a5. Accessed April 2, 2017.

97. Sarigianni M, Liakos A, Vlachaki E, et al. Accuracy of magnetic resonance imaging in diagnosis of liver iron overload: a systematic review and meta-analysis. *Clin Gastroenterol Hepatol.* 2015;13(1):55-63.e5.

98. Tanner MA, Galanello R, Dessi C, et al. A randomized, placebo-controlled, double-blind trial of the effect of combined therapy with deferoxamine and deferiprone on myocardial iron in thalassemia major using cardiovascular magnetic resonance. *Circulation.* 2007;115(14):1876-1884.

99. Pennell DJ, Berdoukas V, Karagiorga M, et al. Randomized controlled trial of deferiprone or deferoxamine in beta-thalassemia major patients with asymptomatic myocardial siderosis. *Blood.* 2006;107(9):3738-3744.

100. Pennell DJ, Porter JB, Cappellini MD, et al. Efficacy of deferasirox in reducing and preventing cardiac iron overload in beta-thalassemia. *Blood.* 2010;115(12):2364

101. Hande KR, Hixson CV, Chabner BA. Postchemotherapy purine excretion in lymphoma patients receiving allopurinol. *Cancer Res.* 1981;41(6):2273-2279.

102. Cortes J, Moore JO, Mariarz RT, et al. Control of plasma uric acid in adults at risk for tumor lysis syndrome: efficacy and safety of rasburicase alone and rasburicase followed by allopurinol compared with allopurinol alone—results of a multicenter phase III study. *J Clin Oncol.* 2010;28(27):4207-4213.

103. Wun T, Hassell K. Best practices for transfusion for patients with sickle cell disease. *Hematol Rev.* 2009;1(2):e22.

104. Ware RE. How I use hydroxyurea to treat young patients with sickle cell anemia. *Blood.* 2010;115(26):5300-5311.

105. Akinsheye I, Alsultan A, Solovieff N, et al. Fetal hemoglobin in sickle cell anemia. *Blood.* 2011;118(1):19-27.

106. Steinberg MH, Forget BG, Higgs DR, Weatherall DJ, eds. *Disorders of Hemoglobin: Genetics, Pathophysiology, Clinical Management.* 2nd ed. Cambridge, United Kingdom: Cambridge University Press; 2009.

107. Novelli EM, Gladwin M. Crises in sickle cell disease. *Chest.* 2016;149(4):1082-1093

108. Warkentin TE. Heparin-induced thrombocytopenia in critically ill patients. *Semin Thromb Hemost.* 2015;41(1):49-60.

109. Warkentin TE. Heparin-induced thrombocytopenia. *Curr Opin Crit Care.* 2015;21(6):576-585.

110. Linkins LA, Dans AL, Moores LK, et al. Treatment and prevention of heparin induced thrombocytopenia. *Chest.* 2012;141(2 Suppl):e495S-e530S.

111. Warkentin TE, Basciano PA, Knopman J, Bernstein RA. Spontaneous heparin-induced thrombocytopenia syndrome: 2 new cases and a proposal for defining this disorder. *Blood.* 2014;123(23):3651-3654.

112. Jay RM, Warkentin TE. Fatal heparin-induced thrombocytopenia (HIT) during warfarin thromboprophylaxis following orthopedic surgery: another example of "spontaneous" HIT? *J Thromb Haemost.* 2008;6(9):1598-1600.

113. Krauel K, Weber C, Brandt S, et al. Platelet factor 4 binding to lipid A of Gram-negative bacteria exposes PF4/heparin-like epitopes. *Blood.* 2012;120(16):3345-3352

114. Warkentin TE, Arnold DM, Nazi I, Kelton JG. The platelet serotonin-release assay. *Am J Hematol.* 2015;90(6):564-572.

115. Warkentin TE, Levine MN, Hirsh J, et al. Heparin-induced thrombocytopenia in patients treated with low-molecular-weight heparin or unfractionated heparin. *N Engl J Med.* 1995;332(20):1330-1335.

116. Warkentin TE, Robers RS, Hirsh J, Kelton JG. An improved definition of immune heparin-induced thrombocytopenia in postoperative orthopedic patients. *Arch Intern Med.* 2003;163(20):2518-2524.

117. Warkentin TE, Sheppard JA, Horsewood P, Simpson PJ, Moore JC, Kelton JG. Impact of the patient population on the risk for heparin-induced thrombocytopenia. *Blood.* 2000;96(5):1703-1708.

118. Greinacher A, Eichler P, Lietz T, Warkentin TE. Replacement of unfractionated heparin by low-molecular-weight heparin for postorthopedic surgery antithrombotic prophylaxis lowers the overall risk of symptomatic thrombosis because of a lower frequency of heparin-induced thrombocytopenia. *Blood.* 2005.106(8):2921-2922.

119. Pouplard C, May MA, Iochmann S, et al. Antibodies to platelet factor 4-heparin after cardiopulmonary bypass in patients anticoagulated with unfractionated heparin or a low-molecular-weight heparin: clinical implications for heparin induced thrombocytopenia. *Circulation.* 1999;99(19): 2530-2536.

120. Selleng S, Malowsky B, Itterman T, et al. Incidence and clinical relevance of anti-platelet factor 4/heparin antibodies before cardiac surgery. *Am Heart J.* 2010;160(2):362-369.

121. Pouplard C, May MA, Regina S, Marchand M, Fusciardi J, Gruel Y. Changes in platelet count after cardiac surgery can effectively predict the development of pathogenic heparin-dependent antibodies. *Br J Haematol.* 2005;128(6):837-841.

122. Girolami B, Prandoni P, Stefani PM, et al. The incidence of heparin-induced thrombocytopenia in hospitalized medical patients treated with subcutaneous unfractionated heparin: a prospective chort study. *Blood.* 2003; 101(8): 2955-2959.

123. Prandoni P, Siragusa S, Girolami B, Fabris F; BELZONI Investigators Group. The incidence of hearpin-induced thrombocytopenia in medical patients treated with low-molecular-weight heparin: a prospective cohort study. *Blood.* 2005;106(9):3049-3054.

124. Prandoni P, Falanga A, Piccioli A. Cancer, thrombosis, and heparin induced thrombocytopenia. *Thromb Res* 2007;120(suppl 2):s137-s140.

125. Stein PD, Hull RD, Matta F, Yaekoub AY, Liang J. Incidence of thrombocytopenia in hospitalized patients with venous thromboembolism. Am J Med. 2009;122(10):919-930.

126. Crowther MA, Cool DJ, Albert M, et al. Canadian Critical Care Trials Group. The 4Ts scoring system for heparin-induced thrombocytopenia in medical-surgical intensive care unit patients. *J Crit Care.* 2010;25(2):287-293.

127. Mayo DJ, Cullinane AM, Merryman PK, Horne MK III. Serologic evidence of heparin sensitization in cancer patients receiving heparin flushes of venous access devices. *Support Care Cancer.* 1999;7(6):425-427.

128. Ellison J, Walkder ID, Greer IA. Antenatal use of enoxaparin for prevention and treatment of thromboembolism in pregnancy. *BJOG.* 2000;107(9):1116-1121.

129. Greer IA, Nelson-Piercy C. Low molecular weight heparins for thromboprophylaxis and treatment of venous thromboembolism in pregnancy: a systematic review of safety and efficacy. *Blood.* 2005;106(2):401-407.

130. Sanson BJ, Lensing AW, Prins MH, et al. Safety of low-molecular-weight heparin in pregnancy: a systematic review. *Thromb Haemost.* 1999;81(5):668-672.

131. Lepercq J, Conard J, Borel-Derlon A, et al. Venous thromboembolism during pregnancy: a retrospective study of enoxaparin safety in 624 pregnancies. *BJOG.* 2001;108(11):1134-1140.

132. Warkentin TE, Elavathil LJ, Hayward CP, Johnston MA, Russett JI, Kelton JG. The pathogenesis of venous limb gangrene associated with heparin-induced thrombocytopenia. *Ann Intern Med.* 1997;127(9):804-812.

133. Hursting MJ, Lewis BE, Macfarlane DE. Transitioning from argatroban to warfarin therapy in patients with heparin-induced thrombocytopenia. *Clin Appl Thromb Hemost.* 2005; 11(3):279-287.

134. Larkin CM, Santos-Martinez MJ, Ryan T, Radomski MW. Sepsis-associated thrombocytopenia. *Thromb Res.* 2016; 141:11-16.

135. Claushuis TAM, Van Vught LA, Scicluna BP, et al. Thrombocytopenia is associated with a dysregulated host response in critically ill sepsis patients. *Blood.* 2016;127(24):3062-3072.

136. Neunert C, Lim W, Crother M, Cohen A, Solberg Jr L, Crowther MA. The American Society of Hematology 2011 evidence-based practice guideline for immune thrombocytopenia. *Blood.* 2011;117(16):4190-4207.

137. Visentin GP, Liu CY. Drug induced thrombocytopenia. *Hematol Oncol Clin N Am.* 2007;21(4):685-696.

138. Arnold DM, Nazi I, Warkentin TE, et al. Approach to the diagnosis and management of drug-induced immune thrombocytopenia. *Transfus Med Rev.* 2013;27(3):137-145.

139. Tsai HM. Thrombotic thrombocytopenic purpura and the atypical hemolytic uremic syndrome: an update. *Hematol Oncl Clin North Am.* 2013;27(3):565-584.

140. Rogers HJ, Allen C, Lichtin AE. Thrombotic thrombocytopenic purpura: the role of ADAMTS13. *Cleve Clin J Med.* 2016;83(8):597-603.

141. Knöbl P. Inherited and acquired thrombotic thrombocytopenic purpura (TTP) in adults. *Semin Thromb Hemost.* 2014;40(4):493-502.

142. Shenkman B, Einav Y. Thrombotic thrombocytopenic purpura and other thrombotic microangiopathic hemolytic anemias: diagnosis and classification. *Autoimmun Rev.* 2014;13(4-5):584-586.

143. Licht C, Greenbaum LA, Muus P, et al. Efficacy and safety of eculizumab in atypical hemolytic uremic syndrome from 2 year extensions of phase 2 studies. *Kidney Int.* 2015;87(5):1061-1073.

Gastroenterology

James F. Crismale, MD, and Thomas Schiano, MD

INTRODUCTION

Myriad gastrointestinal (GI) maladies may affect patients in the intensive care unit (ICU), from GI bleeding to complications from liver cirrhosis. In this chapter, we review several of the most common GI-related clinical scenarios encountered in the ICU.

GASTROINTESTINAL BLEEDING

Upper Gastrointestinal Bleeding

Upper GI bleeding (UGIB) is a common indication for ICU admission. With advances in critical care and endoscopy, the in-hospital mortality of patients admitted for UGIB has modestly decreased over the past several decades, but remains around 2.1%.[1] Etiologies of UGIB can be divided into variceal and nonvariceal hemorrhage; in this section, we will primarily discuss nonvariceal hemorrhage.

Peptic ulcer disease (PUD) is the most common etiology of nonvariceal UGIB, accounting for up to 40% of cases, followed by gastritis or esophagitis, Mallory-Weiss tears, cancer, angiodysplasias, and Dieulafoy lesions.[2] The most common risk factors for PUD are infection with *Helicobacter pylori* and use of nonsteroidal anti-inflammatory drugs (NSAIDs).[3] Ulcer disease may present with epigastric pain but is frequently asymptomatic until a patient presents with signs and symptoms of GI bleeding. If a patient does have pain related to a duodenal ulcer, it typically improves with food and recurs 1 to 3 hours after a meal. In contrast, gastric ulcers are often made worse with eating. Patients with UGIB related to PUD or any etiology typically present either with melena or with hematemesis. If UGI bleeding is very brisk, patients may present with hematochezia. Labs suggestive of an acute UGIB include a decrease of hemoglobin/hematocrit from baseline values, a mildly elevated white blood cell (WBC) count, and an elevated blood urea nitrogen (BUN) out of proportion to creatinine.

The risk of mortality can be estimated using the pre-endoscopic Rockall score (Table 24-1), and the Glasgow-Blatchford score can be utilized to estimate the need for inpatient endoscopic intervention.[4,5] Patients with a Blatchford

score of 0 (BUN < 18.2 mg/dL, hemoglobin [Hgb] ≥ 13 g/dL, systolic blood pressure [SBP] ≥ 100 mmHg, heart rate [HR] < 100 beats/min, no melena, no syncope, no heart disease, no liver failure) have a low likelihood of requiring endoscopic intervention and may be discharged from the emergency department (ED).[6]

Initial therapy for UGIB, as for hemorrhage of any etiology, is timely resuscitation. Patients should have adequate intravenous (IV) access placed with 2 large-bore IVs, infusion of IV fluids to correct volume deficits, and transfusion of packed red blood cells to a goal hemoglobin of 7 g/dL. This transfusion goal has been validated in a large clinical trial comparing a hemoglobin goal of 7 g/dL to a goal of 9 g/dL.[7] Coagulopathy also should be corrected via transfusion of fresh frozen plasma (FFP) and/or platelets, as appropriate. In addition to resuscitation, initial medical therapy should include an IV proton pump inhibitor (PPI). Typically, a PPI is initially given as a high-dose bolus, followed by a continuous infusion.[8] While pre-endoscopic PPI therapy has not been shown to improve mortality or the risk of re-bleeding, it does appear to reduce the incidence of finding ulcers with high-risk stigmata of hemorrhage and, therefore, to reduce the need for endoscopic therapy.[9] Erythromycin may also be given prior to endoscopy to accelerate gastric emptying, so that intragastric blood does not obscure the endoscopist's view. While nasogastric (NG) lavage is frequently attempted to document an upper GI source of bleeding, a negative NG aspirate does not necessarily rule out an upper GI source; therefore, its utility is limited.

Endoscopy should be performed within 24 hours of admission in a patient presenting with an upper GI bleed and should perhaps be performed within 12 hours in high-risk patients (ie, those with hematemesis and hemodynamic instability).[8] Very early endoscopy (within 2 hours of presentation) may actually be deleterious, as there may not be enough time for adequate resuscitation.[10]

Appropriate management of PUD depends in large part upon endoscopic findings. Stigmata of recent hemorrhage (SRH) are utilized to describe the appearance of an ulcer at endoscopy, and to prognosticate the risk of rebleeding and therefore dictate postendoscopic management. The Forrest classification is also used to describe the appearance of an

TABLE 24-1 Pre-endoscopic Rockall Score

Variable	Score			
	0	1	2	3
Age	< 60 y	60–79 y	≥ 80 y	
Shock	None	HR > 100 beats/min, SBP > 100 mmHg	Hypotension (SBP < 100 mmHg)	
Comorbidity	None		Cardiac failure, ischemic heart disease, other major comorbidities	Renal failure, liver failure, disseminated malignancy

HR = heart rate; SBP = systolic blood pressure. Minimum score, 0 (0.2% in-hospital mortality); 3 points, 10% mortality; 5 points, 40% mortality; maximum score, 7 (50% in-hospital morality).

ulcer and corresponds to specific stigmata of recent hemorrhage (Table 24-2). Endoscopic therapy is indicated in the presence of active bleeding, a nonbleeding visible vessel, or an ulcer with overlying clot (if the clot cannot be washed away to reveal lower-risk stigmata underlying it). Endoscopic therapy can be accomplished via cautery or with mechanical clipping of the vessel or bleeding site. Injection of epinephrine may be used as an adjunct to cautery or clipping, but is insufficient to be used alone.[8]

Postendoscopic medical therapy is driven by endoscopic findings and the need for endoscopic therapy. If endoscopic therapy has been applied, then IV PPI should be continued for at least 72 hours. American College of Gastroenterology (ACG) guidelines recommend a continuous infusion of PPI after endoscopic therapy.[8] However, a recent meta-analysis suggests that intermittent dosing of a PPI (eg, pantoprazole every 12 hours) post–endoscopic therapy may be equivalent to continuous dosing, with the advantage of decreased resource utilization.[11] Further data is necessary, and for now, guidelines recommend continuous PPI infusion postendoscopy. If a patient has low-risk stigmata (ie, a flat pigmented spot or clean-based ulcer), he or she may be transitioned to a standard-dose oral PPI and discharged after assuring that he or she is hemodynamically stable and has stable hemoglobin. Routine second-look endoscopy is not recommended in the absence of evidence of ongoing bleeding.[8]

In the setting of ongoing upper GI bleeding not amenable to endoscopic therapy, assistance from interventional radiology may be helpful. Angiography may be performed to identify the vessel from which bleeding is occurring (eg, the gastroduodenal artery in the case of a posterior wall duodenal bulb ulcer), and said vessel may be embolized by interventional radiology with excellent technical success.[12] In the modern era, surgery is less commonly performed for peptic ulcer disease, although it may be necessary in cases where bleeding does not resolve after endoscopic or angiographic therapy. Surgical options include oversewing of the ulcer to ligate the bleeding vessel, coupled with truncal vagotomy in the acute setting. In the nonemergent setting, antrectomy, vagotomy, and gastrojejunal anastomosis (Billroth II) can be performed for the treatment of PUD; however, given the effectiveness of medical therapy with PPIs, the need for this type of surgery is increasingly uncommon.[13]

Lower Gastrointestinal Bleeding

Overt lower GI bleeding (LGIB) accounts for approximately 20% of all cases of GIB.[14] Patients may present with hematochezia or maroon-colored stools. Melena may be seen if there is slow bleeding from the proximal colon. Hemodynamic instability should prompt suspicion for a brisk UGIB, which may occur in up to 15% of patients presenting with hematochezia.[15] Diverticular bleeding accounts for up to 50% of LGIB cases. Other common etiologies include angiodysplasias, colonic ischemia, infectious or inflammatory colitis, radiation proctopathy, and anorectal disorders such as hemorrhoids.[16]

TABLE 24-2 Forrest Classification and Stigmata of Recent Hemorrhage With Risk of Rebleeding Without Endoscopic Therapy

Stigmata of Recent Hemorrhage	Forrest Classification	Risk of Rebleeding	Endoscopic Therapy Indicated?	Postendoscopic PPI Therapy
Active spurting	IA	55%	Yes	IV PPI × 72 h
Active oozing	IB			
Nonbleeding visible vessel	IIA	43%		
Adherent clot	IIB	22%	Yes, if clot cannot be cleared	
Flat red spot	IIC	10%	No	Once daily oral PPI
Clean-based ulcer	III	0%	No	

IV = intravenous; PPI = proton-pump inhibitor.

Data from Laine L, Jensen DM. Management of patients with ulcer bleeding. *Am J Gastroenterol.* 2012;107(3):345-360.

Initial management should focus on appropriate resuscitation, including blood transfusion, if necessary. For patients on systemic anticoagulation, ACG guidelines suggest that endoscopic therapy is safe in patients with an international normalized ratio (INR) of 1.5 to 2.5, so for hemodynamically stable patients, reversal of anticoagulation may not be necessary.[14] Platelets should be transfused in the setting of thrombocytopenia (platelet count $< 50 \times 10^3/\mu L$). For patients requiring massive transfusion (> 3 units packed red blood cells [PRBC] in 1 hour), 1 unit each of platelets and FFP should be transfused per unit of PRBC to prevent transfusion-related coagulopathy.[17] In the great majority of patients (~80%), LGIB will stop spontaneously. However, in patients with ongoing hemorrhage, therapeutic intervention is required to halt bleeding.

In hemodynamically stable patients, colonoscopy should be the first diagnostic and therapeutic procedure attempted. Colonoscopy allows visualization of the colonic mucosa to identify a bleeding site as well as a means for therapeutic intervention. Colonoscopy can identify a definitive or potential bleeding source in 45% to 90% of patients.[18] Early colonoscopy within 8 to 12 hours of presentation (compared with delayed colonoscopy at 36 to 90 hours after presentation) was shown in 1 randomized controlled trial to lead to an increased yield in identification of a bleeding source but did not improve length of stay or rates of rebleeding or surgery.[19,20] Early colonoscopy should be attempted only if the patient is able to tolerate rapid bowel preparation. Nasogastric tube (NGT) placement may facilitate this, as long as the patient is at low risk for aspiration.[16] Endoscopic therapy depends on the bleeding source, and may involve a combination of epinephrine injection, clipping, and/or argon plasma coagulation.[14]

If a patient presents with hemodynamic instability and hematochezia, esophagogastroduodenoscopy (EGD) should be performed first to rule out UGIB. Patients who remain hemodynamically unstable in whom a UGI source of bleeding has been ruled out are unlikely to tolerate bowel preparation for colonoscopy and typically require radiographic intervention to localize and treat the source of bleeding. Radiographic methods for identifying the source of GI bleeding include RBC scintigraphy, computed tomography angiography (CTA), and conventional angiography. Red blood cell scintigraphy can identify bleeding at rates as low as 0.05 to 0.1 mL/min, but it has limited accuracy in identifying a bleeding site (66%).[21] CTA is more accurate, with a sensitivity and specificity of 85% and 92%, respectively. It requires a patient to be bleeding at a rate of 0.3 to 0.5 mL/min. It can also be performed more rapidly than RBC scintigraphy. Its drawbacks include exposure to ionizing radiation and IV contrast media, with attendant risks of contrast allergy as well as contrast-induced nephropathy. If a bleeding site is identified on either RBC scintigraphy or CTA, the patient can be referred for conventional angiography and embolization.[22] Conventional angiography requires a patient to be bleeding at a rate of 0.5 to 1 mL/min to visualize extravasation of contrast media.

Superselective angiographic embolization can control bleeding in 40% to 100% of cases; rebleeding occurs in 0% to 50% of patients. Aside from exposure to radiation and contrast, 1 potential risk of embolization includes bowel ischemia, which may occur in 1% to 4% of patients.[14] Finally, surgical management may be necessary if endoscopic and radiologic intervention fails; if the bleeding source cannot be accurately localized, subtotal colectomy is the procedure of choice.

MESENTERIC ISCHEMIA AND ISCHEMIC COLITIS

Mesenteric Ischemia

Patients with mesenteric ischemia typically present with the acute onset of continuous abdominal pain, the location of which may vary, but it typically begins in the periumbilical region. As symptoms progress, the pain may become more diffuse. While initially patients will present with the classic "pain out of proportion" to physical exam findings, as ischemia progresses, peritonitis develops and patients may have findings consistent with an acute abdomen, including rebound and involuntary guarding. It is important to suspect the diagnosis of mesenteric ischemia in patients presenting with these symptoms and who have a history of ischemic heart disease, atrial fibrillation, hypertension, diabetes, and other cardiovascular risk factors.[23] Mesenteric ischemia most often develops due to embolism of clot into the superior mesenteric artery or as a result of mesenteric artery thrombosis. Patients with mesenteric thrombosis may have a history of chronic mesenteric ischemia, characterized by "mesenteric angina" whenever the patient eats, leading to sitophobia (fear of eating) and weight loss. This pattern of disease may be found in patients with diffuse atherosclerotic disease.[24]

In addition to clinical findings, laboratory studies may show an elevated white blood cell count, amylase, and lactate, although these are nonspecific findings. CTA is especially useful, with a high sensitivity and specificity (93% and 95%, respectively). CTA should be performed without oral contrast, as oral contrast may obscure the mesenteric vessels and reduce sensitivity.[25]

Management of acute mesenteric ischemia involves general supportive measures, including NGT placement, nothing-by-mouth (NPO) status, IV fluids, and initiation of broad-spectrum antibiotics given the risk of bacterial translocation and sepsis. Anticoagulation with unfractionated heparin should be initiated to prevent propagation of clots. Vasopressors should be avoided if possible, as they may exacerbate splanchnic vasoconstriction and worsen ischemia.[26] For patients with clinical or radiographic evidence of peritonitis or for those who are hemodynamically unstable, emergent laparotomy is indicated. For all others, revascularization may be attempted with either open surgical thrombectomy or endovascular therapy with thrombolysis or balloon angioplasty and stenting.[27]

Ischemic Colitis

Of patients hospitalized for LGIB, ischemic colitis (IC) may be the etiology in up to 24% of cases.[28] The most common area of the colon affected is the splenic flexure, where the vascular distributions of the superior and inferior mesenteric arteries form a "watershed" area, leading to increased susceptibility to ischemia during episodes of low blood flow. Although the left colon is most commonly affected, the right colon can be involved in an isolated manner in up to 25% of cases.[29] Risk factors for IC include advanced age, comorbid cardiovascular disease, hypertension, diabetes, hypercoagulable states, and the presence of comorbid GI disease, including irritable bowel syndrome and constipation. Ischemic colitis also can complicate shock, in which hypotension leads to decreased blood flow to watershed areas of the colon. Ischemic colitis may be seen after repair of an abdominal aortic aneurysm if there is occlusion or injury of the inferior mesenteric artery. Numerous medications have been implicated in the etiology of IC, including opiates (vis-à-vis induction of constipation), immunomodulatory drugs, and illicit drugs that induce vasospasm such as cocaine and amphetamines.[28]

The classical presentation of IC is the sudden onset of left lower quadrant (LLQ) cramping abdominal pain, followed within 24 hours by bloody diarrhea or maroon-colored stools Patients may have LLQ tenderness. In cases of right-sided IC, pain is the predominant presenting symptom, and hematochezia is less common. The degree of rectal bleeding in patients with colonic ischemia is usually mild, and transfusion is rarely required. While the diagnosis of IC may be made on clinical findings alone, colonoscopic evaluation and/or imaging studies may be helpful to confirm the diagnosis. A CT scan may show segmental wall thickening, thumb printing (subepithelial hemorrhage/edema), and pericolonic fat stranding. CTA is usually unnecessary, unless a patient presents with severe disease (eg, sepsis, peritoneal signs, isolated right IC), in which it is essential to rule out vascular occlusion.[28] Colonoscopy should be performed within 48 hours to confirm the diagnosis. Typical findings on colonoscopy include erythema, edema, friability, and superficial ulcerations. Deep ulcerations, luminal narrowing, and dusky mucosa are present in more severe disease.[30]

The management of IC varies depending upon its severity. In most cases, symptoms will resolve within 2 to 3 days with supportive care, including bowel rest and intravenous hydration, and up to 80% of patients will require no surgical intervention.[31] In addition to supportive care, ACG practice guidelines recommend the use of broad-spectrum antibiotics for colonic flora in patients with moderate or severe disease.[28] Patients with moderate or severe disease should have a surgical consultation and should be considered for transfer to the ICU. Aside from frank peritonitis, other indications for surgical intervention include the presence of massive hemorrhage, fulminant colitis, or a failure to respond to medical therapy after 2 to 3 weeks. The type of surgery performed depends upon the involved segment of colon, but most commonly requires total or subtotal colectomy. Postoperative mortality can be as high as 48%.[32]

COLON

Diverticular Disease

Colonic diverticuli are sac-like outpouchings of the colon wall that occur at points of weakness where the vasa recta enter the muscle layer of the colon.[33] They develop over time due to increased pressure within the colon lumen and are more common among patients with constipation and abnormalities of colonic motility. Up to 40% of patients undergoing screening colonoscopies may be found to have diverticulosis; 20% of these patients will become symptomatic. The manifestations of diverticular disease include diverticular bleeding, diverticulitis, segmental colitis associated with diverticulosis (SCAD; inflammation of the mucosa surrounding diverticuli, without involvement of the diverticuli themselves), and symptomatic uncomplicated diverticular disease (SUDD).[34] Typically, only management of diverticular bleeding (see "Lower Gastrointestinal Bleeding," discussed previously) and diverticulitis may require ICU-level care; SCAD and SUDD are managed as chronic outpatient conditions.

Similar to appendicitis, diverticulitis occurs when a diverticulum becomes obstructed by a fecalith or other material, leading to bacterial stasis, inflammation, and ultimately microperforation.[35] Patients present with a constellation of symptoms, including LLQ pain, fever, and leukocytosis. In patients with a redundant sigmoid colon, the pain may be on the right side. Nausea and vomiting due to an ileus may be present. Rarely, patients with severe inflammatory changes may present with obstruction. Typical findings on CT, including colonic wall thickening and pericolonic fat stranding in close proximity to colonic diverticuli, are used to support the diagnosis.[36] Ultrasound may be used in patients who have a contraindication to CT, with sensitivity and specificity of 84% and 98%, respectively.[37]

Uncomplicated diverticulitis often can be managed in the outpatient setting with oral antibiotics. Recommended regimens include ciprofloxacin plus metronidazole, trimethoprim-sulfamethoxazole plus metronidazole, amoxicillin-clavulanate, or moxifloxacin, all given for 7 to 10 days.[38] Outpatient treatment is successful in up to 97% of cases.[39] In patients who either fail outpatient therapy or are unable to tolerate oral (PO) therapy, hospitalization and use of IV antibiotics is indicated. Intravenous antibiotic regimens for acute uncomplicated diverticulitis include ciprofloxacin or a third-generation cephalosporin plus metronidazole, or in a patient with risk factors for antimicrobial resistance, piperacillin-tazobactam or a carbapenem.[40] Antibiotics are given for a 7- to 10-day course, although they may be transitioned to oral to complete the course if the patient's condition improves.[41] American Gastroenterological Association guidelines recommend that a colonoscopy should be performed after recovery from an episode of diverticulitis if the patient has not recently undergone a colonoscopy for colorectal cancer screening in order to rule out a concomitant colorectal carcinoma or advanced adenoma.[42]

Complications of diverticulitis include the development of a pericolic abscess, fistulization, obstruction, or free perforation. Although free perforation is a clear indication for emergent surgery, due to a recurrence rate greater than 40%, surgical resection of the involved segment is recommended after any complicated episode of diverticulitis.[43] Abscesses occur in about 15% of patients who develop diverticulitis, and management varies depending upon the size of the abscess. Small (< 3 cm) abscesses may be managed with antibiotics alone if the patient is clinically stable.[44] Larger abscesses require either percutaneous drainage by interventional radiology or, less commonly, by surgical management. Percutaneous drainage also may act as a bridge to surgery, allowing a 1-stage procedure (with primary colocolonic anastomosis) rather than an ostomy with subsequent reanastomosis.[45] Abscesses that are unable to be successfully drained percutaneously require surgical management.[40-42] Fistulae and obstruction also require resection of the involved segment of the colon; if fistulae are complicated (eg, colovesical), multidisciplinary surgical involvement may be required.[43]

Diverticular bleeding is discussed in "Lower Gastrointestinal Bleeding."

Ulcerative Colitis

Ulcerative colitis (UC) is 1 of the 2 forms of idiopathic inflammatory bowel disease (IBD). As opposed to Crohn disease (and as the name implies), only the colon is affected, typically with contiguous inflammation that begins in the rectum at the anal verge. The disease may be isolated to the rectosigmoid in 45% of patients, or it may extend to involve the left colon in 35% of patients. A minority of patients have pancolitis.[35] Patients present with a variety of symptoms, including diarrhea, rectal bleeding, tenesmus, and abdominal pain. Whereas patients usually present with longstanding symptoms, a minority of patients may present acutely with severe or fulminant disease requiring hospitalization. Laboratory findings may include anemia and hypoalbuminemia; serologic evidence of inflammation may be present, including elevations in C-reactive protein (CRP), erythrocyte sedimentation rate (ESR), and platelets.[46] Diagnosis is supported by typical endoscopic findings, which include the presence of inflammation contiguous from the anal verge, ulcerations (superficial or deep), erythema, and friability. Patients with longstanding disease may have pseudopolyps, which are regenerative growths of mucosa that form in response to chronic inflammation. Biopsy findings include cryptitis, crypt abscesses, and a mixed inflammatory infiltrate in the lamina propria. Inflammation is confined to the mucosa, as opposed to Crohn disease where inflammation may be transmural.[35]

As with Crohn disease, the management of UC mainly takes place in the outpatient setting. Treatment includes the use of steroids; topical mesalamine agents; immunomodulators like 6-mercaptopurine, azathioprine, and methotrexate; and biologic agents including anti–tumor necrosis factor (TNF) therapies (infliximab, adalimumab, and golimumab) and integrin inhibitors (vedolizumab). Inpatient management is necessary for patients who fail outpatient therapy or for those with severe or fulminant disease. Severe disease is defined by the Montréal classification as 6 or more bowel movements per day with blood, as well as evidence of systemic toxicity including one of the following: HR greater than 90 beats/min, temperature greater than 37.5°C, hemoglobin less than 10.5 g/dL, or ESR greater than 30 mm/h.[47]

Initial steps in management include general resuscitative measures, including IV hydration and correction of electrolyte abnormalities. Testing for *Clostridium difficile* infection should be performed. If significant abdominal distension or tenderness is present, plain abdominal radiography or CT may be indicated to rule out complications including toxic megacolon or perforation. Flexible sigmoidoscopy should be performed to assess endoscopic grade of disease and to perform biopsies to assess for concomitant cytomegalovirus infection, which requires appropriate antiviral therapy. Despite the presence of mild bleeding, all patients admitted to the hospital with a flare of inflammatory bowel disease should be started on some form of pharmacological venous thromboembolism (VTE) prophylaxis, as the inflammatory state places patients at increased risk for VTE.[48] Initial therapy should include intravenous steroids at a dose of 100 mg IV hydrocortisone every 6 hours or 20 mg IV methylprednisolone every 8 hours. Oral and rectal mesalamine may be continued. The patient should be allowed to eat (or if they are unable to maintain adequate PO intake, supplemental enteral nutrition via nasogastric or nasojejunal tube should be provided), as nourishment of the colonic mucosa may improve outcomes. Bowel rest and parenteral nutrition do not provide any additional benefit and actually may worsen outcomes.[49] Electrolyte abnormalities should be corrected, as hypokalemia or hypomagnesemia may promote the development of toxic megacolon.[50] Antibiotics are not indicated for the treatment of acute UC per se, although they may be appropriate in patients with signs of systemic infection.[51]

Despite aggressive therapy with intravenous steroids, some patients go on to develop complications of disease, including toxic megacolon, refractory hemorrhage, or frank perforation. It is essential for providers to realize when medical therapy with steroids has failed and when an escalation of therapy is appropriate. Multiple scoring systems have been developed to assist providers in decision making regarding the appropriate timing of colectomy. One of the simplest is the Oxford index, in which a stool frequency of more than 8 bowel movements per day on day 3 of intravenous steroids, along with a CRP greater than 45 mg/L, are predictive of requiring a colectomy during admission in 85% of cases.[52]

For patients who do not have toxic megacolon or refractory bleeding but who have not had a good clinical response to 3 to 5 days of IV steroid therapy (defined as a Lichtiger index < 10 for 2 consecutive days; Table 24-3), rescue therapy with IV infliximab or cyclosporine can be considered. The decision of which agent to use depends in large part upon local practice patterns. Two large, open-label trials found no difference in rates of colectomy, mortality, or serious infectious complications between the 2 therapies. Infliximab is given as a single weight-based infusion, followed by further induction infusions at weeks 2 and 6; maintenance therapy is given every 8 weeks. Cyclosporine is given as a continuous, weight-based infusion and is typically administered for 8 days. Monitoring of serum levels of cyclosporine, as well as monitoring of kidney function, blood pressure, and serum electrolytes are required when administering cyclosporine induction therapy. Serum triglycerides should also be monitored, as hypotriglyceridemia is associated with adverse neurologic side effects (including seizures) in patients on IV cyclosporine. Patients who respond to IV cyclosporine must be transitioned to oral cyclosporine and a thiopurine (such as 6-mercaptopurine or azathioprine), as cyclosporine cannot be continued long term as a maintenance therapy.[50] For that reason, patients who have previously failed maintenance therapy with a thiopurine may not be good candidates for salvage therapy with cyclosporine and may benefit more from use of infliximab. If salvage therapy with either infliximab or cyclosporine fails, it is not recommended to again attempt medical salvage therapy with the other agent, as following infliximab with cyclosporine, or vice versa, has been found to significantly increase the risk of infectious complications and mortality.[53]

Crohn Disease

Crohn disease (CD) is a chronic, idiopathic inflammatory bowel disease characterized by transmural inflammation that can affect the entire GI tract. Most commonly, it affects the distal small bowel, with or without involvement of the colon, although occasionally only the colon is affected.[54] Although patients will rarely be admitted to the ICU for management of their Crohn disease per se, management of the complications of CD or its treatment (including sepsis in patients on immunosuppressive therapy) may necessitate ICU-level care. Those on total parenteral nutrition may also be at risk for fungal infections.[46] Patients requiring surgery may be at risk for postoperative complications, including anastomotic leaks and anastomotic bleeding, which may occur in 8% and 5% of patients, respectively.[55,56] Finally, patients with high-output enterocutaneous fistulae that have developed because of refractory CD or postsurgical complications may present with profound hypovolemia, volume depletion, and electrolyte imbalances that may necessitate admission to the ICU. Multidisciplinary care involving gastroenterology, nutrition, and surgery is essential in the management of these complex patients.[57,58]

Sigmoid Volvulus

Sigmoid volvulus is one of the most common etiologies of large bowel obstruction. It develops when a redundant loop of sigmoid colon twists upon its vascular pedicle to cause a closed-loop obstruction, ultimately leading to bowel ischemia. Risk factors include older age, a history of chronic constipation, and a history of colonic dysmotility.[59,60] Patients often present with abdominal pain, obstipation, nausea and vomiting, and abdominal distension. Diagnosis is confirmed radiographically, with abdominal x-ray demonstrating a classic "coffee-bean" sign. Computed tomography may demonstrate a "whirl" pattern around the site of obstruction, with dilated bowel proximal to it.[61]

TABLE 24-3 Lichtiger Index

Symptom	Score
Diarrhea, # daily BMs	
0–2	0
3–4	1
5–6	2
7–9	3
≥ 10	4
Nocturnal diarrhea	
No	0
Yes	1
Visible blood in stool, % of BMs	
0	0
< 50	1
≥ 50	2
100	3
Fecal incontinence	
No	0
Yes	1
Abdominal pain or cramping	
None	0
Mild	1
Moderate	2
Severe	3
General well-being	
Perfect	0
Very good	1
Good	2
Average	3
Poor	4
Terrible	5
Abdominal tenderness	
None	0
Mild/localized	1
Mild-to-moderate/diffuse	2
Severe/rebound	3
Need for antidiarrheal drugs	
No	0
Yes	1

BM = bowel movement.

Reprinted with permission from Lichtiger S, Present DH, Kornbluth A, et al. Cyclosporine in severe ulcerative colitis refractory to steroid therapy. *N Engl J Med.* 1994;330(26):1841-1845. Copyright © 1994 Massachusetts Medical Society.

Treatment for sigmoid volvulus includes IV fluids, naso-gastric decompression, and correction of electrolyte abnormalities. Excluding patients with peritoneal signs who should proceed directly to exploratory laparotomy, flexible sigmoidoscopy should be performed emergently to reduce the volvulus. The sigmoidoscope is inserted past the spiral-shaped area of torsion, and air and stool are suctioned from it. A rectal tube may be placed to allow for continued decompression. Because the recurrence risk is up to 60%, surgical resection of the redundant sigmoid colon is indicated after sigmoidoscopic decompression.[62]

Malignant Large Bowel Obstruction

Colonic adenocarcinoma is the most common etiology of large bowel obstruction, accounting for more than 50% of cases.[63] Non-GI malignancies, such as ovarian and other gynecological cancers, may cause large bowel obstruction via extrinsic compression. In the setting of an obstructing colon cancer, timely relief of the obstruction is indicated to avoid perforation. Options for decompression include emergency surgery with colostomy placement proximal to the point of obstruction (followed by resection of the primary lesion), or endoscopic placement of an uncovered self-expanding metal stent.[64]

Colonic Pseudo-obstruction/Ogilvie Syndrome

Acute colonic pseudo-obstruction (ACPO), also known as Ogilvie syndrome, is characterized by sudden colonic dilatation in absence of a mechanical obstruction. It typically affects older patients, especially those who are immobile or bedbound due to hospitalization or recent surgery. Significant dilatation of the ascending and transverse colon may be seen on abdominal imaging. Bowel ischemia and perforation can occur in 3% to 15% of cases and is associated with a mortality as high as 50%.[65] The risk of perforation is increased with a cecal diameter of more than 10 to 12 cm and when the dilatation has been present for more than 6 days.[66] Conservative management should be initiated with NPO status, IV fluids, NGT decompression, and correction of electrolyte abnormalities. Medications that can contribute to decreased bowel motility (eg, opioids and anticholinergics) should be discontinued. The patient should change positions frequently to encourage bowel motility; prone positioning with hips elevated frequently leads to evacuation of flatus.[66]

If conservative management is unsuccessful after 24 to 48 hours, pharmacologic therapy with neostigmine, an anticholinesterase parasympathomimetic agent, can be attempted. Its side effects include bradycardia, asystole, hypotension, and bronchoconstriction; patients therefore must be on a cardiac monitor while receiving the drug, and atropine must be at the bedside in the case of development of brady-arrhythmias. Administration of neostigmine is successful in approximately 80% of patients, with a rate of recurrence of 10%.[67] If successful, a low-dose polyethylene glycol–based laxative may be started to encourage colonic motility and reduce the risk of recurrence.[68] Colonoscopic decompression is an option if conservative and pharmacologic therapy has failed; success rates range from 61% to 95%.[69] Surgical management with either subtotal colectomy or placement of a tube cecostomy carries a high rate of morbidity and mortality and is reserved for patients who have failed other therapies.[65,66]

GALLBLADDER/BILIARY DISEASE

Up to 20% of patients with gallstones seen on ultrasound may develop symptoms.[70] Classic biliary pain ("biliary colic") results from transient obstruction of the cystic duct with a gallstone and presents as transient right upper quadrant (RUQ) pain that often radiates to the right shoulder. The pain typically lasts for at least 30 minutes to 1 hour, although it may continue for as long as 6 hours and may be associated with nausea and vomiting. Exam findings are often normal, although patients may exhibit mild tenderness in the RUQ. Laboratory results are usually normal, with no elevations in liver enzymes.[71] Diagnosis of cholelithiasis is usually obtained via RUQ ultrasound, which has a sensitivity and specificity of 84% and 99%, respectively.[72] Cholecystectomy is recommended for patients with symptomatic gallstone disease, as the rate of complications, including cholecystitis, cholangitis, and gallstone pancreatitis, increases 1% to 2% per year.[73]

Cholecystitis

Acute calculous cholecystitis is the most common manifestation of gallstone disease. It occurs when a stone becomes lodged in the neck of the gallbladder, leading to sustained obstruction of the cystic duct. Patients present with RUQ pain typically of a greater intensity and longer duration than that which is seen with biliary colic. Fever, RUQ tenderness, and Murphy sign (inspiratory arrest on palpation of the inflamed gallbladder) may be present. Labs may reveal a leukocytosis, with mild elevations in transaminases and bilirubin (although bilirubin will typically be < 2–4 mg/dL; higher values suggest possible bile duct stones with biliary obstruction). Ultrasound may reveal a dilated gallbladder with a thickened gallbladder wall (> 3 mm) and pericholecystic fluid; the presence of a sonographic Murphy sign together with gallstones has a 90% positive predictive value for cholecystitis. If the diagnosis is unclear, cholescintigraphy with a hepatobiliary iminodiacetic acid (HIDA) scan may help to confirm the diagnosis, with nonvisualization of the gallbladder demonstrating sensitivity and specificity greater than 90%.[74,75]

Initial management of uncomplicated cholecystitis includes initiation of pain control, IV fluids, and antibiotics. Recommended antibiotics include a third-generation cephalosporin for patients with mild-to-moderate disease with no known risk factors for resistant organisms. For patients at risk of antimicrobial resistance, or for those with severe disease (suspected empyema of the gallbladder, perforation, or sepsis) broad-spectrum coverage with piperacillin-tazobactam or a carbapenem is recommended.[76] In otherwise healthy patients, early cholecystectomy within 72 hours of symptom onset has been shown to lead to improved outcomes, including shorter length of stay.[77] For patients with multiple comorbidities with a high operative risk, conservative management with antibiotics alone may be more appropriate, with percutaneous cholecystostomy performed in patients who do not improve with nonoperative management alone.[78]

Nonoperative management is also typically necessary for patients with acalculous cholecystitis. The pathophysiology is thought to involve inflammation related to prolonged exposure of the biliary epithelium to bile (owing to a lack of gallbladder contraction in prolonged fasting states, especially in the setting of total parenteral nutrition administration) as well as relative gallbladder ischemia. The diagnosis should be suspected in a critically ill patient with new-onset RUQ pain, leukocytosis, and concerning imaging findings. Ultrasound has a sensitivity and specificity for the diagnosis of acalculous cholecystitis of 67% to 92% and greater than 90%, respectively.[79] The use of HIDA scintigraphy may be less reliable in critically ill patients because of its higher false-positive rate, especially among those with liver enzyme abnormalities. In addition to antibiotics, drainage of the gallbladder with percutaneous cholecystostomy is necessary for successful treatment. Initial technical and clinical success with this technique may be as high as 93%.[80] Elective cholecystectomy is indicated once the patient recovers from the acute critical illness. Of note, percutaneous cholecystostomy should *not* be performed in patients with ascites, as tubes have a high chance of dislodgement from the gallbladder into the peritoneum, leaving a free perforation in the gallbladder wall.

Choledocholithiasis

Choledocholithiasis is defined as the presence of stones within the common bile duct (CBD).[81] Patients with choledocholithiasis may present with biliary colic and/or jaundice owing to extrahepatic biliary obstruction. Pain may be constant if there is persistent blockage at the level of the ampulla, or it may be transient due to a "ball-valve" effect of the stone causing intermittent obstruction. Liver enzymes may be elevated; aminotransferases will elevate first, followed by alkaline phosphatase, γ-glutamyl transferase, and direct and total bilirubin.[82]

Right upper quadrant ultrasound has poor sensitivity for identifying CBD stones (~50%), although it can be helpful in assessing the presence of CBD dilation (> 6 mm).[83] Magnetic resonance cholangiopancreatography (MRCP) has a sensitivity and specificity of 93% and 94%, respectively.[84] Endoscopic ultrasound (EUS), although invasive, provides an excellent view of the CBD, with positive and negative predictive values of 99% and 98%, respectively. When the clinical and noninvasive radiographic picture is equivocal, EUS is often helpful in avoiding unnecessary endoscopic retrograde cholangiopancreatography (ERCP), which is considered the

gold standard for diagnosis and treatment of choledocholithiasis; success rates for stone removal with ERCP range from 87% to 100%.[85] In the absence of cholangitis, ERCP may be performed on a nonurgent basis. Complications of ERCP include post-sphincterotomy bleeding, perforation, and pancreatitis. Post-ERCP pancreatitis may occur in up to 10% of patients; the risk is higher in younger patients, in women, and in patients with prior post-ERCP pancreatitis. Procedure-related risk factors include excessive cannulation time, injection of the pancreatic duct with contrast, and balloon dilation of an intact sphincter.[86] In patients with an intact gallbladder, cholecystectomy should be planned soon after ERCP and stone extraction, as a longer interval between ERCP and cholecystectomy has been associated with an increased risk of biliary complications.[87] Finally, choledocholithiasis can be confirmed on an intraoperative cholangiogram (IOC) performed at the time of cholecystectomy, which should prompt a referral for postoperative ERCP and stone extraction.

The American Society for Gastrointestinal Endoscopy (ASGE) has published criteria[81] to assign risk of choledocholithiasis based on clinical, lab, and imaging parameters (Table 24-4).

After assigning a likelihood of choledocholithiasis, the algorithm in Figure 24-1 can be used to determine the next steps.

Cholangitis

Acute ascending cholangitis is diagnosed when a patient presents with Charcot triad (RUQ pain, jaundice, and fever) in the setting of biliary obstruction. Initial supportive care includes management of sepsis with intravenous fluids and antibiotics.

TABLE 24-4 Predictors of Choledocholithiasis

Predictors of choledocholithiasis
Very strong
CBD stone on transabdominal US
Clinical ascending cholangitis
Bilirubin > 4 mg/dL
Strong
Dilated CBD on US (> 6 mm with gallbladder in situ)
Bilirubin level 1.8–4 mg/dL
Moderate
Abnormal liver biochemical test other than bilirubin
Age older than 55 y
Clinical gallstone pancreatitis
Assigning a likelihood of choledocholithiasis based on clinical predictors
Presence of any very strong predictor: **High**
Presence of both strong predictors: **High**
No predictors present: **Low**
All other patients: **Intermediate**

CBD = common bile duct; US = ultrasound.

Reprinted from ASGE Standards of Practice Committee; Maple JT, Ben-Menachem T, Anderson MA, et al. The role of endoscopy in the evaluation of suspected choledocholithiasis. *Gastrointest Endosc.* 2010;71(1):1-9.

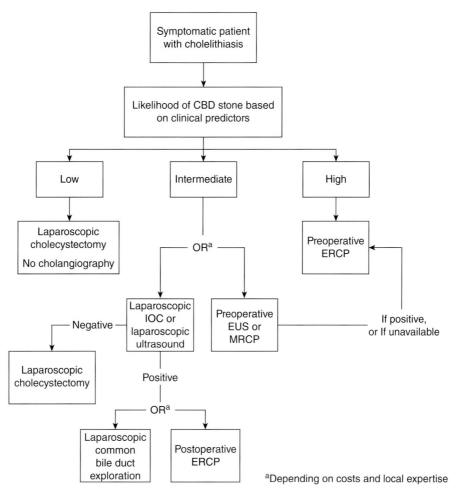

FIGURE 24-1 Choledocholithiasis management algorithm. CBD = common bile duct; ERCP = endoscopic retrograde cholangiopancreatography; EUS = endoscopic ultrasound; IOC = intraoperative cholangiogram; MRCP = magnetic resonance cholangiopancreatography. (Reproduced with permission from ASGE Standards of Practice Committee; Maple JT, Ben-Menachem T, Anderson MA, et al. The role of endoscopy in the evaluation of suspected choledocholithiasis. *Gastrointest Endosc.* 2010;71(1):1-9.)

Reynold pentad is Charcot triad with the addition of shock and altered mental status. Antibiotics are generally continued for 7 to 10 days; if blood cultures are positive, antibiotic therapy should be tailored to the organism(s) recovered. In general, antibiotics that cover Gram-negative organisms and anaerobes should be administered (eg, piperacillin-tazobactam) unless an organism is definitively identified. If the patient does not have any risk factors for antimicrobial resistance, a third-generation cephalosporin in combination with metronidazole may be sufficient.[76] Biliary drainage should be performed as soon as is feasible, but in the absence of persistent abdominal pain, hypotension, and encephalopathy, ERCP need not be performed immediately after presentation (eg, in the middle of the night) but can be performed within 24 hours. However, if the patient decompensates despite adequate antibiotic therapy and fluid resuscitation, urgent decompression is required. This may be performed via ERCP with sphincterotomy and stone extraction or via percutaneous transhepatic cholangiography with placement of an external drain.[85] If sphincterotomy is not able to be performed because of the presence of concomitant coagulopathy,

then endoscopic biliary stent placement may be sufficient for the purposes of biliary decompression, with stone extraction performed at a later date.[88] As with all symptomatic gallstone disease, cholecystectomy is indicated, although not necessarily during the index hospitalization for cholangitis. Cholecystectomy, however, should be performed within 6 weeks of an episode of cholangitis, as data demonstrate reduced rates of recurrence and improved outcomes.[87]

Mirizzi Syndrome

Mirizzi syndrome is an uncommon manifestation of gallstone disease wherein a stone impacted in the cystic duct compresses the extrahepatic bile duct, leading to a syndrome of pain, jaundice, and fever, which may be difficult to distinguish clinically from ascending cholangitis. Laboratory testing may show evidence of obstructive jaundice, and imaging may show a dilated intrahepatic biliary tree but a normal (nondilated) extrahepatic bile duct. Management for Mirizzi syndrome is surgical, with the exact technique depending upon the site of obstruction and the presence of cholecystocholedochal fistula.[89,90]

Bile Leak

Iatrogenic injury to the CBD can occur in up to 1% of cases after laparoscopic cholecystectomy.[91] A bile leak may be suspected in the immediate postoperative period with the appearance of bilious drainage into surgically placed drains, although patients may present up to 4 weeks after cholecystectomy.[92] Patients may complain of RUQ pain, fever, and jaundice. Ultrasound or CT may show a sub- or perihepatic fluid collection. The most sensitive test to confirm the presence of a bile leak is a HIDA scan, which has a sensitivity approaching 100%.[93] Bile leaks can be managed with ERCP, either via placement of a transpapillary biliary stent or via biliary sphincterotomy. Both techniques reduce the transpapillary pressure, allowing bile to drain more easily via the papilla and redirecting bile flow to allow the leak to heal.[91]

PANCREAS

Acute Pancreatitis

Alcohol, along with gallstones, are the 2 most common risk factors for the development of acute pancreatitis.[94] Acute pancreatitis is diagnosed when a patient meets 2 of 3 criteria: (1) typical abdominal pain, (2) serum amylase and/or lipase greater than 3 times the upper limit of normal, and (3) characteristic findings from abdominal imaging. It should be especially noted that imaging is not required to make a diagnosis and is only necessary when either the diagnosis of acute pancreatitis is in question or if a patient who meets clinical and laboratory criteria for acute pancreatitis fails to improve after 48 to 72 hours of therapy (to identify evidence of early local complications).[95]

In acute pancreatitis due to any etiology, the most important aspect of management is prompt fluid resuscitation. Hypovolemia can occur due to impaired oral intake, vomiting, and third-spacing of fluid due to increased vascular permeability from the intense inflammatory state arising in the setting of acute pancreatitis. Inflammation may be exacerbated by low blood flow to the pancreas, worsening activation of pancreatic enzymes and further activation of the inflammatory cascade.[96] Early, aggressive IV hydration (within the first 6 hours of treatment) appears to be the most important treatment; after 24 to 48 hours, the benefit of aggressive fluid resuscitation may be lost. A large, prospective randomized trial demonstrated reduced markers of systemic inflammation (CRP and systemic inflammatory response syndrome [SIRS] criteria) with the use of Ringer lactate solution compared with normal saline in patients with acute pancreatitis.[97] Therefore, guidelines recommend its use for initial resuscitation in acute pancreatitis.[96] After initial correction of hypovolemia via fluid bolus, Ringer lactate should be initiated at 250 to 500 mL/h. If the patient has cardiopulmonary comorbidities, the rate at which fluids are given may need to be lowered, and the patient should be reassessed frequently for evidence of respiratory distress or volume overload. A fall in both the BUN and the hematocrit—reflective of effective fluid resuscitation—should be seen within the first 24 hours. If a decrease in these values is not noted, the rate of fluid may need to be increased.[98] Antibiotics should be reserved only for the presence of concomitant extrapancreatic infection or if a patient subsequently develops evidence of infected pancreatic necrosis. Infected pancreatic necrosis may be suspected if a patient develops clinical deterioration after initial improvement, or in patients who fail to improve after 7 to 10 days of hospitalization. The presence of necrosis is best visualized on an abdominal CT with IV contrast; infection may be confirmed with CT-guided fine-needle aspiration of the necrotic pancreas, although it is also acceptable to treat empirically with antibiotics that penetrate the pancreatic parenchyma, such as meropenem when infected necrosis is suspected. Prophylactic antibiotics and/or antifungals (to prevent the occurrence of infected necrosis) have not been demonstrated to be beneficial in improving mortality.[100] Endoscopic retrograde cholangiopancreatography is indicated in the setting of acute pancreatitis only with concomitant cholangitis, or if there is evidence of ongoing biliary obstruction with persistent jaundice.[96]

While initiating resuscitative measures, the predicted severity of pancreatitis should be determined to assist with triage. There are numerous scoring systems that aim to predict the severity of pancreatitis, and none appears to be superior to another. Ranson criteria has classically been used, but it takes 48 hours to complete the score, by which point the patient's severity of illness will be clinically obvious.[96] A more modern scoring system, the BISAP score (BUN, impaired mental status, SIRS criteria, age, and pleural effusion; Table 24-5) can be performed on initial evaluation, and may be helpful in directing patient triage. Patients with a BISAP score of 3 or greater should be considered for triage to an intensive care unit given

TABLE 24-5 BISAP Score

Score components (1 point each)	**B**UN > 25 **I**mpaired mental status Presence of **S**IRS criteria **A**ge > 60 y **P**leural effusion present
Number of Points	**Mortality**
0	0.1%
1	0.5%
2	1.9%
3	5.3%
4	12.7%
5	22.5%

BISAP = BUN, impaired mental status, SIRS criteria, age, pleural effusion; SIRS = systemic inflammatory response syndrome.

the increased risk of mortality.[101] It should be noted that ACG guidelines do not recommend the use of any single scoring system over another to predict the severity of pancreatitis.[96]

Severity of pancreatitis is described by the modified Atlanta criteria. Patients with mild acute pancreatitis do not have evidence of local complications (eg, necrotizing pancreatitis) or evidence of organ failure. Patients with moderately severe pancreatitis may have local complications or only *transient* organ failure that resolves within 48 hours, while patients with severe pancreatitis have persistent organ failure lasting more than 48 hours. Organ failure is defined as evidence of concomitant GI bleeding, shock with a systolic blood pressure less than 90 mmHg, respiratory failure with Pao_2 of 60% or less, or renal failure with creatinine of 2 mg/dL or greater.[96]

As discussed in Chapter 32, "Nutrition," initiation of early enteral feeding has been shown to improve outcomes via a reduced risk of infectious complications and may accelerate recovery. In mild pancreatitis, feeding may be initiated as soon as the patient wishes to eat.[102] A soft, low-fat diet may be initiated immediately, without a need to "bridge" from NPO status using a clear-liquid diet as an intermediary. There does not appear to be a significant benefit to initiating feeding within 24 hours compared to "on-demand" feeding.[103] For patients with moderately severe or severe pancreatitis who are unable to take in food orally, enteral feeding via nasogastric or nasojejunal tube should be initiated within 3 to 5 days of admission to the ICU. Currently, the data do not strongly support the use of nasojejunal feeding over nasogastric, although these data are evolving.[104] Parenteral nutrition has been demonstrated to increase the risk of infection in patients with acute pancreatitis and should be avoided.[105]

In patients with mild gallstone pancreatitis, early cholecystectomy (performed during the index hospitalization) may significantly reduce the risk of recurrent pancreatitis compared to delayed cholecystectomy (eg, within 30 days of discharge).[106] Surgery should be delayed for patients with moderate to severe pancreatitis or in those with local complications, as cholecystectomy in this setting is technically challenging and may have a higher risk of morbidity and mortality.[107] Patients who have alcoholic pancreatitis should be counseled regarding the severe consequences of further drinking and referred to a structured relapse prevention program.[108]

Pancreatitis may be complicated by the development of local fluid collections. Pseudocysts typically develop more than 4 weeks after an initial bout of pancreatitis. They are simple fluid collections lined with a fibrous capsule. They do not require intervention unless they cause symptoms or biliary obstruction, as in this case. The management of pseudocysts most often involves creation of an endoscopic (less commonly surgical) cystogastrostomy using endoscopic ultrasound-guided insertion of one or many stents through the gastric wall into the pseudocyst, to allow drainage of contents into the gastric lumen.

TABLE 24-6 Pancreatic Fluid Collections

	Necrosis Absent	Necrosis Present
< 4 wk	Acute peripancreatic fluid collection	Necrotizing pancreatitis
> 4 wk	Pseudocyst	Walled-off pancreatic necrosis

There are 4 distinct fluid collections that may develop in the setting of acute pancreatitis, and their management differs. They may be divided by their time course of development (before or after 4 weeks) and by the presence or absence of necrosis (Table 24-6).

Acute peripancreatic fluid collections are a manifestation of interstitial pancreatitis and will typically resolve without intervention. Necrotizing pancreatitis is visualized on CT with IV contrast as a nonenhancing component of the gland and is typically associated with a surrounding fluid collection that consists both of simple fluid and debris. Sterile necrosis does not require specific intervention and will typically resolve spontaneously. As discussed previously, infected pancreatic necrosis typically manifests as a failure of a patient to improve with conservative management and/or clinical worsening after an initial improvement. Up to 60% of patients may respond to therapy with antibiotics alone, but most patients require necrosectomy, which is typically performed endoscopically. The patient is managed conservatively until a stable, walled-off collection organizes, as such collections are technically easier to manage than an unorganized phlegmon. In a patient who is acutely worsening despite antibiotic therapy, and in whom the necrotic tissue is not yet walled off (limiting the likelihood of success of endoscopic necrosectomy), percutaneous drainage of the necrotic collection may be necessary. Open surgery for pancreatic necrosectomy is associated with significant morbidity and mortality and is typically deferred in favor of endoscopic or percutaneous techniques.[99,109]

In addition to pancreatic fluid collections, pancreatitis may be complicated by the development of splenic vein thrombosis, which develops as a reaction to the intense inflammatory response around the pancreas. Splenic vein thrombosis may lead to the development of gastric varices, which can subsequently lead to life-threatening hemorrhage. Doppler ultrasound of the abdomen should be performed in a patient who develops variceal bleeding after a bout of pancreatitis to assess for the presence of splenic vein thrombosis.[110]

Finally, patients may develop a wide range of systemic complications due to pancreatitis. These include organ dysfunction (eg, acute kidney injury and acute respiratory distress syndrome), metabolic disturbances such as hyperglycemia and hypocalcemia, and the abdominal compartment syndrome.[110] Fat necrosis may occur in subcutaneous fat tissue overlying bony prominences, presumably due to circulating lipase.[111]

LIVER DISEASE AND TRANSPLANTATION

Acute Liver Failure

Acute liver failure (ALF) is defined as the development of jaundice, coagulopathy (INR ≥ 1.5), and encephalopathy in a patient without any known preexisting liver condition with a time to disease onset of less than 26 weeks.[112] Without transplantation, acute liver failure carries a mortality of approximately 85%.[113] The King's College criteria (Table 24-7) can be used to prognosticate which patients will require transplantation, with a sensitivity of 68% to 69% and specificity of 82% to 92%.[114] Patients with suspected ALF should be transferred to a liver transplant center as soon as possible and should have a workup initiated to place the patient on the liver transplant (LT) waiting list. Given the extraordinarily high mortality in the absence of LT, patients with ALF are given the highest priority (status 1) on the LT waitlist.

Acetaminophen overdose is the leading cause of acute liver failure in the United States and Europe. Because acetaminophen metabolism may differ among patients, especially if there is concomitant use of alcohol or other drugs, the administration of N-acetylcysteine (NAC) is recommended in all cases of suspected acetaminophen-induced ALF, no matter what the measured serum level of acetaminophen is.[115] N-acetylcysteine works by replenishing intrahepatic glutathione stores, which subsequently allows the conversion of toxic acetaminophen metabolites to nontoxic forms. In cases where there is apparent hepatotoxicity (eg, elevated transaminases) but no evidence of acute liver failure, NAC should be continued until liver enzymes normalize.[116] Data also suggest that NAC is useful in the management of non-acetaminophen-induced ALF; administration is therefore indicated regardless of etiology of liver failure.[117] Other common etiologies for ALF include viral hepatitis (hepatitis A virus [HAV], hepatitis B virus [HBV], varicella zoster virus [VZV], and herpes simplex virus [HSV]), autoimmune hepatitis, Wilson disease, non-acetaminophen drug-induced liver injury (DILI), mushroom (*Amanita phalloides*) poisoning, acute fatty liver

of pregnancy, and vascular disorders (eg, acute Budd-Chiari syndrome).

Aside from disease-directed therapy such as the use of NAC for patients with acetaminophen overdose, penicillin G for *Amanita* toxicity, antiviral therapy (eg, entecavir/tenofovir for fulminant HBV infection, acyclovir for HSV/VZV hepatitis), steroid therapy for autoimmune hepatitis, and prompt delivery of the fetus in acute fatty liver of pregnancy, there are several general management points to consider in patients with ALF. Coagulopathy should generally not be corrected in the absence of overt bleeding or if necessary in the setting of invasive procedures, as progression or recovery of coagulopathy can be utilized to prognosticate the outcome in ALF. As patients with ALF often have leukocytosis, hypotension, and other features of SIRS, it may be difficult to identify patients who also have an underlying infectious process contributing to their clinical syndrome. Blood cultures should be obtained and antibiotics initiated if underlying infection is suspected, although prophylactic antibiotics or antifungals have not been demonstrated to improve outcomes. Empiric antibiotics should also be considered in patients who develop an abrupt clinical deterioration. Hypoglycemia may develop due to hepatic dysfunction, and IV fluids containing dextrose may be necessary to maintain blood glucose. Vasopressor support may be required to maintain mean arterial pressures of at least 75 mmHg to maintain cerebral perfusion pressures. In the setting of acute renal failure, renal replacement therapy may be necessary; given the hemodynamic compromise so often present in ALF, patients will often not tolerate intermittent hemodialysis, and a continuous mode of renal replacement therapy is often necessary.[112] Patients with ALF due to Wilson disease are at especially high risk for AKI, as circulating copper damages renal tubules. Laboratory values, including complete blood count (CBC), chemistries, liver function tests, INR, and fibrinogen should be drawn at least every 4 hours. Phosphate levels should be monitored; hypophosphatemia is a good prognostic marker and is thought to represent a high metabolic demand in a regenerating liver.[118]

The development of hepatic encephalopathy is a cardinal feature of ALF, and because its etiology is somewhat different from that seen in cirrhosis, management differs. Cerebral edema is often present among patients with grade III or IV encephalopathy. It may eventually progress to brainstem herniation, which is universally fatal. A baseline CT of the head should be obtained to rule out alternate causes of altered mental status and to provide baseline neuroimaging. In contrast to patients with cirrhosis, lactulose should *not* be administered to patients with ALF, as gaseous abdominal distension generated by lactulose may ultimately make emergent transplantation more technically challenging. Further, its use has not been shown to improve outcomes. Once patients reach grade III or IV encephalopathy, the likelihood for developing cerebral edema is high, and patients should be intubated and sedated to minimize intracranial pressures (ICP). Measures including keeping the head of the

TABLE 24-7 King's College Criteria

Acetaminophen-Induced ALF	Non-acetaminophen-Induced ALF
Arterial pH < 7.30 **OR** Lactate > 3.5 mmol/L **OR** Grade III or IV encephalopathy **PLUS** • INR > 6.5 • Cr > 3.4 mg/dL	INR > 6.5 with HE of any grade **OR** Any 3 of criteria below with HE • Age < 10 or > 40 y • Bilirubin > 300 mmol/L • Coagulation: INR > 3.5 • Duration of jaundice to HE > 7 d • Etiology: seronegative viral hepatitis, Wilson disease, non-acetaminophen DILI

ALF = acute liver failure; Cr = creatinine; DILI = drug-induced liver injury; HE = hepatic encephalopathy; INR = international normalized ratio.

bed at 30 degrees, minimizing deep suctioning, and minimizing procedures that may be uncomfortable or painful may avoid increases in ICP. Consultation with a neurosurgical team familiar with noninvasive (eg, changes in pupillary size, posturing, changes in peripheral reflexes) and invasive ICP monitoring should be obtained. Invasive ICP monitoring is helpful in identifying early changes in ICP, but it carries associated risks, especially in the setting of ALF in which patients may be coagulopathic. If elevated ICP is detected, specific interventions to reduce ICP are indicated. Such interventions include the use of mannitol (bolus dose of 0.5–1 g/kg, repeated up to a total of 3 doses), hypertonic saline (to maintain serum sodium 145–155 mEq/L), and hyperventilation to a $Paco_2$ of 25 to 30 mmHg.[112]

Patients are able to be listed for top priority (status 1) for liver transplantation when they have fulminant liver failure, and when they are in the ICU requiring ventilatory support, hemodialysis, and have an INR of greater than 2.[119]

Cirrhosis and End-Stage Liver Disease

Cirrhosis is a pathological diagnosis defined by the replacement of normal hepatic parenchyma with nodules of hepatocytes surrounded by fibrous tissue. A variety of insults may lead to this endpoint, many examples of which are listed in Table 24-8. Patients with cirrhosis are at risk of dying due to complications of hepatic dysfunction and portal hypertension. In addition, patients with cirrhosis of any etiology are at a 2% to 4% annual risk of developing hepatocellular carcinoma.[120]

On exam, patients may have obvious clinical ascites, peripheral edema, jaundice, spider angiomata, sarcopenia (muscle wasting), caput medusae, splenomegaly, and palmar erythema. Men may develop gynecomastia and testicular atrophy. On laboratory testing, patients will exhibit thrombocytopenia, hypoalbuminemia, hyperbilirubinemia, and abnormalities in blood coagulation including an elevation in the prothrombin time or INR.

Complications of Portal Hypertension

Patients with cirrhosis typically present to the ICU when complications of portal hypertension lead to hepatic decompensation. Portal hypertension develops due to numerous changes in the normal physiology of portal blood flow. Alterations in the hepatic sinusoidal architecture due to fibrosis leads to increased intrahepatic vascular resistance. At the same time,

splanchnic and systemic vasodilation, along with increased cardiac output leads to a hyperdynamic circulation, which increases portal venous inflow. The increased pressure in the portal system is initially reduced via formation of portosystemic collaterals, of which gastroesophageal varices are one example.[121] As portal pressures increase, complications including variceal hemorrhage, ascites, and portosystemic encephalopathy may develop.

Variceal Hemorrhage

Variceal hemorrhage is a manifestation of decompensated cirrhosis and typically occurs when the hepatic venous pressure gradient (HVPG) exceeds 12 mmHg (normal < 5 mmHg). Its mortality depends on whether variceal hemorrhage develops as an isolated decompensating event or it occurs in conjunction with other complications, including ascites (20% 5-year mortality vs > 80% 5-year mortality). Six-week mortality after a single variceal bleed ranges from 15% to 25%.[121]

Initial management centers around effective resuscitation. As discussed previously in "Upper Gastrointestinal Bleeding," blood should be transfused to a goal hemoglobin of 7 g/dL; patients with Child-Pugh or Child-Turcotte-Pugh classes A and B cirrhosis had significantly lower mortality and rebleeding rates than patients transfused to a higher threshold of 9 g/dL.[7] Correcting coagulopathy using FFP has not been shown to alter outcomes, as the INR in cirrhotics does not accurately reflect the true degree of coagulopathy. Further, transfusion of FFP in addition to blood could contribute to overtransfusion and an increase of portal pressures, perhaps increasing the risk of rebleeding.[122] Antibiotic prophylaxis should be given to patients with cirrhosis and GI bleeding of *any* etiology. Ceftriaxone 1 g every 24 hours for a duration of 7 days has been shown to reduce rates of bacterial infection, rebleeding, and mortality.[123] Vasoactive agents that induce splanchnic vasoconstriction (eg, octreotide or terlipressin) can reduce portal inflow and therefore portal pressures, leading to improved control of bleeding, reduced transfusion requirements, and reduced all-cause mortality.[124] Octreotide is the only agent available in the United States, and it is given at a dose of a 50 μg IV bolus followed by 50 μg/h. An IV proton pump inhibitor is also given as initial therapy when the hemorrhage is not variceal but from a source that would benefit from antisecretory therapy (eg, peptic ulcer disease); the PPI may be discontinued if said alternative etiology is not found.

TABLE 24-8 Common Etiologies of Cirrhosis

Viral	Metabolic	Toxic	Vascular	Autoimmune	Biliary
Hepatitis B	Nonalcoholic fatty liver disease	Alcohol-related liver disease	Chronic Budd-Chiari syndrome	Autoimmune hepatitis Primary biliary cholangitis	Secondary biliary cirrhosis (eg, gallstone disease)
Hepatitis C	α₁-antitrypsin deficiency Hemochromatosis Glycogen storage disorders	Chronic drug-induced liver injury		Primary sclerosing cholangitis	Biliary atresia

Endoscopy should be performed within 12 hours of presentation, and varices ligated if either active bleeding or stigmata of recent hemorrhage (eg, a white nipple or red wale sign) are present.[121] If hemorrhage is controlled with variceal ligation, octreotide should be continued for 5 days and antibiotics continued for a total of 7 days. Antibiotics may be switched to oral if the patient is otherwise ready for discharge. If rebleeding occurs and repeat endoscopic therapy is not successful, or if initial bleeding is refractory to endoscopic therapy, then emergent placement of a transjugular intrahepatic portosystemic shunt (TIPS) is indicated. Balloon tamponade with a Sengstaken-Blakemore tube may be necessary to control hemorrhage while awaiting TIPS.[121] The tube is inserted nasally or orally past the 50 cm mark. Then, suction is applied to the gastric and esophageal ports. The gastric balloon is inflated with 250 to 500 mL of air. It is pulled back up to the resistance from the diaphragm, usually at 30 to 35 cm. Traction is applied via a pulley system with 1 Liter of crystalloid fluid as counterweight. If bleeding occurs via esophageal port, the esophageal balloon is inflated to 30 to 45 mmHg. If bleeding persists despite inflation of esophageal and gastric balloon, traction is increased. If bleeding is controlled, the esophageal balloon is titrated down to 25 mmHg to prevent necrosis. Sengstaken-Blakemore tubes are generally kept in place for 24 hours.

If the patient had bleeding gastric varices, the initial management would be similar, with resuscitation and initiation of IV PPI, octreotide, and ceftriaxone. Hemostatic therapy may differ depending upon the location of the varices and local expertise. Gastric varices that are continuous with esophageal varices (GOV1) may be treated either with band ligation or with injection of cyanoacrylate, if available. Cardiofundal varices must often be treated with TIPS or with balloon-occluded retrograde transvenous obliteration (BRTO), in which the varices are obliterated via injection of a sclerosant into a feeding gastrorenal shunt.[121]

Secondary prophylaxis should be administered to patients who have survived a variceal bleed, as rebleeding rates may be as high as 60%. For patients who have recovered from an initial episode of variceal bleeding, secondary prophylaxis typically involves combination therapy with lowering of portal pressures with a nonselective beta-blocker and local therapy of varices with variceal ligation. Nonselective beta-blockers exert their effect on portal pressures by reducing splanchnic inflow in 2 ways: they reduce cardiac output, and they block β_2 receptors in the splanchnic arterial bed, leading to unopposed α-adrenergic activity and vasoconstriction.[121,125] Either nadolol, propranolol, or carvedilol may be used for prophylaxis. Variceal ligation should be repeated every 2 to 4 weeks until varices are completely eradicated.

For patients who have never bled from varices, recommendations for primary prophylaxis differ. Patients with medium- to large-sized varices should receive prophylaxis, while patients with small varices should only receive prophylaxis if they have Child-Pugh class B or C cirrhosis or if their varices exhibit red wale signs. Primary prophylaxis may include monotherapy with a traditional nonselective beta-blocker (eg, nadolol or propranolol), carvedilol, or serial esophageal variceal ligation.

Hepatic Encephalopathy

Hepatic encephalopathy is a frequent problem affecting patients with end-stage liver disease. It is one of the complications of cirrhosis that defines decompensation.[121] It has a wide range of manifestations, and its presentation ranges from mild impairments in executive functioning to subtle changes in personality to coma. Disturbances of the sleep/wake cycle are common. In addition to confusion, patients may present with clinical exam findings including asterixis, which is defined as a negative myoclonus of the wrists resulting from a loss of postural tone.[126] Diagnosis is made on clinical grounds, and ammonia levels can be helpful when the diagnosis of HE is in question. Encephalopathy can be graded based on clinical presentation:

- Grade 1: trivial lack of awareness, euphoria or anxiety, shortened attention span, altered sleep cycle
- Grade 2: lethargy/apathy, disorientation to time, obvious personality change, asterixis
- Grade 3: somnolence/semistupor, gross confusion, response to stimuli
- Grade 4: coma, not responsive even to painful stimuli

Hepatic encephalopathy may be precipitated by several factors, such as nonadherence to medical therapy, acute GI bleeding, constipation, infection, hypokalemia, hypoxia, hypoglycemia, and renal failure.[127] Any of these acute insults can precipitate HE in a patient whose HE is otherwise well controlled. The presence of occult portosystemic shunts (eg, gastrorenal shunt) may precipitate refractory encephalopathy. The standard of care for treatment of HE remains lactulose, which should be given to achieve 2 to 3 soft bowel movements per day. In the setting of acute encephalopathy, it is given every 1 to 2 hours until 2 soft bowel movements occur, after which it is spaced out to prevent diarrhea and dehydration.[126] In patients who are obtunded, it may be necessary to instill lactulose via nasogastric tube and/or via enemas. In addition to the laxative effect, lactulose is thought to enhance ammonia removal from the body via acidification of the stool by production of lactic acid, which enhances the conversion of ammonia to ammonium; because ammonium is charged and cannot easily be absorbed by the gut, it is excreted in the stool. Lactulose may cause excessive bloating; in patients who are intolerant of lactulose, a polyethylene glycol solution may be substituted with nearly equal efficacy.[128] Rifaximin has good efficacy for the prevention of HE recurrence in combination with lactulose among patients with prior episodes of hospitalization for HE.[129] It is not effective as monotherapy in the acute setting. Numerous studies have investigated the use of other agents for the treatment of HE (eg, L-ornithine L-aspartate, glutaminase inhibitors, and flumazenil); however, none has been found to be superior to the current standard of care.[126]

Ascites

The circulatory dysfunction present in cirrhosis predisposes patients to the development of refractory ascites, hyponatremia, and hepatorenal syndrome (HRS).[130] As portal hypertension progresses, systemic and splanchnic vasodilation worsens, leading to a low effective circulating volume. This activates the renin-angiotensin-aldosterone system, as well as the nonosmotic release of arginine vasopressin (AVP), which results in renal retention of sodium and water, contributing to the development of ascites and edema.[131] A serum ascites–albumin gradient (SAAG) greater than 1.1 g/dL indicates portal hypertension and nonperitoneal causes of ascites, and an SAAG less than 1.1 g/dL indicates nonportal hypertension and peritoneal causes of ascites. While initially managed with dietary sodium restriction and diuretics, ascites may become refractory to medical therapy due to a lack of response to maximum doses (typically 120 mg/d of furosemide and 400 mg/d of spironolactone) or when kidney injury or electrolyte abnormalities occur at submaximal doses.[132] In patients with medically refractory ascites, serial large-volume paracentesis may be necessary to control symptoms. Up to 10 Liters of ascites can typically be removed for symptomatic relief. American Association for the Study of Liver Diseases (AASLD) guidelines recommend giving 6 to 8 g/L of albumin after or during paracentesis that removes more than 4 to 5 Liters of ascites to prevent postparacentesis circulatory dysfunction.[133] Twenty-five percent albumin is usually given, as this provides a lower volume load. A transjugular intrahepatic portosystemic shunt also is effective at controlling refractory ascites in select patients.[134] Patients with ascites are at high risk for the development of umbilical hernias. Elective hernia repair surgery may be risky in patients with significant portal hypertension, although risks of surgery must be weighed against the risks of incarceration, strangulation, and rupture of the hernia. A comprehensive preoperative risk assessment by members of the hepatology and surgical teams would be beneficial in making a decision regarding herniorrhaphy or any other surgical intervention.[135]

Spontaneous Bacterial Peritonitis

Spontaneous bacterial peritonitis (SBP) is common, affecting up to 12% of hospitalized cirrhotic patients. Patients may not present with abdominal pain but may present with encephalopathy or changes in biochemical parameters, including rising bilirubin, creatinine, or INR. Therefore, routine diagnostic paracentesis, even in the absence of clinical peritonitis, is warranted to rule out infection. Spontaneous bacterial peritonitis is diagnosed when polymorphonuclear neutrophil (PMN) count is 250 cells/mm³ or greater, when an ascitic culture is positive, and when there are no secondary causes of peritonitis. In hemorrhagic or traumatic paracentesis, a corrected PMN count is achieved by subtracting 1 PMN for every 250 red cells/mm³. Secondary bacterial peritonitis can be distinguished by its ascitic total protein

of greater than 1 g/dL, ascitic glucose less than 50 mg/dL, ascitic LDH greater than the upper limit of serum, and polymicrobial cultures.

Treatment of SBP is directed at the 3 most common isolates: *Escherichia coli*, *Klebsiella pneumoniae*, and *Streptococcus pneumoniae*, with cefotaxime 2 g every 8 hours as the antibiotic of choice. Other third-generation cephalosporins (eg, ceftriaxone 1 g twice daily) may be substituted if cefotaxime is not available.[133] In addition to antibiotics, the use of IV albumin has been shown to reduce the development of hepatorenal syndrome and subsequent mortality among patients with SBP. The recommended regimen is 1.5 g/kg of IV albumin on day 1, followed by 1 g/kg on day 3 in patients with a creatinine of greater than 1 mg/dL, a BUN of greater than 30 mg/dL, or a total bilirubin of greater than 4 mg/dL.[136] Treatment should be continued for a total of 5 days. In patients who do not improve clinically, repeat diagnostic paracentesis may be advised to determine whether neutrophilia in the ascites is resolving; persistent neutrophilia may indicate the presence of antibiotic resistance or secondary peritonitis. Cross-sectional and imaging analysis of LDH and glucose levels in the ascitic fluid may also be helpful to rule out a secondary source.

Patients should receive prophylaxis to prevent SBP in the following instances:

- Active GI bleeding
- Patients who have survived an episode of SBP
- Ascitic fluid total protein less than 1.5 g/dL PLUS impaired renal function (creatinine > 1.2 mg/dL, BUN > 25 g/dL, or Na < 130 mEq/L) OR liver failure (Child-Turcotte-Pugh Score > 8 or bilirubin > 3 mg/dL)

Recommended regimens for prophylaxis include a quinolone (norfloxacin or ciprofloxacin) or trimethoprim/sulfamethoxazole. American Association for the Study of Liver Diseases guidelines recommend daily administration rather than weekly given the risk of fostering antibiotic resistance with intermittent dosing.[133]

Hepatorenal Syndrome

Hepatorenal syndrome is a form of acute kidney injury that occurs in the context of cirrhosis. A low effective circulating volume combined with inadequate cardiac output and renal vasoconstriction lead to reduced renal blood flow, ultimately causing a reduction in glomerular filtration rate (GFR).[137] Hepatorenal syndrome is divided into 2 types: (1) HRS-1 or HRS-AKI, which is currently defined as acute kidney injury with an increase in serum creatinine of at least 0.3 mg/dL or 1.5- to 2-fold from baseline within 7 days that is unresponsive to 2 days of diuretic withdrawal and volume challenge with 1 g/kg of albumin (up to 100 g), or (2) HRS-2, which is defined by a more gradual reduction in GFR. In all cases, shock must be absent, and there should be no other etiology of kidney disease noted (eg, absence of proteinuria on urinalysis).[138] Urine studies may be helpful to confirm the diagnosis;

a urine sodium of less than 20 mEq/L along with a bland urine sediment is typically seen.

Because many of the clinical and laboratory findings found in HRS may also be seen in patients with prerenal azotemia, diuretic withdrawal and volume expansion with albumin, as noted above, serves both as a diagnostic and therapeutic tool. If these measures do not improve renal function, vasoconstrictor therapy with the combination of midodrine and octreotide has been shown to be successful in improving outcomes in patients with HRS-1.[139] Many patients ultimately require renal replacement therapy (RRT), but this is a temporizing measure; once a patient requires RRT for HRS, the 30-day mortality increases to 73% without liver transplantation.[140] Renal function typically returns to normal after transplantation.

Hyponatremia

Nearly one-third of patients with cirrhosis develop at least mild hyponatremia (Na < 135 mEq/L).[141] Hyponatremia is associated with increased mortality in cirrhosis and now factors into the Model for End-Stage Liver Disease (MELD-Na) score to give increased priority to patients with hyponatremia on the liver transplant waiting list.[142-144] The primary treatment for asymptomatic hyponatremia in cirrhosis is fluid restriction. Patients are typically instructed not to drink more than 1 to 1.5 L/d, although this is often difficult for patients to tolerate.[145] As an adjunct to fluid restriction, infusion of albumin may help to raise serum sodium among patients with cirrhosis and hyponatremia.[146] Because hyponatremia develops chronically among patients with cirrhosis, correction of serum sodium should occur slowly, limiting increases in serum Na to less than 8 to 10 mEq/L in 24 hours and less than 18 mEq/L in 48 hours.[147] In the setting of neurological symptoms (eg, seizures), consultation with nephrology is necessary, and patients may require a more rapid increase in their serum sodium via infusion of hypertonic saline.

Hyponatremia can also be a complication of LT. Patients who are hyponatremic at the time of LT, especially those with pretransplant sodium of less than 125 to 130 mEq/L are at risk for a rapid intraoperative increase in serum sodium, which can predispose patients to osmotic demyelination syndrome.[148,149] Postoperatively, it is essential on the part of the critical care team to closely monitor changes in serum sodium and ensure that sodium does not rise too rapidly from the pretransplant sodium level.

Liver Transplantation

With few exceptions (eg, cure of hepatitis C with direct-acting antiviral therapy, abstinence from alcohol), the clinical course of cirrhosis is almost invariably progressive, with development of complications of portal hypertension or hepatocellular carcinoma. Once these complications develop, liver transplantation is the only true "cure" for many patients. In addition to end-stage liver disease, indications for LT may include acute

TABLE 24-9A   Model for End-Stage Liver Disease Score

Scoring System	Equation
MELD	$0.957 \times \ln(\text{creatinine mg/dL}) + 0.378 \times \ln(\text{bilirubin mg/dL}) + 1.120 \times \ln(\text{INR}) + 0.643$
MELD-Na[a]	$\text{MELD} = \text{MELD(i)} + 1.32 \times (137 - \text{Na}) - (0.033 \times \text{MELD(i)} \times [137\text{-Na}])$

TABLE 24-9B   MELD Score and Associated Mortality

MELD Score	Mortality
< 9	1.9%
10–19	6.0%
20–29	19.6%
30–39	52.6%
≥ 40	71.3%

INR = international normalized ratio; MELD = Model for End-Stage Liver Disease. MELD(i) = Initial MELD. Na = Sodium. Calculator available at https://optn. transplant.hrsa.gov/resources/allocation-calculators/meld-calculator/.

[a] Na < 125 entered as 125, and Na > 137 entered as 137.

liver failure, hepatocellular carcinoma, recurrent cholangitis in a patient with primary sclerosing cholangitis, intractable pruritus in patients with primary biliary cholangitis, hepatopulmonary syndrome, portopulmonary hypertension, or metabolic disease that may be cured by liver transplantation, among others.[150] Patients must undergo an extensive battery of testing prior to being listed for LT, which includes evaluation by hepatology, transplant surgery, cardiology, social work, psychiatry, and infectious disease.[150] Patients are listed in order of priority based on the MELD-Na score (Tables 24-9A and 24-9B). The MELD-Na score incorporates laboratory values including serum bilirubin, creatinine, sodium, and INR, and has been shown to predict 90-day mortality among patients with cirrhosis.[119] Prior to use of the MELD-Na score, the Child-Turcotte-Pugh (CTP) score (which incorporates serum bilirubin, albumin, INR, and degrees of ascites and encephalopathy) was utilized to order patients on the transplant list (Table 24-10). While the CTP score is no longer utilized to determine priority on the LT waiting list, it retains value as a prognostic score for cirrhotic patients, especially those planned to undergo abdominal surgery (although MELD can also provide data on perioperative risk).[151]

Patients who are on the transplant waiting list but are in the ICU are often temporarily too sick to undergo transplant surgery, which is an arduous procedure that involves long operative times and may involve a high levels of blood loss. For a patient to survive transplant surgery, it is essential that he or she be as optimized as possible, which involves treating any acute insults—especially infection—that may compromise a patient's chances of recovering successfully after transplantation.

TABLE 24-10 Child-Turcotte-Pugh Score

	Points		
	1	2	3
Encephalopathy	None	Grade 1–2	Grade 3–4
Ascites	None	Mild-moderate (ie, diuretic responsive)	Severe or refractory
Bilirubin (mg/dL)	< 2	2–3	> 3
Albumin (g/dL)	> 3.5	2.8–3.5	< 2.8
INR	< 1.7	1.7–2.3	> 2.3
Operative Mortality Risk			
5–6 points = CTP class A	10%		
7–9 points = CTP class B	30%		
10–15 points = CTP class C	82%		

CTP = Child-Turcotte-Pugh; INR = international normalized ratio. Calculator available at http://www.hepatitisc.uw.edu/page/clinical-calculators/ctp.

The immediate post-transplant period is a precarious time; close monitoring for the development of complications is essential. Infectious complications in the immediate post-transplant period (< 30 days) are those that may be seen after any major surgery and/or prolonged hospitalization. They include wound infections, intra-abdominal abscesses, and bilomas. Early administration of appropriate empiric antibiotic therapy and consultation with surgical colleagues for intra-abdominal source control (if necessary) is essential. Opportunistic (eg, CMV, herpesviridae, *Pneumocystis* species, and *Candida* species) infections typically occur within 1 to 6 months post-transplant. Patients should be started on a regimen of prophylactic antibiotic, antiviral, and antifungal therapy immediately post-transplantation to prevent these complications. An example regimen might include clotrimazole troches or fluconazole for antifungal prophylaxis, valacyclovir or acyclovir for antiviral prophylaxis (depending upon CMV status of the donor and recipient), and trimethoprim-sulfamethoxazole for *Pneumocystis* prophylaxis. After 6 to 12 months, post-LT patients are no longer on intensive immunosuppression, and their risk of infection is similar to that of the general population. Consultation should be obtained from the transplant hepatology team for assistance in immunosuppression management for any patient in the ICU.[152]

Vascular complications may result in poor graft function. Hepatic artery thrombosis (HAT) may occur early (< 30 days) or late (> 30 days) in the post-transplant course, and the clinical presentations differ depending on the timing with which HAT develops. Early HAT may be characterized by the development of graft dysfunction and possibly fulminant hepatic failure, which may lead to mortality without retransplantation.[153] Risk factors include technical issues related to the initial transplant (including complex arterial reconstruction, the use of arterial conduits, prolonged procedure time) as well as patient-related factors (retransplantation vs primary transplantation, low recipient weight).[153,154]

Diagnosis is typically made via Doppler ultrasonography of the hepatic artery. Graft survival is improved with early detection and revascularization via thrombectomy or stenting, although many patients require retransplantation. Graft and patient survival after retransplantation for early HAT is lower than after primary LT.[153] Late HAT typically presents in a less dramatic fashion, with biliary complications including bilomas and biliary strictures, as the hepatic artery is the primary blood supply to the bile ducts.[155]

Portal vein thrombosis (PVT) may also occur in the immediate post-transplant setting. Its incidence ranges from 0.5% to 15%, and is more common in pediatric patients.[152] It also may be more common among patients with pre-LT PVT.[156] Patients may present with rising aminotransferases, as well as complications of portal hypertension like persistent ascites or variceal hemorrhage. Management includes emergent surgical thrombectomy, but in many cases retransplantation may be required. The presence of PVT may make this technically challenging.[152,156] Routine Doppler ultrasonography in the immediate post-transplant period may be helpful in the early identification of vascular complications.

Due to the high level of immunosuppression administered in the immediate post-transplantation period, acute cellular rejection is relatively rare unless appropriate levels of immunosuppression are not maintained.[152] Hyperacute or antibody-mediated rejection, however, may occur despite appropriate levels of conventional immunosuppression due to the presence of preformed antibodies that deposit in the endothelium of the graft and lead to complement fixation and cell death. It is common in ABO-incompatible transplants but may also occur in patients who receive an ABO-compatible organ. Patients will present with graft dysfunction; biopsy may help confirm the diagnosis.[157] Management may include a combination of high-dose steroids, thymoglobulin, rituximab, plasma exchange, and IV immunoglobulin. Retransplantation may be required.

QUESTIONS

1. A 67-year-old man with a history of hypertension, diabetes, and osteoarthritis presents with a 1-day history of black stool. Since his symptoms began, he endorses about 2 to 3 black bowel movements; he notes that there also appears to be a rim of red around the black stool noted on the toilet paper. He began to feel lightheaded and dizzy at home, so he came to the ED. There, he was found to have the following vital signs: BP of 77/46 mmHg, HR of 110 beats/min, RR of 12 breaths/min, oxygen saturation (Sao$_2$) of 99%, and temperature of 36.4°C (97.5°F). His labs included the following:

WBC	$12 \times 10^3/\mu L$
Hgb	5.5 g/dL (baseline: 12 g/dL)
plt	$197 \times 10^3/\mu L$
Na	138 mEq/L
K	4.0 mEq/L
Cl	107 mEq/L
CO$_2$	24 mEq/L
BUN	35 mg/dL
Creatinine	1.1 mg/dL

On further questioning, a few days prior to the start of his symptoms he tripped and fell, exacerbating the pain from his osteoarthritis. Resuscitation is begun in the ED, and the patient is admitted to the ICU for further monitoring. In addition to large-bore IV access, NPO status, and blood transfusion, what is the most appropriate next step in management?

A. Nasogastric tube placement
B. Pantoprazole 80 mg IV × 1 with initiation of pantoprazole drip at 8 mg/h
C. Pantoprazole 40 mg IV every 12 hours
D. Pantoprazole 40 mg PO every 12 hours

2. A patient admitted for upper GI bleeding has an endoscopy. A clean-based ulcer with a nonbleeding visible vessel is noted in the duodenal sweep. It is treated by the endoscopist with injection of epinephrine and bipolar cautery with excellent hemostasis. What is the most appropriate immediate postendoscopic management and disposition for the patient?

A. Discharge home the following day on a daily dose of PO PPI
B. Keep in ICU and repeat endoscopy in 24 hours to ensure continued hemostasis
C. Transfer to floor and start patient on PO PPI
D. Transfer to floor and continue IV PPI

3. A 72-year-old woman is admitted to the cardiology ward for management of congestive heart failure. During her hospital stay, she was diagnosed with a thrombus in the left ventricle. She was started on anticoagulation with intravenous heparin, with plans to start warfarin prior to discharge. One day prior to her planned discharge, she developed the acute onset of vague abdominal pain. She described the pain as periumbilical. She denies constipation, diarrhea, melena, or hematochezia. On exam, vital signs were as follows: BP of 110/74 mmHg, HR of 90 beats/min, RR of 18, Sao$_2$ of 98%, and temperature of 37.5°C (99.5°F). Her exam revealed no evidence of tenderness, rebound, or guarding. Bowel sounds were diminished. Rectal exam showed brown stool positive for occult blood. Laboratory testing revealed the following:

WBC	$23 \times 10^3/\mu L$
Hgb	8.2 g/dL
plt	$212 \times 10^3/\mu L$
Na	131 mEq/L
K	4.1 mEq/L
Cl	110 mEq/L
CO$_2$	18 mEq/L
BUN	22 mg/dL
Creatinine	0.8 mg/dL
Lactic acid	7.3 mmol/L

What is the most appropriate next step in management?

A. CT with oral contrast
B. Emergent laparotomy
C. Urgent colonoscopy
D. CT angiography without oral contrast

4. A 23-year-old man is admitted to the ICU after drinking a bottle of drain cleaner in a suicide attempt. He is awake and alert but complains of severe chest pain that began shortly after ingestion. He finds it painful to swallow his own secretions. He appears to be breathing comfortably. His vital signs are as follows: BP of 90/68 mmHg, HR of 101 beats/min, RR of 18, Sao$_2$ of 100%, and temperature of 38.1°C (100.6°F). Examination of the oropharynx reveals erythema but no other lesions. Examination of the chest reveals normal heart sounds, a regular rate and rhythm, and clear lungs. No crepitus is noted on palpation of the chest. X-rays of the chest and abdomen are performed and demonstrate no free air in the mediastinum or peritoneum. Which of the following statements is true regarding this patient's caustic ingestion?

A. Vomiting should be induced to expel any remaining foreign material.
B. An NGT should be inserted to remove any remaining foreign material.
C. The patient should be encouraged to drink water to dilute the drain cleaner.
D. Upper endoscopy should be performed as soon as possible.

5. The patient in question 4 returns 3 months later to the ED after eating a steak dinner. He complains of retrosternal discomfort that started during the meal. He is unable to swallow his own secretions, though he is breathing comfortably. What is the most appropriate next step in management?

   A. Barium esophagram
   B. CT chest with IV and oral contrast
   C. Emergent endoscopic evaluation
   D. Chest X-ray

6. A 76-year-old man is admitted to the ICU for management of a multifocal pneumonia. His course has been complicated by the development of ventilator-dependent respiratory failure and hypotension requiring the use of vasopressors. For sedation, he has been receiving fentanyl and midazolam. He is on broad-spectrum antibiotics. For nutritional support, he was receiving nasogastric feeding. However, for the last 24 hours he has not been able to tolerate feeding and has been vomiting when feeding has been attempted. On exam, he has developed significant abdominal distension. He has not had a bowel movement in the last 24 hours. Abdominal x-ray is performed and seen below (Fig. 24-2).

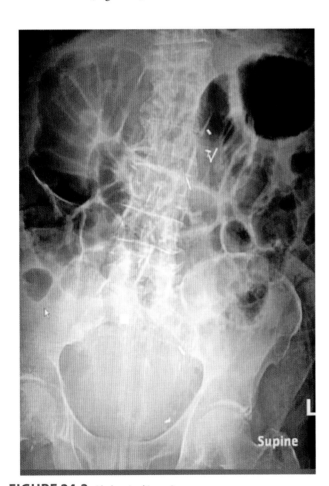

FIGURE 24-2 Abdominal imaging.

What is the most appropriate next step in management?

   A. Emergent laparotomy and exploration
   B. Stop NGT feeds and place NGT to suction
   C. Obtain CT of the abdomen and pelvis with oral and IV contrast
   D. Continue but decrease rate of NGT feeds

7. A 52-year-old woman with a history of hypertension and constipation presents to the ED with LLQ pain. She states that the pain has been present for approximately 3 days. It does not radiate to anywhere else in the abdomen. When the pain first started, she went to her primary care doctor and was prescribed antibiotics. However, the pain has been so bad that she has been unable to tolerate them and her symptoms have progressed. She also believes that she has developed a high fever and had shaking chills. In the ED, she is found to be febrile to 39.7°F (103.4°F), tachycardic to 120 beats/min, with BP of 88/46 mmHg. Her exam is revealing for LLQ tenderness with no rebound or guarding. A CT is performed and is seen below (Fig. 24-3).

Labs demonstrate WBC of $15 \times 10^3/\mu L$, Hgb of 11.2 g/dL, and platelets of $237 \times 10^3/\mu L$; chemistries and liver tests are normal. What is the most appropriate next step in management?

   A. Initiation of intravenous ciprofloxacin and metronidazole
   B. Initiation of oral vancomycin
   C. Exploratory laparotomy
   D. Colonoscopy

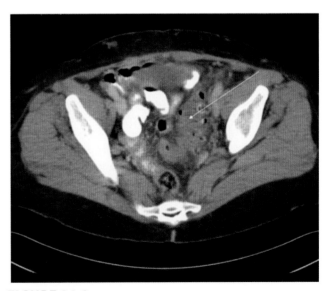

FIGURE 24-3 CT of the abdomen shows sigmoid colonic mural thickening with diverticuli and associated mesocolic fat infiltration. (Reproduced with permission from Cappell MS. Large bowel disorders. In: McKean SC, Ross JJ, Dressler DD, Scheurer DB, eds. *Principles and Practice of Hospital Medicine. 2nd ed.* New York, NY: McGraw-Hill; 2017.)

8. A 50-year-old man was recently discharged from the hospital for sepsis from community-acquired pneumonia. Two weeks later, he returns with profuse, watery diarrhea and abdominal pain. The patient's appetite is reduced, although he can eat and drink normally. Laboratory testing demonstrates the following:

WBC	$23 \times 10^3/\mu L$
Hgb	11.4 g/dL
plt	$525 \times 10^3/\mu L$
Cr	3.7 mg/dL (baseline 1.2 mg/dL)
Albumin	2.3 g/dL

The patient undergoes stool testing and is diagnosed with *C difficile*–associated diarrhea. What is the most appropriate initial antimicrobial therapy?

A. IV vancomycin
B. IV metronidazole
C. PO metronidazole
D. PO vancomycin

9. A 24-year-old woman with a history of ulcerative colitis that was previously well controlled on mesalamine is admitted with 1 week of bloody diarrhea. Previously, her colitis was confined to the left colon and well controlled except for a flare of disease that occurred many years ago and was managed with corticosteroids and topical mesalamine enemas in addition to oral mesalamine. She recently began using NSAIDs for a sports-related injury. Currently, her symptoms include up to 8 bowel movements per day, associated with bleeding and tenesmus but no fever. She called her regular GI doctor when the symptoms began, and she was started on prednisone 40 mg daily. She did not note any improvement in her symptoms and came to the ED. She was initially afebrile, with normal vital signs. Abdominal exam demonstrated mild tenderness in the LLQ but was otherwise normal. Laboratory investigation shows WBC of $12 \times 10^3/\mu L$, Hgb of 8.0 g/dL, and a CRP of 37 mg/L. She undergoes colonoscopy, which shows deep pancolitis that is continuous from the rectum, with deep ulcerations. Biopsies are performed to rule out cytomegalovirus infection. She is admitted to the floor and started on IV steroids. Which of the following statements is true regarding the management of acute severe ulcerative colitis?

A. The patient should be made NPO.
B. The patient should be started on broad-spectrum antibiotics to prevent bacterial translocation from the colon.
C. The patient should be started on low-molecular-weight heparin.
D. Mesalamine should be discontinued.

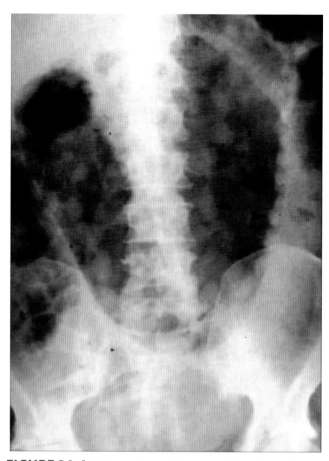

FIGURE 24-4 Abdominal x-ray. (Reproduced from Ahern G, Brygel M. AccessMedicine. *Exploring Essential Radiology*, 2014. Abdomen/Inflammatory Bowel Disease.)

10. The patient in question 9 is admitted for ulcerative colitis exacerbation. Despite 3 days of inpatient treatment, she has persistent diarrhea and bloody bowel movements. She becomes febrile and bleeding progresses; whereas previously bleeding occurred with every other bowel movement, it is now persistent and occurring up to 10 times per day. On exam, she has developed significant abdominal distension. Abdominal x-ray is seen in Figure 24–4.

What is the most appropriate next step?

A. IV infliximab
B. IV cyclosporine
C. Continue trial of IV steroids up to 1 week
D. Proceed to colectomy

11. An 82-year-old man with a history of diabetes, hypertension, hyperlipidemia, coronary artery disease, and COPD is admitted to the ICU was intubated 5 days ago for acute respiratory failure due to a severe COPD exacerbation. Because of an ileus, he was started on TPN for nutritional support. Today, he was noted to become febrile with a

temperature of 39°C (102.2°F). His BP is 90/50 mmHg, with an HR of 102 beats/min. The patient grimaces on palpation of the RUQ. His labs reveal the following:

WBC	22 × 10³/μL
Hgb	7.2 g/dL
plt	350 × 10³/μL
Na	145 mEq/L
K	4.3 mEq/L
Cl	100 mEq/L
CO₂	26 mEq/L
BUN	32 mg/dL
Creatinine	0.92 mg/dL
Lipase	31 U/L
Amylase	55 U/L
AST	75 U/L
ALT	68 U/L
Direct bilirubin	0.6 mg/dL
Total bilirubin	1.2 mg/dL
Albumin	2.7 g/dL

Imaging of the RUQ with US demonstrates no evidence of stones but reveals the presence of a thickened gallbladder wall as well as pericholecystic fluid. Biliary dilatation is not noted. Blood cultures are drawn and antibiotics are started. What is the most appropriate next step in management?

A. Endoscopic retrograde cholangiopancreatography and stent placement
B. Laparoscopic cholecystectomy
C. HIDA scan
D. Percutaneous cholecystostomy

12. A 32-year-old woman with a history of obesity and hypertension presents with 2 days of RUQ pain. She states that the pain came on suddenly and has not abated since it began. She also noted that her skin and eyes began to turn yellow around the same time. Her urine has been darker than usual. In the ED, she was noted to be febrile to 39°C (102.2°F), with a BP of 70/30 mmHg and HR of 112 beats/min. Her physical exam was significant for noticeable jaundice, rigors, and RUQ tenderness. Labs revealed the following:

WBC	6 × 10³/μL
Hgb	11.3 g/dL
plt	298 × 10³/μL
Na	143 mEq/L
K	4.3 mEq/L
Cl	100 mEq/
CO₂	26 mEq/L
BUN	11 mg/dL
Creatinine	0.92 mg/dL
Lipase	31 U/L
Amylase	55 U/L
AST	235 U/L
ALT	168 U/L

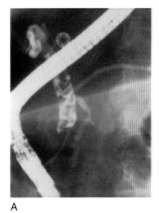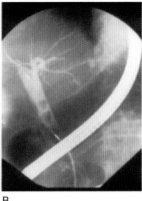

FIGURE 24-5 (A) Bile duct stones in common bile duct. (B) After sphincterotomy, the stone are removed. (Reproduced with permission from Kee Song L, Topazian M. Gastrointestinal endoscopy. In: Kasper D, Fauci A, Hauser S, et al, eds. *Harrison's Principles of Internal Medicine. 19th ed.* New York, NY: McGraw-Hill; 2014.)

Direct bilirubin	3.8 mg/dL
Total bilirubin	6.2 mg/dL
Albumin	3.2 g/dL

Ultrasound revealed dilated intra- and extrahepatic bile ducts, but no stone is seen. She was admitted to the ICU and resuscitation was begun with intravenous fluids. After fluids, her BP improves to 110/80 mmHg and her HR decreases to 88 beats/min. Blood cultures are drawn and the patient is started on broad-spectrum antibiotic therapy. She undergoes endoscopic retrograde cholangiopancreatography (Fig. 24-5).

Sphincterotomy and stone extraction are performed, and the patient's symptoms improve. What is the most appropriate immediate next step in management?

A. Discontinue antibiotics and discharge home with close follow-up
B. Perform urgent laparoscopic cholecystectomy prior to discharge
C. Perform laparoscopic cholecystectomy 3 months after discharge
D. Continue antibiotics to complete a 7- to 10-day course

13. A 32-year-old man with a history of alcohol abuse presents to the ED with abdominal pain. He states that it started the morning of admission, after a long weekend of drinking. He states that he drinks about a "handle" of vodka per day. He describes the pain as epigastric in location and states that the pain extends to his back. He feels nauseated but has not vomited. He notes that the pain is 8/10 in severity. On exam, his vital signs are as follows: BP of 90/60 mmHg, HR of 112 beats/min, RR of

20 breaths/min, Sao$_2$ of 94%, and temperature 38.1°C (100.6°F). He appears visibly uncomfortable. His abdominal exam is concerning for epigastric tenderness with no rebound or guarding. No bruising is notable on his abdomen. Lab findings include the following:

WBC	$18 \times 10^3/\mu L$
Hgb	15.6 g/dL
plt	$350 \times 10^3/\mu L$
Na	145 mEq/L
K	4.3 mEq/L
Cl	100 mEq/
CO$_2$	26 mEq/L
BUN	32 mg/dL
Creatinine	0.87 mg/dL
Lipase	3257 U/L
Amylase	554 U/L
AST	81 U/L
ALT	63 U/L
ALP	78 U/L
Direct bilirubin	0.17 mg/dL
Total bilirubin	0.9 mg/dL
Albumin	3.5 g/dL

The patient is admitted to the ICU for management. The patient receives 3 Liters of IV fluid and his repeat BP and HR are 120/90 mmHg and 88 beats/min, respectively. What is the most appropriate next step in management?

A. Start normal saline at 75 mL/h
B. Start Ringer lactate at 300 mL/h
C. Draw blood cultures and start patient on meropenem
D. Obtain CT abdomen/pelvis with and without IV contrast

14. A 60-year-old man was recently admitted for acute pancreatitis with alcohol abuse. He states that he has stopped drinking, but he returns 1 month later with persistent vague abdominal discomfort. He notes mild scleral icterus. He undergoes CT of the abdomen as seen in Figure 24–6.

His labs are as follows:

WBC	$5 \times 10^3/\mu L$
Hgb	12.0 g/dL
plt	$295 \times 10^3/\mu L$
Na	137 mEq/L
K	4.2 mEq/
Cl	100 mEq/L
CO$_2$	26 mEq/L
BUN	15 mg/dL
Ceatinine	0.8 mg/dL
Lipase	99 U/L
Amylase	32 U/L
AST	137 U/L
ALT	99 U/L
ALP	315 U/L

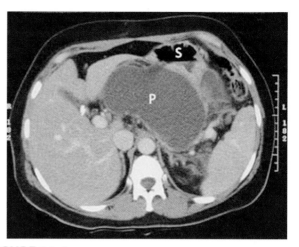

FIGURE 24-6 A CT scan of a pancreatic pseudocyst located in the lesser sac. P, pseudocyst; S, stomach. (Reproduced with permission from Windsor JA, Loveday BT. Chapter 55. Complications of Acute Pancreatitis (Including Pseudocysts). In: Zinner MJ, Ashley SW. eds. *Maingot's Abdominal Operations*, 12e. New York, NY: McGraw-Hill; 2013.)

Direct bilirubin	2.7 mg/dL
Total bilirubin	3.2 mg/dL
Albumin	3.5 g/dL

What is the most appropriate next step in management?

A. ERCP
B. MRCP
C. Cystogastrostomy
D. Discharge and close observation

15. A 25-year-old man presents to the ED with a chief complaint of jaundice. He states that since his girlfriend left him 2 weeks ago, he has been depressed, and admits to wanting to end his life. He states that the previous night he took an entire bottle of extra-strength acetaminophen intentionally in a suicide attempt. He is not sure how many pills he took, but he estimates over 20. He endorses some abdominal discomfort and nausea, but otherwise denies any other complaints. His roommate, however, does endorse that the patient has been somewhat more confused over the last few hours. He is afebrile with normal vital signs. His labs are significant for the following:

WBC	$8 \times 10^3/\mu L$
Hgb	12.3 g/dL
plt	$135 \times 10^3/\mu L$
Na	134 mEq/L
K	4.2 mEq/L
Cl	100 mEq/L
CO$_2$	14 mEq/L
BUN	12 mg/dL
Creatinine	3.8 mg/dL
Phosphate	4.1 mEq/L
Lipase	99 U/L

Amylase	32 U/L
Acetaminophen	120 uGu/L
INR	4.7
pH	7.17
Lactate	7.9 mmol/L
AST	13,258 U/L
ALT	14,286 U/L
ALP	256 U/L
Direct bilirubin	1.2 mg/dL
Total bilirubin	2.7 mg/dL
Albumin	3.5 g/dL

The patient is admitted to the ICU for further monitoring and IV N-acetylcysteine is started. What is the most appropriate next step in management?

A. Transfer to liver transplant center immediately
B. Begin lactulose and rifaximin to treat hepatic encephalopathy
C. Give FFP and vitamin K to correct coagulopathy
D. Keep at local ICU and only transfer if patient's condition does not improve

16. A patient who had liver transplantation 5 days ago was noted to have rising liver tests, with an AST of 5000 U/L, an ALT of 4300 U/L, and a bilirubin of 5.2 mg/dL. His INR increased from 1.3 to 2.7. His tacrolimus levels were noted to be within the therapeutic range. What is the most appropriate next step in management?

A. Liver biopsy
B. Doppler US of liver
C. MRCP
D. Exploratory laparoscopy

17. Which of the following is not a common precipitant of hepatic encephalopathy?

A. Hypokalemia
B. Infection
C. GI bleeding
D. Hyperkalemia

18. A patient with hepatic encephalopathy undergoes a diagnostic paracentesis as part of the workup. Results reveal the following:

Total WBC	2168
Total RBC	3000
% PMN	50
% Lymphs	30
% Mono	20
Gram stain and culture	negative

What is the next step in management?

A. Continue current management, await culture results
B. Cefotaxime 2 g every 8 hours
C. Cefotaxime 2 g every 8 hours and IV albumin 1.5 g/kg
D. CT abdomen/pelvis with and without IV contrast

19. A 47-year-old man with a history of HCV cirrhosis presents with a chief complaint of hematemesis. He states that this has never happened to him before. He began vomiting blood about 2 hours ago, when his wife called emergency medical services (EMS) and brought him to the ED. In the ED, he was found to be hypotensive with a BP of 70/32 mmHg and tachycardic with an HR of 112 beats/min. He was intubated in the ED for airway protection. His labs were as follows:

Hgb	6.7 g/dL (from a baseline of 11 g/dL)
plt	111 × 10³/μL
BUN	32 mg/dL
Cr	1.3 g/dL
AST	63 U/L
ALT	32 U/L
Total bilirubin	1.3 mg/dL
INR	1.8

Two large-bore IVs were placed, and a blood transfusion was initiated. What is the most appropriate initial therapy for this patient?

A. Transfusion of fresh frozen plasma
B. IV pantoprazole, octreotide, and ceftriaxone
C. IV pantoprazole and octreotide
D. Emergent transjugular intrahepatic portosystemic shunt

20. A patient with upper GI bleeding undergoes endoscopy and is found to have 3 large columns of esophageal varices with red wale signs. Ligation bands are placed with good effect and hemostasis is attained. The patient is extubated and does well, with no further rebleeding. What is the recommended approach to prophylaxis against further bleeding in this patient?

A. No prophylaxis recommended as this was the patient's first episode of bleeding
B. Begin nadolol 20 mg once daily
C. Begin nadolol 20 mg once daily and repeat variceal banding in 2 to 4 weeks
D. Place transjugular intrahepatic portosystemic shunt

ANSWERS

1. B. Pantoprazole 80 mg IV × 1 with initiation of pantoprazole drip at 8 mg/h

After appropriate resuscitation with IV fluids and blood products, initial medical therapy should include an IV proton pump inhibitor. Typically, a PPI is initially given as a high-dose bolus followed by a continuous infusion (choice B).[8] Although pre-endoscopic PPI therapy has not been shown to improve mortality or the risk of rebleeding, it does appear to reduce the incidence of finding ulcers with high-risk stigmata of hemorrhage, and therefore reduce the need for endoscopic therapy.[9] Intermittent dosing with an IV PPI (choice C) may be utilized for postendoscopic medical therapy but is not appropriate for pre-endoscopic medical therapy. A PPI should not be given orally prior to endoscopy, as the patient should be NPO; in addition, acid suppression is achieved more rapidly with IV dosing.[8] While nasogastric lavage (choice A) is frequently attempted to document a UGI source of bleeding, a negative NG aspirate does not necessarily rule out an upper GI source; therefore, its utility is limited.

2. D. Transfer to floor and continue IV PPI

Postendoscopic medical therapy is driven by endoscopic findings (eg, stigmata of recent hemorrhage) and the need for endoscopic therapy. If endoscopic therapy has been applied, then IV PPI should be continued for at least 72 hours. American College of Gastroenterology guidelines recommend continuing a continuous infusion of PPI (choice D) after endoscopic therapy, although a recent meta-analysis suggests that intermittent dosing (eg, pantoprazole every 12 hours) of a PPI may lead to equivalent outcomes.[11] If a patient has low-risk stigmata (eg, a flat, pigmented spot or clean-based ulcer), he or she may be transitioned to a standard-dose, oral PPI and discharged after

assuring that he or she is hemodynamically stable and has stable hemoglobin (choices A and C). Routine second-look endoscopy is not recommended in the absence of evidence of ongoing bleeding (choice B).[8] Figure 24-7 shows the different types of endoscopic findings in peptic ulcer disease.

3. D. CT angiography without oral contrast

The patient likely has mesenteric ischemia resulting from embolism of thrombus from the left ventricle. Patients with mesenteric ischemia typically present with the acute onset of abdominal pain, the location of which may vary, but it typically begins in the periumbilical region and may progress to become more diffuse. This patient has evidence of the classic finding of pain out of proportion to the exam. Her laboratory studies point toward ischemia, with an elevated WBC count and high lactate. To confirm the diagnosis, a CT angiogram should be obtained (choice D); this should be performed without oral contrast to ensure excellent contrast between the mesenteric vessels and surrounding structures (choice A). Management may eventually include emergent laparotomy, although this patient is currently hemodynamically stable and does not have peritoneal signs (choice B). Timely endovascular therapy may be sufficient to restore perfusion and salvage her bowel (choice C).

Endoscopic stigmata of bleeding peptic ulcer, classified as high risk or low risk

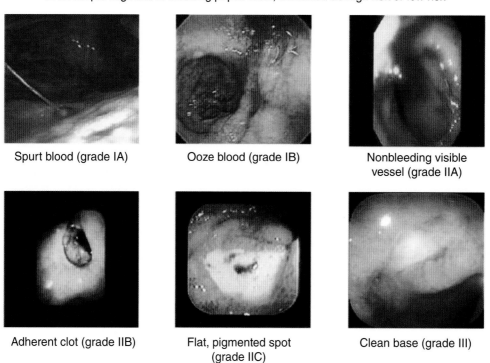

Spurt blood (grade IA)   Ooze blood (grade IB)   Nonbleeding visible vessel (grade IIA)

Adherent clot (grade IIB)   Flat, pigmented spot (grade IIC)   Clean base (grade III)

FIGURE 24-7 Endoscopic findings of peptic ulcer. High risk lesions include active spurting blood (Grade IA), oozing blood (Grade IB), nonbleeding visible vessel called pigmented protuberance (Grade IIA), and adherent clot that is red, maroon, or black and that cannot be dislodged by suction or irrigation (Grade IIB). Low risk lesions include flat pigmented spots (Grade IIC) and clean based ulcers (Grade III).

(Reproduced with permission from Gralnek IM, Barkun A, Bardou M. Management of acute bleeding from a peptic ulcer. *N Engl J Med.* 2008;359(9):928-937.)

TABLE 24-11 Grade of Esophageal Injury

Grade of Injury	Description
Grade 0	Normal
Grade 1	Mucosal edema and hyperemia
Grade 2A	Superficial ulcers, bleeding, exudates
Grade 2B	Deep focal or circumferential ulcers
Grade 3A	Deep ulcers with brown, gray, or black discoloration, localized necrosis
Grade 3B	Extensive necrosis

4. D. Upper endoscopy should be performed as soon as possible.

The patient is presenting with an acute, intentional caustic injury caused by ingestion of drain cleaner. Drain cleaner (eg, Drano) typically has as its active ingredient sodium hydroxide, an alkaline substance that can cause rapid liquefactive necrosis.[158] The liquefactive necrosis caused by alkali ingestion usually causes a deeper injury than that seen with acidic substances, which cause coagulative necrosis and formation of an eschar that prevents deeper tissue injury.[159] After appropriate triage and resuscitation of the patient, upper endoscopy should be performed as soon as possible (typically within 24 hours) to assess the extent of injury (choice D; Table 24-11).[160] Induction of vomiting is not recommended (choice A), as this may re-expose the damaged mucosa to further injury. Similarly, ingestion of water or neutralizing agents is not recommended, as both may cause further spread of the caustic substance and may incite a chemical reaction that may lead to increased thermal injury (choice C). Finally, blind NGT insertion prior to endoscopy is not recommended, as it may induce perforation in patients with extensive necrosis (choice B).[161]

Patients with grade 1 or 2A injury have a good prognosis and can typically begin a clear liquid diet almost immediately after initial endoscopic evaluation. If the patient remains stable, he or she can be advanced to a regular diet within 24 to 48 hours. Patients with grade 2B injuries may be started on clear liquids within 48 hours if they otherwise remain stable. Patients with grade 3 injuries are at high risk of perforation and should be observed for an extended period of time in the intensive care unit, where they can be closely monitored for evidence of perforation. If perforation develops or is imminent, esophagectomy with colonic interposition may be necessary.[160,162]

5. C. Emergent endoscopic evaluation

The patient has likely developed a stricture due to scarring after recovery from his caustic ingestion, and he is now presenting with a food impaction. Given his inability to tolerate his own secretions and the increased risk of aspiration and perforation, he should undergo emergent endoscopic evaluation to remove the impacted food (choice C).[163] A CT scan or chest x-ray may be performed if perforation is suspected, but as most food ingested is not radiopaque, radiographic imaging may not be high yield (choice B and D). Barium swallow is helpful in identifying esophageal strictures but is not indicated in the setting of an acute food impaction and may impair visualization during subsequent endoscopy (choice A).

Strictures may develop in up to one-third of patients following caustic ingestion, with most (> 70%) occurring in patients with grade 2B or 3 injuries. They may be of varying length, depending in part on the initial extent of caustic injury. Strictures are most often treated with serial esophageal dilation. Treatment for strictures refractory to dilation includes endoscopic stenting as well as esophagectomy, although the latter is usually reserved for refractory cases.[164,165]

Caustic ingestion is also a risk factor for the development of esophageal squamous cell carcinoma. Typically, this presents decades after an initial caustic ingestion. Surveillance with EGD every 1 to 3 years is recommended beginning 15 to 20 years after an initial caustic ingestion to identify the development of squamous cell carcinoma.[166]

6. B. Stop NGT feeds and place NGT to suction

The patient is suffering from ileus, likely related to his underlying critical illness, as well the use of an opioid for sedation. Ileus most commonly presents among patients in the postoperative state, although prolonged immobility due to any reason (eg, critical illness) can lead to the development of ileus. Other contributing factors are electrolyte abnormalities including hypercalcemia, hypokalemia, and hypomagnesemia. Use of drugs that have anticholinergic properties may also contribute to the development of ileus. Clinically, patients may present with abdominal pain and distension, nausea, vomiting, and the lack of flatus or bowel movements. In patients who are intubated in the ICU, ileus may also present with an intolerance to enteral feeding. Radiographic findings include diffusely dilated small bowel loops and may also show colonic dilatation. This contrasts with small bowel obstruction, in which no colonic dilatation is present. If the diagnosis is not clear based on abdominal radiographs, then a CT with oral (or nasogastric) contrast may be obtained to rule out the presence of a mechanical small bowel obstruction, but it is not necessary in all cases.

Management for ileus is conservative. The patient's NGT can be placed to suction to relieve the acute abdominal distension. Any electrolyte abnormalities present should be corrected. The patient should be turned frequently to encourage bowel motility. After the bowel is decompressed, slow "trickle" nasogastric feeding may be restarted to encourage small bowel motility.[167] The presence of a prolonged ileus does not necessarily suggest nil per os (NPO) status since NPO status can propogate the ileus. Enteral nutrition is still advocated for patients with ileus unless they have multiple signs of gastrointestinal intolerance such as vomiting, abdominal distention or discomfort, high nasogastric output, reduced bowel movements, and/or worsening or abnormal abdominal radiographs. Due to multiple signs of gastrointestinal intolerance, choice D is wrong.

It is critical to differentiate ileus from small bowel obstruction, as management differs significantly. Cross-sectional imaging with CT may be especially helpful in differentiating ileus from small bowel obstruction, as the identification of a transition point may be easier (choice C). It is possible, however, to differentiate ileus from small bowel obstruction on plain abdominal radiography, with the presence of air-fluid levels and a lack of colonic air or distension suggestive of a transition point in the small bowel.[168] The etiology of small bowel obstruction is intraabdominal adhesions in up to 85% of cases. In the presence of a mechanical small bowel obstruction, NGT suction and bowel rest are indicated, and surgical exploration may be required if the patient fails conservative management (choice B). Up to 73% of patients with a partial small bowel obstruction can be managed nonoperatively, compared with less than 50% of patients with a complete small bowel obstruction.[169] Surgical management involves lysis of adhesions and bowel resection if bowel demonstrates evidence of infarction (choice A).

7. A. Initiation of intravenous ciprofloxacin and metronidazole

The patient appears to be suffering from acute uncomplicated diverticulitis. However, he has failed outpatient therapy with oral antibiotics owing to his inability to take in food orally. Therefore, inpatient therapy with IV antibiotics is indicated (choice A). Intravenous antibiotic regimens for acute uncomplicated diverticulitis include ciprofloxacin or a third-generation cephalosporin plus metronidazole, or in a patient with risk factors for antimicrobial resistance, piperacillin-tazobactam or a carbapenem.[40] Antibiotics are given for a 7- to 10-day course. Initiation of oral vancomycin is not appropriate, as this will not treat the Gram-negative rods and anaerobes typical of intra-abdominal infection (choice B). Exploratory laparotomy is unnecessary for this patient right now but is indicated in the setting of frank peritonitis or perforation, which can occur as a complication of diverticulitis (choice C). Urgent surgery may also be required when medical therapy fails, or if there is a local complication such as an abscess that does not respond to a combination of antibiotic therapy and percutaneous drainage.[41] American Gastroenterological Association guidelines recommend that a colonoscopy be performed after recovery from an episode of diverticulitis if the patient has not

recently undergone a colonoscopy for colorectal cancer screening in order to rule out a concomitant colorectal carcinoma or advanced adenoma (choice D).[42]

8. D. PO Vancomycin

The patient has evidence of severe *C difficile*–associated diarrhea. Initial management depends on the severity of CDAD. If the patient is receiving broad-spectrum antibiotic therapy, this should be discontinued if feasible to allow for more rapid reconstitution of the colonic flora. Patients who meet criteria for mild-to-moderate disease should be started on metronidazole 500 mg PO every 8 hours (choice C). Those who fail to respond to therapy after 3 to 5 days should be switched to PO vancomycin. Those with severe disease should be treated with vancomycin 125 mg PO 4 times daily, even if it is their first infection (choice D). The recommended duration of therapy is 10 days. Patients with fulminant disease and ileus should receive combination therapy with PO vancomycin at 125 mg every 6 hours and IV metronidazole 500 mg every 8 hours. While IV metronidazole does enter the gut via the bile, it is not sufficient to treat severe CDAD alone (choice B). In the setting of ileus (where the PO vancomycin may not reach its intended site of action, the colon), the dose of PO vancomycin may be increased to 500 mg every 6 hours; the addition of vancomycin enemas may also be helpful. Patients with fulminant disease should be referred for surgical evaluation and monitored in the ICU.[170] Intravenous vancomycin has no route of entry into the gut, as it is metabolized almost entirely by the kidneys; it therefore is ineffective in treating *C difficile* infection (choice A).

9. C. The patient should be started on low-molecular-weight heparin.

The patient is admitted with severe acute ulcerative colitis, and as such should be started on venous thromboembolism prophylaxis with low-molecular-weight heparin (choice C). Despite the presence of mild bleeding, all patients admitted to the hospital with a flare of inflammatory bowel disease should be started on some form of pharmacological VTE prophylaxis, as the inflammatory state places patients at increased risk for VTE.[48] The European Crohn's and Colitis Organisation guidelines define severe acute UC as the presence of bloody stools 6 or more times per day *plus* at least one of the following: tachycardia, fever, anemia with hemoglobin less than 10.5 g/dL, or an elevated ESR or CRP. This patient meets criteria for severe acute UC and has failed outpatient therapy with systemic corticosteroids, and therefore requires inpatient admission. Initial therapy should include intravenous steroids at a dose of 100 mg IV of hydrocortisone every 6 hours or 20 mg IV of methylprednisolone every 8 hours. Oral and rectal mesalamine may be continued (choice D). The patient should be allowed to eat (or if she is unable to maintain adequate PO intake, supplemental enteral nutrition via nasogastric or nasojejunal tube should be provided) as nourishment of the colonic mucosa may improve outcomes (choice A). Bowel rest and parenteral nutrition do not provide any additional benefit and may actually worsen outcomes.[49] Electrolyte abnormalities should be corrected, as hypokalemia or hypomagnesemia may promote the development of toxic megacolon.[50] Diagnostic tests that should be performed on admission include stool assay for the presence of *C difficile* (symptoms of which can often mimic or incite a flare of UC), abdominal x-ray or CT if colonic dilatation is suspected, and flexible sigmoidoscopy to assess the endoscopic severity of colitis and perform biopsies to rule out concomitant CMV infection (especially among patients on steroids prior to admission).[50] Antibiotics are not indicated for the treatment of acute UC per se, although they may be appropriate in patients with signs of systemic infection (choice B).[51]

10. D. Proceed to colectomy

The patient in this case has developed 2 indications for urgent colectomy: refractory bleeding and toxic megacolon refractory to medical therapy (choice D). Toxic megacolon is generally defined as a transverse colon diameter of greater than 6 cm or a cecal diameter greater than 9 cm. Continuing IV steroid therapy in this case would not be appropriate, as the patient is at impending risk of colon perforation (choice C). Multiple scoring systems have been developed to assist providers in decision making regarding the appropriate timing of colectomy. One of the simplest is the Oxford index, in which a stool frequency of more than 8 bowel movements per day on day 3 of intravenous steroids, along with a CRP greater than 45 mg/L is predictive of requiring a colectomy during admission in 85% of cases.[52] For patients who do not have toxic megacolon or refractory bleeding but who have not had a good clinical response to 3 to 5 days of IV steroid therapy (defined as a Lichtiger score < 10 for 2 consecutive days), rescue therapy with IV infliximab (choice A) or cyclosporine (choice B) can be considered. The decision of which agent to use depends in large part upon local practice patterns. Two large, open label trials found no difference in rates of colectomy, mortality, or serious infectious complications between the 2 therapies. Infliximab is given as a single, weight-based infusion, followed by further induction infusions at weeks 2 and 6; maintenance therapy is given every 8 weeks. Cyclosporine is given as a continuous, weight-based infusion and is typically administered for 8 days. Monitoring of serum levels of cyclosporine, as well as monitoring of kidney function, blood pressure, and serum electrolytes, is required when administering cyclosporine induction therapy. Serum triglycerides should also be monitored, as hypotriglyceridemia is associated with adverse neurologic side effects (including seizures) in patients on IV cyclosporine. Patients who respond to IV cyclosporine must be transitioned to oral cyclosporine and a thiopurine (such as 6-mercaptopurine or azathioprine), as cyclosporine cannot be continued long term as a maintenance therapy.[50] For that reason, patients who have previously failed maintenance therapy with a thiopurine may not be good candidates for salvage therapy with cyclosporine and may benefit more from use of infliximab. If salvage therapy with either infliximab or cyclosporine fails, it is not recommended to again attempt medical salvage therapy with the other agent, as following infliximab with cyclosporine, or vice versa, has been found to significantly increase the risk of infectious complications and mortality.[53]

11. D. Percutaneous cholecystostomy

The patient is demonstrating signs and symptoms of acute acalculous cholecystitis. The diagnosis should be suspected in a critically ill patient with new onset RUQ pain, leukocytosis, and concerning imaging findings. Ultrasound has a sensitivity and specificity for the diagnosis of acalculous cholecystitis of 67% to 92% and greater than 90%, respectively.[79] The use of HIDA scintigraphy may be less reliable in critically ill patients with a higher false-positive rate, especially among those with liver enzyme abnormalities, and is unnecessary in the presence of convincing clinical and ultrasound findings (choice C). In addition to antibiotics, drainage of the gallbladder with percutaneous cholecystostomy is necessary for successful treatment (choice D). Initial technical and clinical success with this technique may be as high as 93%.[80] Elective cholecystectomy is indicated once the patient recovers from their acute critical illness; patients with acute acalculous cholecystitis are typically too ill to undergo immediate cholecystectomy (choice B). Of note, percutaneous cholecystostomy should not be performed in patients with ascites, as tubes have a high chance of dislodgement from the gallbladder into the peritoneum, leaving a free perforation in the gallbladder wall. Initial surgical management of acalculous cholecystitis is not preferred, as patients are typically too ill to undergo either laparoscopic or open cholecystectomy. Biliary drainage with ERCP or percutaneous transhepatic cholangiography is not indicated at this time as there is no evidence of biliary obstruction (choice A).

12. D. Continue antibiotics to complete a 7- to 10-day course

The patient is suffering from acute cholangitis as evidenced by the presence of Charcot triad (RUQ pain, jaundice, and fever) and requires treatment with urgent biliary decompression with ERCP, sphincterotomy, and stone extraction. Initial supportive care includes management of sepsis with intravenous fluids and antibiotics. Antibiotics are generally continued for 7 to 10 days (choice D); if blood cultures are positive, antibiotic therapy should be tailored to the organism(s) recovered. It would be premature to discontinue antibiotics immediately after ERCP (choice A). In general, antibiotics that cover Gram-negative organisms and anaerobes (eg, piperacillin-tazobactam) should be administered unless an organism is definitively identified. If the patient does not have any risk factors for antimicrobial resistance, a third-generation cephalosporin in combination with metronidazole may be sufficient.[76] As with all symptomatic gallstone disease, cholecystectomy is indicated, although not necessarily during the index hospitalization for cholangitis (choice B). Cholecystectomy, however, should be performed within 6 weeks of an episode of cholangitis, as data demonstrate reduced rates of recurrence and improved outcomes (choice C).[87]

13. B. Start Ringer lactate at 300 mL/h

In acute pancreatitis due to any etiology, the most important aspect of management is prompt fluid resuscitation. Hypovolemia can occur due to impaired oral intake, vomiting, and third-spacing of fluid due to increased vascular permeability from the intense inflammatory state arising in the setting of acute pancreatitis. Inflammation may be exacerbated by low blood flow to the pancreas, worsening activation of pancreatic enzymes, and further activation of the inflammatory cascade.[96] Early, aggressive IV hydration (within the first 6 hours of treatment) appears to be the most important; after 24 to 48 hours, the benefit of aggressive fluid resuscitation may be lost. A large, prospective randomized trial demonstrated reduced markers of systemic inflammation (CRP and SIRS criteria) with the use of Ringer lactate solution compared with normal saline in patients with acute pancreatitis.[97] Therefore, guidelines recommend its use for initial resuscitation in acute pancreatitis.[96] After initial correction of hypovolemia via fluid bolus, Ringer lactate should be initiated at 250 to 500 mL/h (choice B). If the patient has cardiopulmonary comorbidities, the rate at which fluids are given may need to be lowered, and the patient should be reassessed frequently for evidence of respiratory distress or volume overload. This patient does not have any such comorbidities; therefore, a lower rate of IV fluids would be inappropriate (choice A). A fall in both the BUN and the hematocrit—reflective of effective fluid resuscitation—should be seen within the first 24 hours. If a decrease in these values is not noted, the rate of fluid may need to be increased.[98] Antibiotics should be reserved only for the presence of concomitant extrapancreatic infection or if a patient subsequently develops evidence of infected pancreatic necrosis (choice C). Infected pancreatic necrosis may be suspected if a patient develops clinical deterioration after initial improvement, or in patients who fail to improve after 7 to 10 days of hospitalization. The presence of necrosis is best visualized on abdominal CT with IV contrast; infection may be confirmed with CT-guided fine-needle aspiration of the necrotic pancreas, although it is also acceptable to treat empirically with antibiotics that penetrate the pancreatic

parenchyma, such as meropenem.[99] A CT scan performed within the first 72 hours may not show significant changes and, in a patient with classical clinical and laboratory findings, is not necessary to confirm the diagnosis of acute pancreatitis (choice D). Prophylactic antibiotics and/or antifungals (to prevent the occurrence of infected necrosis) have not been demonstrated to be beneficial in improving mortality.[100] Endoscopic retrograde cholangiopancreatography is indicated in the setting of acute pancreatitis only with concomitant cholangitis, or if there is evidence of ongoing biliary obstruction with persistent jaundice.[96]

14. C. Cystogastrostomy

The patient has likely developed biliary obstruction related to a pseudocyst. Pseudocysts typically develop more than 4 weeks after an initial bout of pancreatitis. They are simple fluid collections lined with a fibrous capsule. They do not require intervention unless they cause symptoms or biliary obstruction, as in this case. The management of pseudocysts most often involves creation of an endoscopic (less commonly surgical) cystogastrostomy using endoscopic ultrasound-guided insertion of 1 or many stents through the gastric wall into the pseudocyst, to allow drainage of contents into the gastric lumen (choice C). Endoscopic retrograde cholangiopancreatography with stenting may relieve the biliary obstruction but will not treat the underlying problem (choice A). Magnetic resonance cholangiopancreatography in this case will not add much to what is visible on CT (choice B). Discharge is inappropriate as the patient is symptomatic and jaundiced (choice D). Figure 24-8 shows different morphologic features of pancreatitis.

15. A. Transfer to liver transplant center immediately

The patient has acute liver failure induced by acetaminophen and meets King's College Criteria for liver transplantation referral with an arterial pH of less than 7.30. Acute liver failure is defined as the development of jaundice, coagulopathy (INR ≥ 1.5), and encephalopathy in a patient without any known preexisting liver condition with a time to disease onset of less than 26 weeks.[112] Without transplantation, acute liver failure carries a mortality of approximately 85%.[113] The King's College criteria (see Table 24-7) can be used to prognosticate which patients will require transplantation, with a sensitivity of 68% to 69% and sensitivity of 82% to 92%.[114] Patients with suspected acute liver failure should be transferred to a liver transplant center as soon as possible and initiate workup to be placed on the liver transplant waiting list (choice A). The patient's constellation of clinical and lab findings in this case meet King's College criteria, so keeping him at the local ICU would be inappropriate (choice D). Given the extraordinarily high mortality in the absence of LT, patients with

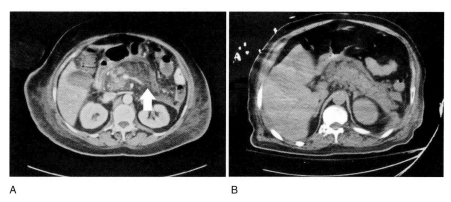

FIGURE 24-8 (A) Acute necrotizing pancreatitis. Notice the decreased enhancement in body and tail (see arrow) on abdominal computed tomography with IV contrast. (B) Acute hemorrhagic pancreatitis. Notice the increased density at the tail of the pancreas.)

ALF are given the highest priority (status 1) on the LT waitlist. In contrast to patients with cirrhosis, lactulose should not be administered to patients with ALF, as gaseous abdominal distension generated by lactulose may ultimately make emergent transplantation more technically challenging. Further, its use has not been shown to improve outcomes (choice B). Coagulopathy should generally not be corrected in the absence of overt bleeding or if necessary in the setting of invasive procedures, as progression or recovery of coagulopathy can be utilized to prognosticate the outcome in ALF (choice C).

16 B. Doppler US of liver

The patient most likely has developed early hepatic artery thrombosis. Hepatic artery thrombosis may occur early (< 30 days) or late (> 30 days) in the post-transplant course, and the clinical presentations differ depending on when HAT develops. Early HAT may be characterized by the development of graft dysfunction and possibly fulminant hepatic failure, possibly leading to mortality without retransplantation.[153] Risk factors include technical issues related to the initial transplant (including complex arterial reconstruction, the use of arterial conduits, and prolonged procedure time) as well as patient-related factors (retransplantation vs primary transplantation, low recipient weight).[153,154] Diagnosis is typically made via Doppler ultrasonography of the hepatic artery. Graft survival may be improved with early detection and revascularization via thrombectomy or stenting, although many patients require retransplantation. Graft and patient survival after retransplantation for early HAT is lower than after primary LT.[153] Late HAT typically presents in a less dramatic fashion, with biliary complications including bilomas and biliary strictures, as the hepatic artery is the primary blood supply to the bile ducts.[155] Liver biopsy (choice A), MRCP (choice C), and exploratory laparoscopy (choice D) are not used in the initial evaluation for HAT.

17. D. Hyperkalemia

Hepatic encephalopathy (HE) is a common problem affecting patients with end-stage liver disease. Hepatic encephalopathy may be precipitated by several factors that must be addressed in order for HE to resolve. In a patient with known HE, nonadherence to medical therapy with lactulose is a common precipitating factor. Other precipitating factors include acute GI bleeding, constipation, infection, hypokalemia, hypoxia, hypoglycemia, and renal failure (choices A–C).[127] Any of these acute insults can precipitate HE in a patient whose HE is otherwise well controlled. Hyperkalemia is not a common precipitant of hepatic encephalopathy (choice D).

18. C. Cefotaxime 2 g every 8 hours and IV albumin 1.5 g/kg

The patient has suspected spontaneous bacterial peritonitis, based on the PMN count in his ascitic fluid, and requires appropriate therapy. Technically, this patient has culture-negative neutrocytic ascites; however, patients with CNNA and SBP clinically behave nearly identically, with similar mortality rates. Therefore, there is no need to wait for culture results prior to initiating treatment (choice A). Treatment of SBP is directed at the 3 most common isolates: *E coli*, *K pneumoniae*, and *S pneumoniae*, with cefotaxime 2 g every 8 hours as the antibiotic of choice. Other third-generation cephalosporins may be substituted if cefotaxime is not available (eg, ceftriaxone 1 g twice daily).[133] In addition to antibiotics, the use of IV albumin has been shown to reduce the development of the hepatorenal syndrome and subsequent mortality among patients with SBP who meet the following criteria: creatinine greater than 1 mg/dL, BUN greater than 30 mg/dL, or total bilirubin greater than 4 mg/dL (choice C). Because the patient in the above scenario has a bilirubin of greater than 4 mg/dL, he meets these criteria and should receive combination therapy with albumin and antibiotics, not albumin alone (choice B). The recommended regimen for patients with SBP is 1.5 g/kg of IV albumin on day 1, followed by 1 g/kg on day 3.[136] Treatment should be continued for a total of 5 days. In patients who do not improve clinically, repeat diagnostic paracentesis may be advised to determine whether neutrophilia in the ascites is resolving; persistent neutrophilia may indicate the presence of antibiotic resistance or secondary peritonitis. Cross-sectional imaging and analysis of LDH and glucose levels in the ascitic fluid may also be helpful to rule out a secondary source. Cross-sectional imaging with CT is not appropriate at this time as there is currently low suspicion for a secondary source of peritonitis (choice D).

19 B. IV pantoprazole, octreotide, and ceftriaxone

The patient is presenting with acute variceal hemorrhage from esophageal varices. After appropriate general resuscitative measures and transfusion of packed red blood cells, initial pharmacotherapy includes initiation of an IV proton pump inhibitor, octreotide (or terlipressin, where it is available), and antibiotic prophylaxis, typically with ceftriaxone (choice B). As discussed previously in "Upper Gastrointestinal Bleeding," blood should be transfused to a goal hemoglobin of 7 g/dL; patients with Child-Turcotte-Pugh class A and B cirrhosis had significantly lower mortality and rebleeding rates than patients transfused to a higher threshold of 9 g/dL.[7] Correcting coagulopathy using fresh frozen plasma has not been shown to alter outcomes, as the INR in cirrhotics does not accurately reflect the true degree of coagulopathy (choice A). Further, transfusion of fresh frozen plasma in addition to blood could contribute to overtransfusion and an increase of portal pressures, perhaps increasing the risk of rebleeding.[122] Antibiotic prophylaxis should be given to patients with cirrhosis and GI bleeding of any etiology. Ceftriaxone 1 g every 24 hours for a duration of 7 days has been shown to reduce rates of bacterial infection, rebleeding, and mortality.[123] Excluding antibiotic prophylaxis would not be appropriate (choice C). If rebleeding occurs and repeat endoscopic therapy is not successful, or if initial bleeding is refractory to endoscopic therapy, then emergent placement of a transjugular intrahepatic portosystemic shunt is indicated (choice D). Balloon tamponade with a Sengstaken-Blakemore tube may be necessary to control hemorrhage while awaiting TIPS.[121]

20. C. Begin nadolol 20 mg once daily and repeat variceal banding in 2 to 4 weeks

This patient requires effective secondary prophylaxis for prevention of recurrent variceal bleeding, as rebleeding rates may be as high as 60% after a first episode of variceal bleeding (choice A). For patients who have recovered from an initial episode of variceal bleeding, secondary prophylaxis typically involves combination therapy with lowering of portal pressures with a nonselective beta-blocker and local therapy of varices with variceal ligation. Nonselective beta-blockers exert their effect on portal pressures by reducing splanchnic inflow in 2 ways: they reduce cardiac output, and they block β_2 receptors in the splanchnic arterial bed, leading to unopposed α adrenergic activity and vasoconstriction.[121,125] Either nadolol or propranolol or carvedilol may be used for prophylaxis. Variceal ligation should be repeated every 2 to 4 weeks until varices are completely eradicated. A beta-blocker alone is insufficient (choice B).

For patients who have never bled from varices, recommendations for primary prophylaxis differ. Patients with medium- to large-sized varices should receive prophylaxis, while patients with small varices should only receive prophylaxis if they have Child-Turcotte-Pugh class B or C cirrhosis or if their varices exhibit with red wale signs. Primary prophylaxis may include monotherapy with a traditional nonselective beta-blocker (eg, nadolol or propranolol), carvedilol, or serial esophageal variceal ligation. It is too early for transjugular intrahepatic portosystemic shunt (choice D).

REFERENCES

1. Abougergi MS, Travis AC, Saltzman JR. The in-hospital mortality rate for upper GI hemorrhage has decreased over 2 decades in the United States: a nationwide analysis. *Gastrointest Endosc.* 2015;81(4):882-888.e1.
2. Gralnek IM, Dumonceau J-M, Kuipers EJ, et al. Diagnosis and management of nonvariceal upper gastrointestinal hemorrhage: European Society of Gastrointestinal Endoscopy (ESGE) Guideline. *Endoscopy.* 2015;47(10):a1-a46.
3. Pérez-Aisa MA, Del Pino D, Siles M, Lanas A. Clinical trends in ulcer diagnosis in a population with high prevalence of *Helicobacter pylori* infection. *Aliment Pharmacol Ther.* 2005;21(1):65-72.
4. Rockall TA, Logan RF, Devlin HB, Northfield TC. Risk assessment after acute upper gastrointestinal haemorrhage. *Gut.* 1996;38(3):316-321.
5. Blatchford O, Murray WR, Blatchford M. A risk score to predict need for treatment for upper gastrointestinal haemorrhage. *Lancet.* 2000;356(9238):1318-1321.
6. Stanley AJ, Ashley D, Dalton HR, et al. Outpatient management of patients with low-risk upper gastrointestinal haemorrhage: multicentre validation and prospective evaluation. *Lancet.* 2009;373(9657):42-47.
7. Villanueva C, Colomo A, Bosch A, et al. Transfusion strategies for acute upper gastrointestinal bleeding. *N Engl J Med.* 2013;368(1):11-21.
8. Laine L, Jensen DM. Management of patients with ulcer bleeding. *Am J Gastroenterol.* 2012;107(3):345-360; quiz 361.
9. Sreedharan A, Martin J, Leontiadis GI, et al. Proton pump inhibitor treatment initiated prior to endoscopic diagnosis in upper gastrointestinal bleeding. *Cochrane Database Syst Rev.* 2010;(7):CD005415.
10. Yen D, Hu SC, Chen LS, et al. Arterial oxygen desaturation during emergent nonsedated upper gastrointestinal endoscopy in the emergency department. *Am J Emerg Med.* 1997;15(7):644-647.

11. Sachar H, Vaidya K, Laine L. Intermittent vs continuous proton pump inhibitor therapy for high-risk bleeding ulcers: a systematic review and meta-analysis. *JAMA Intern Med.* 2014;174(11):1755-1762.

12. Loffroy R, Rao P, Ota S, De Lin M, Kwak B-K, Geschwind J-F. Embolization of acute nonvariceal upper gastrointestinal hemorrhage resistant to endoscopic treatment: results and predictors of recurrent bleeding. *Cardiovasc Intervent Radiol.* 2010;33(6):1088-1100.

13. Abe N, Takeuchi H, Yanagida O, Sugiyama M, Atomi Y. Surgical indications and procedures for bleeding peptic ulcer. *Dig Endosc.* 2010;22(Suppl 1):S35-S37.

14. Strate LL, Gralnek IM. ACG clinical guideline: management of patients with acute lower gastrointestinal bleeding. *Am J Gastroenterol.* 2016;111(4):459-474.

15. Jensen DM. Management of patients with severe hematochezia—with all current evidence available. *Am J Gastroenterol.* 2005;100(11):2403-2406.

16. Strate LL. Lower GI bleeding: epidemiology and diagnosis. *Gastroenterol Clin North Am.* 2005;34(4):643-664.

17. Murphy CH, Hess JR. Massive transfusion: red blood cell to plasma and platelet unit ratios for resuscitation of massive hemorrhage. *Curr Opin Hematol.* 2015;22(6):533-539.

18. Angtuaco TL, Reddy SK, Drapkin S, Harrell LE, Howden CW. The utility of urgent colonoscopy in the evaluation of acute lower gastrointestinal tract bleeding: a 2-year experience from a single center. *Am J Gastroenterol.* 2001;96(6):1782-1785.

19. Green BT, Rockey DC, Portwood G, et al. Urgent colonoscopy for evaluation and management of acute lower gastrointestinal hemorrhage: a randomized controlled trial. *Am J Gastroenterol.* 2005;100(11):2395-2402.

20. Laine L, Shah A. Randomized trial of urgent vs. elective colonoscopy in patients hospitalized with lower GI bleeding. *Am J Gastroenterol.* 2010;105(12):2636-2641; quiz 2642.

21. Strate LL, Naumann CR. The role of colonoscopy and radiological procedures in the management of acute lower intestinal bleeding. *Clin Gastroenterol Hepatol.* 2010;8(4):333-343; quiz e44.

22. Artigas JM, Martí M, Soto JA, Esteban H, Pinilla I, Guillén E. Multidetector CT angiography for acute gastrointestinal bleeding: technique and findings. *Radiographics.* 2013;33(5):1453-1470.

23. Oldenburg WA, Lau LL, Rodenberg TJ, Edmonds HJ, Burger CD. Acute mesenteric ischemia: a clinical review. *Arch Intern Med.* 2004;164(10):1054-1062.

24. Tilsed JVT, Casamassima A, Kurihara H, et al. ESTES guidelines: acute mesenteric ischaemia. *Eur J Trauma Emerg Surg.* 2016;42(2):253-270.

25. Menke J. Diagnostic accuracy of multidetector CT in acute mesenteric ischemia: systematic review and meta-analysis. *Radiology.* 2010;256(1):93-101.

26. Reinus JF, Brandt LJ, Boley SJ. Ischemic diseases of the bowel. *Gastroenterol Clin North Am.* 1990;19(2):319-343.

27. Zhao Y, Yin H, Yao C, et al. Management of acute mesenteric ischemia: a critical review and treatment algorithm. *Vasc Endovascular Surg.* 2016;50(3):183-192.

28. Brandt LJ, Feuerstadt P, Longstreth GF, Boley SJ; American College of Gastroenterology. ACG clinical guideline: epidemiology, risk factors, patterns of presentation, diagnosis, and management of colon ischemia (CI). *Am J Gastroenterol.* 2015;110(1):18-44; quiz 45.

29. Brandt LJ, Feuerstadt P, Blaszka MC. Anatomic patterns, patient characteristics, and clinical outcomes in ischemic colitis: a study of 313 cases supported by histology. *Am J Gastroenterol.* 2010;105(10):2245-2252; quiz 2253.

30. Montoro MA, Brandt LJ, Santolaria S, et al. Clinical patterns and outcomes of ischaemic colitis: results of the Working Group for the Study of Ischaemic Colitis in Spain (CIE study). *Scand J Gastroenterol.* 2011;46(2):236-246.

31. O'Neill S, Yalamarthi S. Systematic review of the management of ischaemic colitis. *Colorectal Dis.* 2012;14(11):e751-e763.

32. Reissfelder C, Sweiti H, Antolovic D, et al. Ischemic colitis: who will survive? *Surgery.* 2011;149(4):585-592.

33. Meyers MA, Alonso DR, Gray GF, Baer JW. Pathogenesis of bleeding colonic diverticulosis. *Gastroenterology.* 1976;71(4):577-583.

34. Peery AF. Recent advances in diverticular disease. *Curr Gastroenterol Rep.* 2016;18(7):37.

35. Bhuket TP, Stollman NH. Chapter 121: Diverticular disease of the colon. In: Feldman M, Friedman LS, Brandt LJ, eds. *Sleisenger and Fordtran's Gastrointestinal and Liver Disease: Pathophysiology/Diagnosis/Management.* 10th ed. Philadelphia, PA: Elsevier/Saunders; 2016: 2123-2138.

36. Goh V, Halligan S, Taylor SA, Burling D, Bassett P, Bartram CI. Differentiation between diverticulitis and colorectal cancer: quantitative CT perfusion measurements versus morphologic criteria—initial experience. *Radiology.* 2007;242(2):456-462.

37. Laméris W, van Randen A, Bipat S, Bossuyt PMM, Boermeester MA, Stoker J. Graded compression ultrasonography and computed tomography in acute colonic diverticulitis: meta-analysis of test accuracy. *Eur Radiol.* 2008;18(11):2498-2511.

38. Salzman H, Lillie D. Diverticular disease: diagnosis and treatment. *Am Fam Physician.* 2005;72(7):1229-1234.

39. Abbas MA, Cannom RR, Chiu VY, et al. Triage of patients with acute diverticulitis: are some inpatients candidates for outpatient treatment? *Colorectal Dis.* 2013;15(4):451-457.

40. Strate LL, Peery AF, Neumann I. American Gastroenterological Association Institute technical review on the management of acute diverticulitis. *Gastroenterology.* 2015;149(7):1950-1976.e12.

41. Morris AM, Regenbogen SE, Hardiman KM, Hendren S. Sigmoid diverticulitis: a systematic review. *JAMA.* 2014;311(3):287-297.

42. Stollman N, Smalley W, Hirano I; AGA Institute Clinical Guidelines Committee. American Gastroenterological Association Institute guideline on the management of acute diverticulitis. *Gastroenterology.* 2015;149(7):1944-1949.

43. Feingold D, Steele SR, Lee S, et al. Practice parameters for the treatment of sigmoid diverticulitis. *Dis Colon Rectum.* 2014;57(3):284-294.

44. Siewert B, Tye G, Kruskal J, et al. Impact of CT-guided drainage in the treatment of diverticular abscesses: size matters. *AJR Am J Roentgenol.* 2006;186(3):680-686.

45. Schechter S, Eisenstat TE, Oliver GC, Rubin RJ, Salvati EP. Computerized tomographic scan-guided drainage of intra-abdominal abscesses. *Dis Colon Rectum.* 1994;37(10):984-988.

46. Ha C, Maser EA, Kornbluth A. Clinical presentation and outcomes of inflammatory bowel disease patients admitted to the intensive care unit. *J Clin Gastroenterol.* 2013;47(6):485-490.

47. Harbord M, Eliakim R, Bettenworth D, et al; European Crohn's and Colitis Organisation [ECCO]. Third European evidence-based consensus on diagnosis and management of

ulcerative colitis. Part 2: current management. *J Crohns Colitis.* 2017;11(7):769-784.

48. Grainge MJ, West J, Card TR. Venous thromboembolism during active disease and remission in inflammatory bowel disease: a cohort study. *Lancet.* 2010;375(9715):657-663.

49. González-Huix F, Fernández-Bañares F, Esteve-Comas M, et al. Enteral versus parenteral nutrition as adjunct therapy in acute ulcerative colitis. *Am J Gastroenterol.* 1993;88(2):227-232.

50. Gomollón F, Dignass A, Annese V, et al. 3rd European evidence-based consensus on the diagnosis and management of Crohn's disease 2016: part 1: diagnosis and medical management. *J Crohns Colitis.* 2017;11(1):3-25.

51. Mantzaris GJ, Hatzis A, Kontogiannis P, Triadaphyllou G. Intravenous tobramycin and metronidazole as an adjunct to corticosteroids in acute, severe ulcerative colitis. *Am J Gastroenterol.* 1994;89(1):43-46.

52. Travis S, Satsangi J, Lémann M. Predicting the need for colectomy in severe ulcerative colitis: a critical appraisal of clinical parameters and currently available biomarkers. *Gut.* 2011;60(1):3-9.

53. Maser EA, Deconda D, Lichtiger S, Ullman T, Present DH, Kornbluth A. Cyclosporine and infliximab as rescue therapy for each other in patients with steroid-refractory ulcerative colitis. *Clin Gastroenterol Hepatol.* 2008;6(10):1112-1116.

54. Sands BE. From symptom to diagnosis: clinical distinctions among various forms of intestinal inflammation. *Gastroenterology.* 2004;126(6):1518-1532.

55. Golda T, Zerpa C, Kreisler E, Trenti L, Biondo S. Incidence and management of anastomotic bleeding after ileocolic anastomosis. *Colorectal Dis.* 2013;15(10):1301-1308.

56. Tilney HS, Constantinides VA, Heriot AG, et al. Comparison of laparoscopic and open ileocecal resection for Crohn's disease: a metaanalysis. *Surg Endosc.* 2006;20(7):1036-1044.

57. Amiot A, Setakhr V, Seksik P, et al. Long-term outcome of enterocutaneous fistula in patients with Crohn's disease treated with anti-TNF therapy: a cohort study from the GETAID. *Am J Gastroenterol.* 2014;109(9):1443-1449.

58. Ravindran P, Ansari N, Young CJ, Solomon MJ. Definitive surgical closure of enterocutaneous fistula: outcome and factors predictive of increased postoperative morbidity. *Colorectal Dis.* 2014;16(3):209-218.

59. Halabi WJ, Jafari MD, Kang CY, et al. Colonic volvulus in the United States: trends, outcomes, and predictors of mortality. *Ann Surg.* 2014;259(2):293-301.

60. Friedman JD, Odland MD, Bubrick MP. Experience with colonic volvulus. *Dis Colon Rectum.* 1989;32(5):409-416.

61. Catalano O. Computed tomographic appearance of sigmoid volvulus. *Abdom Imaging.* 1996;21(4):314-317.

62. Atamanalp SS. Treatment of sigmoid volvulus: a single-center experience of 952 patients over 46.5 years. *Tech Coloproctol.* 2013;17(5):561-569.

63. Deans GT, Krukowski ZH, Irwin ST. Malignant obstruction of the left colon. *Br J Surg.* 1994;81(9):1270-1276.

64. Watt AM, Faragher IG, Griffin TT, Rieger NA, Maddern GJ. Self-expanding metallic stents for relieving malignant colorectal obstruction: a systematic review. *Ann Surg.* 2007;246(1):24-30.

65. Vogel JD, Feingold DL, Stewart DB, et al. Clinical practice guidelines for colon volvulus and acute colonic pseudo-obstruction. *Dis Colon Rectum.* 2016;59(7):589-600.

66. ASGE Standards of Practice Committee; Harrison ME, Anderson MA, Appalaneni V, et al. The role of endoscopy in the management of patients with known and suspected colonic obstruction and pseudo-obstruction. *Gastrointest Endosc.* 2010;71(4):669-679.

67. Saunders MD. Acute colonic pseudo-obstruction. *Best Pract Res Clin Gastroenterol.* 2007;21(4):671-687.

68. Loftus CG, Harewood GC, Baron TH. Assessment of predictors of response to neostigmine for acute colonic pseudo-obstruction. *Am J Gastroenterol.* 2002;97(12):3118-3122.

69. Rex DK. Colonoscopy and acute colonic pseudo-obstruction. *Gastrointest Endosc Clin N Am.* 1997;7(3):499-508.

70. Friedman GD. Natural history of asymptomatic and symptomatic gallstones. *Am J Surg.* 1993;165(4):399-404.

71. Cafasso DE, Smith RR. Symptomatic cholelithiasis and functional disorders of the biliary tract. *Surg Clin North Am.* 2014;94(2):233-256.

72. Shea JA, Berlin JA, Escarce JJ, et al. Revised estimates of diagnostic test sensitivity and specificity in suspected biliary tract disease. *Arch Intern Med.* 1994;154(22):2573-2581.

73. Duncan CB, Riall TS. Evidence-based current surgical practice: calculous gallbladder disease. *J Gastrointest Surg.* 2012;16(11):2011-2025.

74. Q-Y Wang D, Afdhal NH. Chapter 65: Gallstone disease. In: Feldman M, Friedman LS, eds. *Sleisinger's and Fordtran's Gastrointestinal and Liver Disease.* 10th ed. Philadelphia, PA: Elsevier-Saunders; 2016: 1100-1133.

75. Andersson KL, Friedman LS. Chapter 67: Acalculous biliary pain, acute acalculous cholecystitis, cholesterolosis, adenomyomatosis, and gallbladder polyps. In: Feldman M, Friedman LS, eds. *Sleisinger's and Fordtran's Gastrointestinal and Liver Disease.* 10th ed. Philadelphia, PA: Elsevier-Saunders; 2016: 1152-1165.

76. Solomkin JS, Mazuski JE, Bradley JS, et al. Diagnosis and management of complicated intra-abdominal infection in adults and children: guidelines by the Surgical Infection Society and the Infectious Diseases Society of America. *Clin Infect Dis.* 2010;50(2):133-164.

77. Wu XD, Tian X, Liu MM, Wu L, Zhao S, Zhao L. Meta-analysis comparing early versus delayed laparoscopic cholecystectomy for acute cholecystitis. *Br J Surg.* 2015;102(11):1302-1313.

78. Baron TH, Grimm IS, Swanstrom LL. Interventional approaches to gallbladder disease. *N Engl J Med.* 2015; 373(4):357-365.

79. Mirvis SE, Vainright JR, Nelson AW, et al. The diagnosis of acute acalculous cholecystitis: a comparison of sonography, scintigraphy, and CT. *AJR Am J Roentgenol.* 1986;147(6): 1171-1175.

80. Chung YH, Choi ER, Kim KM, et al. Can percutaneous cholecystostomy be a definitive management for acute acalculous cholecystitis? *J Clin Gastroenterol.* 2012;46(3):216-219.

81. ASGE Standards of Practice Committee, Maple JT, Ben-Menachem T, Anderson MA, et al. The role of endoscopy in the evaluation of suspected choledocholithiasis. *Gastrointest Endosc.* 2010;71(1):1-9.

82. Gurusamy KS, Giljaca V, Takwoingi Y, et al. Ultrasound versus liver function tests for diagnosis of common bile duct stones. *Cochrane Database Syst Rev.* 2015;(2):CD011548.

83. Pasanen PA, Partanen KP, Pikkarainen PH, Alhava EM, Janatuinen EK, Pirinen AE. A comparison of ultrasound,

computed tomography and endoscopic retrograde cholangiopancreatography in the differential diagnosis of benign and malignant jaundice and cholestasis. *Eur J Surg.* 1993;159(1):23-29.

84. Kaltenthaler E, Vergel YB, Chilcott J, et al. A systematic review and economic evaluation of magnetic resonance cholangiopancreatography compared with diagnostic endoscopic retrograde cholangiopancreatography. *Health Technol Assess.* 2004;8(10):iii, 1-89.

85. ASGE Standards of Practice Committee; Maple JT, Ikenberry SO, Anderson MA, et al. The role of endoscopy in the management of choledocholithiasis. *Gastrointest Endosc.* 2011;74(4):731-744.

86. ASGE Standards of Practice Committee; Chandrasekhara V, Khashab MA, Muthusamy VR, et al. Adverse events associated with ERCP. *Gastrointest Endosc.* 2017;85(1):32-47.

87. McAlister VC, Davenport E, Renouf E. Cholecystectomy deferral in patients with endoscopic sphincterotomy. *Cochrane Database Syst Rev.* 2007;(4):CD006233.

88. Hui CK, Lai KC, Yuen MF, et al. Does the addition of endoscopic sphincterotomy to stent insertion improve drainage of the bile duct in acute suppurative cholangitis? *Gastrointest Endosc.* 2003;58(4):500-504.

89. Kwon AH, Inui H. Preoperative diagnosis and efficacy of laparoscopic procedures in the treatment of Mirizzi syndrome. *J Am Coll Surg.* 2007;204(3):409-415.

90. Kulkarni SS, Hotta M, Sher L, et al. Complicated gallstone disease: diagnosis and management of Mirizzi syndrome. *Surg Endosc.* 2016;31(5):2215-2222.

91. Canena J, Horta D, Coimbra J, et al. Outcomes of endoscopic management of primary and refractory postcholecystectomy biliary leaks in a multicentre review of 178 patients. *BMC Gastroenterol.* 2015;15:105.

92. Woods MS, Traverso LW, Kozarek RA, et al. Characteristics of biliary tract complications during laparoscopic cholecystectomy: a multi-institutional study. *Am J Surg.* 1994;167(1):27-33; discussion 33.

93. Al Sofayan MS, Ibrahim A, Helmy A, Al Saghier MI, Al Sebayel MI, Abozied MM. Nuclear imaging of the liver: is there a diagnostic role of HIDA in posttransplantation? *Transplant Proc.* 2009;41(1):201-207.

94. Lowenfels AB, Maisonneuve P, Sullivan T. The changing character of acute pancreatitis: epidemiology, etiology, and prognosis. *Curr Gastroenterol Rep.* 2009;11(2):97-103.

95. Arvanitakis M, Delhaye M, De Maertelaere V, et al. Computed tomography and magnetic resonance imaging in the assessment of acute pancreatitis. *Gastroenterology.* 2004;126(3):715-723.

96. Tenner S, Baillie J, DeWitt J, Vege SS; American College of Gastroenterology. American College of Gastroenterology guideline: management of acute pancreatitis. *Am J Gastroenterol.* 2013;108(9):1400-1416.

97. Wu BU, Hwang JQ, Gardner TH, et al. Lactated Ringer's solution reduces systemic inflammation compared with saline in patients with acute pancreatitis. *Clin Gastroenterol Hepatol.* 2011;9(8):710-717.e1.

98. Brown A, Orav J, Banks PA. Hemoconcentration is an early marker for organ failure and necrotizing pancreatitis. *Pancreas.* 2000;20(4):367-372.

99. Mouli VP, Sreenivas V, Garg PK. Efficacy of conservative treatment, without necrosectomy, for infected pancreatic necrosis: a systematic review and meta-analysis. *Gastroenterology.* 2013;144(2):333-340.e2.

100. Jiang K, Huang W, Yang X-N, Xia Q. Present and future of prophylactic antibiotics for severe acute pancreatitis. *World J Gastroenterol.* 2012;18(3):279-284.

101. Wu BU, Johannes RS, Sun X, Tabak Y, Conwell DL, Banks PA. The early prediction of mortality in acute pancreatitis: a large population-based study. *Gut.* 2008;57(12):1698-1703.

102. Eckerwall GE, Tingstedt BBA, Bergenzaun PE, Andersson RG. Immediate oral feeding in patients with mild acute pancreatitis is safe and may accelerate recovery—a randomized clinical study. *Clin Nutr.* 2007;26(6):758-763.

103. Bakker OJ, van Brunschot S, van Santvoort HC, et al. Early versus on-demand nasoenteric tube feeding in acute pancreatitis. *N Engl J Med.* 2014;371(21):1983-1993.

104. Zhu Y, Yin H, Zhang R, Ye X, Wei J. Nasogastric nutrition versus nasojejunal nutrition in patients with severe acute pancreatitis: a meta-analysis of randomized controlled trials. *Gastroenterol Res Pract.* 2016;2016:6430632.

105. Yi F, Ge L, Zhao J, et al. Meta-analysis: total parenteral nutrition versus total enteral nutrition in predicted severe acute pancreatitis. *Intern Med.* 2012;51(6):523-530.

106. da Costa DW, Bouwense SA, Schepers NJ, et al. Same-admission versus interval cholecystectomy for mild gallstone pancreatitis (PONCHO): a multicentre randomised controlled trial. *Lancet.* 2015;386(10000):1261-1268.

107. Uhl W, Müller CA, Krähenbühl L, Schmid SW, Schölzel S, Büchler MW. Acute gallstone pancreatitis: timing of laparoscopic cholecystectomy in mild and severe disease. *Surg Endosc.* 1999;13(11):1070-1076.

108. Nordback I, Pelli H, Lappalainen-Lehto R, Järvinen S, Räty S, Sand J. The recurrence of acute alcohol-associated pancreatitis can be reduced: a randomized controlled trial. *Gastroenterology.* 2009;136(3):848-855.

109. Forsmark CE, Vege SS, Wilcox CM. Acute pancreatitis. *N Engl J Med.* 2016;375(20):1972-1981.

110. Tenner S, Steinberg WM. Chapter 58: Acute pancreatitis. In: Feldman M, Friedman LS, Brandt LJ, eds. *Sleisenger and Fordtran's Gastrointestinal and Liver Disease: Pathophysiology/ Diagnosis/Management.* 10th ed. Philadelphia, PA: Elsevier/ Saunders; 2016: 969-993.

111. Dahl PR, Su WP, Cullimore KC, Dicken CH. Pancreatic panniculitis. *J Am Acad Dermatol.* 1995;33(3):413-417.

112. Lee WM, Stravitz RT, Larson AM. Introduction to the revised American Association for the Study of Liver Diseases position paper on acute liver failure 2011. *Hepatology.* 2012;55(3): 965-967.

113. Ostapowicz G, Fontana RJ, Schiødt FV, et al. Results of a prospective study of acute liver failure at 17 tertiary care centers in the United States. *Ann Intern Med.* 2002;137(12):947-954.

114. Zimmerman HJ, Maddrey WC. Acetaminophen (paracetamol) hepatotoxicity with regular intake of alcohol: analysis of instances of therapeutic misadventure. *Hepatology.* 1995;22(3):767-773.

115. Khandelwal N, James LP, Sanders C, Larson AM, Lee WM; Acute Liver Failure Study Group. Unrecognized acetaminophen toxicity as a cause of indeterminate acute liver failure. *Hepatology.* 2011;53(2):567-576.

116. Wallace CI, Dargan PI, Jones AL. Paracetamol overdose: an evidence based flowchart to guide management. *Emerg Med J.* 2002;19(3):202-205.

117. Lee WM, Hynan LS, Rossaro L, et al. Intravenous N-acetylcysteine improves transplant-free survival in early stage non-acetaminophen acute liver failure. *Gastroenterology.* 2009;137(3):856-864.e1.

118. Baquerizo A, Anselmo D, Shackleton C, et al. Phosphorus as an early predictive factor in patients with acute liver failure. *Transplantation.* 2003;75(12):2007-2014.

119. Organ Procurement and Transplantation Network. Policies. US Department of Health and Human Services Heath Resources and Services Administration Web site. https://optn.transplant.hrsa.gov/governance/policies/. Accessed October 4, 2016.

120. El-Serag HB. Hepatocellular carcinoma. *N Engl J Med.* 2011;365(12):1118-1127.

121. Garcia-Tsao G, Abraldes JG, Berzigotti A, Bosch J. Portal hypertensive bleeding in cirrhosis: Risk stratification, diagnosis, and management: 2016 practice guidance by the American Association for the study of liver diseases. *Hepatology.* 2017; 65(1):310-335.

122. Bosch J, Thabut D, Albillos A, et al. Recombinant factor VIIa for variceal bleeding in patients with advanced cirrhosis: a randomized, controlled trial. *Hepatology.* 2008; 47(5):1604-1614.

123. Chavez-Tapia NC, Barrientos-Gutierrez T, Tellez-Avila F, et al. Meta-analysis: antibiotic prophylaxis for cirrhotic patients with upper gastrointestinal bleeding—an updated Cochrane review. *Aliment Pharmacol Ther.* 2011;34(5):509-518.

124. Wells M, Chande N, Adams P, et al. Meta-analysis: vasoactive medications for the management of acute variceal bleeds. *Aliment Pharmacol Ther.* 2012;35(11):1267-1278.

125. Reiberger T, Ferlitsch A, Payer BA, et al. Non-selective beta-blocker therapy decreases intestinal permeability and serum levels of LBP and IL-6 in patients with cirrhosis. *J Hepatol.* 2013; 58(5):911-921.

126. Vilstrup H, Amodio P, Bajaj J, et al. Hepatic encephalopathy in chronic liver disease: 2014 practice guideline by the American Association for the Study of Liver Diseases and the European Association for the Study of the Liver. *Hepatology.* 2014;60(2):715-735.

127. Khungar V, Poordad F. Hepatic encephalopathy. *Clin Liver Dis.* 2012;16(2):301-320.

128. Rahimi RS, Singal AG, Cuthbert JA, Rockey DC. Lactulose vs polyethylene glycol 3350—electrolyte solution for treatment of overt hepatic encephalopathy: the HELP randomized clinical trial. *JAMA Intern Med.* 2014;174(11):1727-1733.

129. Bass NM, Mullen KD, Sanyal A, et al. Rifaximin treatment in hepatic encephalopathy. *N Engl J Med.* 2010;362(12):1071-1081.

130. Bernardi M, Moreau R, Angeli P, Schnabl B, Arroyo V. Mechanisms of decompensation and organ failure in cirrhosis: From peripheral arterial vasodilation to systemic inflammation hypothesis. *J Hepatol.* 2015;63(5):1272-1284.

131. Ginès P, Guevara M. Hyponatremia in cirrhosis: pathogenesis, clinical significance, and management. *Hepatology.* 2008;48(3):1002-1010.

132. Arroyo V, Ginès P, Gerbes AL, et al. Definition and diagnostic criteria of refractory ascites and hepatorenal syndrome in cirrhosis. International Ascites Club. *Hepatology.* 1996;23(1):164-176.

133. Runyon BA; AASLD. Introduction to the revised American Association for the Study of Liver Diseases Practice Guideline management of adult patients with ascites due to cirrhosis 2012. *Hepatology.* 2013;57(4):1651-1653.

134. Bureau C, Thabut D, Oberti F, et al. Transjugular intrahepatic portosystemic shunts with covered stents increase transplant-free survival of patients with cirrhosis and recurrent ascites. *Gastroenterology.* 2017;152(1):157-163.

135. Im GY, Lubezky N, Facciuto ME, Schiano TD. Surgery in patients with portal hypertension: a preoperative checklist and strategies for attenuating risk. *Clin Liver Dis.* 2014;18(2):477-505.

136. Sort P, Navasa M, Arroyo V, et al. Effect of intravenous albumin on renal impairment and mortality in patients with cirrhosis and spontaneous bacterial peritonitis. *N Engl J Med.* 1999;341(6):403-409.

137. Durand F, Graupera I, Ginès P, Olson JC, Nadim MK. Pathogenesis of hepatorenal syndrome: implications for therapy. *Am J Kidney Dis.* 2016;67(2):318-328.

138. Angeli P, Ginès P, Wong F, et al. Diagnosis and management of acute kidney injury in patients with cirrhosis: revised consensus recommendations of the International Club of Ascites. *J Hepatol.* 2015;62(4):968-974.

139. Esrailian E, Pantangco ER, Kyulo NL, Hu KQ, Runyon BA. Octreotide/midodrine therapy significantly improves renal function and 30-day survival in patients with type 1 hepatorenal syndrome. *Dig Dis Sci.* 2007;52(3):742-748.

140. Witzke O, Baumann M, Patschan D, et al. Which patients benefit from hemodialysis therapy in hepatorenal syndrome? *J Gastroenterol Hepatol.* 2004;19(12):1369-1373.

141. Yun BC, Kim WR, Benson JT, et al. Impact of pretransplant hyponatremia on outcome following liver transplantation. *Hepatology.* 2009;49(5):1610-1615.

142. Biggins SW, Kim WR, Terrault NA, et al. Evidence-based incorporation of serum sodium concentration into MELD. *Gastroenterology.* 2006;130(6):1652-1660.

143. Kim WR, Biggins SW, Kremers WK, et al. Hyponatremia and mortality among patients on the liver-transplant waiting list. *N Engl J Med.* 2008;359(10):1018-1026.

144. Sharma P, Schaubel DE, Goodrich NP, Merion RM. Serum sodium and survival benefit of liver transplantation. *Liver Transpl.* 2015;21(3):308-313.

145. Sinha VK, Ko B. Hyponatremia in cirrhosis—pathogenesis, treatment, and prognostic significance. *Adv Chronic Kidney Dis.* 2015;22(5):361-367.

146. Jalan R, Mookerjee R, Cheshire L, Williams R, Davies N. Albumin infusion for severe hyponatremia in patients with refractory ascites: a randomical trial. *J Hepatol.* 2007; 46(Suppl 1):S95.

147. Spasovski G, Vanholder R, Allolio B, et al. Clinical practice guideline on diagnosis and treatment of hyponatraemia. *Eur J Endocrinol.* 2014;170(3):G1-G47.

148. Romanovsky A, Azevedo LCP, Meeberg G, Zibdawi R, Bigam D, Bagshaw SM. Serum sodium shift in hyponatremic patients undergoing liver transplantation: a retrospective cohort study. *Ren Fail.* 2015;37(1):37-44.

149. Hudcova J, Ruthazer R, Bonney I, Schumann R. Sodium homeostasis during liver transplantation and correlation with outcomes. *Anesth Analg.* 2014;119(6):1420-1428.

150. Martin P, DiMartini A, Feng S, Brown R, Fallon M. Evaluation for liver transplantation in adults: 2013 practice guideline by the American Association for the Study of Liver Diseases and the American Society of Transplantation. *Hepatology.* 2014; 59(3):1144-1165.

151. Kaplan DE, Dai F, Skanderson M, et al. Recalibrating the Child-Turcotte-Pugh Score to improve prediction of transplant-free survival in patients with cirrhosis. *Dig Dis Sci.* 2016;61(11):3309-3320.

152. Razonable RR, Findlay JY, O'Riordan A, et al. Critical care issues in patients after liver transplantation. *Liver Transpl.* 2011;17(5):511-527.

153. Bekker J, Ploem S, de Jong KP. Early hepatic artery thrombosis after liver transplantation: a systematic review of the incidence, outcome and risk factors. *Am J Transplant.* 2009;9(4):746-757.

154. Mourad MM, Liossis C, Gunson BK, et al. Etiology and management of hepatic artery thrombosis after adult liver transplantation. *Liver Transpl.* 2014;20(6):713-723.

155. Lucey MR, Terrault N, Ojo L, et al. Long-term management of the successful adult liver transplant: 2012 practice guideline by the American Association for the Study of Liver Diseases and the American Society of Transplantation. *Liver Transpl.* 2013;19(1):3-26.

156. Chen H, Turon F, Hernández-Gea V, et al. Nontumoral portal vein thrombosis in patients awaiting liver transplantation. *Liver Transpl.* 2016;22(3):352-365.

157. Del Bello A, Danjoux M, Congy-Jolivet N, et al. Histological long-term outcomes from acute antibody-mediated rejection following ABO-compatible liver transplantation. *J Gastroenterol Hepatol.* 2017;32(4):887-893.

158. Gumaste VV, Dave PB. Ingestion of corrosive substances by adults. *Am J Gastroenterol.* 1992;87(1):1-5.

159. Fisher RA, Eckhauser ML, Radivoyevitch M. Acid ingestion in an experimental model. *Surg Gynecol Obstet.* 1985; 161(1):91-99.

160. Zargar SA, Kochhar R, Mehta S, Mehta SK. The role of fiberoptic endoscopy in the management of corrosive ingestion and modified endoscopic classification of burns. *Gastrointest Endosc.* 1991;37(2):165-169.

161. Kirsh MM, Peterson A, Brown JW, Orringer MB, Ritter F, Sloan H. Treatment of caustic injuries of the esophagus: a ten year experience. *Ann Surg.* 1978;188(5):675-678.

162. Zhou JH, Jiang YG, Wang RW, et al. Management of corrosive esophageal burns in 149 cases. *J Thorac Cardiovasc Surg.* 2005;130(2):449-455.

163. ASGE Standards of Practice Committee; Ikenberry SO, Jue TL, Anderson MA, et al. Management of ingested foreign bodies and food impactions. *Gastrointest Endosc.* 2011; 73(6):1085-1091.

164. Evrard S, Le Moine O, Lazaraki G, Dormann A, El Nakadi I, Devière J. Self-expanding plastic stents for benign esophageal lesions. *Gastrointest Endosc.* 2004;60(6):894-900.

165. Broor SL, Raju GS, Bose PP, et al. Long term results of endoscopic dilatation for corrosive oesophageal strictures. *Gut.* 1993;34(11):1498-1501.

166. Kochhar R, Sethy PK, Kochhar S, Nagi B, Gupta NM. Corrosive induced carcinoma of esophagus: report of three patients and review of literature. *J Gastroenterol Hepatol.* 2006; 21(4):777-780.

167. Venara A, Neunlist M, Slim K, et al. Postoperative ileus: pathophysiology, incidence, and prevention. *J Visc Surg.* 2016;153(6):439-446.

168. Lappas JC, Reyes BL, Maglinte DD. Abdominal radiography findings in small-bowel obstruction: relevance to triage for additional diagnostic imaging. *AJR Am J Roentgenol.* 2001; 176(1):167-174.

169. Fevang BT, Jensen D, Svanes K, Viste A. Early operation or conservative management of patients with small bowel obstruction? *Eur J Surg.* 2002;168(8-9):475-481.

170. McDonald LC, Gerding DN, Johnson S, et al. Clinical Practice Guidelines for Clostridium difficile infection in Adults and Children: 2017 Update by the Infectious Diseases Society of America (IDSA) and Society for Healthcare Epidemiology of America (SHEA). *Clinical Infectious Disease.* 2018;66(7):e1-e48.

Obstetrics

Anna Collo Go, MD, Ronaldo Collo Go, MD, and
Evangeline Collo Go, MD

INTRODUCTION

The prevalence of obstetric patients in critical care is 1 to 9 in 1000 pregnancies, with a 12% to 20% mortality.[1-4] The majority of puerperium cases are related to hemorrhage or hypertension, while the majority of postpartum cases are due to hemorrhage and postsurgical complications.[5] Physiologic changes associated with pregnancy affect diagnostics and treatment.

MATERNAL PHYSIOLOGIC CHANGES

Maternal cardiovascular changes occur in the first trimester, may manifest as early as 5 weeks, peak by the end of the second trimester, plateau up to term, and normalize 2 to 12 weeks postpartum.[6] This is primarily mediated by estrogen effecting uterine blood flow and progesterone and prostaglandin E2 causing vasodilation of uteroplacental vessels.[1] Cardiac output (CO) increases by 30% to 50% from 8 to 28 weeks.[3,6] Central venous pressure (CVP) and pulmonary capillary wedge pressure (PCWP) are unchanged secondary to reduced systemic vascular resistance (SVR; 20-30%) and pulmonary vascular resistance (PVR; 20-30%).[7] After 24 weeks, supine hypotension syndrome is characterized by hypotension, 5 to 10 mmHg below normal, and bradycardia secondary to decrease in cardiac output from compression of the inferior vena cava (IVC) by the gravid uterus. This can be alleviated by a left lateral tilt positioning.[3,6,7] During labor, there is an increase of 10% to 20% in CO due to a return of 300 to 500 mL of blood to the maternal circulation with each uterine contraction.[3,7]

Prothrombogenic effects include changes with coagulation factors such as increased fibrinogen, factor VII, and factor X and decreased factor XI, factor XIII, and platelets.[1] The patient's ability to tolerate up to 1 Liter of blood loss during labor counteracts the effects of physiologic anemia (ie, increased plasma volume by up to 50% by term with a much lower increase in red blood cells) and decrease in colloid oncotic pressure (by 14%).[3,6,7] There is an increased lower extremity venous pressure from compression of the uterus on the inferior vena cava, causing varicose veins and hemorrhoids.

Pulmonary changes are progesterone mediated, causing an increase in tidal volume (30-35%), minute ventilation (20-40%), and respiratory alkalosis ($Paco_2$ of 28-32 mmHg) with compensatory renal excretion of bicarbonate (CO_2 of 18-21 mEq/L) by term.[3,6] The gravid uterus causes a 10% to 25% decrease in functional residual capacity with a 4-cm elevation of diaphragm, and much less decrease in total lung capacity secondary to compensation of the thoracic cage.[3,6,7] Chest wall and total respiratory compliance decrease with no effect on total lung compliance.[3] Maternal-to-fetal oxygen exchange is enhanced by the ability of the fetus to extract oxygen better at higher hemoglobin (Hgb) concentrations, a higher oxygen saturation of fetal hemoglobin (HgbF) (80-90%) compared to that of HgbA (50-55%) at a Po_2 of 30 to 35 mmHg, and the presence of a patent ductus arteriosus.[1,3]

Renal changes include a 45% to 50% increase in glomerular filtration rate (GFR) and creatinine clearance resulting in a decrease in the following: serum creatinine (< 0.8-0.9 mg/dL), blood urea nitrogen (< 15 mg/dL), and uric acid levels (< 6 mg/dL).[1,6] Decreased blood pressure and wide pulse pressure in the late second and early third trimester are partly due to the decreased serum osmolarity and reduced sensitivity to increasing levels of aldosterone, estrogen, and plasma renin. Acute kidney injury is defined in a pregnant patient as having a serum creatinine of greater than 1 mg/dL.[1] Beginning in the sixth week, the right ureter is compressed secondary to the growing uterus, which increases urinary stasis and therefore infection.

Gastrointestinal changes are linked to progesterone-related smooth muscle relaxation and the displacement of organs. Nutrient adsorption may be increased, but at the same time, the patient may experience increased constipation, obstipation, or exacerbated gastroesophageal reflux disease (GERD). There will also be decreased utility of diagnostic physical signs such as Murphy sign and McBurney point.[1] Decreased gallbladder tone and emptying, biliary stasis secondary to progesterone, and increased cholesterol and lithogenicity of bile secondary to estrogen increase cholelithiasis. Alkaline phosphate maybe increased from 2 to 15 times normal.

PREGNANCY-SPECIFIC DISEASES

Rheumatologic Diseases

Pregnant patients with systemic lupus erythematosus (SLE) have a higher incidence of spontaneous abortions, intrauterine growth restriction, preterm labor, premature rupture of membranes, and preeclampsia. There is also an additional challenge in differentiating between SLE nephritis and preeclampsia, although elevated anti–double stranded DNA (anti-dsDNA) could suggest active SLE and normal or slightly elevated complement C3 and C4 could suggest preeclampsia. Other autoimmune diseases may show improvement, such as rheumatoid arthritis, especially in the second and third trimester, although the reason has not been definitively established.[8]

Neurologic Diseases

Headaches are common during pregnancy and in the postpartum period. Headache frequency and characteristics should prompt the clinician to investigate for secondary causes. Thunderclap headache, described as having an abrupt onset of severe unusual headaches, may be due to preeclampsia, posterior reversible encephalopathy syndrome (PRES), or cerebral vein thrombosis. Multiple episodes of migraine headaches (5 or more) or tension headaches (10 or more) should be considered in diagnosing primary headache disorders. Migraines with auras can manifest with transient positive or negative neurologic deficits that typically resolve after 30 minutes. Prompt evaluation for other causes such as cerebrovascular accident (CVA), preeclampsia, HELLP (hemolysis, elevated liver enzymes, low platelet count), cervicoarterial dissection, orbital hemorrhage, and pituitary apoplexy should be considered. Bilateral throbbing headaches that may be accompanied by blurred vision and scotomata are typical in preeclamptics. Postdural headaches secondary to low cerebrospinal fluid (CSF) pressure from the administration of spinal anesthesia can occur up to 1 week postpartum. These headaches, typically nuchal and occipital, that are exacerbated by standing up and relieved by sitting down, may be accompanied by tinnitus, diplopia, and hyperacusis, and can resolve in 48 hours after a blood patch.[9]

Patients with multiple sclerosis have reduced exacerbations during the third trimester but increased risk of exacerbations up to 3 months postpartum.[8,10] The cause of this is unclear but may be due to decreased cell-mediated immunity, increased production of tolerance promoting signals, and interferon γ.[10] Forty percent of patients with myasthenia gravis will experience an exacerbation.[11]

The incidence of cardiovascular disease is as follows: Ischemic CVA occurs more frequently than intracerebral hemorrhage (ICH), which occurs more frequently than subarachnoid hemorrhage (SAH), which occurs more frequently than cerebral venous thrombosis.[12,13] Diagnosis is via computed tomography (CT) of the head with abdominal shield or magnetic resonance imaging (MRI) with iodine, but avoiding gadolinium.[12,13] Thrombolysis with recombinant tissue plasminogen activator can be given to patients with ischemic CVA within 3 to 4.5 hours of onset, since it does not cross the placenta.[14-21] Aspirin can be used as

thromboprophylaxis, although there is an association with gastroschisis in the first trimester.[22]

Patients with epilepsy do not have an increased frequency of seizures during pregnancy.[23] Antiepileptic medications are associated with fetal complications. Phenytoin is associated with cleft palate and lip, and nail and distal phalangeal hypoplasia. Phenobarbital is associated with congenital heart defects and facial defects. Valproic acid is associated with spina bifida and cardiovascular and urogenital malformations.

Pulmonary Diseases

In acute respiratory distress syndrome (ARDS) and other pulmonary diseases, a plateau pressure of greater than 30 cm H_2O may not be applicable in pregnant patients where normal intra-abdominal pressures increase to 14 mmHg; therefore monitoring of transpulmonary pressures is required. Maintenance of a maternal Pao_2 greater than 70 mmHg is required to ensure adequate fetal oxygenation. The normal $Paco_2$ is 28 to 32 mmHg, but hypocapnia and hypercapnia must be avoided in pregnancy. Hypocapnia causes decreased uteroplacental blood flow and fetal alkalosis. Hypercapnia, Pao_2 greater than 60 to 70 mmHg, can lead to elevated intracranial pressure. Termination of pregnancy is recommended if ARDS is secondary to specific obstetric causes.[12]

For patients with thromboembolic disease, deep vein thrombosis (DVT) is more common than pulmonary edema (PE). Eighty-five percent of DVT cases occur in the left lower extremity due to compression of the left iliac vein by the uterus. The initial test for DVT is ultrasound, although there is a high false-negative rate in pelvic vein thrombosis; if the initial test is negative, it may be repeated in 1 week. A chest radiograph should be used to rule out other cases of hypoxia with abdominal shielding. Computed tomography angiography (CTA) is indicated if the patient presents with severe hypoxia, hemodynamic compromise, or ventilation/perfusion (V/Q) scan with negative results but high suspicion. A V/Q scan is preferred if the patient is hemodynamically stable so as to expose breast milk to less carcinogenic radiation. Treatment with low-molecular-weight heparin (LMWH) is preferred over unfractionated heparin (UFH), except in the cases of obesity, renal dysfunction, and high risk of bleeding. If patient is on long term LMWH, after 36 to 37 weeks, it is recommended that the patient be switched to UFH for massive DVT, massive PE, or thrombolysis.[12]

Cardiac Diseases

Pregnancy is contraindicated in the following cases: pulmonary hypertension, systolic ejection fraction less than 30%, New York Heart Association (NYHA) class III/IV, previous peripartum cardiomyopathy with residual deficit, severe mitral or aortic stenosis, severe coarctation of aorta, aortic dilation greater than 45 mm in Marfan syndrome, or aortic dilation greater than 50 mmHg with bicuspid aortic valve. Balloon valvotomy for severe mitral or aortic stenosis is tolerated after 20 weeks age of gestation (AOG). If the patient presents with resistant heart failure for aortic stenosis, delivery via cesarean section and then valvotomy are recommended.[12]

If cardiac arrest occurs after 20 weeks AOG, delivery via cesarean section is recommended if return of spontaneous circulation (ROSC) is not achieved within 4 minutes. Neurological fetal outcome is better if delivery is within 5 minutes of cardiac arrest.[12]

Endocrinologic Diseases

Diabetic ketoacidosis can occur in glucose as low as 180 mg/dL.[12]

Gastrointestinal Diseases

For acute abdomen, ultrasound is preferred, but MRI is preferred if the patient is greater than 35 weeks AOG or the ultrasound is nonconclusive.[24-26] Laparoscopy is safe at any trimester, although fetal demise has been reported.[27-29]

Infectious Diseases

Generalized blanching erythema suggests streptococcal toxic shock syndrome.[12,30,31] Culture should be obtained from both sides of the placenta, and ultrasound should be performed to monitor for retained products, pyometra, or abscess.[12,30,31] Intramyometrial gas on ultrasound suggests *Clostridium perfringens* and warrants surgical intervention.[12,30,31] Preferred antibiotic is clindamycin with aminoglycoside.[12,30,31]

Table 25-1 defines and describes the United States Food and Drug Administration (FDA) drug categories regarding safety during pregnancy.

TABLE 25-1 FDA Drug Categories, Definition, Medications, and Side Effects

Category	Definition	Medications	Side Effects
A	Adequate and well-controlled human studies on pregnant women fail to demonstrate fetal risk in first trimester and subsequent trimesters	Milk of magnesia	None
B	Animal studies fail to demonstrate fetal risk, but there are no well-controlled human studies and benefits outweigh risks OR animal studies have not been conducted and there are no human studies	Methyldopa Piperacillin-Tazobactam Cefepime Metronidazole Erythromycin Azithromycin Amphotericin B Meropenem Daptomycin Fosfomycin Enoxaparin Hydrochlorothiazide Dobutamine Bromocriptine	None
C	Animal studies have shown adverse effect to fetus but there are no well-controlled, randomized human studies and benefits may outweigh risks OR animal studies have not been conducted and there are no well-controlled human studies	Cyclosporine[32] or Tacrolimus[32] Prednisolone[32] Hydralazine Labetalol ACEI (first trimester) Nifedipine Milrinone Dopamine Digoxin Metoprolol Epinephrine Norepinephrine Heparin Haldol (third trimester) Vancomycin Clarithromycin Trimethoprim Fluoroquinolones Chloramphenicol Imipenem Fluconazole Echinocandins	Premature labor, hyperkalemia, low birth weight, renal dysfunction[32] Intrauterine growth retardation, cleft palate, premature rupture of membranes, fetal adrenal hypoplasia[32] IUGR, fatigue, sleep disturbance, bronchoconstriction[33] Cardiac and central nervous system fetal abnormalities[33] Reflex tachycardia[33] Gasping syndrome, osteoporosis, seizures, intracranial hemorrhage Feeding disorder, respiratory depression, hyper- or hypotonia, tremor

(Continued)

TABLE 25-1 FDA Drug Categories, Definition, Medications, and Side Effects (Continued)

Category	Definition	Medications	Side Effects
D	There is human fetal risk based on investigational and marketing studies in humans BUT there are potential benefits in life-threatening situations or serious disease in which safer medications are ineffective	Azathioprine[32]	Lymphopenia, hypogammaglobulinemia, thymic hypoplasia[32]
		Mycophenolate[32]	Microtia, congenital malformation, first trimester loss[32]
		ACEI (second and third trimesters)	Renal failure, oligohydramnios, pulmonary hypoplasia, calvarial abnormalities, fetal growth restriction[7]
		Lisinopril	
		Losartan	
		Lorazepam	Neonatal flaccidity, feeding and respiratory difficulties, hypothermia
		Midazolam	
		Diazepam	
		Aminoglycosides	
		Tetracyclines	
		Tigecycline	
X	Animal and human studies show fetal abnormalities OR positive evidence of fetal risk from investigational or marketing studies AND risks outweigh potential benefits	Coumadin	

ACEI = angiotensin-converting enzyme inhibitors; IUGR = intrauterine growth restriction.

QUESTIONS

1. A 29-year-old woman at 8 weeks age of gestation has been having intractable nausea and vomiting for the last 2 weeks and was admitted to the hospital. She was started on antiemetic medications and dextrose ½ normal saline for intravenous fluids. After 2 weeks, she failed to improve and her neurologic status appeared to change. Her cognition appeared to have slowed down and she was noted to have vertical and horizontal nystagmus. Her labs show the following:

WBC	$15 \times 10^3/\mu L$
Hgb	16 g/dL
Hct	45%
plt	$150 \times 10^3/\mu L$
Na	135 mEq/L
K	2.2 mEq/L
Cl	88 mEq/L
CO$_2$	34 mEq/L
BUN	40 mg/dL
Crea	1.2 mg/dL
Ca	8 mg/dL
Glucose	90 mg/dL
Albumin	3.5 g/dL
AST	150 U/L
ALT	150 U/L
Alk phos	100 U/L
Total Bili	3.5 mg/dL
Lipase	200

Her CT head was negative. Her video electroencephalography (VEEG) is pending. What is the likely diagnosis?

A. Wernicke encephalopathy from hyperemesis gravidarum
B. Subclinical status epilepticus from HELLP syndrome
C. Hepatic encephalopathy from intrahepatic cholestasis of pregnancy
D. Hyperparathyroidism

2. A 35-year-old woman at 30 weeks age of gestation was complaining of nausea, vomiting, and abdominal pain. Her vital signs include blood pressure (BP) of 160/100 mmHg, heart rate (HR) of 120 beats/min, respiratory rate (RR) of 22 breaths/min, O$_2$ saturation of 95% on room air, and a temperature of 36.7°C. She has icteric sclerae and no jugular vein distension (JVD). Her lungs are clear to auscultation. Her cardiac sounds are tachycardic with no murmurs. Her abdomen is distended with right upper quadrant tenderness. Fetal heart sounds are present at 155 beats/min. Lower extremity edema is noted. Neuro examination shows the patient is awake and alert, and tremors are noted in her upper extremities. Her labs show the following:

WBC	$4.5 \times 10^3/\mu L$
Hgb	8 g/dL
Hct	28%
plt	$98 \times 10^3/\mu L$
Na	138 mEq/L
K	3.8 mEq/L

Cl	101 mEq/L
CO$_2$	28 mEq/L
BUN	35 mg/dL
Crea	0.9 mg/dL
Ca	6.8 mg/dL
Glucose	100 mg/dL
Albumin	2.8 g/dL
AST	1000 U/L
ALT	1000 U/L
Alk phos	100 U/L
Total bili	3.5 mg/dL
Indirect bili	2.5 mg/dL
Haptoglobin	20 mg/dL

Her peripheral smear shows schistocytes. What is the next step?

A. Delivery
B. Magnesium sulfate
C. Corticosteroids
D. Platelet transfusion

3. A 35-year-old woman with a body mass index (BMI) of 26, at 36 weeks age of gestation of a twin pregnancy, was complaining of nausea, vomiting, and abdominal pain. Her vital signs are BP of 140/90 mmHg, HR of 120 beats/min, RR of 22 breaths/min, and O$_2$ sat of 98% on room air. She has icteric sclerae. Her pupils are reactive to light. Her lungs are clear to auscultation. Her cardiac sounds show tachycardia and no murmur. Her abdomen is distended and tender, and fetal heart sounds are 155 beats/min. Her neuro examination shows a slight resting tremor. The patient is lethargic. Her labs show the following:

WBC	16 × 10^3/μL
Hgb	8.9 g/dL
Hct	27%
plt	70 × 10^3/μL
Na	137 mEq/L
K	3 mEq/L
Cl	98 mEq/L
CO$_2$	30 mEq/L
BUN	50 mg/dL
Crea	3 mg/dL
Ca	6.8 mg/dL
Glucose	50 mg/dL
Albumin	2.8 g/dL
AST	400 U/L
ALT	500 U/L
Alk phos	200 U/L
Total bili	8.5 mg/dL
Direct bili	6 mg/dL
Haptoglobin	50 mg/dL
Ammonia	70 μmol/L
INR	2
Fibrinogen	100 mg/dL
FDP	300 μg/mL

HBsAg	negative
Anti-HBs	positive
Anti-HBc IgM	negative
Anti-HBc IgG	positive
HBeAg	negative
Anti-HBe	negative
Hep E IgM	negative
Hep A IgM	negative

Dextrose was administered in the intravenous fluids and coagulopathies were corrected. What is the next step?

A. Delivery
B. Acyclovir
C. Ursodeoxycholic acid
D. Corticosteroids

4. Which of the following is true?

A. Acute cholecystitis should be managed with percutaneous drainage.
B. Endoscopy should be performed during the first trimester.
C. Pregnant women with autoimmune hepatitis should be continued on corticosteroids and/or azathioprine.
D. Hepatitis B is a contraindication to pregnancy.

5. A 40-year-old woman at 33 weeks age of gestation was complaining of nausea, vomiting, shortness of breath, and right upper quadrant pain. Her vital signs are BP of 90/60 mmHg, HR of 101 beats/min, RR of 18 breaths/min, and O$_2$ sat of 94% on room air. She has icteric sclerae. Her pupils are reactive to light. Her lungs are clear to auscultation. Her cardiac sounds show tachycardia and no murmur. Her abdomen is distended, with a tender right upper quadrant, bowel sounds present, and fetal heart sounds of 145 beats/min. Her neurologic examination shows a slight resting tremor. The patient is lethargic. Her labs show the following:

WBC	16 × 10^3/μL
Hgb	6.8 g/dL
Hct	21%
plt	200 × 10^3/μL
Na	130 mEq/L
K	3.3 mEq/L
Cl	100 mEq/L
CO$_2$	27 mEq/L
BUN	25 mg/dL
Crea	1.5 mg/dL
Ca	6.8 mg/dL
Glucose	90 mg/dL
Albumin	3.8 g/dL
AST	400 U/L
ALT	500 U/L
Alk phos	300 U/L
Total bili	5.5 mg/dL
Direct bili	2 mg/dL

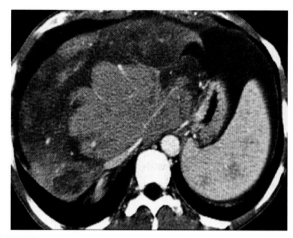

FIGURE 25-1 CT of the abdomen shows enhanced and enlarged caudate lobe with atropy of the periphery. (Reproduced with permission from Alessandrino F, Mortele KJ. State-of-the-art imaging of the gastrointestinal system. In: Greenberger NJ, Blumberg RS, Burakoff R, eds. *CURRENT Diagnosis & Treatment: Gastroenterology, Hepatology, & Endoscopy. 3rd ed.* New York, NY: McGraw-Hill; 2015.)

CT of the abdomen is shown below in Figure 25-1. What is the next step?

A. Heparin drip
B. Enoxaparin renal dose
C. Transjugular intrahepatic portosystemic shunt
D. Liver transplantation

6. A 42-year-old obese woman at 22 weeks age of gestation was complaining of nausea. She had in vitro fertilization. Her vitals were BP of 150/90 mmHg, HR of 90 beats/min, RR of 22 breaths/min, and temperature of 37°F. Her physical examination is otherwise unremarkable. Her labs include the following:

Hgb	15 g/L
plt	200 × 10³/µL
crea	1.0 mg/dL
Urine protein	350 mg/dL
AST	50 U/L
ALT	50 U/L

After 4 hours, her vitals were repeated and they were unchanged. What is the diagnosis?

A. Gestational hypertension
B. Preeclampsia
C. Chronic hypertension
D. Chronic hypertension with superimposed preeclampsia

7. For the patient in question 6, what is the treatment?

A. Emergent delivery
B. Labetalol
C. Supportive
D. Magnesium sulfate

8. A 24-year-old woman at 19 weeks age of gestation was noted to have BP of 160/110 mmHg. She has been compliant with her outpatient visits and was noted to have 3+ in her urine dipstick at least twice in the last month. What is the diagnosis?

A. Preeclampsia
B. Chronic hypertension
C. Gestational hypertension
D. Chronic hypertension with superimposed preeclampsia

9. A 32-year-old woman at 32 weeks age of gestation was complaining of frontal headaches, nausea, vomiting, and abdominal pain for the last 2 days. Her vitals are BP of 160/90 mmHg, HR of 98 beats/min, RR of 22 breaths/min, O₂ sat of 98% on room air, and temperature 36.6°C. Her physical examination shows anicteric sclerae, lungs clear to auscultation, heart sounds regularly regular with no murmurs, distended abdomen, right upper quadrant tenderness, and bowel sounds and fetal heart sounds present. Her labs show the following:

WBC	11 × 10³/µL
Hgb	10 g/dL
Hct	30%
plt	350 × 10³/µL
Na	135 mEq/L
K	4 mEq/L
Cl	108 mEq/L
CO₂	26 mEq/L
BUN	10 mg/dL
Crea	0.9 mg/dL
Ca	6.8 mg/dL
Glucose	100 mg/dL
Albumin	3 g/dL
AST	250 U/L
ALT	250 U/L
Alk phos	175 U/L
Total bili	1.2 mg/dL
Direct bili	0.8 mg/dL

She was given 1 dose of intramuscular (IM) magnesium sulfate 5 mg. Her urine output is 100 mL/h. Her magnesium level is 5 mEq/L. A repeat physical examination shows ankle clonus and hyperreflexic patellar reflex. What is the next step?

A. Dexamethasone 6 mg IV every 6 hours for 48 hours and then delivery
B. Solumedrol 60 mg IV every 6 hours for 24 hours and then delivery
C. Calcium gluconate 1 g IV
D. Magnesium sulfate 4 mg IV

10. A 25-year-old woman who is primigravida and 48 hours postpartum was complaining of headache and blurring of vision, followed by unresponsiveness, backward eye rolling, and symmetrical tonic clonic movements of her upper and lower extremities. She has a history myasthenia gravis and preeclampsia. Her vitals are systolic BP (SBP) of 160/90 mmHg, HR of 100 beats/min, RR of 18 breaths/min, O_2 sat of 88% on room air, and temperature of 36.6°C. Her physical examination shows anicteric sclerae with nystagmus. Her lungs have right lower lobe rhonchi. Her heart sounds are regularly regular. Her abdomen is soft, with normoactive bowel sounds, and nontender. Her extremities have good pulses, no cyanosis, and no edema. The neuro exam shows that the patient is responsive to pain. Her labs show the following:

WBC	$10 \times 10^3/\mu L$
Hgb	7 g/dL
Hct	30%
plt	$50 \times 10^3/\mu L$
Na	135 mEq/L
K	4 mEq/L
Cl	108 mEq/L
CO_2	26 mEq/L
BUN	10 mg/dL
Crea	0.9 mg/dL
Ca	7 mg/dL
Glucose	100 mg/dL
Albumin	3 g/dL
AST	100 U/L
ALT	100 U/L
Alk phos	175 U/L
Total bili	2 mg/dL
Direct bili	1 mg/dL

Her CT head shows cerebral edema with petechial hemorrhage. What is the next step?

A. Magnesium sulfate 6 mg IV
B. Ativan 2 mg IV
C. Labetalol 200 mg IV
D. Levetiracetam 1000 mg IV

11. A 35-year-old woman, with past medical history of migraines, in her first trimester of pregnancy, complains of recurrent progressive headaches in the last few weeks. She had a sudden thunder-clap–like episode that prompted further evaluation. She had a lumbar puncture prior to the onset of headaches because she had fever and nuchal rigidity. She also complains of auras, which are not atypical for her history of migraines. Her vitals are BP of 140/90 mmHg, HR of 80 beats/min, RR of 18 breaths/min, and O_2 sat of 95% on room air. Her physical examination is otherwise unremarkable. Her CT was unremarkable except for the posterior portion of superior sagittal sinus, which has a dense triangle. What is your diagnosis?

A. Migraines
B. Posterior reversible encephalopathy syndrome
C. Reversible cerebral vasoconstriction syndrome
D. Cerebral venous thrombosis

12. A 38-year-old African American woman with history of preeclampsia had an uneventful cesarean section. Forty-eight hours after delivery, a rapid response was called after she complained of shortness of breath. She was found to have an O_2 saturation of 84% on room air. Her oxygenation improved to 88% with nonrebreather mask. Her lungs had diffuse crackles bilaterally. She subsequently became confused, and her blood pressure was 60/40 mmHg. Her abdomen was soft and slightly tender. Her arterial blood gas showed a pH of 7.22/Pco_2 80 mmHg/Po_2 50 mmHg/HCO_3 26 mmol/L/O_2 saturation 88% on room air. The patient was emergently intubated, and a right internal jugular vein catheter was placed. A CTA of the chest showed no pulmonary embolism with diffuse ground glass opacities. Her labs showed the following:

WBC	$9 \times 10^3/\mu L$
Hgb	10 g/dL
Hct	30%
plt	$100 \times 10^3/\mu L$
Na	140 mEq/L
K	4 mEq/L
Cl	108 mEq/L
CO_2	26 mEq/L
BUN	10 mg/dL
Crea	1.9 mg/dL
Ca	6.8 mg/dL
Glucose	90 mg/dL
Albumin	3 g/dL
AST	250 U/L
ALT	250 U/L
Alk phos	175 U/L
Total bili	1.2 mg/dL
Direct bili	0.8 mg/dL
LDH	200 u/L
Fibrinogen	50 mg/dL
INR	3
PTT	90 seconds
FDP	50 Ug/mL

Which of the following is true regarding this patient's disease?

A. Diagnosis is made via finding amniotic fluid in a specimen obtained from right heart catheterization regardless of clinical scenario.
B. It is an immunologic response to fetal products.
C. A V/Q scan is need for diagnosis.
D. It is related to prior terbutaline use.

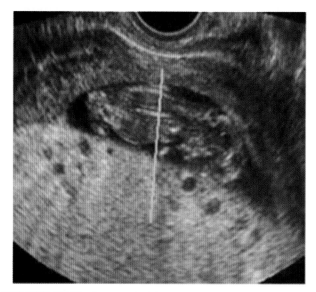

FIGURE 25-2 Ultrasound of this patient. (Reproduced with permission from Gestational Trophoblastic Disease. In: Cunningham F, Leveno KJ, Bloom SL, et al., eds. *Williams Obstetrics*, Twenty-Fourth Edition New York, NY: McGraw-Hill; 2013. Image contributed by Dr. Elysia Moschos.)

13. A 45-year-old woman with no significant past medical history was complaining of abdominal distention and vaginal bleeding. The patient claims that her last sexual partner was 3 months ago. She had a serum human chorionic gonadotropin (HCG) which showed 125,000 mIU/mL. No fetal heart sounds were detected. She had pelvic ultrasound, as in Figure 25-2. What is the next step?

A. Repeat serum HCG
B. Dilatation and curettage
C. Administer tocolytics
D. Methotrexate

14. A 35-year-old African American woman with history of diabetes mellitus and preeclampsia was complaining of

shortness of breath. She is in her 36th week age of gestation. She denies any sick contacts or recent travel. Her chest radiograph shows bilateral infiltrates with pleural effusions. Her labs are as follows:

WBC $11 \times 10^3/\mu L$
plt $150 \times 10^3/\mu L$
Crea 1.4 mg/dL

Her B-type natriuretic peptide (BNP) is 1400 pg/mL, and her echocardiogram shows an ejection fraction (EF) of 35% with no wall motion abnormalities. Which is the correct pathophysiology of this patient's disease?

A. Maternal response to hydrops fetalis
B. Overexaggerated response to overstimulation of ovaries
C. Prolactin
D. Vasodilation leading to hypotension, increased cardiac output, and subsequent decreased atrial filling time

15. Regarding the patient in question 14, which of the following is true regarding the management of her disease?

A. Anticoagulation with heparin should be continued for at least 2 months postpartum
B. Atrial fibrillation is the most common arrhythmia
C. Neurohormonal treatment is also advocated
D. All of the above

16. A 40-year-old woman at 36 weeks age of gestation was complaining of vaginal bleeding. Transabdominal ultrasound is seen below (Fig. 25-3). What is your diagnosis?

A. Placenta previa
B. Placental abruption
C. Placenta accreta
D. Retained placenta

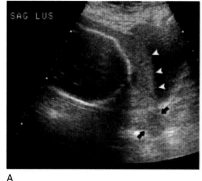
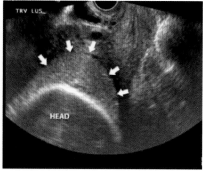

FIGURE 25-3 Transabdominal ultrasound. **Obstetrical hemorrhage.** (Reproduced with permission from Obstetrical Hemorrhage. In: Cunningham F, Leveno KJ, Bloom SL, et al., eds. *Williams Obstetrics*, Twenty-Fourth Edition New York, NY: McGraw-Hill; 2013.)

17. For the patient in question 16, she was given a medication that promoted myometrial contraction. This was followed with bronchospasm. What medication was given?

   A. Oxytocin
   B. Carboprost
   C. Ergometrine
   D. Magnesium sulfate

ANSWERS

1. A. Wernicke encephalopathy from hyperemesis gravidarum

   When evaluating liver function tests during pregnancy, the physiologic hepatic changes must be taken into account. Physiologic hepatic changes include (1) serum albumin, which may be lowered due to dilutional effects of increased plasma volume; (2) serum alkaline phosphatase, which may be produced in the bone, liver, intestine, kidney, and leukocytes, can be elevated up to 2-15 times due to placental production, particularly during the third trimester; and (3) decreased bile salts, increased biliary cholesterol, and decreased gallbladder emptying. Elevated levels of AST, ALT, γ-glutamyl transferase, and bilirubin would warrant further investigation.[32]

   Hyperemesis gravidarum (HG) is defined as persistent vomiting that is associated with a 5% weight loss and ketosis. It can lead to Wernicke encephalopathy, central pontine myelinolysis, and death. The direct correlation between levels of HCG and severity of vomiting has suggested a causal relationship, although other theories include starvation, placenta cytokines, and abnormal mitochondrial fatty acid oxidation.[33-36] Hyperemesis gravidarum begins in the first trimester, peaks at 8 to 12 weeks, and usually resolves by 20 weeks' age of gestation. Labs may show hemoconcentration, hypokalemia, metabolic alkalosis, transaminitis of 100 to 1600 U/L, and total bilirubin less than 4 mg/dL, and amylase and lipase may be elevated 5-fold as opposed to 5- to 10-fold in acute pancreatitis. Biopsy shows necrosis, steatosis, and bile plugs.[35] Risk factors include multiple gestations, molar pregnancies, hydrops fetalis, and trisomy 21.[35] Treatment includes hydration, thiamine supplementation, antiemetics, small meals, and psychotherapy.[35] If refractory, then hydrocortisone and total parenteral nutrition may be used.[35] HELLP syndrome and intrahepatic cholestasis of pregnancy are associated with nausea and vomiting during the third trimester, hypertension, and thrombocytopenia (choices B and C). Hyperparathyroidism is less likely due normal calcium levels corrected for albumin (choice D).

2. C. Corticosteroids

   The patient has HELLP syndrome. A variant of preeclampsia, HELLP syndrome occurs between 27 and 37 weeks of gestation in 70% of patients, and within 48 hours of delivery.[37] There are elevated liver enzymes (usually ≥ 500 U/L), hemolysis with microangiopathic anemia with schistocytes, elevated uric acid, elevated bilirubin, elevated LDH, and thrombocytopenia. Genetic variants, such as GCCR, TLR4, vascular endothelial growth factor gene, FAS gene, cluster of differentiation 95 (CD95) and factor V Leiden mutation, and inadequate vascular placental implantation, are proposed pathogeneses.[37] Right upper quadrant pain occurs in 90% of patients. Other symptoms are nausea, vomiting, and weight gain (4 kg). There are 2 classifications for the diagnosis of HELLP. The Tennessee classification involves platelets of $100 \times 10^3/\mu L$ or less, AST of 70 U/L or greater, and LDH of 600 U/L or greater. The Mississippi classification involves class I: platelets of $50 \times 10^3/\mu L$ or less, AST or ALT of 70 U/L or greater, and LDH of 600 U/L or greater; class II: platelets of 50 to $100 \times 10^3/\mu L$, AST or ALT of 70 U/L or greater, and LDH of 600 U/L or greater; or class III: platelets of 100 to $150 \times 10^3/\mu L$, AST or ALT of 70 U/L or greater, and LDH of 600 U/L or greater.[37] Treatment includes magnesium sulfate. Delivery is warranted if the patent is 34 weeks' AOG or there are other complications such as multiple organ failure, disseminated intravascular coagulation (DIC), infarct, renal failure, or abruptio placenta.[37]

   Corticosteroids are given to decrease respiratory distress syndrome, to help fetal lung development, and to improve circulatory stability for 23 to 34 weeks' age of gestation and anticipation of delivery within 7 days. Given that the patient and the fetus appear to be hemodynamically stable and there is no evidence of maternal complications such as DIC, pulmonary infarction, pulmonary edema, or multiorgan failure, delivery can be momentarily delayed. Magnesium sulfate can be given prior to delivery for neuroprotection (choice B). There is no indication for platelet transfusion (goal is > $40 \times 10^3/\mu L$) (choice D).

3. A. Delivery

   Acute fatty liver of pregnancy (AFLP) usually occurs in the third trimester, is associated with mitochondrial long-chain 3-hydroxyacyl-CoA dehydrogenase (LCHAD) deficiency, and is more common in the primiparae, in twin pregnancies, and in patients with low BMI. This causes metabolites to accumulate in the liver, leading to toxicity. Right upper quadrant pain, nausea, vomiting, and jaundice are found. Laboratories show markers of DIC, AST, and ALT (typically 300–1000 U/L), alkaline phosphatase 3 to 10 times the normal limit (44-147 IU/L), total bilirubin less than 5 mg/dL, thrombocytopenia, and hypoglycemia. It is difficult to distinguish AFLP from HELLP syndrome, and clues to suggest AFLP are lack of hemolysis, coagulation abnormalities, hypoglycemia, and/or encephalopathy. Definitive diagnosis is based on a liver biopsy that shows

TABLE 25-2 Swansea Diagnostic Criteria for Acute Fatty Liver of Pregnancy

6 or more of the following:
- Vomiting
- Abdominal pain
- Polydipsia/polyuria
- Encephalopathy
- Bilirubin > 14 µmol/L
- Hypoglycemia
- Urea > 340 µmol/L
- Leukocytosis
- Ascites or bright liver on ultrasound
- AST/ALT > 42 IU/L
- Ammonia > 46 µmol/L
- Creatinine > 150 µmol/L
- Prothrombin time > 14 s or aPPT > 34 s
- Microvascular steatosis on liver biopsy

ALT = alanine aminotransferase; aPPT = activated prothrombin time; AST = aspartate aminotransferase.

microvascular hepatic steatosis, although clinical diagnosis is most common. Swansea criteria is used (Table 25-2).[38-40] Prevention can include dietary modification. Treatment is delivery (Strong Recommendation).[38] Laboratory abnormalities normalize 7 to 10 days postpartum.[37]

The hepatitis panel suggests that the patient does not have hepatitis A, B, or E (Tables 25-3 and 25-4). Hepatitis E and herpes simplex virus (HSV), 2 of the causes of acute hepatitis in pregnancy, can lead to acute liver failure, especially in the second and third trimesters, respectively.[41] In addition to derangement in the liver profile and coagulopathy, HSV hepatitis usually is accompanied by fever, leukopenia,

TABLE 25-4 Comparison of Hepatitis A, B, and C Serologies

HAV IgM	HBsAg	HBsAb	Anti-HBcAg	HBcAb IgM	HBcAb IgG	Anti-HCV	Interpretation
+	−	−				−	Acute hepatitis A
−	+		+			−	Acute hepatitis B
				+			Acute hepatitis B
					+		Vaccinated for hepatitis B
		+					Resolved hepatitis B
−	+		−			−	Chronic hepatitis B
−	−		+			−	Acute hepatitis B
−	−					+	Acute or chronic hepatitis C

+ = positive; − = negative; cAb = core antibody; cAg = core antigen; HAV = hepatitis A virus; Hb = hepatitis B; HCV = hepatitis C virus; IgG = immunoglobulin G; IgM = immunoglobulin M; sAb = surface antibody; sAg = surface antigen.

Data from Acute viral hepatitis panel. LabTestsOnline. © 2017 American Association for Clinical Chemistry (AACC). https://labtestsonline.org/understanding/analytes/hepatitis-panel/tab/test/. Accessed May 6, 2017.

and visible dermatologic lesions. Definitive diagnosis is based on culture, polymerase chain reaction, and serologies. Acyclovir (choice B) and valacyclovir, both category B, can be used to treat HSV in pregnancy. Given the

TABLE 25-3 Hepatitis B Serologies

Serologic Markers	Characteristic	Immunity from Infection	Immunity from Vaccination	Acute Infection	Chronic Infection
Hepatitis B Surface Antigen (HBsAg)	• 1-10 weeks after exposure • Prior to symptoms or elevated ALT	−	−	−/+	+
Hepatitis B Surface antibody (anti-HBs)	• Follows disappearance of HBsAg • Confirm immunity • Carriers have both HBsAg and anti-HBs	+	+	−	−
IgM against Hepatitis B core antigen (IgM anti-HBc)	• Presence may precede HBsAg and anti-HBs	−	−	+	−/+
IgG against Hepatitis B core antigen		+	−	−	+
Hepatitis B e antigen (HBeAg)	• Marker of replication and infection	−	−	+	−/+
Hepatitis B e antibody (HBeAb)		−/+	−		
Serum HBV DNA	• Disappearance marks recovery from acute hepatitis B but may remain detectable via PCR	−/+ if PCR	−	+	+

+ = detectable; − = undetectable; −/+ = may be detectable; c = core; eAg = e antigen; IgG = immunoglobulin G; IgM = immunoglobulin M; HB = hepatitis B; HBV = hepatitis B virus; sAg = surface antigen.

Adapted from Staros EB, Mekaroonkamol P, Hashemi N. Hepatitis B test. MedScape Web site. http://emedicine.medscape.com/article/2109144-overview#a2. Accessed. July 15, 2017.

clinical presentation and laboratory findings, the patient does not have HSV hepatitis. Biopsy after delivery confirms the presence of microvascular steatosis.

Intrahepatic cholestasis of pregnancy is the second most common cause of jaundice in pregnancy, the first being hepatitis.[42,43] It is a triad of pruritis, elevated aminotransferases, and bile levels late in the second and third trimesters with spontaneous resolution within 2 to 3 weeks postpartum. Pathogenesis revolves around estrogen, progesterone, multiparity, and environmental factors. The pruritis can be mild to debilitating, having a predilection for the hands and soles of the feet. Jaundice may follow 1 to 4 weeks later but sometimes may be the initial presentation.[43] Steatorrhea and cholecystitis can result. Total fasting bile acid levels can exceed 40 µmol/L. Cholic acid is higher than chenodeoxycholic acid. Glycine to taurine conjugated bile acids decrease.[42,43] Another entity called asymptomatic hypercholanemia of pregnancy has elevated bile acids above 11 µmol/L with normal liver function tests.[42] In intrahepatic cholestasis of pregnancy, serum aminotransferases are elevated up to 2 to 10 times normal and can even be 1000 U/L.[43] It is common in South America, Europe, and South Asia.[42,43] Ursodeoxycholic acid (choice C) is the initial treatment. Corticosteroids (choice D) have no role in acute fatty liver of pregnancy. See Table 25-5 for pharmacologic treatment of intrahepatic cholestasis of pregnancy.[42]

TABLE 25-5 Drugs for Intrahepatic Cholestasis of Pregnancy

Drug	Dose	Clinical Effect
Ursodeoxycholic acid	15 mg/kg per day or 500 mg BID	Decreases pruritis, liver enzymes and bile acids by replacing more cytotoxic bile acids
Cholestyramine	8-16 g/day	Decrease pruritis via binding bile salts and increase their fecal excretion; constipation
S-adenoxyl methionine	1000 mg/day	Decreases pruritis by affecting fluid composition of hepatic membranes and increases excretion of hormonal metabolites
Dexamethasone	12 mg/day	Decreases pruritis and bile acids
Phenobarbital	2-5 mg/kg per day	Decreases pruritis
Antihistamines	25-50 mg per day	Decreases pruritis

Data from Ozkan S, Ceylan Y, Ozkan OV, Vildirim S. Review of a challenging clinical issue: intrahepatic cholestasis of pregnancy. *World J Gastroenterol.* 2015;21(23):7134-7141.

4. C. Pregnant women with autoimmune hepatitis should be continued on corticosteroids and/or azathioprine

Pregnant women with chronic liver disease can continue their medications. Pregnant women with autoimmune hepatitis can continue corticosteroids and/or azathioprine, pregnant women with primary biliary cirrhosis can continue ursodeoxycholic acid, and pregnant women with Wilson disease can continue penicillamine, trientine, or zinc, but with a dose reduction.[38] Acute cholecystitis should be managed with laparoscopic cholecystectomy due to high rates of recurrent symptoms, hospitalization, preterm labor and deliveries, and spontaneous abortions if intervention is deferred (choice A).[38,44,45] Endoscopy should be performed during the second trimester (choice B).[38] Hepatitis is not a contraindication to pregnancy (choice D). Patients with a high viral load (200,000 U/mL or 10⁶ log copies/mL) can be given antivirals such as tenofovir or telbivudine in the third trimester to reduce perinatal transmission.[38]

Flares of hepatitis B can occur intrapartum and postpartum, occasionally accompanied by loss of the hepatitis B e antigen. Risk of vertical transmission is high if there is no prophylaxis and the patient is HBeAg-positive or if there are high hepatitis B virus DNA levels. Telbivudine and tenofovir, both category B agents, can be administered during the third trimester, 28 to 32 weeks, when HBV DNA levels are greater than 7 to 8 $\log_{10}$ IU/mL. Hepatitis C normally poses no maternal threat, but there is a high rate of vertical transmission in the presence of coinfection with HIV and hepatitis C virus RNA. Treatment of hepatitis C should be avoided because ribavirin is category X and interferon is category C.

5. C. Transjugular intrahepatic portosystemic shunt

The patient has Budd-Chiari syndrome (BCS) is an obstruction of hepatic venous outflow from the hepatic veins to the cavoatrial junction that causes abdominal pain, hepatosplenomegaly, and ascites.[46] Etiology of the obstruction can be intraluminal (primary) such as thrombosis, thrombophlebitis, or webs, or extraluminal (secondary), such as abscess, and inferior vena cava membranous webs. This obstruction can lead to perisinusoidal necrosis of hepatocytes in Rappaport zone 3 and liver failure.[46,47] Occlusion of 3 hepatic veins occurs in two-thirds of cases, and caudate hypertrophy occurs in half of cases.[46,48] Imaging modalities include Doppler ultrasound (usually the initial study), CT scan (which may help delineate ascites and the patency of the hepatic vein and inferior vena cava), and MRI (which can delineate acute versus chronic BCS, where acute has divergent signal intensities and decreased peripheral enhancement and chronic has heterogeneous signals throughout the liver).[46] Although sampling error may occur, liver biopsy will show extravasation of red cells into the liver-cell plate and space of Disse is suggestive of BCS.[46]

Treatment may include anticoagulation (LMWH is preferred to UFH in the earlier weeks of pregnancy) and even tissue plasminogen activators (choices A and B). However, this patient most likely has developed portal hypertension, and it would be prudent to rule out varices or subclinical gastrointestinal hemorrhage prior to initiating anticoagulation since the patient is anemic. Transjugular intrahepatic portosystemic shunt (TIPPS) might be the best choice for this patient.[49-51] Accepted ionizing radiation during pregnancy is 5 rad, and the maximum risk is between 8 and 25 weeks.[49] Liver transplantation can be considered if all other treatment fails (choice D).

6. B. Preeclampsia

Preeclampsia is defined as SBP of 140 mmHg or greater or diastolic BP (DBP) of 90 mmHg or greater on 2 occasions 4 hours apart after 20 weeks' AOG *or* SBP of 160 mmHg or greater or DBP of 110 mmHg or greater and repeated after a few minutes *with* proteinuria defined as 300 mg or greater in a 24-hour collection, a protein/creatinine ratio of greater than 0.3, or dipstick 1+ in a patient who is previously normotensive.[33] Risk factors for preeclampsia include primiparity, previous preeclampsia, chronic hypertension, chronic renal disease, thrombophilia, multifetal pregnancy, in vitro fertilization, family history of preeclampsia, diabetes, obesity, systemic lupus erythematosus, and age over 40 years.[33] Uterine arterial Doppler increased resistance, placental growth factor, vascular endothelial growth factor, or soluble fms-like tyrosine kinase I have been evaluated as potential biomarkers but none has been validated.[33,44-49] In preeclampsia, the shallow implantation results in incomplete invasion of the cytotrophoblasts, resulting in the native arterioles retaining their ability to vasoconstrict.[52] In normal pregnancy, cytotrophoblasts invade the decidua tunica media of the maternal spiral arteries and replace the endothelium, which is called pseudovascularization.[52] Other types of pregnancy-related hypertension disorders are listed in Table 25-6.[33] American College of Obstetrics and Gynecology (ACOG) stratified their recommendations and quality of evidence based on the GRADE system. High is defined as high confidence that true effect lies close to that of estimate of effect. Moderate is defined as true effect is close to estimate of effect but there is possibility that it is different. Low is the confidence of effect is limited and that true effect maybe

TABLE 25-6 Pregnancy-Related Hypertension Disorders, Diagnosis, and Treatment

Name	Diagnosis	Treatment
Chronic hypertension (choice C)	HTN before 20 wk AOG *or* Gestational HTN that fails to improve postpartum	• Treat with antiHTN to maintain SBP of 120–160 mmHg or DBP of 80–105 mmHg (low evidence) • AntiHTN includes methyldopa, nifedipine, and/or labetalol (moderate evidence) • Avoid ACEI, ARB, mineralocorticosteroid-receptor antagonists (moderate evidence) • Initiate low-dose aspirin daily late in patients at great risk for adverse effects (preterm, preeclampsia) • Ultrasound for intrauterine fetal growth restriction and, if positive, fetoplacental assessment with umbilical artery Doppler (low and moderate evidence, respectively)
Preeclampsia	In a previously normotensive patient with SBP ≥ 140 mmHg or DBP ≥ 90 mmHg on 2 occasions 4 h apart after 20 wk AOG *or* SBP ≥ 160 mmHg or DBP ≥ 110 mmHg and repeated after a few minutes *With* Proteinuria defined as ≥ 300 mg in 24-h collection, > 0.3 protein/creatinine ratio, or dipstick 1+ *Or if no proteinuria,* New onset HTN with platelets < 100,000/μL, serum creatinine > 1.1 mg/dL or doubling of baseline creatinine, liver transaminases doubled, pulmonary edema, or cerebral or visual defects Can develop postpartum	• For preeclampsia without severe features and no indication for delivery at < 37 0/7 wk, expectant management (low evidence) • Preeclampsia without severe features > 37 0/7 wk, delivery (moderate evidence) • Preeclampsia with SBP < 160 mmHg or DBP < 110 mmHg with no maternal symptoms, no magnesium sulfate prophylaxis (low evidence) • Aspirin as prophylaxis • Avoid NSAIDs

(Continued)

TABLE 25-6 **Pregnancy-Related Hypertension Disorders, Diagnosis, and Treatment (Continued)**

Name	Diagnosis	Treatment

Preeclampsia with severe features (any of the following)	SBP ≥ 160 mmHg or DBP ≥ 110 mmHg and repeated at least 4 h apart while on bedrest, platelets < 100,000/μL, serum creatinine > 1.1 mg/dL or doubling of baseline creatinine, liver transaminases doubled, pulmonary edema, or cerebral or visual defects	• At ≤ 34 0/7 wk in patients with stable maternal and fetal vital signs, expectant management (moderate evidence)
		• These patients should also receive corticosteroids for fetal lung maturity (high evidence)
		• At ≥ 34 0/7 wk with unstable maternal or fetal vital signs, delivery (moderate evidence)
		• Administer antiHTN in patients with preeclampsia with severe features (SBP ≥ 160 mmHg or DBP ≥ 110 mmHg)
		• Administer corticosteroids and delay delivery for 48 h if VS stable, ≤ 33 6/7 wk AOG, and any of the following:
		  • Preterm premature rupture of membranes
		  • Platelets < 100,000/μL
		  • Persistently abnormal LFT (transaminase ≥ 2 × normal)
		  • Fetal growth restriction (< 5th percentile)
		  • Severe oligohydramnios (amniotic fluid index < 5 cm)
		  • Reverse end diastolic flow on umbilical artery via Doppler
		  • New-onset renal dysfunction or increasing renal dysfunction (moderate evidence)
		• Delivery should not be delayed after initial maternal stabilization regardless of age of gestation in severe preeclampsia complicated by the following:
		  • Uncontrolled HTN
		  • Eclampsia
		  • Pulmonary edema
		  • Abruptio placentae
		  • DIC
		  • Interpartum fetal demise
		  • Nonreassuring of fetal status (moderate evidence)
		• Type of delivery should be dictated by fetal age of gestation, presentation, cervical status, and maternal and fetal conditions (moderate evidence)
		Magnesium sulfate is recommended for intrapartum and postpartum severe preeclampsia (moderate evidence)

Chronic HTN with superimposed preeclampsia (choice D)	Patient with HTN early in gestation and develop proteinuria > 20 wk AOG *or* Patient with proteinuria < 20 wk AOG and one of the following: 1. Sudden onset of HTN or escalation of medications for previously controlled HTN 2. Increased liver function tests 3. Platelets < 100,000/μL 4. Right upper quadrant pain and headaches 5. Renal insufficiency (creatinine ≥ 1.1 mg/dL or doubled from baseline) 6. Pulmonary edema or congestion 7. Sudden and substantial increase in proteinuria	
Gestational HTN (Choice A)	HTN after 20 wk AOG without proteinuria	
Postpartum HTN	Mild HTN developing 2–6 mo and resolving within 1 y postpartum	

ACEI = angiotensin-converting enzyme inhibitor; AOG = age of gestation; ARB = angiotensin-receptor blocker; DBP = diastolic blood pressure; DIC = disseminated intravascular coagulation; HTN = hypertension; LFT = liver function tests; NSAIDs = nonsteroidal anti-inflammatory drugs; SBP = systolic blood pressure.

substantially different. Very low is very little confidence in the effect estimate and more likely true effect is different from estimate effect.

In postpartum hypertension, regardless of etiology (gestational, previously preeclamptic, or superimposed preeclampsia), blood pressure should be monitored for up to 10 days after delivery.[33] If the patient is symptomatic, her blood pressure should be monitored earlier.[33] In the case of persistent SBP of 150 mmHg or greater, or DBP of 100 mmHg or greater on 2 occasions, 4 to 6 hours apart, antihypertensives should be initiated.[33] If the SBP is 160 mmHg or greater or the DBP is 110 mmHg or greater, treatment should be initiated within 1 hour.[33]

7. C. Supportive

The patient has preeclampsia with no severe features. Management would be supportive care. The blood pressure is at goal for preeclampsia and there is no need for labetalol (choice B). Emergent delivery would be disastrous for the fetus at 22 weeks age of gestation (choice A). Magnesium sulfate is recommended for severe preeclampsia (choice D).

8. D. Chronic hypertension with superimposed preeclampsia

Proteinuria is defined as urinary excretion of protein of 150 mg/d.[53-55] The excretion may consist of 20% low-molecular-weight proteins such as immunoglobulin, 40% high-molecular-weight albumin, and 40% Tamm-Horsfall mucoproteins.[53-55] The barrier to protein excretion begins at the glomerular capillaries, which are permeable to fluid and solutes but not to proteins, and the adjacent basement membrane and epithelial cells covered by negatively charged heparin sulfate proteoglycans.[51] Proteinuria can be further categorized as (1) glomerular, secondary to increased permeability of proteins at the glomerular level; (2) tubular, which is decreased protein reabsorption; and (3) overflow, which is increased production of low-molecular-weight proteins.[53-55] Protein excretion of 0.15 to 2 g can be either type, but protein excretion of greater than 2 g usually is glomerular. Preeclampsia has the glomerular type of proteinuria.

Determination of proteinuria begins with a urine dipstick with or without sulfosalicylic acid (SSA) turbidity test, which can detect Bence Jones proteins. For urine dipstick, a negative result means less than 10 mg/dL, a trace means 10 to 20 mg/dL, 1+ means 30 mg/dL, 2+ means 100 mg/dL, 3+ means 300 mg/dL, and 4+ means 1000 mg/dL.[53] If the persistent proteinuria (3+ to 4+ in 2 different readings in 1 month) is identified and no correlation is determined with the rest of the urinalysis, a 24-hour urine protein measurement or urine protein/creatinine ratio is performed.[53] Table 25-7 shows false positive and false negative results of dipstick tests.[53]

The patient has chronic hypertension with superimposed preeclampsia because of the presence of proteinuria at less than 20 weeks' AOG and the sudden onset of hypertension. Other scenarios that fit this definition include a patient with hypertension early in gestation who develops proteinuria at more than 20 weeks AOG or a patient with proteinuria at less than 20 weeks AOG having one of the following: increased liver function tests, platelet levels less than 100,000/mL, right upper quadrant pain and headaches, renal insufficiency (creatinine ≥ 1.1 mg/dL or doubled from baseline), pulmonary edema or congestion, or sudden and substantial increase in proteinuria.[37] To see why the answers are wrong, see Table 25-6.

TABLE 25-7 False Positive and False Negative Dipstick Test Results

	False Positive	False Negative
Proteinuria dipstick analysis	pH >7.5, concentrated urine, prolonged immersion of dipstick, hematuria, penicillin, sulfonamides, tolbutamide, pus[53]	Dilute urine (specific gravity > 1.015)[53]
Sulfosalicylic acid test (rarely used now)	Radiographic dyes, penicillin, sulfonamides[53]	Dilute urine, alkaline pH[53]

9. A. Dexamethasone 6 mg IV every 6 hours for 48 hours and then delivery

The patient has severe preeclampsia, and she is a risk for preterm delivery. Antenatal corticosteroids are considered for pregnant women during 23+0 and 23+6 weeks AOG who are at risk of preterm delivery within the next 7 days and have been shown to reduce the risk of respiratory distress syndrome, intraventricular hemorrhage, necrotizing enterocolitis, neonatal mortality, and systemic infection in the first 48 hours.[56,57] Betamethasone 12 mg IM daily or dexamethasone 6 mg IM every 12 hours are considered because they are less metabolized by placental 11-β-hydroxysteroid dehydrogenase type 2 enzyme. Solumedrol is not the preferred corticosteroid (choice B). The patient is also at risk for seizures from eclampsia. The current recommended use of magnesium sulfate in pregnancy is (1) prevention and treatment of seizures in preeclampsia and eclampsia; (2) fetal neuroprotection before anticipated early preterm (< 32 weeks of gestation) delivery; and (3) short-term prolongation of pregnancy (< 48 hours) to allow administration of antenatal corticosteroids in patients at risk for preterm delivery within 7 days.[58-62] Magnesium can be delivered IM or IV. The IM regimen consists of 4 g IM followed by 10 g IM and 5 g IM via alternating buttock. The IV regimen consists of 4 g IV loading dose followed by 1 to 2 g via continuous infusion. Therapeutic plasma concentrations are 3.5 to 7 mEq/L (4.2–8.4 mg/dL).[58,63] At 8 to 10 mEq/L, patellar reflexes are lost. Respiratory failure occurs at levels over 13 mEq/L.[28] Cardiac arrest can occur at higher levels.[63] Despite the magnesium level being elevated, she is still not at risk for magnesium toxicity, given that her patellar reflexes are preserved, she is not in respiratory distress, and she has no arrhythmias. The patient should be started on a magnesium maintenance infusion and not a repeat bolus (choice D). The patient does not have signs of magnesium toxicity and there is no need to reverse magnesium levels with calcium gluconate (choice C).

10. B. Ativan 2 mg IV

Eclampsia is suggested by the proteinuria, the mildly elevated uric acid, the thrombocytopenia, and the petechial hemorrhages and cerebral edema on CT. Eclampsia usually occurs by the 28th week of gestation but has been seen at least 48 hours postpartum.[13] The associated symptoms and physical findings include frontal headaches, visual disturbances, right upper quadrant pain, mental status changes, blood pressure greater than 160/110 mmHg, edema, proteinuria, and hyperactive reflexes.[13,64] Eclampsia can be associated with HELLP, PRES, and reversible cerebral vasoconstriction syndrome (RCVS). Postpartum eclampsia has higher incidences of ICH and cerebral venous thrombosis (CVT).

The initial treatment for eclampsia is seizure control with a 48-hour course of magnesium sulfate with a 4- to 6-g loading dose over 15 to 20 minutes followed by a 1- to 2-g/h maintenance infusion with level goal of 3 to 5 meq (choice A). Blood pressure control usually improves as well. If not, antihypertensives are given with an SBP goal of 140 to 160 mmHg and DBP goal of 90 to 110 mmHg (choice C). However, the patient has a recent history of myasthenia gravis, and magnesium sulfate can precipitate an exacerbation. In this instance or if the seizure is refractory to magnesium sulfate, benzodiazepines are advocated over other antiepileptics (choices B and D).

11. D. Cerebral venous thrombosis

Dural sinus or cerebral venous thrombosis accounts for 0.51% of CVAs.[65,66] Cerebral venous sinus thrombosis occurs in the first trimester in patients with known thrombophilia, but 75% occur postpartum.[13] Risk factors include pregnancy; thrombophilia, such as antithrombin III deficiency; protein C deficiency; protein S deficiency; antiphospholipid and anticardiolipin antibodies; activated protein C resistance; factor V Leiden resistance; factor II mutation; hyperhomocysteinemia; oral contraceptives; androgens; danazol; lithium; IVIG; ecstasy; cancer; infection, particularly parameningeal; blood patch; spontaneous intracranial hypotension; lumbar puncture; paroxysmal nocturnal hemoglobinuria; iron deficiency anemia; nephrotic syndrome; polycythemia; systemic lupus erythematosus; Behçet disease; inflammatory bowel disease; thyroid disease; and sarcoidosis.[65] Thrombosis is most common in superior sagittal sinus 62%, transverse sinus 41% to 45%, straight sinus 18%, cortical veins 17%, internal jugular vein 12%, and deep venous system 11%.[65]

Clinical manifestations typically occur as a result of increased intracranial pressure from decreased venous drainage or focal brain injury from ischemia or hemorrhage.[65] Headache, which occurs in 90% of patients, can be diffuse and progressive for weeks. It can also be described as a sudden, severe thunderclap headache and have associated papilledema and/or diplopia.[65] Seizures occur in 40% of patients, and neurologic, sensory, and motor deficits are often bilateral.[65]

The American Heart Association Stroke Council Recommendations define Classes as: Class I if there is evidence that procedure is effective; Class IIa if there is conflicting evidence about the efficacy of procedure or treatment and weight of evidence is in favor; Class IIb is the efficacy of procedure or treatment is less well established; and Class III where there is evidence that the treatment or procedure is not useful and/or can be harmful.[65] Level of Evidence is A if data is from multiple randomized clinical trials or meta-analysis, Level B if from a single randomized trial or nonrandomized studies; and Level of Evidence C if from consensus opinion of experts, cases studies, or standard of care.[65] Initial diagnostics should include routine labs and evaluation for prothrombotic conditions (Class I, LOE C).[65] Lumbar puncture is generally not helpful, although patients generally have elevated open pressures, 50% have elevated WBC, and 35% have elevated protein.[67] D-dimer may be used to exclude patients with low probably of CVT (Class IIb; LOE B). Patients with CVT can have atypical presentations, such as intracerebral hemorrhage, evidence of intracranial hypertension, and somnolence and confusion in the elderly.[36] Imaging studies are key (Class I; LOE C). Although CT is reported to have 95% sensitivity and 91% specificity, with 90% to 100% accuracy depending on whether imaging the sinus or vein, it is only positive in 30% of cases of CVT.[65] Thrombosed sinuses or veins appear as hyperdensities. The posterior portion of the superior sagittal sinus can have a dense triangle or delta sign, ischemia or hemorrhage shown near a sinus, or a contrast-enhanced dural lining of the sinus with a filling defect in a vein or sinus.[65] Magnetic resonance imaging appears to be more sensitive than CT. Central venous thrombosis can appear as isointense to parenchyma on T1 MRI but hypointense on T2 secondary to deoxyhemoglobin during the first week. During the second week with formation of methemoglobin, it appears hyperintense on T1 and T2 and further evolution shows a low signal on gradient-echo and susceptibility-weighted images.[65] Secondary changes such as edema and hemorrhage have the same pattern as on CT. Computed tomography venography is equivalent to MRI venography in diagnosis and appears to be for subacute and chronic thrombosis. Variable structures and inadequate resolution of veins and sinuses, and inconclusive results from hypoplasia or atresia of cerebral veins, may warrant the use of cerebral angiography or direct cerebral venography. Failure of sinus appearance; venous congestion with dilated cortical, scalp, or facial veins; enlargement of collateral vessels; and reversal of venous flow suggest CVT in angiography. In direct cerebral venography, direct injection of dye reveals luminal filling defects and can also measure sinus pressure, typically less than 10 mm H_2O.[65]

Reversible cerebral vasoconstriction syndrome is characterized by severe, thunderclap-type headaches that peak within seconds, with each episode lasting 1 to 3 hours; reoccur within 1 to 2 weeks; are associated with acute neurologic symptoms; and are suggested by diffuse segmental cerebral artery vasoconstriction that resolves within 3 months (choice C).[13,68] Visual deficits usually occur but so can sensory and motor deficits. Seizures rarely recur. Diagnostic criteria include (1) acute and severe headache with or without focal deficits or seizures; (2) uniphasic course without new symptoms more than 1 month from onset; (3) segmental vasoconstriction of cerebral arteries via CT, MRI, or direct catheter angiography; (4) no evidence of aneurysmal subarachnoid hemorrhage; (5) normal or near normal CSF (protein < 100 mg/dL, WBC < 15/μL); and (6) complete or near complete resolution of arteries with follow-up angiography within 12 weeks of onset.[68] Neuroimaging may be initially normal except for convexity subarachnoid hemorrhage, which can occur within 1 week; intracerebral hemorrhage; cerebral infarction; and reversible brain edema.[13,68] Angiography would reveal the segmental vasoconstriction, which can also be seen in aneurysmal subarachnoid hemorrhage and primary angiitis of the central nervous system, except that there would be constriction, it would be secondary to vasospasm, and it would be localized near an aneurysm with no convexity bleeding in aneurysmal SAH, and irregular, eccentric, and asymmetrical narrowings in primary angiitis.[68] Primary angiitis also appears to have an insidious onset with stepwise deterioration, the CSF has an inflammatory pattern, and MRI can show infarcts of various ages.[68] Treatment is to avoid triggers, including vasoactive drugs, analgesics, antiepileptic drugs, sexual activity, nimodipine, magnesium sulfate, or verapamil.

Posterior reversible encephalopathy syndrome is reversible ischemia, usually on the posterior lobes of the brain secondary to decreased sympathetic innervation and secondary to disruption of cerebral blood flow and the blood–brain barrier (choice B).[68,69] Normally, the cerebral blood flow (CBF) varies directly with cerebral perfusion pressure (CPP) and inversely with cerebral vascular resistance (CVR): CBF = CPP/CVR.[69] From a mean arterial pressure of 50 to 150 mmHg, cerebral arterioles constrict to maintain constant CBF. The muscular media hypertrophies in chronic hypertension, leading to higher tolerance for high BP but low tolerance for low BP.[69] In PRES, there is a breakdown of autoregulation; when MAP exceeds the limit of contraction of the vessel wall, CBF increases unimpeded, and plasma extravasates, leading to edema. However, it has also been suggested that this phenomenon is not necessarily dependent on the absolute blood pressure but the rapid change in blood pressure and can also occur in lower blood pressures if there is associated endothelial dysfunction leading to blood–brain barrier failure.[69,70] Although the parietal and occipital lobes are the most commonly involved, other areas of involvement include the posterior frontal, temporal, thalamus, cerebellum, brainstem, and basal ganglia.[69] Risk factors include

hypertension; eclampsia; preeclampsia; drugs such as cocaine, amphetamines, and LSD; tricyclic antidepressants; monoamine oxidase inhibitors (MAOIs); bronchodilators; erythropoietin; midodrine; fludrocortisone; hypertension, hypervolemia, and hemodilution (triple-H) therapy; IVIG; cyclosporine; tacrolimus; interferons; indinavir; cisplatin; cytarabine; gemcitabine; systemic lupus erythematosus; scleroderma; vasculitis; thrombotic thrombocytopenic purpura; Henoch-Schönlein purpura; hemolytic-uremic syndrome; tumor lysis syndrome; sepsis; hypomagnesemia; hypercalcemia; hypocholesterolemia; Guillain-Barré syndrome; and renal failure.[69-71] Posterior reversible encephalopathy syndrome is not necessarily mutually exclusive, as it can occur with other disorders, such as eclampsia and RCVS.[67-69] Clinical presentation includes headache, visual disturbances, mental status changes, seizures, dysarthria, limb incoordination, and brisk deep tendon reflexes.[69] Diagnosis is further enhanced particularly with MRI via T2 flair images, although it may initially be normal. There is symmetrical white matter edema in the posterior lobes, particularly in the parietal and occipital regions. The calcarine and paramedian portions of the occipital lobe are spared. The cerebellum, brainstem, and basal ganglia might be involved. Cerebrospinal fluid is usually normal but can have mild pleocytosis if there is severe blood–brain barrier breakdown, and serum von Willebrand factor may be elevated because it is continuously produced by endothelial cells.[69] Treatment includes a 20% reduction in blood pressure and treating the underlying disease.

An abnormal radiographic image makes migraines less likely (choice A).

12. **B. It is an immunologic response to fetal products.**

The patient most likely has amniotic fluid embolism (AFE). The maternal mortality ratio is 0.5 to 1.7 per 100,000 births.[72] The clinical presentation is sudden cardiovascular collapse with arrhythmias, hypotension, pulmonary edema, respiratory failure, DIC, and altered mental status during labor, delivery, or 48 hours postpartum.[72] Most patients will have hypotension and respiratory distress, 50% will have DIC, and 20% will have seizures.[72] Risk factors vary per study and geographic location but include maternal age younger than 20 or older than 35 years of age, cesarean delivery, forceps delivery, vacuum delivery, placenta previa, abruptio placentae, eclampsia, cervical laceration, uterine rupture, African American race, dystocia, and preeclampsia.[72-75] Pathophysiology is multifactorial and controversial. Generally, it is believed that there is breach of physical barriers, followed by a pressure gradient that allows entry of amniotic fluid into the maternal circulation at the level of the endocervical veins, uterine trauma, or placental attachment sites.[72-79] The amniotic fluid is believed to travel to the maternal pulmonary circulation causing activation of the complement system and anaphylactoid or immune response, since there is a lag time between entry of amniotic fluid into maternal circulation and inflammatory response.[72] There is increased pulmonary vascular resistance and right heart failure, followed by left heart failure.[72] Amniotic fluid tissue factor triggers the extrinsic coagulation pathway by binding to factor VII, activates factor X, and develops consumptive coagulopathy.[72,80-82] This also leads to microthrombosis in the pulmonary vasculature, in turn leading to vasoconstriction.[72,80-83]

Diagnosis is clinical and by exclusion. Laboratory findings are nonspecific with leukocytosis, DIC (prolonged prothrombin time and partial thromboplastin time and decreased fibrinogen), thrombocytopenia, hypoxemia on arterial blood gas, pulmonary edema on chest radiograph, and a dilated right ventricle with leftward deviation of the interatrial and interventricular septa, and cavity obliteration of the left ventricle.[72] Diagnostic markers such as increased zinc coproporphyrin, serum sialyl-Tn antigen greater than 50 μ/mL, increased levels of tryptase, and decreased levels of C3 and C4 have been proposed as markers but are not routinely available.[72] Treatment is largely supportive with the priority of hemodynamic stability. Cryoprecipitate contains fibronectin, which can help facilitate the removal of amniotic fluid via the monocyte and macrophage systems.[72,84]

Finding amniotic fluid in the blood specimen from a right heart catheterization is nonspecific for diagnosis without the appropriate clinical scenario (choice A). A V/Q scan will not help in diagnosis (choice C). The associated DIC is not typically associated with tocolytic-induced pulmonary edema (choice D).

13. B. Dilatation and curettage

Human chorionic gonadotrophin is produced by the trophoblast, which is a layer outside the blastocyst that provides nutrition for the embryo and can develop as part of the placenta and fetal membranes.[85] There are 2 forms: HCG and hyperglycosylated HCG (HCG-H). Human chorionic gonadotrophin contains an α subunit that is common also to other glycoprotein hormones such as luteinizing hormone (LH) and thyroid-stimulating hormone (TSH), and a β subunit.[86] The test for serum HCG levels is an immunoassay that uses 2 antibodies to sites on the β subunit. Levels of HCG are elevated in pregnancy and gestational trophoblastic diseases (GTD). A GTD should be considered in any woman of reproductive age with abnormal bleeding. They are more common in Asia then in the United States or Europe and have a bimodal age distribution with women younger than 16 years of age and older than 45 years of age.[86] In GTD, the levels may be extremely elevated, to the point that there can be a false-negative serum HCG test called a "hook effect."[85] The hook effect is when the serum HCG immunoassays fail to capture and bind to the elevated levels of HCG due to oversaturation and are washed away. This creates a false negative. High suspicion should alert the laboratory to dilute the specimen (choice A).

Elevated HCG levels (> 100,000 mIU/mL) should prompt evaluation via pelvic ultrasound. A complete hydatidiform mole (CHM) generally contains no fetal tissue and has a snowstorm appearance on ultrasound. A partial hydatidiform mole (PHM) can have a snow storm appearance on ultrasound but also has some fetal tissue, such as fetal erythrocytes and vessels in the villi, as seen in this patient (see Fig. 25-4).

A CHM is diploid and results from duplication of the haploid genome of a single sperm or fertilization of 1 ova with 2 sperms.[86] A PHM is triploid and results from fertilization of 1 ovum with 2 sperms or a diploid sperm.[86] Pathologically, a CHM has abnormal trophoblastic hyperplasia, karyorrhectic debris, and collapsed vessels, whereas a PHM has patchy villous hydropic changes with irregularly shaped villi and trophoblastic pseudoinclusions, and patchy trophoblastic hyperplasia.[86] They can present with abnormal first trimester bleeding and can have a snowstorm

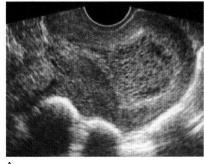
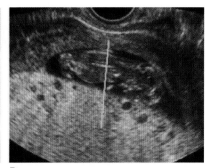

A   B

FIGURE 25-4 Sonograms of hydatidiform moles. **(A) Complete mole. (B) Partial mole.** (Reproduced with permission from Gestational Trophoblastic Disease. In: Cunningham F, Leveno KJ, Bloom SL, et al., eds. *Williams Obstetrics,* Twenty-Fourth Edition New York, NY: McGraw-Hill; 2013. Image contributed by Dr. Elysia Moschos.)

appearance on ultrasound during the second trimester. Treatment is dilation and curettage.

Hydatidiform moles are at risk for gestational trophoblastic neoplasia (GTN). Other risk factors include CHM with trophoblastic proliferation as defined by uterine size greater than gestational age, HCG greater than 100,000 mIU/mL, ovarian theca lutein cysts greater than 6 cm in diameter, and age greater than 35 years old. Gestational trophoblastic neoplasia include choriocarcinoma, which have abnormal villous components, and placental site trophoblastic tumors and epithelioid trophoblastic tumors, which have abnormal extravillous components. Choriocarcinoma (CC) are epithelial-based HCG/human placental lactogen–producing germ tumors with villous trophoblasts, central necrosis, cytotrophoblastic cells, and multinucleated synthiotrophoblastic areas.[86] It occurs in men and women. In women, 50% occur after HM, 25% after spontaneous abortions, and 22.5% after normal pregnancies. It can arise in the mediastinum or pineal gland and tends to metastasize early, particularly into the lung and from the lungs into the brain.[78] Symptoms are based on location. It is chemoresponsive, particularly with methotrexate, actinomycin, cyclophosphamide, and etoposide. A placental site trophoblastic tumor (PSTT) is the extravillous equivalent of CC with less necrosis and less hemorrhage.[86] The patient does not have GTN and is at a lower risk than CHM, therefore methotrexate is not indicated (choice D). There is no role for tocolytics for this patient (choice C).

14. C. Prolactin

Maternal factors that predispose to pulmonary edema include increased maternal volume, decreased peripheral resistance, and hyperaldosteronism.[87] Even preeclampsia can manifest with cardiogenic pulmonary edema from uncontrolled hypertension with diastolic dysfunction and preserved EF.[88] Peripartum cardiomyopathy (PPCM) is defined as development of heart failure in the last month of pregnancy and up to 5 months postpartum in a patient with no known preexisting heart disease and echocardiographic findings of left ventricular end-diastolic dimension greater than 2.7 cm/m^2 and M-mode fractional shortening less than 30% and/or left ventricular EF less than 45%.[88,89] In the United States, the incidence is 1 in 4000 births. and risk factors include age greater than 30 years, African American race, preeclampsia, multiple gestations, substance abuse, prolonged use of tocolytics, diabetes mellitus, obesity, asthma, anemia, genetics (*TTN*), and malnutrition.[88] During the first and second trimesters, there is increased blood volume, leading to increased preload, a 20% to 50% increase in cardiac output from increased HR by 15% to 40% and stroke volume of 15% to 25%, and a 30% decrease in peripheral vascular resistance. It seems unlikely that they influence the development of PCCM.[88] Myocarditis with positive myocardial biopsies

for Coxsackievirus, Echovirus, parvovirus, and selenium deficiency have all been proposed as possible causes, although with conflicting data.[88,90] Recent mouse models showed a decrease in antioxidant production via downregulation of STAT3 transcription factor, leading to unopposed cathepsin cleavage of prolactin, and that, in turn, leads to packaging of MiR-146a into cardiac myocytes.[91,92] This leads to cardiac apoptosis and manifestations of cardiomyopathy. MiR-146a has been proposed as a biomarker, and administration of bromocriptine to block prolactin has reversed the cardiomyopathy in animal models.[88,91,92] Another hormone-related pathogenesis involves the deletion of proliferator-activated receptor-γ coactivator-1α, which in turn can promote the prolactin-mediated pathway and loss of the provascular vascular endothelial growth factor (VEGF) pathway.[88-99] Inhibition of VEGF is secondary to a soluble variant of VEGF receptor 1, soluble FMS-like tyrosine kinase 1 (sFlt1), which is elevated in patients with multiple gestations and preeclampsia.[100]

β-Agonists, which have been used as tocolytics to prevent premature labor, increase arginine vasopressin and activate the renin-angiotensin system, which causes water and sodium retention, respectively, and cause vasodilation with hypotension and compensatory rise in cardiac output (choice D).[87] Prolonged use can trigger shortened left atrial emptying, decreased diastolic filling, and reduced systolic ejection time.[87] This can lead to cardiogenic pulmonary edema. Other tocolytics (eg, calcium channel blockers such as nifedipine or magnesium sulfate) have also caused pulmonary edema.

Ovarian hyperstimulation syndrome (OHSS) is a consequence of an exaggerated response to ovulation stimulation from gonadotropin, clomiphene citrate, and gonadotropin-releasing hormone (choice B).[100,101] Risk factors include age greater than 30 years, polycystic ovaries or high basal antral follicle count, estradiol, previous OHSS, large number of small follicles (8–12 mm), use of HCG for luteal phase support after intravenous fertilization, greater than 20 oocytes retrieved, and early pregnancy.[100,101] The pathophysiology is an increase in vascular permeability from vasoactive peptides released from granulosa cells of hyperstimulated ovaries, and serum VEGF correlates with severity of disease.[93] This results in fluid shifts from intravascular space to extravascular space, such as peritoneal, pleural, and pericardial spaces. Symptoms such as bloating, weight gain, fatigue, and decreased urine output can begin 24 hours but mostly 7 to 10 days after HCG administration.[100,101] Treatment is largely supportive and intended to provide symptomatic relief.

Mirror syndrome, also called Ballantyne syndrome, is the development of preeclampsia-like manifestations between 16 and 34 weeks' AOG and is associated with anasarca and pulmonary edema[6] (choice A). It is the maternal complication from the shedding of trophoblastic debris by the hydropic placenta.[102] It can be distinguished from preeclampsia by visualization of hydrops fetalis on ultrasound. It is also associated with rhesus alloimmunization, nonimmune hydrops, fetal arrhythmias, twin-twin transfusion syndrome, viral infections, tumors, and malformations.[6,103] Treatment involves resolution of fetal issues.

15. D. All of the above

Treatment includes optimizing volume status and neurohormonal status, and preventing arrhythmias and thromboembolic events. With the implications of prolactin in the pathogenesis of PPCM, suppression via bromocriptine is currently being investigated[88] (choice C). Immunotherapy via intravenous immunoglobulin and pentoxifylline are not yet universally accepted.[89] Thromboembolism carries a 6.6% morality, and it is advised to start anticoagulation with heparin during pregnancy and 2 months postpartum[88] (choice A). Other recommendations have suggested to continue anticoagulation until there is echographic evidence of recovery.[89] Atrial fibrillation is the most common arrhythmia in PCCM and can be treated with quinidine, procainamide, and digoxin[82] (choice B). Sudden cardiac death secondary to ventricular arrhythmias is a common cause of mortality and an automated implantable cardioverter defibrillator is advocated when the EF is less than 30%.[88] Recovery, defined as left ventricular (LV) EF of greater than 0.5 or improvement by more than 0.20 occurs for most patients and should be evident by 6 months but can be as late as 48 months.[89] Delayed recovery is likely in African American patients, delayed diagnosis, high NYHA functional class, LV thrombus, multiparity, and coexisting disease. Five percent of patients receiving cardiac transplantation were from PPCM.[88,89]

16. A. Placenta previa

Obstetric hemorrhage is a leading cause of ICU admission.[104,105] Antepartum hemorrhage occurs between 24 weeks' AOG and full term, prior to delivery. Postpartum hemorrhage occurs within 24 hours of delivery up to 6 weeks postpartum.[104,105] Minor bleeding is between 500 and 1000 mL of blood loss, while major bleeding is more than 1000 mL.[104] Risk factors for postpartum hemorrhage include placental abruption, placenta previa, multiple pregnancies, preeclampsia, previous PPH, Asian ethnicity, BMI greater than 35, hemoglobin less than 9 g/dL, cesarean section, labor induction, retained placenta, mediolateral episiotomy, operative vaginal delivery, prolonged labor (> 12 hours), baby weighing more than 4 kg, pyrexia, and age greater than 40 years.[6,104,105] Separation of the placenta exposes the terminal portion of the uterine arteries and the spiral arteries and causes bleeding. The uterus contracts, which stops the bleeding. The Kleihauer-Betke test is a diagnostic test for fetal-maternal hemorrhage that detects fetal red blood cells in a maternal blood sample. The maternal blood sample is exposed to an acidic pH, and adult red blood cells (hemoglobin A) becomes pale, or "ghosts," while fetal red blood cells (hemoglobin F) remain pink. The percentage of fetal to maternal red blood cells is determined by counting 2000 cells. False positives are seen in sickle cell trait. Ultrasound findings help distinguish the different causes of antepartum hemorrhage, as seen in Figures 25-5 to 25-7 and Table 25-8.

17. B. Carboprost

Management of the postpartum hemorrhage should include evacuation of the uterus, uterus contraction via massage, uterotonics, extrinsic myometrial compression, ligation of vessels, or surgical removal of the uterus. Uterotonics (choices A and C) are not without complications, as seen in Table 25-9. Magnesium sulfate (choice D) is not associated with bronchospasm.

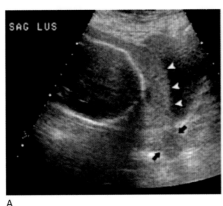
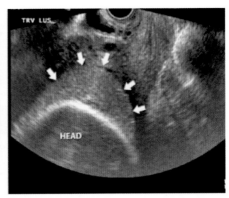

FIGURE 25-5 Total placenta previa. (A) Placenta (white arrow heads) cover the cervix (black arrows). (B) Placenta (arrows) is between cervix and fetal head. (Reproduced with permission from Obstetrical Hemorrhage. In: Cunningham F, Leveno KJ, Bloom SL, et al. eds. *Williams Obstetrics,* Twenty-Fourth Edition New York, NY: McGraw-Hill; 2013.)

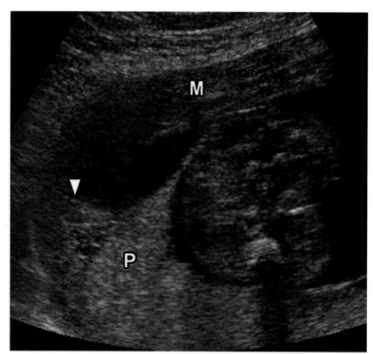

FIGURE 25-6 Placenta abruptio. The placenta (P) is pushed away from the myometrium (M) by an hypoechoic fluid, that appears to be layered (arrowhead) suggestive of blood. (Reprinted with permission from Elsayes KM, Trout AT, Friedkin AM, et al. *Imaging of the placenta: a multimodality pictorial review.* RadioGraphics. 2009;29:1371-1391.)

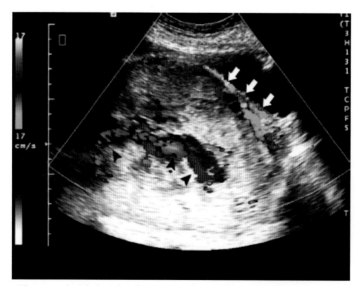

FIGURE 25-7 Placenta accreta. Ultrasound with doppler shows retroplacental vessels (white arrows) within the myometrium. The black arrows represent intraplacental venous lakes which are abnormal. (Reproduced with permission from Obstetrical Hemorrhage. In: Cunningham F, Leveno KJ, Bloom SL, et al. eds. *Williams Obstetrics,* Twenty-Fourth Edition New York, NY: McGraw-Hill; 2013.)

TABLE 25-8 Platental Disorders, Definition, Types, and Ultrasound Findings

Placental Disorders	Definition	Types	Ultrasound
Placenta previa (choice A)	Abnormal placental placement near or on the internal cervical os	• Partial: 2 cm from cervical os • Complete: placenta covering the entire cervical os	Placenta 2 cm from os or covering the os
Placental abruption (choice B)	Premature separation of the placenta from the uterus with hemorrhage into the decidua basalis	• Class 0: asymptomatic • Class 1: no to mild bleeding, slight uterine tenderness, no fetal or maternal distress, no coagulopathy • Class 2: no to moderate bleeding, moderate uterine tenderness, maternal orthostatic, fetal distress, fibrinogen 50–250 mg/dL • Class 3: no to severe bleeding, painful uterus, shock, fetal death, fibrinogen < 50 mg/dL	Retroplacental clot Concealed hemorrhage Expanding hemorrhage
Placenta accreta (choice C)	Placenta invades the uterine wall	• Placenta increta: invades only myometrium • Placenta percreta: invades myometrium, serosa, and sometimes other organs	Irregularly shaped lacunae with turbulent blood flow, protrusion of placenta into bladder, increased vascularity in serosa and bladder, thinning of myometrium, loss of retroplacental space
Retained placenta (choice D)	No placental expulsion within 30 min of birth		Heterogeneous material noted within endometrial cavity that may be avascular and has calcifications

TABLE 25-9 Uterotonics, Mechanisms of Action, Dose, Side Effects, and Contraindications

Drug Name	Action	Dose and Frequency	Side Effects	Contraindications
Oxytocin (choice A)	A naturally occurring polypeptide Acts on oxytocin-specific receptors in uterine myometrium promoting uterine smooth muscle contraction	Maximum bolus dose 5 IU slow intravenous (IV) (bolus can be repeated if needed); short acting, so often administered as 10 IU/h infusion over 4 hours 500 µg IV or intramuscularly (IM)	Reflex tachycardia Hypotension	Caution in hypovolemic and cardiac patients due to vasodilatation and hypotension
Ergometrine (choice C)	Acts on α-adrenergic, dopaminergic and serotonin 5-HT$_2$ receptors Uterine smooth muscle contraction not clearly associated with a specific receptor		Tachycardia Hypertension Nausea Vomiting	Avoid in patients with preeclampsia and cardiovascular disease
Carboprost (choice B)	Prostaglandin F$_{2\alpha}$ analog Profound smooth muscle contractor	250 µg IM Dose can be repeated every 15 min (maximum of 8 doses)	Bronchospasm Intrapulmonary shunting Hypoxia Vomiting Diarrhea Shivering Pyrexia	Avoid in asthmatics and preexisting respiratory and cardiac disease (not for IV administration)
Misoprostol	Prostaglandin E$_1$ analog	800–1000 µg rectally/vaginally		Allergy to misoprostol or other prostaglandins

REFERENCES

1. Naylor DF, Olson MM. Critical care obstetrics and gynecology. *Crit Care Clin.* 2003;19(1):127-149.

2. Baskett TF, Sternadel J. Maternal intensive care and near-miss mortality in obstetrics. *Br J Obstet Gynaecol.* 1998;105(9):981-984.

3. Lapinsky SE, Kruczynski K, Slutsky AS. Critical care in the pregnant patient. *Am J Respir Crit Care Med.* 1995;152(2):427-455.

4. Kilpatrick SJ, Matthay MA. Obstetric patients requiring critical care. A five-year review. *Chest.* 1992;101(5):1407-1412.

5. Martin SR, Foley MR. Intensive care in obstetrics: an evidence-based review. *Am J Obstet Gynecol.* 2006;195(3):673-689.

6. Guntupalli KK, Hall N, Karnad DR, Bandi V, Belfort M. Critical illness in pregnancy: part I: an approach to a pregnant patient in the ICU and common obstetric disorders. *Chest.* 2015;148(4):1093-1104.

7. Price LC, Slack A, Nelson-Piercy C. Aims of obstetric critical care management. *Best Pract Res Clin Obstet Gynaecol.* 2008;22(5):775-799.

8. Waldorf KMA, Nelson JL. Autoimmune disease during pregnancy and the microchimerism legacy of pregnancy. *Immunol Invest.* 2008;37(5):631-644.

9. Edlow JA, Caplan LR, O'Brien K, Tibbles CD. Diagnosis of acute neurologic emergencies in pregnant and post-partum women. *Lancet Neurol.* 2013;12(2):175-185.

10. Kevat D, Mackillop L. Neurological diseases in pregnancy. *J R Coll Physicians Edinb.* 2013;43(1):49-58.

11. Pascuzzi R. *Medications and Myasthenia Gravis.* New York, NY: Myasthenia Gravis Foundation; 2000: 1-46.

12. Guntupalli KK, Karnad DR, Bandi V, Hall N, Belfort M. Critical illness in pregnancy: part ii: common medical conditions complicating pregnancy and puerperium. *Chest.* 2015; 148(5):1333-1345.

13. Edlow JA, Caplan LR, O'Brien K, Tibbles CD. Diagnosis of acute neurological emergencies in pregnant and post-partum women. *Lancet Neurol.* 2013;12(2):175-185.

14. Wanderer JP, Leffert LR, Mhyre JM, Kuklina EV, Callaghan WM, Bateman BT. Neurologic disorders in obstetric practice. In: Powrie RO, Greene MF, Camann W, eds. *De Swiet's Medical Disorders in Obstetric Practice.* 5th ed. Chichester, England: Blackwell Publishing; 2010: 371-403.

15. Karnad DR, Guntupalli KK. Neurologic disorders in pregnancy. *Crit Care Med.* 2005;33(Suppl 10):S362-S371.

16. Grear KE, Bushnell CD. Stroke and pregnancy: clinical presentation, evaluation, treatment, and epidemiology. *Clin Obstet Gynecol.* 2013;56(2):350-359.

17. Johnson D, Kramer D, Cohen E, et al. Thrombolytic therapy for acute stroke in late pregnancy with intra-arterial recombinant tissue plasminogen activator. *Stroke.* 2005;36(6):E53-E55.

18. Murugappan A, Coplin W, Al-Sadat A, et al. Thrombolytic therapy of acute ischemic stroke during pregnancy. *Neurology.* 2006;66(5):768-770.

19. Elford K, Leader A, Wee R, Stys P. Stroke in ovarian hyper-stimulation syndrome in early pregnancy treated with intra-arterial rt-PA. *Neurology.* 2002;59(8):1270-1272.

20. Wiese K, Talkad A, Mathews M, Wang D. Intravenous recombinant tissue plasminogen activator in a pregnant woman with cardioembolic stroke. *Stroke.* 2006;37(8):2168-2169.

21. Dapprich M. Fibrinolysis with alteplase in a pregnant woman with stroke. *Cerebrovasc Dis.* 2002;13(4):290.

22. Grear KE, Bushnell CD. Stroke and pregnancy: clinical presentation, evaluation, treatment and epidemiology. *Clin Obstet Gynecol.* 2013;56(2):350-359.

23. Harden CL, Hopp J, Ting TY, et al. Practice parameter update: management issue for women with epilepsy-focus on pregnancy (an evidence-based review): obstetrical complications and change in seizure frequency: report of the Quality Standards Subcommittee and Therapeutics and Technology Assessment Subcommittee of the American Academy of Neurology and American Epilepsy Society. *Neurology.* 2009;73(2):126-132.

24. Puylaert JB, Rutgers PH, Lalisang RI, et al. A prospective study of ultrasonography in the diagnosis of appendicitis. *N Engl J Med.* 1987;317(11):666-669.

25. Lim HK, Bae SH, Seo GS. Diagnosis of acute appendicitis in pregnant women: value of sonography. *AJR Am J Roentgenol.* 1992;159(3):539-542.

26. Pedrosa I, Lafornara M, Pandharipande PV, Goldsmith JD, Rofsky NM. Pregnant patients suspected of having acute appendicitis: effect of MR imaging on negative laparotomy rate and appendiceal perforation rate. *Radiology.* 2009;250(3):749-757.

27. Guidelines Committee of the Society of American Gastrointestinal and Endoscopic Surgeons, Yumi H. Guidelines for diagnosis, treatment, and use of laparoscopy for surgical problems during pregnancy: this statement was reviewed and approved by the Board of Governors of the Society of American Gastrointestinal and Endoscopic Surgeons (SAGES), September 2007. It was prepared by the SAGES Guidelines Committee. *Surg Endosc.* 2008;22(4):849-861.

28. Gurbuz AT, Peetz ME. The acute abdomen in the pregnant patient. Is there a role for laparoscopy? *Surg Endosc.* 1997;11(2):98-102.

29. Carver TW, Antevil J, Egan JC, Brown CV. Appendectomy during early pregnancy: what is the preferred surgical approach? *Am Surg.* 2005;71(10):809-812.

30. Sriskandan S. Severe peripartum sepsis. *J R Coll Physicians Edinb.* 2011;41(4):339-346.

31. Barton JR, Sibai BM. Severe sepsis and septic shock in pregnancy. *Obstet Gynecol.* 2012;120(3):689-706.

32. Ryan JM, Heneghan MA. Pregnancy and the liver. *Clin Liver Dis.* 2014;4(3):51-54.

33. Roberts JM, August PA, Bakris G, et al. Hypertension in pregnancy. Washington DC: American College of Obstetrics and Gynecology; 2013:1-89.

34. Jamjute P, Ahmad A, Ghosh T, Banfield P. Liver function test and pregnancy. *J Matern Fetal Neonatal Med.* 2009; 22(3):274-283.

35. Neill AM, Nelson-Piercy C. Hyperemesis gravidarum. *Obstet Gynaecol.* 2003;5:204-207.

36. Outlaw WM, Ibdah JA, Koch KL. Hyperemesis gravidarum and maternal liver disease. Madame Curie Bioscience Database. https://www.ncbi.nlm.nih.gov/books/NBK5974/. Accessed February 9, 2017.

37. Hammoud GH, Ibdah JA. Preeclampsia-induced liver dysfunction, HELLP syndrome, and acute fatty liver of pregnancy. *Clin Liver Dis.* 2014;4(3):69-73.

38. Tran TT, Ahn J, Reau NS. ACG clinical guideline: liver disease and pregnancy. *Am J Gastroenterol.* 2016;111(11):1-19.

39. Goel A, Ramakrishna B, Zachariah U, et al. How accurate are the Swansea criteria to diagnose acute fatty liver of pregnancy in predicting hepatic microvescicular steatosis? *Gut.* 2011;60(1):138-139.

40. Treem WR, Shoup ME, Hale DE, et al. Acute fatty liver of pregnancy, hemolysis, elevated liver enzymes, and low platelets syndrome, and long chain 3-hydroxyacyl-coenzyme A dehydrogenase deficiency. *Am J Gastroenterol.* 1996;91(11): 2293-2300.

41. Kwon H, Lok AS. Viral hepatitis and pregnancy. *Clin Liver Dis.* 2014;4(3):55-57.

42. Ozkan S, Ceylan Y, Ozkan OV, Vildirim S. Review of a challenging clinical issue: intrahepatic cholestasis of pregnancy. *World J Gastroenterol.* 2015;21(23):7134-7141.

43. Pusl T, Beuers U. Intrahepatic cholestasis of pregnancy. *Orphanet J Rare Dis.* 2007;2:26.

44. Steinbrook RA, Brooks DC, Datta S. Laparoscopic cholecystectomy during pregnancy. Review of Anesthetic management, surgical considerations. *Surg Endosc.* 1996;10(5):511-515.

45. Date RS, Kaushal M, Ramesh A. A review of the management of gallstone disease and its complications in pregnancy. *Am J Surg.* 2008;196(4):599-608.

46. Horton JD, San Miel FL, Ortiz JA. Budd-Chiari syndrome: illustrated review of current management. *Liver Int* 2008;28(4):455-466.

47. Khuroo MS, Datta DV. Budd-Chiari syndrome following pregnancy. Report of 16 cases, with roentgenologic, hemodynamic and histologic studies of the hepatic outflow tract. *Am J Med.* 1980;68(1):113-121.

48. Chung RT, Iafrate AJ, Amrein PC, Sahani DV, Misdraji J. Case records of the Massachusetts general hospital. Case 15-2006. A 46-year-old woman with sudden onset of abdominal distention. *N Engl J Med.* 2006;354(20):2166-2175.

49. Grant WJ, McCashland T, Botha JF, et al. Acute Budd-Chiari syndrome during pregnancy: surgical treatment and orthotopic liver transplantation with successful completion of the pregnancy. *Liver Transpl.* 2003;9(9):976-979.

50. Ingraham CR, Padia SA, Johnson GE, et al. Transjugular intrahepatic portosystemic shunt placement during pregnancy: a case series of five patients. *Cardiovasc Intervent Radiol.* 2015;38(5):1205-1210.

51. Nicolas C, Ferrand E, d'Alteroche L, et al. Pregnancies after transjugular intrahepatic portosystemic shunt for noncirrhotic portal hypertension. *Eur J Gastroenterol Hepatol.* 2014;26(4):488-490.

52. Zhou Y, Damsky CH, Fisher SJ. Preeclampsia is associated with failure of human cytotrophoblasts to mimic a vascular adhesion phenotype. One cause of defective endovascular invasion in this syndrome? *J Clin Invest.* 1997;99(9):2152-2164.

53. Carroll MF, Temte JL. Proteinuria in adults: a diagnostic approach. *Am Fam Physician.* 2000;62(6):1333-1340.

54. Simerville JA, Maxted WC, Pahira JJ. Urinalysis: a comprehensive review. *Am Fam Physician.* 2005;71(6):1153-1162.

55. Naderi ASA, Reilly RF. Primary care approach to proteinuria. *J Am Board Fam Med.* 2008;21(6):569-574.

56. Liggins GC, Howie RN. A controlled trial of antepartum glucocorticoid treatment for prevention of the respiratory distress syndrome in premature infants. *Pediatrics.* 1972;50(4):515-525.

57. Roberts D, Brown J, Medley N, Dalziel SR. Antenatal corticosteroids for accelerating fetal lung maturation for women at risk of preterm birth. *Cochrane Database Syst Rev.* 2017;3: CD004454.

58. Lu JF, Nightingale CH. Magnesium sulfate in eclampsia and pre-eclampsia: pharmacokinetic principles. *Clin Pharmacokinet.* 2000;38(4):305-314.

59. Eclampsia Trial Collaborative Group. Which anticonvulsant for women with eclampsia? Evidence from the collaborative eclampsia trial. *Lancet.* 1995;345(8963):1455-1463.

60. Altman D, Carroli G, Duley B, et al; Magpie Trial Collaboration Group. Do women with pre-eclampsia, and their babies, benefit from magnesium sulphate? The Magpie Trial: a randomised, placebo-controlled trial. *Lancet.* 2002;359(9321):1877-1890.

61. Duley L, Almeric M, Hall D. Alternative magnesium sulphate regimens for women with pre-eclampsia and eclampsia. *Cochrane Database Syst Rev.* 2010;8:CD007388.

62. American College of Obstetricians and Gynecologists, Society for Maternal-Fetal Medicine. *Magnesium Sulfate Use in Obstetrics.* Committee Opinion 652; January 2016. https://www.acog.org/Resources-And-Publications/Committee-Opinions/Committee-on-Obstetric-Practice/Magnesium-Sulfate-Use-in-Obstetrics. Accessed August 30, 2017.

63. Euser AG, Cipolla MJ. Magnesium sulfate for the treatment of eclampsia: a brief review. *Stroke.* 2009;40(4):1169-1175.

64. Gilbert JS, Ryan MK, LaMarca BB, Sedeek M, Murphy SR, Granger JP. Pathophysiology of hypertension during preeclampsia: linking placental ischemia with endothelial dysfunction. *Am J Physiol Heart Circ Physiol.* 2008;294(2):H541-H550.

65. Saposnik G, Barinagarrementeria F, Brown RD, et al; American Heart Association Stroke Council and the Council on Epidemiology and Prevention. Diagnosis and management of cerebral venous thrombosis: a statement for healthcare professionals from the American Heart Association/American Stroke Association. *Stroke.* 2011;42(4):1158-1192.

66. Stam J. Thrombosis of the cerebral veins and sinuses. *N Engl J Med.* 2005;352(17):1791-1798.

67. Ferro JM, Canhão P, Stam J, Bousser MG, Barinagarrementeria F; ISCVT Investigators. Prognosis of cerebral vein and dural sinus thrombosis: results of the International Study on Cerebral Vein and Dural Sinus Thrombosis (ISCVT). *Stroke.* 2004;35(3):664-670.

68. Ducros A. Reversible cerebral vasoconstriction syndrome. *Lancet Neurol.* 2012;11(10):906-917.

69. Feske SK. Posterior reversible encephalopathy syndrome: a review. *Semin Neurol.* 2011;31(2):203-214.

70. Schwartz RB, Feske SK, Polak JF, et al. Preeclampsia-eclampsia: clinical and neuroradiographic correlates and insights into the pathogenesis of hypertensive encephalopathy. *Radiology.* 2000;217(2):371-376.

71. Bartynski WS. Posterior reversible encephalopathy syndrome, part 1: fundamental imaging and clinical features. *AJNR Am J Neuroradiol.* 2008;29(6):1036-1042.

72. Conde-Agudelo A, Romero R. Amniotic fluid embolism: an evidence-based review. *Am J Obstet Gynecol.* 2009;201(5): 445.e1-445.13.

73. Kramer MS, Rouleau J, Baskett TF, Joseph KS. Maternal Health Study Group of the Canadian Perinatal Surveillance System. Amniotic-fluid embolism and medical induction of labour: a retrospective, population-based cohort study. *Lancet.* 2006; 368(9545):1444-1448.

74. Abenhaim HA, Azoulay L, Kramer MS, Leduc L. Incidence and risk factors of amniotic fluid embolisms: a population-based study on 3 million births in the United States. *Am J Obstet Gynecol.* 2008;199(1):49.e1-49.e8.

75. Knight M; UKOSS. Amniotic fluid embolism: active surveillance versus retrospective database review. *Am J Obstet Gynecol.* 2008;199(4):e9.

76. Cheung AN, Luk SC. The importance of extensive sampling and examination of cervix in suspected cases of amniotic fluid embolism. *Arch Gynecol Obstet.* 1994;255(2):101-105.

77. Bastien JL, Graves JR, Bailey S. Atypical presentation of amniotic fluid embolism. *Anesth Analg.* 1998;87(1):124-126.

78. Thomson AJ, Greer IA. Non-haemorrhagic obstetric shock. *Baillieres Best Pract Res Clin Obstet Gynaecol.* 2000;14(1):19-41.

79. Masson RG, Ruggieri J, Siddiqui MM. Amniotic fluid embolism: definitive diagnosis in a survivor. *Am Rev Respir Dis.* 1979;120(1):187-192.

80. Courtney LD, Allington M. Effect of amniotic fluid on blood coagulation. *Br J Haematol.* 1972;22(3):353-355.

81. Lockwood CJ, Bach R, Guha A, Zhou XD, Miller WA, Nemerson Y. Amniotic fluid contains tissue factor, a potent initiator of coagulation. *Am J Obstet Gynecol.* 1991;165(5 Pt 1): 1335-1341.

82. McDougall RJ, Duke GJ. Amniotic fluid embolism syndrome: case report and review. *Anaesth Intensive Care.* 1995; 23(6):735-740.

83. Uszyński M, Zekanowska E, Uszyński W, Kuczyński J. Tissue factor (TF) and tissue factor pathway inhibitor (TFPI) in amniotic fluid and blood plasma: implications for the mechanism of amniotic fluid embolism. *Eur J Obstet Gynecol Reprod Biol.* 2001;95(2):163-166.

84. Rodgers GP, Heymach GJ 3rd. Cryoprecipitate therapy in amniotic fluid embolization. *Am J Med.* 1984;76(5):916-920.

85. Goff B. Human Chorionic Gonadotropin: Testing in pregnancy and gestational trophoblastic disease and causes of low persistent levels. https://www.uptodate.com/contents/human-chorionic-gonadotropin-testing-in-pregnancy-and-gestational-trophoblastic-disease-and-causes-of-low-persistent-levels?source=search_result&search=hcg&selectedTitle=3~150. Accessed September 8, 2017.

86. Seckl MJ, Sebire NJ, Fisher RA, et al; ESMO Guidelines Working Group. Gestational trophoblastic disease: ESMO clinical practice guidelines for diagnosis, treatment, and follow-up. *Ann Oncol.* 2013;24(Suppl 6):vi39-50.

87. Lamont RF. The pathology of pulmonary oedema with the use of beta-agonists. *Brit J Obstet Gynaecol.* 2000;107(4):439-444.

88. Arany Z, Elkayam U. Peripartum cardiomyopathy. *Circulation.* 2016;133(14):1397-1409.

89. Bhattacharyya A, Basra SS, Sen P, Kar B. Peripartum cardiomyopathy. *Tex Heart Inst J.* 2012;39(1):8-16.

90. Cenac A, Gaultier Y, Devillechabrolle A, Moulias R. Enterovirus infection in peripartum cardiomyopathy. *Lancet.* 1988; 2(8617):968-969.

91. Bultmann BD, Klingel K, Nabauer M, Wallwiener D, Kandolf R. High prevalence of viral genomes and inflammation in peripartum cardiomyopathy. *Am J Obstet Gynecol.* 2005;193(2):363-365.

92. Fett JD. Viral particles in endomyocardial biopsy tissue from peripartum cardiomyopathy patients. *Am J Obstet Gynecol.* 2006;195(1):330-331; author reply 331-332.

93. Pearson GD, Veille JC, Rahimtoola S, et al. Peripartum cardiomyopathy: National Heart, Lung, and Blood Institute and Office of Rare Diseases (National Institutes of Health) workshop recommendations and review. *JAMA.* 2000;283(9): 1183-1188.

94. Karaye KM, Yahaya IA, Lindmark K, Henein MY. Serum selenium and ceruloplasmin in Nigerians with peripartum cardiomyopathy. *Int J Mol Sci.* 2015;16(4):7644-7654.

95. Kara RJ, Bolli P, Karakikes I, et al. Fetal cells traffic to injured maternal myocardium and undergo cardiac differentiation. *Circ Res.* 2012;110(1):82-93.

96. Cenac A, Sacca-Vehounkpe J, Poupon J, et al. [Serum seleniumand dilated cardiomyopathy in Cotonou, Benin]. *Med Trop (Mars).* 2009;69(3):272-274.

97. Homans DC. Peripartum cardiomyopathy. *N Engl J Med.* 1985;312(22):1432-1437.

98. Bajou K, Herkenne S, Thijssen VL, et al. PAI-1 mediates the antiangiogenic and profibrinolytic effects of 16K prolactin. *Nat Med.* 2014;20(7):741-747.

99. Patten IS, Rana S, Shahul S, et al. Cardiac angiogenic imbalance leads to peripartum cardiomyopathy. *Nature.* 2012;485(7398):333-338.

100. Shmorgun D, Claman P; Joint SOGC-CFAS Clinical Practice Guidelines Committee. The diagnosis and management of ovarian hyperstimulation syndrome. *J Obstet Gynaecol Can.* 2011;33(11):1156-1162.

101. Practice Committee for American Society of Reproductive Medicine. Ovarian hyperstimulation syndrome. *Fertil Steril.* 2008;90(3):S188-S193.

102. Redman CW, Sargent IL. Placental debris, oxidative stress and pre-eclampsia. *Placenta.* 2000;21(7):597-602.

103. Midgley DY, Harding K. The mirror syndrome. *Eur J Obstet Gynecol Reprod Biol.* 2000;88(2):201-202.

104. James AH, McLintock C, Lockhart E. Postpartum hemorrhage: when uterotonics and sutures fail. *Am J Hematol.* 2012: 87(Suppl 1):S16-S22.

105. Committee on Obstetric Practice. Committee opinion 529: placenta accreta. *Obstet Gynecol.* 2012;120(1):207-211.

Acute Kidney Injury and Renal Replacement Therapy

26

Saad A. Bhatti, MD, Karen Braich, MD, and Vijay Lapsia, MD

INTRODUCTION

The incidence of dialysis-requiring acute kidney injury (AKI-D) has increased in the past decade in the United States. From 2000 to 2009, there were 1.09 million hospitalizations (95% confidence interval [CI], 1.04–1.15 million) with AKI-D in the United States. From 2007 to 2009, the population incidence of AKI-D increased by 11% per year (95% CI, 1.07–1.16; $P < 0.001$).[1] Hospitalized patients with AKI-D were older than their counterparts who did not have AKI-D (63.4 vs 47.6 years), were more likely to be male (57.3% vs 41.1%), to be black (15.6% vs 10.2%), to have sepsis (27.7% vs 2.6%), to have heart failure (6.2% vs 2.7%), and to undergo cardiac catheterization (5.2% vs 4.4%) and mechanical ventilation (29.9% vs 2.4%).[1] The temporal trend in the 6 diagnoses—septicemia, hypertension, respiratory failure, coagulation/hemorrhagic disorders, shock, and liver disease—sufficiently and fully accounted for the temporal trend in AKI-D.[2] This chapter will discuss the diagnosis of acute kidney injury and types of renal replacement therapy.

DIAGNOSIS OF ACUTE KIDNEY INJURY

Acute kidney injury is considered when there is an abrupt decrease in urine output. Diagnostic criteria have gone through an evolution, from RIFLE (risk, injury, failure, loss of kidney function, and end-stage kidney disease) criteria, AKIN (Acute Kidney Injury Network) criteria, and now KDIGO (Kidney Disease: Improving Global Outcomes) criteria.[3-5] This was deemed necessary for research, clinical, and prognostication purposes. See Tables 26-1 and 26-2.

Investigation of the etiology of AKI begins with the characterization of the urinalysis with or without urine culture and serum and urine electrolytes. Fractional excretion of sodium (FE_{Na}) is represented by the following relationship: (Urine Sodium × Serum Creatinine)/(Serum Sodium × Urine Creatinine) × 100. An FE_{Na} less than 1 suggests prerenal and an FE_{Na} greater than 2 suggests acute tubular necrosis (ATN). Limitations to an FE_{Na} less than 1 is that it is also seen in chronic diseases such as liver cirrhosis, congestive heart failure, vasculitis, acute glomerulonephritis, nonoliguric

ATN, and contrast-induced nephropathy. An alternative is fractional excretion of urea (FE_{urea}), which represents the relationships among urine urea nitrogen, blood urea nitrogen (BUN), serum creatinine, and urine creatine and can help distinguish the 2 main causes of renal failure regardless of recent diuretic use. An FE_{urea} greater than 0.4 indicates an intrinsic cause of renal failure, while an FE_{urea} less than 0.3 indicates a prerenal cause.[6] A BUN-to-creatinine ratio of 20:1 can suggest prerenal causes of AKI, although this might be erroneous in the setting of elevated BUN from gastrointestinal bleeding or corticosteroid use. Urine eosinophils can suggest acute interstitial nephritis but can also be seen in transplant rejection, pyelonephritis, atheroembolic disease, and rapidly progressive glomerulonephritis. Imaging studies such as renal ultrasound or CT scan are sometimes considered.

INDICATIONS FOR RENAL REPLACEMENT THERAPY

Acute kidney injury treated with renal replacement therapy (AKI-RRT) occurs in approximately 13% of ICU patients.[7] Indications for renal replacement therapy include refractory hyperkalemia, metabolic acidosis, uremic pericarditis, encephalopathy, refractory volume overload, and drug intoxications (aspirin, lithium, metformin, ethylene glycol, methanol, and Amanita). Delays in initiating RRT can result in serious preventable complications and even death.[8-10]

LOGISTICS INVOLVED IN RENAL REPLACEMENT THERAPY

The right internal jugular vein is the preferred site for a temporary hemodialysis (HD) catheter, but the femoral vein is a viable alternative.[5,11] Subclavian access is not preferred due to kinking and/or the risk of stenosis. A hemodialysis catheter may be needed in end-stage renal disease (ESRD) patients undergoing continuous low-flow modalities, as such low blood flow rates may result in clotting of a preexisting arteriovenous fistula (AVF) or arteriovenous graft (AVG).

TABLE 26-1 RIFLE and AKIN Criteria

RIFLE Category	Serum Creatinine Criteria	Urine Output Criteria
A. The acute dialysis quality initiative (ADQI) criteria for the definition and classification of AKI (ie, RIFLE criteria)		
Risk	Increase in serum creatinine ≥ 1.5 × baseline or decrease in GFR ≥ 25%	< 0.5 mL/kg/h for ≥ 6 h
Injury	Increase in serum creatinine ≥ 2.0 × baseline or decrease in GFR ≥ 50%	< 0.5 mL/kg/h for ≥ 12 h
Failure	Increase in serum creatinine ≥ 3.0 × baseline or decrease GFR ≥ 75% or an absolute serum creatinine ≥ 354 µmol/L with an acute rise of at least 44 µmol/L	< 0.3 mL/kg/h > 24 h or anuria ≥ 12 h
B. The acute kidney injury network (AKIN) criteria for the definition and classification of AKI		
Stage 1	Increase in serum creatinine ≥ 26.2 µmol/L or increase to ≥ 150–199% (1.5- to 1.9-fold) from baseline	< 0.5 mL/kg/h for ≥ 6 h
Stage 2	Increase in serum creatinine to 200–299% (> 2- to 2.9-fold) from baseline < 0.5 mL/kg/h for ≥ 12 h	< 0.5 mL/kg/h for ≥ 12 h
Stage 3	Increase in serum creatinine to ≥ 300% (≥ 3-fold) from baseline or serum creatinine ≥ 354 µmol/L with an acute rise of at least 44 µmol/L or initiation of RRT	< 0.3 mL/kg/h ≥ 24 h or anuria ≥ 12 h

AKI = acute kidney injury; GFR = glomerular filtration rate; RIFLE = risk, injury, failure, loss of kidney function, and end-stage kidney disease; RRT = renal replacement therapy.

From Bagshaw SM, George C. A comparison of the RIFLE and AKIN criteria for acute kidney injury in critically ill patients. *Nephrology Dialysis Transplantation*, 23(5),2008;1570; by permission of Oxford University Press.

TABLE 26-2 KDIGO Criteria

Stage	Serum Creatinine	Urine Output
1	1.5 to 1.9 × baseline or ≥ 0.3 mg/dL (≥ 26.5 µmol/L) increase	< 0.5 mL/kg/h for 6–12 h
2	2.0 to 2.9 × baseline	< 0.5 mL/kg/h for ≥ 12 h
3	3.0 × baseline or increase in serum creatinine to ≥ 4.0 mg/dL (≥ 353.6 µmol/L) or initiation of renal replacement therapy or in patients < 18 y, a decrease in eGFR to < 35 mL/min per 1.73 m²	< 0.3 mL/kg/h for ≥ 24 h or anuria for ≥ 12 h

eGFR = estimated glomerular filtration rate.

Data from Kellum JA, Lameire N; KDIGO AKI Guideline Work Group. Diagnosis, evaluation, and management of acute kidney injury: a KDIGO summary. *Crit Care.* 2013;17(1):204.

Renal replacement machines have a blood pump with an adjustable speed that determines blood flow rates (BFR) and a filter. In case of intermittent hemodialysis (IHD) or sustained low-efficiency dialysis (SLED), the dialysate flows in a countercurrent direction to maintain the gradient for diffusion of particles across the semipermeable membrane of the filter. Composition of the dialysate can be adjusted for patient-specific needs (eg, calcium, bicarbonate, and potassium concentrations). Dialysate flow can be interrupted with blood flowing through the filter resulting in pure ultrafiltration using principle of convection; pure ultrafiltration (PUF) and slow continuous ultrafiltration (SCUF) differ in the blood-flow rates they use. Dialysis filters have various sizes and UF coefficients depending on the surface area and porosity (eg, high flux and low flux).

For continuous venovenous hemofiltration (CVVH), blood flows through a filter generating ultrafiltrate. This removes plasma water containing solutes. The replacement fluids (RF) are added either before (predilution/inflow) the blood flows through the filter or after (postdilution/outflow). Effluent flow is reported as mL/kg/h. The difference between the effluent flow and volume of RF determines the net fluid removal. Addition of RF and removal of plasma water via convection through the filter results in changes in blood composition requiring periodic monitoring of blood chemistry. Replacement fluids are adjusted based on results of blood chemistry.

INTENSITY OF RENAL REPLACEMENT THERAPY

A Cochrane review assessed the effects of different intensities (intensive and less intensive) of continuous RRT (CRRT) on mortality and on recovery of kidney function in critically ill AKI patients.[12] It included all randomized controlled trials (RCTs) of patients with AKI in the ICU regardless of age, comparing intensive (usually a prescribed dose ≥35 mL/kg/h) versus less intensive CRRT (usually a prescribed dose < 35 mL/kg/h). More intensive CRRT did not demonstrate beneficial effects on mortality or recovery of kidney function in critically ill patients with AKI. There was an increased risk of hypophosphatemia with more intense CRRT. Intensive CRRT reduced the risk of mortality in patients with postsurgical AKI.

Two large multicenter randomized control trials investigated whether there is a correlation with intensity of RRT with improved patient outcomes: the Randomized Evaluation of Normal versus Augmented Level of Renal Replacement (RENAL) trial, which compared postdilution effluent flow of 40 mL/kg/h to 25 mL/kg/h[13]; and the Acute Renal Failure Trial Network (ATN) studies,[14] which compared IHD, SLED, or CVVH 35 mL/kg/h 6 times per week, representing the intensive renal support protocol, versus IHD, SLED, or CVVH 20 mL/kg/h 3 times per week, regarded as the less intensive renal support. These studies demonstrated that increased intensity of RRT was not associated with improved patient outcomes.

MODALITY

Modalities differ by utilizing either diffusion (dialysis) or convection (filtration) or a combination (diafiltration).

Pump speed determines the blood flow across the machine, which is 350 mL/min in the conventional mode of hemodialysis and can be lowered in hemodynamically unstable patients to 200 mL/min. The lowering of blood flow results in a longer duration of treatment to achieve clearance and/or ultrafiltration and uses modalities such as SLED, CVVH, or continuous venovenous hemodiafiltration (CVVHDF) (see Fig. 26-1). These forms of hemodialysis use low blood-flow rates to avoid abrupt changes in hemodynamics and body milieu. Additionally, removal of solutes by conventional IHD can result in rapid changes in serum osmolality. Low blood-flow rates allow for more gradual shifts in osmolality, which is preferred in patients with central nervous system (CNS) injury (eg, stroke or traumatic brain injury) to avoid sudden changes in intracranial pressure. Peritoneal dialysis uses the patient's peritoneal membrane to achieve clearance (both convection and diffusion) and ultrafiltration.

Modalities of CRRT

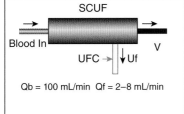

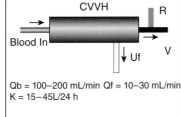

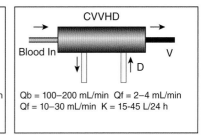

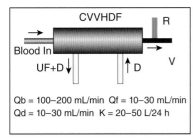

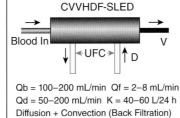

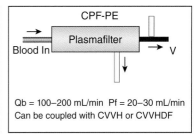

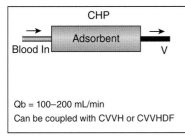

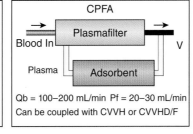

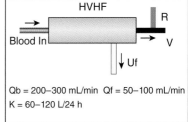

FIGURE 26-1 Modalities of continuous renal replacement therapies (CRRT). Techniques available today for renal replacement in the intensive care unit. CAVH = continuous arteriovenous hemofiltration; CHP = continuous hemoperfusion; CPFA = plasma filtration coupled with adsorption; CPF-PE = continuous plasma filtration–plasma exchange; CVVH = continuous venovenous hemofiltration; CVVHD = continuous venovenous hemodialysis; CVVHDF = continuous venovenous hemodiafiltration; CVVHDF = continuous high-flux dialysis; D = dialysate; HVHF = high-volume hemofiltration; K = clearance; Pf = plasma filtrate flow; Qb = blood flow; Qd = dialysate flow; Qf = ultrafiltration rate; R = replacement; SCUF = slow continuous ultrafiltration; SLED = sustained low-efficiency daily dialysis; UFC = ultrafiltration control system. UF = ultrafiltration; V = vein (Reprinted with permission from Cerda J, Ronco C. Modalities of continuous renal replacement therapy: technical and clinical considerations. *Semin Dial.* 2009;22(2):114-122.)

ANTICOAGULATION FOR RENAL REPLACEMENT THERAPY

Except for peritoneal dialysis, all modalities of RRT result in blood flowing through the circuit with resultant activation of the clotting cascade, which inevitably causes clotting of the circuit, resultant blood loss, and interruption of RRT. Clotted circuits can be flushed with IV fluids to minimize blood loss with an undesirable increase in the patient's intravascular volume. An IV bolus of heparin (30 IU/kg) can be given at the beginning of IHD for ESRD patients to prevent clotting of the circuit in dialysis units. Continuous RRT requires hourly administration of heparin (5–10 IU/kg/h) depending on the duration of the treatment session, with a target partial thromboplastin time (PTT) 1.5 times the control. Frequent circuit clotting despite heparin should raise the possibility of heparin induced thrombocytopenia (HIT) and heparin induced thrombocytopenia with thrombosis (HITT). When HITT is suspected or confirmed, all heparin products must be stopped and replaced by an alternative. Patients with AKI requiring RRT in the ICU may have contraindications for heparin (bleeding risk, CNS injury, HIT). Low-molecular-weight heparins (LMWHs) have several advantages over unfractionated heparin (UFH), including a lower incidence of HIT, less affinity for antithrombin, less platelet (and polymorphonuclear cell) activation, less inactivation by platelet factor-4, greater and more consistent bioavailability, and no metabolic side effects.[15] However, LMWHs are eliminated by CRRT. Although some studies have used fixed doses of LMWH, continuous intravenous administration of LMWH adjusted to achieve systemic anti-factor Xa levels of 0.25 to 0.35 U/mL may be the safer option, resulting in improved filter survival as compared with UFH.[16]

Another option is the use of citrate with CVVH. Regional citrate is more efficacious in prolonging circuit lifespan and reducing the risk of bleeding and should be recommended as the priority anticoagulant for critically ill patients who require CRRT.[17] In adult patients with AKI, there is no difference in mortality between the groups treated with regional citrate and those treated with heparin.[18] Citrate is infused before the blood enters the circuit to chelate calcium. The ratio of total calcium to ionized calcium (iCa) guides the infusion rate, as citrate accumulation may occur in liver failure, altering the ratio to greater than 2.5. Calcium citrate complexes are metabolized into bicarbonate in the muscles, liver, and kidney; thus, citrate toxicity causes both a metabolic alkalosis and a severe hypocalcemia.

EFFECTS OF MODALITY: DIALYSIS VERSUS HEMOFILTRATION

No survival benefit is associated with choosing dialysis (diffusion) over hemofiltration (convection). A systematic review and meta-analysis compared extended daily dialysis (EDD; defined as extended hemodialysis or hemodiafiltration for more than 6 but less than 24 hours per session using a conventional HD machine) with CRRT in patients with AKI. It included 17 studies from 2000 to 2014: 7 RCTs and 10 observational studies involving 533 and 675 patients, respectively. In both RCTs and observational studies, there were no significant differences in recovery of kidney function, fluid removal, or days in the ICU.[19] Extended daily dialysis showed a similar biochemical efficacy to CRRT during treatment (via serum urea, serum creatinine, and serum phosphate). A meta-analysis of RCTs showed no difference in mortality rates between EDD and CRRT. Observational studies showed survival benefit with EDD that might have been affected by allocation or selection bias.[19]

A meta-analysis compared the rate of dialysis dependence among severe AKI survivors according to the choice of initial RRT modality applied (CRRT or IRRT).[20] Twenty-three studies (7 RCTs and 16 observational studies involving 472 and 3499 survivors, respectively) reporting dialysis dependence among survivors from severe AKI requiring RRT were included. Pooled analyses of RCTs showed no difference in the rate of dialysis dependence among survivors.[20] Pooled analyses of observational studies suggested a higher rate of dialysis dependence among survivors who initially received IRRT as compared with CRRT.[20] The speed of correction of metabolic anomalies is greater with intermittent HD, but the advantage of IHD over continuous techniques has not been specifically assessed. There are no data indicating a superiority or inferiority of diffusive versus convective modalities. Pooled data from a few randomized trials suggest that hemofiltration increases the clearance of medium to larger molecules without improving clinical outcomes, although confidence intervals are wide[21] (Table 26-3). Hemofiltration may also reduce filter life. This latter finding, together with the increased RF requirements to achieve equivalent small-molecule clearance when pre-filter replacement is used, suggests that hemofiltration may be more expensive than hemodialysis.[21] There is a broad consensus that, compared with standard IHD, CRRT may be the optimal treatment for hemodynamically unstable patients,[5] and IHD may be a more suitable option when patients have left or are soon to leave the ICU.

TIMING OF RENAL REPLACEMENT THERAPY INITIATION

Despite several studies comparing early versus late renal replacement therapy, there is no general agreement on the optimal time to initiate renal replacement therapy in acute kidney injury.

A large, multicenter, observational study called the Beginning and Ending Supportive Therapy for the Kidney (BEST Kidney) study included 1238 patients in the ICU who developed AKI requiring RRT in 23 countries and stratified

TABLE 26-3 Comparison of the Renal Replacement Therapy Modalities

Modality	Primary Mode of Clearance	BFR(mL/min)	Dialysate	RF	Anticoagulation	Time
IHD	Diffusion	250–400	Yes	No	Short, heparin	3–4 h
SLED	Diffusion	100–200	Yes	No	Long, heparin	8–24 h
CVVH	Convection	200–300	No	Yes	Continuous heparin/citrate	24 h
CVVHD	Both	200–300	Yes	Yes	Continuous heparin/citrate	24 h
SCUF	Convection	100–200	No	No	Long, heparin/citrate	varies

BFR = blood-flow rate; CVVH = continuous venovenous hemofiltration; CVVHD = continuous venovenous hemodialysis; IHD = intermittent hemodialysis; RF = replacement fluid; SCUF = slow continuous ultrafiltration; SLED = sustained low-efficiency dialysis.

patients into early (median urea < 67.8 mg/dL, creatinine < 3.48 mg/dL, and < 2 days from ICU admission) and late (median urea > 67.8 mg/dL, creatinine > 3.48 mg/dL, and > 5 days from ICU admission) RRT initiation. Late RRT initiation on the basis of creatinine was associated with lower adjusted mortality, whereas late RRT initiation on the basis of days from ICU admission was associated with higher adjusted mortality.[8]

In a multicenter randomized trial (Artificial Kidney Initiation in Kidney Injury, or AKIKI) involving critically ill patients (n = 620) with severe AKI, there was no significant difference in mortality between the early and the delayed strategies for the initiation of RRT.[22] With the early strategy, RRT was started immediately after randomization. With the delayed strategy, RRT was initiated if at least one of the following criteria was met: severe hyperkalemia, metabolic acidosis, pulmonary edema, BUN more than 112 mg/dL, or oliguria more than 72 hours after randomization. Forty-nine percent of patients in the delayed-strategy group did not receive RRT. The primary outcome was overall survival at day 60 (48.5% early group vs 49.7% delayed strategy). More catheter-related bloodstream infections were seen in the early group (10% vs 5%). Diuresis occurred earlier in the delayed strategy group.

The single center Early versus Late Initiation of Renal Replacement Therapy in Critically Ill Patients with Acute Kidney Injury (ELAIN) RCT (n = 231) showed that early (within 8 hours of diagnosis of KDIGO stage 2; n = 112) initiation of RRT compared with delayed (within 12 hours of stage 3 AKI or no initiation; n = 119) initiation of RRT reduced mortality over the first 90 days.[23] Duration of RRT (9 days vs 25 days) and length of hospital stay (51 days vs 82 days) were significantly shorter in the early group than in the delayed group. There was no significant effect on requirement of RRT after day 90, organ dysfunction, and length of ICU stay. Given the lack on conclusive data supporting either late vs early RRT, there is still no consensus about the optimal time to initiate RRT in the setting of an AKI. Thus, an approach to the initiation of the RRT should be based on the clinical picture. The latest KDIGO guidelines suggest that renal replacement therapy should be initiated in the setting of life-threatening electrolyte, fluid, and/or acid–base balance.[5]

MEDICATION ADMINISTRATION DURING RENAL REPLACEMENT THERAPY

Determinants of drug removal during RRT include molecular size, ionic charge, volume of distribution (Vd) and protein binding with more effective removal of high-molecular-weight substances during convection. A high-flux membrane, with increased permeability of medium-sized molecules, presents a greater capacity to remove drugs with a high molecular weight compared to low-flux membranes. Hydrophobic synthetic membranes have a high adsorption capacity, whereas cellulose acetate membranes show less adsorption with effecting drug removal. Pharmacokinetics (PK) is altered with accumulation of drugs in AKI. Increasing evidence suggests that antibiotic dosing in critically ill patients with AKI often does not achieve pharmacodynamics (PD) goals, and the continued high mortality rate due to infectious causes appears to confirm these findings.[24] Sampling Antibiotics in Renal Replacement Therapy (SMARRT) is a multinational, observational pharmacokinetic study in critically ill patients requiring RRT that should help develop some consensus about dosing of vancomycin, linezolid, piperacillin/tazobactam, and meropenem.[25] The application of RRT significantly complicates antibiotic dosing with factors such as altered protein binding and antibiotic hydrophilicity affecting PK. In addition, the operational characteristics of RRT, such as mode, filter type, BFR, membrane fouling, fluid replacement site, and total effluent rate, all can influence drug disposition. Volume of distribution is the PK parameter that determines antibiotic loading dose requirements. Hydrophilic antibiotics are usually confined to the intravascular and interstitial fluid in tissues and have a lower Vd than more lipophilic antibiotics (like many quinolones). In the acute phase of critical illness, fluid resuscitation coupled with reduced protein binding can increase the Vd. Increased Vd has been demonstrated for penicillins,[26] carbapenems,[27] and glycopeptides.[28] The maintenance dose of antibiotic is primarily determined by clearance (CL). For antibiotics such as vancomycin, piperacillin/tazobactam, and meropenem, CL is predominantly by the kidneys; RRT modalities have varying effects on antibiotic removal with effluent flow rate being a reliable predictor of antibiotic clearance in critically ill patients despite significantly altered pharmacokinetics in these patients.[29] In data analyzed from 30 published studies, current dosing regimens achieved target concentrations for meropenem (89%), piperacillin (83%), and vancomycin (60%) against susceptible pathogens.[29] Recent studies have shown that under modern CRRT, the extent of elimination of antibiotics is regularly underestimated so that nowadays, the risk of antibiotic underdosing is higher than toxicity due to overdosing.[30]

EFFECTS OF FLUID ACCUMULATION

Positive fluid balance has been associated with an increased risk for mortality in critically ill patients with AKI with or without RRT.[31] The Finnish Acute Kidney Injury (FINNAKI) study was a prospective, multicenter, observational cohort study in 17 Finnish ICUs during a 5-month period collected data on patient characteristics, RRT timing, and parameters at RRT initiation. Association of parameters at RRT initiation, including fluid overload (defined as cumulative fluid accumulation > 10% of baseline weight) with 90-day mortality was studied. The crude 90-day mortality of patients with or without fluid overload was 59.2% versus 31.4% (P < 0.001). In logistic regression, fluid overload was associated with an increased risk for 90-day mortality (odds ratio 2.6) after adjusting for disease severity, time of RRT initiation, initial RRT modality, and sepsis. Similar findings were seen in prospectively collected registry data on patients older than 16 years who received RRT for at least 2 days in an ICU at 2 university-affiliated hospitals,[32] 251 of the 494 (51%) patients died during that hospitalization while 25.3% of hospital survivors were dialysis dependent at discharge. Mean daily fluid balance (odds ratio, 1.36 per 1000 mL positive; 95% CI, 1.18–1.57) was among independent risk factors for mortality but not with RRT dependence at discharge among survivors. In the Randomized Evaluation of Normal versus Augmented Level (RENAL) replacement therapy study (n = 1453, 35 ICUs in Australia and New Zealand), a negative mean daily fluid balance was consistently associated with improved clinical outcomes.[13]

DISCONTINUING RENAL REPLACEMENT THERAPY

There is limited data regarding discontinuing RRT for AKI. The KDIGO AKI practice guidelines recommends to discontinue RRT when kidney function has recovered to meet needs of the patient or is no longer consistent with goals of care.[5,33,34] A post hoc analysis of a multicenter observational study of 529 survivors of AKI showed urine output as the most successful predictor of cessation of RRT.[34]

OUTCOMES AFTER RENAL REPLACEMENT THERAPY

Acute kidney injury is a risk factor for developing chronic kidney disease (CKD).[35] In a cohort of 1292 patients requiring RRT for AKI, mortality increased from 59.7% at hospital discharge to 72.1% at 3 years. Dialysis dependence was reported in 19.0% and was associated with age, diabetes, CKD, and oliguria at the time of initiation of RRT.[36] There was no significant difference in hazards for nonrecovery or reasons for nonrecovery (mortality or ESRD) with IHD versus CRRT among survivors (n = 638) to hospital discharge at 90 and 365 days.[37] In a monocentric RCT (The Effect of Continuous versus Intermittent Renal Replacement Therapy on the Outcome of Critically Ill Patients with Acute Renal Failure, or CONVINT), patients (n = 252) were randomized to receive either daily IHD or CVVH. The primary outcome measure was survival at 14 days after the end of RRT. No statistically significant differences were observed between the investigated treatment modalities regarding mortality, renal-related outcome measures, or survival at 14 days after RRT.[38]

BIOMARKERS

Biomarkers are utilized and are undergoing testing for early detection and prognosis of AKI[39]. Secondary analysis of the 1219 adults in the Translational Research Investigating Biomarker Endpoints in AKI (TRIBE-AKI) trial showed that using several biomarkers in patients with AKIN stage I AKI could predict development of severe progressive AKI.[40] Biomarkers included urinary interleukin (IL)-18, urinary albumin-to-creatinine ratio (ACR), and urinary and plasma neutrophil gelatinase-associated lipocalin (NGAL).

A large multicenter study was conducted to identify novel biomarkers for AKI in critically ill adults.[41] The top 2 biomarkers among a panel of 300 markers tested earlier were validated in 728 critically ill adult subjects without evidence of AKI at the time of enrollment. Urine insulin-like growth factor-binding protein 7 (IGFBP7) and tissue inhibitor of metalloproteinases-2 (TIMP-2), both inducers of G1 cell cycle arrest, a key mechanism implicated in AKI, were significantly superior to all previously described markers of AKI. The Topaz study showed that critically ill patients with a product of urinary TIMP-2 and IGFBP7 of greater than 0.3 had 7 times the risk for AKI (95% CI, 4–22) compared with critically ill patients with a test result less than 0.3; the relative risk increased by 17-fold in those with values greater than 2.0.[41] It validated the value of single measurement of urinary TIMP-2 × IGFBP7 to predict moderate to severe AKI within 12 hours in a prospective study of critically ill adults (n = 420).

Cutoff values greater than 0.3 (high risk) and greater than 2.0 (very high risk) with imminent moderate to severe AKI were also validated in the Opal study (n = 154).[42] The Biologic Markers of Recovery for the Kidney study (BioMaRK) examined the ability of blood and urine biomarkers to predict recovery among patients with dialysis-requiring AKI.[43] Among 817 patients requiring RRT, 50.8% died and 36.8% were RRT independent. After adjusting for variables, increased concentrations of plasma IL-8 and IL-18 and tumor necrosis factor 1 (TNFR1) were independently associated with slower renal recovery. Higher concentrations of IL-6, IL-8, IL-10, and IL-18; macrophage migration inhibitory factor (MIF); TNFR1; and death receptor 5 (DR5) were associated with mortality.

PREVENTION

Avoidance of conditions and medications that can induce acute kidney injury is the primary method of prevention. The current guidelines from KIDGO stratified their recommendations based on the GRADE System. Level 1 is a strong recommendation while Level 2 is a weak recommendation.[5] Quality of supporting evidence is further stratified into A (high), B (moderate), C (low), and D (very low).[5] KIDGO guidelines does not recommend diuretics in the prevention (Grade 1B) or diuretics for the treatment of AKI except in the setting of volume overload (Grade 2C).[5]

There have been inconsistent reports that show that low-dose dopamine (1–3 μg/kg/min) provides renal protection by causing vasodilatation, natriuresis, and improved GFR, and 1 study even suggested that dopamine causes vasoconstriction in AKI; therefore, it is not recommended (Grade 1A).[5,44-47] Fenoldopam (Grade 2C) and atrial natriuretic peptide (Grade 2B) are also not recommended for the prevention or treatment of AKI.[5]

Iatrogenic causes of AKI, such as medications or procedures, should be limited. Aminoglycosides have concentration-dependent bactericidal activity with prolonged postantibiotic effect; therefore, they can be administered as a single dose rather than in multiple doses per day to prevent AKI (Grade 2B).[5] Levels should be obtained if multiple daily doses are given for more than 24 hours (Grade 1A) or if single daily dosing is given for more than 48 hours (Grade 2C).[5] For amphotericin B, lipid formulations should be used (Grade 2A) or other azole antifungal agents and/or echinocandins (Grade 1A).[5] To prevent contrast-induced AKI, N-acetylcysteine (NAC) has not be shown to be of benefit (Grade 1A).[5] A nonpharmacologic approach to prevent contrast-induced AKI is to use the lowest possible dose of contrast. Volume expansion with isotonic sodium chloride or sodium bicarbonate solutions are recommended to prevent contrast-induced AKI (Grade 1A).[5]

QUESTIONS

1. A 70-year-old man presents with peritonitis from a ruptured diverticulum and has an urgent partial colectomy. Postoperatively, he requires vasopressors and multiple liters of IV fluid.

His medical history includes stage 4 CKD from hypertension. His usual medications include lisinopril 20 mg daily, amlodipine 10 mg daily, and furosemide 80 mg twice daily.

On the first postoperative day, his temperature is 101°F, heart rate (HR) is 90 beats/min, and his blood pressure (BP) is 120/60 mmHg. His urine output declines to 5 mL/h despite continued IV fluids and repeat doses of IV furosemide boluses. His abdomen is mildly distended, quiet, and tender to palpation. He has pitting edema of the hands and lower legs. Bladder pressure is 10 cm H_2O. His labs showed the following:

Na	125 mEq/L
K	6.4 mEq/L
Cl	100 mEq/L
BUN	50 mg/dL
CO_2	18 mEq/L
Crea	4.5 mg/dL

His urine sediment shows granular casts and cellular debris. An electrocardiogram (ECG) shows tall T waves in precordial leads and a shortened QT interval.

In addition to intravenous calcium, insulin, and dextrose, which the following is the next most appropriate treatment?

A. Furosemide drip at 10 mg/h
B. Sodium zirconium cyclosilicate
C. Sodium polystyrene sulfonate
D. Hemodialysis

2. A 37-year-old cirrhotic woman undergoes esophagogastroduodenoscopy after developing significant hematemesis and melena at home. The patient was given approximately 2 units of packed red blood cells (PBRCs), 1 unit of fresh frozen plasma (FFP), and 2 Liters of intravenous (IV) fluids. After experiencing a repeat episode of hematemesis in the emergency department (ED) and desaturating to 80%, the patient was emergently intubated in the EDR and started on octreotide and somatostatin and given another 2 units of PRBCs. The patient's blood pressure began to drop during the intubation, and she required pressor support. She underwent esophageal band ligation and was subsequently admitted to the medical ICU. She remained mechanically ventilated with an oxygen saturation (Sao_2) of 90% on a fraction of inspired oxygen (Fio_2) of 0.6 with a positive end-expiratory pressure of 15 cm H_2O. Her chest x-ray showed bilateral pulmonary edema. The patient's urine output is approximately 10 mL/h. Her labs show the following:

Hgb	6.5 g/dL
Hct	19%
plt	$50 \times 10^3/\mu L$
crea	3 mg/dL
K	4.5 mEq/L
BUN	60 mg/dL
CO_2	17 mEq/L

The patient is given an additional 2 units of PRBCs and started on CVVH to prevent further volume overload. She was noted to have twitching in her upper extremities. Subsequent labs show the following:

Na	138 mEq/L
K	4.5 mEq/L
Cl	100 mEq/L
CO_2	10 mEq/L
BUN	45 mg/dL
Creat	2.5 mg/dL
Ionized Ca	0.8 mEq/L
Phos	1.4 mEq/L
Lactic acid	2.5 mmol/L
INR	1.30
AST	14 U/L
ALT	20 U/L
Ammonia	32

What is the most likely reason for her further deterioration?

A. Septic shock
B. Alcohol withdrawal
C. Citrate toxicity
D. Fulminant liver failure

3. A 76-year-old woman was found unresponsive in the street. She is emergently intubated on the field and brought to the ED. Her vitals are BP of 86/45 mmHg, HR of 109 beats/min, respiratory rate (RR) set by the ventilator at 16 breaths/min, and O_2 saturation (sat) of 100%. The patient is given approximately 2 Liters of fluids with no change in BP, so she is started on vasopressors, given 1 dose of empiric antibiotics, and admitted to the ICU. A computed tomography (CT) scan of the head is negative for an acute pathology. Her bloodwork returns showing potassium of 6.5 mEq/L, creatine phosphokinase (CPK) of 15,000 U/L, creatinine of 3 mg/dL, and BUN of 50 mg/dL, and there is no more than 20 mL of urine in her Foley bag. Renal is consulted for renal replacement therapy, and the patient is started on CVVH. The system clots after a few hours, the filter is replaced, and CVVH is continued. After another hour, the nurse notes the filter pressure is rising again. The ICU nurse calls you to help correct the problem. Which of the following is not a reasonable recommendation?

A. Add citrate to the CVVH circuit while carefully monitoring the calcium level.
B. Switch the replacement fluid from postdilution to predilution.
C. Start the patient on a heparin drip for systemic anticoagulation.
D. Check the catheter for kinks and reposition patient.

4. A 72-year-old man with past medical history of CKD stage 4 (baseline creatinine, 2.5–3 mg/dL), diabetes mellitus (DM), hypertension (HTN), and history of cerebrovascular accident (CVA) was admitted to the neurosurgery ICU after he was found to have a significant subarachnoid hemorrhage with slight mass effect on computed tomography of the head. The patient is currently intubated and sedated. His vitals are labile with BP of 90/56 mmHg, HR of 92 beats/min, and O_2 sat of 100% on mechanical ventilation and on low-dose vasopressors. The patient was noted to have no urine output for the last 12 hours. His labs show the following:

Na	136 mEq/L
K	5.8 mEq/L
CO_2	13 mEq/L
BUN	100 mg/dL
Crea	6.4 mg/dL

Which is the best mode of RRT for this patient?

A. Intermittent HD (same prescription as outpatient schedule)
B. SLED
C. CVVH
D. B or C

5. A 55-year-old patient with past medical history of ESRD on hemodialysis, DM, HTN, HIV (noncompliant with medications), and IV drug use was discharged back to his outpatient dialysis unit after a prolonged hospital course where he was treated for an epidural abscess. The patient was admitted with lower back pain and lower extremity weakness that imaging confirmed was a significant infection. The patient was started on vancomycin and will be continuing the antibiotics for another 2 weeks while outpatient. The patient is seen today with complaints of 6 new fibrous areas of skin on both his lower extremities. The skin appears hardened, stretched, and mildly tender to palpation, with some erythema but no drainage. The patient states the first plaque soon after his discharge. The patient has also noted worsening stiffness in of both ankles and knees. What could be the cause of these plaques?

A. Amyloidosis with skin involvement
B. Kaposi sarcoma
C. Gadolinium contrast used for magnetic resonance imaging
D. Systemic lupus erythematous

6. A 72-year-old man with past medical history of CKD stage 4, HTN, and hypersensitivity lung disease (HLD) was referred to a cardiologist for vague chest discomfort both with exercise and at rest. A nuclear stress test was done and found to be positive. The patient was scheduled for cardiac catheterization. Which of the following measures could help prevent progression of the patient's CKD?

A. IV hydration at 100 mL/h starting the day prior and until an hour before cardiac catheterization
B. Starting weight-based IV hydration an hour before cardiac catheterization and then depending on a measured left ventricular end-diastolic pressure (LVEDP) during the procedure, an increase or decrease in hydration for 4 hours after the procedure
C. Mucomyst (N-acetylcysteine) 1200 mg every 11 hours × 4 doses, starting the day prior to the procedure
D. Use of high-osmolar contrast media

7. A 75-year-old woman with past medical history of CKD stage 3, HTN, HLD, DM, coronary artery disease (CAD) status post–coronary artery bypass graft was admitted to the ICU after developing sepsis due to community-acquired pneumonia requiring both vasopressors and intubation. The patient was noted to have decreased urine output on day 3 of admission, approximately 40 mL/h, and her creatinine rose from 1.6 mg/dL to 2 mg/dL. Her BUN was 40 mg/dL, her potassium was 4 mEq/L, and her CO_2 was 23 mEq/L. Additionally, the patient started to develop upper extremity and sacral edema. Which of the following measures could help improve the patient's survival?

A. Initiation of RRT now
B. Wait to initiate RRT until there is a clear clinical parameter, such as an electrolyte abnormality, severe volume overload, or acidemia
C. Start IV furosemide at 10 mg/h
D. None of the above

8. A 50-year-old man is being evaluated for an AKI. The patient was started on cefazolin 7 days ago for cellulitis on his lower extremity. The patient began to note that he developed worsening bilateral extremity edema in addition to decreased urination. Blood tests revealed creatinine of 2.2 mg/dL. Urinalysis showed 5 to 10 erythrocytes, 10 to 20 leukocytes, and trace protein. His vitals were stable, and his physical exam revealed no new rashes and the cellulitis had mostly healed. The patient did not report taking any other medications. Which of the following is the next best step?

A. Renal biopsy
B. Oral steroids
C. Urine eosinophils
D. Different antibiotic

9. A 62-year-old man is hospitalized with acute onset of shortness of breath. In the ED, he coughed up a large quantity of blood and subsequently developed hypoxic respiratory failure requiring intubation. On physical exam, the patient has coarse crackles in both lung fields, no jugular vein distension (JVD), trace lower extremity edema, and vitals within normal limits. Pertinent labs show the following:

Crea	3.2 mg/dL
BUN	58 mg/dL
Hgb	10 g/dL
U/A	3+ blood, 2+ protein, 20–30 RBC, 5–10 WBC
Urine protein-to-creatinine ratio	2.2

His antineutrophil cytoplasmic antibody (ANCA) serology is negative. His complement levels are within normal limits. His antinuclear antibodies (ANA) and double-stranded DNA (dsDNA) are negative. A renal biopsy reveals necrotizing crescentic glomerulonephritis. What is the most likely diagnosis?

A. Membranous nephritis
B. Microscopic polyangiitis
C. Cardiorenal syndrome
D. Anti–glomerular basement membrane antibody disease

ANSWERS

1. D. Hemodialysis

Emergent indications for hemodialysis are severe metabolic acidosis, hyperkalemia, significant uremia causing altered mental status, pericardial rub and uremic frost, hypervolemia, and toxin removal. Hemodialysis is the most reliable way to address life-threatening hyperkalemia in a patient with severely impaired renal function. Other methods to lower serum potassium are temporary, delayed, and/or require intact renal or gastrointestinal function to be effective.

A furosemide (Lasix) drip would be ineffective (choice A). The patient is almost anuric despite receiving multiple doses of IV furosemide without increase of urine output. Sodium zirconium cyclosilicate is a novel cation exchanger that appears to be effective and have a reasonable onset of action (within 4 hours) but has not been extensively studied, particularly in patients with severe hyperkalemia and ECG changes (choice B). Its safety and efficacy in a patient with recent bowel surgery have not been established. Currently, this agent is approved only for chronic hyperkalemia.[48] Sodium polystyrene sulfonate (Kayexalate) can be given orally or rectally to remove potassium via the gastrointestinal tract (choice C). It is contraindicated in patients with recent bowel surgery due to an increased risk for intestinal necrosis.

2. C. Citrate toxicity

Citrate toxicity is characterized by low ionized calcium concentration and normal or elevated total serum calcium due to measurement of serum citrate-calcium in addition to just total serum calcium. Although citrate toxicity can occur at lower ratios, it is likely if ratio of total serum calcium to ionized calcium concentration >2.5. It is usually seen with high anion gap metabolic acidosis but can be seen in metabolic alkalosis. The developing hypocalcemia can become life threatening.[49]

Citrate is commonly used in CVVH to provide local anticoagulation of the hemofilter. The citrate is infused into the hemocircuit prefilter and chelates ionized calcium, leading to inhibition of the coagulation cascade. Within the hemofilter, the majority of the citrate and chelated calcium enters the dialysate and is removed from the hemocircuit. Calcium chloride therefore must be infused centrally to replace the lost calcium. The remaining portion of citrate that is not dialyzed through the filter enters the patient's systemic circulation and is metabolized in the liver. In general, citrate should be avoided in patients who cannot metabolize citrate effectively and therefore are at a high risk for development of citrate accumulation, such as those with severe liver failure and lactic acidosis.[49]

Lastly, while the other options are likely, they are less likely given the presentation.

The patient has no signs or symptoms that would point to infection and thus indicate sepsis (choice A). There is no mention of the patient having alcoholic cirrhosis and no recent mention of alcohol consumption (choice B). The patient does not have fulminant liver failure as per laboratories (choice D).

3   C. Start the patient on a heparin drip for systemic anticoagulation.

Initiation of systemic anticoagulation in a critically ill patient who still has no clear diagnosis and could potentially be bleeding is not recommended.

Regional anticoagulation can be achieved by the prefilter infusion of citrate (choice A). Citrate chelates calcium, decreasing ionized calcium (iCa) in the extracorporeal circuit, thus requiring close monitoring of calcium to avoid citrate buildup and life-threatening hypocalcemia.

In predilution CRRT, substitution fluids are administered before the filter, thus diluting the blood in the filter, decreasing hemoconcentration, and improving blood and filtrate flow conditions (choice B). However, this is done at the expense of clearance, so there is a need to assess risk versus benefit.

Vascular access is a major determinant of circuit survival (choice D). Both high arterial and venous pressures are detrimental. Access failure causes blood flow reductions, which are associated with early circuit clotting.[15,16]

4.   D. B or C

Critically ill adults with acute kidney injury experience considerable morbidity and mortality, and there has always been controversy regarding the optimal renal replacement intervention. In the setting of hemodynamic instability, the use of intermittent hemodialysis can lead to more hemodynamic instability (choice A). Most studies have shown no clear advantage of CVVH over SLED (choices B and C); both have similar mortality and time to renal recovery.[50] Both CVVH and SLED use lower blood flows for a longer duration to achieve the same amount of clearance and ultrafiltration as intermittent HD.[50] These forms of hemodialysis avoid abrupt changes in hemodynamics and body milieu.

5.   C. Gadolinium contrast used for magnetic resonance imaging

Nephrogenic systemic fibrosis (NSF) is an iatrogenic fibrosing disorder that primarily affects individuals with chronic kidney disease following exposure to gadolinium-based contrast agents (GBCAs) during imaging procedures.[51] Gadodiamide is almost exclusively excreted renally and therefore has a markedly prolonged half-life in renal failure patients, including dialysis patients. Nephrogenic systemic fibrosis is characterized by skin thickening, tethering, and hyperpigmentation; flexion contractures of joints; and extracutaneous fibrosis. The pathogenesis is not clearly understood but skin lesions tend to develop 2 to 4 weeks after exposure. Clinically, NSF resembles scleroderma and eosinophilic fasciitis, and histopathologically, it resembles scleromyxedema. Fibrosis can be limited to the skin but at its worse can involve internal organs such as the lungs, muscles, myocardium, even cardiac valves. No definitive treatment is available.[51]

Given the patient's time of presentation, recent exposure and lack of other symptoms that are commonly seen with the other options, NSF is the most likely option. Amyloidosis can present in any number of ways but patients usually have constitutional signs, and associated lesions can have many different forms but not the thickness/shininess described in this patient (choice A).[52] Kaposi sarcoma can present in AIDS patients but lesions are brown, red, purple and usually papular (choice B). Kaposi sarcoma can present with only lesions or be associated with constitutional signs; diagnosis is confirmed with biopsy. Lesions associated with systemic lupus erythematosus (SLE) tend to be the known macular/papular facial rash, in addition to erythematous patches across the body (choice D). Light microscopy of NSF would show expansion of the dermis with fibrosis, and special stains would confirm increased collagen, mucin, and elastic fiber deposition, and occasionally gadolinium deposits.[53]

6.   B. Starting-weight based IV hydration an hour before cardiac catheterization and then depending on a measured left ventricular end-diastolic pressure (LVEDP) during the procedure, an increase or decrease in hydration for 4 hours after the procedure

While the use of IV hydration continues to be debated and re-evaluated, consensus still stands on IV hydration as being preferred to no prophylaxis at all. The Prevention of Contrast Renal Injury with Different Hydration Strategies (POSEIDON) trial, the best evidence in favor of hydration so far, helped create an easy-to-follow algorithm as specified in the answer above. The overall incidence of acute kidney injury in the POSEIDON trial was 11.4%, but with a striking difference of 16.3% in control versus 6.7% in the intervention arm, resulting in a relative risk of 0.41 with a number needed to treat of 11. The major adverse event rates showed a similar beneficial trend, which were significant at 6 months.[54] As per the study, IV hydration is started an hour before the procedure at a rate of 3 mL/kg/h. During the procedure, LVEDP is established and used to guide post-procedure fluid administration:

1. An LVEDP less than 8 mmHg: increase IV hydration to 5 mL/kg/h
2. An LVEDP between 8 and 13 mmHg: no change
3. An LVEDP more than 13 mmHg: decrease IV hydration to 1 mL/kg/h

Intravenous hydration should be continued for 4 hours after the procedure.[54]

As noted above, while IV hydration is preferred, LVEDP is a better guide to optimize post-procedure hydration in patients undergoing cardiac catheterization (choice A). Mucomyst has repeatedly been shown to have no effect on prevention of contrast-induced nephropathy (choice C) and the use of high-osmolar contrast media is more likely to cause contrast-induced nephropathy (choice D).[54]

7. D. None of the above

Several studies have looked at the benefit of early (choice A) versus late (choice B) initiation of HD in the setting of AKI and there is still no consensus. Some studies concluded that early initiation improves mortality, while others recommend waiting to initiate HD (AKIKI and ELAINE trials).[22,23]

The use of furosemide to treat patients with AKI has not been shown to decrease blood transfusion requirements, decrease duration of RRT, or improve survival (choice C). Furosemide use has not translated into decreased severity of clinical AKI. Controlled trial of loop diuretics in patients who had late AKI and were simultaneously being started on dialysis showed no outcome benefits.[55]

Since the use of a loop diuretic does not prevent the progression of AKI or decrease the need for RRT and since there is no consensus on when hemodialysis should be initiated, the decision to proceed with hemodialysis versus a trial of diuretics should depend on the individual needs of the patient at that time, taking into consideration hemodynamic instability, electrolyte imbalance, mental status, etc.

8. D. Different antibiotic

The patient has acute interstitial nephritis (AIN), which can be caused by infections, multiple drugs, malignancy, and even autoimmune conditions. In this case, the patient has no other apparent cause for AKI except for the use of this new medication, and penicillins are well known to cause AIN. Discontinuation of the offending agent is the mainstay therapy for drug-induced AIN.

Renal biopsy is best utilized in the conditions were the diagnosis is less clear (choice A); in this case, stopping the offending agent would be the best option. If the patient's AKI still does not improve/resolve, then proceeding with a biopsy would be an option.[56] The role of steroids in AIN is controversial, evidence is conflicting, and they are usually reserved for patients who cannot discontinue the offending agent (choice B). Very rarely do patients present with the triad of fever, rash, and urine eosinophils, thus checking for urine eosinophils will not help make the diagnosis of AIN (choice C).

9. D. Anti–glomerular basement membrane antibody disease

Anti–glomerular basement membrane (GBM) antibody disease is an autoimmune process that is caused by antibodies directed at type IV collagen that binds to the glomerular basement membrane. This patient is presenting with a pulmonary renal syndrome with both hemoptysis and hypoxic respiratory failure and renal failure with active urine sediment containing protein, leukocytes, and erythrocytes. The necrotizing crescents on the renal biopsy are consistent with rapidly progressive glomerulonephritis (RPGN), which can be broken down into 3 categories: (1) immune (SLE, immunoglobulin A, cryoglobulinemia), (2) pauci-immune (ANCA-associated vasculitis), and (3) anti-GBM antibody disease. Pulmonary involvement can be seen in all 3 categories. Given that complements were mostly normal, ANCA, ANA, and dsDNA were negative, the most likely diagnosis is anti-GBM. While the information was not provided in the stem, the biopsy can usually be diagnostic. Anti-GBM will show necrotizing crescents with linear staining of immunoglobulin G along the glomerular basement.[57]

Membranous nephropathy requires nephrotic range proteinuria more than 3 g of protein in the urine but without blood in the urine (choice A). Cardiorenal syndrome tends to have bland urine, and there would not likely be significant blood and/or protein in the urine. Additionally, the patient's physical exam should be more consistent with overload, such as positive JVD and LE edema (choice C). Lastly, the patient is noted to be ANCA negative, making MPA unlikely also (choice B).

REFERENCES

1. Hsu RK, McCulloch CE, Dudley RA, et al. Temporal changes in incidence of dialysis-requiring AKI. *J Am Soc Nephrol*. 2013; 24(1):37-42.
2. Hsu RK, McCulloch CE, Heung M, et al. Exploring potential reasons for the temporal trend in dialysis-requiring AKI in the United States. *Clin J Am Soc Nephrol*. 2016;11(1):14-20.

3. Brochard L, Abroug F, Brenner M, et al; ATS/ERS/ESICM/ SCCM/SRLF Ad Hoc Committee on Acute Renal Failure. An official ATS/ERS/ESICM/SCCM/SRLF statement: prevention and management of acute renal failure in the ICU patient. *Am J Respir Crit Care Med.* 2010;181(10):1128-1155.

4. Kellum JA, Lameire N; KDIGO AKI Guideline Work Group. Diagnosis, evaluation, and management of acute kidney injury: a KDIGO summary. *Crit Care.* 2013;17(1):204.

5. KDIGO clinical practical guideline for acute kidney injury. *Kidney Int.* 2012;2(1):1-141.

6. Carvounis CP, Nisar S, Guro-Razuman S. Significance of the fractional excretion of urea in the differential diagnosis of acute renal failure. *Kidney Int.* 2002;62(6):2223-2229.

7. Hoste EA, Bagshaw SM, Bellomo R, et al. Epidemiology of acute kidney injury in critically ill patients: the multinational AKI-EPI study. *Intensive Care Med.* 2015;41(8):1411-1423.

8. Bagshaw SM, Uchino S, Bellomo R, et al; Beginning and Ending Supportive Therapy for the Kidney (BEST Kidney) Investigators. Timing of renal replacement therapy and clinical outcomes in critically ill patients with severe acute kidney injury. *J Crit Care.* 2009;24(1):129-140.

9. Mendu ML, Ciociolo GR Jr, McLaughlin SR, et al. A decision-making algorithm for initiation and discontinuation of RRT in severe AKI. *Clin J Am Soc Nephrol.* 2017;12(2):228-236.

10. Vaara ST, Reinikainen M, Wald R, Bagshaw SM, Pettilä V; FINNAKI Study Group. Timing of RRT based on the presence of conventional indications. *Clin J Am Soc Nephrol.* 2014;9(9): 1577-1585.

11. Parienti JJ, Mégarbane B, Fischer MO, Lautrette A, Gazui N; Cathedia Study Group. Catheter dysfunction and dialysis performance according to vascular access among 736 critically ill adults requiring renal replacement therapy: a randomized controlled study *Crit Care Med.* 2010;38(4):1118-1125.

12. Fayad AI, Buamscha DG, Ciapponi A. Intensity of continuous renal replacement therapy for acute kidney injury. *Cochrane Database Syst Rev.* 2016;10:CD010613.

13. RENAL Replacement Therapy Study Investigators, Bellomo R, Cass A, Cole L. An observational study fluid balance and patient outcomes in the randomized evaluation of normal vs. augmented level of replacement therapy trial. *Crit Care Med.* 2012;40(6):1753-1760.

14. VA/NIH Acute Renal Failure Trial Network; Palevsky PM, Zhang JH, O'Connor TZ, et al. Intensity of renal support in critically ill patients with acute kidney injury. *N Engl J Med.* 2008;359(1):7-20.

15. Joannidis M, Oudemans-van Straaten HM. Clinical review: patency of the circuit in continuous renal replacement therapy. *Crit Care.* 2007;11(4):218.

16. Joannidis M, Kountchev J, Rauchenzauner M, et al. Enoxaparin vs. unfractionated heparin for anticoagulation during continuous veno-venous hemofiltration: a randomized controlled crossover study. *Intensive Care Med.* 2007;33(9):1571-1579.

17. Gattas DJ, Rajbhandari D, Bradford C, Buhr H, Lo S, Bellomo R. A randomized controlled trial of regional citrate versus regional heparin anticoagulation for continuous renal replacement therapy in critically ill adults. *Crit Care Med.* 2015; 43(8):1622-1629.

18. Liu C, Mao Z, Kang H, Hu J, Zhou F. Regional citrate versus heparin anticoagulation for continuous renal replacement therapy in critically ill patients: a meta-analysis with trial sequential analysis of randomized controlled trials. *Crit Care.* 2016;20(1):144.

19. Zhang L, Yang J, Eastwood GM, Zhu G, Tanaka A, Bellomo R. Extended daily dialysis versus continuous renal replacement therapy for acute kidney injury: a meta-analysis. *Am J Kidney Dis.* 2015;66(2):322-330.

20. Schneider AG, Bellomo R, Bagshaw SM, Glassford NJ. Choice of renal replacement therapy modality and dialysis dependence after acute kidney injury: a systematic review and meta-analysis. *Intensive Care Med.* 2013;39(6):987-997.

21. Friedrich JO, Wald R, Bagshaw SM, Burns KE, Adhikari NK. Hemofiltration compared to hemodialysis for acute kidney injury: systematic review and meta-analysis. *Crit Care.* 2012;16(4):R146.

22. Gaudry S, Hajage D, Schortgen F, et al. Initiation strategies for renal-replacement therapy in the intensive care unit. *N Engl J Med.* 2016;375(2):122-133.

23. Zarbock A, Kellum JA, Schmidt C, et al. Effect of early vs delayed initiation of renal replacement therapy on mortality on critically ill patients with acute kidney injury: the ELAIN randomized controlled trial. *JAMA.* 2016;315(20):2190-2199.

24. Lewis SJ, Mueller BA. Antibiotic dosing in patients with acute kidney injury: "enough but not too much." *J Intensive Care Med.* 2016;31(3):164-176.

25. Roberts JA, Choi GY, Joynt GM, et al. SaMpling Antibiotics in Renal Replacement Therapy (SMARRT): an observational pharmacokinetic study in critically ill patients. *BMC Infect Dis.* 2016;16:103

26. Varghese JM, Jarrett P, Boots RJ, et al. Pharmacokinetics of piperacillin and tazobactam in plasma and subcutaneous interstitial fluid in critically ill patients receiving continuous venovenous haemodiafiltration. *Int J Antimicrob Agents.* 2014;43(4): 343-348.

27. Roberts JA, Udy AA, Bulitta JB, et al. Doripenem population pharmacokinetics and dosing requirements for critically ill patients receiving continuous venovenous haemodiafiltration. *J Antimicrob Chemother.* 2014;69(9):2508-2516.

28. DelDot ME, Lipman J, Tett SE. Vancomycin pharmacokinetics in critically ill patients receiving continuous venovenous haemodiafiltration. *Br J Clin Pharmacol.* 2004;58(3):259-268.

29. Jamal JA, Udy AA, Lipman J, Roberts JA. The impact of variation in renal replacement therapy settings on piperacillin, meropenem, and vancomycin drug clearance in the critically ill: an analysis of published literature and dosing regimens. *Crit Care Med.* 2014;42(7):1640-1650.

30. Michael E, Kindgen-Milles D. [Antibiotic dosing for renal function disorders and continuous renal replacement therapy]. *Anaesthesist.* 2015;64(4):315-323.

31. Vaara ST, Korhonen AM, Kaukonen KM, et al. Fluid overload is associated with an increased risk for 90-day mortality in critically ill patients with renal replacement therapy: data from the prospective FINNAKI study. *Crit Care.* 2012:16(5):R197.

32. Silversides JA, Pinto R, Kuint R, et al. Fluid balance, intradialytic hypotension, and outcomes in critically ill patients undergoing renal replacement therapy: a cohort study. *Crit Care.* 2014;18(6): 624.

33. Katayama S et al. Factors predicting successful discontinuation of continuous renal replacement therapy. *Anaesth Intensive Care.* 2016;44(4):453-457.

34. Uchino S, Bellomo R, Morimatsu H, et al. Discontinuation of continuous renal replacement therapy: a post hoc analysis of a prospective multicenter observational study. *Crit Care Med.* 2009;37(9):2576-2582.

35. Heung M, Steffick DE, Zivin K, et al. Acute kidney injury recovery pattern and subsequent risk of CKD: an analysis of Veterans Health Administration Data. *Am J Kidney Dis.* 2016;67(5):742-752.

36. De Corte W, Dhondt A, Vanholder R, et al. Long-term outcome in ICU patients with acute kidney injury treated with renal replacement therapy: a prospective cohort study. *Crit Care.* 2016; 20(1):256.

37. Liang KV, Sileanu FE, Clermont G, et al. Modality of RRT and recovery of kidney function after AKI in patients surviving to hospital discharge. *Clin J Am Soc Nephrol.* 2016;11(1):30-38.

38. Schefold JC, von Haehling S, Pschowski R, et al. The effect of continuous versus intermittent renal replacement therapy on the outcome of critically ill patients with acute renal failure (CONVINT); a prospective randomized controlled trial. *Crit Care.* 2014;18(1):R11.

39. Malhotra R, Siew ED. Biomarkers for the early detection and prognosis of acute kidney injury. *Clin J Am Soc Nephrol.* 2017; 12(1):149-173.

40. Koyner JL, Garg AX, Coca SG, et al; TRIBE-AKI Consortium. Biomarkers predict progression of acute kidney injury after cardiac surgery. *J Am Soc Nephrol.* 2012;23(5):905-914.

41. Bihorac A, Chawla LS, Shaw AD, et al. Validation of cell-cycle arrest biomarkers for acute kidney injury using clinical adjudication. *AJRCCM.* 2014;189(8):932-939.

42. Hoste EA, McCullough PA, Kashani K; Sapphire Investigators. Derivation and validation of cutoffs for clinical use of cell cycle arrest biomarkers. *Nephrol Dial Transplant.* 2014;29(11): 2054-2061.

43. Murugan R, Wen X, Shah N, et al; Biological Markers for Recovery of Kidney (BioMaRK) Study Investigators. Plasma inflammatory and apoptosis markers are associated with dialysis dependence and death among critically ill patients receiving renal replacement therapy. *Nephrol Dial Transplant.* 2014; 29(10):1854-1864.

44. Bellomo R, Chapman M, Finfer S, et al. Low-dose dopamine in patients with early renal dysfunction: a placebo-controlled randomised trial. Australian and New Zealand Intensive Care Society (ANZICS) Clinical Trials Group. *Lancet.* 2000; 356(9248):2139-2143.

45. Murray PT. Use of dopaminergic agents for renoprotection in the ICU. In: Vincent JL, ed. *Yearbook of Intensive Care and Emergency Medicine.* Berlin, Germany: Springer-Verlag; 2003: 637-648.

46. Lauschke A, Teichgraber UK, Frei U, et al. "Low-dose" dopamine worsens renal perfusion in patients with acute renal failure. *Kidney Int.* 2006;69(9):1669-1674.

47. Kellum JA, M Decker J. Use of dopamine in acute renal failure: a meta-analysis. *Crit Care Med.* 2001;29(8):1526-1531.

48. Weisberg LS. Management of severe hyperkalemia. *Crit Care Med.* 2008;36(12):3246-3251.

49. Meier-Kriesche HU, Gitomer J, Finkel K, DuBose T. Increased total to ionized calcium ratio during continuous venovenous hemodialysis with regional citrate anticoagulation. *Crit Care Med.* 2001;29(4):748-752.

50. Kovacs B, Sullivan KJ, Hiremath S, Patel RV. Effect of sustained low efficient dialysis versus continuous renal replacement therapy on renal recovery after acute kidney injury in the intensive care unit: a systematic review and meta-analysis. *Nephrology (Carlton).* 2017;22(5):343-353.

51. Galan A, Cowper SE, Bucala R. Nephrogenic systemic fibrosis (nephrogenic fibrosing dermopathy). *Curr Opin Rheumatol.* 2006;18(6):614-617.

52. Hazenberg BP. Amyloidosis: a clinical overview. *Rheum Dis Clin North Am.* 2013;39(2):323-345.

53. Nijssen EC, Rennenberg RJ, Nelemans PJ, et al. Prophylactic hydration to protect renal function from intravascular iodinated contrast material in patients at high risk of contrast-induced nephropathy (AMACING): a prospective, randomised, phase 3, controlled, open-label, non-inferiority trial. *Lancet.* 2017;389(10076):1312-1322.

54. Brar SS, Aharonian V, Mansukhani P, et al. Haemodynamic-guided fluid administration for the prevention of contrast-induced acute kidney injury: the POSEIDON randomised controlled trial. *Lancet.* 2014;383(9931):1814-1823.

55. Cantarovich F, Rangoonwala B, Lorenz H, Verho M, Esnault VL; High-Dose Furosemide in Acute Renal Failure Study Group. High-dose furosemide for established ARF: a prospective, randomized, double-blind, placebo-controlled, multicenter trial. *Am J Kidney Dis.* 2004;44(3):402-409.

56. Raghavan R. Acute interstitial nephritis—a reappraisal and update. *Clin Nephrol.* 2014;82(3):149-162.

57. McAdoo S, Pusey CD. Anti-glomerular basement membrane disease. *Clin J Am Soc Nephrol.* 2017;12(7):1162-1172.

Surgical Intensive Care Unit

Khalid Sherani, MD, Jennifer Cabot, MD, and Stephen M. Pastores, MD

INTRODUCTION

Surgical procedures constitute a sudden insult to the body, which can result in a myriad of life-threatening complications.[1] While most postoperative complications occur 1 to 3 days after surgery, others can take weeks to present.[2]

Some complications may occur after any type of operation and have predictable time courses (Table 27-1). Others are more specific to the operation performed and the patient's medical history (Table 27-2). Postoperative fever is one of the most common complications encountered after any type of operation and requires a systematic approach to identify the etiology (Table 27-3).

In this chapter, we will first outline the main postoperative complications that a critical care provider is likely to encounter in the intensive care unit (ICU), followed by a more in-depth discussion of particularly common or serious complications.

MAJOR GASTROINTESTINAL SURGERY

Abdominal Compartment Syndrome

Abdominal compartment syndrome (ACS) is a life-threatening complication defined as sustained intra-abdominal pressure (IAP) greater than 20 mmHg *with new organ dysfunction*.[3] Risk factors for ACS include (1) decreased abdominal wall compliance due to abdominal surgery, major trauma, burns, or prone positioning; (2) increased volume of intraluminal bowel contents due to gastroparesis, ileus, pseudo-obstruction, or volvulus; (3) increased volume of peritoneal free fluid due to hemoperitoneum, infection, carcinomatosis, or ascites; and (4) capillary leak due to massive fluid resuscitation or transfusion therapy, acidosis, hypothermia, or acute pancreatitis.[2–4]

The frequency of ACS is estimated at 5% of critically ill patients.[3] This diagnosis requires a high level of suspicion and is easily missed. Unfortunately, untreated ACS carries an extremely high mortality rate. The 3 hallmark signs of ACS are (1) a sudden increase in plateau pressures on the ventilator due to extrinsic compression from the abdomen, (2) hypotension due to impaired venous return, and (3) oliguria/anuria due to hypotension and compression of the renal vessels.[4] The physical exam will reveal a distended and tense abdomen, hypotension, tachycardia, jugular venous distension, peripheral edema, and evidence of hypoperfusion. Bladder pressure, which is an estimation of the IAP, will be greater than 20 mmHg.[3]

Treatment includes supportive care (nasogastric and rectal tube decompression, pain control, supine position, and chemical paralysis) and/or abdominal decompression via laparotomy.[5]

Pancreatitis

One to three percent of patients undergoing a peripancreatic operation will develop pancreatitis. Of all cases of acute pancreatitis, postoperative pancreatitis accounts for approximately 10%.[6] Secondary infection and pancreatic necrosis are 3-fold more common in the setting of postoperative pancreatitis than biliary or alcoholic pancreatitis. Both infection and necrosis are associated with a high mortality rate (30–40%). Diagnosis of postoperative pancreatitis requires a high index of suspicion, as the clinical exam is nonspecific and amylase/lipase levels may be normal.[7] Abdominal computed tomography (CT) showing pancreatic edema and peripancreatic fluid collections may help to establish the diagnosis. Close monitoring and management in the ICU are recommended for patients with end-organ dysfunction, and early enteral nutrition may limit injury and decrease the rate of infection. The use of prophylactic antibiotics is not recommended in patients with pancreatic necrosis without evidence of infection. Severe cases of pancreatitis may result in fluid collections that require percutaneous drainage or endoscopic transgastric necrosectomy.

Cholecystitis

Postoperative cholecystitis is mostly acalculous (70–80%) and occurs more commonly in males (75%).[6] Risk factors include critical illness, endoscopic sphincterotomy, and parenteral nutrition.[6] Postoperative cholecystitis progresses rapidly to necrosis and is less likely to respond to conservative management. The diagnosis may be confirmed via ultrasound or CT demonstrating pericholecystic fluid, intramural gas, and/or gallbladder wall thickening. Critically ill patients, who are often too unstable to undergo surgery, may undergo percutaneous cholecystostomy tube placement for decompression.

TABLE 27-1 General Postoperative Complications

- Immediate (hours to days)
  - Complications of anesthesia: malignant hyperthermia, allergic reaction, arrhythmia, hypotension, hypertension
  - Hemorrhage: primary (cut ends of vasculature), secondary (congenital bleeding diathesis, consumptive coagulopathy, anticoagulant-related)
  - Hypoxia: aspiration pneumonitis, atelectasis, pulmonary edema, transfusion reaction
  - Oliguria: inadequate fluid replacement, bladder atony secondary to anesthetics, acute tubular necrosis secondary to medications, hypotension, or rhabdomyolysis
  - Shock: hypovolemic (blood or fluid loss), distributive (sepsis, side effect of anesthesia), cardiogenic (post-surgical MI), obstructive (acute PE)
  - Thromboembolic events: cerebrovascular accident, MI, PE

- Early (days)
  - Acute kidney injury: prerenal, intrinsic, obstructive
  - Anastomotic breakdown/wound dehiscence
  - Dehydration
  - Delirium
  - Electrolyte imbalance
  - Hypoxic respiratory insufficiency: acute respiratory distress syndrome, pneumonia, PE
  - Ileus/Ogilvie syndrome
  - Infection: local wound infection or systemic infection (pneumonia, urinary, intravascular catheters, abscess)
  - Thromboembolic events: deep venous thrombosis, PE
  - Urinary retention
  - Transfusion-associated reactions

- Late (weeks to months)
  - Abscess
  - Fistula
  - Hernia: incisional, internal

MI = myocardial infarction; PE = pulmonary embolism.

TABLE 27-2 Procedure-Specific Complications

Type of Procedure	Specific Complications

Gastrointestinal surgery	- Bowel operations
	  - Anastomotic complications/leak
	  - Bowel obstruction
	  - Fluid collections
	  - Ileus/Ogilvie syndrome
	  - Nerve damage (presacral plexus)
	- Gallbladder operations
	  - Common bile duct injury/leak
	  - Pancreatitis

Thoracic surgery	- Air leak, pneumothorax, and bronchopleural fistula - Lobar torsion - Pleural effusions and hemothorax - Postpneumonectomy syndrome - Postpneumonectomy pulmonary edema
Cardiac surgery	- Arrhythmias (bradycardia, supraventricular, ventricular) - Myocardial ischemia - Shock (blood loss, vasodilation due to warming, cardiopulmonary bypass–induced inflammation and capillary leak, decrease in ventricular compliance due to ischemia-reperfusion injury)

Vascular surgery	- Cerebrovascular accident
	- Compartment syndrome due to
	  - Bleeding
	  - Reperfusion edema
	- Cranial nerve injuries
	- Graft-related complications
	  - Fistula formation
	  - Hemorrhage
	  - Infection
	  - Ischemia
	  - Rethrombosis
	- Multisystem organ failure

Urological surgeries	- Bleeding/hematuria - Electrolyte abnormalities (most commonly hyponatremia) - Retrograde ejaculation - Sphincter damage/incontinence - Urinary tract infections (urethritis, cystitis, pyelonephritis, prostatitis)
Neck surgeries	- Airway obstruction secondary to compression from hematoma - Electrolyte abnormalities (most commonly hypocalcemia due to parathyroid gland damage/removal) - Facial or recurrent laryngeal nerve damage

Anastomotic Leak

Anastomotic leak is the most common complication following gastrointestinal surgery, with an incidence of 2.9% to 15.3%.[8] Small bowel and ileocolic anastomoses have the lowest leak rates, while coloanal anastomoses have the highest.[9] Approximately one-third of deaths after colorectal procedures are attributed to leaks.[8] Anastomotic leaks commonly present with increased or persistent discharge from drains, abscess formation, or peritonitis. Leaks may manifest as late as 12 days postprocedure and even following hospital discharge.[10] Abdominal CT imaging may show a localized abscess and/or contrast extravasation. Treatment includes broad-spectrum antibiotics, bowel rest, re-exploration, and abdominal washout. The anastomotic breakdown itself may be addressed in a number of ways, commonly via primary re-anastomosis with or without proximal stoma creation.

Bowel Obstruction

About 50% of postoperative bowel obstructions occur in the setting of colorectal surgery.[8] The most common etiologies are adhesions and internal hernias. Most patients have a period of normal bowel function after the procedure before developing symptoms of obstruction. Symptomatically, it can be difficult to differentiate bowel obstruction from postoperative ileus. Radiologic studies including abdominal CT may be helpful. Treatment options include conservative management, such as nasogastric tube decompression and bowel rest, as well as surgical exploration. Strangulation is uncommon but is associated with a 15% mortality rate.[9]

TABLE 27-3 Etiologies of Postoperative Fever

- Immediate
  - Drug fever
  - Malignant hyperthermia (rare)
  - Transfusion reaction

- Acute
  - Catheter-associated infections
  - Skin and soft tissue infections
  - Urinary tract infection
  - Ventilator-associated pneumonia/aspiration pneumonia/pneumonitis

- Subacute
  - Antibiotic-associated fever
  - Catheter-associated infections/thrombophlebitis
  - *Clostridium difficile* colitis
  - Skin and soft tissue infections, wound-related complications
  - Urinary tract infection
  - Ventilator-associated pneumonia/aspiration pneumonia/pneumonitis

- Delayed
  - Blood-product-related infections (parasitic, viral)
  - Chylothorax, chyloperitoneum, lymphedema
  - Late wound-related complications (fistulae/leaks)
  - Postpericardiotomy syndromes

THORACIC SURGERY

Air Leak and Pneumothorax

Small air leaks and pneumothoraces are common after thoracotomy.[11] Most resolve spontaneously without intervention, but large, bilateral, or tension pneumothoraces may result in hemodynamic collapse. Therefore, prompt aspiration of pneumothoraces is crucial in the later situations.

Bronchopleural Fistula

Bronchopleural fistula (BPF) develops in approximately 2% of pneumonectomy cases.[12,13] It often is associated with hemodynamic and respiratory instability and carries a mortality rate of 5% to 20%.[12] Bronchopleural fistula may be addressed via bronchial stump revision and patching with a flap.

Pleural Effusion and Hemothorax

Small effusions are common post-thoracotomy and are mostly exudative in nature. The majority of these effusions resolve without any specific management. However, large effusions associated with a drop in hemoglobin or those failing to resolve warrant further investigation. The presence of hemothorax requires prompt evacuation via a chest tube or a washout to prevent secondary infection and trapped lung.

Lobar Torsion

Lobar torsion is a rare but serious complication following lobectomy. This diagnosis requires a high index of suspicion. Delayed or missed diagnosis often lead to fatal outcomes.[12,13]

Clinically, lobar torsion presents with rapid hemodynamic deterioration and complete opacification of the infarcted area on imaging studies. Treatment involves early resection of gangrenous areas, antibiotics, and supportive care.

Postpneumonectomy Syndrome

Postpneumonectomy syndrome is an extremely rare complication characterized by a mediastinal shift toward the side of the resected lung and herniation of the overinflated lung in the same direction.[14] Symptoms include dyspnea, stridor, dysphagia, and reflux resulting from compression of central airways and the esophagus. Treatment includes mediastinal repositioning and prosthesis implantation.

Postpneumonectomy Pulmonary Edema

Postpneumonectomy pulmonary edema (PPPE) is a serious complication characterized by acute hypoxemic respiratory failure after pneumonectomy, more commonly after a right-sided resection.[15] It carries a very high mortality rate.[15] Symptoms typically appear 2 to 4 days following lung resection.[15,16] Management includes low-tidal-volume ventilation, diuretics, and judicious fluid management.[14] In select cases, low-dose corticosteroids, pulmonary vasodilators, inhaled nitric oxide, and extracorporeal membrane oxygenation (ECMO) may be helpful.[17,18]

CARDIAC SURGERY

Shock

Hemodynamic instability is very common during the immediate perioperative period following cardiac surgery.[19] Etiologies include blood loss, warming-induced vasodilation, cardiopulmonary bypass–related inflammation and endothelial cell leak, transient decrease in ventricular compliance due to ischemia-reperfusion injury, cardiac tamponade, valvular dysfunction, and tension pneumothorax.[20,21] Volume resuscitation and inotropic and/or vasopressor support are often required to maintain systemic perfusion.[22] In cases requiring significant inotropic support, placement of an intra-aortic balloon pump (IABP) should be considered. Absolute contraindications to an IABP include severe aortic valve insufficiency, aortic dissection, and severe aortoiliac occlusive disease.[23]

Myocardial Ischemia

Myocardial ischemia following cardiac surgery is associated with a poor prognosis. Ischemia due to graft thrombosis, stenosis, or unbypassed territory may require a return to the operating room or percutaneous intervention in the cardiac catheterization suite.

Dysrhythmias

Atrial fibrillation accounts for 50% of postoperative dysrhythmias and usually resolves spontaneously within 24 hours.[22]

Reversible causes, including electrolyte imbalances, fluid overload, dehydration, and infections, should be identified and treated. Since beta-blockers and calcium channel blockers are negative inotropes, amiodarone is used frequently for pharmacologic cardioversion. Patients who are hemodynamically unstable require electrical cardioversion. Although premature ventricular contractions are common after cardiac surgery, sustained ventricular dysrhythmias are rare. Electrical cardioversion is required in cases of sustained ventricular tachycardia and ventricular fibrillation. A permanent pacemaker should be considered for patients who develop symptomatic sick sinus syndrome or complete atrioventricular block lasting longer than 5 to 7 days postoperatively.[23]

VASCULAR SURGERY

Cerebrovascular Infarction

Stroke occurs in 1% to 3% of patients after carotid endarterectomy (CEA).[24] The most common causes are embolization from atherosclerotic plaques, hypotension-related ischemia, and thrombosis at the site of the arteriotomy. Previous stroke and postoperative atrial fibrillation increase the risk of stroke. Aspirin and preoperative administration of a statin may decrease the incidence.

Cranial Nerve Injuries

Cranial nerve deficits, particularly of the hypoglossal and recurrent laryngeal nerves, occur in up to 12% of cases.[25] The most common etiology is excessive traction during the operation.

Multisystem Organ Failure

Multisystem organ failure (MSOF) occurs most frequently after vascular procedures involving the great vessels, such as repair of a ruptured aortic aneurysm. Patients with respiratory, hepatic, and/or renal failure following such procedures have an extremely high mortality.[26]

Graft Infection

A graft infection can be a devastating complication, particularly following procedures involving the aorta. Treatment involves a prolonged course of antibiotics and graft replacement or removal, if possible. Some patients might require lifelong suppressive antibiotics, especially if the graft must remain in place.

Lymphatic Fistulas

Lymphatic fistulas have an incidence of up to 18% following vascular procedures.[26] They may impair wound healing and lead to wound or graft infections. Conservative treatment includes compression dressings, local wound care, drainage of lymphatic collections, and antibiotics. Persistent lymph drainage of more than 100 mL/d requires surgical intervention.

ORTHOPEDIC SURGERY

Fat Embolism

About 90% of patients with long bone fractures and joint replacements are found to have fat particles in their pulmonary vasculature.[27] Blood transfusions, intravenous fat emulsions, and bone marrow manipulation may also lead to fat embolism.[28] Clinical manifestations include the triad of neurologic dysfunction, respiratory insufficiency, and petechial rash on the chest and upper extremities.[29,30] Symptoms usually manifest within 12 to 72 hours following the injury but may be delayed for several days.[31] Diagnosis is based in clinical suspicion, as the presence of fat droplets in sputum and urine is nonspecific. Treatment is mainly supportive.[27] Prognosis depends on the degree of respiratory compromise.

Compartment Syndrome

Long bone fractures account for 75% of cases of compartment syndrome.[32] Signs and symptoms include the 5 Ps: pain out of proportion to apparent injury (earliest sign), paresthesias (also early), pallor, paralysis (very rare), and pulselessness (almost never seen).[33] The physical exam also may reveal a tense compartment, diminished sensation, and pain with passive muscle movement. Clinical suspicion and measurement of compartment pressures establishes the diagnosis. An intracompartmental pressure of 30 mmHg or higher, or a delta pressure (diastolic blood pressure − intracompartmental pressure ≤ 30 mmHg) in a patient with a concerning history and physical exam is strongly suggestive of acute compartment syndrome.[32,33] However, serious athletes such as triathlon runners may have compartment pressures far above 30 mmHg without clinical compartment syndrome.[32] Laboratory findings include markedly elevated creatine kinase levels and myoglobinuria due to muscle ischemia and breakdown. Definitive treatment consists of immediate fasciotomy. Hyperbaric oxygen may serve as an adjunctive therapy.

Venous Thromboembolism

Deep venous thrombosis (DVT) and pulmonary edema (PE) are especially common after pelvic or hip operations. A blood clot can form within the deep veins of the upper or lower extremities, particularly in the presence of Virchow triad: endothelial injury (due to the initial injury, the operation, or central line placement), venous stasis, or hypercoagulability.[34] The physical exam may reveal swelling, pain, tenderness, or discoloration of the involved extremity, as well as palpable firmness of the vein. Duplex ultrasound confirms the diagnosis. Therapeutic anticoagulation is the mainstay of treatment, but if there is a high concern for bleeding or recurrent DVT while on anticoagulation, an inferior vena cava filter may be considered. Prophylactic measures to prevent DVT/PE include early ambulation, sequential compression devices, and prophylactic doses of anticoagulants.

QUESTIONS

1. A 55-year-old African American man with a history of hypertension, a 30-pack-year history of smoking, alcohol use, and peripheral vascular disease was complaining of nausea, vomiting, abdominal pain, and melanic stools. Two weeks ago, he had an endovascular repair of his abdominal aortic aneurysm. In the emergency department (ED), his vital signs were blood pressure (BP) of 90/60 mmHg, heart rate (HR) of 122 beats/min, respiratory rate (RR) of 22 breaths/min, oxygen saturation of 95% on room air, and temperature of 97.8°F. His physical examination was unremarkable except for a tender, distended abdomen. He had a CT of the abdomen and pelvis which showed inflammatory stranding and gas between the aorta and the small intestine.

   What is the most common area of involvement with this disease?

   A. Duodenum
   B. Stomach
   C. Large intestine
   D. Cecum

2. For the patient in question 1, which type of endoleak is self-limited?

   A. Type I
   B. Type II
   C. Type III
   D. Type IV

3. A 54-year-old woman with no significant past medical history underwent a mastectomy for stage IIA ductal adenocarcinoma. Three days after the operation, she developed progressively worsening shortness of breath and worsening hypotension. An arterial blood gas revealed hypoxemia with a high A-a gradient and respiratory alkalosis. The electrocardiogram (ECG) showed sinus tachycardia. A bedside echocardiogram shows McConnell sign. The cardiac care unit (CCU) team decides to start the patient on vasopressor support. Which of the following medications is least likely to worsen the underlying problem?

   A. Norepinephrine
   B. Vasopressin
   C. Epinephrine
   D. Dopamine

4. An 81-year-old man with a history of hypertension and coronary artery disease underwent a wide resection of a melanoma on his right lower extremity. On postoperative day 2, he was found to have a left lower extremity deep vein thrombosis. He was started on a heparin infusion at 1000 U/h. That evening, he began to complain of severe groin and back pain and became hypotensive to

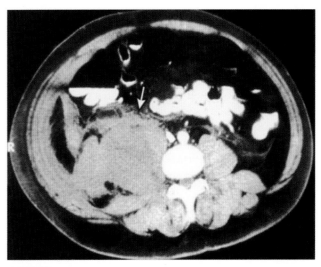

FIGURE 27-1 CT scan of abdomen and pelvis. (Reproduced with permission from Escobar MA, Key NS. Hemophilia A and hemophilia B. In: Kaushansky K, Lichtman MA, Prchal JT, et al. eds. *Williams Hematology. 9th ed.* New York, NY: McGraw-Hill; 2015.)

60/40 mmHg. His CT scan of the abdomen and pelvis is shown above (Fig. 27-1).

What is the most likely cause of the patient's acute decompensation?

A. Retroperitoneal hematoma
B. Inferior vena cava thrombosis
C. Massive pulmonary embolus
D. Intraperitoneal aortic dissection/rupture

5. What risk factors did the patient in question 4 have that would predispose him to this complication?

   A. History of cancer and immobilization
   B. Age and anticoagulation
   C. Cardiac history
   D. The recent operative procedure

6. Use of noninvasive positive pressure ventilation is known to decrease the rate of which of the following in postoperative patients?

   A. Rate of intubation
   B. Hospital mortality
   C. Atelectasis
   D. All of the above

7. Which of the following is a contraindication to the use of noninvasive mechanical ventilation?

   A. Impaired swallow or cough
   B. Poor respiratory drive
   C. Facial, esophageal, or gastric surgery
   D. All of the above

8. A 70-year-old alcoholic man underwent an elective inguinal hernia repair. The patient had an uneventful postoperative course for the intial 24 hours but developed tachycardia and altered mental status on postoperative day 1, followed by a tonic-clonic seizure. The patient was given benzodiazapines for presumed alcohol withdrawal and a one-time dose of phenytoin. Twelve hours later, he was noted to be febrile with a maximum temperature of 101°F. His physical examination did not reveal any obvious source of infection. Laboratory data was significant for a leukocyte count of $12 \times 10^3/\mu L$. Urine analysis showed 1 to 2 white blood cells with negative nitrite and leukocyte esterase. Imaging studies showed clear lungs without any gross effusion or consolidation. The patient had no further seizures and denied any complaints. He had no further occurrence of fever. Which of the following is the most likely cause of patient's fever?

A. Atelectasis
B. Surgical site infection
C. Drug fever
D. *C difficile* colitis

9. A 66-year-old man underwent a total hip replacement for osteoarthritis. On postoperative day 2, the patient developed a new oxygen requirement and became confused. He then developed the rash shown below on his left axilla (Fig. 27-2). By postoperative day 3, the patient was intubated and transferred to the ICU.

What is the most likely diagnosis?

A. Acute respiratory distress syndrome
B. Pulmonary embolism
C. Fat embolism
D. Toxic shock syndrome

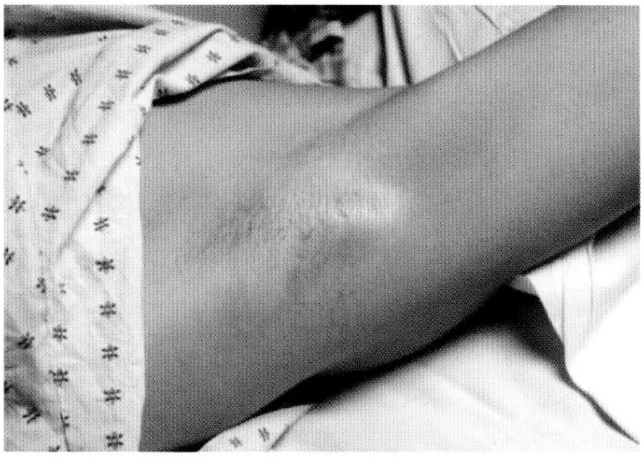

10. For the patient in question 9, what is the most appropriate initial treatment?

A. Broad-spectrum antibiotics
B. Supportive measures, including oxygen supplementation and airway protection
C. Corticosteroids
D. Anticoagulation

11. A 65-year-old man with a history of hypertension, hyperlipidemia, and diabetes mellitus was admitted for a cerebral vascular accident. The patient was noted to have an 80% right carotid artery stenosis and underwent a right carotid endarterectomy. Estimated blood loss was minimal. Postoperatively, the patient's nurse noted swelling around the site and marked it with black marker. One hour later, the nurse states that the swelling has decreased. However, the ecchymosis has spread beyond the margins she marked (Fig. 27-3). The patient's vital signs are BP of 130/80 mmHg, HR of 80 beats/min, RR of 18 breaths/min, and oxygen saturation of 95% on room air. Besides the discoloration, the physical examination is otherwise unremarkable.

Laboratories include white blood cell count of $12 \times 10^3/\mu L$, hemoglobin of 12 g/dL, and platelet count of $230 \times 10^3/\mu L$.

What is the next step?

A. No further treatment
B. Mechanical ventilation
C. Surgery
D. Protamine

FIGURE 27-2 Patient's left axilla. (Reproduced with permission from Drew JM, Demos HA, Pellegrini Jr. VD. Management of common perioperative complications in orthopedic surgery. In: McKean SC, et al., eds. *Principles and Practice of Hospital Medicine. 2nd ed.* New York, NY: McGraw-Hill; 2016.)

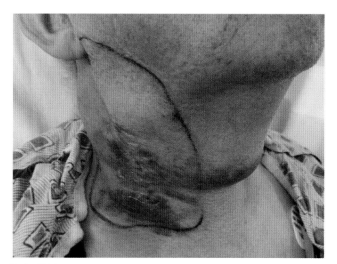

FIGURE 27-3 Patient's right neck after surgery.

12. What approach will prevent reperfusion syndrome after carotid endarterectomy?

    A. Blood pressure control
    B. Heparin infusion
    C. Aspirin
    D. Simvastatin

13. A 50-year-old man with a 35-year history of alcohol abuse was complaining of hematemesis. In the ED, he was noted to have a systolic BP of 72 mmHg and HR of 135 beats/min. He continued to have hematemesis and was subsequently intubated for airway protection. His hemoglobin was 5 g/dL, his platelet count was $105 \times 10^3/\mu L$, and his INR was 4. An introducer and 2 18-gauge needles were placed. Massive blood transfusion protocol was initiated. Gastroenterology was called, and they noticed an active Dieulafoy arterial bleed. Two clips were placed, and 30 units of packed red blood cells, 10 units of fresh frozen plasma, 5 pools of platelets, and 7 Liters of crystalloid boluses were given.

    His current labs include the following:

Hgb	10 g/dL
plt	$150 \times 10^3/\mu L$
INR	1.2
Na	150 mEq/L
Cl	119 mEq/L
K	4.9 mEq/L
Crea	3.9 mg/dL (from a baseline of 0.9 mg/dL)
Ca	6.8 mg/dL

    He was noted to have a distended abdomen. His abdominal pressure, estimated via the bladder pressure, was 25 mmHg. What is the next step?

    A. Change to a larger Salem Sump and place on continuous low-wall suction
    B. Laparotomy

C. Continuous neuromuscular blocking agent
D. Furosemide 40 mg IV

14. A 72-year-old woman with history of Parkinson disease and a total abdominal hysterectomy presented to the ED with 24 hours of nausea, vomiting, and abdominal pain. Her initial vital signs were BP of 130/60 mmHg, HR of 108 beats/min, RR of 22 breaths/min, oxygen saturation of 98% on room air, and temperature of 97.7°F. Her physical examination was otherwise unremarkable except for a distended abdomen.

    Her laboratory values included the following:

WBC	$23 \times 10^3/\mu L$
Hgb	15.4 g/dL
plt	$360 \times 10^3/\mu L$
Na	145 mEq/L
K	5 mEq/L
Cl	98 mEq/L
Bicarbonate	25 mEq/L
Crea	1.49 mg/dL (from a baseline of 0.89 mg/dL)
Ca	7 mg/dL
Lactic acid	4.8 mg/dL

    Computed tomography scans of her abdomen and pelvis are shown below (Fig. 27-4).

    Her abdominal pressure was 22 mmHg. A nasogastric tube was inserted and placed on continuous low-wall suction. Abdominal pressure remained 22 mmHg. What is the next best step?

    A. Exploratory laparotomy
    B. Rectal tube for continuous low-wall suction
    C. Antibiotics
    D. Normal saline

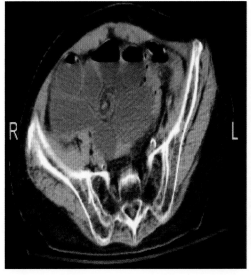
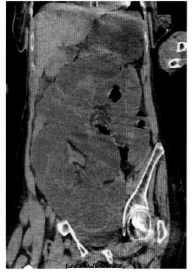

FIGURE 27-4 CT abdomen and pelvis.

15. A 76-year-old man with myelodysplastic syndrome, arthritis, and hypertension who was recently admitted for a blast crisis is complaining of bilateral 10/10 lower extremity pain (right greater than left) over the past 4 hours. On physical examination, he is noted to have discoloration and crepitus of the right lower extremity. A surgeon made lateral incisions on the lower extremity (Fig. 27-5). Purulent material was expressed, and he was able to place a digit between the fascial planes. The patient's vital signs were unremarkable except for a fever of 103°F.

Lower extremity Doppler ultrasounds were negative. His labs were as follows:

WBC	$22.5 \times 10^3/\mu L$
Hgb	6.2 g/dL
INR	1.44
Crea	1.67 mg/dL (from a baseline of 1.10 mg/dL)
Lactic acid	6 mg/dL
pH	6.98
Guaiac	negative

The patient received a 2-Liter bolus of normal saline and 1 unit of packed red blood cells. Bedside ultrasound showed an inferior vena cava diameter of 1.99 cm at baseline and 1.56 cm with inspiration. Wound culture grew *Clostridium septicum*. What is the next step?

A. Wide excision and debridement
B. 1-L bolus of normal saline
C. CT with IV contrast of leg
D. MRI of leg

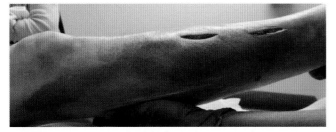

FIGURE 27-5 Right lower extremity with lateral surgical incisions.

16. Another patient is admitted on the same day. He is a 50-year-old man with a history of diabetes mellitus on insulin and diabetic nephropathy. He drinks 4 to 5 beers a day and is a current smoker. He had a mechanical fall earlier in the day and was noted to have bruising on his left lower extremity. In the ED, his vital signs were BP of 140/90 mmHg, HR of 101 beats/min, RR of 18 breaths/min, and oxygen saturation of 95% on room air. His leg was warm and nontender with good capillary refill and good pulses (Fig. 27-6). Labs showed the following:

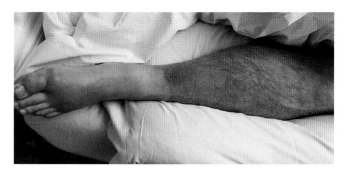

FIGURE 27-6 Left lower extremity.

WBC	$14 \times 10^3/\mu L$
Hgb	12 g/dL
Crea	1.6 mg/dL
Lactic acid	4.0 mg/dL
Creatinine kinase	25,000 U/L

A manometer revealed a compartment pressure of 35 mmHg.

What is the next step?

A. 1-Liter bolus of normal saline
B. Fasciotomy
C. CT with IV contrast
D. Antibiotics

17. A 51-year-old woman with Crohn disease underwent a laparoscopic small bowel resection. Most of the incisions healed, but there is one that appears to be leaking bowel contents. A slice of her CT scan of the abdomen and pelvis is shown below (Fig. 27-7).

What is the etiology of the leakage?

A. Abscess
B. Enterocutaneous fistula
C. Wound dehiscence
D. Seroma

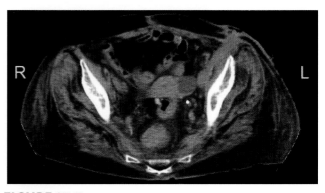

FIGURE 27-7 CT of the abdomen and pelvis.

ANSWERS

1. A. Duodenum

The patient has an aortoenteric fistula, which is an abnormal connection between the aorta and the gastrointestinal tract. It is considered primary when the abnormal connection is caused by compression of the abdominal aortic aneurysm against the gastrointestinal tract (usually the duodenum). It is considered secondary when the abnormal connection is due to erosion of a prosthetic aortic graft into the intestinal tract. The pathogenesis of a secondary aortoenteric fistula includes the following: mechanical pulsation of the aortic graft against the intestine, failure to suture all aortic layers, failure to separate the graft from the intestine, and endoleak.[35,36] Aortoenteric fistulas can also occur in the stomach (choice B), large intestine (choice C), and cecum (choice D).

Diagnosis is difficult, and the triad of abdominal mass, gastrointestinal bleeding, and abdominal pain occurs only in 10% to 12% of patients.[35] Other presentations include thrombosis with ischemia, weight loss, and sepsis. Gastrointestinal bleeding may temporarily cease (known as a "sentinel bleed') and then be followed by severe decompensation. Computed tomography angiography without oral contrast has been suggested as the first-line imaging modality, with sensitivity and specificity as high as 94% and 85%, respectively. Ectopic gas adjacent to or in the aorta, bowel thickening, discontinuation of the aortic wall, and contrast extravasation into the bowel lumen can suggest an aortoenteric fistula. Fifty percent of diagnostic laparotomies are falsely negative.

Treatment includes resuscitation, tissue debridement, intestinal repair or resection, ostomy, and revascularization. This is achieved via open aortic repair or endovascular aneurysm repair.

2. D. Type IV

Endoleak is another complication that can follow endovascular repair of an abdominal aortic aneurysm. It can be clinically silent or cause aortic rupture, and it can be identified immediately after completion of arteriography or in a delayed fashion during surveillance follow-up (Table 27-4).[36]

3. B. Vasopressin

McConnell sign is right ventricular dilation with leftward bowing of the interventricular septum. This echocardiogram finding is 77% sensitive and 96% specific for acute pulmonary embolism.[31] Massive pulmonary embolism blocks pulmonary artery outflow, causing pulmonary hypertension, obstructive shock, and hemodynamic compromise. Vasopressin selectively vasodilates pulmonary vasculature through V1 receptor–mediated nitric oxide release and, therefore, does not worsen pulmonary hypertension. The other vasopressors listed cause pulmonary vasoconstriction and would thus worsen pulmonary hypertension (choices A, C, and D).

4. A. Retroperitoneal hematoma

The computed tomography scan in this question shows a right retroperitoneal hematoma (RPH). There is no sign of inferior vena cava thrombosis (choice B), massive pulmonary embolus (choice C), or intraperitoneal aortic dissection/rupture (choice D).

Right peritoneal hematoma is difficult to diagnose and carries a mortality of 7%.[37] Death in the immediate term is due to exsanguination, while death in the intermediate/long term is due to abdominal compartment syndrome. Right peritoneal hematoma most commonly presents with unexplained hypotension and tachycardia (from blood loss), and less commonly with femoral neuropathy (sudden severe groin pain radiating to the anteromedial thigh and lumbar region), iliopsoas spasm (flexion and/or external rotation of the hip), or abdominal distension. Rarely, and late in the course, a patient may develop Grey Turner sign (flank hematoma) or Cullen sign (periumbilical hematoma).

5. B. Age and anticoagulation

A myriad of risk factors may predispose a patient to retroperitoneal hematoma. These include, but are not limited to, anticoagulation, advanced age, ruptured aortic aneurysm, ruptured renal aneurysm, acute pancreatitis, malignancy, and iatrogenic causes (such as kidney biopsy, bone marrow biopsy, and common femoral artery canalization for cardiac catheterization or other vascular procedures). History of cancer and immobilization (choice A), cardiac history

TABLE 27-4 Types of Endoleak, Description, and Treatment

Endoleak	Description	Treatment
Type Ia (choice A)	Leak at proximal attachment	Reballooning, reversal of anticoagulation, aortic extender cuff, or balloon stent
Type Ib (choice A)	Leak at distal attachment	Reballooning, reversal of anticoagulation, iliac limb extensions
Type II (choice B)	Presence of patent inferior mesenteric artery, lumbar tributaries, or intercostal arteries	For most cases, observation greater than 6 months Rupture is rare, but if expansion occurs, can cause embolization; treatment via embolization or ligation indicated based on symptoms, ≥ 5 mm expansion, and patent inflow and outflow vessels
Type III (choice C)	Junctional leak	Deployment of additional stent graft components
Type IV (choice D)	Graft wall porosity	Self-limited

(choice C), and the recent operative procedure (choice D) would not place the patient at increased risk for RPH.[37]

Treatment of RPH is usually supportive, with blood transfusion, correction of coagulopathy, fluid resuscitation, and close monitoring. Rarely, a patient may require endovascular treatment such as selective intra-arterial embolization or stent grafting. Evacuating the hematoma may cause more harm than benefit, as this will remove the tamponade effect on the bleeding vessel. Thus, open repair is reserved for cases in which the patient is unstable and conservative/endovascular repair attempts have failed.

6. D. All of the above

Postoperative respiratory failure is a common complication and is associated with a high mortality. There are no predictable scoring systems to predict who will develop postoperative respiratory failure.[38] Prevention strategies include the use of low intraoperative tidal volume, which has been proven to decrease the incidence of lung injury and respiratory failure. Treatment strategies for those who do develop postoperative respiratory failure include the use of noninvasive mechanical ventilation.[39] This modality has been shown to decrease the rate of reintubation, hospital mortality, pneumonia, atelectasis, infection, and sepsis; it also decreases the overall risk of complications in postoperative patients.[39,40]

7. D. All of the above

Despite the usefulness of noninvasive mechanical ventilation in many clinical situations, there are several contraindications to its implementation. Impaired swallow or cough (choice A) would predispose a patient to aspiration. Noninvasive mechanical ventilation will not increase a patient's respiratory rate, and therefore, it is not useful in a patient with poor respiratory drive (choice B). Recent surgery or trauma to the face (choice C) prevents mask application, and inadvertent gastrointestinal tract insufflation secondary to increased ventilation pressures would put new esophageal and gastric anastamoses at risk for disruption.[40]

8. C. Drug fever

Postoperative fever should be evaluated with a systematic approach. A helpful pneumonic is the 4 Ws:

- Wind: pneumonia, pulmonary embolism, and aspiration; controversy regarding atelectasis[41-43]
- Water: urinary tract infection[41-43]
- Wound: surgical site infection, cellulitis[41-43]
- What did we do?: iatrogenic causes such as hospital-acquired infections, transfusions, drugs, intravenous line site infections[41-43]

In this scenario, the patient was given phenytoin, a drug known to cause fever. The diagnosis is reached by (1) ruling out other causes, and (2) establishing a temporal relationship of fever following drug administration and

defervescence following drug cessation.[7] This patient has clear lungs on imaging studies ruling out atelectasis (choice A) and has no evidence of wound infection (choice B), diarrhea (choice D), or any other infection, and his fever curve corresponds to phenytoin administration.

9. C. Fat embolism

This vignette describes a case of fat embolism syndrome (FES), which most commonly occurs following long bone and pelvic fractures. It may also occur following orthopedic procedures such as joint replacements and internal fixations that produce high bone marrow pressures. The risk increases along with the number of bones fractured, and FES has been identified in more than 30% of patients with bilateral femur fractures.[28]

The mechanism of FES is not well understood. Proposed mechanisms include (1) translocation of fat globules from adipose tissue or the bone marrow to the bloodstream, and (2) the breakdown of fat into toxic substances including free fatty acids and C-reactive protein.[29]

Furthermore, FES does not have a pathognomonic laboratory or radiological diagnostic feature and is a clinical diagnosis. Fat embolism syndrome typically presents with the triad of hypoxia, neurologic disturbances, and a petechial rash. Hypoxia usually occurs first, and a clinical picture indistinguishable from acute respiratory distress syndrome may develop. Shortly thereafter, the majority of patients become confused and then become obtunded. Finally, a petechial rash can develop in the anterior chest, arms, head, neck, axillae, and conjunctiva, but it only occurs in 20% to 50% of patients.[30] This triad typically occurs 24 to 72 hours after the inciting event. Rarely, a patient may present within 12 hours or several weeks following the insult.

Acute respiratory distress syndrome (choice A) and pulmonary embolism (choice B) would not usually present with a rash or confusion, and toxic shock syndrome (choice D) would more typically present with high fever, hypotension, and a diffuse sunburn-like rash that can also involve the palms and soles.

10. B. Supportive measures, including oxygen supplementation and airway protection

Treatment for FES is supportive. Antibiotics (choice A) and anticoagulation (choice D) do not have a role in FES treatment. Steroids (choice C) may be of benefit in preventing FES in high-risk patients, but they are not part of the typical treatment of FES once it has occurred.[28] Despite the lack of tailored treatments for FES, it is usually self-limited, and the majority of patients recover.

11. A. No further treatment

Carotid endarterectomy reduces the risk of cerebrovascular accident (CVA). However, complications of this procedure include cerebrovascular accident, myocardial infarction, hemotoma, nerve injury, restenosis, infection such as parotitis and infected patch, and hyperperfusion syndrome.[24-26]

Risk factors for hematoma include uncontrolled hypertension and anticoagulation. One of the initial concerns for cervical hematoma is airway compromise. In this patient, the hematoma is receding and redistributing, with the ecchymosis surpassing the demarcation. The patient appears comfortable and therefore does not require mechanical ventilation (choice B). Since the patient has stabilized, there is no need for surgical exploration, which would be the treatment of choice for an expanding hematoma (choice C). Protamine is used to reverse heparin but is not needed in this patient with a stable/receding hematoma (choice D).

12. A. Blood presure control

Patients with high-grade stenosis develop chronic cerebral hypoperfusion, dilation of small blood vessels, and impairment of cerebral autoregulation.[25] With correction of stenosis via endarterectomy, these small blood vessels fail to vasoconstrict, which can lead to hyperperfusion syndrome. Hyperperfusion syndrome can result in seizures, cerebral edema, and hemorrhage. The risk of hemorrhage, which is the most dreaded complication of hyperperfusion syndrome, persists for up to 2 weeks after surgery. One characteristic finding of hyperperfusion syndrome is a headache that improves with an upright position.[25] Blood pressure control is key in amioliorating this complication.

Heparin (choice B), aspirin (choice C), and simvastatin (choice D) do not prevent this complication.

13. D. Furosemide 40 mg IV

The patient has abdominal compartment syndrome in the setting of massive fluid resuscitation. Abdominal compartment syndrome (ACS) is defined as sustained IAP greater than 20 mmHg (with or without abdominal perfusion pressure [APP] < 60 mmHg) and new organ dysfunction or damage.[3,4] Abdominal perfusion pressure (APP) is calculated as Mean Arterial Pressure – Intra-abdominal Pressure. The bladder pressure, measured via instillation of 25 mL of sterile saline, is the usual indirect measure of intra-abdominal pressure. A normal IAP is 5 to 7 mmHg; intra-abdominal hypertension is defined as an IAP of 12 mmHg or greater.[3,4]

Risk factors for ACS include the following:

1. Diminished abdominal wall compliance secondary to abdominal surgery, major trauma, burns, and prone positioning
2. Increased intraluminal contents from gastroparesis, ileus, pseudo-obstruction, and volvulus
3. Increased intra-abdominal contents from acute pancreatitis, hemoperitoneum, infection; tumors; excessive insufflation pressures with laparoscopy, ascites, and peritoneal dialysis; and capillary leak from acidosis, hypothermia, massive fluid resuscitation, or polytransfusion.[3,4]

TABLE 27-5 Interventions for Secondary Abdominal Compartment Syndrome

Purpose of Intervention	Intervention
Improve abdominal wall compliance	Sedation, neuromuscular blockade avoid head of bed > 30°
Evacuation of intraluminal contents	Nasogastric and rectal tube decompression, prokinetics
Evacuation of abdominal contents	Paracentesis, percutaneous drainage
Improvement of positive fluid balance	Diuretics
Organ support	Alveolar recruitment

Abdominal compartment syndrome may be divided into primary and secondary cases. Primary ACS is due to a condition that requires early surgical or radiologic intervention, whereas secondary ACS may be addressed, at least initially, with the medical interventions listed in Table 27-5.[3-5]

Due to the volume overload from fluid resuscitation, diuretics would seem appropriate to improve abdominal compartment syndrome. Laparotomy (choice B) is premature at this point. Neuromuscular blockade (choice C) might aide in improving the pressures but will not remove the fluid volume overload. Inserting a Salem Sump might be counterproductive because it can dislodge the clips placed on the Diulefoy lesion (choice A).

14. A. Exploratory laparotomy

This patient has primary ACS due to a bowel obstruction. Surgical intervention is paramount. Medical conservation treatment such as rectal decompression (choice B) might temporarily decrease the abdominal pressures, but ultimately she would need an exploratory laparotomy. Antibiotics (choice C) and fluid resuscitation (choice D) without additional interventions to decrease abdominal pressure are inappropriate treatments for ACS.

15. A. Wide excision and debridement

The patient has a necrotizing soft tissue infection (NSTI) extending into the dermis, subcutaneous tissue, fascia, adipose tissue, and muscle. Immediate diagnosis is paramount, because even with treatment, mortality is 25% to 30%.[44,45] Clinical markers that suggest NSTI include swelling, erythema, pain out of porportion to appearance, discoloration, blisters, necrosis, crepitus, and/or subcutaneous gas. Wall et al have suggested that leukocytosis of greater than 15.3×10^3 cells/μL and serum sodium greater than 135 mEq/L increase the likelihood of NSTI.[46-48]

The 3 types of NSTI are described in Table 27-6. Radiographic images demonstrating subcutaneous air or increased thickness of the fascial layer with or without

TABLE 27-6 Types of Necrotizing Soft Tissue Infection

	Pathogen	Characteristics
Type I	• Polymicrobial • *Clostridium perfringens* • *Clostridium septicum* • *Clostridium sordellii*	• Onset: hours • Purulent drainage • From *Clostridium* species, toxins A and 0
Type II	• β-Hemolytic streptococci (group A streptococci)	• Young and healthy patients • > 2 d before symptomatic • M proteins to manifest superantigen activity
Type III	• Gram-negative, such as *Vibrio vulnificus*	

enhancement suggest NSTI, but surgical intervention is often necessary to establish definitive diagnosis. Surgical incisions showing clear separation of fascial layers confirm necrotizing fasciitis but not necrotizing adipositis or necrotizing myositis.[45]

In the current case, the patient's necrotizing infection was confirmed surgically; thus, obtaining a CT scan (choice C) or MRI (choice D) before proceeding to the operating room for definitive management would be inappropriate. Treatment of NSTI involves wide excision and debridement of the infected tissues (choice A) as early as possible. Antibiotics and fluid resuscitation (choice B) are required adjuncts but are not the curative treatment. Data for hyperbaric oxygen and IV immunoglobulin are variable.[44,45]

16. B. Fasciotomy

Acute compartment syndrome of the limb most often occurs in the setting of long bone fractures of the lower extremities but can also involve the upper extremities in the setting of trauma or burns. Elevated compartment pressures result in decreased venous outflow, a decreased arteriovenous pressure gradient, and collapse of arterioles. There are also nontraumatic causes of acute compartment syndrome of the limb, including postischemic compartment syndrome after revascularization procedures. In this syndrome, the reperfusion of previously ischemic compartments leads to edema and increased pressures. Measurement of the compartment pressure via manometer may be indicated to confirm the diagnosis and determine which patients will benefit from fasciotomy (choice B). Indications for immediate surgical intervention via fasciotomy include: less than or equal to 30 mmHg difference between diastolic pressure and measured compartment pressure with clinical correlation or measured compartment pressure more than or equal to 30 mmHg clinical correlation. Amputation is indicated when the muscle is believed to be dead since fasciotomy would not be beneficial.

A CT scan (choice C) is relatively contraindicated due to the patient's history of diabetic nephropathy and the potential for acute kidney injury in the setting of compartment-syndrome induced rhabdomyolysis. Antibiotics (choice D) and crystalloid boluses (choice A) should not delay fasciotomy.

17. B. Enterocutaneous fistula

The CT scan shows an enterocutaneous fistula (ECF; choice B). There is no sign of abscess (choice A), wound dehiscence with free intraperitoneal air (choice C), or seroma (choice D). Enterocutaneous fistulae are abnormal connections between the gastrointestinal tract and the skin.[49] They carry high morbidity, and mortality ranges from 5% to 20%. Spontaneous closure is rare, especially for high-output ECF (> 500 mL/24 h), and persistent ECF usually requires operative intervention. Other factors that influence spontaneous closure include etiology, size, distal flow, and tract epithelization.[49]

Conservative treatments include bowel rest, with total parenteral nutrition to decrease secretions, octreotide to decrease output, fibrin glue, and negative pressure wound therapy (also known as a "wound vac").[49]

REFERENCES

1. Hallman M, Treggiari M, Deem S. Chapter 55: Critical care medicine. In: Barash P, Cullen B, Stoelting R, eds. *Clinical Anesthesia.* 7th ed. Philadelphia, PA: Lippincott-Williams & Wilkins; 2013: 918-941.
2. Taylor S, Kirton OC, Staff I, Kozol RA. Postoperative day one: a high risk period for respiratory events. *Am J Surg.* 2005;190(5):752-756.
3. Kirkpatrick AW, Roberts RJ, DeWaele J, et al. Intra-abdominal hypertension and the abdominal compartment syndrome: updated consensus definitions and clinical practice guidelines from the World Society of the Abdominal Compartment Syndrome. *Intensive Care Med.* 2013;39(7):1190-1206.
4. Hunt L, Frost SA, Hillman K, et al. Management of intraabdominal hypertension and abdominal compartment syndrome: a review. *J Trauma Manag Outcomes.* 2014;8(1):2.
5. Walker K, Criddle LM. Pathophysiology and management of abdominal compartment syndrome. *Am J Crit Care.* 2003;12(4):367-371.
6. To KB, Napolitano LM. Common complications in the critically ill patient. *Surg Clin North Am.* 2012;92(6):1519-1557.
7. Thompson JS, Baxter BT, Allison JG, Johnson FE, Lee KK, Park WY. Temporal patterns of postoperative complications. *Arch Surg.* 2003;138(6):596-602; discussion 602-603.
8. Kirchhoff P, Clavien PA, Hahnloser D. Complications in colorectal surgery: risk factors and preventive strategies. *Patient Saf Surg.* 2010;4(1):5.
9. Behm B, Stollman N. Postoperative gastrointestinal complications. In: Lubin MF, Smith III RB, Dodson TF, Spell NO, Walker HK, eds. *Medical Management of the Surgical Patient: A Textbook of Perioperative Medicine.* 4th ed. Cambridge: Cambridge University Press; 2006: 199-206.

10. Hyman N, Manchester TL, Osler T, Burns B, Cataldo PA. Anastomotic leaks after intestinal anastomosis: it's later than you think. *Ann Surg.* 2007;245(2):254-258.

11. Agostini P, Cieslik H, Rathinam S, et al. Postoperative pulmonary complications following thoracic surgery: are there any modifiable risk factors? *Thorax.* 2010;65(9):815-818.

12. Brooks-Brunn JA. Predictors of postoperative pulmonary complications following abdominal surgery. *Chest.* 1997;111(3):564-571.

13. Canet J, Gallart L. Predicting postoperative pulmonary complications in the general population. *Curr Opin Anaesthesiol.* 2013;26(2):107-115.

14. Blum JM, Stentz MJ, Dechert R. Preoperative and intraoperative predictors of postoperative acute respiratory distress syndrome in a general surgical population. *Anesthesiology.* 2013;118(1):19-29.

15. Arieff AI. Fatal postoperative pulmonary edema: pathogenesis and literature review. *Chest.* 1999;115(5):1371-1377.

16. American Thoracic Society; Infectious Diseases Society of America. Guidelines for the management of adults with hospital-acquired, ventilator-associated, and healthcare-associated pneumonia. *Am J Respir Crit Care Med.* 2005;171(4):388-416.

17. Sun Z, Sessler DI, Dalton JE, et al. Postoperative hypoxemia is common and persistent: a prospective blinded observational study. *Anesth Analg.* 2015;121(3):709-715.

18. Fisher BW, Majumdar SR, McAlister FA. Predicting pulmonary complications after nonthoracic surgery: a systematic review of blinded studies. *Am J Med.* 2002;112(3):219-225.

19. Stephens RS, Whitman GJ. Postoperative critical care of the adult cardiac surgical patient. Part I: routine postoperative care. *Crit Care Med.* 2015;43(7):1477-1497.

20. Farouque HM, Tremmel JA, Raissi Shabari F, et al. Risk factors for the development of retroperitoneal hematoma after percutaneous coronary intervention in the era of glycoprotein IIb/IIIa inhibitors and vascular closure devices. *J Am Coll Cardiol.* 2005;45(3):363-368.

21. Trimarchi S, Smith DE, Share D, et al; BMC2 Registry. Retroperitoneal hematoma after percutaneous coronary intervention: prevalence, risk factors, management, outcomes, and predictors of mortality: a report from the BMC2 (Blue Cross Blue Shield of Michigan Cardiovascular Consortium) registry. *JACC Cardiovasc Interv.* 2010;3(8):845-850.

22. Grimm JC, Whitman G Jr. Postoperative care of the cardiac surgical patient. In: O'Donnell JM, Nacul FE, eds. *Surgical Intensive Care Medicine.* 3rd ed. Cham, Switzerland: Springer; 2016: 653-668.

23. Hernandez AF, Whellan DJ, Stroud S, Sun JL, O'Connor CM, Jollis JG. Outcomes in heart failure patients after major noncardiac surgery. *J Am Coll Cardiol.* 2004;44(7):1446-1453.

24. Biller J, Feinberg WM, Castaldo JE, et al. AHA Scientific Statement: Guidelines for Carotid Endarterectomy. *Circulation.* 1998;97:501-509.

25. Comerota AJ, DiFiore R, Tzilinis A, Chahwan S. Cervical hematoma following carotid endarterectomy is morbid and preventable: a 12-year case-controlled review. *Vasc Endovascular Surg.* 2012;46(8)610-616.

26. Ricotta JJ, Aburahma A, Ascher E, Eskandari M, Faries P; Society for Vascular Surgery. Updated society for vascular surgery guidelines for management of extracranial carotid disease. *J Vasc Surg.* 2011;54(3):e1-e31.

27. Bederman SS, Bhandari M, McKee MD, Schemitsch EH. Do corticosteroids reduce the risk of fat embolism syndrome in patients with long-bone fractures? A meta-analysis. *Can J Surg.* 2009;52(5):386-393.

28. Eriksson EA, Pellegrini DC, Vanderkolk WE, Minshal CT, Fakhry SM, Cohle SD. Incidence of pulmonary fat embolism at autopsy: an undiagnosed epidemic. *J Trauma.* 2011;71(2):312-315.

29. Julman G. Pathogenesis of non-traumatic fat embolism. *Lancet.* 1988;1(8599):1366-1367.

30. Kaplan RP, Grant JN, Kaufman AJ. Dermatologic features of the fat embolism syndrome. *Cutis.* 1986;38(1):52-55.

31. Kind MB, Harmon KR. Unusual forms of pulmonary embolism. *Clin Chest Med.* 1994;15(3):561-580.

32. Elliott KG, Johnstone AJ. Diagnosis of acute compartment syndrome. *J Bone Joint Surg Br.* 2003;85(5):625-632.

33. Peters CL, Scott SM. Compartment syndrome in the forearm following fractures of the radial head or neck in children. *J Bone Joint Surg Am.* 1995;77(8):1070-1074.

34. Patel KP, Hale K, Pastores SM. Critical care issues in oncologic surgery patients. In: O'Donnell JM, Nacul FE, eds. *Surgical Intensive Care Medicine.* 3rd ed. Cham, Switzerland: Springer; 2016: 759-770.

35. Kim H. Abdominal hemorrhage: a review of aortoenteric fistula. http://rwjms.rutgers.edu/radiology/education/documents/AortoentericfistulabyHansolKim.pdf. Accessed February 1, 2017.

36. Chaikof EL et al. The Society of Vascular Surgery Practice Guidelines on the Care of Patients with an Abdominal Aortic Aneurysm. *J Vasc Surg.* 2018;67(1):2-77.

37. Chan YC, Morales JP, Reidy JF, Taylor PR. Management of spontaneous and iatrogenic retroperitoneal haemorrhage: conservative management, endovascular intervention or open surgery? *Int J Clin Pract.* 2008;62(10):1604-1613.

38. Smith PR, Baig MA, Brito V, Bader F, Bergman MI, Alfonso A. Postoperative pulmonary complications after laparotomy. *Respiration.* 2010;80(4):269-274.

39. Montravers P, Veber B, Auboyer C, et al. Diagnostic and therapeutic management of nosocomial pneumonia in surgical patients: results of the Eole study. *Crit Care Med.* 2002;30(2):368-375.

40. Mace SE. Bilevel positive airway pressure ventilation. *J Clin Outcomes Med.* 1999;6(9):41-48.

41. O'Grady NP, Barie PS, Bartlett JG. Guidelines for evaluation of new fever in the critically ill adult patient: 2008 update from the American College of Critical Care Medicine and the Infectious Disease Society of America. *Crit Care Med.* 2008;36(4):1330-1349.

42. Moore LJ, McKinley BA, Turner KL, et al. The epidemiology of sepsis in general surgery patients. *J Trauma.* 2011;70(3):672-680.

43. Badillo AT, Sarani B, Evans SR. Optimizing the use of blood cultures in the febrile postoperative patient. *J Am Coll Surg.* 2002;194(4):477-487.

44. Hakkarainen TW, Kopari NM, Pham TN, Evans HL. Necrotizing soft tissue infections: review and current concepts in treatment, systems of care and outcomes. *Curr Probl Surg.* 2013;51(8):344-362.

45. Delinger EP, Anaya DA. Necrotizing soft-tissue infection: diagnosis and management. *Clin Infect Dis.* 2007;44(5):705-710.

46. Beilman GC, Dunn DL. Surgical infections. In: Brunicardi F, Andersen DK, Billiar TR, Dunn DL, Hunter JG, Matthews JB, Pollock RE, eds. *Schwartz's Principles of Surgery. 10th ed.* New York, NY: Mc-Graw-Hill; 2015. http://accessmedicine.mhmedical.com/content.aspx?bookid=980&sectionid=59610847. Accessed May 25, 2018.

47. Wall D, Klein S, Black S, de Virgilio C. A simple model to help distinguish necrotizing from non-necrotizing soft-tissue infections. *J Am Coll Surg.* 2000;191(3):227-231.

48. Wall D, de Virgilio C, Black S, Klein S. Objective criteria may assist in distinguishing necrotizing fasciitis from nonnecrotizing soft tissue infections. *Am J Surg.* 2000;179(1):17-21.

49. Taggarshe D, Bakston D, Jacobs M, McKendrick A, Mittal VK. Management of enterocutaneous fistulae: a 10 years experience. *World J Gastrointest Surg.* 2010;2(7):242-246.

Transplantation

Sakshi Dua, MD

INTRODUCTION

Organ transplantation is an established treatment for patients with a wide variety of end-stage diseases. It is essential for physicians to familiarize themselves with the field of transplant medicine since an encounter with a transplant candidate or recipient is inevitable.[1]

PHYSIOLOGY OF THE IMMUNE SYSTEM

The immune system distinguishes self from nonself to eliminate potentially harmful molecules and cells. The immune system also has the capacity to recognize and destroy abnormal cells that derive from host tissues. Any molecule capable of being recognized by the immune system is considered an antigen (Ag). The skin, cornea, and mucosa of the respiratory, gastrointestinal (GI), and genitourinary (GU) tracts form a physical barrier that is the body's first line of defense.[2]

Breaching of anatomic barriers can trigger 2 types of immune response: innate and acquired. Many molecular components (eg, complement factors, cytokines, acute phase proteins) participate in both innate and acquired immunity.[2]

Innate immunity

Innate (natural) immunity does not require prior exposure to an Ag (ie, immunologic memory) to be effective. Thus, it can respond immediately to an invader. It recognizes mainly Ag molecules that are broadly distributed rather than specific to 1 organism or cell. Components include phagocytic cells, natural killer (NK) cells, and polymorphonuclear leukocytes. Phagocytic cells (neutrophils in blood and tissues, monocytes in blood, macrophages in tissues) ingest and destroy invading Ags. Attack by phagocytic cells can be facilitated when an Ag is coated with an antibody (Ab), which is produced as part of acquired immunity, or when complement proteins opsonize Ags.

Natural killer cells kill virus-infected cells and some tumor cells. Polymorphonuclear leukocytes (neutrophils, eosinophils, basophils, mast cells) and mononuclear cells (monocytes, macrophages) release multiple inflammatory mediators.[2]

Acquired immunity

Acquired (adaptive) immunity requires prior exposure to an Ag and thus takes time to develop after the initial encounter with a new invader. This system remembers past exposures and is Ag specific. Components include cell-mediated immunity from T-cell responses and humoral immunity from B-cell responses (B cells secrete Ag-specific Ab).[2]

B cells and T cells work together to destroy foreign Ag. Ag-presenting cells (such as dendritic cells) are needed to present Ags to T cells.[2] The immune system is activated when circulating Abs or cell surface receptors recognize a foreign Ag. These receptors may be highly specific (Ab expressed on B cells or T-cell receptors) or broadly specific (such as pattern-recognition receptors called toll-like receptors). Immune activation occurs when Ab-Ag complexes or complement-coated molecules bind to surface receptors for the crystallizable fragment (Fc) region of immunoglobulin G (FcγR) and for C3b and iC3b.[2]

Once recognized, an Ag, Ag-Ab complex, or complement-molecule complex is phagocytosed. T cell–derived cytokines, particularly interferon-γ (IFN-γ), stimulate the phagocyte to produce more lytic enzymes and other bactericidal products and thus enhance its ability to kill or sequester the foreign Ag.[2] Unless Ag is rapidly phagocytosed and entirely degraded (an uncommon event), the acquired immune response is recruited. This response begins in the spleen for circulating Ag, regional lymph nodes for tissue Ag, and mucosa-associated lymphoid tissues (eg, tonsils, adenoids, Peyer patches) for mucosal Ag.[2]

The immune response in transplantation is a form of adaptive immunity. The principal targets are the major histocompatibility complex (MHC) molecules expressed on the surface of donor cells (allo-MHC). T-cell recognition of antigen is the primary event that initiates the immune response. This key step requires the interaction of the T-cell receptor (TCR) with antigen presented as a peptide by the antigen-presenting cell (APC) and a costimulatory receptor/ligand interaction on the T-cell/APC cell surface. Activated T cells are directly cytotoxic and provide help for B-cell antibody production and macrophage-induced delayed-type hypersensitivity (DTH) responses. Proteins encoded by the MHC are the principal antigenic determinants of graft rejection. Organs transplanted between MHC-identical individuals are readily accepted, whereas organs transplanted between MHC antigen-mismatched individuals are inevitably rejected in the absence of immunosuppressive agents.[2]

The antigen-presenting protein products of the MHC have been classified into class I and II groups that are characterized by structure, expression, and the cellular compartment from which they obtain antigenic peptides to present to T cells. Class I MHC molecules include human leukocyte antigen (HLA)-A, HLA-B, and HLA-C molecules and are found on all cell types except red blood cells. Class I molecules present cytoplasm-derived peptide antigens to CD8-positive T cells, which induce cell lysis.[2]

Class II MHC molecules include HLA-DP, HLA-DQ, and HLA-DR molecules. Class II MHC molecules are constitutively expressed on interstitial dendritic cells, macrophages, and B cells, but expression may be upregulated on epithelial cell and vascular endothelial cell after exposure to proinflammatory cytokines. Class II molecules present peptides derived from extracellular proteins to CD4-positive T cells.[2]

The activation of costimulatory pathways is required for T-cell entry into the cell cycle. Multiple costimulatory molecules have been identified including CD28 and CD40. Chemokine-regulated attraction of leukocytes to sites of tissue injury, infection, or allo-transplantation is essential for the induction of the acute inflammatory response.[2]

T helper cells are divided into 2 distinct populations, type 1 (Th1) and type 2 (Th2) cells. Type 1 T helper cells produce interleukin-2 (IL-2) and interferon-γ and induce macrophage activation, leading to DTH responses. Acute allograft rejection is predominantly mediated by a Th1 immune response. T-cell activation results in intracellular signaling that activates cytokine DNA promoter regions permitting transcription of mRNA.[2]

All allograft recipients are at risk of graft rejection; the recipient's immune system recognizes the graft as foreign and seeks to destroy it. Recipients of grafts containing immune cells (particularly bone marrow, intestine, and liver) are at risk of graft-versus-host disease. Pretransplantation screening and immunosuppressive therapy minimize risk of these complications during and after transplantation.[2]

UNITED NETWORK FOR ORGAN SHARING AND ORGAN ALLOCATION

Transplantation uses allografts from living related, living unrelated, or deceased donors. Deceased donor organs can be recovered from heart-beating or so-called "brain dead" donors and from non–heart-beating or so-called "cardiac death" donors.[1]

The United Network for Organ Sharing (UNOS) is a national, private, nonprofit organization that develops policies and guidelines, maintains data on wait lists, runs organ matches, and records all transplants. In the United States and Puerto Rico, 58 organ procurement organizations (OPOs) coordinate organ procurement in designated service areas.[1]

Allocation of organs depends on disease severity for some organs (liver, heart) and on disease severity plus the time spent on waiting list for others (lung, kidney, and bowel).

Pretransplantation Screening

Due to the scarcity of donor organs, potential organ transplant recipients are thoroughly screened for medical and nonmedical factors to improve the likelihood of success given the risk and expense of transplantation.[2]

Tissue Compatibility

Both donors and recipients are universally tested for ABO antigens to ensure blood type compatibility and to prevent hyperacute rejection. Recipients are also tested for presensitization to donor antigens by checking panel reactive antibodies (PRA) against human leukocyte antigen. Human leukocyte antigen tissue typing is most important for hematopoietic stem cell and kidney transplantation. However, due to time constraints, HLA tissue typing is not typically performed prior to heart, lung, liver, and pancreas transplantation.[2]

Infection

To diminish the risk of donor-transmitted infections and reactivation of latent infections in recipients, several tests are performed pretransplant. These include serologic tests for cytomegalovirus (CMV), Epstein-Barr virus (EBV), herpes simplex virus (HSV), varicella-zoster virus (VZV), hepatitis B and C virus, and human immunodeficiency virus (HIV), and a tuberculin skin test (TST).[2]

Financial and Psychosocial

Given the expense and emotional burden of going through organ transplantation, candidates undergo consultations with financial coordinators and social workers for psychosocial screening.[2]

Indications and Contraindications

Indications and Contraindications are listed in Table 28-1.

In addition to organ-specific contraindications, there are general contraindications such as ABO incompatibility, active uncontrolled infection or sepsis, cancer (except for certain neuroendocrine, skin, and brain tumors or hepatocellular cancer confined to the liver), and the presence of advanced acquired immunodeficiency syndrome (AIDS) if human immunodeficiency virus positive. Relative contraindications include psychosocial morbidities such as substance addiction, known nonadherence with follow-up visits and medications, and active psychiatric problems. Extremes of body weight, poor functional status, and HIV status are considered contraindications on an individual basis.[2]

TABLE 28-1 Types of Transplantation, Indications, and Contraindications

Type of Transplantation[2]	Indications	Contraindications
Lung transplant	ILD, CF, COPD, PAH	Mechanical ventilation for > 7 d, lung cancer
Cardiac transplant	CHF, CAD, cardiomyopathy, congenital heart disease	Pulmonary hypertension unresponsive to preoperative medical treatment
Liver transplant	Cirrhosis, fulminant hepatic necrosis, hepatocellular cancer (HCC), primary sclerosing cholangitis	Uncontrolled extrahepatic malignancy, advanced cardiopulmonary disease, sepsis, active alcohol abuse, malnutrition, multisystem organ failure, compensated cirrhosis
Hematopoietic stem cell transplant	Leukemia, lymphoma, myeloma, aplastic anemia, myelodysplasia	Sepsis
Renal transplant	End-stage renal disease	Severe heart disease, cancer
Small bowel transplant	Autoimmune enteritis, congenital enteropathy, Hirschsprung disease, short bowel syndrome, secondary cholestatic liver disease	Sepsis

CAD = coronary artery disease; CF = cystic fibrosis; CHF = congestive heart failure; COPD = chronic obstructive pulmonary disease; HCC = hepatocellular cancer; ILD = interstitial lung disease; PAH = pulmonary arterial hypertension.

INDUCTION IMMUNOSUPPRESSION

Immunosuppressants control graft rejection and are primarily responsible for the success of transplantation. Induction immunosuppression is practiced in many solid organ transplants. The rationale is that the risk of acute cellular rejection (ACR) is highest immediately after transplantation (donor leukocyte load), and the quickest way to maximize the level of immunosuppression at a time when risk of ACR is the greatest is with induction immunosuppression. This also allows a delay in initiating maintenance immunosuppression (which is often nephrotoxic).[2]

Corticosteroids

A high dose is usually given at the time of transplantation, and then is reduced gradually to a maintenance dose, which is given indefinitely.

Immunoglobulins

Antilymphocyte globulin (ALG) and antithymocyte globulin (ATG) are fractions of animal antisera directed against human cells: lymphocytes (ALG) and thymus cells (ATG). Both ALG and ATG suppress cellular immunity while preserving humoral immunity. They are used with other immunosuppressants to allow those drugs to be used in lower, less toxic doses.[2]

Monoclonal Antibodies

Monoclonal antibodies (mAbs) directed against T cells provide a higher concentration of anti-T-cell antibodies and fewer irrelevant serum proteins than do ALG and ATG.

- OKT3 (a mouse antibody) inhibits T-cell receptor (TCR)–antigen binding, resulting in immunosuppression. OKT3 was used primarily to control episodes of acute rejection; it was also used at the time of transplantation to reduce incidence or delay onset of rejection episodes. However, the drug is no longer available.
- Anti–IL-2 receptor monoclonal antibodies inhibit T-cell proliferation by blocking the effect of IL-2, secreted by activated T cells. Basiliximab is a humanized anti–IL-2 receptor antibody.
- Alemtuzumab (Campath-1H) is a humanized rat monoclonal antibody that targets the CD52 antigen expressed on both T and B cells.[2]

MAINTENANCE IMMUNOSUPPRESSIVE AGENTS

Maintenance immunosuppressive drugs can be divided into the following categories: calcineurin inhibitors (CNI) such as tacrolimus (TAC) and cyclosporine A (CsA), anti-metabolites such as mycophenolate mofetil (MMF) and azathioprine (AZA), and mammalian target of rapamycin (mTOR) inhibitors such as sirolimus (SRL) and corticosteroids.

Calcineurin Inhibitors

Calcineurin dephosphorylates cytoplasmic nuclear factor of activated T cells (NFAT), permitting its translocation to the nucleus where it binds to the IL-2 promoter sequence and then stimulates transcription of IL-2 mRNA. Interleukin-2 produced by type 1 helper T cells is the predominant mediator of acute allograft rejection.[2] Calcineurin is the ultimate target of CsA and TAC (or FK506) and its inhibition by these medications leads to immune tolerance. Cyclosporine A binds to an intracellular protein, cyclophilin, and this complex ultimately binds to and inhibits the phosphatase activity of calcineurin. Tacrolimus binds to the FK506 binding protein (FKBP), which inhibits calcineurin in a similar manner.[3]

Drug Interactions

Calcineurin inhibitors are metabolized in the liver by the cytochrome p450 family. Some common drugs that cause an increase in TAC or CsA levels include cytochrome p450 inhibitors such as the following[3]:

- Diclofenac, doxycycline, imatinib, isoniazid, propofol, protease inhibitors, quinidine, telithromycin
- Calcium channel blockers such as diltiazem, verapamil, and nicardipine
- Macrolides such as clarithromycin and erythromycin
- Azole antifungals, especially voriconazole, for which a TAC dose must be decreased by 66%
- Metoclopramide

Some common drugs that cause a decrease in TAC or CsA levels include cytochrome p450 inducers such as the following[3]:

- Nafcillin, nevirapine
- Anticonvulsants: carbamazepine, phenobarbital, phenytoin, primidone
- Rifamycins: rifabutin, rifampin
- St John's wort

Other interactions worth mentioning are the following[3]:

- Synergistic nephrotoxic effects with ganciclovir
- Increased risk of hemolytic uremic syndrome (HUS) or thrombotic thrombocytopenic purpura (TTP) with SRL
- Hyperkalemia when used in conjunction with K+-sparing diuretics or angiotensin converting enzyme inhibitors (ACEI)
- Synergistic nephrotoxicity in conjunction with gentamicin, tobramycin, vancomycin, sulfamethoxazole/trimethoprim, and nonsteroidal anti-inflammatory drugs (NSAIDs)
- Synergistic neurotoxicity can be seen with CsA and imipenem (seizures)
- Histamine-2 blockers and allopurinol both increase CsA levels/toxicity

Side Effects

Side effects of calcineurin inhibitors include the following:

- Nephrotoxicity, which may range from mild renal dysfunction to end-stage renal disease requiring hemodialysis (often dose dependent but may be idiosyncratic; renal dysfunction may be reversible if the drug is stopped early; both acute and chronic renal insufficiency can be seen)
- Hypertension (HTN)
- Dyslipidemia
- Electrolyte disturbances such as hypokalemia and hypomagnesemia
- HUS
- Neurologic complications including seizures, tremors, and headaches
- Post-transplant diabetes (specific to TAC)
- Hirsutism and gingival hyperplasia (specific to CsA)[3]

Antimetabolites

The antimetabolites, or antiproliferative agents, interfere with the synthesis of nucleic acids and exert their immunosuppressive effects by inhibiting the proliferation of both T and B lymphocytes.[2]

Mycophenolate Mofetil

Mycophenolate mofetil is a reversible inhibitor of inosine monophosphate dehydrogenase, a critical enzyme for the de novo synthesis of guanine nucleotides. Lymphocytes lack a key enzyme in the guanine salvage pathway and are dependent upon the de novo pathway for the production of purines necessary for RNA and DNA synthesis. Therefore, both T- and B-lymphocyte proliferation is selectively inhibited.[3]

Drug Interactions

Drug interactions with MMF include the following:

- Valganciclovir: both drugs increase each other's effects, hence concurrent use can worsen myelosuppression
- Metronidazole: not recommended with MMF
- Fluoroquinolones: norfloxacin not recommended with MMF
- Rifamycins: not recommended with MMF
- Magnesium salts: separate doses by 2 hours
- CsA: interferes with its enterohepatic circulation; the usual dose of MMF when used in conjunction with CsA should be 1500 mg twice daily (BID)[3]

Side Effects

Side effects of MMF use include the following:

- Gastrointestinal distress is the most notable side effect, with manifestations such as nausea, vomiting, and diarrhea
- Leucopenia, anemia, and general bone marrow suppression[3]

Azathioprine

Azathioprine is a prodrug that first is hydrolyzed rapidly in the blood to its active form, 6-mercaptopurine, and subsequently converted to a purine analogue, thioinosine monophosphate. This antimetabolite is incorporated into DNA and inhibits further nucleotide synthesis, thereby preventing mitosis and proliferation of rapidly dividing cells, such as activated T and B lymphocytes.[3]

Drug Interactions

Drug interactions with AZA include the following:

- Allopurinol: potentially fatal toxicity from pancytopenia; if coadministration cannot be avoided, then AZA should be administered at 20% to 30% of normal dose
- Sulfamethoxazole/trimethoprim: concurrent use may lead to exaggerated leucopenia
- ACEI: concurrent use can induce anemia and severe leucopenia
- Warfarin: AZA may interfere with anticoagulant effect[3]

Side Effects

Side effects of AZA use include the following:

- Dose-dependent myelosuppression resulting in thrombocytopenia, leucopenia, and macrocytic anemia
- Hepatotoxicity, hepatic veno-occlusive disease
- Nausea, vomiting, diarrhea, pancreatitis
- Skin rashes, alopecia
- Interstitial pneumonitis[3]

Mammalian Target of Rapamycin Inhibitors

Sirolimus is structurally similar to TAC and also binds to the FK binding protein. However, it exerts its immunosuppressive effects via a calcineurin-independent mechanism. The drug-immunophilin complex inhibits a protein kinase in the cytoplasm called mammalian target of rapamycin. This protein kinase, mTOR, is involved in the transduction signals from the IL-2 receptor to the nucleus, causing cell cycle arrest at the G1 to S phase. The consequence of mTOR inhibition is inhibition of both T- and B-cell proliferation in response to cytokine signals.[3]

Drug Interactions

Mammalian target of rapamycin inhibitors are also metabolized by the cytochrome p450 family of enzymes and are subject to the same drug interactions as CNI. Their use with voriconazole is not approved since it causes 11-fold increase in area under the curve (AUC) of SRL.[3] AUC reflects total drug exposure over time and is used to compare two drug formulations and drug monitoring with narrow therapeutic index.

Side Effects

Side effects of mTOR inhibitor use include the following:

- SRL does not independently cause renal insufficiency but can potentiate CNI-induced nephrotoxicity by both increasing levels and potentiating mechanisms of nephropathy
- Dyslipidemia
- Hypertension
- Myelosuppression (especially thrombocytopenia)
- Thrombotic microangiopathy
- Lymphoceles and pleural/pericardial effusions
- Pulmonary toxicity ranging from interstitial pneumonitis to organizing pneumonia, lymphocytic alveolitis, alveolar hemorrhage, and pulmonary vasculitis
- Poor wound healing and anastomotic site complications, including fatal airway dehiscence in the perioperative period due to antifibroproliferative effect[3]

POST-TRANSPLANT COMPLICATIONS

Hyperacute Rejection

Hyperacute rejection occurs within 48 hours of transplantation and is caused by preexisting complement fixing antibodies to graft antigens (presensitization). It is rare due to pretransplant screening. It is characterized by small vessel thrombosis and graft infarction. No treatment is effective other than graft removal.[2]

Accelerated rejection occurs 3 to 5 days after transplantation and is caused by pre-existing non–complement fixing antibodies to graft antigens. It is also rare and is characterized by cellular infiltrate with or without vascular changes. Treatment is with high-dose steroids or antilymphocyte preparations. Plasmapheresis can clear circulating antibodies rapidly.[2]

Acute Rejection

Acute rejection is caused by a T-cell-mediated delayed hypersensitivity reaction to allograft histocompatibility antigens. It is characterized by a mononuclear infiltrate with varying degrees of edema, hemorrhage, and necrosis. Vascular endothelium is the primary target. Treatment includes high-dose steroids, antilymphocyte preparations, or both. After the resolution of acute rejection, the severely damaged parts of the graft heal by fibrosis, whereas the rest of the graft functions normally. Mortality is low and the graft can survive for long periods thereafter.[2]

Chronic Rejection

Chronic rejection leads to graft dysfunction occurring months to years after transplant. Causes are varied and include early acute rejection episodes, periprocedural ischemia, graft reperfusion injury, and infections such as CMV. The histopathology is organ specific, so it is an airway-based lesion in lung transplant recipients (obliterative bronchiolitis [OB]) and a vessel-based lesion in others (transplantation atherosclerosis). Regardless, it is characterized by extracellular matrix deposition, intimal and smooth muscle proliferation, and fibrotic obliteration of structures. Chronic rejection usually progresses insidiously despite immunosuppression, and no effective treatment exists.[2]

INFECTIONS

The increased susceptibility of the immunosuppressed organ transplant recipient broadens the possible spectrum of microorganisms infecting them. Preventive antimicrobial strategies have reduced the incidence and altered the timing of infections from different microbes after transplantation. The sequence with which different organisms appear in the post-transplantation course is dependent on time since transplant (Table 28-2).

- The first month after transplants is influenced by the infectious risks posed by surgery and the intensive care unit. Nosocomial bacterial pathogens predominate in this period.
- The second to sixth month after transplant is a period of sustained intense immunosuppression characterized by emergence of opportunistic infections.
- Beyond 6 months, most patients with stable graft function have slightly lowered immunosuppression. This period is characterized by community-acquired pathogens.

TABLE 28-2 Types of Infection Expected Per Month After Transplantation

0–1 Months	1–6 Months	> 6 Months
Bacterial infections: Gram-negative bacilli, Gram-positive cocci	Viral infections: cytomegalovirus, Epstein-Barr virus, varicella-zoster virus	Viral infections: Epstein-Barr virus, varicella-zoster virus, respiratory viruses
Fungal infections	Opportunistic infections: *Pneumocystis, Toxoplasma, Nocardia*	Bacterial infections: Gram-negative bacilli, *Pseudomonas* spp
Viral infections: herpes simplex, respiratory viruses	Bacterial infections: Gram-negative bacilli, *Pseudomonas* spp	Fungal infections: *Aspergillus* spp

During periods of enhanced immunosuppression for episodes of acute rejection or for the treatment of chronic rejection, opportunistic infections can be anticipated and appropriate precautions taken.[4-6]

ISCHEMIA TIME

Warm ischemic time refers to the amount of time that an organ remains at body temperature after its blood supply has been stopped or reduced. In the event of brain-dead organ recovery, the warm ischemic time is very minimal because the time that the heart stops is virtually the same time that the organs are cooled. For organ recovery from a donation after circulatory death (DCD), warm ischemic time includes the amount of time that the organ is not being properly perfused prior to death, the 5-minute waiting period following death, and the time that it takes for cannulation to occur and to get the flushes and icing started. Acceptable warm ischemic times for DCD vary from transplant center to transplant center and from patient to patient.[2]

Cold ischemic time refers to the amount of time that an organ is chilled or cold and not receiving a blood supply. Cold ischemic time varies widely by organ, but in general, it is best to transplant an organ as soon as possible.

Below is a list of generally accepted cold ischemic times[2]:

- Heart: 4 hours
- Lungs: 4 to 6 hours
- Liver: 6 to 10 hours
- Pancreas: 12 to 18 hours
- Intestines: 6 to 12 hours
- Kidneys: 24 hours

QUESTIONS

1. During which phase of HSCT is the patient at most risk for encapsulated bacterial and varicella-zoster virus infections?

   A. Pre-engraftment phase
   B. Postengraftment phase
   C. Late engraftment phase
   D. All of the above

2. Which of the following can be seen 3 months post HSCT?

   A. Diffuse alveolar hemorrhage
   B. Idiopathic pneumonia syndrome
   C. Cardiogenic pulmonary edema
   D. Bronchiolitis obliterans

3. A 65-year-old man with idiopathic pulmonary fibrosis is being listed for lung transplant. Which of the following is the most likely cause of death within the first week of lung transplant?

   A. CMV pneumonia
   B. Primary graft failure
   C. Post-transplant lymphoproliferative disorder
   D. Bronchiolitis obliterans syndrome

4. What is most likely to be the largest contributor to a patient's mortality at 5 years after lung transplant?

   A. CMV pneumonia
   B. Primary graft failure
   C. Post-transplant lymphoproliferative disorder
   D. Bronchiolitis obliterans syndrome

5. A 59-year-old woman with idiopathic cardiomyopathy underwent an uneventful orthotopic heart transplant. Following transplant, when is the patient at highest risk for CMV disease?

   A. 0 to 1 month
   B. 1 to 6 months
   C. More than 6 months
   D. All the above

6. Following transplant, when is the patient at highest risk for *Pseudomonas* infection?

   A. 0 to 1 month
   B. 1 to 6 months
   C. More than 6 months
   D. All the above

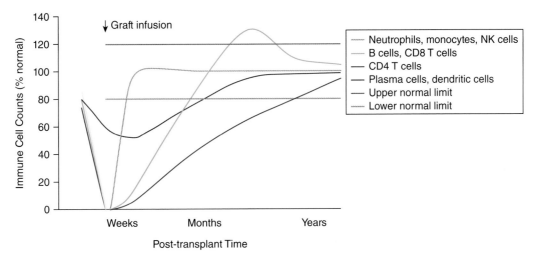

FIGURE 28-1 Immune cell counts peri and post myeloablative regimen of hematopoietic cell transplantation. (From Storek J (2008). Immunological reconstitution after hematopoietic cell transplantation-its relation to the contents of the graft, *Expert Opinion on Biological Therapy*, 8:5, 583-597. Reprinted by permission of the publisher (Taylor & Francis Ltd.) NK = natural killer.

7. A 45-year-old man with alcoholic liver cirrhosis is being listed for a liver transplant. What is the most likely explanation for this patient's severe hypoxemia that does not correct completely with supplemental O$_2$?

    A. Hepatopulmonary syndrome
    B. Severe portopulmonary hypertension
    C. Massive ascites
    D. Large hepatic hydrothorax

8. Which of the following is a contraindication to immediate listing for liver transplant?

    A. Hepatopulmonary syndrome
    B. Severe portopulmonary hypertension
    C. Massive ascites
    D. Large hepatic hydrothorax

9. A 49-year-old woman with end-stage lung disease due to pulmonary Langerhans cell histiocytosis (PLCH) undergoes a bilateral lung transplant. What is the likely cause if, on postoperative day 8, the patient's chest tube thoracostomy shows a persistent air leak?

    A. Recurrence of PLCH
    B. Severe pulmonary hypertension
    C. Bronchial dehiscence
    D. Acute cellular rejection

10. When is the patient at the *highest* risk for acute cellular rejection?

    A. In the first year post-transplant
    B. After the first year post-transplant
    C. After the second year post-transplant
    D. All of the above

ANSWERS

1. C. Late engraftment phase

    Hematopoietic cell transplantation is the transfer of stem cells from the same individual (autologous) or another (allogenic) with the goal of lifelong engraftment of the administered cells, leading to cure or improved outcomes for hematologic malignancies, bone marrow failure, and immunodeficiencies.[7] The preparative myeloablative regimen for HSCT causes a prolonged recovery of the immune system (Fig. 28-1). Neutrophil recovery is dependent on the graft type and can take 2 to 4 weeks. Lymphocyte recovery takes months (with natural killer T cells followed by B cells and CD8 T cells and then CD4 T cells).[7]

    Due to this sequence of immune recovery, the risk of infections of HSCT is divided into 3 sections: pre-engraftment phase, or phase I (< 15–45 days after HSCT), during which infection results from profound neutropenia and mucocutaneous breakdown; postengraftment phase, or phase II (30–100 days after HSCT), during which infection results from impaired cell-mediated immunity; and late phase, or phase III (> 100 days after HSCT), during which chronic GVHD plays a role[7] (Fig. 28-2).

    In the pre-engraftment phase, infections result from Gram-negative bacilli, Gram-positive organisms, gastrointestinal streptococcal species, *Aspergillus* species, and *Candida* species (choice A).

    In the postengraftment phase, infections from *Pneumocystis jirovecii*, CMV, and EBV-associated PTLD appear (choice B). In the late engraftment phase, infections from encapsulated bacteria and varicella-zoster virus appear (choice C).

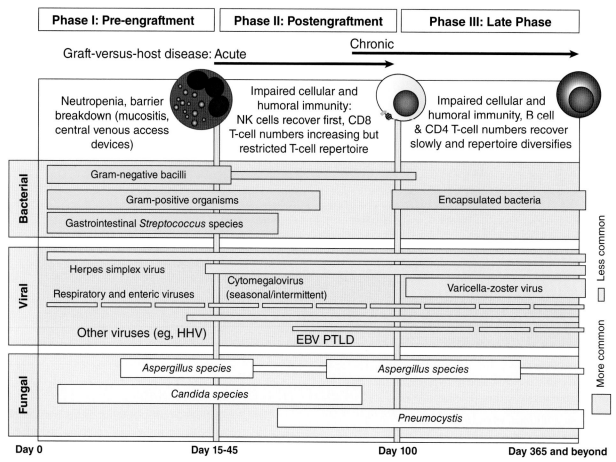

Phase I: Pre-engraftment   **Phase II: Postengraftment**   **Phase III: Late Phase**

FIGURE 28-2 Phases of opportunistic infections. (Reprinted with permission from Tomblyn M, Chiller T, Einsele H, et al. Guidelines for preventing infectious complications among hematopoietic cell transplantation recipients: a global perspective. *Biol Blood Marrow Transplant.* 2009;15(10):1143-1238.) EBV = Epstein-Barr virus; HHV = human herpesvirus; PTLD = post-transplant lymphoproliferative disorder.

Infections from *Aspergillus*, HSV reactivation, and community-acquired respiratory viruses are possible in all 3 phases (choice D). Timing from transplant and presence of graft-versus-host disease are the 2 main risk factors for infection. Other risk factors include HLA match, disease status, donor type, graft type, type and duration of pre- and post-immunosuppression, conditioning intensity, and neutrophil engraftment.[7]

2. D. Bronchiolitis obliterans

Chronic airflow obstruction is the most common late complication of allogeneic HSCT, typically occurring beyond the third month and associated with underlying chronic GVHD in the majority of cases (choice D).[8]

Diffuse alveolar hemorrhage (DAH; choice A) is most commonly observed within the first month after HSCT, often during the periengraftment phase, but with a slightly later onset encountered in up to 42% of cases. Patients can have dyspnea, nonproductive cough, fever, and diffuse pulmonary infiltrates, but hemoptysis is rare. Intensive care unit admission and mechanical ventilation

are required by the majority of patients with mortality rates of 80% to 100%.[4] Death is usually a result of superimposed multisystem organ failure or sepsis rather than respiratory failure from refractory hemorrhage. Anecdotally, high-dose corticosteroids (500–1000 mg/d of methylprednisolone for 3–4 days followed by tapering) may improve the survival rate.[4] While pathogenesis of DAH in HSCT recipients remains obscure, it is likely that DAH is part of a spectrum of acute lung injury induced by conditioning chemotherapy, radiation, and occult infection. The fact that many cases occur at the time of engraftment suggests that neutrophil influx into the lung may accentuate the injury and in some way precipitate hemorrhage.[4]

The term *idiopathic pneumonia syndrome* (IPS; choice B) is suggested to reflect the diversity of clinical presentations and likely multifactorial etiologies of "diffuse lung injury occurring after marrow transplant for which an infectious etiology is not identified."[4] The median time to onset is 21 days after transplantation, but also, more delayed median onset, between 42 and 49 days, is reported. Bronchoalveolar lavage, rather than lung biopsy, is recommended as the primary diagnostic approach to exclude infection.[4] Risk factors for development of IPS include transplantation for a malignancy other than leukemia, high-intensity conditioning regimens, older patient age, and high-grade acute GVHD. Patients with IPS present with dyspnea, fever, nonproductive cough, increasing oxygen requirements, and diffuse radiographic infiltrates. Pathology demonstrates diffuse alveolar damage and interstitial pneumonitis.[4] The course is typically rapid, with up to two-thirds of patients progressing within several days to respiratory failure requiring mechanical ventilation. Collective mortality is 74%. Idiopathic pneumonia syndrome likely arises from diverse etiologies. A sequence of events likely involves chemokine-driven recruitment of inflammatory and immune-effector cells to the lung, release of oxidants and proinflammatory cytokines, and, in the case of allogeneic transplantation, a second wave of injury mediated by alloreactive T lymphocytes. Beyond supportive care, there is no proven treatment for IPS, including high-dose corticosteroid therapy.[4]

Pulmonary edema (choice C) is the most common early post-transplantation complication. Administration of large volumes of intravenous fluid as well as chemotherapy- and radiation-induced cardiac dysfunction are important etiologic factors in the genesis of hydrostatic pulmonary edema. Noncardiogenic pulmonary edema can result from drug-induced pulmonary toxicity, sepsis, aspiration, transfusion of blood products, or acute GVHD.[4] Several acute lung injury syndromes—idiopathic pneumonia syndrome, engraftment syndrome, and diffuse alveolar hemorrhage—occur in the overlapping period of pre- and postengraftment phase (choice B).

3. B. Primary graft failure

Mild, transient pulmonary edema (ie, reimplantation response, reperfusion pulmonary edema) is a nearly universal feature of the freshly transplanted lung allograft. It is presumed to be a consequence of ischemia–reperfusion injury and increase in microvascular permeability, with surgical trauma and lymphatic disruption being contributing factors.[4] In about 12% to 22% of cases, injury is sufficiently severe to cause a form of acute respiratory distress syndrome termed *primary graft failure*. Risk factors include donor female sex, donor African American ethnicity, donor age (less than 21 or more than 45 years), and a recipient diagnosis of idiopathic pulmonary hypertension. An association between prolonged graft ischemic time and primary graft failure has been observed. The diagnosis of primary graft failure rests on the development of widespread radiographic infiltrates and markedly impaired oxygenation within the initial 72 hours of transplantation, and the exclusion of other causes of early graft dysfunction, such as volume overload, pneumonia, rejection, atelectasis, and pulmonary venous outflow obstruction. Histologic examination of lung tissue reveals a prevailing pattern of diffuse alveolar damage.

Treatment is supportive, relying on conventional mechanical ventilation utilizing low tidal volume strategies, extracorporeal life support, and retransplantation.[4] With an associated in-hospital mortality rate of 42% to 60%, primary graft failure is the leading cause of perioperative deaths among transplant recipients (choice B). Cytomegalovirus pneumonia after lung transplantation is most likely to occur *after* the first month of transplantation in the absence of antiviral prophylaxis (choice A). Post-transplant lymphoproliferative disorder (PTLD) has an onset *after* 6 months of lung transplant in most cases, with a majority related to EBV (choice C). The onset of bronchiolitis obliterans syndrome (BOS) almost always occurs after 6 months after lung transplant (choice D).

4. D. Bronchiolitis obliterans syndrome

Bronchiolitis obliterans syndrome affects 50% or more of recipients who survive beyond 5 years and accounts for a considerable proportion of cases of lung allograft loss and recipient death post-transplant. It is the leading cause of death for recipients who survive beyond 1 year post-transplant[8] (choice D). Bronchiolitis obliterans syndrome is frequently equated with the term *chronic rejection*. However, various interventions, including intensified immunosuppression, have little or no effect on progressive loss of allograft function in patients with BOS. Additionally, many nonimmune mechanisms have also been implicated or suggested as playing a role in BOS pathogenesis. These include airway injury due to primary graft dysfunction (PGD), gastroesophageal reflux (GER), various infections, and airway ischemia due to disruption of the bronchial circulation. These "nonimmune" factors may promote tissue damage and inflammation that in turn initiates and intensifies an alloimmune recipient response. Established obliterative bronchiolitis displays variable evidence of inflammation, alloimmune reactions, autoimmunity, and fibroproliferation with airway obliteration that leads to allograft airway remodeling and loss of function. Obliterative bronchiolitis may represent a final common endpoint for a variety of forms of allograft injury.[7]

Cytomegalovirus is the most common viral pathogen encountered in all solid organ recipient populations.[4] Cytomegalovirus infection typically emerges 1 to 3 months after transplantation, although onset may be delayed in patients receiving prophylaxis (choice A). Infection can occur by transfer of virus with the allograft or by reactivation of a latent virus remotely acquired by the recipient. Seronegative recipients who acquire organs from seropositive donors are at greatest risk for developing infection, and these primary infections tend to be the most severe. The use of antilymphocyte antibody therapy for immunosuppression also enhances the likelihood and severity of infection in susceptible recipients. An incidence of 15% to 55% has been reported after lung transplantation. The higher frequency of CMV pneumonitis in the lung transplant population is consistent with the notion that the lung is a major site of CMV latency. The efficacy of ganciclovir in the treatment of CMV disease is well established. Ganciclovir reduces the overall mortality associated with CMV pneumonitis from 50% to 20% and mortality in the subset requiring mechanical ventilation from more than 90% to 60%. Some advocate the addition of CMV hyperimmune globulin in treatment of severe disease. The presence of ganciclovir-resistant disease is associated with decreased survival in lung transplant recipients.[4]

Primary graft failure is a cause of mortality in the immediate postoperative period (choice B).

Post-transplant lymphoproliferative disorder (PTLD) is a term applied to a spectrum of abnormal B-cell proliferative responses ranging from benign polyclonal hyperplasia to more commonly encountered malignant lymphomas.[4] Lung transplant recipients have a 37% mortality rate directly attributable to PTLD over a median observation period of 3 years (choice C).

Epstein-Barr virus has been identified as the stimulus for B-cell proliferation, which proceeds in an unchecked fashion because of the muted cytotoxic T-cell response in the immunosuppressed host. EBV-naïve recipients who acquire primary infection at the time of organ transplantation are at greatest risk of developing PTLD. A higher intensity of immunosuppression and, in particular, the use of antilymphocyte antibody preparations have also been implicated as risk factors. The incidence of PTLD is greatest within the first year post-transplantation.

5. **B. 1 to 6 months**

The intermediate period (31–180 days after transplant) is the typical time of onset of infections attributable to latent pathogens transmitted from donor organs and blood products and those reactivated within the recipient. This is also the period during which classical opportunistic infections will present. In the absence of prophylaxis, CMV infection peaks during this time period (choice B).[6] The first month after solid organ transplant is characterized by bacterial (Gram-negative and Gram-positive) infections, fungal infections, and HSV (choice A). A period of more than 6 months after transplant places the patients also at risk for varicella-zoster infection (choice C). *Aspergillus* and HSV play a role in all of the post-transplantation periods (choice D).

6. **D. All the above**

Some infections occur irrespective of time. These may reflect nosocomial acquisition, which is seen more commonly in the presence of invasive devices (eg, intravenous catheters, urinary catheters, endotracheal intubation, and surgical procedures). *Pseudomonas* infections are an example of these infections (choice D). The first month after solid organ transplant is characterized by Gram-negative and Gram-positive bacterial, fungal, and HSV infections (choice A). Months 1 to 6 see the emergence of opportunistic pathogens such as *Pneumocystis jirovecii* and CMV (choice B). At more than 6 months after transplant, patients are at risk for additional viruses including VZV infections (choice C).

7. **A. Hepatopulmonary syndrome**

Hepatopulmonary syndrome is defined as the triad of liver disease, arterial hypoxemia, and abnormal intrapulmonary vascular dilatation.[4] Proof of the presence of intrapulmonary vascular abnormalities is provided by demonstration of systemic uptake of technetium-labeled macroaggregated albumin on standard radionuclide perfusion imaging or the delayed appearance of bubbles in the left atrium by contrast echocardiography. Due to intrapulmonary shunting, this process can only be *partially* corrected with administration of 100% oxygen, which serves to increase the pressure gradient favoring transfer of oxygen from the alveolus to the bloodstream (choice A). An unusual feature of hepatopulmonary syndrome is the tendency for oxygenation to worsen in the erect position as opposed to supine position (orthodeoxia), presumably due to basilar predominance of the vascular abnormalities.[4]

Severe portopulmonary hypertension in itself does not cause hypoxemia unless there is concomitant right heart failure, which by virtue of ventricular interdependence can impact left ventricular output and cause a cardiogenic shock (choice B). Massive ascites can cause basilar lung atelectasis and a restrictive lung physiology, which can cause hypoxemia that can be amenable to correction with supplemental O_2 (choice C). Large hepatic hydrothorax can similarly cause a shunt physiology due to compressive atelectasis of the underlying lung, which can be corrected with supplemental O_2 (choice D).

8. **B. Severe portopulmonary hypertension**

Although mild pulmonary hypertension does not appear to adversely impact liver transplantation, more significant elevations in pressure are associated with excessive post-transplantation mortality rates of 60% to 100% for liver transplant recipients with a preoperative mean pulmonary artery pressure of or exceeding 50 mmHg (choice B). Most deaths occur intraoperatively or in the immediate postoperative period and are largely attributable to progressive right heart failure and hemodynamic collapse. Portopulmonary hypertension diagnosis rests on demonstration of a mean pulmonary artery pressure exceeding 25 mmHg, and a normal pulmonary capillary wedge pressure and is encountered in 1% to 2% of patients with chronic liver disease and in up to 12.5% of patients referred for liver transplant evaluation.[4] The demonstration that intravenous prostacyclin (epoprostenol) significantly improves pulmonary hemodynamics in patients with portopulmonary hypertension provides a strategy for optimizing the condition of some patients who would otherwise be excluded from consideration for transplantation.[4]

Although hepatopulmonary syndrome was once considered an absolute contraindication to liver transplantation, subsequent demonstration of its resolution after transplantation has led to the reversal of this stance (choice A). Massive ascites is not a contraindication to liver transplantation (choice C). Similarly, large hepatic hydrothorax is not a contraindication to liver transplantation (choice D).

9. C. Bronchial dehiscence

Major dehiscence of the bronchial anastomosis was once a leading cause of perioperative mortality, but refinements in surgical technique, tissue preservation, and immunosuppression have reduced the risk of life-threatening dehiscence to a negligible level. Focal dehiscence, incidentally detected on bronchoscopy or heralded by the appearance of a spontaneous pneumothorax, is still encountered in 1% to 6% of patients (choice C). Tube thoracostomy may be required for evacuation of pneumothoraces, but focal dehiscence usually heals without surgical intervention.[4]

Recurrence of PLCH, while can occur post–lung transplant, will not be expected to happen in this timeframe of the immediate postoperative period (choice A).

Severe pulmonary hypertension, while well established as a consequence of PLCH, will not be responsible for a bronchopleural fistula (choice B).

Acute cellular rejection is commonly seen in a majority of lung transplant recipients; however, it is not expected to cause prolonged postoperative air leak (choice D). Approximately 55% to 75% of transplant recipients experience at least 1 episode of acute rejection within the first year. Beyond this period, the frequency of acute rejection declines to a low level.[4]

10. A. In the first year post-transplant

Lung transplant recipients are uniquely predisposed to pulmonary injury mediated by alloreactive T lymphocytes in the form of acute allograft rejection. Approximately 55% to 75% of transplant recipients experience at least 1 episode of acute rejection within the first year (choice A). Beyond this period, the frequency of acute rejection declines to a low level (choice B).

Factors that influence the likelihood of developing acute rejection include degree of HLA discordance between donor and recipient, polymorphisms in toll-like receptor 4, primary graft dysfunction, and viral infections. Symptoms of acute rejection are nonspecific and include malaise, low-grade fever, dyspnea, and cough. Radiographic infiltrates, a decline in arterial oxygenation at rest or with exercise, and an abrupt fall of greater than 10% in spirometric values are important clues to the possible presence of rejection, but similar findings accompany infectious episodes. Transbronchial lung biopsy has emerged as the gold standard for diagnosis of acute rejection. The histologic hallmark of acute rejection is the presence of perivascular lymphocytic infiltrates that, in more severe cases, spill over into the adjacent interstitium and alveolar airspaces. Conventional treatment of acute rejection consists of a 3-day pulse of high-dose intravenous methylprednisolone. A transient increase in oral prednisone and subsequent tapering over several weeks is advocated for histologically mild episodes.[4]

REFERENCES

1. United Network For Organ Sharing. https://unos.org/transplantation/ Accessed May 25, 2018.
2. Hertl M, Smith JF. Overview of transplantation. *Merck Manual.* https://www.msdmanuals.com/professional/immunology-allergic-disorders/transplantation/overview-of-transplantation. Accessed May 25, 2018.
3. Bhorade SM, Stern E. Immunosuppression for lung transplantation. *Proc Am Thorac Soc.* 2009;6(1):47-53.
4. Kotloff RM, Ahya VN, Crawford SW. Pulmonary complications of solid organ and hematopoietic stem cell transplantation. *Am J Respir Crit Care Med.* 2004;170(1):22-48.
5. Remund KF, Best M, Egan JJ. Infections relevant to lung transplantation. *Proc Am Thorac Soc.* 2009;6(1):94-100.
6. Green M. Introduction: infections in solid organ transplantation. *Am J Transplant.* 2013;13(Suppl 4):3-8.
7. Tomblyn M, Chiller T, Einsele H, et al; Center for International Blood and Marrow Research; National Marrow Donor program; European Blood and Marrow Transplant Group; American Society of Blood and Marrow Transplantation; Canadian Blood and Marrow Transplant Group; Infectious Diseases Society of America; Society for Healthcare Epidemiology of America; Association of Medical Microbiology and Infectious Disease Canada; Centers for Disease Control and Prevention. Guidelines for preventing infectious complications among hematopoietic cell transplantation recipients: a global perspective. *Biol Blood Marrow Transplant.* 2009;15(10):1143-1238.
8. Meyer KC, Raghu G, Verleden GM, et al; ISHLT/ATS/ERS BOS Task Force Committee; ISHLT/ATS/ERS BOS Task Force Committee. An International ISHLT/ATS/ERS clinical practice guideline: diagnosis and management of bronchiolitis obliterans syndrome. *Eur Respir J.* 2014;44(6):1479-1503.

Trauma and Warfare

Ronaldo Collo Go, MD

INTRODUCTION

This chapter discusses trauma resuscitation, burns, organ-specific trauma, chemical warfare, and biological warfare.

RESUSCITATION

Trauma is the leading cause of death for those younger than 40 years of age, with the majority of death secondary to bleeding within the first few hours of injury.[1-3] Damage-control resuscitation has become the standard of care for battlefield resuscitation and now is becoming more common in civilian trauma.[4] The goal is rapid hemorrhagic control with administration of balanced whole products in a plasma, platelet, and red blood cell at 1:1:1 ratio that mimic fresh whole blood, treat coagulopathy, and minimize colloid administration in patients requiring massive transfusion ($\geq$ 10 units packed red blood cells [pRBC] in 24 hours).[4]

The European Guidelines on management of major bleeding and coagulopathy following trauma stratified their recommendation as such: Grade 1A for strong recommendation, high quality of evidence due to benefits clearly outweigh risks and quality of evidence is from randomized controlled trials (RCTs) without important limitations or from overwhelming evidence from observational studies; Grade 1B for strong recommendation moderate quality of evidence due to benefits clearly outweigh risks and quality of evidence is from randomized controlled trials with limitations; Grade 1C strong recommendation, low quality or very low quality of evidence due to benefits clearly outweigh risks and support is from observational studies; Grade 2A weak recommendation, high quality of evidence due to benefits balance risks and evidence is from randomized control trials without important limitations or from overwhelming evidence from observational studies; Grade 2B weak recommendation and moderate quality of evidence due to benefits balance risks with randomized control trials with important limitations; and Grade 2C weak recommendation and low quality of evidence due to uncertainty in estimates of benefits and risks and evidence is from observational studies or case series.[5] Time between injury and control of bleeding needs to be minimized, since most fatalities occur within 24 hours of injury (Grade 1A).[5] Management bundles have been created to expedite care (Table 29-1). Tourniquets need to be applied to presurgical open extremity injuries and can be left in place for up to 6 hours (Grade 1B).[5] Major bleeding may not always be obvious and clinical presentation may correlate to the degree of blood loss (Table 29-2). Mechanisms of injury that suggest major bleeding include falling from a height of 20 feet or more, high-energy deceleration impact, and high-velocity gunshot wounds.[5] Radiographic studies of the head, chest, abdominal cavity, and pelvis are often needed, and hemodynamic instability would warrant emergent surgery.[5]

Acute Traumatic Coagulopathy

Acute traumatic coagulopathy (ATC) consists of derangements in prothrombin time (PT), partial thromboplastin time (PTT), and thrombin time (TT); thrombocytopenia; low fibrinogen; and a disseminated intravascular coagulation (DIC) score of 4 or greater, associated with trauma.[6] Although the true pathogenesis is unknown, ATC is believed to occur within 30 minutes of injury secondary to anticoagulation effects of protein C with inhibition of factors VIIIa and Va, profibrinolytic effects from inhibition of plasminogen activator inhibitor-1, and tissue factor expression with exposure of collagen, localized coagulation, platelet activation, and thrombin generation.[6-8] Acute traumatic coagulopathy is an independent predictor of massive transfusion, protracted intensive care unit (ICU) stay, multiorgan failure, and death.[7,9-14]

Acute traumatic coagulopathy is worsened by the consumption of coagulation factors and platelets; the dilutional effect secondary to replacement of lost whole blood with replacement fluids and blood products; hormonal and cytokine changes that lead to endothelial cell activation; dysfunction of platelets and coagulation proteases secondary to hypothermia and acidosis; and continued bleeding causing lost axial flow (red cells flow in the middle while platelets and plasma are in proximity to endothelium) and little contact of platelets and plasma with endothelium.[9]

Hypothermia

Hypothermia is caused by heat loss at the scene and from treatments such as intravenous (IV) fluids.[4] Coagulation protease activity and dysfunction with platelet activation, aggregation,

TABLE 29-1 Suggested Management Bundles

Prehospital Bundle	Intrahospital Bundle	Coagulation Bundle
• Prehospital time minimized • Tourniquet employed in case of life-threatening bleeding from extremities • Damage-control resuscitation concept applied • Trauma patient transferred directly to an adequate trauma specialty center	• Full blood count, prothrombin time, fibrinogen, calcium, viscoelastic testing, lactate, and pH assessed within the first 15 min • Immediate intervention applied in patients with hemorrhagic shock and an identified source of bleeding unless initial resuscitation measures are successful • Immediate further investigation undertaken using focused assessment with sonography for trauma (FAST), computed tomography (CT), or immediate surgery if massive intra-abdominal bleeding is present in patients presenting with hemorrhagic shock and an unidentified source of bleeding • Damage-control surgery concept applied if shock or coagulopathy is present • Damage-control resuscitation concept continued until the bleeding source is identified and controlled • Restrictive erythrocyte transfusion strategy (hemoglobin, 7–9 g/dL) applied	• Tranexamic acid administered as early as possible • Acidosis, hypothermia, and hypocalcemia treated • Fibrinogen maintained at 15–2 g/L • Platelets maintained at > 100 × 10⁹/L • Prothrombin complex concentrate administered in patients pretreated with warfarin or direct-acting oral coagulants (until antidotes are available)

Source: Rossaint R, Bouillon B, Cerny V, et al. The European guideline on management of major bleeding and coagulopathy following trauma: fourth edition. *Crit Care.* 2016;20:100.

and adhesion are seen when temperatures decrease from 37°C to 33°C.[4] Acidosis secondary to injury, hypoxia, hyperperfusion, and subsequently lactic acidosis contributes to coagulopathy, with protease dysfunction as suggested by a 50% reduction of prothrombinase activity with a pH less than 7.2, decreased thrombin generation, and increased fibrinolysis.[4,15-17]

Dilutional Effects

Dilutional effects are suggested by 1 study when coagulopathy is induced in 40% of trauma patients receiving 2 Liters of crystalloid and in 70% of trauma patients receiving 4 Liters of crystalloid.[10] Starch-based colloids coat von Willebrand factor (vWF) and fibrinogen, causing them to be dysfunctional and

to cause falsely high fibrinogen readings in assays.[8,11] It has been suggested that dilutional effects prolonged PT secondary to a reduction of factor VII and starch colloids, leading to fibrinogen dysfunction and worsening clot stability.[4,8,18]

Damage Control Resuscitation

To control acidosis, hypothermia, hypoperfusion, and coagulopathy, damage control resuscitation (DCR) is recommended for severe hemorrhagic shock, particularly in abdominal trauma and orthopedic surgery (Grade 1B).[4,5] Known triggers for DCR include hypothermia (≤ 34°C), pH less than or equal to 7.2, inaccessible major venous injury, extensive surgery, and coagulopathy.[5] In abdominal and orthopedic trauma, DCR

TABLE 29-2 American College of Surgeons Advanced Trauma Life Support (ATLS) Classification of Blood Loss Presentation

	Class 1	Class II	Class III	Class IV
Blood loss (mL)	Up to 750	750–1500	1500–2000	> 2000
Blood loss (% blood volume)	Up to 15%	15–30%	30–40%	> 40%
Pulse rate (beats/min)	< 100	100–120	120–140	> 140
Systolic blood pressure	Normal	Normal	Decreased	Decreased
Pulse pressure (mmHg)	Normal or increased	Decreased	Decreased	Decreased
Respiratory rate	14–20	20–30	30–40	> 35
Urine output (mL/h)	> 30	20–30	5–15	Negligible
Central nervous system/mental status	Slightly anxious	Mildly anxious	Anxious, confused	Confused, lethargic
Initial fluid replacement	Crystalloid	Crystalloid	Crystalloid and blood	Crystalloid and blood

Reprinted with permission from American College of Surgeons Committee on Trauma. *ATLS® Student Manual.* 9th ed. Chicago, IL: American College of Surgeons; 2012. https://www.44c.in.ua/files/book11.pdf. Accessed May 24, 2018.

consists of 3 parts. The first part involves control of bleeding and decontamination. Packing for at least 48 hours and temporal closure are performed. The second part involves rewarming, correction of coagulopathy, improvement of acid–base status, and any other procedures.[5] The third part involves definitive surgery.[5]

In patients with no traumatic brain injury (TBI) nor spinal injury, tissue oxygenation, prevention of dislodgement of clot, dilutional effects on coagulation factors by over-resuscitation, and hypothermia are achieved via permissive hypotension (systolic blood pressure [SBP] goal, 80–90 mmHg).[5] The recommendation is grade 1C, since there are no good randomized trials, although this approach showed improved survival in penetrating trauma and penetrating and blunt trauma.[19,20] Dutton et al randomized patients with hemorrhagic shock to target SBP greater than 100 mmHg or SBP of 70 mmHg until hemostasis is achieved.[21] The study showed no difference in injury severity score (19.65±11.8 vs 23.64±13.8; $P = 0.11$), duration of active hemorrhage (2.97±1.75 hours vs 2.57±1.46 hours; $P = 0.20$), or overall survival.[21]

Despite the recommendation that crystalloids, particularly normal saline (NS), may be used as the initial form of resuscitation in trauma patients (Grade A1), it is limited to 1 to 1.5 Liters due to dilutional and hypothermia effects, and normal saline can induce acute kidney injury (AKI) with hyperchloremic metabolic acidosis.[5,22,23] In addition to fibrinogen and von Willebrand factor dysfunction and dilutional effects of starch-based colloids, they can also induce renal failure and have not been shown to improve survival compared to crystalloids.[5] With hypertonic saline (HS), a randomized controlled trial comparing it to dextran and Ringer lactate had improved acute respiratory distress syndrome (ARDS)-free survival in patients requiring 10 or more units of pRBC[24], and another study showed a more effective reduction in elevated intracranial pressure.[25] However, Cooper et al failed to show any improvement in neurologic function in 6 months in patients treated with hypertonic saline compared to normal saline, and in 2 large prospective trials, Bulger et al failed to show any advantage with HS compared to NS.[26-28] The composition of crystalloids and colloids in comparison to the composition of blood is shown in Table 29-3.

Resuscitation with blood products is preferred over crystalloids and colloids with a goal hemoglobin of 7 to 9 g/dL (Grade 1C), platelets of 50×10^9/L (Grade 1C) or 100×10^9/L with ongoing bleeding or traumatic brain injury (Grade 2B), PT and aPTT less than 1.5 times normal (Grade 1C), and fibrinogen of 1.5 to 2 g/L (Grade 1C).[5] Blood work may not be available during the initial phase of resuscitation and should not preclude the use of blood products. These transfusion goals become more important during the goal-directed phase of resuscitation.

Fresh whole blood has been split to its components for storage purposes. Packed RBCs can be stored for 42 days at 4°C, platelets can be stored for 5 days at 22°C, cryoprecipitate can be stored for 1 year at –20°C, and fresh frozen plasma (FFP) can be stored for 1 year at –20°C. Glycerol is used to protect cells. With component transfusion, some of the blood products are lost. There is a 20% reduction in RBCs. There is 70% diminished of factor function from FFP, with factor V and VII affected the most. Dried plasma has been used, and it can be stored for up to 15 months. Liquid plasma is the best, and it is not frozen. It is available for use within 28 days. Type O is the universal donor. The Prospective, Observational, Multicenter Major Trauma Transfusion (PROMMTT) prospective cohort study suggested that trauma patients who received less than a 1:2 ratio of pRBC to platelets or pRBC to FFP were 3 to 4 times more likely to die compared to a 1:1 ratio or higher within the first 24 hours.[12] A decreased 6-hour mortality was found with increased ratios of plasma to RBCs (adjusted hazard ratio [aHR], 0.31; 95% confidence

TABLE 29-3 Composition of Crystalloid and Colloid Compared to Blood

	pH	Na	K	Cl	Ca	Mg	Lactate	Acetate	Gluconate	Dextrose	Osmolarity
Normal in Blood	7.35	140	4	104	2.3	1					285
Crystalloid											
Ringer lactate		130	4	109	1.5		28				273
PlasmaLyte	7.4	140	5			1.5		27	23		295
Normal saline	5.7	154		154							308
3% Saline	5	513		513							1025
D5W	4.3									278	272
Colloid											
Albumin	6.9	130-160									310
Dextran		154		154							310
Hetastarch		154		154							310

D5W = 5% dextrose in water.

interval [CI], 0.16–0.58), and platelets to RBCs (aHR, 0.55; 95% CI, 0.31–0.98).[12] The Pragmatic, Randomized Optimal Platelet and Plasma Ratios (PROPPR) study showed no significant 24-hour and 30-day mortality in trauma patients given plasma, platelets, and pRBC at a 1:1:1 ratio compared to a 1:1:2 ratio (12.7% vs 17%; 95% CI, −9.6% to 1.1%; *P* = 0.12; and 22.4% vs 26.1%; 95% CI, −10.2% to 2.7%; *P* = 0.26, respectively).[29] However, exsanguination, which is the most common cause of death within the first 24 hours, was significantly decreased in the 1:1:1 ratio compared to the 1:1:2 ratio (9.2% vs 14.6%; 95% CI, −10.4% to −0.5%).[29] A retrospective study of trauma patients who were transfused with warm frozen whole blood (FWB) versus component therapy at a 1:1:1 ratio showed improved 24-hour and 30-day survival in the warm FWB compared to component therapy (96% vs 88%, *P* = 0.018; and 95% to 82%, *P* = 0.002).[30] The volume of warm FWB was less than component therapy because of a lack of additives and anticoagulants, and it was associated with improved 30-day survival.[30] Virology may prohibit fresh whole blood use in civilian trauma.

It has been suggested that a platelet count less than 50×10^9/L or a fibrinogen level less than 0.5 g/L and a platelet count less than 100×10^9/L are predictors of microvascular bleeding, and those levels represent the threshold for transfusing and the predictor of progression of intracerebral hemorrhage, respectively.[5,31,32] Initial thrombocytopenia may not be obvious in the initial phase due to release of platelets from bone marrow and the spleen.[5,33,34] Thrombocytopenia as low as 50×10^9/L is found when 2 Liters of blood loss are replaced by crystalloids or red cells.[5,35] Furthermore, there is growing evidence to support that qualitative dysfunction of platelets, particularly platelet aggregation, can have as much or more impact on mortality as quantitative function.[5,35-39] There is evidence that qualitative dysfunction of platelets is evident in acute traumatic coagulopathy.[5] Platelet transfusions also are recommended for patients who are receiving antiplatelet therapy with intracerebral hemorrhage, and platelet function should be monitored (Grade 2C).[5] Five units of platelets are required to normalize platelet activity in patients taking aspirin, and 10 to 15 units of platelets are required to normalize platelet activity in patients taking aspirin and clopidogrel.[5,40] This may be repeated. Desmopressin, at a dose 0.3 μg/kg diluted in 50 mL of normal saline and given over 30 minutes, enhances platelet aggregation and adherence and is recommended for trauma patients on antiplatelet agents or who have von Willebrand disease (Grade 2C).[5] It has been suggested that administration of desmopressin with platelet transfusions improve platelet dysfunction, but it has not been shown to decrease radiographic progression of intracerebral hemorrhage or mortality.[41-49] Recombinant factor VIIa and fibrinogen have been shown to improve hemostasis in patients receiving APA.[5]

Fibrinogen is the most essential substrate in clot formation and is the earliest and most affected factor in ATC.[5] Recently, it has been recommended that transfusion of 2 g of fibrinogen to mimic the first 1:1 ratio of the first 4 units pRBC has improved survival with fibrinogen correction (Grade 1C).[5,50]

Cryoprecipitate that contains fibrinogen, factors VIII and XIII, vWF, and fibronectin is given when fibrinogen is 1 g/L to 1.5 g/L, since fibrinogen is activated by thrombin to form insoluble fibrin.[9]

Prothrombin complex concentrates (PCC) are produced from the cryoprecipitate supernatant after removal of antithrombin and factor XI. They are used to correct congenital or acquired vitamin K–dependent coagulation factor defects. There are 2 types: PCC 3 contains factor II, IX, and X, and PCC 4 contains factors II, VII, IX, and X, all at concentrations 25 times higher than in plasma. They also may contain heparin, protein C, and protein S. Half-lives differ, at 6 hours for factor VII and 60 to 72 hours for factor II.[51] Prothrombin complex concentrates are in small volumes and can be administered rapidly.[51] Therefore, the advantages of PCC over FFP in correcting vitamin K–factor coagulopathy include (1) faster correction of the international normalized ratio (INR); (2) smaller volumes: 15 mL/kg of FFP versus 1 to 2 mL/kg of PCC; and (3) faster preparation.[51] Complications include heparin-induced thrombocytopenia and thrombogenic events.[51] It has been recommended to administer PCC in patients who need early reversal of vitamin K–dependent oral anticoagulants (Grade 1A).[5]

Tranexamic acid (TXA) is an antifibrinolytic agent that is a competitive inhibitor of plasminogen with a plasma half-life of 120 minutes.[5] The Clinical Randomisation of Antifibrinolytic Therapy in Significant Haemorrhage (CRASH-2) trial studied adult trauma patients who were given TXA (1 g loading dose followed by an 8-hour infusion dose) compared to placebo.[52] Administration of TXA reduced all-cause mortality, risk of bleeding deaths, and exsanguination within the first 24 hours.[52-58] There was no increased risk of venous or arterial thrombotic events, such as deep venous thrombosis and myocardial infarctions, respectively.[52-58] Tranexamic acid should be given within 3 hours of injury, since there is a 1.3% increase of bleeding if given after 3 hours.[5,52-59] One potential complication is seizure in cardiac pulmonary bypass patients.[58] Aminocaproic acid is 10-fold weaker than TXA and is administered with a loading dose of 150 mg/kg followed by a continuous infusion of 15 mg/kg/h.

Additional interventions are necessary to achieve hemostasis in patients on direct oral anticoagulants. There are 2 groups: direct thrombin inhibitors such as dabigatran, and factor Xa inhibitors such as apixaban, rivaroxaban, and edoxaban[60] (see Fig. 29-1). Dabigatran has been approved for treatment of nonvalvular atrial fibrillation, deep vein thrombosis (DVT), and pulmonary embolism (PE). It peaks 2 to 3 hours after administration, and 80% is eliminated through the kidneys and 20% through the liver.[60] It binds to thrombin (factor IIa).[61] Thrombin time and ecarin clotting time (ECT) are used to monitor levels.[62-66] There are 3 available factor Xa inhibitors that directly inhibit free and clot-bound factor Xa. Rivaroxaban is approved for nonvalvular atrial fibrillation (AF) and DVT. It peaks at 2 to 4 hours after oral administration, and two-thirds undergoes metabolic degradation and one-third is unchanged and eliminated via the kidneys.[60,67-70] Apixaban is approved for nonvalvular AF and DVT. It has

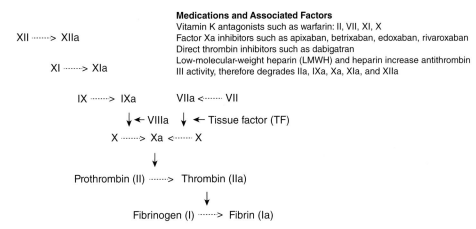

Medications and Associated Factors
Vitamin K antagonists such as warfarin: II, VII, XI, X
Factor Xa inhibitors such as apixaban, betrixaban, edoxaban, rivaroxaban
Direct thrombin inhibitors such as dabigatran
Low-molecular-weight heparin (LMWH) and heparin increase antithrombin
III activity, therefore degrades IIa, IXa, Xa, XIa, and XIIa

FIGURE 29-1 Medications and their target factors in the coagulation cascade.

a 15-hour half-life, and 35% is removed via the kidneys.[60,71,72] Edoxaban and betrixaban are other factor Xa inhibitors. Generally, Factor Xa assays are needed to monitor levels and activity.[60,73,74]

Nonspecific reversal agents for dabigatran include charcoal, if administered within 1 to 2 hours of ingestion; desmopressin, by stimulating release of factor VIII and vWF, PCC; and hemodialysis, because of dabigatran's low protein binding.[60] Idarucizumab is a humanized monoclonal antibody fragment that binds to both free and thrombin-bound dabigatran with an affinity 350 times greater than for thrombin.[60,75-79] Idarucizumab 5 g IV reverses dabigatran in a dose-dependent manner with normalization of ECT, TT, and aPPT values.[75-79] Andexanet alfa is a recombinant modified human factor Xa decoy that binds to factor Xa inhibitors with a high affinity, allowing factor Xa activity. It is administered as a bolus followed by infusion.[60,80-83] Reversal is assessed via decrease in antifactor Xa, unbound factor Xa inhibitors, and restoration of thrombin generation.[60,80-83] Reversal was noted within 2 to 5 minutes after bolus and was maintained with continuous infusion.[60,80-83] Reversal stopped after 1 to 3 hours after cessation of continuous infusion.[60,83-86]

The European Task Force for Advanced Bleeding Care from Major Trauma recommends routine monitoring of coagulopathy such as PT/INR, PT, and fibrinogen.[5] These laboratory studies are limited by (1) an inability to monitor quantities of coagulation factor and thrombin potential; (2) a lack of monitoring interactions between coagulation proteases and phospholipids; and (3) the length of time (at least an hour) to obtain results.[5,6] Therefore, viscoelastic studies such as thromboelastography (TEG) and rotational thromboelastometry (ROTEM) have been suggestive as valuable tools in understanding coagulopathy and guiding transfusions in trauma. (Grade 1C).[5,6] If they are not available during the initial phase of resuscitation, they are still important during the goal-directed resuscitation phase. Serial lactic acid may also serve as surrogate markers for bleeding and shock (Grade 1B).[5] Hypocalcemia can occur during massive transfusion secondary to citrate

binding and should be monitored and maintained at normal levels (Grade 1C).[5]

Despite this discussion of controlling hemorrhage, trauma patients are at high risk for thromboembolism. It is recommended that pharmacologic thromboprophylaxis be initiated within 24 hours of control of hemorrhage (Grade 1B).[5] Pneumatic compression (Grade 1C) and stockings (Grade 2C) are also recommended. Inferior vena cava filters as prophylaxis are not recommended. (Grade 1C)[5]

BURNS

Every year in the United States, there are 40,000 hospitalizations and 3400 deaths from burns.[84-89] Survival is 97% for patients admitted to burn centers.[84-89] The etiology of burns includes thermal, electrical, and chemical burns, and depth of burns includes superficial, superficial dermal, and full thickness (Tables 29-4 and 29-5).[84]

There are 3 zones of burns. The zone of coagulation is exposed to the greatest amount of heat and has irreversible tissue damage.[84-86] The tissue must be exposed to temperatures greater than 41.1°C (106°F), which is needed for protein to be denatured.[85] The zone of stasis surrounds the zone of coagulation. It is associated with decreased tissue perfusion and is potentially salvageable. However, continued hypoxia and ischemia can lead to tissue necrosis if no intervention is done within 48 hours.[85] The mechanism is secondary to autophagy within the first 24 hours and followed by apoptosis in the next 24 hours.[85] The zone of hyperemia is the outermost area where there is increased perfusion; tissue in the zone of hyperemia will likely recover.[84-86] Burn healing is a dynamic process with overlapping stages of inflammation, proliferation, and remodeling.[85]

Severe burns affecting 20% total body surface area (TBSA) can result in *burn shock*, which is a combination of hypovolemic, distributive, and cardiogenic shock.[84,90,91] Intravascular volume is depleted secondary to increased capillary permeability, and only 30% of the body surface area can be

TABLE 29-4 Types of Burns and Description

Type	Causes	Description
Thermal burns	Scalds: 70% of burns in children and also in elderly	Superficial burns
	Flame: 50% of burns in adults, sometimes with inhalation injury	Deep dermal or full thickness
	Contact	Deep dermal or full thickness
Electrical	3–4% of burns Entry and exit points Voltage strength directly proportional to extent of tissue damage	
	Low voltage or domestic electricity	Small contact burns at entry and exit sites, can cause arrhythmias
	True high-tension injuries if ≥ 1000 V	Tissue bone necrosis, rhabdomyolysis, fatal if > 70,000 V
	Flash injury: arc current from high-tension voltage	Superficial burns, although clothes can be set on fire; no current passing through body
Chemical	Alkalis are worse than acids	Deep burns; can continue to cause necrosis even after agent is removed
	Chromic acids	
	Dichromatic acid	
	Hydrofluoric acid	

resuscitated due to reduced sodium ATPase activity, disruption of the cellular transmembrane ionic gradient, and protein loss and secondary to microvascular injury from inflammatory mediators.[91] There is increased systemic vascular resistance and decreased cardiac output.[89]

Mortality is increased if resuscitation is delayed by 2 hours, and hypovolemic shock occurs if resuscitation is delayed in patients with burns of greater than 15% to 20% TBSA. The goal is to provide fast resuscitation while avoiding the sequela of over-resuscitation, as suggested by the phenomenon called *fluid creep*, which can lead to pulmonary edema and compartment syndrome. This has led to exploration of other fluid resuscitation methods, such as albumin and hypertonic saline.

In burn patients, the primary survey starts with airway evaluation followed by vascular access and monitoring devices.[90,91] Primary injury occurs from direct thermal injury and secondary injury results from systemic inflammatory response. The secondary survey includes determination of mechanism of injury; evaluation for inhalation injury and carbon monoxide intoxication, corneal burns, and abuse; and then a detailed assessment of burns.[90,91]

Resuscitation with crystalloid fluids within the first 24 hours is key, using the Parkland formula or modified Brooke formula generally is reserved for second- or third-degree burns. The Parkland formula calculates the amount of crystalloid fluids as 4 mL/kg multiplied by the percentage of TBSA burned. The first half is given over the first 8 hours and the second half is given over the next 16 hours. Fluid resuscitation is crystalloid, usually lactated Ringer over isotonic saline because its more physiologic, and after 18 to 24 h when capillary integrity is restored, colloids can be used (5% albumin with lactated Ringer).

The rule of nines or the palm rule can be used to calculate body surface area. Burns less than 15% BSA are not associated with extensive capillary leak. Pulse, blood pressure (BP),

TABLE 29-5 Types of Burns and Their Characteristics

Burns	Depth	Characteristic
First Degree	Superficial epidermis	Red, good capillary refill, painful, healing with no scar after 5-10 days
Second Degree	Partial dermis	Red with blisters, edema, good capillary refill, painful, healing with minimal scarring after 2-3 weeks
Second Degree	Deep dermis	Pinkish to white, thick skin texture, poor or no capillary refill, healing with dense scar after 1-2 months
Third Degree	Full thickness	White, black or brown, leathery with no capillary, painless, no spontaneous healing
Fourth Degree	Involvement of subcutaneous tissue, tendon, and / or bone	Variable, no capillary refill, painless, no spontaneous healing

and urine output (0.5-1 mL/kg) are monitored to measure adequate perfusion. Urine output goals are 30 to 50 mL/h, and higher goals should be avoided in order to prevent over-resuscitation. Gradual increases in maintenance fluids instead of boluses prevent worsening edema. Pigmented urine, such as in high voltage or deep thermal injury, should be cleared. Glycosuria also can elevate urine output falsely, and some patients might require diuresis. Urinalysis should be obtained at least 8 hours after resuscitation.

Although it has been hypothesized that capillary leak is improved at 18 to 24 hours, this is not certain. One test involves administering equal portions of albumin and Lactated Ringer, and if urine output improves, this could suggest that capillary leak has resolved. An infusion of 5% albumin is given over 24 hours at a dose of 0.5 mL/kg/% TBSA burned; free water in mL/h is determined by the following equation: (25 + % TBSA burned) × BSA (mm²). Sodium must be monitored since the albumin is rich in protein. Unlike crystalloids, of which only 20% to 30% remain in the intravascular space, 50% of colloids remain in the intravascular space. Other centers prefer FFP at 0.5 to 1 mL/kg for the first 24 hours. Dextran has twice the oncotic pressure of albumin and reduces erythrocyte aggregation. This reduces edema formation in nonburned areas, although removal of dextran leads to edema if capillary leak still present. Hypertonic saline (180–300 mEq/L Na), with a serum goal of 160 mEq/L or less, theoretically mobilizes extravascular fluid into the vascular space by increasing the osmotic gradient. A compromise is to use lactated Ringer with 50 mEq sodium bicarbonate. The greatest benefit is seen in inhalation injury and in burns involving 40% TBSA or more.

Burn depth can be underestimated, since tissue may initially appear viable, but appearance changes over time. The Lund and Browder chart or the rule of nines is employed for adults (9% TBSA for the head, neck, and each arm; 18% TBSA for the anterior thorax, posterior thorax, and each leg; 1% TBSA for the perineum).

First-degree burns are limited to the epidermis and are similar to a sunburn without blisters. They are red, dry, and painful. There are 2 types of second-degree burns. Superficial partial-thickness burns involve papillary dermal elements and are pink, moist, and painful. There is blister formation and heal well without skin graft. Deep partial-thickness burns involve deeper reticular dermis and have a variable appearance from pink to white, with a dry surface, diminished sensation, and sluggish or absent capillary refill. Third-degree burns are leathery, dry, and waxy. They will contract but not heal. Blisters occur in second- and third-degree burns. Fourth-degree burns involve subcutaneous tissue, tendon, or bone. Circumferential or near-circumferential burns should be noted because they can progress to ischemia or interfere with ventilation.

High doses of ascorbic acid (vitamin C) during the initial 24 hours post-burn reduced fluid requirements by 40%, tissue water by 50%, and ventilator days.[91]

Early nutritional support is important and is associated with shorter hospital stays, increased wound healing, and decreased infections.[91] Carbohydrates and fat supplementation might be minimized, since hyperglycemia leads to increase in systemic inflammatory response syndrome (SIRS), and fat can cause further immunosuppression.[85] Amino acids and vitamins are key, and it is hypothesized that insulin administration delays the catabolic state and increases protein synthesis.[85,92-96]

Virtually every patient will meet criteria for SIRS. Early excision and skin graft is now the accepted practice. In adults, there is no role for prophylactic antibiotics. Human tetanus immunoglobulin (250–500 IU) is administered regardless of immune status to prevent tetanus.[86] Tetanus toxoid 0.5 mL is also given intramuscularly (IM) if the patient has not received complete primary immunization or has not received a booster in the last 10 years.[86] Patients partially immunized or never immunized should also receive the vaccine.[86]

Early excision, 24 to 48 hours from injury, is associated with decreased blood loss, length of stay, infection, graft take, and mortality.[85,96-100] Full-thickness burns are treated with an autograft, which is a split-thickness skin graft from the patient's uninjured skin.[85] With an autograft, risk of rejection is low, although pain and the wound healing burden on donor sites are high.[87] Temporary coverage can also be achieved with allografts, tissue from other living or dead donors; xenografts, tissue from different species; skin substitutes; and dermal analogs.[85] The traditional dressing approach is mafenide acetate in the morning and a silver sulfadiazine cream at night covered with gauze.[85] There are some dressings impregnated with silver, although it has been suggested that silver delays wound healing. Topical antibiotics have been used to prevent the development of infection, to reduce microbial load, and to decrease conversion from a partial to a full-thickness burn (Table 29-6).[86,101-103] It is an adjunct to early debridment.[86,101-103]

Infections are serious complications in burns, and it might be difficult to distinguish colonization from infection. Increasing inflammation (edema, redness, pain), purulent discharge, and fever and leukocytosis can determine true infection.[86] Wound swabs may show purulence but true infection will have elevated polymorphonuclear neutrophil (PMN) count with moderate to heavy growth from pathogenic organisms.[86] Tissue quantitative cultures for infection would have 10^4 or more CFU/g or 10^5 or more colony-forming units (CFU)/g of tissue, and predicted potential of sepsis, and can have 75% mortality.[86,104] A polymerase chain reaction (PCR) may be able to identify the organism, but the infection will still need culture to help determine antibiotic sensitivities.[86]

There are 4 types of burn-related infections: (1) burn impetigo with loss of epithelium from previously epithelized surface not related to trauma, which is treated with cleaning of debris and exudates, topical antistaphylococcal antibiotics, and grafting of unstable areas; (2) burn-related surgical wound infection that is surgically created in nonepithelized skin with loss of overlying graft or membrane, which is treated in a similar way to burn impetigo; (3) burn wound cellulitis, which is an infection of uninjured skin surrounding the wound with local progression, is treated with antibiotics against *Streptococcus pyogenes*; and (4) invasive burn wound infection with infection in unexcised burn and invasion into underlying

TABLE 29-6 Types of Topical Agent and Associated Preparation, Penetration, Type of Antibacterial Activity, and Toxicity

Topical Agent	Preparation	Eschar Penetration	Antibacterial Activity	Major Toxicity
Silver nitrate (AgNO$_3$)	0.5% solution	None	Bacteriostatic against aerobic Gram-negative bacilli, *Pseudomonas aeruginosa*, limited antifungal	Electrolyte imbalance
Silver sulfadiazine (Silvadene, Flamazine, Thermazine, Burnazine)	1% water-soluble cream (oil-in-water emulsion)	None	Bactericidal against aerobic Gram-negative bacilli, *P aeruginosa*, some *Candida albicans*	Leukopenia
Mafenide acetate (Sulfamylon)	10% water-soluble cream (oil-in-water emulsion), 5% solution	Limited	Broad spectrum against aerobic Gram-negative bacilli, *P aeruginosa*, anaerobes	Metabolic acidosis
Nanocrystalline silver dressings (ACTICOAT A.B. dressing, Silverlon)	Dressing consisting of 2 sheets of high-density polyethylene mesh coated with nanocrystalline silver	Moderate	Potent activity against aerobic Gram-negative bacilli, *P aeruginosa*, aerobic Gram-positive bacilli, MRSA, VRE, multidrug-resistant *Enterobacteriaceae*	Limited toxicity

MRSA = methicillin-resistant *Staphylococcus aureus*; VRE = vancomycin-resistant enterococci

From Church D, Elsayed S, Reid O, et al. Burn wound infections. *Clin Microbiol Rev.* 2006;19(2):403-434. With permission from American Society for Microbiology.

tissue that is diagnosed by histology or cultures and that is treated with systemic antibiotics and wound excision.[86]

ORGAN-SPECIFIC CONSIDERATIONS

Traumatic Brain Injury

Traumatic brain injury encompasses many forms, which are not mutually exclusive. In addition to intracerebral hemorrhage, there are 4 types of hemorrhage associated with traumatic brain injury. An epidural hematoma is an arterial bleed, usually from the middle meningeal artery at the level of the foramen spinosum, from rupture of the anterior meningeal artery, or from a dural arteriovenous fistula. Bleeding occurs between the dura and the skull and radiographically appears as concave. A subdural hematoma is usually secondary to torn bridging veins between the surface of the brain and the dural sinuses, but it may occur from the small cortical arteries. Bleeding occurs between the dura and arachnoid spaces radiographically appears as a crescent. A subarachnoid hemorrhage has many etiologies that may directly or indirectly lead to trauma, such as arteriovenous (AV) malformation, cocaine use, cavernous sinus thrombosis, cerebral amyloid angiopathy, sickle cell disease, pituitary apoplexy, arterial dissection, or moyamoya. An associated skull fracture and contusion may suggest that the subarachnoid hemorrhage is a direct consequence of trauma. A diffuse axonal injury is the result of deceleration and acceleration and/or rotational injury and radiographically appears as areas of focal 5- to 15-mm intraparenchymal hemorrhage.

Linear skull fractures extend through the thickness of the calvarium and have no clinical significance unless they cross the middle meningeal groove or dural sinuses.[105] Depressed skull fractures occur below the adjacent skull and are usually associated with traumatic brain injury.[106] A basilar skull fracture involves the plate of the ethmoid bone, the orbital plate of the frontal bone, the petrous and squamous portions of the temporal bone, and the sphenoid and occipital bones.[107,108] It can lead to epidural hematomas, dural tears leading to cerebrospinal fluid (CSF) leaks, and cranial nerve palsies. A Battle sign or retroauricular or mastoid ecchymosis, periorbital ecchymosis or raccoon eyes, clear rhinorrhea or otorrhea, and hemotympanum may appear 1 to 3 days after the event and are clinical signs of a basilar skull fracture. Penetrating fractures usually occur from bullets, knives, and explosives and are usually associated with traumatic brain injury.[109]

The central nervous system is encompassed in a fixed, nearly incompressible space. The skull has a total volume of 1450 mL, with the brain comprising 1300 mL (85%), CSF comprising 65 mL (5%), and blood comprising 110 mL (10%).[110,111] Cerebrospinal fluid is continuously produced at the rate of 20 mL/h (total of 500 mL/24 h) in the choroid plexus and is absorbed in the arachnoid granules in venous circulation. According to the Monro-Kellie hypothesis, these components are constant and an increase in one means a decrease in another.[111] Otherwise, pressure increases and herniation can occur. Intracranial pressure (ICP) varies with age, but generally, in adults is 5 to 15 mmHg (7.5–20 cm H$_2$O) and positional, with lower values obtained if the head is elevated.[111] Intracranial pressure also is important in that it influences cerebral perfusion pressure (CPP) and oxygen delivery to the brain, using the following formula:

$$CPP = MAP - ICP \text{ or } CPP = (1/3 \text{ SBP} + 2/3 \text{ DBP}) - ICP$$

where MAP is the mean arterial pressure, SBP is the systolic blood pressure, and DBP is the diastolic blood pressure. Normally, there is pressure autoregulation that maintains CPP at 50 to 150 mmHg. Arterioles dilate in response to elevated pressure or constrict in response to low pressure. In pathologic states, this autoregulation is impaired and CPP passively follows cerebral blood flow (CBF), a process called *pressure passive flow*.[111]

In trauma, there is a heterogeneous group of causes for initial elevated ICP, which includes trauma-induced masses such as fractures, hemorrhage, and foreign bodies; cerebral edema; hyperemia; cerebral vasodilatation from hypercapnia from hyperventilation; hydrocephalus from CSF drainage obstruction; and increased intrathoracic and intra-abdominal pressures.[111] Traumatic brain injury is a unique catalyst for elevated ICP, since there can be a secondary increase 3 to 10 days after trauma, secondary to delayed hematoma formation and vasospasm.[111]

Physical examination and radiographic evidence can suggest increased intracranial pressure, but their absence does not definitively exclude its absence.[111] Intracranial pressure monitoring is indicated for patients with a Glasgow coma score (GCS) of less than or equal to 8 after resuscitation and an abnormal computed tomography (CT) of the head on admission and for patients with a GCS of 8 or less with normal head CT on admission plus 2 or more of the following: age greater than 40 years, motor posturing, and SBP less than 90 mmHg.[111-113] Management via ICP monitoring and indirect measure of CPP is advocated to reduce 2-week postinjury mortality.[113] It can be performed via intraventricular catheters or intraparenchymal microtransducer sensors, but the former is therapeutic as well.[112] An intraventricular catheter is inserted through the frontal horn of the lateral ventricle into a burr hole at the Kocher point on the nondominant side and at a depth of 5 to 6 cm, aiming at the medial epicanthus and external auditory meatus until CSF is reached. The head is positioned at 30 degrees and zeroed at the level of the tragus (equivalent to the foramen of Monro). Drainage is typically performed when ICP reaches 10 cm H_2O, but for a ruptured aneurysm, drainage occurs when ICP reaches 20 cm H_2O. Threshold goals are for an ICP less than 22 cm H_2O and a CPP of 60 to 70 mmHg.[113] Patients with intact autoregulation might be able to tolerate higher CPP, although it has been suggested that patients with CPP greater than 70 mmHg have worse outcomes and higher incidence of acute respiratory distress syndrome.[114] If the CPP is less than 50 mmHg, vasopressors and fluids are indicated.[110,115] With head elevation, BP and ICP must be zeroed at the same level (foremen of Munro) to get an accurate CPP measurement.[110] Intraventricular catheters allow administration of medications such as tissue plasminogen activator (tPA), since it can facilitate resolution of intraventricular hemorrhage (IVH).[116] In TBI, once the ICP is normal for 48 to 72 hours, the drain is clamped, and if there are no signs of elevated ICP for 12 to 24 hours, the drain can be removed.

Advanced cerebral monitoring includes transcranial Doppler to measure hypo- and hyperperfusion and vasospasm, such as in subarachnoid hemorrhage; measurements of local tissue oxygen via invasive brain tissue oxygen tension (PbtO$_2$) and jugular arteriovenous oxygen difference (AVDO$_2$); microdialysis to measure brain metabolism of glucose, lactate, pyruvate, and glutamate; and electrocorticography, but only jugular bulb monitoring of AVDO$_2$ is recommended to reduce mortality and improve outcomes at 3 to 5 months postinjury.[113] Jugular bulb venous oximetry is an indirect measure of cerebral oxygen use and is contraindicated in cervical spine injury, tracheostomy, and coagulopathy. Transcranial Doppler is often utilized to differentiate vasospasm from subarachnoid hemorrhage.

Other treatment thresholds include jugular venous O$_2$ saturation (SjvO$_2$) less than 50% or brain oxygen tension less than 15 mmHg. The jugular bulb is the dilated portion below the base of skull; the catheter is inserted in the dominant side. Determination of the dominant side can be obtained by monitoring ICP with compression of the internal jugular vein, CT assessment of jugular foremen, or comparison via ultrasound. Under sterile technique and ultrasound guidance, needle, Guidewire, and catheter are inserted in the cephalad direction, advancing the Guidewire 2 to 3 cm from the puncture site and advancing the catheter until it meets resistance, usually at 15 cm. Then, the catheter is pulled back 0.5 to 1 cm to prevent vascular injury from the movement. Complications include infection, pneumothorax, thrombosis, and carotid artery puncture. A normal SjvO$_2$ is 50% to 75%. An SjvO$_2$ less than 50% without falling arterial O$_2$ saturation suggests a fall in cerebral blood flow or increased cerebral metabolic rate of oxygen (CMRO$_2$); if CPP is maintained, there is decreased cerebral blood flow secondary to increased resistance from vasospasm or hyperventilation. An SjvO$_2$ greater than 85% indicates hyperemia, a rise in cerebral blood flow, shunting of blood, or decreased CMRO$_2$, which can suggest cell death. Limiting factors to SjvO$_2$ monitoring include (1) poor correlation of concomitant values for cerebral oximetry to internal jugular venous sample; (2) extracerebral contamination if the sample is not obtained within 2 cm of the jugular bulb at a rate less than 2 mL/min; (3) measurement of only global cerebral oxygenation and not focal areas of ischemia; (4) the Bohr effect, falsely high values of SjVO$_2$ during alkalosis; (5) limitations occurring from brainstem injuries; and (6) irregularities on vein wall, kinking, or fibrin formation.

The difference in oxygen content between arterial and jugular venous (AjvDO$_2$) is based on the equation CMRO$_2$/CBF:

$$CMRO_2 = CBF \times OEF \times Sao_2,$$

where OEF is the oxygen ejection fraction and Sao$_2$ is the arterial oxygen saturation. A normal AjvDO$_2$ is 4 to 8 mL O$_2$/100 mL blood. An AjvDO$_2$ less than 4 mL O$_2$/100 mL blood indicates that oxygen supplementation is greater than demand. An AjvDO$_2$ greater than 8 mL O$_2$/100 mL blood can mean ischemia. Hyperperfusion stage (day 0) means, normal AVDO$_2$, and normal SjvO$_2$. Hyperemic stage (days 1–3) means increased CBF, decreased AVDO$_2$, increased SjvO$_2$, increased hyperglycolysis, and decreased microvascular resistance. Vasospasm stage (days 4–15) means decreased AVDO$_2$, increased SjvO$_2$ secondary to decreased CMRO$_2$, or cell death.

Hyperosmolar therapy via mannitol and hypertonic saline reduces blood viscosity and constriction of pial arterioles leading to decreased intracranial pressure, but no specific recommendation is made due to insufficient evidence on clinical outcomes.[113] Early (within 2.5 hours) and short-term hypothermia is not recommended due to conflicting data.[113] A continuous external ventricular drain (EVD) may be used to lower ICP in patients with a GCS less than 6 during the first 12 hours of TBI, starting at 1 to 2 mL/min. The EVD may be removed if there is no neurological change or no worsening pressures for 24 hours. Hyperventilation should only be considered in impending herniation but otherwise avoided during the first 24 hours when cerebral blood flow is critical.[5,113] If utilized, jugular venous oxygen saturation and brain tissue oxygen partial pressure should be monitored. Corticosteroids are associated with high mortality and are not recommended.[113] Patients are at risk for early (within 7 days) or late (after 7 days) seizures. Patients at risk for early seizure include those with any of the following: a GCS of 10 or less; amnesia for more than 30 minutes; a linear or depressed skull fracture; immediate seizures; penetrating head injury; subdural, epidural, or intracerebral hematoma; cortical contusion; age of 65 years or less; chronic alcoholism; and depression.[114] Seizure prophylaxis is intended to prevent chronic epilepsy, herniation, and death. Phenytoin or valproic acid with levetiracetam as an alternative is recommended for early seizure prophylaxis. Deep vein thrombosis prophylaxis is recommended after 24 hours if there is no worsening hemorrhage.

Surgical evacuation of a subdural hematoma is indicated if the clot thickness is greater than 10 mm, it has a midline shift greater than 5 mm regardless of GCS, GCS has decreased 2 or more points since admission, or pupils are fixed, asymmetrical, and dilated.[115] The ABC/2 score is used in epidural hematomas and intracerebral hemorrhages to help with prognosis and treatment approaches. In this assessment, A is the greatest diameter on the CT slice with the largest area of hemorrhage, B is the largest diameter 90 degrees to A on the same CT slice, and C is number of CT slices of hemorrhage times the slice thickness in centimeters.[116] Surgery is indicated in epidural hematoma if the volume is greater than 30 cm³ or a GCS is less than 9 with pupillary abnormalities.[117] Surgery may also be indicated for cerebellar hemorrhage greater than 3 cm in diameter, brainstem compression, and/or hydrocephalus or supratentorial hemorrhage greater than 30 mL within 1 cm of the surface.[118]

Craniotomy considerations include the following: (1) decompressive (unilateral) craniotomy for severe TBI, malignant middle cerebral artery infarction, and aneurysmal subarachnoid hemorrhage; (2) bifrontal craniotomy for refractory ICP secondary to diffuse cerebral edema for post-TBI within 48 hours; (3) subtemporal decompression, temporal lobectomy, and decompressive craniotomy for refractory ICP and impending herniation; (4) infections such as subdural empyema, meningitis, and encephalitis; (5) severe subdural and venous sinus thrombosis; and (6) intracranial hemorrhage greater than 50 cm³ in volume, or a GCS less than 8

with frontal or temporal hemorrhage 20 cm³ or greater with a midline shift of 5 mm or more or cisternal compression.[119-133]

Blunt and Penetrating Chest Trauma

The initial survey of a patient with chest trauma involves identification of tension pneumothorax, hemothorax, flail chest, and cardiac tamponade. Evacuation of air or blood from the pleural space is necessary to prevent tension pneumothorax or lung entrapment and trapped lung, respectively. Tube thoracotomy is often performed and left in place until pneumothorax is no longer seen or drainage is less than 150 mL in 24 hours with pleural effusions. The size of the chest tube is a topic of debate. In nontraumatic situations, small-bore chest tubes (10–14F) have been used to drain pneumothoraces, pleural effusions, malignant effusions, and hemothoraces. Small studies have suggested the same benefit in traumatic uncomplicated pneumothorax and traumatic hemothorax.[134,135]

Flail chest is the paradoxical movement of the chest secondary to 3 or more rib fractures with both anterior and posterior fractures in each rib, posterior flail segments, anterior flail segments, or the sternum and both sides of the thorax. Respiratory insufficiency is secondary to pulmonary contusion. Treatment is primarily supportive and includes pain management via oral, IV, or epidural medications. There is a current trend that surgical fixation results in decreased morbidity, ventilator days, ICU stay, and mortality.[136,137]

Blast injury to the lung results in tissue damage from the blast wave (primary), from material propelled (secondary), from the patient being propelled to other objects (tertiary), and from heat and chemicals from the devices (quaternary).[138-140] The injury from a blast wave is from spallation, implosion, and inertia. Treatment is supportive and if the patient develops respiratory failure, ARDS protocol should be initiated. Table 29-7 lists the blast lung injury severity score.[139]

Cardiac penetrating and blunt trauma can result in commotio cordis, intramural hematoma, valvular damage, septal damage, myocardial infarction, arrhythmias, and tamponade. The right ventricle often is damaged due to its location.[141] Commotio cordis involves no anatomical or structural damage but results in sudden cardiac death secondary to ventricular fibrillation and vasospasm from blunt trauma.[142] Intramural hematoma is usually in the right ventricle, which may cause premature ventricular contractions or blocks. It

TABLE 29-7 Blast Injury Severity Score

	Severe	Moderate	Mild
Pao₂/Fio₂ mmHg	< 60 mmHg	60–200 mmHg	> 200 mmHg
Chest x-ray	Massive bilateral infiltrates	Bilateral or unilateral infiltrates	Localized infiltrates
Bronchial pleural fistula	Yes	Yes/No	No

Fio₂ = fraction of inspired oxygen; Pao₂ = partial pressure of oxygen.

is usually transient and resolves after 4 to 12 weeks. Coronary artery dissection, usually in the left main or left anterior descending artery, usually starts at a diseased portion of the vessel and leads to myocardial infarction. For penetrating cardiac trauma, immediate thoracotomy is indicated.[143] For tamponade, evacuation via pericardiocentesis is needed.[143]

Blunt traumatic aortic injury (BTAI) is the second most common cause of death from trauma.[144] A CT scan with IV contrast is preferred for diagnosis. Endovascular repair is preferred over open repair to minimize blood loss, paraplegia, and mortality.[145-148] Delayed treatment after a period of medical management via blood pressure control is preferred, except in patients who are at high risk for rupture, including active extravasation and pseudoaneurysm.[144]

Blunt and Penetrating Abdominal Trauma

Patients who are hemodynamically unstable warrant a focused assessment with sonography in trauma (FAST) examination and/or a CT scan, surveillance blood work, and surgical intervention.[149] Patients who are hemodynamically stable warrant surveillance blood work, imaging studies, and serial physical examination. A laparotomy is not indicated for patients with penetrating abdominal trauma from stab wounds or gunshot wounds without signs of peritonitis or diffuse abdominal tenderness.[150] Laparoscopy may be used to evaluate concomitant diaphragmatic or peritoneal damage. Selective nonoperative management of abdominal gunshot wounds reduces the rates of negative and nontherapeutic laparotomies and reduces overall length of stay.[151]

Extremity Trauma

The initial goal of treatment of penetrating or blunt trauma to the extremities is to control hemorrhage, via manual compression, clips for visible vessels, or tourniquet.[152] Imaging should include areas above and below the injury. Antibiotics are prescribed if there is an open wound, and tetanus prophylaxis should be administered. In the event of an amputation, the amputated part is wrapped in sterile saline and indirectly cooled. Reimplantation is contraindicated if warm ischemia time is 6 hours or more for major extremities or 10 hours or more for digits.[153] Nerve damage is assessed via a thorough physical examination for neuropathy. Vascular injury can also be assessed via physical examination. Patients with active extravasation, absent pulses, or bruit should go to the operative room without surgery.[154] Patients with unexplainable hematoma, a wound next to an artery, and neurological deficit may prompt further imaging. An ankle-brachial index (ABI) less than 0.9 has a 87% sensitivity and 97% specificity for arterial injury.[155] An ABI greater than 0.9 has a 100% specificity of predicting safe discharge.[156]

CHEMICAL WARFARE

When chemicals are involved, responders must wear personal protective equipment (PPE).[157] First responders should wear level A PPE and first receivers (at the decontamination unit) should wear level C PPE (Table 29-8). First receivers in the hospital (postdecontamination) should wear work clothes (such as surgical scrubs), a mask, and surgical gloves, and may wear PPE.

Decontamination includes removal of contaminated clothes and irrigation with lukewarm water and soap, if available. Spot decontamination may be performed with reactive skin decontamination lotion, activated charcoal, flour, clay, or bread for nerve gas and blistering agents.

Chemical agents are categorized as pulmonary agents, blood agents, vesicants, nerve agents, and incapacitating agents.[158] Prompt recognition is key. There may be unusual scents and smoke. Chlorine is a yellow-green gas with chlorine odor; phosgene is colorless or seen as a white cloud, with a hay, grass,

TABLE 29-8 Levels of Personal Protective Equipment

Level A	Level B	Level C	Level D
Highest level of skin, respiratory, and eye protection required	*Highest level of respiratory but lower level of skin protection*	*Concentration and type of airborne substances are known and criteria for air purifying respirators are met*	*Work uniform, affording minimal protection*
• Positive-pressure self-contained breathing apparatus • Totally encapsulated chemical protective suit • Coveralls (optional) • Long underwear (optional) • Gloves (outer), chemical resistant • Gloves (inner), chemical resistant • Boots, chemical resistant • Hard hat (optional) • Disposable protective suit, gloves, and boots	• Positive-pressure self-contained breathing apparatus • Totally encapsulated chemical protective suit • Coveralls (optional) • Gloves (outer), chemical resistant • Gloves (inner), chemical resistant • Boots, chemical resistant (optional) • Hard hat (optional) • Face shield (optional)	• Full-face or half-face mask, air purifying respirators • Hooded chemical-resistant clothing • Coveralls (optional) • Gloves (outer and inner), chemical resistant • Boots, chemical resistant (optional) • Boot-covers, chemical resistant (optional) • Hard hat (optional) • Escape mask (optional) • Face shield (optional)	• Coveralls • Gloves (optional) • Boots/shoes, chemical resistant • Boots (outer), chemical resistant (optional) • Safety glasses or chemical splash goggles (optional) • Hard hat (optional) • Escape mask (optional) • Face shield (optional)

Source: Occupational Safety and Health Administration. Occupational safety and health standards: hazardous materials. Regulations (standards—29 CFR). https://www.osha.gov/pls/oshaweb/owadisp.show_document?p_table=STANDARDS&p_id=9767. Accessed May 24, 2018.

or corn odor; cyanide has the odor of bitter almonds; sulfur mustard has a yellow-brown vapor that is odorless or has an onion, garlic, mustard, or asphalt odor; tabun has a fruit odor; and VX (nerve gas) has an amber color.[158-161]

Chlorine and Phosgene

Chlorine and phosgene have an acrid smell and are respiratory irritants. Chlorine combines with reactive oxygen species and other airway constituents to form reactive oxidants.[162] At 40 to 60 parts per million (ppm), reactive airway disease, pneumonitis, or acute pulmonary edema can develop. At 400 ppm, it can be fatal in over 30 minutes. Phosgene ($COCl_2$) has 3 phases: the initial phase (bioprotective) causes a vagal reflex action; the second phase (clinical latent) lasts for several hours postexposure with no signs or symptoms despite progression of airway edema; and the third phase (terminal) leads to noncardiogenic pulmonary edema.[163] Treatment for both is supportive.

Cyanide

Cyanide binds to the trivalent iron of cytochrome oxidase and inhibits catalytic function.[164] This histotoxic hypoxia leads to metabolic acidosis, hyperlactatemia, and reduced arteriovenous oxygen difference. It leads to confusion, convulsions, coma, and cardiorespiratory arrest.[164] Treatment consists of sodium thiosulphate (1250 mg IV over 10 minutes) to convert cyanide to thiocyanate; sodium nitrite (300 mg IV over 10 minutes) to convert hemoglobin to methemoglobin, which binds cyanide; and hydroxocobalamin 400 m IV over 20 minutes, which forms cyanocobalamin with cyanide.[164]

Mustard Gas

Mustard gas forms sulfonium ions, which causes nicotinamide adenine dinucleotide (NAD^+) depletion, glycolysis, and release of proteases. Diffuse erythema, edema, and burns are seen. Eye pain, blurred vision, lacrimation, bronchiolitis, and bone marrow suppression may occur.[164] Sodium thiosulphate, vitamin E, and dexamethasone have been suggested to improve survival and reduce organ failure.[164,165]

Nerve Gas

Nerve gases, such as sarin, Soman, VX, and tabun, are high-potency anticholinesterases.[164] Their mechanism of action is inactivation of acetylcholinesterase, leading to accumulation of acetylcholine at muscarine, nicotine, and central synapses. It has a triphasic syndrome. The first cholinergic phase lasts for 1 to 2 days and consists of a depolarizing neuromuscular blockade that results from accumulation of acetylcholine that can lead to bronchoconstriction, bradycardia, seizures, and neuromuscular respiratory failure.[164] The second phase lasts for 4 to 18 days and consists of a nondepolarizing blockade due to downregulation of acetylcholine receptors, which causes muscle weakness, cranial nerve palsies, and respiratory failure.[164] The third phase involves inactivation of the neuropathy target esterase enzyme

and occurs 7 to 14 days after exposure. It is characterized by sensation disturbances in addition to weakness.[164]

Pretreatment consists of nerve agent pyridostigmine pretreatment (NAPP) that reversibly inhibits 30% of the acetylcholinesterase. This prevents the nerve gas from binding to the acetylcholinesterase. Later on, pyridostigmine-induced inhibition is reversed, allowing the activity of acetylcholinesterase to resume. Treatment consists of atropine (2 mg IV every 2 minutes until pupillary dilatation and heart rate [HR] is greater than 80 beats/min), which antagonizes muscarinic side effects and pralidoxime (15–30 mg/kg IV or IM over 20 minutes and can be repeated every 4 hours for a therapeutic level of 4 μ/mL), which antagonizes nicotinic side effects.[164]

BIOLOGICAL WARFARE

Anthrax is caused by the Gram-positive bacteria *Bacillus anthracis* and has cutaneous, gastrointestinal, inhalation, and injectional forms.[164,166] Diagnosis and treatment are based on the clinical presentation, cultures, lumbar puncture, and radiographs. The cutaneous form has a 1- to 12-day incubation period and manifests as a pruritic papule that progresses to a pustule, and then to an eschar with associated edema, fever, and adenopathy.[166,167] Mortality is 1%.[168] Treatment is a 7- to 10-day course of quinolone, doxycycline, or penicillin for isolated cutaneous anthrax that does not involve the head or neck.[166] The gastrointestinal form consists of esophageal ulcers, adenopathy, dysphagia, and fever followed by abdominal pain, nausea and vomiting, diarrhea, and ascites.[166] Mortality is 60%.[169,170] The inhalation form has an incubation period of 1 day to 9 weeks and consists of constitutional symptoms, shock, respiratory distress leading to ARDS with hemorrhagic mediastinitis, pleural effusions, and pericardial effusions.[166] Mortality is 45% to 90%.[166,171] The injectional form is not associated with eschar and can progress to meningitis and shock. Mortality is 34%.[168] In injectional, gastrointestinal, and inhalation forms when meningitis has not been ruled out, a 60-day treatment consisting of quinolone, linezolid, and meropenem is warranted.[166] Glucocorticoid is recommended for meningitis or extensive cutaneous anthrax with edema involving the head and neck. If meningitis is ruled out, a quinolone with linezolid or clindamycin is advised.[166] It has been advocated to also administer an antitoxin such as raxibacumab, obiltoxaximab, and anthrax immunoglobulin.[166,172,173] For postexposure prophylaxis, anthrax vaccine is given along with ciprofloxacin and doxycycline for 60 days.[166]

Ricin is a protein derivative of castor beans. The toxin has 2 subunits connected by a disulfide bridge. It is internalized, where it depurinates the adenine residue of 28S ribosomal RNA within the 60S subunit, irreversibly inactivates the elongation of polypeptides, and causes cell death.[164,174] It can be inhaled, ingested, or absorbed through the skin.[175] Symptoms include shortness of breath, cough, abdominal pain, diarrhea, drowsiness, confusion, coma, weakness, and cardiovascular collapse, leading to death within 36 to 72 hours.[164] Treatment is supportive and an avian antitoxin has been developed for use in animals.[164]

Smallpox is caused by the variola virus. The incubation period of 10 to 14 days is followed by constitutional symptoms, and then an infectious period characterized by a rash starting in the mouth and spreading centrifugally, progressing to macules, papules, vesicles, and scabs in 2 weeks.[166] The mortality rate is 25%.[176] Diagnosis is based on culture, PCR, and serologic testing.[166] Airborne precautions are warranted. There is currently no available treatment, although there are investigational drugs such as cidofovir and tecovirimat.[166,177] A smallpox vaccine, ACAM2000, is given after exposure but before the rash appears.[166] It is contraindicated in immunocompromised patients and is associated with side effects such as pericarditis, myocarditis, eczema vaccinatum, generalized vaccinia, progressive vaccinia, and vaccinia encephalitis.[178-182]

Plague is caused by bacterium *Yersinia pestis* and is transmitted via fleas.[166] There are 3 presentations: (1) bubonic plague, which consists of constitutional symptoms, lymphadenopathy, and intense pain near adenopathy; (2) septicemic plague with gastrointestinal symptoms and leading to multiorgan failure; and (3) pneumonic plague, which can be primary but is usually secondary to hematogenous spread, leading to dyspnea, fever, chest pain, and hemoptysis. Diagnosis is via culture and serology. Treatment consists of a 10-day course of streptomycin, gentamicin, or doxycycline.[183,184] Postexposure prophylaxis consists of a 7-day course of doxycycline or a 10-day course of a quinolone.[183,184]

Botulism is caused by the Gram-positive spore forming bacillus *Clostridium botulinum*, which produces neurotoxins, the most toxic being neurotoxin A. These toxins bind to presynaptic receptors at cholinergic synapses, internalize, and permanently inhibit acetylcholine release.[165] There are several forms, such as infantile, wound, gastrointestinal, and inhalational, which is the worst form.[164] Six hours after inhalation, there is descending paralysis and cranial nerve dysfunction.[164] Diagnosis is based on culture, mouse assays, and detection of the toxin.[164] Treatment consists of administration of the heptavalent A-G antitoxin.[164,184] Due to the risk of polymicrobial infection with wound botulism, antibiotics such as metronidazole or penicillin are used as adjunct.

Shellfish poisoning is secondary to dinoflagellates, which include *Alexandrium tamarense*, *Gymnodinium catenatum*, and *Pyrodinium bahamense*.[164] It is an inhibitor of voltage-gated sodium channels with ingestion, leading to nausea and diarrhea, paralysis, and respiratory and cardiovascular failure.[164] A guinea pig antitoxin has been developed.

QUESTIONS

1. A 30-year-old woman was in a motor vehicle accident in which his car exploded. She has sustained burns on her anterior and posterior chest and abdomen and circumferential burns around her right upper extremity. What percentage of burns does the patient have?

   A. 27%
   B. 36%
   C. 45%
   D. 54%

2. A 59-year-old woman is pulled out of a burning building and arrives in the emergency department (ED). Her past medical history is unknown. Her vital signs are as follows: BP of 120/80 mmHg, HR of 80 beats/min, respiratory rate (RR) of 18 breaths/min, and oxygen saturation of 98% on nonrebreather. She is arousable to painful stimulation and her clothes have some charred edges. No burns are noted. Her oral pharynx shows some redness but no edema. Her lungs are clear to auscultation. What would you do next?

   A. Intubate
   B. Watch and observe
   C. Administer steroids
   D. Administer antibiotics

3. Carbon monoxide and cyanide poisoning can be found in patients with smoking injury. Which of the following is true?

   A. Cyanide is not found in cassava.
   B. A lactic acid level can be a surrogate for cyanide poisoning.
   C. Hemolytic anemias can have elevated carboxyhemoglobin.
   D. All of the above

4. A 24-year-old man was exposed to a colorless gas with an odor like that of hay. After a couple of hours, the patient denies any symptoms and appears to be hemodynamically stable. What is the next step?

   A. Continue monitoring
   B. Start oral prednisone 40 mg daily
   C. Discharge patient home
   D. Start ipratropium bromide/albuterol every 6 hours

5. A 30-year-old man had a head-on collision with a truck. On physical examination, his right eye is dilated but both eyes are reactive to light. He has some facial lacerations to his forehead. A cervical collar is in place. His lungs are clear to auscultation. His heart sounds are regular. His abdomen is soft and nontender. Bowel sounds are present. A neurologic examination showed that the patient is arousable to his name but falls asleep right away. His head CT shows a subdural hemorrhage. Which of the following would be the most effective in improving increased intracranial pressure?

   A. Elevating his head 30 degrees
   B. Administering hypertonic saline
   C. Administering mannitol
   D. Hyperventilation

6. For the patient in question 5, what is the next step?

    A. Phenytoin 100 mg IV every 8 hours
    B. Therapeutic hypothermia
    C. Enoxaparin
    D. Dexamethasone 10 mg IV every 6 hours

7. Which is true regarding cranial hemorrhage?

    A. Early (within 48 hours) evacuation of intracerebral hemorrhage is beneficial compared to conservative management.
    B. There is no role for evacuation for cerebellar hemorrhage.
    C. Deep intracerebral hemorrhage should be removed.
    D. None of the above.

8. A 20-year-old woman fell from a second-floor window. She was found unconscious. She had a cervical collar placed, and she was subsequently intubated for airway protection. In the ED, she had a high quality CT of her entire body, which showed some rib fractures. What is the next step?

    A. Remove the cervical collar.
    B. Wait for the patient to awaken and then have her perform maneuvers.
    C. Order a cervical MRI.
    D. Order an x-ray.

9. A 56-year-old woman was complaining of headache and neck pain in the ED. She was discharged on an NSAID. Her daughter found her unresponsive in her bathroom. Emergency medical services (EMS) arrived and she was subsequently intubated and sent to the ED. Laboratory and computed tomography (Fig. 29-2) findings from the ED are as follows:

WBC $10 \times 10^3/\mu L$
Hgb $12.1 \times 10^6/\mu L$

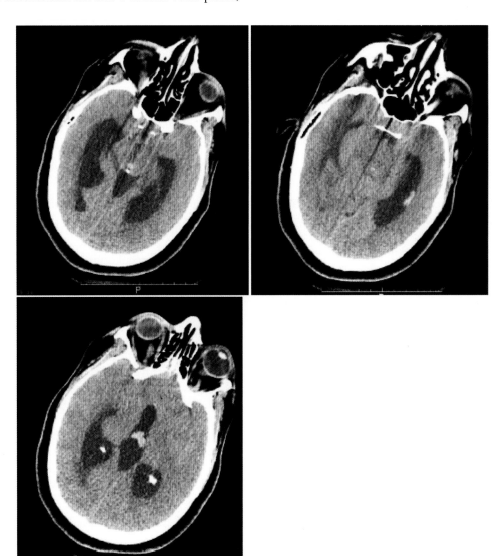

FIGURE 29-2 CT head obtained in the emergency department.

plt	$246 \times 10^3/\mu L$
Na	138 mEq/L
K	3.2 mEq/L
Cl	105 mEq/L
CO_2	25 mEq/L
BUN	13 mg/dL
Crea	0.80 mg/dL
Ca	9.2 mg/dL
INR	1.01

An external ventricular drain was placed. A CT angiogram of the brain showed no aneurysm or AV malformation. What would be the next step?

A. FFP
B. PCC 3
C. Lumbar puncture
D. Intraventricular tPA

10. A 70-year-old man with diabetes, chronic obstructive pulmonary disease, hypertension, sick sinus syndrome status post–permanent pacemaker implantation had a mechanical fall. He was noted to have posterior and lateral fractures of left ribs 3 through 8 and a left-sided pneumothorax. (Fig. 29-3). A left-sided chest tube was placed. Patient is on IV dilaudid for pain but still complains of inadequate pain control. What is the next step?

A. Mechanical ventilation
B. Surgical fixation
C. Epidural anesthesia
D. Continue current management

11. A passenger involved in a motor vehicle accident sustained a hemothorax. A surgical chest tube has been placed. After two days, the repeat chest radiograph shows persistent effusion. What is the next step?

A. Insert another chest tube
B. Administer thrombolytics

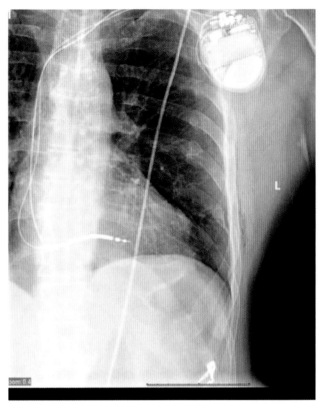

FIGURE 29-3 Chest radiography.

C. Perform video-assisted thoracoscopic surgery
D. Continue current management

12. This is the TEG of a patient admitted for hemorrhagic shock secondary to motor vehicular accident (Fig. 29-4). What is the next step?

A. Platelet transfusion
B. Fresh frozen plasma
C. Observation
D. Tranexamic acid

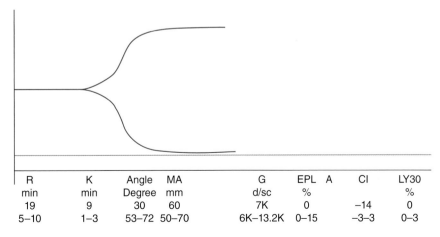

R min	K min	Angle Degree	MA mm		G d/sc	EPL %	A	CI	LY30 %
19	9	30	60		7K	0		−14	0
5–10	1–3	53–72	50–70		6K–13.2K	0–15		−3–3	0–3

FIGURE 29-4 TEG.

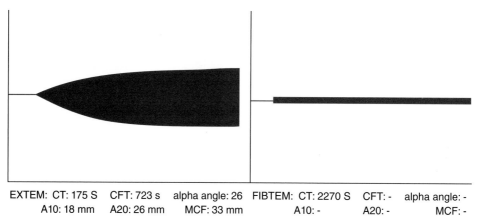

EXTEM: CT: 175 S   CFT: 723 s   alpha angle: 26   FIBTEM: CT: 2270 S   CFT: -   alpha angle: -
        A10: 18 mm   A20: 26 mm   MCF: 33 mm   A10: -   A20: -   MCF: -

FIGURE 29-5 Initial ROTEM.

13. A 30-year-old soldier sustained trauma after a bomb exploded. His initial ROTEM is shown in Figure 29-5. What would be the next best step?

    A. Fibrinogen and platelets
    B. Platelets
    C. Fibrinogen
    D. Tranexamic acid, fibrinogen concentrate, PCC, factor XIII

14. A 21-year-old man was complaining of severe right arm pain. He was bitten by a rattle snake 45 minutes ago. What is the next step?

    A. Give 1 vial of antivenom
    B. Give 2 to 3 vials of antivenom
    C. Give 4 to 6 vials of antivenom
    D. Apply a tourniquet

15. A 60-year-old morbidly obese woman with obstructive sleep apnea compliant to continuous positive airway pressure (CPAP), hypertension, and diabetes was involved in a motor vehicle accident. On physical examination, her vital signs were as follows: BP of 140/90 mmHg, HR of 122 beats/min, RR of 24 breaths/min, and oxygen saturation of 85% on room air. She has multiple facial wounds, and blood appears to be gushing out of her mouth. Her chest is nontender and her lungs are clear to auscultation. Heart sounds are tachycardia with no murmurs. Her abdomen was soft and slightly tender, with hypoactive bowel sounds and ecchymoses noted on the left upper quadrant. Her extremities showed good pulses with no edema or cyanosis. Which approach is best to secure airway?

    A. Macintosh laryngoscope
    B. Miller laryngoscope
    C. GlideScope
    D. Needle cricothyroidectomy

16. A 65-year-old woman with diabetes and a prior cerebro-vascular accident but with no residual deficits had a mechanical fall, sustaining left-sided trochanteric hip fracture. What is the next step?

    A. Surgery after 72 hours
    B. No surgical intervention
    C. Antibiotic prophylaxis after surgery
    D. DVT prophylaxis initiated 48 hours after surgery and when hemoglobin is stable

17. An 80-year-old man sustained a mechanical fall while getting out of the shower. He was found to have a right non-displaced cervical fracture of the middle portion on anteroposterior chest radiograph. What would be the next step?

    A. Observation
    B. Sling and ice
    C. Order a CT chest
    D. Surgical evaluation

18. Which of the following statements is true regarding bioterrorism?

    A. Rocky Mountain spotted fever has eschar formation prior to onset of lymphadenopathy.
    B. Q fever has ulcerative glands as a clinical presentation.
    C. Plague, tularemia, Rocky Mountain spotted fever, and Q fever have ticks as vectors.
    D. Plague, tularemia, Rocky Mountain spotted fever, and Q fever can be treated with doxycycline.

19. A 25-year-old man was involved in a motor vehicular accident. His CT with IV contrast is shown in Figure 29-6. What is the grade of traumatic aortic injury and what is the next step?

    A. Grade 1 and BP control
    B. Grade 2 and endovascular aneurysm repair
    C. Grade 3 and endovascular aneurysm repair
    D. Grade 4 and open repair

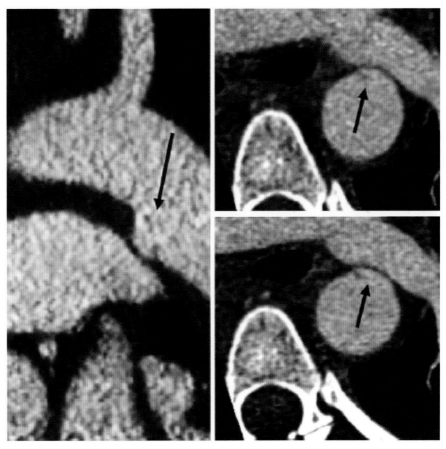

FIGURE 29-6 Traumatic aortic injury marked by arrow. (Reprinted with permission from Cullen EL, Lantz EJ, Johnson CM, Young PM. Traumatic aortic injury: CT findings, mimics, and therapeutic options. *Cardiovasc Diagn Ther.* 2014;4(3):238-244.)

20. A 35 year old man presents with symptoms of fever, headache, and rash about 48 hours after being bitten by a spider (Fig. 29-7). What is the type of spider?

A. *Loxosceles*
B. *Latrodectus* spp
C. *Atrax* and *Hydronyche spp*
D. *Centruroides*

ANSWERS

1. C. 45%

   As shown in Figure 29-8, the anterior trunk represents 18%, the posterior trunk represents 18%, and anterior and posterior right upper extremities represent 9%. The patient has a total of 45% TBSA burned. Choices A, B, and D are incorrect.

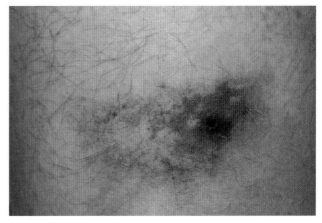

FIGURE 29-7 Patient presents with discoloration on right arm and diffuse rash. (Reproduced with permission from Zafren K, Thurman R, Jones ID. Environmental conditions. In: Knoop KJ, Stack LB, Storrow AB, Thurman R. eds. *The Atlas of Emergency Medicine.* 4th ed. New York, NY: McGraw-Hill; 2016.)

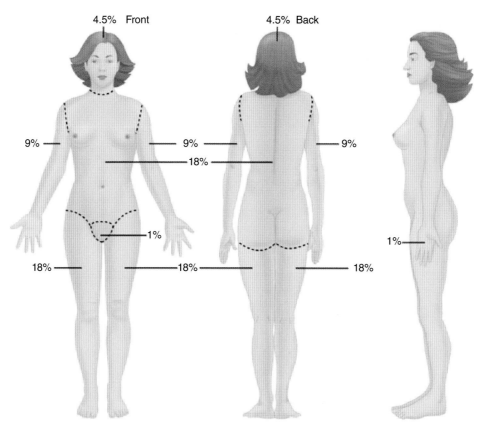

4.5% Front

4.5% Back

9% — 9% — 9%

18%

— 1%

1% —

18% — 18% — 18%

FIGURE 29-8 Body diagram for estimation of total burned surface area (% TBSA) in adults, using the rule of nines (numbers are for anterior only and posterior only). (Reproduced with permission from Friedstat J, Endorf FW, Gibran NS. Burns. In: Brunicardi F, Andersen DK, Billiar TR, Dunn DL, Hunter JG, Matthews JB, Pollock RE, eds. *Schwartz's Principles of Surgery. 10th ed.* New York, NY: McGraw-Hill; 2015.)

2. **A. Intubate**

Inhalation injury is found in 8% to 15% of burn patients with a mean mortality rate of 56% in 2 series.[185-189] The history and physical findings of smoke exposure, facial burns, singed nasal vibrissae, and carbonaceous secretions can suggest but not confirm inhalation injury. Fiberoptic bronchoscopic (FOB) inspection can confirm injury with the presence of erythema, mucosa edema, gray mucosal discoloration, erosions, or desquamation.[185] However, a negative FOB finding does not exclude the presence of inhalation injury, since this is a dynamic process, and a repeat FOB is sometimes warranted to see progression of disease and/or to exclude the presence of parenchymal disease.[185-193] Acute upper airway obstruction can be suggested by serial nasopharyngeal examination revealing edematous obliteration of aryepiglottic fold, arytenoid eminences, and interarytenoid areas.[193] Nebulized heparin (5000–10,000 units every 4–6 hours) with normal saline has been shown to decrease cast formation in animal models, and heparin with N-acetylcysteine has been shown to decrease reintubation and mortality in children.[185-187,193] Bronchial hygiene therapy (coughing, chest physiotherapy, ambulation, suctioning, bronchoscopy, and pharmacologic agents) and lung protective strategy are usually employed.[193] Although it has been hypothesized that corticosteroids are an attractive option to decrease inflammation

and edema, they can also delay wound healing (choice C). Antibiotics should be reserved for when there is evidence of true infection (choice D). Inhalation injury is a dynamic process, and watching and waiting can lead to catastrophic results (choice B).

3. **B. A lactic acid level can be a surrogate for cyanide poisoning.**

Smoke inhalation is associated with carbon monoxide and cyanide poisoning. In pure smoke inhalation, cyanide is the leading cause of mortality.[194] In inhalation injury, concomitant carbon monoxide poisoning has a higher rate of mortality.[195,196] Cyanide is found with the combustion of synthetic materials, but also in the pits of apricots, bitter almonds, cherries, and peaches; in cassava root; and in the medication sodium nitroprusside[195] (choice A). Cyanide binds and inhibits cytochrome oxidase a_3 in the mitochondrial electron transport chain, resulting in anaerobic generation of ATP and profound acidosis with lactate generation.[195] Cyanide is eliminated by its hepatic conversion to thiocyanate via the enzyme rhodanese and subsequent renal excretion.[196] Patients with acute renal failure are predisposed to cyanide poisoning.

Carbon monoxide is the result of combustion of fuels. Carbon monoxide has an affinity greater for hemoglobin

TABLE 29-9 Comparison Between Carbon Monoxide Poisoning and Cyanide Poisoning

Carbon Monoxide Poisoning	Cyanide Poisoning
• Mild: headache, dizziness, nausea, vomiting, flu-like symptoms, fatigue, confusion • Severe: delirium, ataxia, coma, chest pain, SOB, MI, CVA	• Mild: headache, nausea, vertigo, HTN • Severe: SOB, bradycardia, HTN, arrhythmias, coma

CVA = cerebrovascular accident; HTN = hypertension; MI = myocardial infarction; SOB = shortness of breath.

compared to oxygen (200 to 1) and causes a leftward shift in the hemoglobin-oxygen dissociation curve, which results in hypoxia.[195] 10% to 15% of carbon monoxide binds to myoglobin and impairs oxygen delivery to myocardial mitochondria, which can lead to ischemia.[197] Symptom comparison between carbon monoxide poisoning and cyanide poisoning is seen in Table 29-9.

Diagnosis of carbon monoxide poisoning begins with a high degree of suspicion. Standard pulse oximetry will not be able to differentiate the different wavelengths of hemoglobin, carboxyhemoglobin, and methemoglobin.[195] Carbon monoxide symptoms are only present in 30% of patients, and cherry red lips are only present in 40% of patients.[193] Serum carboxyhemoglobin can aid in the diagnosis of carbon monoxide poisoning but can also be seen in methylene chloride, hemolytic anemia, and newborns (choice C). Normal levels are 2% to 3% in nonsmokers and 5% to 13% in chronic smokers.[195] Serum carboxyhemoglobin levels fall by one-half in 4 hours in patients breathing in room air and in 1 hour in patients breathing 100% oxygen.[193] This can lead to falsely normal levels, since most burn patients are immediately placed on 100% oxygen regardless of levels (choice D).[193] Neurologic sequelae are not uncommon, and age greater than 36 years and 24-hour exposure are independent risk factors.[196] These sequelae include cognitive decline such as disorientation, amnesia, and visual and spatial skills; delayed onset parkinsonism; dystonia; chorea; myoclonus; anxiety; depression; and irritability.[197] Standard treatment is oxygen supplementation. Hyperbaric oxygen therapy (100% at 2.4–3 atm) may be used in patients with loss of consciousness, pregnancy, duration of exposure of 24 hours, hemodynamic instability, acidosis, and/or a carboxyhemoglobin level of 25%, since it can lower the carbon monoxide elimination half-life to 20 minutes.[196,198,199]

Just like with carbon monoxide poisoning, diagnosis for cyanide poisoning begins with a high degree of suspicion. Elevated lactic acid can be a surrogate for cyanide poisoning since aerobic metabolism is shifted toward anaerobic metabolism, reaching 8 mmol/L in nonsmokers and 10 mmol/L in smokers (choice B).[197] Cyanide levels may be obtained but are often delayed (choice A). Toxic levels start at 1 mg/L.[197,200] Treatment consists of amyl nitrite, sodium nitrite, and sodium thiosulfate. Elevated levels of Pao$_2$ on venous blood gas are highly suggestive of cyanide poisoning, since the cells are not able to extract oxygen (choice C).[197] Potential complications include hypotension and hypoxia from nitrites displacing oxygen from hemoglobin-producing methemoglobin. Hydroxocobalamin, however, is an alternative that does not carry these side effects (Table 29-10).[198]

4. A. Continue monitoring

The patient was most likely exposed to phosgene. Patients develop delayed-onset cardiogenic pulmonary edema, and it would be best to continue monitoring this patient. Corticosteroids (choice B) and albuterol (choice D) would not be able to prevent the development of this complication. Discharging the patient will not allow acute response once cardiogenic pulmonary edema develops (choice C).

TABLE 29-10 Cyanide Poisoning Treatment

Antidote	Mechanism of Action	Administration	Notes
• Cyanide kit • Amyl nitrite • Sodium nitrite • Sodium thiosulfate	• Oxides iron in hemoglobin to cyanmethemoglobin, which draws cyanide away from mitochondrial cytochrome a$_3$ • Acts as a sulfur donor to form thiosulfate	• Amyl nitrite: inhaled for 15–30 sec • Sodium nitrite: IV over 3–5 min • Sodium thiosulfate IV over 30 min	• Methemoglobin should not exceed 20% • Avoid in pregnancy • Contraindicated in smoke inhalation
• Hydroxocobalamin	• Binds to cyanide to form cyanocobalamin	• 5 g IV over 15 minutes	• Red color in skin and urine within 2–3 d • Interferes with tests for magnesium, liver function, creatinine, iron, carboxyhemoglobin, methemoglobin, oxyhemoglobin

IV = intravenous.

5. B. Administering hypertonic saline

Medical management to reduce ICP includes adequate sedation—since coughing, agitation, and posturing can elevate ICP—and elevation of the head to least 45 to 90 degrees at the midline to facilitate venous drainage (choice A). Hypertonic saline (7.5–23.4%) has been shown to improve ICP better and has fewer treatment failures compared to mannitol.[201-210] The sodium goal is 145 to 155 mEq/L every 4 to 6 hours. Hypertonic saline draws fluid from the cerebral parenchyma and reduces intracranial volume and ICP. Complications include hypokalemia, hyperchloremic acidosis, and bleeding from platelet aggregation dysfunction and prolonged coagulation times.[110] Mannitol (choice C), at a dose of 0.25 to 1.4 g/kg (for herniation), lowers ICP in 1 to 5 minutes, peaks at 20 to 60 minutes, and lasts for 1.5 to 6 hours.[110] Long-term reduction in ICP requires 0.25 to 0.5 g/kg every 4 to 6 hours. Mannitol is a volume expander that decreases blood viscosity and improves cerebral blood flow and oxygenation in a manner that is more pronounced with an intact pressure autoregulation.[110] It draws fluid from the cerebral parenchyma, and this process takes about 15 to 30 minutes.[110] For maximal effect, the serum osmolarity goal is 310 to 320 mOsm/L but must remain at or below 320 mOsm/L to prevent hypovolemia, renal failure, and hyperosmolarity. Because it can cross the blood–brain barrier and worsen vasogenic edema by drawing fluid into the CNS, it should be tapered over 2 to 3 days to prevent rebound edema and increased ICP.[110,112] Hyperventilation (mild hypocapnia with goal PCO_2 of 30–35 mmHg) decreases ICP by causing alkalosis, which can cause vasoconstriction of cerebral arterioles (choice D). Cerebral blood flow is already compromised in the first 24 hours, so hyperventilation should be reserved for spikes in ICP after that period. This effect is short lived, lasting 11 to 20 hours. The CSF pH will eventually normalize, which will cause cerebral arterioles to dilate, which in turn increases ICP. Hyperventilation can decrease cerebral blood flow, but it is uncertain if it can trigger ischemia. Barbiturates are used in refractory elevated ICP despite medical and/or surgical treatment. They decrease metabolic demand, blood flow, and ICP. Complications include hypotension, hypoxia, and secondary ischemia. Pentobarbital is loaded at 10 mg/kg over 30 minutes with maintenance dose of 1 mg/kg/h.

6. A. Phenytoin 100 mg IV every 8 hours

Use of prophylactic antiepileptics such as phenytoin for posttraumatic seizures (PTS) is advocated within the first 7 days.[113] However, PTS has not been associated with worse outcomes. There is insufficient evidence to recommend prophylactic hypothermia because it has not been shown to improve mortality compared to normothermia (choice B).[113,211,212] Compression stockings or intermittent pneumatic compression to prevent deep vein thrombosis

has been advocated over the use chemoprophylaxis because of the risk of hematoma expansion.[113] Since then, further investigations have suggested safety with chemoprophylaxis after 24 hours or after 48 hours of radiographic stability of the hemorrhage.[113,213,214] Risk for DVT increases if chemoprophylaxis is withheld after 7 days.[214] Although this patient would benefit from DVT prophylaxis, he would have to be re-evaluated after 24 hours and the hemorrhage would have to be stable (choice C). Corticosteroids are generally avoided in TBI because they are associated with worse outcomes (choice D).[113]

7. D. None of the above

In the Surgical Trial in Intracerebral Hemorrhage (STITCH), there was no overall benefit from early surgery (choice A), defined as within 48 hours (468 patients), versus conservative treatment (496 patients) ($P = 0.414$ with a 6-month mortality of 36% vs 37%).[124] However, there was a trend toward favorable outcomes with surgical intervention for superficial ICH that were 1 cm or less from the cortical surface compared to deeper hematomas (choice C).[124] A cerebellar hemorrhage should be removed if the size is 3 cm with worsening neurological status, there is a risk of brainstem compression, or there is obstructive hydrocephalus (choice B).

8. A. Remove the cervical collar.

For intubated and unconscious patients, a high-quality CT of the cervical spine is sufficient for clearance, with a negative predictive value of 91% and with a 0% incidence of unstable injuries after initial negative CT.[215] The patient does not need to be awake for cervical clearance (choice B). No further imaging is necessary for cervical spine clearance in patients who are awake and alert, with no neck pain or head trauma, no drugs or alcohol, no abnormal neurologic finding, and no other "distracting" injury. Physical examination findings of no bruises, deformities, or tenderness, and pain-free active movements clear the patient. For symptomatic conscious patients, an x-ray with lateral, anteroposterior, and open mouth views are needed (choice D). An anteroposterior x-ray should be able to evaluate the spinous process of the C2 through T1 vertebrae. The open-mouth view should be able to see C1 and the odontoid peg. A CT scan should be used to evaluate areas that are not seen on x-ray. Areas above and below the area should be investigated, since they need to be undamaged for internal fixation. An MRI is warranted if an abnormality is found (choice C).

9. D. Intraventricular tPA

Intraventricular hemorrhage is rarely seen alone but usually is seen with intracerebral hemorrhage or subarachnoid hemorrhage. Recurrence of bleeding is possible, particularly if there is an associated coagulopathy or vascular malformation, or an obstructing hydrocephalus.

The patient does not have an associated aneurysm or coagulopathy, so giving her fresh frozen plasma (choice A) or PCC 3 (choice B) would not be helpful. This patient has obstructive hydrocephalus, and therefore, intraventricular tPA is needed. In several studies, it has been shown to increase clot resolution, reduce need for repeat EVD, reduce shunting, decrease ventriculitis, and decrease mortality.[216-221] The procedure entails (1) withdrawal of a volume of CSF equivalent to the drug dosage; (2) injection of tPA through the ventriculostomy at a dose of 3 to 8 mg, with a higher dose given when all ventricles are affected; (3) flushing the catheter with 1 to 1.5 mL of preservative-free normal saline; (4) clamping the EVD for 2 hours and unclamping if ICP is greater than 25 mmHg to allow 1 to 2 mL of CSF to drain; (5) after 2 hours, alternating EVD from open to zero gravity to closed every 1 hour for 12 hours; (6) repeating head CT at 12 to 24 hours; and (7) repeating tPA, as necessary, depending on results.[221,222] CLEAR III is a randomized double-blinded placebo-controlled multiregional trial of patients with an EVD with stable, nontraumatic ICH less than 30 mL, with intraventricular hemorrhage obstructing the third or fourth ventricle, and with intracerebral hemorrhage.[222] The study showed that patients given 12 doses of 1-mg alteplase versus 0.9% saline had lower case fatality (46 [18%] vs 73 [29%]; hazard ratio, 0.60; 95% CI, 0.41–0.86; $P = 0.006$), but a greater proportion had a modified Rankin scale (mRS) score of 5 after 180 days (42 [17%] vs 21 [9%]; RR, 1.99; 95% CI, 1.22–3.26; $P = 0.007$).[222] This patient had an isolated intraventricular hemorrhage.

Patients with intraventricular hemorrhage can progress to intracranial hypertension as a result of obstructive hydrocephalus. Decompressive craniectomy versus medical management for refractory intracranial hypertension resulted in decreased mortality (26.9% vs 48.9%) but increased vegetative state (8.5% vs 2.1%), higher rates of lower severe disability (21.9% vs 14.4%), higher upper severe disability (15.4% versus 8%), and less good recovery (4% vs 6.9%) at 6 months.[223] Since it is rarely seen in isolation, it has been hypothesized that the poor prognosis from IVH is from associated injuries.[224] Lumbar puncture is not indicated, since the patient had an external ventricular drain placed (choice C).

10. C. Epidural anesthesia

Twenty-five percent of mortality in blunt trauma is related to thoracic injury, which can result in flail chest with or without pulmonary contusion.[225,226] Pulmonary contusions are usually accompanied by chest wall injury, such as flail chest, but can occur alone in explosion injuries.[225] Flail chest is defined by 3 or more ribs with 2 or more fractures and is the result of significant kinetic trauma or mild trauma in patients with osteoporosis, multiple myeloma, or other pathologies. There are 3 variations: posterior flail segments, anterior flail segments, and bilateral flail

segments with sternal involvement. Animal studies have shown that contusions are lung parenchymal lacerations with leakage of blood and plasma into the alveoli, resulting in increased blood flow and increased vascular resistance.[227,228] Uninjured lung tissue also was noted to have delayed capillary leak with development of thickened septa, increased vacuolation, and edema within 8 hours postinjury.[229] There are long term sequelae resulting in persistent obstruction and restriction, persistent chest wall pain, and therefore persistent dyspnea.[230] Pulmonary fibrosis may appear on CT 1 to 6 years after injury. Mainstay treatment includes adequate pain control. Epidural anesthesia might be preferred if other forms of pain medication are inadequate, since it has little respiratory compromise. Studies have shown that ventilator support to overcome chest wall instability has not been beneficial and has not improved mortality (choice A).[230,231] Continuing current management (choice D) with inadequate pain control could lead to pulmonary splinting and compromised work of breathing. There is data to support surgical fixation of flail chest (choice B). Small, observational studies have shown improvement in vent days, ICU days, and overall mortality, although most surgeons are waiting for adequate data from randomized controlled trials to put this in practice.[232-242]

11. C. Perform video-assisted thoracoscopic surgery

Hemothoraces should be evaluated for drainage, and initial drainage should be with a tube thoracostomy.[243] Although it has been debated whether a hemothorax less than 1.5 cm on chest CT can be treated with observation, there have been studies that suggest drainage within 7 days prevents empyema and fibrothorax (choice D).[244-248] However, tube thoracostomy is a risk factor for empyema in 33% of patients.[244-248] The threshold for drainage for most physicians is 500 mL.[244] Although there is data to support the use of fibrinolytics, it is difficult to gauge its actual contribution over tube thoracotomy.[243] Therefore, it is a second-line treatment (choice B). Persistent hemothorax on chest radiograph, more than 1500 mL of hemothorax evacuated on tube thoracostomy, persistent bleeding from chest at a rate of 150 to 200 mL/h for 2 to 4 hours, and a persistent need for blood transfusions for hemodynamic instability warrant video-assisted thoracotomy.[243] A prospective randomized study by Meyer et al showed early video-assisted thoracoscopic surgery instead of a second chest tube (choice A) after retained hemothorax after initial chest tube placement had shorter duration of chest tube drainage, fewer hospital days, and lower hospital costs than second chest tube.[249]

12. B. Fresh frozen plasma

It is difficult to determine whether bleeding is secondary to surgical causes or to an underlying coagulopathy based on standard coagulation tests such as PTT or PT.

Limitations of these tests include the following: (1) the tests stop upon fibrin formation; (2) they do not assess the quality of the clot; (3) they do not assess hyperfibrinolysis, which is an independent predictor of mortality in trauma; (4) coagulation factor use is heterogeneous; (5) artificial colloids impair the analysis of fibrinogen; and (5) it takes more than 1 hour to get results.[250]

Therefore, viscoelastic tests such as rotational thromboelastometry and thromboelastography are often utilized. They provide dynamic information on clot formation and strength, and they break down within 15 minutes.[250] Rotational thromboelastometry has a plastic pin in a blood sample cup that rotates backs and forth.[250] Thromboelastography uses a stationary wire, and the cup is rotated.[250]

A normal TEG is shown below and illustrates the 3 phases of hemostasis: initiation (R), amplification (K), and propagation (α) (see Table 29-11 and Figure 29-9). Conventional TEG uses kaolin to activate the intrinsic pathway or R time, whereas rapid thromboelastography uses kaolin and tissue factor and produces activated clotting time (ACT).[251-268] Coagulopathy will have a prolonged R time or TEG-ACT, whereas a hypercoagulable state will have a shortened R time or TEG-ACT.[251-268] The next step is the K time and α angle, which reflects the levels of fibrinogen and the cross-linking of fibrin to the initial phase of clot formation.[251-268] Platelet aggregation occurs until the clot reaches its maximum strength at the maximum amplitude. Clot lysis soon follows and is expressed as LY-30.[251-268] For this patient, the R time is prolonged, suggesting coagulopathy or depletion of coagulation factors. Fresh frozen plasma is warranted. The K time is prolonged, and the α angle is less than 53 degrees, which would indicate the use of cryoprecipitate, which is not a choice. The maximum amplitude is within range, so platelets are not indicated (choice A). Tranexamic acid would be indicated if LY30 more than 3% due to marker for hyperfibrinolysis, but the patient's LY30 is 0% (choice D). Observation (choice C) is not indicated because the patient would continue to bleed.

13. D. Tranexamic acid, fibrinogen concentrate, PCC, factor XIII

Rotational thromboelastometry is another viscoelastic test, and its variables have similar counterparts to TEG. An activator is added to initiate the clotting time (measured in seconds) at 2 mm.[250] It is used to determine the substitution of clotting factors via FFP or to provide anticoagulant antidotes such as protamine. Clotting time (CT) is start of measurement until initiation of clotting. It involves thrombin formation and start of clot polymerization. Clotting formation time (CFT) is time of initiation of clot until the clot firmness of 20 mm is detected. It involves clot stabilization with fibrin polymeration, platelets and factor XIII. If the CFT is shortened, it suggests a hypercoagulable state. The α angle describes the kinetics of the clot. A larger angle reflects rapid clot formation and a smaller angle reflects thrombocytopenia or hypofibrinogenemia. The amplitude at 10 minutes (A10) is a surrogate for maximum clot firmness (MCF) or amplitude at 20 minutes (A20). A low MCF suggests decreased clot firmness, and an elevated MCF suggests hypercoagulable state. The lysis index measures the remaining clot firmness at 30 minutes (LI30) and 60 minutes (LI60). Intrinsic screening test (INTEM) where CT is sensitive to heparin, extrinsic screening test (EXTEM) where CT is not sensitive to heparin, APTEM where hyperfibrinolysis is identified via aprotinin, and FIBTEM, which determines contribution of fibrinogen to clot firmness, are routinely tested.[250] HEPTEM is an additional test. HEPTEM uses heparinase to inhibit heparin and identifies heparin effects (Fig. 29-10).

In EXTEM, the clotting time is prolonged at 175 seconds (43–82 seconds). The CFT is prolonged 723 seconds (normal range, 48–127 seconds). The MCF is low at 33 mm (normal range, 52–70 mm). The A20 is low at 18 mm (normal range, 50–70 mm). The α angle is low at 26 degrees (normal range, 65–80°). The FIBTEM shows an MCF of 0 (normal range, 7–24 mm). The patient needs tranexamic acid, fibrinogen concentrate, PCC, and factor XIII

TABLE 29-11 Thromboelastography

	Definition	Normal Values	Measures	Interpretation
R	Reaction time: time from start of test to formation of fibrin (initiation)	5–10 min	Intrinsic pathway	If R > 10 min, give fresh frozen plasma
K	Kinetics (s): time to achieve clot strength (amplification)	1–3 min	Fibrinogen, platelet number	If K time > 3 min, give cryoprecipitate
α angle	Slope between R and K, measures speed of clot formation (thrombin burst)	53–72 degrees	Fibrinogen, platelet number	If α angle < 53 degrees, give cryoprecipitate ± platelets
MA	Maximum amplitude (mm): strength of clot (stability of clot)	50–70 mm	Platelet number and function	If MA < 50 mm, give platelets
A30 or LY30	Amplitude at 30 min, degree of fibrinolysis	0–3%	Fibrinolysis	If LY30 > 3%, give tranexamic acid

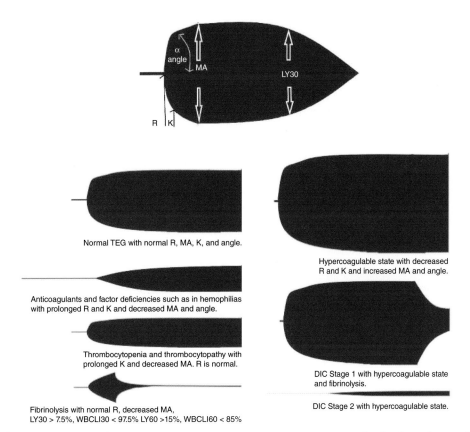

FIGURE 29-9 Different morphologies of TEG. R = Reaction Time; K = Kinetics; MA = maximum amplitude; LY30 = degree of fibrinolysis at 30 min

Normal TEG with normal R, MA, K, and angle.

Anticoagulants and factor deficiencies such as in hemophilias with prolonged R and K and decreased MA and angle.

Thrombocytopenia and thrombocytopathy with prolonged K and decreased MA. R is normal.

Fibrinolysis with normal R, decreased MA, LY30 > 7.5%, WBCLI30 < 97.5% LY60 >15%, WBCLI60 < 85%

Hypercoagulable state with decreased R and K and increased MA and angle.

DIC Stage 1 with hypercoagulable state and fibrinolysis.

DIC Stage 2 with hypercoagulable state.

(choice D). Platelets are not indicated (choices A and B). Fibrinogen concentrate is not enough (choice C). After the products are administered, the ROTEM is as follows (Fig. 29-11).

14. C. Give 4 to 6 vials of antivenom

In the United States, there are 2 groups of venomous snakes: coral snakes with red, yellow, and black bands, and crotaline

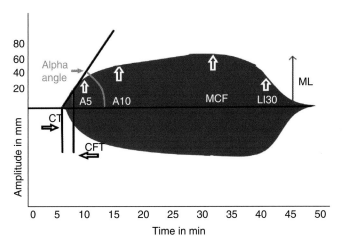

FIGURE 29-10 Rotational thromboelastometry. CT = clotting time; CFT= clotting formation time; A5 = smplitude 5 minutes after CT; A10 = amplitude 10 minutes after CT; MCF = maximum clot firmness; LI30 = clot lysis index at 30 minutes; ML = maximum lysis %.

snakes.[267] An approach to snake bites would begin with stabilization of the patient and an attempt to identify the snake. Envenomation is graded (Table 29-12).[267] Twenty-five percent of crotaline snake bites might be "dry bites"; however, envenomation is dynamic and the grade can progress. Observation for 6 to 8 hours is warranted, and if there is no progression, the patient can be discharged. Routine labs include complete blood count, complete metabolic profile, PTT, PT, urinalysis, urine myoglobin, and if the grade is 2 or higher, a DIC panel. Evidence of envenomation warrants IV and normal saline administration. Prophylactic antibiotics, a compression band or tourniquet, and incision and suction of fang marks, unless occurring within 15 to 30 minutes, are not advocated (choice D).[267] The extremity is held at the level of the heart. Compartment syndrome is a complication of rattlesnake envenomation and fasciotomy may be indicated.[267]

There are 2 types of antivenom therapy. For coral snake bites, *Micrurus* antivenin, and for crotaline snake bites, *Crotalidae* polyvalent immune fab (CroFab). For CroFab, an initial dose of 4 to 6 vials over 60 minutes is given and the patient is monitored for allergic reactions (choices A and B). If control is not achieved, an additional 4 to 6 vials can be given. If control is achieved, 3 maintenance doses of 2 vials each are given. Recurrence is when symptoms of envenomation has returned. In recurrence, 2 vials are given IV. Contraindications to CroFab include dry bite, allergic reaction, allergic reaction to sheep serum, and a history of hypersensitivity to papaya or papain.[267] Washing

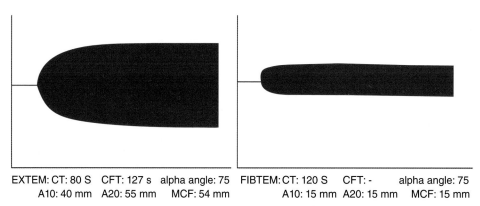

EXTEM: CT: 80 S   CFT: 127 s   alpha angle: 75   FIBTEM: CT: 120 S   CFT: -   alpha angle: 75
A10: 40 mm   A20: 55 mm   MCF: 54 mm   A10: 15 mm   A20: 15 mm   MCF: 15 mm

FIGURE 29-11 ROTEM after administration of tranexamic acid, fibrinogen, PCC, and Factor XIII.

the wound with soap is recommended but application of tourniquet (choice D), sucking the venom or slicing the wound with a knife are not recommended. A tourniquet reduces blood flow which can lead to gangrene.

15. D. Needle cricothyroidectomy

Emergent cricothyroidectomy is a temporary airway indicated in patients who cannot be ventilated due to facial trauma, oral obstruction from bleeding, vomiting, angioedema, epiglottitis, Ludwig angina, or upper airway chemical or thermal burns.[268-271] Contraindications include laryngeal or tracheal injury or anomaly and anterior neck swelling.

Preparation in adults for needle cricothyroidectomy include sterile technique, lidocaine, and a 12–16 gauge catheter over needle attached to a 10-mL saline syringe.[270-271] Landmarks from cephalad to caudad include hyoid cartilage, thyroid cartilage, cricothyroid membrane, cricoid cartilage, and

TABLE 29-12 Envenomation Grade With Associated Signs and Symptoms

Grade	Signs and Symptoms of Envenomation
0	Fang marks; swelling and erythema around the fang mark < 2.5 cm; minimal pain and tenderness; no systemic symptoms
1	Fang marks; history of immediate pain with the bite; swelling and erythema 5–15 cm; no systemic signs or symptoms
2	Fang marks; history of immediate severe pain; swelling and erythema 15–40 cm; mild systemic symptoms; and/or abnormal laboratory findings
3	Fang marks; history of immediate severe pain; swelling and erythema > 40 cm; petechiae and bullae; moderate systemic symptoms; bleeding or DIC; abnormal laboratory values
4	Fang marks; signs of multiple envenomation sites; history of immediate severe pain; severe systemic signs; possibly coma, shock, bleeding, DIC, and paralysis

DIC = disseminated intravascular coagulation.

tracheal rings. Left and right cricothyroid arteries and veins meet at the superior portion of the cricothyroid membrane. Therefore, the needle is inserted at the inferior portion of the cricothyroid membrane, caudally, at a 30 to 45 degrees angle. Once bubbling is noted in the syringe, the catheter is advanced to the hub. Then, the needle is removed and the catheter is connected to oxygen tubing. Ventilation is titrated to 10 to 16 breaths/min. A definitive airway needs to be performed.

A Macintosh laryngoscope has a curve blade and is designed to go to the angle at the base of the tongue and epiglottis (choice A). A Miller laryngoscope has a straight blade and is designed to go beneath the laryngeal surface of the epiglottis. It is designed for a floppy epiglottis or anterior larynx (choice B). A GlideScope is a video-assisted laryngoscope, usually with a Macintosh blade (choice C). Due to the facial trauma and oral bleeding, none of these is indicated and may delay securing an airway in this patient.

16. B. No surgical intervention

Early surgical intervention (24–48 hours) is associated with fewer medical complications and mortality rates compared to delayed surgical intervention (> 72 hours; choice A).[272-274] There are 3 locations of hip fracture. A femoral head fracture is at a high risk for vascular necrosis and warrants open reduction with internal fixation (ORIF) or arthroplasty. Conservative treatment may be reserved for severely debilitated patients, patients over 70 years of age, or stable impacted fractures. Intertrochanteric fractures are extracapsular and at a low risk for avascular necrosis but at a high risk for displacement. Open reduction with internal fixation or arthroplasty may be recommended, but again, in certain populations, medical management might be sufficient. Trochanteric fractures are related to the bony prominence on the lateral aspect of the proximal femur. It usually is treated via medical management (non–weight bearing for 3–4 weeks), but surgery can be an option if it is displaced more than 1 cm. Antibiotic prophylaxis should be initiated within 60 to 120 minutes prior to surgery to prevent surgical site infection (choice C).[275-278] Orthopedic patients are at a high risk for deep venous thrombosis, and the American College of Chest Physicians guidelines suggest pharmacologic prophylaxis 12 hours preoperatively or 12 hours postoperatively for a duration of 35 days (choice D).[279]

17. B. Sling and ice

Most clavicular fractures occur in the middle portion, then the distal portion, and lastly, the proximal portion.[280,281] Surgical intervention is warranted if there is neurovascular compromise, the fracture is open, there is tenting of the skin, or there is a floating shoulder (ipsilateral clavicle and glenoid neck fracture) (choice D).[280] For this patient with a nondisplaced fracture of the middle portion of the clavicle, restriction of motion to less than 30 degrees of abduction, forward flexion, or extension via sling or figure-8 bandage, and intermittent icing for 2 to 3 days would be the initial treatment. Observation is incorrect (choice A). Performing another radiographic study to confirm diagnosis is not necessary (choice C).

18. D. Plague, tularemia, Rocky Mountain spotted fever, and Q fever can be treated with doxycycline.

Rocky Mountain spotted fever has no eschar formation prior to adenopathy (choice D). Tularemia, not Q fever, has ulcerative glands (choice B). Although tularemia, Rocky Mountain spotted fever, and Q fever can be transmitted by ticks, plague is transmitted by fleas (choice C). See Table 29-13.[282-287]

19. A. Grade 3 and endovascular aneurysm repair

The patient has a traumatic grade 3 aortic injury with an intimal flap and a small pseudoaneurysm. The injury warrants endovascular aneurysm repair (EVAR).

Traumatic blunt aortic injury is associated with high mortality. The current guidelines recommend CT with contrast for the initial evaluation.[288-290] Per Starnes et al, there are 4 types.[289] Grade 1 (choice A) has an intimal tear with an absence of an aortic external contour abnormality and intimal defect and/or a thrombus less than 10 mm in length or width. Grade 2 (choice B) has a large intimal flap with an absence of an aortic external contour abnormality and intimal defect and/or a thrombus of 10 mm or more in length or width. Grade 3 (choice C) has pseudoaneurysms with an aortic external contour abnormality with a contained rupture. Grade 4 (choice D) is a rupture with an aortic external contour abnormality and free contrast extravasation or hemothorax. The current guidelines also recommend endovascular repair for patients with no contraindication. Delayed surgical repair and blood pressure control are recommended for grade 1 and grade 2 but urgent surgical repair is warranted for grade 3 and grade 4.

20. A. *Loxosceles*

The patient was bitten by a spider from the genus *Loxosceles*, also known as recluse, fiddle-back, or brown spider.

They are nocturnal and found in dark places outdoors but also can be seen at home. Its venom has phospholipase D that leads to dermonecrosis, direct hemolytic effects on red blood cells that can cause complement activation and platelet aggregation and hyaluronidase that can increase the size of lesion.[291,292] Initial manifestations includes mild pain and erythema that can progress to irregular areas of ecchymosis, ischemia, edema, and painful hemorrhagic blisters after more than 12 hours. After 24 to 48 hours, there can be generalized rash, fever, headaches, nausea and vomiting.[292] The hemolytic anemia is positive for direct antiglobulin test to complement C3 and IgG.[292] Acute renal failure, DIC, and rhabdomyolysis have also been reported. Necrosis of the lesion occurs after 72 hours and after more than or equal to 5 days the lesion becomes a dry necrotic eschar with well formed borders.[292] It can take weeks to months to heal, depending on the lesion's depth. Treatment includes antivenom, corticosteroids, dapsone, antihistamine, analgesics, hyperbaric oxygen therapy, and surgical excisions.[291,292]

Latrodectus spp. (choice B) includes the black widow spiders, which are distinguished by black shiny body with red hourglass marking.[291,292] Most of the bites are from the larger female spiders. Its venom consists of neurotoxin Alpha-latrotoxin. Clinical presentation varies per species but includes gradual and continuous pain for hours to day, diaphoresis often at the bite site or below the knee, and/or asymmetrical regional diaphoresis.[291] Paralysis, myocardial injury, and priapism has also be reported.[292] Treatment includes antivenom and analgesics, with benzodiazepines for muscle spasms.[292]

Atrax and *Hydronyche spp* are types of spiders found mostly in Eastern Australia.[292] When envenomation occurs, autonomic dysfunction occurs with bradycardia or tachycardia, hypotension or hypertension. Cholinergic symptoms includes miosis or mydriasis, diaphoresis, lacrimation, and hypersalivation. Neurologic symptoms includes paresthesias, fasciculations, and coma. First aid includes immobilization with pressure bandage and antivenom.[292] Patient is monitored after 2 hours and antivenom can be repeated if there is lack of response.[292]

Centruroides is a family of scorpions found in North America.[291] They are yellow to brown with variable tooth underneath the stinger. Symptoms range for pain and localized paresthesias (Grade I) to remote paresthesias (Grade II). Somatic or autonomic nerve dysfunction (Grade III) include tachycardia, nausea, blurred vision, shortness of breath, dysphagia, restlessness, and involuntary shaking.[291] Combined somatic and autonomic symptoms is considered Grade IV. Pain and localized and remote paresthesias maybe treated with ice, oral analgesics, and tetanus immunization.[291] Somatic and autonomic dysfunction would require more aggressive supportive care including intubation and antivenom.[291]

TABLE 29-13 Agents of Bioterrorism: Characteristics, Diagnosis, and Treatment

	Characteristics	Diagnosis	Treatment
Rocky mountain spotted fever	• Intracellular, Gram-negative coccobacilli *Rickettsia rickettsii* • Reservoirs are hard ticks from family *Ixodidae* • Fever, headache, photophobia, myalgias, anorexia, vomiting, abdominal pain, and rash 2–5 d after fever • Rash begins on wrists and ankles with centrifugal progression to palms and soles then centripetal from wrists and ankles to arms, legs, and trunk • Rash begins as small, blanching, erythematous macules that can progress to maculopapular and then to skin necrosis and gangrene • Rash may be absent in elderly or African Americans	• Clinical • Antibodies are not detected until after 7 d of infection • Gold standard is indirect fluorescent antibody test with 4-fold increase in titers or convalescent titer > 1/64 but indistinguishable from other *Rickettsia* species • Immunohistochemical staining of tissue biopsies	• Doxycycline • Chloramphenicol

Q fever	• Gram-negative pleomorphic coccobacillus *Coxiella burnetii*, which lives in macrophages
	• Inhalation or ingestion
	• Reservoirs are ticks, cattle, goats, sheep, cats, rabbits, pigeons, dogs
	• Flu-like symptoms with high fever (> 40°C) and retro-orbital headaches, pneumonia, hepatitis, endocarditis, maculopapular or purpuric rash, and aseptic meningitis or encephalitis
		• IFA with antiphase I and II of IgA, IgM, and IgG
		  • Acute infection: phase II IgM > 1:64 or phase II IgG > 1:256
		  • Past infection: IgG ≤ 200, no IgM or IgA
		• PCR
		• Cultures
			• Doxycycline (first choice)
			• Clarithromycin or azithromycin, erythromycin, minocycline, trimethoprim-sulfamethoxazole

Plague	• Gram-negative coccobacillus ("closed safety pin" shape) Yersinia pestis
	• Reservoirs are fleas
	• 3 clinical presentations
	  • Bubonic plague: skin eschar, plaques, or necrosis near lymph nodes before lymph adenopathy most commonly seen in cervical, axilla, and groin area
	  • Pneumonia plague
	  • Septic plague
		• 4-fold rise of at least 1:16 in antibody titers of F1 antigen
		• Culture
			• Streptomycin (first choice) or gentamicin
			• Doxycycline
			• Quinolones
			• Chloramphenicol

Tularemia	• Caused by small, nonmotile aerobic Gram-negative coccobacillus Francisella tularensis, which multiplies in macrophages and infects lungs, lymph nodes, kidneys, and liver
	• From rodents or insects such as fleas
	• Clinical presentation depends on route of infection
	  • Ulceroglandular if skin contact with initial papule, to pustule, to ulcer, and then tender regional adenopathy
	  • Oculoglandular with ulcer in conjunctiva, chemosis, vasculitis, and regional adenopathy
	  • Oropharyngeal
	  • Pneumonia with bilateral lobar and pleural involvement and hilar adenopathy
	  • Systemic
		• Clinical
		• DFA, PCR
		• Culture with cysteine-enriched medium
		• Biopsy of suppurative necrosis with granulomas
			• Streptomycin (first choice) or gentamicin for 10 d
			• Tetracyclines or chloramphenicol for 14 d
			• Fluoroquinolones for 10 d

DFA = direct fluorescent antibody; IFA = immunofluorescence assay; Ig = immunoglobulin; PCR = polymerase chain reaction.

REFERENCES

1. Chapter 2: Status of health related SDGs. In World Health Statistics 2018: Monitoring Health for SDGs. World Health Organization, Geneva: 2018: 4-11. http://www.who.int/gho/publications/world_health_statistics/2018/EN_WHS2018_Part2.pdf?ua=1. Accessed April 4, 2018.

2. Sauaia A, Moore FA, Moore EE, et al. Epidemiology of trauma: a reassessment. *J Trauma.* 1995;38(2):185-193.

3. Centers for Disease Control and Prevention. 10 Leading causes of death in the United States. https://webappa.cdc.gov/cgi-bin/broker.exe. Accessed May 25, 1018.

4. Curry N, Davis PW. What's new in resuscitation strategies for the patient with multiple trauma? *Injury.* 2012;43(7):1021-1028.

5. Rossaint R, Bouillon B, Cerny V, et al. The European guideline on management of major bleeding and coagulopathy following trauma: fourth edition. *Crit Care.* 2016;20:100.

6. Curry NS, Davenport RA, Hunt BJ, Stanworth SJ. Transfusion strategies for traumatic coagulopathy. *Blood Rev.* 2012;26(5):223-232.

7. Brohi K, Singh J, Heron M, Coats T. Acute traumatic coagulopathy. *J Trauma.* 2003;54(6):1127-1130.

8. Fenger-Eriksen C, Tønnesen E, Ingerslev J, Sørensen B. Mechanisms of hydroxyethyl starch-induced dilutional coagulopathy. *J Thromb Haem.* 2009;7(7):1099-1105.

9. Poole D. Coagulopathy and transfusion strategies in trauma. Overwhelmed by literature, supported by weak evidence. Blood Transfusion. 2016;14(1):3-7.

10. Rossaint R, Bouillon B, Cerny V, et al. Management of bleeding following major trauma: an updated European guideline. *Crit Care.* 2010;14(2):R52.

11. Frith D, Goslings JC, Gaarder C, et al. Definition and drivers of acute traumatic coagulopathy: clinical and experimental investigations. *J Thromb Haemost.* 2010;8(9):1919-1925.

12. Holcomb JB, Junco DJ, Fox EE, et al. The prospective, observational, multicenter major trauma transfusion (PROMMTT) study: comparative effectiveness of a time-varying treatment with competing risks. *JAMA Surg.* 2013;148(2):127-136.

13. Simmons JW, Powell MF. Acute traumatic coagulopathy: pathophysiology and resuscitation. *BJA: British Journal of Anaesthesia.* 2016;117(3):iii31-iii43.

14. Macleod JB, Lynn M, McKenney MG, Cohn SM, Murtha M. Early coagulopathy predicts mortality in trauma. *J Trauma.* 2003;55(1):39-44.

15. Meng ZH, Wolberg AS, Monreo DM 3rd, Hoffman M. The effect of temperature and pH on the activity of factor VIIa: implications for the efficacy of high-dose factor VIIa in hypothermic and acidotic patients. *J Trauma.* 2003;55(5):886-891.

16. Martini WZ, Pusateri AE, Uscilowicz JM, Delgado AV, Holcomb JB. Independent contributions of hypothermia and acidosis to coagulopathy in swine. *J Trauma.* 2005;58(5):1002-1010.

17. Martini WZ, Holcomb JB. Acidosis and coagulopathy: the differential effects on fibrinogen synthesis and breakdown in pigs. *Ann Surg.* 2007;246(5):851-853.

18. Shaz BH, Winkler AM, James AB, Hillyer CD, MacLeod JB. Pathophysiology of early trauma-induced coagulopathy: emerging evidence for hemodilution and coagulation factor depletion. *J Trauma.* 2011;70(6):1401-1407.

19. Bickell WH, Wall MJ Jr, Pepe PE, et al. Immediate versus delayed fluid resuscitation for hypotensive patients with penetrating torso injuries. *N Engl J Med.* 1994;331(17):1105-1109.

20. Sampalis JS, Tamim H, Denis R, et al. Ineffectiveness of on-site intravenous lines: is prehospital time the culprit? *J Trauma.* 1997;43(4):608-615; discussion 615-617.

21. Dutton RP, Mackenzie CF, Scalea TM. Hypotensive resuscitation during active hemorrhage: impact on in-hospital mortality. *J Trauma.* 2002;52(6):1141-1146.

22. Chowdhury AH, Cox EF, Francis ST, Lobo DN. A randomized, controlled, double-blind crossover study on the effects of 2-L infusions of 0.9 % saline and plasma-lyte(R) 148 on renal blood flow velocity and renal cortical tissue perfusion in healthy volunteers. *Ann Surg.* 2012;256(1):18-24.

23. Yunos NM, Bellomo R, Hegarty C, Story D, Ho L, Bailey M. Association between a chloride-liberal vs chloride-restrictive intravenous fluid administration strategy and kidney injury in critically ill adults. *JAMA.* 2012;308(15):1566-1572.

24. Bulger EM, Jurkovich GJ, Nathens AB, et al. Hypertonic resuscitation of hypovolemic shock after blunt trauma: a randomized controlled trial. *Arch Surg.* 2008;143(2):139-148.

25. Battison C, Andrews PJ, Graham C, Petty T. Randomized, controlled trial on the effect of a 20% mannitol solution and a 7.5% saline/6% dextran solution on increased intracranial pressure after brain injury. *Crit Care Med.* 2005;33(1):196-202.

26. Cooper DJ, Myles PS, McDermott FT, et al. Prehospital hypertonic saline resuscitation of patients with hypotension and severe traumatic brain injury: a randomized controlled trial. *JAMA.* 2004;291(11):1350-1357.

27. Bulger EM, May S, Brasel KJ, et al. Out-of-hospital hypertonic resuscitation following severe traumatic brain injury: a randomized controlled trial. *JAMA.* 2010;304(13):1455-1464.

28. Bulger EM, May S, Kerby JD, et al. Out-of-hospital hypertonic resuscitation after traumatic hypovolemic shock: a randomized, placebo-controlled trial. *Ann Surg.* 2011;253(3):431-441.

29. Holcomb JB, Tilley BC, Baraniuk S, et al. Transfusions of plasma, platelets, and red blood cells in a 1:1:1 vs 1:1:2 ratio and mortality in patients with severe trauma. *JAMA.* 2015;315(5):471-482.

30. Spinella PC, Perkins JG, Grathwohl KW, Beekley AC, Holcomb JB. Warm Fresh whole blood is independently associated with improved survival for patients with combat-related traumatic injuries. *J Trauma.* 2009;66(4 suppl):S69-S76.

31. Counts RB, Haisch C, Simon TL, Maxwell NG, Heimbach DM, Carrico CJ. Hemostasis in massively transfused trauma patients. *Ann Surg.* 1979;190(1):91-99.

32. Ciavarella D, Reed RL, Counts RB, et al. Clotting factor levels and the risk of diffuse microvascular bleeding in the massively transfused patient. *Br J Haematol.* 1987;67(3):365-368.

33. Brown LM, Call MS, Margaret Knudson M, et al. A normal platelet count may not be enough: the impact of admission platelet count on mortality and transfusion in severely injured trauma patients. *J Trauma.* 2011;71(2 Suppl 3):S337-S342.

34. Floccard B, Rugeri L, Faure A, et al. Early coagulopathy in trauma patients: an on-scene and hospital admission study. *Injury.* 2012;43(1):26–32.

35. Hiippala ST, Myllyla GJ, Vahtera EM. Hemostatic factors and replacement of major blood loss with plasma-poor red cell concentrates. *Anesth Analg.* 1995;81(2):360-365.

36. Nekludov M, Bellander BM, Blomback M, Wallen HN. Platelet dysfunction in patients with severe traumatic brain injury. *J Neurotrauma.* 2007;24(11):1699-1706.

37. Wohlauer MV, Moore EE, Thomas S, et al. Early platelet dysfunction: an unrecognized role in the acute coagulopathy of trauma. *J Am Coll Surg.* 2012;214(5):739-746.

38. Jacoby RC, Owings JT, Holmes J, Battistella FD, Gosselin RC, Paglieroni TG. Platelet activation and function after trauma. *J Trauma.* 2001;51(4):639-647.

39. Kutcher ME, Redick BJ, McCreery RC, et al. Characterization of platelet dysfunction after trauma. *J Trauma Acute Care Surg.* 2012;73(1):13-19.

40. Vilahur G, Choi BG, Zafar MU, et al. Normalization of platelet reactivity in clopidogrel-treated subjects. *J Thromb Haemost.* 2007;5(1):82-90.

41. Reiter RA, Mayr F, Blazicek H, et al. Desmopressin antagonizes the in vitro platelet dysfunction induced by GPIIb/IIIa inhibitors and aspirin. *Blood.* 2003;102(13):4594-4599.

42. Leithauser B, Zielske D, Seyfert UT, Jung F. Effects of desmopressin on platelet membrane glycoproteins and platelet aggregation in volunteers on clopidogrel. *Clin Hemorheol Microcirc.* 2008;39(1-4):293-302.

43. Coppola A, Di Minno G. Desmopressin in inherited disorders of platelet function. *Haemophilia.* 2008;14(Suppl 1):31-39.

44. Laupacis A, Fergusson D. Drugs to minimize perioperative blood loss in cardiac surgery: meta-analyses using perioperative blood transfusion as the outcome. The International Study of Peri-operative Transfusion (ISPOT) Investigators. *Anesth Analg.* 1997;85(6):1258-1267.

45. Powner DJ, Hartwell EA, Hoots WK. Counteracting the effects of anticoagulants and antiplatelet agents during neurosurgical emergencies. *Neurosurgery.* 2005;57(5):823-831; discussion 823-831.

46. Kapapa T, Rohrer S, Struve S, et al. Desmopressin acetate in intracranial haemorrhage. *Neurol Res Int.* 2014;2014:298767.

47. Naidech AM, Maas MB, Levasseur-Franklin KE, et al. Desmopressin improves platelet activity in acute intracerebral hemorrhage. *Stroke.* 2014;45(8):2451-2453.

48. Reiter R, Jilma-Stohlawetz P, Horvath M, Jilma B. Additive effects between platelet concentrates and desmopressin in antagonizing the platelet glycoprotein IIb/IIIa inhibitor eptifibatide. *Transfusion.* 2005;45(3):420-426.

49. Kim D, O'Leary M, Nguyen A, et al. The effect of platelet and desmopressin administration on early radiographic progression of traumatic intracranial hemorrhage. *J Neurotrauma.* 2015;32(22):1815-1821.

50. Stinger HK, Spinella PC, Perkins JG, et al. The ratio of fibrinogen to red cells transfused affects survival in casualties receiving massive transfusions at an army combat support hospital. *J Trauma.* 2008;64(2 Suppl):S79-S85; discussion S85.

51. Franchini M, Lippi G. Prothrombin complex concentrates: an update. *Blood Transfus.* 2010;8(3):149-154.

52. Shakur H, Roberts I, Bautista R, et al. Effects of tranexamic acid on death, vascular occlusive events, and blood transfusion in trauma patients with significant haemorrhage (CRASH-2): a randomised, placebo-controlled trial. *Lancet.* 2010;376(9734):23-32.

53. Roberts I, Shakur H, Ker K, Coats TJ. Antifibrinolytic drugs for acute traumatic injury. *Cochrane Database Syst Rev.* 2012;12:CD004896.

54. Roberts I, Prieto-Merino D, Manno D. Mechanism of action of tranexamic acid in bleeding trauma patients: an exploratory analysis of data from the CRASH-2 trial. *Crit Care.* 2014;18(6):685.

55. Harvin JA, Peirce CA, Mims MM, et al. The impact of tranexamic acid on mortality in injured patients with hyperfibrinolysis. *J Trauma Acute Care Surg.* 2015;78(5):905-911.

56. Cole E, Davenport R, Willett K, Brohi K. Trancxamic acid use in severely injured civilian patients and the effects on outcomes: a prospective cohort study. *Ann Surg.* 2015;261(2):390-394.

57. Kalavrouziotis D, Voisine P, Mohammadi S, Dionne S, Dagenais F. High-dose tranexamic acid is an independent predictor of early seizure after cardiopulmonary bypass. *Ann Thorac Surg.* 2012;93(1):148-154.

58. Roberts I, Shakur H, Afolabi A, et al. The importance of early treatment with tranexamic acid in bleeding trauma patients: an exploratory analysis of the CRASH-2 randomised controlled trial. *Lancet.* 2011;377(9771):1096-1101.

59. Roberts I, Perel P, Prieto-Merino D, et al; CRASH-2 Collaborators. Effect of tranexamic acid on mortality in patients with traumatic bleeding: prespecified analysis of data from randomised controlled trial. *BMJ.* 2012;345:e5839

60. Tummala R, Kavtaradze A, Gupta A, Ghosh RK. Specific antidotes against direct oral anticoagulants: a comprehensive review of clinical trials data. *Int J Cardiol.* 2016;214:292-298.

61. Stangier J, Rathgen K, Stähle H, Gansser D, Roth W. The pharmacokinetics, pharmacodynamics and tolerability of dabigatran etexilate, a new oral direct thrombin inhibitor, in healthy male subjects. *Br J Clin Pharmacol.* 2007;64(3):292-303.

62. Van Ryn J, Baruch L, Clemens A. Interpretation of point-of-care INR results in patients treated with dabigatran. *Am J Med.* 2012;125(4):417-420.

63. Baruch L, Sherman O. Potential inaccuracy of point-of-care INR in dabigatran treated patients, *Ann Pharmacother.* 2011;45(7-8):e40.

64. Van Ryn J, Stangier J, Haertter S, et al. Dabigatran etexilate—a novel, reversible, oral direct thrombin inhibitor: interpretation of coagulation assays and reversal of anticoagulant activity. *Thromb Haemost.* 2010;103(6):1116-1127.

65. Lindahl TL, Baghaei F, Blixter IF, et al; Expert Group on Coagulation of the External Quality Assurance in Laboratory Medicine in Sweden. Effects of the oral, direct thrombin inhibitor dabigatran on five common coagulation assays. *Thromb Haemost.* 2011;105(2):371-378.

66. Douxfils J, Mullier F, Robert S, Chatelain C, Chatelain B, Dogné JM. Impact of dabigatran on a large panel of routine or specific coagulation assays. Laboratory recommendations for monitoring of dabigatran etexilate. *Thromb Haemost.* 2012;107(5):985-997.

67. Patel MR, Mahaffey KW, Garg J, et al; ROCKET AF Investigators. Rivaroxaban versus warfarin in nonvalvular atrial fibrillation. *N Engl J Med.* 2011;365(10):883-891.

68. Kristensen SD, Le Heuzey JY, Mavrakis H, et al. 2012 focused update of the ESC Guidelines for the management of atrial fibrillation: an update of the 2010 ESC Guidelines for the management of atrial fibrillation. Developed with the special contribution of the European Heart Rhythm Association. *Eur Heart J.* 2012;33(21):2719-2747.

69. January CT, Wann LS, Alpert JS, et al. 2014 AHA/ACC/HRS guideline for the management of patients with atrial

fibrillation: executive summary: a report of the American College of Cardiology/American Heart Association Task Force on Practice Guidelines and the Heart Rhythm Society. *Circulation.* 2014;130(23):2071-2104.

70. Harder S, Graff J. Novel oral anticoagulants: clinical pharmacology, indications, and practical considerations. *Eur J Clin Pharmacol.* 2013;69(9):1617-1633.

71. Granger CB, Alexander JH, McMurray JJ, et al; ARISTOTLE Committees and Investigators. Apixaban versus warfarin in patients with atrial fibrillation. *N Engl J Med.* 2011;365(11):981-992.

72. Gallego P, Roldán V, Lip GY. Novel oral anticoagulants in cardiovascular disease. *J Cardiovasc Pharmacol Ther.* 2014;19(1):34-44.

73. Samama MM, Martinoli JL, LeFlem L, et al. Assessment of laboratory assays to measure rivaroxaban—an oral, direct factor Xa inhibitor. *Thromb Haemost.* 2010;103(4):815-825.

74. Kubitza D, Becka M, Wensing G, Voith B, Zuehlsdorf M. Safety, pharmacodynamics, and pharmacokinetics of BAY 59-7939—an oral, direct factor Xa inhibitor—after multiple dosing in healthy male subjects. *Eur J Clin Pharmacol.* 2005;61(12):873-880.

75. Schiele F, van Ryn J, Canada K. A specific antidote for dabigatran: functional and structural characterisation. *Blood.* 2013;121(18):3554-3562.

76. Honickel M, Grottke O, van Ryn J. Use of a specific antidote to dabigatran (idarucizumab) reduces blood loss and mortality in dabigatran-induced and trauma-induced bleeding in pigs. *Crit Care.* 2014;18(Suppl 1):99.

77. van Ryn J, Litzenburger T, Schurer J. Reversal of anticoagulant activity of dabigatran and dabigatran-induced bleeding in rats by a specific antidote (antibody fragment). *Circulation.* 2012;126:A9928.

78. Glund S, Stangier J, Schmohl M, et al. Safety, tolerability, and efficacy of idarucizumab for the reversal of the anticoagulant effect of dabigatran in healthy male volunteers: a randomised, placebo-controlled, double-blind phase 1 trial. *Lancet.* 2015;386(9994):680-690.

79. Pollack CV Jr, Reilly PA, Eikelboom J, Glund S, Verhamme P, Bernstein RA. Idarucizumab for dabigatran reversal. *N Engl J Med.* 2015;373(6):511-520.

80. Crowther M, Lu G, Conley PB. Reversal of factor Xa inhibitors-induced anticoagulation in healthy subjects by andexanet alfa. *Crit Care Med.* 2014;42(12):A1469.

81. Crowther MA, Levy G, Lu G. A phase 2 randomized, double-blind, placebo-controlled trial demonstrating reversal of edoxaban-induced anticoagulation in healthy subjects by andexanet alfa (PRT064445), a universal antidote for factor Xa (fXa) inhibitors. Paper presented at: 56th annual meeting of the American Society of Hematology; December 6-9, 2014; San Francisco, CA.

82. Crowther MA, Mathur V, Kitt M. A phase 2 randomized, double-blind, placebo-controlled trial demonstrating reversal of rivaroxaban-induced anticoagulation in healthy subjects by andexanet alfa (PRT064445), an antidote for Fxa inhibitors. Paper presented at: 55th annual meeting of the American Society of Hematology; December 7-10, 2013; New Orleans, LA.

83. Siegal DM, Curnutte JT, Connolly SJ, et al. Andexanet alfa for the reversal of factor Xa inhibitor activity. *N Engl J Med.* 2015;373(25):2413-2424.

84. Hettiarachy S, Dziewulski P. ABC of burns: pathophysiology and types of burns. *BMJ.* 2004;328(7453):1427-1429.

85. Rowan MP, Cancio LC, Elster EA, et al. Burn wound healing and treatment: review and advancements. *Crit Care.* 2015;19:243.

86. Church D, Elsayed S, Reid O, Winston B, Lindsay R. Burn wound infections. *Clin Microbiol Rev.* 2006;19(2):403-434.

87. Gibran NS, Wiechman S, Meyer W, et al. American Burn Association consensus statements. *J Burn Care Res.* 2013;34(4):361-385.

88. Mann R, Heimbach D. Prognosis and treatment of burns. *West J Med.* 1996;165(4):215-220.

89. American Burn Association. Burn incidence and treatment in the United States: 2013 fact sheet. 2013. http://www.ameriburn.org/resources_factsheet.php. Accessed May 12, 2017.

90. Snell JA, Loh N, Mahambrey T, Shokrollai K. Clinical review: The critical care management of the burn patient. *Crit Care.* 2013;17(5):241.

91. Latenser BA. Critical care of the burn patient. The first 48 hours. *Crit Care Med.* 2009;37(10):2819-2826.

92. Ferrando AA, Chinkes DL, Wolf SE, Matin S, Herndon DN, Wolfe RR. A submaximal dose of insulin promotes net skeletal muscle protein synthesis in patients with severe burns. *Ann Surg.* 1999;229(1):11-8.

93. Hrynyk M, Neufeld RJ. Insulin and wound healing. *Burns.* 2014;40(8):1433-1446.

94. Pidcoke HF, Baer LA, Wu X, Wolf SE, Aden JK, Wade CE. Insulin effects on glucose tolerance, hypermetabolic response, and circadian-metabolic protein expression in a rat burn and disuse model. *Am J Physiol Regul Integr Comp Physiol.* 2014;307(1):R1-R10.

95. Pidcoke HF, Wade CE, Wolf SE. Insulin and the burned patient. *Crit Care Med.* 2007;35(9 Suppl):S524-S530.

96. Sakurai Y, Aarsland A, Herndon DN, et al. Stimulation of muscle protein synthesis by long-term insulin infusion in severely burned patients. *Ann Surg.* 1995;222(3):283-294.

97. Desai MH, Herndon DN, Broemeling L, Barrow RE, Nichols Jr RJ, Rutan RL. Early burn wound excision significantly reduces blood loss. *Ann Surg.* 1990;211(6):753-759; discussion 759-762.

98. Herndon DN, Barrow RE, Rutan RL, Rutan TC, Desai MH, Abston S. A comparison of conservative versus early excision. Therapies in severely burned patients. *Ann Surg.* 1989;209(5):547-552; discussion 552-553.

99. Saaiq M, Zaib S, Ahmad S. Early excision and grafting versus delayed excision and grafting of deep thermal burns up to 40% total body surface area: a comparison of outcome. *Ann Burns Fire Disasters.* 2012;25(3):143-147.

100. Vinita P, Khare NA, Chandramouli M, Nilesh S, Sumit B. Comparative analysis of early excision and grafting vs delayed grafting in burn patients in a developing country. *J Burn Care Res.* 2014;37(5):278-282.

101. Monafo WW, West MA. Current treatment recommendations for topical burn therapy. *Drugs.* 1990;40(3):364-373.

102. Heggers JP, Hawkins H, Edgar P, Villarreal C, Herndon DN. Treatment of infections in burns. In: Herndon DN, ed. *Total Burn Care.* London, England: Saunders; 2002: 120-169.

103. Murphy KD, Lee JO, Herndon DN. Current pharmacotherapy for the treatment of severe burns. *Expert Opin Pharmacother.* 2003;4(3):369-384.

104. Pruitt BA, Foley FD. The use of biopsies in burn care. *Surgery.* 1973;73(6):887-897.

105. Golfinos JG, Cooper PR. Skull fracture and post-traumatic cerebrospinal fluid fistula. In: Cooper PR, Golfinos JG, eds, *Head Injury.* 4th ed. New York: McGraw-Hill; 2000: 155.

106. Bullock MR, Chesnut R, Ghajar J, et al; Surgical Management of Traumatic Brain Injury Author Group. Surgical management of depressed cranial fractures. *Neurosurgery.* 2006; 58(3 Suppl):S56-S60.

107. Yilmazlar S, Arslan E, Kocaeli H, et al. Cerebrospinal fluid leakage complicating skull base fractures: analysis of 81 cases. *Neurosurg Rev.* 2006;29(1):64-71.

108. Dahiya R, Keller JD, Litofsky NS, Bankey PE, Bonassar LJ, Megerian CA. Temporal bone fractures: otic capsule sparing versus otic capsule violating clinical and radiographic considerations. *J Trauma.* 1999;47(6):1079-1083.

109. Anglin D, Hutson HR, Luftman J, Qualls S, Moradzadeh D. Intracranial hemorrhage associated with tangential gunshot wounds to the head. *Acad Emerg Med.* 1998;5(7):672-678.

110. Rangel-Castillo L, Gopinath S, Robertson CS. Management of intracranial hypertension. *Neurol Clin.* 2008;26(2): 521-541.

111. Doczi T. Volume regulation of the brain tissue—a survey. *Acta Neurochir (Wien).* 1993;121(1-2):1-8.

112. El Ahmadieh TY, Adel JG, El Tecle NE, et al. Surgical treatment of elevated intracranial pressure: decompressive craniectomy and intracranial pressure monitoring. *Neurosurg Clin N Am.* 2013;24(3):375-391.

113. Carney N, Totten AM, O'Reilly C, et al. *Guidelines for the Management of Severe Traumatic Brain Injury.* 4th ed. Braintrauma. org. 2016: 1-244. https://braintrauma.org/uploads/03/12/ Guidelines_for_Management_of_Severe_TBI_4th_Edition .pdf. Accessed June 4, 2017.

114. Robertson CS, Valadka AB, Hannay HJ, et al. Prevention of secondary ischemic insults after traumatic brain injury. *Crit Care Med.* 1999;27(10):2086-2095.

115. Brain Trauma Foundation; American Association of Neurological Surgeons; Congress of Neurological Surgeons. Guidelines for the management of severe traumatic brain injury. *J Neurotrauma.* 2007;24(Suppl 1):S1-S106.

116. Webb AJ, Ullman NL, Mann S, Muschelli J, Awad IA, Hanley DF. Resolution of intraventricular hemorrhage varies by ventricular region and dose of intraventricular thrombolytic: the Clot Lysis: Evaluating Accelerated Resolution of IVH (CLEAR IVH) program. *Stroke.* 2012;43(6):1666-1668.

117. Schell RM, Cole DJ. Cerebral monitoring: jugular venous oximetry. *Anesth Analog.* 2000;90(3):449-466.

118. Torbic H, Forni AA, Anger KE, Degrado JR, Greenwood BC. Use of antiepileptics for seizure prophylaxis after traumatic brain injury. *Am J Health Syst Pharm.* 2013;70(9):759-766.

119. Bullock MR, Chesnut R, Ghajar J, et al; Surgical Management of Traumatic Brain Injury Author Group. Surgical management of acute subdural hematomas. *Neurosurgery.* 2006; 58(3 Suppl):S16-S24.

120. Kothari RU, Brott T, Broderick JP, et al. The ABCs of measuring intracerebral hemorrhage volumes. *Stroke.* 1996;27(8): 1304-1305.

121. Bullock MR, Chesnut R, Ghajar J, et al; Surgical Management of Traumatic Brain Injury Author Group. Surgical management of acute epidural hematomas. *Neurosurgery.* 2006;58 (3 Suppl):S7-S15.

122. Morgenstern LB, Hemphill JC 3rd, Anderson C, et al; American Heart Association Stroke Council; Council on Cardiovascular Nursing. Guidelines for the management of spontaneous intracerebral hemorrhage: a guideline for healthcare professionals from the American Heart Association/American Stroke Association. *Stroke.* 2010;41(9):2108-2129.

123. Bullock MR, Chesnut R, Ghajar J, et al. Surgical management of traumatic parenchymal lesions. *Neurosurgery.* 2006; 58(Suppl 3):S25-S46

124. Gregson BA, Rowan EN, Mitchell PM, et al. Surgical trial in traumatic intracerebral hemorrhage (STITCH(Trauma)): study protocol for a randomized controlled trial. *Trials.* 2012;13:193.

125. Mendelow AD, Gregson BA, Fernandes HM, et al. Early surgery versus initial conservative treatment in patients with spontaneous supratentorial intracerebral haematomas in the international surgical trial in intracerebral haemorrhage (STICH): a randomized trial. *Lancet.* 2005;365(9457):387-389.

126. Murthy JM, Chowdary GV, Murthy TV, et al. Decompressive craniectomy with clot evacuation in large hemispheric hypertensive intracerebral hemorrhage. *Neurocrit Care.* 2005;2(3):258-262.

127. Maira G, Anile C, Colosimo C, et al. Surgical treatment of primary supratentorial intracerebral hemorrhage in stuporous and comatose patients. *Neurol Res.* 2002;24(1):54-60.

128. Wada Y, Kubo T, Asano T, et al. Fulminant subdural empyema treated with a wide decompressive craniectomy and continuous irrigation–case report. *Neurol Med Chir.* 2002;42(9):414-416.

129. Baussart B, Cheisson G, Compain M, et al. Multimodal cerebral monitoring and decompressive surgery for the treatment of severe bacterial meningitis with increased intracranial pressure. *Acta Anaesthesiol Scand.* 2006;50(6):762-765.

130. Schwab S, Junger E, Spranger M, et al. Craniectomy: an aggressive treatment approach in severe encephalitis. *Neurology.* 1997;48(2):412-417.

131. Agrawal D, Hussain N. Decompressive craniectomy in cerebral toxoplasmosis. *Eur J Clin Microbiol Infect Dis.* 2005;24(11):772-773.

132. Ausman JI, Rogers C, Sharp HL. Decompressive craniectomy for the encephalopathy of Reye's syndrome. *Surg Neurol.* 1976;6(2):97-99.

133. Keller E, Pangalu A, Fandino J, et al. Decompressive craniectomy in severe cerebral venous and dural sinus thrombosis. *Acta Neurochir Suppl.* 2005;94:177-183.

134. Kulvatunyou N, Erickson L, Vijayasekaran A, et al. Randomized clinical trial of pigtail catheter versus chest tube in injured patients with uncomplicated traumatic pneumothorax. *Br J Surg.* 2014;101(2):17-22.

135. Kulvatunyou N, Joseph B, Friese RS, et al. 14 French pigtail catheters placed by surgeons to drain blood on trauma patients: is 14Fr too small? *J Trauma Acute Care Surge.* 2012;73(6):1423-1427.

136. Doban AR, Eriksson EA, Denlinger CE, et al. Surgical rib fixation for flail chest deformity improves liberation from mechanical ventilation. *J Crit Care.* 2014(1):139-143.

137. Slobogean GP, MacPherson CA, Sun T, Pelletier ME, Hameed SM. Surgical fixation vs nonoperative management of flail chest: a meta-analysis. *J Am Coll Surg.* 2013;216(2):302-311.

138. Mackenzie IMJ, Tunnicliffe B. Blast injuries to the lung: epidemiology and management. *Phil Trans R Soc B.* 2011;366(1562):295-299.

139. Pizov R, Oppenheim-Eden A, Malot I, et al. Blast lung injury from an explosion on a civilian bus. *Chest.* 1999;115(1):165-172.

140. Dante D, Lee J. Trauma and blast injuries. In: Broaddus VC, Mason RJ, Ernst JD, et al, eds. *Murray and Nadel's Textbook of Respiratory Medicine*. 6th ed. Philadelphia, PA: Elsevier Saunders; 2016: 1354-1366.

141. Lateef Wani M, Ahangar AG, Wani SN, Irshad I, Ul-Hassan N. Penetrating cardiac injury: a review. *Trauma Mon*. 2012;17(1): 230-232.

142. Yousef R, Carr JA. Blunt cardiac trauma: a review of the current knowledge and management. *Ann Thorac Surg*. 2014;98(3):1134-1140.

143. Lee TH, Quellet JH, Cook M, Schreiber MA, Kortbeek JB. Pericardiocentesis in trauma: a systematic review. *J Trauma Acute Care Surg*. 2013;75(4):543-549.

144. Akowuah E, Baumbach A, Wilde P, Angelini G, Bryan AJ. Emergency repair of traumatic aortic rupture: endovascular versus conventional open repair. *J Thorac Cardiovasc Surg*. 2007;134(4):897-901.

145. Amabile P, Rollet G, Vidal V, Collart F, Bartoli JM, Piquet P. Emergency treatment of acute rupture of the descending thoracic aorta using endovascular stent-grafts. *Ann Vasc Surg*. 2006;20(6):723-730.

146. Andrassy J, Weidenhagen R, Meimarakis G, Lauterjung L, Jauch KW, Kopp R. Stent versus open surgery for acute and chronic traumatic injury of the thoracic aorta: a single-center experience. *J Trauma*. 2006;60(4):765-771.

147. Arthurs ZM, Starnes BW, Sohn VY, Singh N, Martin MJ, Andersen CA. Functional and survival outcomes in traumatic blunt thoracic aortic injuries: an analysis of the National Trauma Databank. *J Vasc Surg*. 2009;9(4):988-994.

148. Azizzadeh A, Charlton-Ouw KM, Chen Z, et al. An outcome analysis of endovascular versus open repair of blunt traumatic aortic injuries. *J Vasc Surg*. 2013;57(1):108-114.

149. Hoff WS, Holevar M, Nagy KK, et al; Eastern Association for the Surgery of Trauma. Practice management guidelines for the evaluation of blunt abdominal trauma: the EAST Practice Management Guidelines Work Group. *J Trauma*. 2002;53(3):602-615.

150. Como JJ, Bokhari F, Chiu WC, et al. Practice management guidelines for selective nonoperative management of penetrating abdominal trauma. *J Trauma*. 2010;68(3):721-733.

151. Lamb CM, Garner JP. Selective nonoperative management of civilian gunshot wounds to the abdomen: a systematic review of the evidence. *Injury*. 2014;45(4):659-666.

152. Bulger EM, Snyder D, Schoelles K, et al. An evidence-based prehospital guideline for external hemorrhage control: American College of Surgeons Committee on Trauma. *Prehosp Emerg Care*. 2014;18(2):163-173.

153. Sapega AA Heppenstall RB, Sokolow DP, et al. The bioenergetics of preservation of limbs before replantation. The rationale for intermediate hypothermia. *J Bone Joint Surg Am*. 1988;70(10):1500-1513.

154. Fox N, Rajani RR, Bokhari F, et al; Eastern Association for the Surgery of Trauma. Evaluation and management of penetrating lower extremity arterial trauma: an Eastern Association for the Surgery of Trauma practice management guideline. *J Trauma Acute Care Surg*. 2012;73(5 Suppl 4): S315-S320.

155. Lynch K, Johansen K. Can Doppler pressure measurement replace "exclusion" arteriography in the diagnosis of occult extremity arterial trauma? *Ann Surg*. 1991;214(6):737-741.

156. Sadjadi J, Cureton E, Dozier K, et al. Expedited treatment of lower extremity gunshot wounds. *J Am Coll Surg*. 2009;209(6):740-745.

157. Occupational Safety and Health Administration. Occupational safety and health standards: hazardous materials. Regulations (standards—29 CFR). Available at https://www.osha.gov/pls/oshaweb/owadisp.show_document?p_table=STANDARDS&p_id=9767. Accessed June 29, 2017.

158. Madsen JM. Chemical terrorism: rapid recognition and initial management. In: Post TW, ed. UpToDate, Waltham, MA: UpToDate, Inc. http://www.uptodate.com. Accessed May 13, 2017.

159. Tuorinsky SD, Sciuto AM. Toxic inhalational injury and toxic industrial chemicals. In: Tuorinsky SD, ed. *Medical Aspects of Chemical Warfare*. 2nd ed. Washington, DC: Office of the Surgeon General, TMM Publications; 2008: 339-370.

160. Hurst CG, Petrali JP, Barillo DJ, et al. Vesicants. In: Tuorinsky SD, ed. *Medical Aspects of Chemical Warfare*. 2nd ed. Washington, DC: Office of the Surgeon General, TMM Publications; 2008: 259-310.

161. Busl KM, Bleck TP. Treatment of neuroterrorism. *Neurotherapeutics*. 2012;9(1):139-157.

162. White CW, Martin JG. Chlorine gas inhalation: human clinical evidence of toxicity. *Proc Am Thorac Soc*. 2010;7(4):257-263.

163. Vaish AK, Consul S, Agrawal A, et al. Accidental phosgene gas exposure: a review with background study of 10 cases. *J Emerg Trauma Shock*. 2013;6(4):271-275.

164. White SM. Chemical and biological weapons. Implications for anaesthesia and intensive care. *Br J Anaesth*. 2002;89(2):306-324.

165. Borak MD, Sidell FR. Agents of chemical warfare: sulfur mustard. *Ann Emerg Med*. 1992;21(3):300-308.

166. Adalja AA, Toner E, Inglesby TV. Clinical management of potential bioterrorism-related conditions. *New Engl J Med*. 2015;372(10):954-962.

167. Martin GJ, Friedlander AM. Bacillus anthracis (anthrax). In: Bennett JE, Dolin R, Blaser MJ, eds. *Mandell, Douglas, and Bennett's Principles and Practice of Infectious Diseases*. 8th ed. Philadelphia, PA: Elsevier; 2014: 2391-2409.

168. Sweeney DA, Hicks CW, Cui X, Li Y, Eichacker PQ. Anthrax infection. *Am J Respir Crit Care Med*. 2011;184(12): 1333-1341.

169. Centers for Disease Control and Prevention. Gastrointestinal anthrax after an animal-hide drumming event—New Hampshire and Massachusetts, 2009. *MMWR Morb Mortal Wkly Rep*. 2010;59(28):872-877.

170. Christian MD. Biowarfare and bioterrorism. *Crit Care Clin*. 2013;29(3):717-756

171. Jernigan DB, Raghunathan PL, Bell BP, et al. Investigation of bioterrorism-related anthrax, United States, 2001: epidemiologic findings. *Emerg Infect Dis*. 2002;8(10):1019-1028.

172. Migone TS, Subramanian GM, Zhong J, et al. Raxibacumab for the treatment of inhalational anthrax. *N Engl J Med*. 2009;361(2):135-144.

173. Mytle N, Hopkins RJ, Malkevich NV, et al. Evaluation of intravenous anthrax immune globulin for treatment of inhalation anthrax. *Antimicrob Agents Chemother*. 2013;57(11): 5684-5692.

174. Prigent J, Panigai L, Laourette P, et al. Neutralising antibodies against ricin toxin. *PLoS One*. 2011;6(5):1-10.

175. Centers for Disease Control. Facts about ricin. CDC Emergency Preparedness and Response. https://emergency.cdc.gov/agent/ricin/facts.asp. Accessed June 27, 2017.

176. Peterson BW, Damon IK. Orthopoxviruses: vaccinia (smallpox vaccine), variola (smallpox), monkeypox, and cowpox. In: Bennett JE, Dolin R, Blaser MJ, eds. *Mandell, Douglas, and Bennett's Principles and Practice of Infectious Diseases.* 8th ed. Philadelphia, PA: Elsevier; 2014: 1694-1702.

177. Smee DF. Orthopoxvirus inhibitors that are active in animal models: an update from 2008 to 2012. *Future Virol.* 2013;8(9):891-901.

178. Nalca A, Zumbrun EE. ACAM2000: the new smallpox vaccine for United States Strategic National Stockpile. *Drug Des Devel Ther.* 2010;4:71-79.

179. ACAM 2000 [package insert]. Gaithersburg, MD: Emergent BioSolutions; 2007.

180. Adverse reactions following smallpox vaccination. Morbidity and /mortality Weekly Report. https://www.cdc.gov/mmwr/preview/mmwrhtml/mm5213a4.htm. Updated May 3, 2013. Accessed May 25, 2018.

181. Casey C, et al. Medical management of smallpox (vaccinia) adverse reactions: vaccinia immune globulin and cidofovir. Morbidity and /mortality Weekly Report. https://www.cdc.gov/mmwr/preview/mmwrhtml/rr5501a1.htm . Updated January 19, 2006. Accessed May 25, 2018.

182. Lederman ER, Davidson W, Groff HL, et al. Progressive vaccinia: case description and laboratory-guided therapy with vaccinia immune globulin, ST-246, and CMX001. *J Infect Dis.* 2012;206(9):1372-1385.

183. Mead PS. *Yersinia* species (including plague). In: Bennett JE, Dolin R, Blaser MJ, eds. *Mandell, Douglas, and Bennett's Principles and Practice of Infectious Diseases.* 8th ed. Philadelphia, PA: Elsevier; 2014: 2607-2618.

184. Mwengee W, Butler T, Mgema S, et al. Treatment of plague with gentamicin or doxycycline in a randomized clinical trial in Tanzania. *Clin Infect Dis.* 2006;42(5):614-621.

185. Cancio LC, Batchinsky AI, Dubick MA, et al. Inhalation injury: pathophysiology and clinical care proceedings of a symposium conducted at the trauma institute of San Antonio, TX, USA on 28 March 2006. *Burns.* 2007;33(6):681-692.

186. Shimazu T, Yukioka T, Ikeuchi H, Mason AD Jr, Wagner PD, Pruitt BA Jr. Ventilation–perfusion alterations after smoke inhalation injury in an ovine model. *J Appl Physiol.* 1996;81(5):2250-2259.

187. Hubbard GB, Langlinais PC, Shimazu T, Okerberg CV, Mason AD Jr, Pruitt BA Jr. The morphology of smoke inhalation injury in sheep. *J Trauma.* 1991;31(11):1477-1486.

188. Thompson PB, Herndon DN, Traber DL, Abston S. Effect on mortality of inhalation injury. *J Trauma.* 1986;26(2):163-165.

189. Silverstein P, Dressler DP. Effect of current therapy on burn mortality. *Ann Surg.* 1970;171(1):124-129.

190. Cox CS, Zwischenberger JB, Traber DL, Traber LD, Haque AK, Herndon DN. Heparin improves oxygenation and minimizes barotrauma after severe smoke inhalation in an ovine model. *Surg Gynecol Obstet.* 1993;176(4):339-349.

191. Desai MH, Mlcak R, Richardson J, Nichols R, Herndon DN. Reduction in mortality in pediatric patients with inhalation injury with aerosolized heparin/N-acetylcystine therapy. *J Burn Care Rehabil.* 1998;19(3):210-212.

192. Brown M, Desai M, Traber LD, Herndon DN, Traber DL. Dimethylsulfoxide with heparin in the treatment of smoke inhalation injury. *J Burn Care Rehabil.* 1988;9(1):22-25.

193. Mlcak RP, Suman OE, Herndon DN. Respiratory management of inhalation injury. *Burns.* 2007;33(1):2-13.

194. Baud FJ, Barriot P, Toffis V, et al. Elevated blood cyanide concentrations in victims of smoke inhalation. *N Engl J Med* 1991;325(25):1761-1766.

195. Stevens J, El-Shammaa E. Carbon monoxide and cyanide poisoning in smoke inhalation victims. *Trauma Reports.* January 1, 2015.

196. Baud FJ, Borron SW, Mégarbane B, et al. Value of lactic acidosis in the assessment of the severity of acute cyanide poisoning. *Crit Care Med.* 2002;30(9):2044-2050.

197. Hamel J. A review of acute cyanide poisoning with a treatment update. *Crit Care Nurse.* 2011;31(1):72-80.

198. Quinn DK, McGahee SM, Politte LC, et al. Complications of carbon monoxide poisoning: a case discussion and review of the literature. *Prim Care Companion J Clin Psychiatry.* 2009;11(2):74-79.

199. Hampson NB, Piantadosi CA, Thom SR, Weaver LK. Practice recommendations in the diagnosis, management and prevention of carbon monoxide poisoning. *Am J Respir Crit Care Med.* 2012;186(11):1095-1101.

200. Fortin JL, Waroux S, Giocanti JP, et al. Hydroxocobalamin for poisoning caused by ingestion of potassium cyanide: a case study. *J Emerg Med.* 2010;39(3):320-324.

201. Battison C, Andrews PJ, Graham C, Petty T. Randomized, controlled trial on the effect of a 20% mannitol solution and a 7.5% saline/6% dextran solution on increased intracranial pressure after brain injury. *Crit Care Med.* 2005;33(1):196-202.

202. Vialet R, Albanese J, Thomachot L, et al. Isovolume hypertonic solutes (sodium chloride or mannitol) in the treatment of refractory posttraumatic intracranial hypertension: 2 mL/kg 7.5% saline is more effective than 2 mL/kg 20% mannitol. *Crit Care Med.* 2003;31(6):1683-1687.

203. Kamel H, Navi BB, Nakagawa K, Hemphill JC 3rd, Ko NU. Hypertonic saline versus mannitol for the treatment of elevated intracranial pressure: a meta-analysis of randomized clinical trials. *Crit Care Med.* 2011;39(3):554-559.

204. Marko NF. Hypertonic saline, not mannitol, should be considered gold-standard medical therapy for intracranial hypertension. *Crit Care.* 2012;16(1):113-115.

205. Hinson HE, Stein D, Sheth KN. Hypertonic saline and mannitol therapy in critical care neurology. *J Intensive Care Med.* 2013;28(1):3-11.

206. Rickard AC, Smith JE, Newell P, Bailey A, Kehoe A, Mann C. Salt or sugar for your injured brain? A meta-analysis of randomized controlled trials of mannitol versus hypertonic sodium solutions to manage raised intracranial pressure in traumatic brain injury. *Emerg Med J.* 2014;31(8):679-683.

207. Burgess S, Abu-Laban RB, Slavik RS, Vu EN, Zed PJ. A systematic review of randomized controlled trials comparing hypertonic sodium solutions and mannitol for traumatic brain injury: implications for emergency department management. *Ann Phamacother.* 2016;50(4):291-300.

208. Prabhakar H, Singh GP, Anand V, Kalaivani M. Mannitol versus hypertonic saline for brain relaxation in patients undergoing craniotomy. *Cochrane Database Syst Rev.* 2014;(6):CD010026.

209. Mirski M, Denchev DI, Schnitzer MS, Hanley DF. Comparison between hypertonic saline and mannitol in the reduction of elevated intracranial pressure in a rodent model of acute cerebral injury. *J Neurosurg Anesthesiol.* 2000;12(4):334-344.

210. Mortazavi MM, Romeo AK, Deep A, et al. Hypertonic saline for treating raised intracranial pressure: literature review with meta-analysis. *J Neurosurg.* 2012;116(1):210-221.

211. Muizelaar JP, van der Poel HG, Li ZC, et al. Pial arteriolar vessel diameter and CO_2 reactivity during prolonged hyperventilation in the rabbit. *J Neurosurg.* 1988;69(6):923-927.

212. Kuroda Y. Neurocritical care update. *J Intensive Care.* 2016;4:36.

213. Saadeh Y, Gohil K, Bill C, et al. Chemical venous thromboembolic prophylaxis is safe and effective for patients with traumatic brain injury when started 24 hours after the absence of hemorrhage progression on head CT. *J Trauma Acute Care Surg.* 2012;73(2):426-430.

214. Abdel-Aziz H, Dunham CM, Malik RJ, Hileman BM. Timing for deep vein thrombosis chemoprophylaxis in traumatic brain injury: an evidence-based review. *Crit Care.* 2015;19:96.

215. Patel MB, Humble SS, Cullinane DC, et al. Cervical spine collar clearance in the obtunded adult blunt trauma: a systemic review and practice management guideline from the Eastern Association for the Surgery of Trauma. *J Trauma Acute Care Surg.* 2015;78(2):430-441.

216. Andrews CO, Engelhard HH. Fibrinolytic therapy in intraventricular hemorrhage. *Ann Pharmacother.* 2001; 35(11):1435-1438.

217. Engelhard HH, Andrews CO, Slavin KV, Charbel FT. Current management of intraventricular hemorrhage. *Surg Neurol.* 2003;60(1):15-21.

218. Nyquist P, Hanley DF. The use of intraventricular thrombolytics in intraventricular hemorrhage. *J Neurol Sci.* 2007; 261(1-2):84-88.

219. Huttner HB, Tognoni E, Bardutzky J, et al. Influence of intraventricular fibrinolytic therapy with rt-PA on the long-term outcome of treated patients with spontaneous basal ganglia hemorrhage: a case-control study. *Eur J Neurol.* 2008;15(4):342-349.

220. Naff N, Williams MA, Keyl PM, et al. Low-dose recombinant tissue-type plasminogen activator enhances clot resolution in brain hemorrhage: the intraventricular hemorrhage thrombolysis trial. *Stroke.* 2011;42(11):3009-3016.

221. Morgan T, Awad I, Keyl P, Lane K, Hanley D. Preliminary report of the clot lysis evaluating accelerated resolution of intraventricular hemorrhage (CLEAR-IVH) clinical trial. *Acta Neurochir Suppl.* 2008;105:217-220.

222. Hanley DF, Lane K, McBee N, et al; CLEAR III Investigators. Thrombolytic removal of intraventricular haemorrhage in treatment of severe stroke: results of the randomised, multicentre, multiregion, placebo-controlled CLEAR III Trial. *Lancet.* 2017;389(10069):603-611.

223. Hutchinson PJ, Kolias AG, Timofeev IS, et al; RESCUEicp Trial Collaborators. Trial of decompressive craniectomy for traumatic intracranial hypertension. *New Engl J Med.* 2016;375(12):1119-1130.

224. Atzema C, Mower WR, Hoffman JR, et al; National Emergency X-Radiography Utilization Study (NEXUS) II Group. Prevalence and prognosis of traumatic intraventricular hemorrhage in patients with blunt head trauma. *J Trauma.* 2006; 60(5):1010-1017.

225. Simon B, Ebert J, Bokhari F, et al; Eastern Association for the Surgery of Trauma. Management of pulmonary contusion and flail chest: an Eastern Association for the Surgery of Trauma for practice management guideline. *J Trauma Acute Care Surg.* 2012;73(5 Suppl 4):s351-s361.

226. Allen GS Coates NE. Pulmonary contusion: a collective review. *Am Surg.* 1996;62(11):895-900.

227. Oppenheimer L, Craven KD, Forkert L, Wood LD. Pathophysiology of pulmonary contusion in dogs. *J Appl Physiol.* 1979;47(4):718-728.

228. Wagner RB, Slivko B, Jamieson PM, Dills MS, Edwards FH. Effect of lung contusion on pulmonary hemodynamics. *Ann Thorac Surg.* 1991;52(1):51-57; discussion 57-58.

229. Craven KD, Oppenheimer L, Wood LD. Effects of contusion and flail chest on pulmonary perfusion and oxygen exchange. *J Appl Physiol.* 1979;47(4):729-737.

230. Shackford SR, Smith DE, Zarins CK, Rice CL, Virgilio RW. The management of flail chest. A comparison of ventilatory and nonventilatory treatment. *Am J Surg.* 1976;132(6): 759-762.

231. Shackford SR, Virgilio RW, Peters RM. Selective use of ventilator therapy in flail chest injury. *J Thorac Cardiovasc Surg.* 1981;81(2):194-201.

232. Mouton W, Lardinois D, Furrer M, Regli B, Ris HB. Long-term follow-up of patients with operative stabilization of a flail chest. *J Thorac Cardiovasc Surg.* 1997;45(5):242-244.

233. Mayberry JC, Terhes JT, Ellis TJ, Wanek S, Mullins RJ. Absorbable plates for rib fracture repair: preliminary experience. *J Trauma.* 2003;55(5):835-839.

234. Galan G, Peñalver JC, París F, et al. Blunt chest injuries in 1696 patients. *Eur J Cardiothorac Surg.* 1992;6(6):284-287.

235. Balci AE, Eren S, Cakir O, Eren MN. Open fixation in flail chest: review of 64 patients. *Asian Cardiovasc Thorac Ann.* 2004;12(1):11-15.

236. Tanaka H, Yukioka T, Yamaguti Y, et al. Surgical stabilization of internal pneumatic stabilization? A prospective randomized study of management of severe flail chest patients. *J Trauma.* 2002;52(4):727-732; discussion 732.

237. Voggenreiter G, Neudeck F, Aufmkolk M, et al. Operative chest wall stabilization in flail chest—outcomes of patients with or without pulmonary contusion. *J Am Coll Surg.* 1998;187(2):130-138.

238. Engel C. Operative fixation with osteosynthesis plates. *J Trauma.* 2006;58:181-186.

239. Nirula R, Allen B, Layman R, Falimirski ME, Somberg LB. Rib fracture stabilization in patients sustaining blunt chest injury. *Am Surg.* 2006;72(4):307-309.

240. Campbell N, Conaglen P, Martin K, Antippa P. Surgical stabilization of rib fractures using Inion OTPS wraps—techniques and quality of life follow-up. *J Trauma.* 2009;67(3):596-601.

241. Marasco S, Cooper J, Pick A, Kossmann T. Pilot study of operative fixation of fractured ribs in patients with flail chest. *ANZ J Surg.* 2009;79(11):804-808.

242. Mayberry JC, Ham LB, Schipper PH, Ellis TJ, Mullins RJ. Surveyed opinion of American trauma, orthopedic, and thoracic surgeons on rib and sternal fracture repair. *J Trauma.* 2009;66(3):875-879.

243. Mowery NT, Gunter OL, Collier BR, et al. Practice management guidelines for management of hemothorax and occult pneumothorax. *J Trauma.* 2011;70(2):510-518.

244. Bilello JF, Davis JW, Lemaster DM. Occult traumatic hemothorax: when can sleeping dogs lie? *Am J Surg.* 2005;190(6):841-844.

245. Heniford BT, Carrillo EH, Spain DA, Sosa JL, Fulton RL, Richardson JD. The role of thoracoscopy in the management of retained thoracic collections after trauma. *Ann Thorac Surg.* 1997;63(4):940-943.

246. Fabbrucci P, Nocentini L, Secci S, et al. Video-assisted thoracoscopy in the early diagnosis and management of post-traumatic pneumothorax and hemothorax. *Surg Endosc.* 2008;22(5):1227-1231.

247. Karmy-Jones R, Holevar M, Sullivan RJ, Fleisig A, Jurkovich GJ. Residual hemothorax after chest tube placement correlates with increased risk of empyema following traumatic injury. *Can Respir J.* 2008;15(5):255-258.

248. Vassiliu P, Velmahos GC, Toutouzas KG. Timing, safety, and efficacy of thoracoscopic evacuation of undrained post-traumatic hemothorax. *Am Surg.* 2001;67(12):1165-1169.

249. Meyer DM, Jessen ME, Wait MA, Estrera AS. Early evacuation of traumatic retained hemothoraces using thoracoscopy: a prospective, randomized trial. *Ann Thorac Surg.* 1997;64(5):1396-1400.

250. Schöchl H, Maegele M, Solomon C, Gorlinger K, Voelckel W. Early and individualized goal-directed therapy for trauma-induced coagulopathy. *Scand J Trauma Resusc Emerg Med.* 2012;20:15.

251. Enriquez LJ, Shore-Lesserson L. Point-of-care coagulation testing and transfusion algorithms. *Br J Anaesth.* 2009;103 (Suppl 1):i14-i22.

252. Luddington RJ. Thromboelastography/thromboelastometry. *Clin Lab Haematol.* 2005;27(2):81-90.

253. Wang SC, Shieh JF, Chang KY, et al. Thromboelastography-guided transfusion decreases intraoperative blood transfusion during orthotopic liver transplantation: randomized clinical trial. *Transfusion.* 2010;47(7):2590-2593.

254. Speiss BD, Gilles BS, Chandler W, Verrier E. Changes in transfusion therapy and reexploration rate after institution of a blood management program in cardiac surgical patients. *J Cardiothoracic Vasc Anesth.* 1995;9(2):168-173.

255. Ak K, Isbir CS, Tetik S, et al. Thromboelastography-based transfusion algorithm reduced blood product use after elective CABG: a prospective randomized study. *J Card Surg.* 2009;24(4):404-410.

256. Niles SE, McLaughlin DF, Perkins JG, et al. Increased mortality associated with the early coagulopathy of trauma in combat casualties. *J Trauma.* 2008;64(6):1459-1463.

257. Brohi K, Singh J, Heron M, Coats T. Acute traumatic coagulopathy. *J Trauma.* 2003;54(6):1127-1130.

258. Cotton BA, Gunter OL, Isbell J, et al. Damage control hematology: the impact of a trauma exsanguination protocol on survival and blood product utilization. *J Trauma* 2008;64(5):1177-1182.

259. Cohen MJ, Call M, Nelson M, et al. Critical role of activated protein C in early coagulopathy and later organ failure, infection and death in trauma patients. *Ann Surg.* 2012;255(2):379-385.

260. Cohen MK, Kutcher M, Redick B, et al; PROMMTT Study Group. Clinical and mechanistic drivers of acute traumatic coagulopathy. *J Trauma Acute Care Surg.* 2013;75(1 Suppl 1):S40-S47.

261. Kaufmann CR, Dwyer KM, Crews JD, et al. Usefulness of thromboelastography in assessment of trauma patient coagulation. *J Trauma.* 1997;42(4):716-720.

262. Martini WZ, Cortez DS, Dubick MA, et al. Thromboelastography is better than PT, aPTT, and activated clotting time in detecting clinically relevant clotting abnormalities after hypothermia, hemorrhagic shock, and resuscitation in pigs. *J Trauma.* 2008;65(3):535-543.

263. Holcomb JB, Minei KM, Scerbo ML, et al. Admission rapid thromboelastography can replace conventional coagulation tests in the emergency department: experience with 1975 consecutive trauma patients. *Ann Surg.* 2012;256(3):476-486.

264. Cotton BA, Faz G, Hatch QM, et al. Rapid thromboelastography delivers real-time results that predict transfusion within 1 hour of admission. *J Trauma.* 2011;71(2):407-417.

265. Vogel AM, Radwan ZA, Cox CS, Cotton BA. Admission rapid thromboelastography delivers real-time "actionable" data in pediatric trauma. *J Ped Surg.* 2013;48(6):1371-1376.

266. Tapia NM, Chang A, Norman M, et al. TEG-guided resuscitation is superior to standardized MTP resuscitation in massively transfused penetrating trauma patients. *J Trauma Acute Care Surg.* 2012;74(2):378-386.

267. Cribari C. Management of poisonous snakebites. American College of Surgeons. https://www.facs.org/~/media/files/ quality%20programs/trauma/publications/snakebite.ashx. Updated 2004. Accessed May 25, 2018.

268. Fikkers BG, van Vugt S, van der Hoeven JG, van den Hoogen FJA, Marres HAM. Emergency cricothyrotomy: a randomised crossover trial comparing the wire-guided and catheter-over-needle techniques. *Anaesthesia.* 2004;59(10):1008-1011.

269. Gillespie MB, Eisele DW. Outcomes of emergency surgical airway procedures in a hospital-wide setting. *The Laryngoscope.* 1999;109(11):1766-1769.

270. Hsiao J, Pacheco-Fowler V. Cricothyroidotomy. *NEJM.* https:// www.nejm.org/doi/full/10.1056/nejmvcm0706755. Accessed May 25, 2018.

271. Khan H. Cricothyroidotomy. *Emedicine.* https://emedicine. medscape.com/article/1830008-overview. Updated July 30, 2015. Accessed June 17, 2017.

272. Simunovic N, Devereaux PJ, Sprague S, et al. Effect of early surgery after hip fracture on mortality and complications: systematic review and meta-analysis. *CMAJ.* 2010;182(15): 1609-1616.

273. Grimes JP, Gregory PM, Noveck H, Butler MS, Carson JL. The effects of time-to-surgery on mortality and morbidity in patients following hip fracture. *Am J Med.* 2002;112(9):702-709.

274. Vidán MT, Sánchez E, Gracia Y, Marañón E, Vaquero J, Serra JA. Causes and effects of surgical delay in patients with hip fracture: a cohort study. *Ann Intern Med.* 2011;155(4): 226-233.

275. Southwell-Keely JP, Russo RR, March L, Cumming R, Cameron I, Brnabic AJ. Antibiotic prophylaxis in hip fracture surgery: a metaanalysis. *Clin Orthop Relat Res.* 2004;(419):179-184

276. Gillespie WJ, Walenkamp GH. Antibiotic prophylaxis for surgery for proximal femoral and other closed long bone fractures. *Cochrane Database Syst Rev.* 2001;(1):CD000244.

277. Bratzler DW, Dellinger EP, Olsen KM, et al. Clinical practice guidelines for antimicrobial prophylaxis in surgery. *Surg Infect (Larchmt).* 2013;14(1):73-156.

278. Steinberg JP, Braun BI, Hellinger WC, et al; Trial to Reduce Antimicrobial Prophylaxis Errors (TRAPE) Study Group. Timing of antimicrobial prophylaxis and the risk of surgical site infections: results from the Trial to Reduce Antimicrobial Prophylaxis Errors. *Ann Surg.* 2009;250(1):10-16.

279. Falck-Ytter Y, Francis CW, Johanson NA, et al; American College of Chest Physicians. Prevention of VTE in orthopedic surgery patients: Antithrombotic Therapy and Prevention of Thrombosis, 9th ed: American College of Chest Physicians evidence-based clinical practice guidelines. *Chest.* 2012; 141(2 Suppl):e278S-e325S.

280. Allman FL Jr. Fractures and ligamentous injuries of the clavicle and its articulation. *J Bone Joint Surg Am.* 1967;49(4):774-784.

281. Robinson CM. Fractures of the clavicle in the adult. Epidemiology and classification. *J Bone Joint Surg Br.* 1998;80(3):476-484.

282. Dantas-Torres F. Rocky Mountain spotted fever. *Lancet Infect Dis.* 2007;7(11):724-732.

283. Dennis DT, Inglesby TV, Henderson DA, et al; Working Group on Civilian Biodefense. Tularemia as a biological weapon: medical and public health management. *JAMA.* 2001;285(21):2763-2773.

284. Marrie TJ. *Coxiella burnetii* pneumonia. *Eur Respir J.* 2003;21(4):713-719.

285. Powell OW, Kennedy KP, McIver M, Silverstone H. Tetracycline in the treatment of "Q" fever. *Australas Ann Med.* 1962;11:184-188.

286. Gikas A, Spyridaki I, Scoulica E, Psaroulaki A, Tselentis Y. In vitro susceptibility of *Coxiella burnetii* to linezolid in comparison with its susceptibilities to quinolones, doxycycline, and clarithromycin. *Antimicrob Agents Chemother.* 2001;45(11):3276-3278.

287. Raoult D, Marrie T, Mege J. Natural history and pathophysiology of Q fever. *Lancet Infect Dis.* 2005;5(4):219-226.

288. Fox N, Schwartz D, Salazar JH, et al. Evaluation and management of blunt traumatic aortic injury: a practice management guideline from the Eastern Association for the Surgery of Trauma. *J Trauma Acute Care Surg.* 2015;78(2): 136-146.

289. Starnes BW, Lundgren RS, Gunn M, et al. A new classification scheme for treating blunt aortic injury. *J Vasc Surg.* 2012;55(1):47-54.

290. Cullen EL, Lantz EJ, Johnson CM, Young PM. Traumatic aortic injury: CT findings, mimics, and therapeutic options. *Cardiovasc Diagn Ther.* 2014;4(3):238-244.

291. Zafren K, Thurman R, Jones ID. ENVIRONMENTAL CONDITIONS. In: Knoop KJ, Stack LB, Storrow AB, Thurman R, eds. *The Atlas of Emergency Medicine. 4th ed.* New York, NY: McGraw-Hill; . http://accessmedicine.mhmedical.com/content.aspx?bookid=1763&sectionid=125436840. Accessed May 28, 2018.

292. Isbister GK, Fan HW. Spider bite. *Lancet.* 2011;378: 2039-2047.

30

Toxicology

Ronaldo Collo Go, MD, Rania Esteitie, MD, Faisal Tamimi, MD,
Han Yu, MD, and Ronni Levy, MD

INTRODUCTION

Toxicology represent a clinical dilemma for clinicians worldwide and impart a diagnostic challenge, particularly in the intensive care unit (ICU) setting. A poisoned patient typically cannot provide a history; therefore, an adequate diagnosis relies on laboratory data and an astute clinician identifying specific toxidromes and having a high index of suspicion.

EPIDEMIOLOGY

Poisoning is the leading cause of injury-related death in the United States.[1] In 2015, 47% of exposure cases involved children younger than 6 years of age, but as in previous years, many of the more serious cases occurred among adolescents and adults. A total of 57% of human exposures involved medications or pharmaceuticals. Other exposures were to household products, plants, mushrooms, pesticides, animal bites and stings, carbon monoxide, and many other types of nonpharmaceutical substances.[2] The majority of exposures were ingestions or aspirations in 79% (Fig. 30-1) and were unintentional (Fig. 30-2). The categories of substances or toxins with the largest number of exposures in all ages included analgesics (11.1%), cleaning substances (7.6%), and sedative–hypnotics (5.8%).[2]

PHYSIOLOGY

Pharmacologic Considerations

1. **Absorption:** The degree of absorption of medications is highly dependent on the environment at the site of administration. Shock states decrease perfusion and shunt blood to the vital organs reduce systemic absorption of drugs from the intestines and intramuscular and subcutaneous tissues.[3] Intestinal atrophy can begin after only 3 days of starvation and is not prevented by parenteral nutrition (see Figure 30-3).[4]
2. **Distribution:** Sepsis, shock, burn injury, pancreatitis, and alterations in plasma protein binding are just a few examples of disease entities influencing the volume of distribution (Vd). Alternatively, fluid resuscitation, as frequently necessary in critically ill patients, will also lead to increased Vd.

3. **Metabolism:** Drug metabolism occurs predominantly in the liver and is driven mainly by the cytochrome P450 enzyme system. Critical illness affects metabolic activity by alterations in plasma protein concentration, hepatic enzymatic activity, and blood flow. Many drugs used in critically ill patients may either induce or inhibit the activity of the various isoenzymes included in the cytochrome P450 complex.
4. **Elimination:** Augmented renal clearance can be driven by sepsis, burn injury, or use of inotropic agents. On the other hand, acute kidney injury may complicate clearance of drugs, necessitating renal replacement therapy or dialysis.[5]

DIAGNOSIS

The diagnosis is often clinical, and it is common that multiple toxicities occur at the same time.[6-10] (Tables 30-1 to 30-4)[7,11-16] Treatment is not necessarily dependent on confirmation of the diagnosis because it may delay an opportunity to prevent further damage.

Urine drug tests are immunoassays in which antibodies bind to a particular structure[6] (Table 30-5). False negatives and false positives are common. After detection, gas chromatography–mass spectrometry can be used for confirmation.[6] Serum levels should also be obtained such as acetaminophen, carbamazepine, digoxin, metals, lithium, phenytoin, salicylate, theophylline, caffeine, toxic alcohol, and valproic acid.[6] Cooximetry may aid in diagnosis with detection of elevated levels of carboxyhemoglobin, methemoglobin, and sulfhemoglobin. Low anion gap is found in lithium, bromide, iodine, lipidemia, or hypoalbuminemia. Osmolal gap is elevated in ethanol, ethylene glycol, methanol, isopropanol, propylene glycol, ketones, and shock.

TREATMENT

Gastrointestinal Decontamination

Gastrointestinal decontamination is performed with activated charcoal and whole-bowel irrigation (WBI). Syrup of

Routes of exposure

■ Ingestion   ■ Dermal   ■ Inhalation or nasal
■ Ocular   ■ Bite or sting   ■ Unknown
■ Parenteral

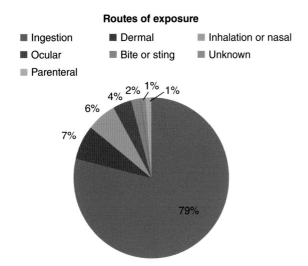

FIGURE 30-1 Routes of exposure for a total of 2,279,087 reported exposure cases. (Data from Gummin DD, Mowry JB, Spyker DA, et al. (2017) 2016 Annual Report of the American Association of Poison Control Centers' National Poison Data System (NPDS): 34th Annual Report, *Clin Toxicol*, 55(10), 1072-1254.)

ipecac and gastric lavage are not recommended because of side effects and no proven benefit. Activated charcoal binds to drugs and creates diffusion gradient between circulation and gut that prevents absorption and decreases serum levels.[7] The dose of activated charcoal is 25 to 100 g in adults and is of maximal benefit if given within 1 hour of ingestion.[6] Side effects include vomiting, constipation, diarrhea, and aspiration. WBI is performed with administration of 1.5 to 2 L/H of polyethylene glycol solution to improve transit of toxins such

■ Unintentional   ■ Intentional
■ Adverse reaction   ■ Unknown   ■ Other

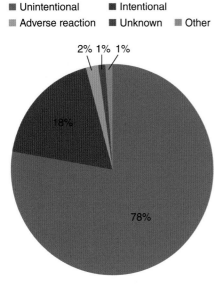

FIGURE 30-2 Reasons for exposures for a total of 2,168,371 exposure cases. (Data from Gummin DD, Mowry JB, Spyker DA, et al. (2017) 2016 Annual Report of the American Association of Poison Control Centers' National Poison Data System (NPDS): 34th Annual Report, *Clin Toxicol*, 55(10), 1072-1254.)

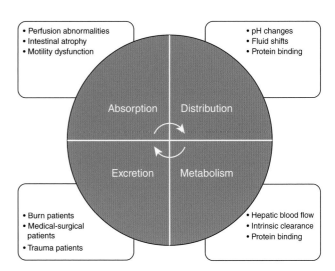

FIGURE 30-3 Pharmacokinetics in critical illness.

as enteric-coated aspirin, sustained-release lithium, extended-release verapamil, or iron or in "drug packers."[6] Endoscopy is used to remove drug bezoars, and laparotomy is used to remove illicit drug packets.

TABLE 30-1   Toxidrome and Clinical Characteristics

Toxidrome	Clinical Characteristics
Anticholinergic (antihistamines, atropine, baclofen, benztropine, tricyclic antidepressants, phenothiazine, scopolamine)	Fever, dry skin, flushing, mydriasis, ileus, urinary retention, tachycardia, hypertension, psychosis, myclonus, seizures, coma
Cholinergic (carbamate, organophosphates, physostigmine, pilocarpine)	Salivation, lacrimation, urination, diarrhea, emesis wheezing, diaphoresis, bradycardia, miosis
β adrenergic (albuterol, theophylline)	Tachycardia, hypotension, tremor
α adrenergics (phenylephrine, phenylpropanolamine)	Hypertension, bradycardia, mydriasis
β and α adrenergics (amphetamines, cocaine, ephedrine, phencyclidine, pseudoephedrine)	Hypertension, tachycardia, mydriasis, diaphoresis, dry mucous membranes
Hallucinogenic (amphetamines, cocaine, cannabinoids, lysergic acid diethylamide, pnecyclidine)	Hallucinations, psychosis, panic, fever, mydriasis, hyperthermia, synesthesia
Serotinin (fluoxetine, meperidine, paraoxetine, sertraline, trazodine, clomipramine)	Irritability, hyperreflexia, flushing, diarrhea, diaphoresis, fever, trismus, tremor, myoclonus
Extrapyramidal (haloperidol, phenothiazines, resperidone olanzapine)	Rigidity, trismus, hyperreflexia, choreoasthetosis, opisthothonas
Narcotics (opiates, propoxyphene)	Miosis, altered metal status, hypotension, hypothermia, decreased bowel sounds, shallow breaths

TABLE 30-2 Plant Name and Clinical Characteristics

Plant Name	Clinical Characteristics
Jimsonweed, angel's trumpet, deadly nightshade, mandrake, black henbane	Anticholinergic symptoms including agitation, hallucinations, hyperthermia, tachycardia, rhabodmyolysis, renal failure
Tobacco, betel nut, hemlock	Paresthesias, nausea, vomiting, seizures, autonomic instability bronchospasm, bronchorrhea, salivation
Morning glory and Hawaiian baby woodrose	Hallucinations, agitation, tachycardia, rhabdomyolysis
Water hemlocks / dropwarts from genera *Cicuta* and *Oenanthe*	Vomiting, seizures, rhadomyolysis
Strychnine	Hyperreflexia, rigidity, opisthotonus, rhabomyolysis, acute renal injury, respiratory failure
Foxglove, common oleander, yellow oleander, lily of the valley	Vomiting, bradycardia, AV blocks, increase automaticity
Monkshood, genus *Veratrum*, Rhododendron	Sinus bradycardia, heart blocks, paraesthesias, vomiting
Pyrrolizidine alkaloids like groundsel and comfrey	Liver failure
Ackee fruit	Hyperammonia, hepatic microvascular steatosis, vomiting, abdominal pain, hypotonia, seizures, coma
Amanita phalloides, *Lepiota* species, and *Galerina* species	Gastroenteritis, encephalopathy, liver failure
Gyromitrin	Gastroenteritis, hemolytic anemia, methemoglobinemia
Amanita muscaria, *Amanita pantherina*	Nausea, vomiting, CNS abnormalities such as depression, stimulation, seizures, ataxia

TABLE 30-3 Animal Bites and Clinical Characteristics

Animal	Clinical Characteristics
Scorpion (*Centruroides sculpturatus*)	Pain and parathesias that can lead to cranial nerve palsies including loss of pharyngeal tone
Brown Recluse Spider (*Loxosceles reclusa*)	Erythema to large ulceration on site of bite that can progress to necrosis resulting in eschar, hemolytic anemia, diarrhea
Black Widow (*Latrodectus mactans*)	Painful target like lesion, intermittent muscle spasms, diaphoresis (local or diffuse), fever, priapism, acute cardiomyopathy
Pit vipers	Pain and edema with formation of hemorrhagic bullae around bite stie, tachycardia, vomiting, paresthesia, fasciculations, diarrhea, shock
Stingrays (*Chondrichthyes*)	Hemorrhage, pain, edema, wound necrosis
Stone fish and Lion Fish (*Scorpaenidae* family)	Hemorrhage, pain, edema, wound necrosis
Portugese-man-of-war (*Physalia physalis*)	Pain, edema, redness, wound necrosis, delayed hypersensitivity reaction, shock
Sea sponge	Wound necrosis
Sea urchin	Pain, arthritis, nausea, vomiting, muscular paralysis

TABLE 30-4 Heavy Metal and Clinical Characteristics

Heavy Metal	Clinical Characteristics
Aresenic	Acute toxicity includes hemorrhagic gastroenteritis, shock, acute tubular necrosis, hemolysis, cardiomyopathy Chronic toxicity includes pigmentation, keratosis, cancer of skin, lung, liver, bladder, and kidney, diabetes, gangrene, peripheral neuropathy, peripheral vascular disease
Cadmium	Acute toxicity includes symptoms related to acute pneumonitis and symptoms related to gastroenteritis, bone pain Chronic toxicity includes yellowish discoloration of teeth, microcytic hypochromic anemia, transaminitis, osteomalacia, chronic renal failure
Lead	Acute toxicity leads to loss of appetite, abdominal pain, central and peripheral nervous system symptoms including headache, hallucinations, vertigo, acute encephalopathy with seizures and coma, impaired hematopoiesis, and renal failure Chronic toxicity can lead to decrease libido, impaired reaction time, hypertension, conduction abnormalities
Aluminium	Contact dermatitis, mouth ulcers, nausea, vomiting, diarrhea, arthritic pain
Mercury	Acute toxicity if inhaled can cause pneumonitis and cardiogenic pulmonary edema, irritability, depression, shyness, tremors, memory problems, polyneuropathy, gastroenteritis, acute kidney injury, hair loss, arrthymias Exposure during pregnancy can cause fetal abnormalities such as mental retardation

TABLE 30-5 Drug and Approximate Detection Period

Drug	Approximate Detection Period
Amphetamine, methamphetamine	4 d
Barbiturate	
Short acting (eg, pentobarbital)	24 h
Long acting (phenobarbital)	3 wk
Benzodiazepines	
Short acting (eg, lorazepam)	3 d
Long acting (eg, diazepam)	4 wk
Cocaine metabolite (benzoylecgonine)	3 d
Marijuana (cannabinoids)	
Single use	3 d
Long-term use	4 wk
Opiates (varies by agent)	4 d
Phencyclidine	8 d

Data from Levine M, Brooks DE, Truitt CA, et al. Toxicology in the ICU: general overview and approach to treatment. Chest. 2011;140(3):795-806; Chattergoon DS, Verjee Z, Anderson M, et al. Carbamazepine interference with an immune assay for tricyclic antidepressants in plasma. J Toxicol Clin Toxicol. 1998;36(1-2):109-113; McQuillen KK, Anderson AC. Osmol gaps in the pediatric population. Acad Emerg Med. 1999;6(1):27-30.

Extracorporeal Elimination Technique

Low-molecular-weight, low Vd, high water solubility, and low protein-binding xenobiotics are removed effectively via hemodialysis.[6] These include salicylates, phenobarbital, theophylline, methanol, ethylene glycol, lithium, propylene glycol, isopropyl alcohol, valproic acid, and carbamazepine.[6]

Urinary Alkalinization

Urine alkalinization (urine pH ≥ 7.5, but in salicylates, the goal is pH ≥ 8.5) traps drugs in the urine that have undergone ionization and limits reabsorption.[6] These medications include salicylates, chlorpropamide, 2-4-dichlorophenoxyacetic acid, diflunisal, fluoride, mecoprop, methotrexate, and phenobarbital.[6]

Hyperinsulinemia Euglycemia

Hyperinsulinemia euglycemia (HIE) is suggested for calcium channel blocker poisoning. Calcium channel blockers impair insulin release and cause insulin resistance, and causes myocardial cells to change energy substrate from fatty acids to glucose.[17] It is believed that HIE promotes uptake of glucose into adipose and muscles, reduces cytosolic calcium concentrations, and moves potassium intracellularly.[6,17] It works within 30 minutes and may improve blood pressure (BP) but

not conduction defects. The regimen is 1 unit/kg intravenous (IV) bolus followed by 0.5 to 1 unit/kg/h with a glucose infusion of 0.5 g/kg/h.[6]

Lipid Emulsion

Lipid emulsion is believed to decrease the Vd of toxins, inhibit mitochondrial metabolism, impair fatty acid delivery to mitochondria, and activate potassium and calcium channels involved with anesthetic toxicity.[6] Medications include bupivacaine, clomipramine, verapamil, and propranolol.[6] The regimen is 20% lipid emulsion at 1.5 mL/kg over 1 minute followed by 0.25 mL/kg/min for 60 minutes.[18] The maintenance infusion is increased to 0.5 mL/kg/min if hypotension is present.[19]

Antidotes

Some toxins have specific antidotes as listed in the table below (Table 30-6).

TABLE 30-6 Drug and Antidote

Drug	Antidote
Acetaminophen	N-acetylcysteine
Anticholinergics	Physostigmine
Anticholinesterases	Atropine
Benzodiazepines	Flumazenil
Black widow spider	Equine derived antivenom
Carbon monoxide	Oxygen
Coral snake	Equine derived antivenom
Cyanide	Amyl nitrite, sodium nitrite, sodium thiosulfate, hydroxycobalamin
Digoxin	Digoxin-specific antibodies
Ethylene glycol	Ethanol/fomepizole, thiamine, and pyridoxine
Heavy metals (arsenic, copper, gold, lead, and mercury)	Dimercaprol (BAL), Ethylenediamie tetra-acetic acid, penicillamine
Hypoglycemic agents	Dextrose, glucagon, octreotide
Iron	Deferoxamine mesylate
Isoniazid	Pyridoxine
Methanol	Ethanol or fomepizole, folic acid
Methemoglobinemia	Methylene blue
Opioids	Naloxone
Organophosphate	Atropine, pralidoxamine
Rattlesnake bite	Equine-derived antivenom

Reprinted with permission from Mokhlesi B, Leiken JB, Murray P, et al. Adult toxicology in critical care: Part I: general approach to the intoxicated patient. Chest. 2003;123(2):577-592.

QUESTIONS

1. A 50-year-old man with a history of atrial fibrillation on anticoagulation, systolic heart failure with an ejection fraction of 35%, diabetes mellitus, and depression was found unresponsive by his wife. The patient was complaining of blurring of vision the past few days. Home medications include paroxetine, diltiazem, and digoxin. He was rushed to the emergency department (ED), where he was found to have the following vital signs: blood pressure 80/60 mmHg; heart rate (HR) 140 beats/min; respiratory rate (RR) 22 breaths/min; oxgen saturation (O_2 sat) greater than 95% on room air, and temperature, 97.5°F. Laboratory results showed the following:

White blood cell (WBC)	$8 \times 10^3/\mu L$
Hemoglobin (Hgb)	10 mg/dL
Platelets (plt)	$90 \times 10^3/\mu L$
Na	134 mEq/L
K	6 mEq/L
Cl	109 mEq/L
CO_2	25 mEq/L
Glucose	100 mEq/L
Creatine (Cr)	0.9 mg/dL
Blood urea nitrogen (BUN)	20 mg/dL

The digoxin level was 2 ng/mL. The electrocardiogram (ECG) shows biventricular tachycardia.
What is the next step?

A. Digoxin immune fab
B. Activated charcoal
C. Hemodialysis
D. Insulin and glucose drips

2. A 24-year-old woman who recently broke up with her boyfriend decided to ingest a bottle of aspirin. After 2 hours, she started complaining of abdominal pain and went to the ED for consultation. Her laboratory test results showed the following:

WBC	$10 \times 10^3/\mu L$
Hgb	14 mg/dL
plt	$90 \times 10^3/\mu L$
Na	145 mEq/L
K	5.0 mEq/L
Cl	109 mEq/L
CO_2	25 mEq/L
Glucose	90 mEq/L
Cr	0.5 mg/dL
Lactic acid	5 mmol/L
BUN	15 mg/dL

Arterial blood gas analysis showed pH 7.50/22/160/25/99%. Salicylate serum level was 50 mg/dL. She was started on activated charcoal but her abdominal pain worsened. Radiography of the kidneys, ureters, and bladder showed an ileus. What is the next step?

A. Activated charcoal
B. Sodium bicarbonate drip
C. Acetazolamide
D. Hemodialysis

3. A 50-year-old man was found unresponsive in his home by his housekeeper. Next to his body was an open bottle of metoprolol. He was intubated for airway protection and transferred to the ED. His blood pressure was 70/50 mm Hg, and his HR was 30 beats/min, and he was given a 2-Liter crystalloid bolus and started on dopamine infusion. He was given glucagon bolus but had no response. What is the next step?

A. Repeat glucagon bolus
B. Calcium chloride
C. Lipid emulsion therapy
D. High insulin euglycemia

4. A 60-year-old man with history of atrial fibrillation on diltiazem, lower extremity spasticity after a motor vehicular accident now on a baclofen pump, and bipolar disorder on lithium was found unresponsive at his home. Before this, his baclofen pump was recently filled, and his lithium dosage was recently increased. Current vital signs show BP, 78/55 beats/min; HR, 45 beats/min; O_2 sat, 80%; and RR, 10 breaths/min. Physical examination was otherwise unremarkable. The patient was started on dopamine and intubated for airway protection. The ECG showed sinus bradycardia. Urine toxicology was negative. Computed tomography (CT) of the head was negative. Serum levels of calcium channel blocker, digoxin, and baclofen were still pending. Lithium level was 0.8 mEq/L. Glucose level was 90 mmol/L. What is the next step?

A. Perform lumbar puncture and stop the baclofen pump
B. Calcium chloride drip, high insulin euglycemia therapy, and change dopamine to norepinephrine
C. Glucagon
D. Whole-bowel irrigation and hemodialysis

5. A 56-year-old male nursing home resident with a long history of psychiatric issues, including schizophrenia and depression; recent prolonged hospitalization for septic shock; and vancomycin-resistant enterococcus (VRE) presented with acute respiratory failure requiring intubation. Chest radiography showed consolidation of the right lung base consistent with pneumonia, which was confirmed by CT of the chest. The patient was started on linezolid and piperacillin–ticarcillin.

The patient's respiratory status improved during his first hospital day, but then the intensivist was notified by the nurse because the patient developed sudden jerking movements and appeared to have an altered mental state. On examination, the patient's temperature was 39.0°C, RR was 30 breaths/min, HR was 106 beats/min, blood pressure was 190/100 mmHg, and Sao$_2$ was 95% on room air. The patient appeared agitated and alert only to person. On physical examination, his lungs were clear to auscultation with a regular rate and rhythm. His pupils were 7 mm and reactive, but ocular clonus was present. His neurologic examination was notable for hyperreflexes and inducible clonus in both upper extremities. What is the likely antidote?

A. Cyproheptadine
B. Bromocriptine
C. Physostigmine
D. Dantrolene

6. An 89-year-old man with a history of dementia was hospitalized for pneumonia. His hospital stay was unremarkable until his fifth hospital day, when he developed extreme agitation and required one-to-one supervision. On day 6, at the request of his family, he was given three doses of Ativan equaling 10 mg, which did not work. He was then given one dose of Haldol 5 mg with some effect. He was started on Haldol as needed. He subsequently became nauseous and was started on metoclopramide. Symptoms persisted, and he was subsequently intubated for aspiration. The patient was kept on sedation via fentanyl and propofol. After 1 week, the patient was placed on pressure support. He continued to have temperatures of 104° to 105°F, HRs of 130 to 140 beats/min, and BPs of 140 to 150 mm Hg and was noted to have diaphoresis, depressed reflexes, and muscle rigidity. Laboratory results showed WBC count, $13 \times 10^3/\mu L$; Hgb, 12 g/dL; plt, 300 $10^3/\mu L$; lactic acid, 3 mmol/L; creatine phosphokinase (CPK), 13,000 U/L; BUN, 30 mg/dL; triglycerides 20 mg/dL and Cr 2.5 mg/dL. What is his diagnosis?

A. Neuroleptic malignant syndrome
B. Serotonin syndrome
C. Anticholinergic syndrome
D. Propofol infusion syndrome

7. A 67-year-old woman with stage IV vaginal cancer was admitted to the ICU for sepsis, worsening renal failure thought to be caused by obstruction, and acute respiratory failure from volume overload. The patient's home medications included dilantin, acetaminophen as needed, and zolpidem. Bilateral stents were placed for her hydronephrosis, her Cr stabilized at 5.0 mg/dL, and she began to produce good urine. She remained hemodynamically stable, and her liver enzymes and lactic acid levels normalized. The patient received IV bicarbonate and was placed on hemodialysis but continued to have a high anion gap

metabolic acidosis. The patient was sedated with fentanyl and Versed drip. What was the cause of her high anion gap metabolic acidosis?

A. Propylene glycol
B. 5-Oxoprolinuria
C. Acute renal failure
D. D-Lactic acidosis

8. Which ingestion causes an osmolar gap but not a metabolic acidosis or high anion gap?

A. Ethylene glycol
B. Methanol
C. Isopropyl acid
D. None of the above

9. A 40-year-old man with a history of hypertension and bipolar disorder was found unresponsive on the floor of his house. He was found with an empty bottle of lithium next to him. He was recently started on lisinopril for hypertension. The patient was rushed to the ED, where he was intubated. CT of the head was negative. He was starting to wake up, and sedation was initiated. Laboratory results included WBC count, $15 \times 10^3/\mu L$; Hgb, 14 g/L; plt, $300 \times 10^3/\mu L$; Na, 145 mEq/L; K, 3 mEq/L; Cl, 106 mEq/L; Cr, 1 mg/dL; Ca, 8 mg/dL; and glucose, 100 mg/dL. His lithium level was 3.5 mEq/L. In-vitro fertilization (IVF) was initiated. What is the next step?

A. Activated charcoal
B. Whole-bowel irrigation
C. Extracorporeal treatment
D. Sodium polystyrene

10. A 30-year-old man was found unresponsive in the garden. He was diaphoretic and foaming at the mouth and noted to have tonic-clonic movements. Emergency medical services arrived, and they noted that he was hypotensive and bradycardic to the 30s. His pupils were pinpoint. He had diffuse wheezes bilaterally. He had hyperactive bowel sounds. IV access was obtained, and he was initiated on fluid bolus and atropine. ECG showed sinus bradycardia. A family member said he was last seen responsive 4 hours ago. He is a farmer, and he has been spraying some crops with insecticide. What would be the next step?

A. Intubate with etomidate and succinylcholine.
B. Give atropine until the wheezes improve with pralidoxime.
C. Give atropine until the tachycardia improves then give pralidoxime.
D. Remove clothing and wash body with soap and administer activated charcoal.

11. A 30-year-old woman was found unresponsive in her bedroom. She had an open bottle of medications next to her. She had a history of hypertension and depression.

On physical examination, she was noted to have BP, 60/40 mm Hg; HR, 134 beats/min; RR, 18 breaths/min; O$_2$ sat, 98%; and temperature, 104°F. Physical examination showed dilated pupils that were reactive to light. Her lungs were clear to auscultation. Her heart sounds were tachycardic with no murmurs. Her abdomen was distended with hypoactive bowel sounds. A crystalloid fluid bolus was started and the patient was intubated. The was is intubated for airway protection. The ECG shows QRS greater than 100 sec, QRS complex with terminal rightward deflection, deep S wave in leads I, AVL, tall R wave in lead AVR, R wave in AVR greater than 3 mm.

What is the next treatment?

A. Sodium bicarbonate
B. Activated charcoal
C. Hypertonic saline
D. Lipid emulsion

12. A 25-year-old woman complains of being bitten by a scorpion 6 hours ago on her right arm. She feels numbness at the sting site and appears to have involuntary jerking movements at that extremity. She is also complaining of blurring of vision and she has hypersalivation. She was already given antivenom and after 2 hours her symptoms have not improved. What is the severity of her envenomation and what should be the next step?

A. Grade II and patient should just receive analgesics
B. Grade III and the patient should just be monitored for another 6 hours
C. Grade IV and the patient should receive another dose of antivenom
D. Grade IV and the patient should just be monitored for another 6 hours

13. Which of the following is true regarding iron poisoning?

A. Bowel obstruction can occur 4 weeks after ingestion
B. Latent phase occurs before 6 hours of ingestion
C. Serum level 100 mcq/dL is associated with serious systemic toxicity
D. Reddish color urine during chelation is an indication to stop chelation therapy

14. Which of the following is true regarding heavy metal poisoning?

A. Blood lead level more than 100 mcq/dL is an indication for chelation treatment
B. Chelation therapy is indicated in lead poisoning, arsenic poisoning, mercury poisoning, and cadmium poisoning
C. Aluminum is not found in hemodialysis fluid
D. Free erythrocyte protoprophyrin (FEP) or zinc protoporphyrin (ZPP) might not be indicated for blood lead level less than or equal to 10 mcq/gL

ANSWERS

1. A. Digoxin immune fab

Digoxin inhibits the sodium potassium adenosine triphosphate pump, increasing sodium and extracellular potassium, leading to increased intracellular calcium and contractility.[20,21] This can lead to automaticity and cardiac blocks.[22] Symptoms depend on chronicity, with acute toxicity presenting as nausea, vomiting, and other symptoms related to conduction abnormalities. These symptoms include shortness of breath; palpitations; drowsiness; headaches; altered mental status; paresthesias; disturbances such as yellow-green distortion, photophobia, decreased visual acuity, scotomata, and transient halos; nausea; vomiting; abdominal pain; and diarrhea.[20,21] Concomitant use of verapamil, diltiazem, erythromycin, tetracycline, and paroxetine can increase digoxin levels.[20,21] There are supraventricular tachycardia from increased automaticity and slow ventricular response caused by decreased atrioventricular conduction.[20] The most common nontoxic digitalis effects on ECG are a sagging ST segment; flattened, inverted, or biphasic T wave; and shortened QT interval. However, this patient has a bidirectional ventricular tachycardia (beat-to-beat alteration of the QRS axis), and digitalis poisoning is one of the few causes.

Hyperkalemia is associated with acute toxicity caused by inhibition of sodium–potassium ATPase. Hypokalemia, hypomagnesemia, and hypercalcemia are concerning in chronic toxicity and may be caused by medications for congestive heart failure. The digoxin therapeutic level (0.5–0.8 ng/mL or 0.65–1 nmol/L) should be obtained 4 hours after an IV dose and 6 hours after an oral dose. Toxicity does not necessarily correlate with serum levels, but digoxin levels can help distinguish digitalis toxicity from other poisonings with similar presentations of hypotension and bradycardia.

First-line treatment for this patient with arrhythmias secondary to digitalis toxicity or hyperkalemia (≥ 5.5 mEq/L) is digoxin immune fab (40-mg vial in 4 mL of sterile water) IV over 30 minutes followed by 0.5 mg/min for 8 hours and then 0.1 mg/min for 6 hours. Repeat serum digoxin levels will be false high for up to 2 weeks after treatment with digoxin immune fab.

Gastrointestinal decontamination is most effective if given within 1 hour of ingestion but can also be effective up to 6 to 8 hours after ingestion (choice B).

Because of the large Vd and molecular weight, hemodialysis or hemoperfusion is not beneficial in digitalis toxicity (choice C). Insulin and glucose drips would be indicated if there is calcium channel blocker toxicity, which is not the case for this patient (choice D).

2. B. Sodium bicarbonate drip

This patient has aspirin toxicity, which can occur at levels greater than 30 mg/dL. Aspirin causes platelet dysfunction because of inhibition of cyclooxygenase; nausea, vomiting, and hyperventilation caused by stimulation of the medulla; and metabolic acidosis caused by interference with metabolic processes.[22,23] Alkalinization of urine pH is indicated regardless of the respiratory alkalosis. This is often achieved via sodium bicarbonate drip to maintain a pH greater than 7.5.[24,25]

Activated charcoal (choice A) minimizes the absorption of salicylate. Repeated doses maybe encouraged until the serum peak levels are reached. However, this patient has an ileus, and repeat doses are contraindicated. Acetazolamide (choice C) alkalinizes urine and improves salicylate excretion but also lowers serum pH. This allows salicylate to enter the blood–brain barrier, worsening neurotoxicity. Hemodialysis (choice D) is indicated in altered mental status, pulmonary edema, renal failure, severe systemic acidosis with a pH less than 7.20, and a salicylate concentration of 90 mg/dL with normal kidney function or 80 mg/dL in renal insufficiency.[16] The patient does not need dialysis yet.

3. A. Repeat glucagon bolus

Glucagon acts on adenylate cyclase, releasing cyclic adenosine monophosphate, which increases intracellular calcium and augments contractility. It is given as an IV bolus; if there is a response, an infusion is initiated. If there is no response, the bolus may be repeated [26,27] (choice A). Complications include vomiting and tachyphylaxis. Calcium salts can be added if glucagon does not work by improving inotropy (choice B). Lipid emulsion therapy and high insulin euglycemia can be initiated if the patient is still refractory to these measures (choices C and D).[28-30]

4. A. Perform lumbar puncture and stop the baclofen pump

Baclofen is the drug of choice for spasticity from the central nervous system (CNS). Oral baclofen does not cross the blood–brain barrier, and often a baclofen pump is placed. Symptoms of toxicity occur during filling procedures and includes hypotension, bradycardia, respiratory depression, or paralysis or may even mimic brain death.[31,32] In such situations, a lumbar puncture might be indicated and the pump held for up to 48 hours.[32]

Calcium channel blocker poisoning may be associated with hyperglycemia, which helps differentiate it from beta-blocker poisoning. The current guidelines suggest for calcium channel blocker poisoning as first-line treatment (1) calcium supplementation via 10% calcium chloride 10 to 20 mL (1–2 g) every 10 to 20 minutes; 0.2 to 0.4 mL/kg/h; 10% calcium gluconate 30 to 60 mL (3–6 g) every 10 to 20 minutes; or 0.6 to 1.2 mL/kg/h or (2) high insulin euglycemia therapy and pressors via norepinephrine and/or epinephrine if there is shock[33] (choice B).

Glucagon maybe indicated if the patient has overdosed on metoprolol. However, this patient was not taking metoprolol (choice C).

Therapeutic lithium serum levels are 0.8 to 1.2 mEq/L but often do not correlate with clinical symptoms of toxicity such as nausea, vomiting, diarrhea, ataxia, myoclonus, fasciculations, altered mental status, seizures, and encephalopathy. Whole-bowel irrigation might be used in patients with suspected lithium poisoning, but it is contraindicated in patients who have altered mental status and do not have a secure airway. Hemodialysis is an effective treatment. The hemodynamic instability and low normal serum lithium levels make lithium toxicity less likely (choice D).

5. A. Cyproheptadine

As an outpatient, the patient had been taking the selective serotonin reuptake inhibitor (SSRI) escitalopram, which was overlooked. Because of the patient's psychiatric history and physical examination findings, it is important to rule out serotonin syndrome even if an SSRI is not listed as one of his home medications. After placing a phone call to his pharmacy, it was confirmed that he had been taking an SSRI. When SSRIs are combined with monoamine oxidase (MAO) inhibitors, such as linezolid, serotonin syndrome may result. Serotonin syndrome is diagnosed clinically, and guided via the Hunter criteria. This criteria include (1) inducible clonus plus agitation or diaphoresis, (2) ocular clonus plus agitation or diaphoresis, (3) tremor plus hyperreflexia, and (4) hypertonia and a temperature above 38°C plus ocular or inducible clonus.[34] Usually, serotonin syndrome will stop within 24 hours from the discontinuation of the inciting agent. However, if the patient's condition does not improve, cyproheptadine is an antidote for serotonin syndrome.[35] It acts as a potent antihistamine and serotonin antagonist with anticholinergic effects. It may, however, cause CNS depression and hypotension, so patients need to be closely monitored.

Serotonin syndrome may be confused with other syndromes such as neuroleptic malignant syndrome (NMS) or sepsis. Serotonin syndrome can be distinguished by several key features. Serotonin syndrome usually occurs within 24 hours of the start of a monoamine oxidase inhibitor and resolves within 24 hours after the triggering medication is withdrawn. However, NMS takes days to weeks to resolve and is characterized by rigidity and depressed reflexes. Bromocriptine is a dopaminergic agonist used for NMS (choice B). Malignant hyperthermia (MH) should also be in the differential diagnosis with serotonin syndrome. MH occurs, however, after patients are exposed to halogenate volatile anesthetics or depolarizing agents such as succinylcholine. Increased end-tidal CO_2 levels, high temperatures, hyperthermia, and rigidity are characteristic of this syndrome.

Dantrolene acts on skeletal muscles and inhibits the release of calcium from the sarcoplasmic reticulum and reduces calcium levels associated with MH (choice D). Physostigmine is an acetylcholinesterase inhibitor that increases the levels of acetylcholine. It is used with anticholinergic toxicities (choice C).

6. **A. Neuroleptic malignant syndrome**

The patient developed NMS secondary to the neuroleptic agent Haldol. NMS is associated with three symptoms: (1) mental status change; (2) autonomic instability such as tachycardia, hypertension, and tachypnea; and (3) muscle rigidity.[36,37] Mortality rates can be as high as 10% to 20% with NMS.[36,37] Thus, it is important to diagnose early. Any neuroleptic agent may trigger NMS, including the new atypical antipsychotic drugs. Antiemetic agents have also been associated with NMS. These include metoclopramide, promethazine, and droperidol.

Serotonin syndrome (choice B) usually occurs within 24 hours of the initiation of an MAO inhibitor. It is also associated with hyperreflexia, clonus, and shivering, which are not normally seen with NMS.

Anticholinergic toxicity (choice C) can lead to hyperthermia, change of mental status, and tachycardia but should not usually lead to muscle rigidity.

Propofol-related infusion syndrome (PRIS) (choice D) is a life-threatening condition with no specific treatment other than supportive care, and it can mimic many other disorders. Predisposing risk factors include severe critical illness, use of vasopressors, and carbohydrate depletion. It is characterized by refractory bradycardia and ultimately asystole. PRIS lacks specific signs and symptoms but is often associated with metabolic acidosis, lactic acidosis, hyperlipidemia, rhabdomyolysis, and an enlarged liver.[38-40] High doses of propofol have been linked to PRIS, but low doses have also been reported. It requires a high index of suspicion when patients are taking propofol. This patient has low triglycerides and is febrile, which are not seen in PRIS.

7. **B. 5-Oxoprolinuria**

Critically ill patients who take acetaminophen, are malnourished, and have renal failure are at risk for elevated levels of 5-oxoproline (pyroglutamic acid).[41] Chronic acetaminophen ingestion has been associated with reduced plasma glutathione levels and elevation of 5-oxoproline levels in serum and urine. With renal failure, there is the addition of reduced urine excretion of 5-oxoproline. All of this leads to an increased level of 5-oxoproline and subsequently high anion gap metabolic acidosis.

High anion gap metabolic acidosis occurs frequently in ICU patients. Often it is attributable to liver or renal failure or lactic acidosis. However, in some cases, the high anion gaps cannot be explained. In some cases, high levels of 5-oxoproline levels can explain the high anion gap metabolic acidosis when acetaminophen levels are normal,

no liver necrosis exists, and an overdose cannot explain the situation.

The patient has no evidence of intentional overdose. The patient is on bicarbonate and hemodialysis, which contains high doses of bicarbonate. Patients on hemodialysis and bicarbonate should not have large anion gap metabolic acidosis. D-Lactic acidosis is associated with abdominal surgery and fistulas, which this patient does not have (choice D). Propylene glycol is associated with Ativan drip, not Versed drip.

8. **C. Isopropyl acid**

Isopropyl alcohol has similar effects as alcohol. It is found in many disinfectants and makes up to 70% of rubbing alcohol. Individuals without access to alcohol can use it to get inebriated.

When quantitative testing for alcohols such as isopropyl alcohol, ethylene glycol, or methanol is not accessible, checking the osmolar gap is important. The osmolar gap cannot distinguish among isopropyl, ethylene glycol, or methanol, but it will demonstrate their presence.

In contrast to ethylene glycol (choice A) and methanol (choice B) toxicity, toxic ingestions of isopropyl will not lead to an elevated anion gap or metabolic acidosis. Isopropyl is metabolized to ketones via alcohol dehydrogenase, which cannot be oxidized to acids and lead to a metabolic acidosis or high anion gap. Acetone is its main metabolite and leads to low toxicity.

9. **C. extracorporeal treatment**

Lithium has a narrow therapeutic index, and the most common complication of chronic ingestion is nephrogenic diabetes insipidus. Diuretics, angiotensin-converting enzyme inhibitors, and nonsteroidal antiinflammatory drugs can potentiate lithium toxicity. Lithium accumulation can decrease the urine-concentrating ability of the kidneys and increase serotonin metabolites, leading to serotonin-like syndrome. Clinical manifestations include tremors, altered mental status, seizures, nausea, vomiting, abdominal pain, diarrhea, and cardiovascular collapse.

Treatment includes stabilization, cessation of lithium administration or removal of medications that will reduce elimination, hydration to promote lithium removal, decontamination, and enhanced elimination.[42] Activated charcoal (choice A) does not bind lithium ions and is useless unless there is suspicion for other agents involved. WBI (choice B) might be helpful in early phase of poisoning because it restricts absorption, decreases bioavailability, and removes residual lithium. The Poisoning Workgroup recommends extracorporeal treatment (choice C) if lithium is greater than 4 mEq/L or the patient has an altered mental status, seizures, or life-threatening dysrhythmias irrespective of lithium level (grade ID).[43-45] Extracorporeal treatment is continued until clinical improvement or the lithium level is less than 1 mEq/L for more than 36 hours.[43] Sodium polystyrene sulfonate has been proposed to remove lithium, but it can cause hypokalemia, which is not ideal for this patient[44-45](choice D).

10. B. Give atropine until the wheezes improve with pralidoxime

Organophosphate (OP) inhibits acetylcholinesterase and pseudocholinesterase activities, causing acetylcholine to accumulate.[46,47] Acetylcholinesterase is found in synaptic junctions and red blood cells. Pseudocholinesterase via butyrylcholinesterase is found to the plasma. Aging is the irreversible binding of OP to acetylcholinesterase, and the degree is related to the type of OP. Dimethyl compounds age more than Diethyl compounds.

The effects of acetylcholine buildup are related to the location of the blockade—muscarinic (cholinergic) and nicotinic (skeletal muscle and autonomic ganglia). SLUDGE/BBB and DUMBELS are the mnemonics for the muscarinic effects. SLUDGE/BBB stands for salivation, lacrimation, urination, defecation, gastric emesis, bronchorrhea, bronchospasm, and bradycardia. DUMBELS stands for defecation; urination; miosis; bronchorrhea, bronchospasm or bradycardia; emesis; lacrimation; and salivation.[46,47] Nicotinic effects includes fasciculations, muscle weakness, and paralysis.[46,47] These manifestations can be categorized according to acute cholinergic crisis that can manifest within minutes to hours, with an intermediate syndrome within 24 to 96 hours and OP-induced delayed neuropathy occurring 2 to 3 weeks after exposure.

The intermediate syndrome consists of neck flexion weakness, decreased deep tendon reflexes, cranial nerve abnormalities proximal muscle weakness, and respiratory failure.[46-48] Delayed and long-term neuropathy are independent of acute cholinergic toxicity and are characterized by painful stocking glove paresthesias followed by symmetrical motor polyneuropathy with flaccid weakness of the lower extremities.[46-48] The initial approach is to remove the patient's clothing and wash the skin with soap and water. If ingested, activated charcoal might be used (choice D). Atropine is given at 0.5 to 2 mg IV and doubled every 5 minutes until secretions decrease, heart rate improves, and wheezing improves. Improvement of tachycardia is not an indication to discontinue atropine and generally can be continued until the rest of the symptoms have improved (choice C). The improvement of bronchoconstriction is the primary reason to discontinue atropine. Atropine is usually not given alone. Pralidoxime is given to reverse muscular weakness and fasciculations at a 1- to 2-g initial bolus followed by infusion and until at least 24 hours of being asymptomatic. Intubation is necessary, but succinylcholine is metabolized by acetylcholinesterase and can lead to prolonged blockade (choice A).

11. A. Sodium bicarbonate

The patient has tricyclic antidepressant (TCA) poisoning. TCAs block fast sodium channels and antagonize muscarinic acetylcholine receptors, peripheral α_1-adrenergic receptors, histamine (H1) receptors, and CNS γ-aminobutyric acid (GABA) A receptors.[49] They are absorbed in the gut and reach maximum plasma concentrations in 2 to 8 hours. Clinical presentation includes anticholinergic symptoms such as dilated pupils, flushed skin, dry mouth, hypomotility of bowels, hyperthermia, and urinary retention. CNS findings include altered metal status, seizures, and coma. ECG shows QRS greater than 100 sec, QRS complex with terminal rightward deflection, deep S wave in leads I, AVL, tall R wave in lead AVR, R wave in AVR greater than 3 mm, and R/S ratio in AVR greater than 0.7 seconds.[49,50] Other ECG findings include sinus tachycardia, ventricular tachycardia, and ventricular fibrillation. Although the definitive diagnosis is based on serum TCA levels, it is not always available in time. Therefore, the clinical presentation with ECG findings should prompt treatment. If the patient was seen within 2 hours of ingestion, activated charcoal would be useful (choice B). Sodium bicarbonate is the primary treatment for cardiotoxicity, particularly if QRS is greater than 100 msec or the patient has ventricular arrhythmia. Sodium bicarbonate is given as a 1- to 2-mEq/Kg bolus and repeated if there is no initial response. Whether QRS narrows or not, sodium bicarbonate drip is initiated. The pH goal is 7.5 to 7.55. The patient should be monitored for hypokalemia, hypernatremia, and volume overload. The rationale of sodium bicarbonate is that the increase in extracellular sodium and alkalotic pH make sodium less available to sodium channels. If symptoms are refractory, hypertonic saline maybe used. Other therapies suggested for refractory symptoms includes vasopressors and lipid emulsion (choices C and D).

12. C. Grade IV and the patient should receive another dose of antivenom

Grade I is pain or paresthesia at the sting site; Grade II is pain or paresthesia locally and remote from the sting site; Grade III is cranial nerve dysfunction OR somatic dysfunction; and Grade IV is cranial nerve and somatic dysfunction.[11] The cranial nerve dysfunction includes blurred vision, opsoclonus which is similar to nystagmus except there is no associated rhythmic movement, tongue fasciculations, dysponia and dysphagia, and somatic dysfunction includes restlessness and involuntary limb movements.[11] The patient has Grade IV envenomation. Therefore, choice A and B are wrong. Antivenom (3 vials reconstituted in 50 mL NS and administered over 10 minutes) is reserved for Grade III and IV. Response should be seen by 1 to 2 hours. If no response, this could be the antivenom is unable to reach the venom or amount of venom exceeds antivenom.[11,12] Another dose of antivenom can be given at a lower dose (1 vial) for two additional occurances.[11]

Waiting up to 6 hours is not appropriate; therefore choice D is wrong. Antivenom side effects including vomiting, pyrexia, rash, nausea, and pruritis.

13. A. Bowel obstruction can occur 4 weeks after ingestion

There are 4 phases of iron toxicity.[10] The first phase has gastrointestinal symptoms such as nausea, vomiting, abdominal pain, hematemesis, and melena within 6 hours. The second phase is quiescent or latent phase where there is resolution of gastrointestinal symptoms but metabolic acidosis can continue to progress (choice B). Third phase is sometimes divided into two phases: (1) shock and metabolic acidosis with coagulopathy starting at 6 to 72 hours after ingestion and (2) hepatic necrosis from 12 to 96 hours after ingestion. Fourth phase is bowel obstruction which occurs after 2-8 weeks from ingestion (choice A). Iron preparations include ferrous gluconate with 12% elemental iron, ferrous sulfate with 20% elemental iron, and ferrous fumarate with 33% elemental iron.[51] Risk of life threatening toxicity occurs with ingestion of more than 60 mg/kg of elemental iron.[10] Serum level of less than 350 mcq/dL has minimal toxicity where as serum levels of more than 500 mcq/dL can lead to serious systemic toxicity. Therefore, choice C is wrong. Chelation is performed with Deferoxamine which binds ferrix iron (Fe^{3+}) to form ferrioxamine, which is water soluable and indicated if: (1) symptomatic with serum iron level > 350 mcq/dL; (2) evidence of lethargy, abdominal pain, hypovolemia, or acidosis; (3) all symptomatic patients with multiple emesis, altered mental status, and acidosis; and (4) positive radiographic evidence of multiple iron pill fragments.[52] Chelation is continued until the reddish-orange urine color created by ferrioxamine is clear, asymptomatic and serum iron level is less than 150 ug/dL.[52] Therefore, choice D is wrong.

14. D. Free erythrocyte protoprophyrin (FEP) or zinc protoporphyrin (ZPP) might not be indicated for blood lead level less than or equal to 10 mcq/gL

Blood lead level (BLL) more than 80 mcg/dL is an indication for chelation treatment with 2,3 dimercaptosuccinic acid (DMSA) or calcium disodium ethylenediaminetetraacetate (Ca Na$_2$EDTA).[15,52] However, chelation treatment can be an indication if BLL is 40 to 80 mcq/dL, if presence of symptoms and duration of exposure, and underlying medical problems (choice A). Chelation therapy is indicated in lead poisoning, arsenic poisoning, mercury poisoning but not cadmium poisoning[15,16] (choice B). Sources of aluminum toxicity includes hemodialysis fluid, phosphate binders, and antacids[15,16] (choice C). Free erythrocyte protoprophyrin or zinc protoporphyrin are indicators for lead exposure since lead causes inhibition of enzymes involved in hemoglobin synthesis.[15,52] However, BLL less than or equal to 25 mcq/dL does not inhibit the enzymes for hemoglobin synthesis, therefore, FEP or ZZP would not be increased[15,52] (choice D).

REFERENCES

1. Warner M, Chen LH, Makuc DM, et al. Drug poisoning deaths in the United States, 1980-2008. *NCHS Data Brief.* 2011;(81):1-8.

2. 2015 Annual Report of the American Association of Poison Control Centers' National Poison Data System (NPDS): 32nd Annual Report. *Clin Toxicol (Phila).* 2017;55(10):1072-1252.

3. Beale RJ, Hollenberg SM, Vincent JL, et al. Vasopressor and inotropic support in septic shock: an evidence-based review. *Crit Care Med.* 2004;32(11 Suppl):S455-S465.

4. Hernandez G, Velasco N, Wainstein C, et al. Gut mucosal atrophy after a short enteral fasting period in critically ill patients. *J Crit Care.* 1999;14(2):73-77.

5. Boucher BA, Wood GC, Swanson JM. Pharmacokinetic changes in critical illness. *Crit Care Clin.* 2006;22(2):255-271, vi.

6. Levine M, Brooks DE, Truitt CA, et al. Toxicology in the ICU: part 1: general overview and approach to treatment. *Chest.* 2011;140(3):795-806.

7. Mokhlesi B, Leiken JB, Murray P, Corbrdige TC. Adult toxicology in critical care: Part I: General approach to the intoxicated patient. *Chest.* 2003;123(2):577-592.

8. Alapat PM, Zimmerman JL. Toxicology in the critical care. *Chest.* 2008;133(4):1006-1013.

9. Brooks DE, Levine M, O'Connor AD, French RNE, Curry SC. Toxicology in the ICU: Part 2: specific toxins. *Chest.* 2011;140(4):1072-1085.

10. Levine M, Ruha AM, Graeme K, Brooks DE, Canning J, Curry SC. Toxicology in the ICU. Part 3: natural toxins. *Chest.* 2011;140(5):1357-1370.

11. Quan D. North American poisonous bites and stings. In: Kruse J, ed. Toxicology, An Issue of Critical Care Clinics. 2012;28(4):277-327.

12. Haque ZK, Stefanec T. Environmental injuries and toxic exposures. In: Oropello JM, Pastores SM, Kvetan V, eds. *Critical Care.* New York, NY: McGraw-Hill; http://accessmedicine.mhmedical.com/content.aspx?bookid=1944&sectionid=143520525. Accessed June 04, 2018.

13. Lei C, Badowski NJ, Auerbach PS, Norris RL. Disorders caused by venomous snakebites and marine animal exposures. In: Kasper D, Fauci A, Hauser S, Longo D, Jameson J, Loscalzo J, eds. *Harrison's Principles of Internal Medicine, 19e* New York, NY: McGraw-Hill; 2014. http://accessmedicine.mhmedical.com/content.aspx?bookid=1130&sectionid=79757620. Accessed June 04, 2018.

14. Lank P, Corbridge T, Murray PT. Toxicology in adults. In: Hall JB, Schmidt GA, Kress JP, eds. *Principles of Critical Care.* 4th ed. New York, NY: McGraw-Hill; 2014. http://accessmedicine.mhmedical.com/content.aspx?bookid=1340&sectionid=80027807. Accessed June 04, 2018.

15. Hu H. Heavy metal poisoning. In: Jameson J, Fauci AS, Kasper DL, Hauser SL, Longo DL, Loscalzo J, eds. *Harrison's Principles of Internal Medicine.* 20th ed. New York, NY: McGraw-Hill;. http://accessmedicine.mhmedical.com/content.aspx?bookid=2129&sectionid=181951155. Accessed June 05, 2018.

16. Jiashankar M, Tseten T, Albalagan N, Mathew BB, Beeregowda K. Toxicity, mechanism, health effects of some heavy metals. *Interdiscip Toxicol.* 2014;7(2):60-72.

17. Lheureux PE, Zahir S, Gris M, et al. Bench-to-bedside review: hyperinsulinaemia/euglycaemia therapy in the management of overdose of calcium-channel blockers. *Crit Care.* 2006;10(3):212.

18. American College of Medical Toxicology. Interim guidance for the use of lipid resuscitation therapy. http://www.acmt.net/cgi/page.cgi?aid53384&_id552&zine5show.

19. Felice KL, Schumann HM. Intravenous lipid emulsion for local anesthetic toxicity: a review of the literature. *J Med Toxicol.* 2008;4(3):184-191.

20. Moorman JR, Pritchett LC. The arrhythmias of digitalis intoxication. *Arch Intern Med.* 1985;145:1289-1292.

21. Patel V, James PA. Digitalis toxicity and management. http://emedicine.medscape.com/article/154336.

22. Juurlink DN, Gosselin S, Kielstein JT, et al; Extrip Workgroup. Extracorporeal treatment for salicylate poisoning: systematic review and recommendations from EXTRIP Workgroup. *Ann Emerg Med.* 2015;66(2):165-181.

23. Hill JB. Salicylate intoxication. *N Engl J Med.* 1973;288(21):1110.

24. Proudfoot AT, Krenzelok EP, Vale JA. Position paper on urine alkalinization. *J Toxicol Clin Toxicol.* 2004;42(1):1.

25. Prescott LF, Balali-Mood M, Critchley JA, et al. Diuresis or urinary alkalinisation for salicylate poisoning? *Br Med J (Clin Res Ed).* 1982;285(6352):1383.

26. Bailey B. Glucagon in beta-blocker and calcium channel blocker overdoses: a systematic review. *J Toxicol Clin Toxicol.* 2003;41(5):595.

27. Boyd R, Ghosh A. Towards evidence based emergency medicine: best BETs from the Manchester Royal Infirmary. Glucagon for the treatment of symptomatic beta blocker overdose. *Emerg Med J.* 2003;20(3):266.

28. Cole JB, Stellpflug SJ, Ellsworth H, et al. A blinded, randomized, controlled trial of three doses of high-dose insulin in poison-induced cardiogenic shock. *Clin Toxicol (Phila).* 2013;51(4):201-207.

29. Jovic-Stosic J, Gligic B, Putic V, et al. Severe propranolol and ethanol overdose with wide complex tachycardia treated with intravenous lipid emulsion: a case report. *Clin Toxicol (Phila).* 2011;49(5):426-430.

30. Stellpflug SJ, Harris CR, Engebretsen KM, et al. Intentional overdose with cardiac arrest treated with intravenous fat emulsion and high-dose insulin. *Clin Toxicol (Phila).* 2010;48(3):227-229.

31. Sullivan R, Hodgman MJ, Kao L, Tormoehlen LM. Baclofen overdose mimicking brain death. *Clin Toxicol.* 2012;50:141-144.

32. Watve SV, Sivan M, Raza WA, Jamil FF. Management of acute overdose or withdrawal in intrathecal baclofen therapy. *Spinal Cord.* 2012;50:107-111.

33. St-Onge M, Anseeuw K, Cantrell FL, et al. Expert consensus recommendations for the management of calcium channel blocker poisoning in adults. *Crit Care Med.* 2017;45(3):e306-e316.

34. Dunkley EJ, Isbister GK, Sibbritt D, et al. The Hunter serotonin toxicity criteria: a simple and accurate diagnostic decision rules for serotonin toxicity. *QJM.* 2003;96(9):635-642.

35. Lappin RI, Auchincloss EL. Treatment of the serotonin syndrome with cyproheptadine. *N Engl J Med.* 1995;331(15):1021.

36. Berman BD. Neuroleptic malignant syndrome: a review for neurohospitalists. *Neurohospitalist.* 2011;1(1):41-47.

37. Tse L, Barr AM, Scarapicchia V, Vila-Rodriguez F. Neuroleptic malignant syndrome: a review from a clinically oriented perspective. *Curr Neuropharmacol.* 2015;13:395-406.

38. Kam PCA, Cardone D. Propofol infusion syndrome. *Anaesthesia.* 2007;62:690-701.

39. Honore PK, Spapen HD. Propofol infusion syndrome: early blood purification to the rescue? *Crit Care.* 2016;20:197.

40. Krajcova A, Waldauf P, Duska F. Propofol infusion syndrome: a structured review of experimental studies and 153 published case reports. *Crit Care.* 2015;19(298):1-9.

41. Duewell JL, Fenves AZ, Richey DS, et al. 5-Oxoproline (pyroglutamic) acidosis associated with chronic acetaminophen use. *Proc (Bayl Univ Med Cent).* 2010;23(1):19-20.

42. Altschul E, Craig Grossman, Renee Dougherty, et al. Lithium toxicity: a review of pathophysiology, treatment, and prognosis. *Pract Neurol.* 2016;42-45.

43. Decker BS, Goldfarb DS, Dargan PI, et al; EXTRIP Workgroup. Extracorporeal treatment for Lithium Poisoning: Systematic Review and Recommendations from EXTRIP Workgroup. *Clin J Am Soc Nephrol.* 2015;10(5):875-887.

44. Bretaudeau DM, Hamel JF, Boels D, Harry P. Lithium poisoning: the value of early digestive tract decontamination. *Clin Toxicol (Phila).* 2013;51(4):243-248.

45. Bretaudeau DM, Hamel JF, Boels D, Harry P. Lithium poisoning: the value of early digestive tract decontamination. *Clin Toxicol (Phila).* 2013;51(4):243-248.

46. Eddleston M, Buckley NA, Eyer P, Dawson AH. Management of acute organophosphate pesticide poisoning. *Lancet.* 2008;371:597-607.

47. Sungar M, Guven M. Intensive care management of organophosphate insecticide poisoning. *Crit Care.* 2001;5:211-215.

48. Sidell FR. Clinical effects of organophosphorus cholinesterase inhibitors. *J Appl Toxicol.* 1994;14(2):111.

49. Kerr GW, McGuffie AC, Wilkie S. Tricyclic antidepressant overdose: a review. *Emerg Med J.* 2001;18:236-241.

50. Burns E. Tricyclic overdose (sodium-channel blocker toxicity). https://lifeinthefastlane.com/ecg-library/basics/tca-overdose/.

51. Tenenbein M. Toxicokinetics and toxicodynamics of iron poisoning. *Toxicol Let.* 1998;102-103:653-656.

52. Willams RH, Erickson T. Evaluating lead and iron intoxication in an emergency setting. *Laboratory Medicine.* 1998;29(4):1-8.

Critical Care Ultrasound

Jason Filopei, MD, Young Im Lee, MD, and Samuel Acquah, MD

INTRODUCTION

Critical care ultrasound (CCUS) is an extension of the physical examination. The front-line clinician performs, interprets, and applies goal-directed examinations to rapidly diagnose and manage life-threatening conditions, including acute respiratory failure and undifferentiated shock. The American College of Chest Physicians/La Société de Ré animation de Langue Francaise Statement on Competence in Critical Care Ultrasonography (ACCP/SRLF Statement) highlights five areas of focus for intensivists: cardiac, thoracic (consisting of both the lungs and the pleura), vascular (consisting of both diagnostic and vascular access), and abdominal ultrasound.[1] CCUS examinations are not comprehensive examinations that evaluate all anatomic structures and measurements of an organ or body region.

This chapter serves as a brief overview of the most common uses of CCUS. In no way is it meant to be completely comprehensive; however, it serves as an adequate introductory tool and covers the material most frequently tested on the American Board of Internal Medicine Pulmonary and Critical Care board examinations.

Equipment

It is imperative to have an easily accessible and portable machine that allows for rapid and repeated use. Machines ideally should have a high-frequency vascular probe (Fig. 31-1A) and low-frequency phased array probe (Fig. 31-1B). Appropriate manufacturer warranty and technical support should be included in the purchase because of heavy use and the high likelihood for maintenance.

Operator Position, Marker Orientation, and Knobology

It is imperative to develop a consistent approach when obtaining, describing, and interpreting ultrasound images. If possible, the operator should always be positioned immediately down- or upstream (adjacent) to the system console, allowing for ease of image acquisition and manipulation. When appropriate (if possible), patient position should be optimized for the current examination (eg, when possible, goal-directed echocardiography GDE should be performed with the patient in the left lateral decubitus position).

Operators should familiarize themselves with the various functions of the ultrasound interface. For basic CCUS, one must master the functions that manipulate image position (depth) and brightness (gain). Depth should be adjusted so that the structure of interest (eg, the heart) occupies the center of the screen. Gain can be increased or decreased to make structures brighter or darker, respectively. Machines often have near, far, and full screen gain adjustment.

Probe Manipulation

Operators should hold the ultrasound probe similar to how they hold a pen, allowing the base of the hand to rest on the patient to provide added stability. The probe indicator should always be uniform for various examinations (eg, for lung or pleural ultrasound, the indicator should always be cephalad, with vascular diagnostics and access to the patient's left). Operators should slide the probe across the surface of interest (eg, thorax) either medial lateral or cephalocaudal to obtain the appropriate window for the structure being examined (eg, lung). Rotating the probe clock or counterclockwise, fanning medial lateral, or angling the probe toward or away from the indicator all allow for optimizing or adjusting a scanning plane. These maneuvers are best appreciated with hands-on training.

Basic Critical Care Echocardiography

Basic critical care echocardiography is a qualitative "eyeball" assessment of global cardiac function done in a systematic fashion to answer a particular question. A goal-directed echocardiogram consists of five views: parasternal long-axis (PSLA), midventricular parasternal short-axis (PSSA), apical four-chamber (A4C), subcostal long-axis (SCLA), and longitudinal inferior vena cava (IVC).[1] It has been shown that with focused training, these combined views performed in a goal-directed fashion can differentiate a critically ill patient's shock state, including hypovolemic, obstructive, vasodilatory, or cardiogenic shock.[2]

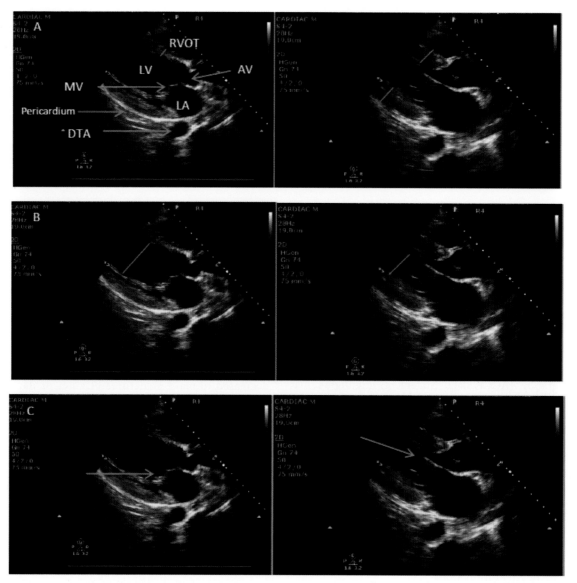

FIGURE 31-1 (A) Note the difference in length of blue lines in diastole and systole indicating the change in thickness of myocardial wall of the interventricular septum. Arrow points to the descending thoracic aorta. (B) Note the difference in LV cavity size in systole and diastole. **(C)** Note the close approximation of the anterior leaflet of mitral valve to the interventricular septum (arrow). AV, aortic valve; DTA, descending thoracic aorta; LA, left atrium; LV, left ventricle; MV, mitral valve; RVOT, right ventricular outflow tract.

The PSLA (Fig. 31-1) is obtained by placing the probe in an intercostal space (second to fifth depending on patient anatomy) immediately adjacent to the left side of sternum and rotating the probe indicator toward the patient's right shoulder (10 o'clock position). Left ventricular function (LVF) is assessed looking for myocardial thickening, endocardial excursion, and anterior mitral valve leaflet excursion (Table 31-1). The presence of a pericardial effusion is assessed by observing fluid tracking anterior to the descending thoracic aorta (DTA). Aortic and mitral valve catastrophe can be assessed in the PSLA by applying two-dimensional color. An on-axis image will show the right ventricular outflow tract (RVOT), aortic valve (AV), and left atrium all midline, and the left ventricle (LV) apex should be just out of the image window.

The PSSA (Fig. 31-2) is obtained by rotating the probe indicator 90 degrees clockwise from the PSLA to face the patient's left shoulder (2 o'clock position). The operator should fan the probe until the LV is visualized at the midventricular–papillary muscle level. LVF, right ventricle (RV) and LV septum kinetics, pericardial effusions, and regional wall motion abnormalities can all be assessed in the PSSA. An on-axis image will show a circular left ventricular cavity (as opposed to off-axis, yielding an oval-shaped LV) and small crescentic shaped RV at the LV anteroseptal wall.

The A4C view (Fig. 31-3) is obtained by sliding the probe slightly inferolateral to the nipple line. (In women, the probe must be positioned under the breast tissue.) The orientation marker should be rotated perpendicular to

TABLE 31-1 Left Ventricular Function and Associated Ultrasound Findings

Ultrasound findings	Left Ventricular Function
Myocardial thickening [A]	Increase in heart muscle wall thickness; Normal values varies per age and sex
Endocardial excursion [B]	LV cavity shrinking by > 40%
Mitral valve excursion [C]	Approximation of MV < 1 cm to the interventricular septum (no presence of severe mitral/aortic valvular regurgitation)

LV = left ventricle; MV = mitral valve.

A, B, and C refers to images in Figure 31-1.

the patient's left shoulder (3 o'clock position). If a patient can safely be turned to the left lateral decubitus position, this often yields a higher quality image. An on-axis view elongates the heart into a "football" shape compared with a foreshortened "basketball" shape, leading to gross over-assessments of RV and LV size. To correct an off-axis "basketball" shape, the operator often must slide the probe one intercostal space caudad. The A4C view allows comparison of the RV-to-LV ratio to assess for shock caused by acute cor pulmonale. LVF can be underestimated in this view because of difficulty in assessing myocardial thickness and endocardial excursion.

The SCLA view (Fig. 31-4) is obtained by laying the probe flat on the patient's abdomen just inferior to the xiphoid process with the indicator rotated to the 3 o'clock position. The liver edge is the most anterior structure and is used as an acoustic window. The SCLA view is sometimes the only view obtainable because of barriers in critically ill patients such as chest wall drains, dressings, obesity, or increased air artifact caused by chronic lung disease and use of mechanical ventilation. The SCLA view can be used to assess for shock caused by pericardial effusion in the clinical context of cardiac

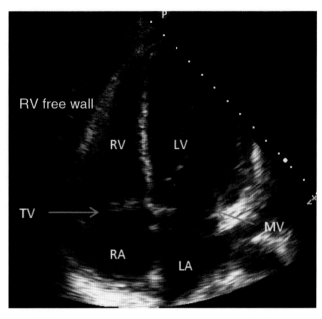

FIGURE 31-3 Apical four chamber. LA, left atrium; LV, left ventricle; MV, mitral valve; RA, right atrium; RV, right ventricle; TV, tricuspid valve.

tamponade, LVF, and RV-to-LV ratio and for cardiac standstill during advanced cardiac life support.

The longitudinal IVC view (Fig. 31-5) is obtained with a counterclockwise rotation and slight angling of the probe caudad from the SCLA with the indicator facing 12 o'clock. Although often used to indiscriminately evaluate "volume status," it has only been validated when certain criteria are met (eg, passive mechanical ventilation with 10 cc/kg of tidal volume while in sinus rhythm). Current expert opinion suggests that IVC size is useful in extreme cases such as smaller than 1 cm or larger than 2.5 cm to assess fluid responsiveness.[3,4] Two common imaging pitfalls should be avoided. First, if the IVC is imagined off-axis, it will create the "cylinder effect," underestimating its diameter. Second, it can be confused

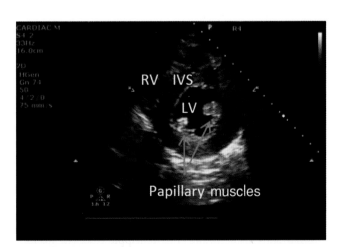

FIGURE 31-2 Parasternal short axis. IVS, interventricular septum; LV, left ventricle; RV, right ventricle.

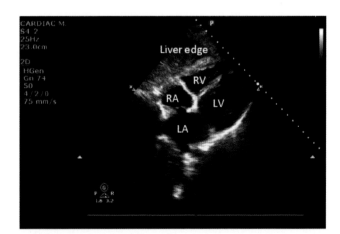

FIGURE 31-4 Subcostal long axis. LA, left atrium; LV, left ventricle; RA, right atrium; RV, right ventricle.

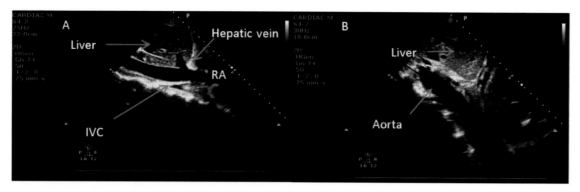

FIGURE 31-5 (A) On-axis IVC view; (B) Abdominal aorta. IVC, inferior vena cava; RA, right atrium.

with the aorta. The course of the IVC is intrahepatic, and the aorta is extrahepatic.

Thoracic Ultrasound: Lung and Pleura

Thoracic ultrasound (TUS) encompasses both lung and pleural ultrasound. TUS is essential to CCUS in the diagnosis and management of respiratory failure, pleural effusions, and shock. TUS is superior to the portable chest radiographs, which are often rotated, hypoinflated, and under- or overpenetrated.[4] There are no data to recommend abdominal over lung preset; however, the abdominal preset is favored. The linear probe is best used in children to examine the pleural line and in the setting of evaluation before and after vascular access placement.

Traditionally, air was the sonographer's enemy. However, lung ultrasound (LUS) uses an air–fluid continuum that generates artifacts and patterns created by apposition and movement of the pleura and the presence or absence of fluid within the interstitial space. The operator places a phased array probe in any thoracic rib interspace perpendicular to the pleural line to generate these artifacts or patterns. It is important to distinguish the edge of each rib, which are found superior to the pleural line and cause complete drop-off of ultrasound beams (ie, black immediately inferior to them) as opposed to the pleura, which creates a horizontal echogenic line (ie, A-line). A normal aerated lungs shows lung sliding, which is a predictable repetition of normal pleura undergoing horizontal movement throughout the respiratory cycle. Lung that becomes "wet" shows B-lines that originate from the pleural line; move horizontally with lung sliding; travel vertically, often obliterating the A-line pattern; and reach the end of the imaged field. As a lung fills with more fluid, an alveolar consolidation pattern (C pattern) will develop similar in appearance to the liver. Lung point is seen in the presence of a pneumothorax and is the loss of lung sliding within the same interspace being examined. Daniel Lichenstein developed the Bedside Lung Ultrasound in Emergency (BLUE) Protocol (Fig. 31-6) combining LUS artifacts into different patterns to define pathologic states. These patterns are pictured and defined in Table 31-2.[5-7]

Pleural effusions are a common finding in critically ill patients. Pleural ultrasound should be performed as part of every evaluation of a patient with dyspnea or respiratory failure.[8] Although pleural ultrasound should be performed as part of a systematic evaluation of the thorax, a focused examination to evaluate a suspected or known effusion is acceptable in certain cases. Pleural ultrasound has superior diagnostic accuracy compared with chest radiography for the detection of pleural effusions and an enhanced ability to characterize an effusion's complexity.[9] It is imperative to identify three findings to confirm the presence of a pleural effusion, which is an anechoic (black) space surrounded by the following anatomic boundaries: the chest wall, the diaphragm, the subdiaphragmatic organ (liver or spleen), and the atelectatic or consolidated lung.

Lower Extremity Ultrasound

Critically ill patients experience an increased prevalence of venous thromboembolic (VTE) disease. There is a significant increase in morbidity and mortality in these patients, particularly if treatment is withheld because of a delay in diagnosis. Bedside triplex ultrasound examination is considered the gold standard for diagnosis; however, sonographic technicians are not readily available to perform comprehensive examinations. Existing literature shows that intensivists with focused training can perform compression ultrasound to diagnose deep vein thrombosis with a high degree of accuracy.[10] Images are acquired using a high-frequency linear transducer with a patient in the supine position with the leg externally rotated and the knee flexed. The examination can be categorized into five points in two separate regions, namely the femoral and popliteal. The probe is placed in transverse orientation perpendicular to the vein as high up toward inguinal ligament as possible. Compressions are performed every 1 to 2 cm (Table 31-3). The following key landmarks must be visualized: the common femoral vein, the confluence of the greater saphenous vein and common femoral vein, the confluence of the lateral perforator and common femoral vein where the femoral artery splits into the superficial and deep femoral artery, the confluence of

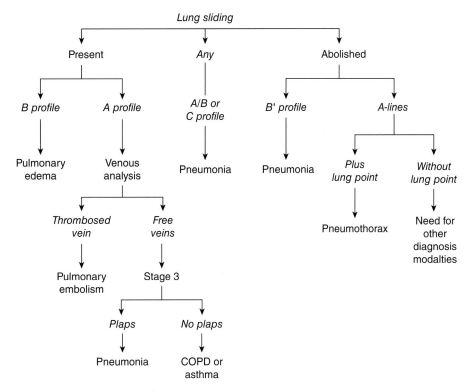

FIGURE 31-6 The BLUE protocol. (Reprinted with permission from Lichtenstein DA, Mezière GA. Relevance of lung ultrasound in the diagnosis of acute respiratory failure: the BLUE protocol. *Chest.* 2008;134(1):117-125.)

the common and deep femoral veins, and the popliteal vein. The examination can be continued distal to the superficial femoral vein and deep vein branch point with compressions every 1 to 2 cm on the medial portion of the thigh.

Vascular Access Ultrasound

Ultrasound guidance increases success rates for safely obtaining central venous access in the internal jugular position. It

has been shown to reduce complication rates caused by pneumothorax and arterial punctures.[11] Its use is considered the standard of care and is recommended by multiple regulatory agencies as well as various professional societies. A complete examination starts with preprocedural scanning of both the left and right neck to identify the safest site for insertion. The internal jugular vein's position is noted in relation to the carotid artery (vein lateral to the artery rather than directly anterior to it) and the distance from the surface and to rule out

TABLE 31-2 The Three Common Lung Ultrasound Patterns

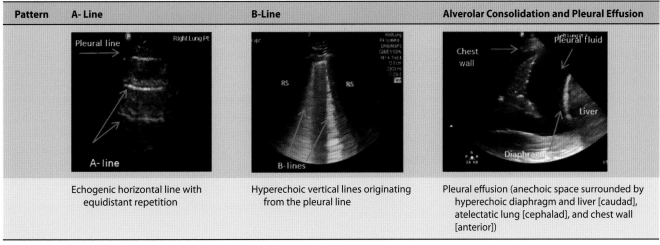

Pattern	A- Line	B-Line	Alverolar Consolidation and Pleural Effusion
	Echogenic horizontal line with equidistant repetition	Hyperechoic vertical lines originating from the pleural line	Pleural effusion (anechoic space surrounded by hyperechoic diaphragm and liver [caudad], atelectatic lung [cephalad], and chest wall [anterior])

RS = rib shadow.

TABLE 31-3 Lower Extremity Vascular Anatomy

Zone 1- Femoral	
Common femoral vein (CFV) and common femoral artery (CFA) just at the inguinal ligament (above are the external iliac artery and iliac vein; below would be the greater saphenous vein [GSV] junction)	
CFA and GSV merging into the CFV	
Branch of superficial femoral artery (SFA) and deep femoral artery (DFA) with lateral perforator vein (LPV)	
Common femoral artery and confluence of femoral and deep femoral vein (DFV)	
Femoral artery (FA) and femoral vein (FV; formerly superficial femoral vein [SFV])	
Zone II: Popliteal	
Popliteal artery (PA) and popliteal vein (PV) within the popliteal fossa	

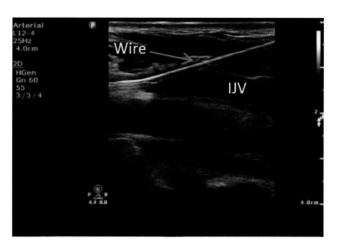

FIGURE 31-7 Wire insertion longitudinal into the internal jugular vein (IJV).

the presence of thrombus or distal stenosis before insertion by scanning the vein in the transverse position. After an operator has chosen an ideal site, confirming the presence of lung sliding on the anterior chest of the ipsilateral side to confirm is encouraged when there is concern for postprocedure pneumothorax. The procedure should be performed under standard sterile technique (sterile ultrasound probe cover) using dynamic needle guidance visualizing in real time the insertion of the needle tip into the lumen of the vein. After the wire is inserted, its appropriate placement should be reconfirmed with ultrasound in both the transverse and longitudinal planes (Fig. 31-7). Postprocedure, pneumothorax can be effectively ruled out by again checking for the presence of lung sliding (only if it had been present before the procedure). Various line placement techniques using saline injections to confirm venous location at the superior vena cava or right atrium have been studied and show a high degree of accuracy for appropriate line placement.

Abdominal Ultrasound

Abdominal ultrasound is most useful in the emergency department (ED) in the setting of trauma cases; however, it still has many uses in the critical care setting. Computed tomography will undoubtedly remain the gold standard for diagnosing abdominal pathology; however, abdominal ultrasound can be used in various trauma-related protocols to evaluate for a source of renal failure and the presence of ascitic fluid and to guide diagnostic paracentesis. Finally, intra-abdominal vascular pathology, including abdominal aortic aneurysms and dissections, should be evaluated for trauma and unexplained shock states.

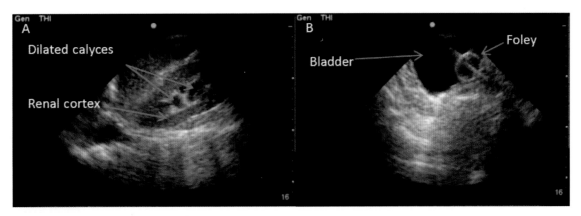

FIGURE 31-8 (A) Mild hydronephrosis. (B) Bladder with small amount of urine and Foley balloon in place.

Abdominal ultrasound, like all other Point of Care Utrasound (POCUS), is approached in a systematic way. If it is not being done in the setting of a FAST (focused assessment with sonography for trauma) or EFAST (extended focused assessment with sonography for trauma) protocol, the approach should be systematically to evaluate the genitourinary and gastrointestinal (GI) systems. First, the operator can evaluate the kidney in both the transverse and longitudinal views to assess for the presence of hydronephrosis (Fig. 31-8A), free fluid in the hepato- or splenorenal recesses, or a kidney stone. Then an assessment of the bladder can be done to assess anuria and Foley catheter placement (Fig. 31-8B).

The GI system should be evaluated by assessing the anterior and paracolic gutters of the abdomen. The presence of peristalsis and gut sliding often is suggestive of a normal GI tract; however, these signs have not been systematically evaluated. The presence of ascitic fluid (Fig. 31-9) is often seen in the dependent areas of the abdomen if the patient is in the supine position.

QUESTIONS

1. A 23-year-old woman presents with worsening of right-sided pleuritic chest pain, intermittent episodes of night-time chills, and a cough productive of yellow sputum. She received a 5-day oral course of azithromycin without relief. Her initial vital signs are temperature of 97.8°F, heart rate of 141 beats/min, respiratory rate of 34 breaths/min, and oxygen saturation of 86% on room air. A chest radiograph is performed and is pictured in Figure 31-10.

A medical intensive care unit (ICU) consultation is called for evaluation of multilobar and impending respiratory failure. A lung ultrasound of the right lung base is performed and is pictured in Figure 31-11.

This image is highly suggestive of what process?

A. Ascites
B. Complex pleural effusion
C. Pleural mass
D. Atelectasis

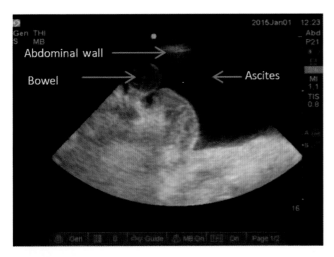

FIGURE 31-9 Abdominal ascites.

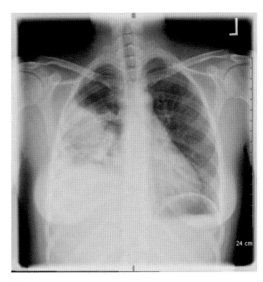

FIGURE 31-10 Portable chest radiograph.

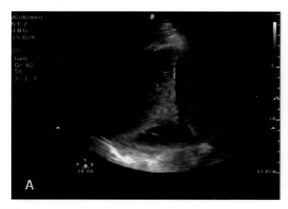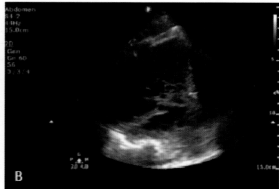

FIGURE 31-11 Thoracic ultrasound obtained in the midaxillary scan line.

2. Regarding the patient in question 1, what would be the next step?

   A. Catheter insertion via landmark use only with instillation of streptokinase
   B. Ultrasound-guided catheter insertion with instillation of dornase and alteplase
   C. Thoracic surgery consult for evaluation of video-assisted thoracoscopic surgery
   D. Both B and C

3. A 52 year-old obese woman is admitted to the intensive care unit during the night for septic shock caused by a urinary tract infection. The patient has received 30 cc/kg of crystalloid but remains in a shock state. The patient is intubated for increased work of breathing, and the on-call resident performs an ultrasound-guided triple-lumen catheter insertion of the right internal jugular vein under your supervision for vasopressor use. The trainee requires three sticks for completion of the procedure because of excessive soft tissue at the neck; however, the procedure is seemingly completed without event. Twenty minutes after the procedure, despite vasopressor infusion, the patient's shock state worsens with rising oxygen requirements. You suspect an iatrogenic pneumothorax from line insertion; however, the x-ray technician has not returned any pages. You perform a lung ultrasound with the phased array probe to assist with your suspected diagnosis. Which of the following statements is true about the sensitivity and specificity of lung ultrasound for the diagnosis of pneumothorax?

   A. The presence of lung sliding rules in pneumothorax at that location.
   B. The presence of lung point rules out pneumothorax at that location.
   C. The absence of lung sliding rules in pneumothorax at that location.
   D. The presence of lung sliding rules out pneumothorax at that location.

4. You suspect pneumothorax and lung ultrasound is performed. With the probe located on the anterior chest wall at the midclavicular line, your two-dimensional and M-mode image are pictured in Figure 31-12. Which of the following images support your suspicion?

5. A 28-year-old man with AIDS presents to the ED with acute right-sided pleuritic chest pain. Three days before in the same ED, the patient had a bedside incision and drainage of a 3 × 4 cm buttock wound. Examination showed a cachectic-appearing man with a T_{max} of 96.8, blood pressure 88/44 mmHg, heart rate of 119 beats/min, respiratory rate of 28 breaths/min, and oxygen saturation of 87% on room air. Laboratory studies show a white blood cell count of $14.2 \times 10^3/\mu L$, creatinine of 1.92 mg/dL, and lactic acid of 4.2 mmol/L. CXR shows a possible right lower lobe opacity. A diagnosis of severe sepsis with shock is made, prompting initiation of a sepsis protocol. The patient receives 30 cc/kg of crystalloid and broad-spectrum antibiotics; however, his shock state worsens, prompting intensive care unit evaluation. A goal-directed echocardiogram is performed to evaluate the patient's shock state. The following representative images are shown (Fig. 31-13).

   These images are supportive of which type of shock?

   A. Cardiogenic shock from left ventricular failure from acute myocardial infarction
   B. Obstructive shock from a massive pulmonary embolism
   C. Vasoplegic shock in sepsis
   D. Obstructive shock from a pericardial effusion

6. A 65-year-old man recently diagnosed with metastatic colon cancer with significant disease burden in the liver and omentum is admitted because of 1 day of acute-onset weakness and general malaise. The patient is brought to the ED by his wife and syncopizes before reaching the ED. He is rushed to the trauma bay and found to be afebrile, tachycardic, hypotensive, and tachypneic. He is diaphoretic

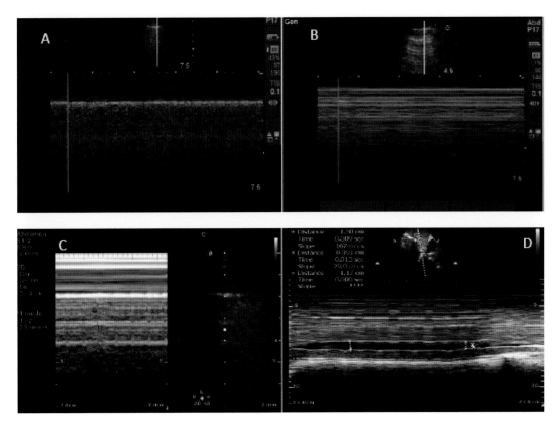

FIGURE 31-12 Answer choices for Question 4.

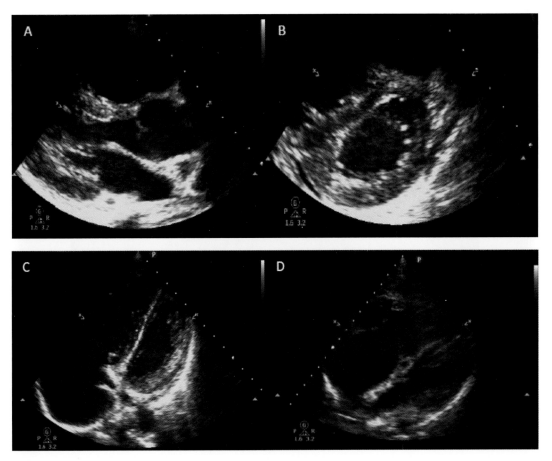

FIGURE 31-13 Echographic findings of shock.

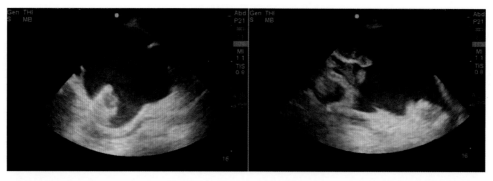

FIGURE 31-14 Abdominal ultrasound.

and pale appearing on examination. He receives 2 Liters of crystalloid with some improvement in his blood pressure and heart rate. He is sent for computed tomography of the chest and abdomen, which reveals a new subsegmental pulmonary embolism, omental and hepatic metastases, and newfound ascitic fluid in the abdomen. He is given Lovenox for the pulmonary emboli and admitted to the general medical floor. Six hours after admission at 3 AM, the patient becomes acutely tachycardic and hypotensive again and complains of acute abdominal pain. An ICU consult is called, and a bedside abdominal ultrasound examination is performed, which shows the following images in the right paracolic gutter (Fig. 31-14).

The image in the clinical context is most consistent with

A. ascites.
B. hemoperitoneum.
C. small bowel obstruction.
D. sarcoma.

7. A 62-year-old man is postoperative day 2 from coronary artery bypass surgery. He was extubated from mechanical ventilation this morning and was doing well. While he is eating lunch, he becomes acutely diaphoretic and dyspneic, his blood pressure decreases from 110/80 to 70/40 mmHg, and his heart rate increases from 82 to 125 beats/min. There is jugular venous distention. As part of your evaluation of undifferentiated shock, you perform a goal-directed echocardiogram. An apical four-chamber view could not be obtained because of chest wall dressings (Fig. 31-15).

Based on these images and the clinical scenario, what would be the appropriate treatment choice?

A. Intravenous diuretics
B. Pericardiocentesis
C. Thoracentesis
D. Phenylephrine

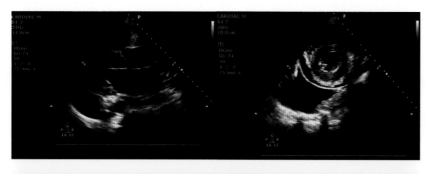

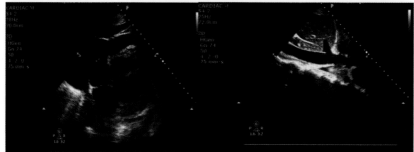

FIGURE 31-15 Goal directed echocardiogram with PSLA, PSSA, SCLA, and IVC.

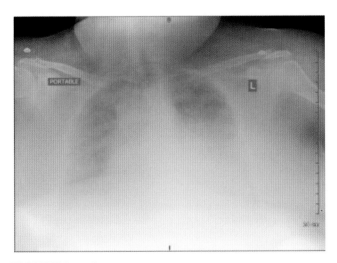

FIGURE 31-16 Portable chest radiograph.

and respiratory rate of 25 beats/min. She cannot complete a full sentence, has bilateral wheezing in all the posterior lung fields, and has 3+ pitting edema in both legs with chronic venous stasis changes. An arterial blood gas is performed and shows 7.29/68/61. A portable chest radiograph is pictured in Figure 31-16.

A diagnosis of COPD exacerbation is made, and the patient is given intravenous methylprednisolone and three rounds of inhaled bronchodilator nebulizers. The patient remains dyspneic, so an ICU consult is called for impending respiratory failure. A lung ultrasound is performed, and representative images are shown in Figure 31-17.

This lung ultrasound pattern is most consistent with

A. COPD exacerbation.
B. acute pulmonary embolism.
C. acute pulmonary edema.
D. bacterial pneumonia.

8. A 74-year-old obese woman with systolic heart failure with an ejection fraction of 35% and severe chronic obstructive pulmonary disease (COPD) presents to the ED with gradual worsening of dyspnea over the past 3 days. She reports a productive cough but is unclear whether it is any worse. On examination, the patient has a temperature of 97.8°F, pulse rate of 98 beats/min, blood pressure of 142/88 mmHg,

9. A 68-year-old woman with diabetes mellitus and chronic stage IV kidney disease is admitted to ICU with severe diabetic ketoacidosis caused by a urinary tract infection. She receives appropriate treatment with volume resuscitation, insulin, and antibiotics. On her fourth day of admission, the patient develops new bilateral lower extremity edema, right slightly greater than left. Her platelets drop

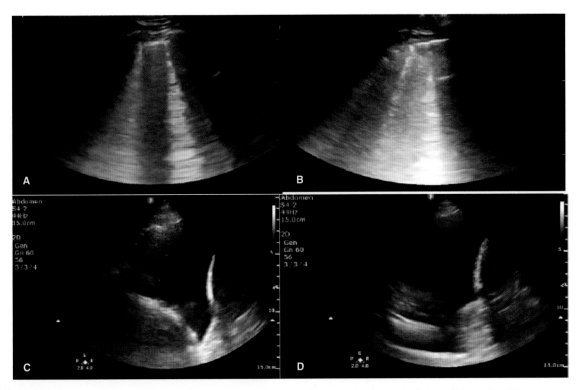

FIGURE 31-17 Thoracic ultrasound images A and B are representative of Zones 1 and 2 on the bilateral chest. C and D are representative of Zones 3 and 4.

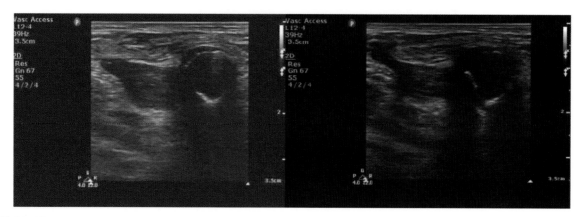

FIGURE 31-18 Bilateral lower extremity compression ultrasound.

from 180 to 90 × 10³/uL. You perform a bilateral lower extremity compression ultrasound and obtain the following image (Fig. 31-18).

What would be your next treatment decision?

A. Call for an official lower extremity Doppler examination.
B. Start a heparin drip.
C. Start an argatroban drip.
D. Continue with current management because the examination findings were normal.

10. A 61-year-old obese woman with COPD and systolic heart failure presents with 3 days of dyspnea on exertion. She states she also has been experiencing cough, wheezing, orthopnea, and worsening swelling in her legs. She reports compliance with a low-salt diet and her furosemide daily. Her initial vital signs are temperature of 97.8°F, heart rate of 85 beats/min, blood pressure of 182/78 mmHg, respiratory rate of 38 breaths/min, and oxygen saturation of 82%. Her physical examination reveals both bibasilar crackles and inspiratory and expiratory wheezing in all lung fields. A chest radiograph shows bilateral ground glass opacities. An arterial blood gas shows respiratory acidosis. The patient is placed on non-invasive positive pressure ventilation with settings of IPAP 15 EPAP 8 FIO2 of 100%. An intensive care unit consult is called for respiratory failure. A lung ultrasound is performed as part of the assessment shows the following image in all 8 fields (Fig. 31-19).

The above pattern is most consistent with which of the following diagnosis?

A. Acute pulmonary edema
B. Obstructive airways disease exacerbation
C. Pneumothorax
D. Pneumonia

11. An 82-year-old woman with severe COPD, coronary artery disease, type 2 diabetes, hypertension, and hyperlipidemia is sent in from a nursing home because of altered mental status. On arrival in the ED, the patient is in severe respiratory distress, and her initial vitals are T_{max} of 97.5, heart rate of 120 beats/min, blood pressure of 145/82 mmHg, respiratory rate of 36 breaths/min, and room air saturation of 88%. Laboratory studies and urinalysis are done and show a leukocytosis and white blood cells and nitrites, respectively. A lung ultrasound is performed and shown in Figure 31-20.

The above pattern is classified as

A. A-line pattern.
B. B-line pattern.
C. Lung point.
D. Consolidation pattern and pleural effusion.

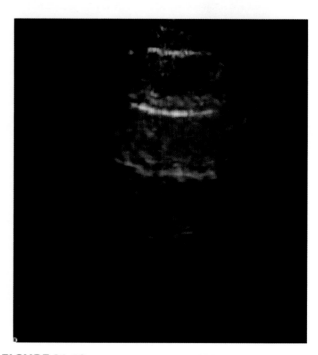

FIGURE 31-19 Lung ultrasound.

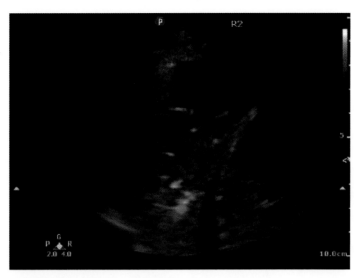

FIGURE 31-20 Lung ultrasound.

12. You are preparing to perform a right-sided internal jugular catheter insertion under ultrasound guidance. After scanning both sides of the neck, evaluating it for both venous thromboembolism and stenosis, you have chosen the right side based on one of the images in Figure 31-21.

Which of the following images represents an appropriate placement site on the right side?

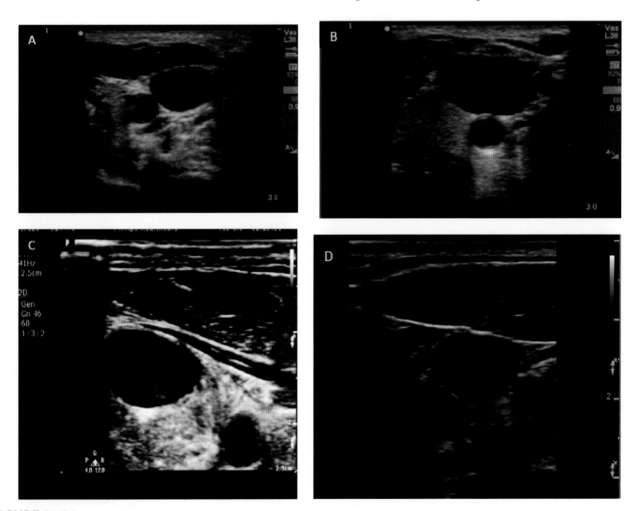

FIGURE 31-21 Answer choices for Question 12.

ANSWERS

1. B. Complex pleural effusion

The image shown was acquired on the lateral thorax in the midaxillary line using a low-frequency convex probe with the indicator pointed cephalad. The key anatomic boundaries for defining a pleural effusion are shown: the chest wall (anterior), diaphragm (caudad), liver (caudad) pleural surface, and lung (cephalad). Identification of the diaphragm is imperative to avoid an intra-abdominal tap. Choice A is incorrect because there is no fluid seen below the diaphragm in this image. Choice C is incorrect because there is no pleural mass noted. Choice D is incorrect because atelectasis would appear simple without septations or loculations often with a small tail at the lung edge, known as the plankton sign. The prevalence of pleural effusions in IUCs can range as high as 60% to 90%.[12] Pleural ultrasound can detect as little as 3 to 5 mL of fluid and has been shown to have a higher sensitivity for detecting and characterizing pleural effusions than chest radiographs.[13] Compared with chest computed tomography, pleural ultrasound had a sensitivity and specificity of 93%.[14] The presence of septations seen in part B on pleural ultrasound is highly suggestive of empyema[15] (Fig. 31-22).

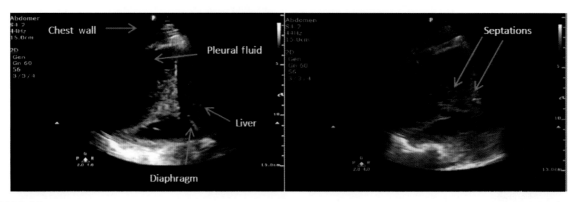

FIGURE 31-22 Complex pleural effusion with appropriate landmarks. Septations of a complex pleural effusion.

2. D. Both B and C

The patient would undergo ultrasound-guided catheter insertion with instillation of dornase and alteplase and thoracic surgery consult for evaluation of video-assisted thoracoscopic surgery.

After a multidisciplinary discussion between the pulmonary critical care and thoracic surgery service, a chest tube using ultrasound guidance is inserted given the clinical findings. Pus was aspirated, and pleural fluid studies showed a pH of 6.8, cell count and differential of 4700 polymorphonuclear leukocytes, 82% neutrophils, 10% lymphocytes, glucose level less than 20 mg/dL, lactate dehydrogenase of 180 u/L, and total protein of 4g/dL. Gram stain and culture grew resistant *Streptococcus pneumoniae*. Thoracostomy tube insertion should be performed under either direct ultrasound guidance or using appropriate interspace based on ultrasound imaging.[16]

Based on the Multicenter Intrapleural Sepsis Trial (MIST) II trial, an appropriate next step in management could be to insert a chest drain to allow for appropriate source control and instillation of alteplase and dornase.[17] In the trial, the alteplase and dornase group showed a significant decrease in rate of surgical referral and hospital length of stay. We advocate for an interdisciplinary approach to empyema given the various treatment modalities and heterogeneous evidence base. Choice A is incorrect because the patient has complex pleural effusion causing sepsis and impending respiratory failure and requires appropriate source control with immediate drainage; antibiotics alone would not be sufficient. Choice B is incorrect because ultrasound should be used either for direct guidance or appropriate interspace selection. Also, streptokinase alone should not be used given the results of the MIST II trial.

3. D. The presence of lung sliding rules out pneumothorax at that location.

The pleural line is generated by the apposition of the parietal and visceral pleura. It is abolished if air comes between the two because ultrasound waves cannot propagate through air (ie, pneumothorax). The presence of lung sliding on thoracic ultrasound rules out pneumothorax in the region being scanned with 100% specificity.[17] This has been shown in numerous papers in the literature, including the original BLUE protocol.[6] It is imperative to note that PTX is ruled out where lung sliding is present and does not rule out a PTX in another location or a loculated PTX. Choice B is incorrect because the presence of lung point rules in pneumothorax with a high degree of accuracy rather than ruling it out.[18] Choice C is incorrect because the absence of lung sliding does not rule in pneumothorax; other lung pathologies can abolish lung sliding, including pneumonia, preexisting bullous lung disease or scarring, apnea (ie, right or left mainstem intubation), and previous pleurodesis.

4. C.

This image shown is acquired using a low-frequency convex probe placed in an intercostal space in the midclavicular line on the anterior chest perpendicular to the pleural surface with the indicator pointed cephalad. Choice A is incorrect because it shows a two-dimensional and M-mode image of normal lung sliding. This can be appreciated in the M-node image as the seashore sign, with the near field showing soft tissue that is wavy ("ocean") and the far field showing lung movement and appearing "sandlike."[19] Choice B is a more challenging image of lung ultrasound and shows lung pulse. Lung pulse is the rhythmic movement of the pleura caused by vibrations being transmitted from the cardiac rhythm. Some literature suggests that lung pulse also rules out pneumothorax, but this remains controversial.[20] Choice D is a cardiac ultrasound and M-mode image of the inferior vena cava and should not be confused with lung ultrasound.

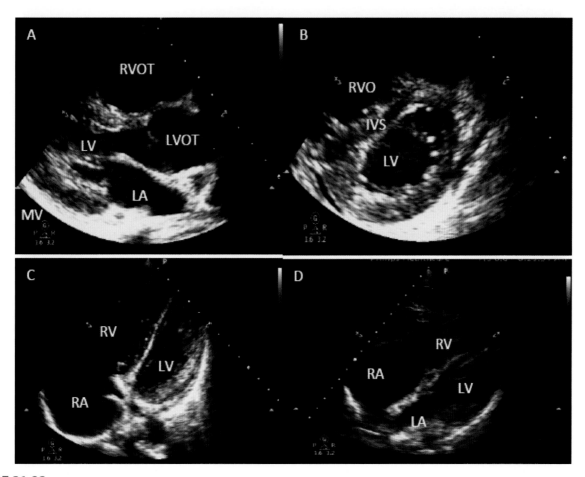

FIGURE 31-23 Shock due to acute cor pulmonale. LA, left atrium; LV, left ventricle; LVOT, left ventricular outflow tract; MV, mitral valve; RA, right atrium; RV, right ventricle; RVOT, right ventricular outflow tract.

5. B. Obstructive shock from a massive pulmonary embolism

The images show the PSLA, PSSA, off-axis A4C, and SCLA views. Image acquisition tips are described in this chapter. In all images, there is evidence of right-sided volume and pressure overload (Fig. 31-23). Assessing the right ventricle is best performed in the PSSA, A4C, and SCLA views. The PSLA is not used to assess the RV size qualitatively because it shows the RVOT; however, in cases of severe dilation, the RVOT is often obviously enlarged. A normal RV in the PSSA is crescentic shape and is barely visible, and all walls of the LV should move outward at end-diastole. In this case, there is a "D-shaped" septum during end-diastole, which is highly suggestive of right-sided volume and pressure overload. In the A4C view, the RV-to-LV ratio can be defined as normal (< 0.6; moderate dilation is > 0.6 and < 1; severe dilation is ≥ 1). Some advanced measurements to evaluate RV function in the A4C view such as an M-mode evaluation of tricuspid annular plane systolic excursion (TAPSE) can be performed, with a value of less than 1.6 highly predictive of reduced systolic function.[21] The SCLA view can be used to evaluate the RV-to-LV ratio qualitatively; however, it often can underestimate right ventricular size. Choice A is incorrect because there is a clear alternate diagnosis. LVF is best assessed in the parasternal views and cannot be depicted with still images for the purposes of this chapter. Choice C is incorrect because vasodilatory shock is more

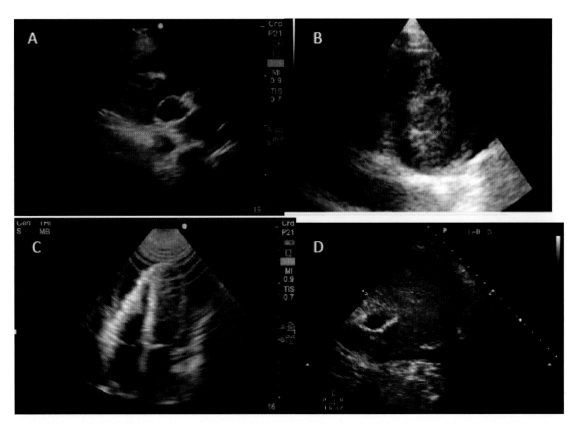

FIGURE 31-24 Typical POCUS findings in vasodilatory shock. (A) PSLA showing collapse of LV cavity, (B) PSSA showing effacement of LV walls, (C) A4C showing same, (All indicating hyperdynamic LV), (D) showing intra-hepatic virtual IVC.

often characterized by a normal, hyperdynamic, and or severely decreased left ventricle. Images would show end-systolic obliteration and a "virtual" IVC. Choice D is incorrect because there is no pericardial effusion present.

Volume resuscitation was halted after ultrasound evaluation. Because a bedside deep vein thrombosis study did not yield a lower extremity clot, a CTPA was performed showing a saddle embolus, and thrombolytics were administered with good outcome. At 6-month follow-up, the patient was asymptomatic with normal RV size and function.

6. B. Hemoperitoneum

The image shows intraperitoneal fluid suggestive of hemorrhagic ascites. Ultrasound has been found to be very useful as a screening tool in trauma cases for detecting free fluid in the abdomen; however, differentiating the type of fluid based solely on the ultrasound characteristics is challenging. The images show a slightly hyperechoic layering ultrasound dust, suggesting that the fluid being imaged is complicated and possibly blood. One technique to be more precise to ensure the image is truly hyperechoic and not just an overgained image would be to downgain the entire image and slowly increase the gain to see if the "dust" is not gain artifact. Although choice A could be correct, in applying the images to the clinical setting at the bedside, it is more likely to be blood than simple fluid. A subsequent diagnostic tap revealed a bloody tap, and anticoagulation

was held. Choice C is incorrect because evidence supportive of a small bowel obstruction would be dilated loops of bowel without peristalsis, which cannot be appreciated on the still images provided. Choice D is incorrect because there is no identifiable mass seen on the still images provided.

7. B. Pericardiocentesis

A pericardial effusion is defined as greater than 50 cc of fluid present between the parietal and visceral layers of the pericardium. The differential diagnosis for a pericardial effusion is broad and includes trauma, infectious, malignant, uremia, and inflammatory. Although it is uncommon, pericardial effusions can cause acute obstructive shock with high mortality rates when unrecognized.[22] Detection of pericardial fluid with GDE is one of the most important applications of GDE and has been shown to be done reliably by non–cardiology-trained physicians with high degrees of accuracy.[23] However, several pitfalls must be noted. First, echocardiographic signs of cardiac tamponade require advanced Doppler and M-mode maneuvers that are outside the scope of practice of basic critical care echocardiographers. All findings must be applied to the clinical situation because a pericardial effusion could be large and chronic without significant hemodynamic effect or small and acute with significant hemodynamic effect. Second, the operator must be able to differentiate pericardial fluid from both pleural and ascitic fluid. The presented images show a large pericardial effusion that has rapidly accumulated in the postoperative setting. In addition, a pleural effusion is also noted. The PSLA view must include the DTA because pericardial fluid will accumulate and track anteriorly to the DTA while pleural fluid tracks posteriorly to it.[23] The PSSA clearly shows the hyperechoic pericardium that distinguishes between pericardial and pleural fluid. The SCLA4 view uses the liver as an acoustic window and is often the best view to assess a pericardial effusion and observe for diastolic collapse initially of the right atrium and then the right ventricle. Ascitic fluid will always be anterior in the SCLA view and often separated by the falciform ligament.[24] The IVC view in tamponade physiology will show a distended and nondistensible vessel invariably.[25] This view is particularly helpful in patients who have hyperdynamic LV in whom a nonsignificant pericardial effusion may appear to cause collapse. Answer choices A and D are not correct because diuretics and inotropes do not treat patients with obstructive shock. Answer choice C is not correct because although there is pleural effusion present, it will not appropriately treat the patient's shock state.

8. C. Acute pulmonary edema

The presence of B-lines bilaterally anteriorly with the loss of A-lines is nearly diagnostic for pulmonary edema.[6] A multiple but distinct versus coalesced B-line pattern has been correlated with moderate and severe interstitial syndromes, respectively. To differentiate from an inflammatory process such as acute respiratory distress syndrome, some literature supports the presence of a smooth pleural line without spared areas as more suggestive of pulmonary edema.[26] The presence of simple-appearing bilateral pleural effusions at the bases further supports a diagnosis of acute pulmonary edema. Effusions are present in up to 90% of patients presenting with decompensated heart failure.[27] Answer choices A and B are both incorrect because the predominant lung ultrasound finding in COPD and pulmonary vascular disease causing respiratory failure is lung sliding with bilateral A-lines. Answer choice D is incorrect because lung ultrasound in bacterial pneumonia would show signs of asymmetry, abolition of lung sliding, or dense consolidations at the bases.

9. C. Start an argatroban drip.

The image was obtained using a high-frequency linear probe with the indicator facing the patient's left and placing the probe just below the inguinal ligament perpendicular to the vascular structures. Shown is a hyperechoic well-formed deep venous thrombosis that was not compressible upon application of pressure (see Fig. 31-18). Choice D is wrong. DVT is a highly prevalent disease in ICU patients, and if left untreated, it can have catastrophic complications.[28] The existing literature shows that bedside

diagnostic vascular ultrasound using the compression technique alone can be performed by emergency and critical care physicians with focused training with a high degree of accuracy.[10] Timely access to expert sonographers and radiology reading may not be present around the clock and often leads to significant delays in diagnosis. Examination of the venous system of the legs should be approached as a two-zone and five or more compression examination identifying key landmarks. The focus of the examination should be to go as high up into the groin as possible before the iliac vein dives deep into abdomen. There is a possibility of heparin-induced thrombocytopenia, so starting heparin drip is incorrect (choice B). Obtaining official lower extremity dopplers (choice A) is good for documentation but will not treat the problem.

10. B. Obstructive airways disease exacerbation

An A-line pattern with lung sliding represents a normal aeration pattern (Fig. 31-25). This pattern is seen in a patient with acute dyspnea and respiratory failure caused by obstructive airways disease (eg, asthma, COPD) or pulmonary vascular disease (eg, pulmonary embolus). Choice A is incorrect because acute pulmonary edema is most often characterized as bilateral B-lines. Choice C is incorrect because pneumothorax is best characterized by the presence of lung point. Choice D is incorrect because pneumonia is best characterized as an alveolar consolidation pattern.

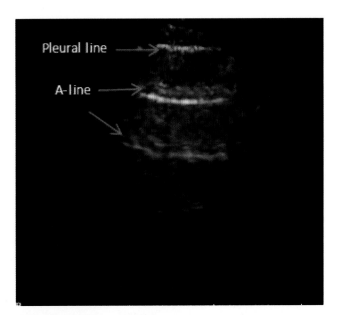

FIGURE 31-25 A line pattern.

11. D. Consolidation pattern and pleural effusion

TUS findings consistent with pneumonia are consolidation patterns with the presence of dynamic air bronchograms and basal pleural effusion.[29] In the BLUE protocol, whereas asymmetric B-lines and abolition of lung sliding

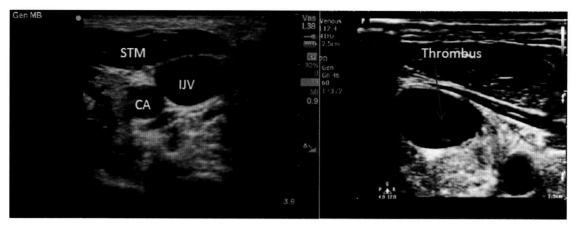

FIGURE 31-26 Thrombus in the IJV. CA = carotid artery; IJV = internal jugular vein; STM = sternothoracic muscle.

can also be suggestive of pneumonia, B-lines associated with consolidation are suggestive of pneumonia. Community-acquired pneumonia (CAP) is one of the most common worldwide diseases and is diagnosed in an appropriate clinical setting in the presence of an infiltrate on chest radiography or chest computed tomography. Although a high-quality posteroanterior and lateral film has a good sensitivity for CAP, in the ICU, the practitioner is often left with low-quality portable films in which sensitivity wanes significantly.[30] Choice A is incorrect because the most common lung ultrasound findings for pulmonary embolism causing respiratory failure are a normal bilateral A-line pattern or the presence of subpleural infarcts in the setting of known VTE or right ventricular failure. Choice B is incorrect because lung ultrasound findings for acute pulmonary edema causing respiratory failure are normally bilateral B-lines. Choice C is incorrect because the lung ultrasound finding most consistent with pneumothorax is lung point.

12. A.

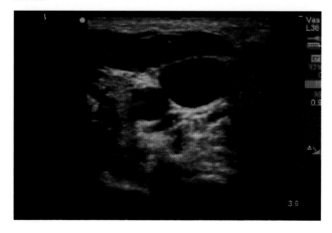

Dynamic needle guidance for venous catheter insertion using a high-frequency linear probe with the indicator pointing toward the patient's left side is the gold standard for internal jugular vein cannulation. Complication rate is reduced, including pneumothorax and carotid cannulation, compared with using landmarks. A transverse (preferred) or longitudinal approach can be used for cannulation. The procedure should always start with prescanning both sides of the neck and evaluating the ideal site of insertion based on the size, compressibility, and depth of the vessel. This is particularly important in critically ill patients who are immobilized and may have already undergone prior vascular access insertion. The site and machine are prepped under sterile conditions for insertion. The needle should be inserted at a 45- to 60-degree angle just proximal to the probe. The probe should then be tilted toward the head to find the needle tip and traced toward the center of the vessel by slowly tilting the probe cephalad and tracking the needle tip through the soft tissue into the vessel lumen. Of the images provided, only answer choice A fulfills these criteria. Choice C is incorrect because there is a VTE at the posterior wall of the vessel. On compression ultrasound, the anterior and posterior walls did not come together. Next, an optimal image with the vein in the center of the screen not overlying the carotid artery should be obtained. This should be done to minimize the risk of a carotid stick in the event the needle is pushed through the posterior wall of the vein. This is best seen in choice A because it is the only one that fits the stated criteria (Fig. 31-26).

REFERENCES

1. Mayo PH, Beaulieu Y, Doelken P, et al. American College of Chest Physicians/La Société de Réanimation de Langue Française statement on competence in critical care ultrasonography. *Chest.* 2009;135(4):1050-1060.
2. Jones AE, Tayal VS, Sullivan DM, Kline JA. Randomized, controlled trial of immediate versus delayed goal-directed ultrasound to identify the cause of nontraumatic hypotension in emergency department patients. *Crit Care Med.* 2004;32(8):1703-1708.
3. Kory P. Counterpoint: should acute fluid resuscitation be guided primarily by inferior vena cava ultrasound for patients in shock? No. *Chest.* 2017;151(3):533-536.

4. Lee CW, Kory PD, Arntfield RT. Development of a fluid resuscitation protocol using inferior vena cava and lung ultrasound. *J Crit Care*. 2016;31(1):96-100.

5. Lichtenstein D, Goldstein I, Mourgeon E, et al. Comparative diagnostic performances of auscultation, chest radiography, and lung ultrasonography in acute respiratory distress syndrome. *Anesthesiology*. 2004;100(1):9-15.

6. Lichtenstein DA, Mezière GA. Relevance of lung ultrasound in the diagnosis of acute respiratory failure: the BLUE protocol. *Chest*. 2008;134(1):117-125.

7. Lichtenstein DA, Lascols N, Mezière G, Gepner A. Ultrasound diagnosis of alveolar consolidation in the critically ill. *Intensive Care Med*. 2004;30(2):276-281.

8. Maslove DM, Chen BT, Wang H, Kuschner WG. The diagnosis and management of pleural effusions in the ICU. *J Intensive Care Med*. 2013;28(1):24-36.

9. Lichtenstein DA. Lung ultrasound in the critically ill. *Ann Intensive Care*. 2014; 4(1):1.

10. Kory PD, Pellecchia CM, Shiloh AL, et al. Accuracy of ultrasonography performed by critical care physicians for the diagnosis of DVT. *Chest*. 2011;139(3):538-542.

11. Leung J, Duffy M, Finckh A. Real-time ultrasonographically-guided internal jugular vein catheterization in the emergency department increases success rates and reduces complications: a randomized, prospective study. *Ann Emerg Med*. 2006;48(5):540-547.

12. Mattison LE, Coppage L, Alderman DF, et al. Pleural effusions in the medical ICU: prevalence, causes, and clinical implications. *Chest*. 1997;111(4):1018-1023.

13. Kelbel C, Börner N, Schadmand S, et al. [Diagnosis of pleural effusions and atelectases: sonography and radiology compared]. *Rofo*. 1991;154(2):159-163.

14. Lichtenstein D, Goldstein I, Mourgeon E, et al. Comparative diagnostic performances of auscultation, chest radiography, and lung ultrasonography in acute respiratory distress syndrome. *Anesthesiology*. 2004;100(1):9-15.

15. Tu CY, Hsu WH, Hsia TC, et al. Pleural effusions in febrile medical ICU patients: chest ultrasound study. *Chest*. 2004;126(4):1274-1280.

16. Havelock T, Teoh R, Laws D, Gleeson F. Pleural procedures and thoracic ultrasound: British Thoracic Society Pleural Disease Guideline 2010. *Thorax*. 2010;65(Suppl 2):ii61-ii76.

17. Rahman NM, Maskell NA, West A, et al. Intrapleural use of tissue plasminogen activator and DNase in pleural infection. *N Engl J Med*. 2011;365(6):518-526.

18. Lichtenstein DA, Mezière G, Lascols N, et al. Ultrasound diagnosis of occult pneumothorax. *Crit Care Med*. 2005;33(6):1231-1238.

19. Lichtenstein DA. Lung ultrasound in the critically ill. *Ann Intensive Care*. 2014;4(1):1.

20. Lichtenstein DA, Lascols N, Prin S, Mezière G. The "lung pulse": an early ultrasound sign of complete atelectasis. *Intensive Care Med*. 2003;29(12):2187-2192.

21. Rudski LG, Lai WW, Afilalo J, et al. Guidelines for the echocardiographic assessment of the right heart in adults: a report from the American Society of Echocardiography endorsed by the European Association of Echocardiography, a registered branch of the European Society of Cardiology, and the Canadian Society of Echocardiography. *J Am Soc Echocardiogr*. 2010;23(7): 685-713.

22. Vincent JL, De backer D. Circulatory shock. *N Engl J Med*. 2013;369(18):1726-1734.

23. Mandavia DP, Hoffner RJ, Mahaney K, Henderson SO. Bedside echocardiography by emergency physicians. *Ann Emerg Med*. 2001;38(4):377-382.

24. Blanco P, Volpicelli G. Common pitfalls in point-of-care ultrasound: a practical guide for emergency and critical care physicians. *Crit Ultrasound J*. 2016;8(1):15.

25. Himelman RB, Kircher B, Rockey DC, Schiller NB. Inferior vena cava plethora with blunted respiratory response: a sensitive echocardiographic sign of cardiac tamponade. *J Am Coll Cardiol*. 1988;12:1470-1477.

26. Copetti R, Soldati G, Copetti P. Chest sonography: a useful tool to differentiate acute cardiogenic pulmonary edema from acute respiratory distress syndrome. *Cardiovasc Ultrasound*. 2008;6:16.

27. Kataoka H, Takada S. The role of thoracic ultrasonography for evaluation of patients with decompensated chronic heart failure. *J Am Coll Cardiol*. 2000;35(6):1638-1646.

28. Minet C, Potton L, Bonadona A, et al. Venous thromboembolism in the ICU: main characteristics, diagnosis and thromboprophylaxis. *Crit Care*. 2015;19:287.

29. Reissig A, Copetti R, Mathis G, et al. Lung ultrasound in the diagnosis and follow-up of community-acquired pneumonia: a prospective, multicenter, diagnostic accuracy study. *Chest*. 2012;142(4):965-972.

30. Ye X, Xiao H, Chen B, Zhang S. Accuracy of lung ultrasonography versus chest radiography for the diagnosis of adult community-acquired pneumonia: review of the literature and meta-analysis. *PLoS One*. 2015;10(6):e0130066.

Nutrition

Ronaldo Collo Go, MD

INTRODUCTION

Critical illness is associated with a systemic inflammatory response and catabolic state that leads to increased infections, multiorgan dysfunction, prolonged hospitalization, and death. The individual's adaptive response aims to increase energy provision to vital organs by increasing release of pituitary hormones, increasing sympathetic nervous system stimulation, and increasing peripheral resistance to anabolic hormones. Society of Critical Care Medicine (SCCM) and American Society of Parenteral and Enteral Nutrition (ASPEN)'s approach to nutritional is designed to preserve lean body mass, attenuate stress response, prevent oxidative injury, and modulate immune response.[1] The current nutritional bundle includes (1) assess patients for nutritional risk and calculate energy and protein requirements to determine goals; (2) initiate enteral nutrition (EN) within 24 to 48 hours after the onset of critical illness and admission to the intensive care unit (ICU) and increase to goal within the first week of the ICU stay; (3) reduce the risk of aspiration or improve tolerance to gastric feeding with the use of prokinetic agents, continuous infusion, chlorhexidine mouthwash, elevation of the head of the bed, and diverted level of feeding in the gastrointestinal (GI) tract; (4) implement enteral feeding protocols with institution-specific strategies to promote delivery of enteral nutrition; (5) do not use gastric residual volumes as part of routine care to monitor ICU patients on EN; and (6) start parenteral nutrition (PN) early when EN is not feasible or sufficient in high-risk poorly nourished patients.[1]

NUTRITIONAL ASSESSMENT

The patient population in the ICU is heterogeneous, and objective markers such as albumin, prealbumin, transferrin, and retinol binding protein participate in the acute phase response and do not accurately reflect the nutritional status of a critically ill patient.[1] Other markers are still under investigation; these include calcitonin, C-reactive protein, interleukin-1, interleukin-6, citrulline, ultrasound with measurement of muscle mass, and computed tomography.[1] Nutritional risk assessment such as the Nutritional Risk Score (NRS-2002)

helps to identify patients who will likely benefit from early enteral therapy because they will reduce nosocomial infection, complications, and mortality risk.[1] Patients with an NRS-2002 greater than 3 are at risk, and those with scores of 5 or greater are at high nutritional risk.[1-4]

Energy needs are determined via indirect calorimetry (low evidence), but when this is unavailable, a weight-based equation of 25 to 30 kcal/kg/d can be used.[1] The accuracy of this equation varies from 40% to 75% and becomes less accurate with obese and underweight patients.[1] Other considerations for this calculation include using dry weight and including energy provided by dextrose-containing fluids and lipid-based medications.[1] Because of protein's role in wound healing, immune function, and maintaining lean body mass, protein requirements are higher in critically ill patients, and most EN has a high ratio of nonprotein calorie to nitrogen.[1] When nitrogen balance studies are not available, 1.2 to 2 g/kg/d can be used to monitor adequate protein provision, although requirements maybe higher in patients with burns or trauma.[1] There is low-level evidence suggesting that protein provision is more closely linked to better outcomes than total energy provision, although two subsequent small randomized controlled trials (RCTs) showed no difference.[1,5-9]

Early Initiation of Enteral Nutrition

Although the quality of evidence is poor, it is recommended that EN be initiated within 24 to 48 hours of critical illness in patients who are unable to maintain volitional intake because it is believed that EN maintains gut functional integrity via maintaining blood flow; releases trophic endogenous agents such as cholecystokinin, gastrin, bombesin, and bile salts; and maintains tight junctions and structural integrity via maintaining villous height and support IgA producing immunocytes that make up gut-associated tissue and in turn mucosal-associated lymphoid tissue.[1-4,10-16] Heyland and colleagues[14] showed a trend toward reduced mortality (relative risk [RR] = 0.52; 95% confidence interval [CI] 0.25–1.09; $P = 0.08$), Mark and coworkers[15] showed a reduction in infectious morbidity (RR = 0.45; 95% CI 0.30–0.66; $P = 0.00006$), and Doig and colleagues[16] showed reductions in pneumonia (odds ratio [OR] = 0.31; 95% CI 0.12–0.78; $P = 0.02$) and mortality (OR = 0.34; 95% CI 0.14–0.85; P = 0.02) but no difference in multiorgan failure (MOF).

Enteral nutrition is generally preferred over PN because of reduced infectious and noninfectious complications and hospital length of stay.[1,14-20] Although assessment of contractility should not be a prerequisite for initiating EN, reduced or absent bowel sounds are associated with greater symptoms of intolerance and higher mortality rates (11.3% vs 22.6% vs 36.0%).[21-23] Although in most critically ill patients, EN is safely initiated in the stomach, there is a moderate to high level of evidence for diverting EN lower in the GI tract for those who are at high risk of aspiration or have intolerance.[1] Davies and coworkers[24] found no difference in clinical outcomes such as length of stay, mortality rate, nutrient delivery, or pneumonia between gastric and small bowel EN, but aggregates of the RCTs showed improved nutrient delivery with small bowel feeding and reduced risk of pneumonia.[1,24-35]

Patients with low nutrition risk with normal baseline nutrition status (NRS-2000 ≤ 3 or Nutrition Risk in the Critically Ill [NUTRIC] score ≤ 5) do not need specialized nutritional therapy over the first ICU week because it does not improve mortality rates. Those who are at high nutrition risk (NRS-2000 > 5 or NUTRIC score ≥ 5 or severely malnourished) should be advanced toward goal within 24 to 48 hours and should receive more than 80% of estimated goal within 48 to 72 hours to achieve clinical benefit.[1] Fewer than 50% of critically ill patients meet their nutritional goal, and it is recommended to limit NPO (nothing by mouth) status, avoid using gastric residual volume (GRV) less than 500 mL in the absence of other signs of intolerance as a limiting factor to EN, use enteral feeding protocols, and use top-down or volume-based feeding protocols.[1] Volume-based feeding use 24-hour volume targets instead of hourly targets. Top-down protocols use a volume-based strategy, prokinetics, and postpyloric tube feeding.

There are three complications from EN: bowel ischemia, aspiration, and diarrhea. Bowel ischemia is a rare complication, and EN is generally avoided in patients who have a mean arterial pressure of less than 50 mmHg, those in whom pressors are being initiated, and those who require escalating pressor doses.[1] If a patient has been initiated on EN and has signs of intolerance such as abdominal distention, increasing nasogastric output, decreased stool or flatus, hypoactive bowel sounds, or increasing metabolic acidosis, EN should be held because these can be early signs of bowel ischemia.[1]

Aspiration is another complication, and the patient population at high risk includes those who have an inability to protect their airways, nasoenteric enteral access devices, mechanical ventilation, altered mental status, gastroesophageal reflux disease, or poor oral care; who are older than 70 years of age or are supine; who undergoing bolus feeding; or who are in facilities with inadequate nurse-to-patient ratios.[1,36] Efforts to attenuate this risk include postpyloric feeding if the patient is at high risk for aspiration with a moderate to high level of evidence, continuous infusion rather than bolus feeding, prokinetics such as metoclopramide or

erythromycin, keeping the head of the bed elevated by 30 to 45 degrees, use of chlorhexidine mouthwash twice a day, reducing sedation, and minimizing transport out of the ICU.[1,36-56]

Diarrhea is defined as two to three liquid stools or more than 250 g of liquid stool per day, and contributing factors include fiber; osmolality of EN; high content of fermentable oligosaccharides, disaccharides, and monosaccharides and polyols (FODMAPS); delivery mode; contamination; medications such as antibiotics, proton pump inhibitors, oral hypoglycemics, nonsteroidal anti-inflammatory drugs, and sorbitol; and infections.[1]

Adjunctive Therapy

There are three types of adjunctive therapy: prebiotic fiber, probiotics, and multivitamins. A total of 10 to 20 mg in divided doses of prebiotic fiber or fermentable soluble fiber, such as fructo-oligosaccharides, is given over 24 hours in patients with diarrhea because they are fermented in the colon into short-chain fatty acids, which provide nutrition to colonocytes, increase blood flow and stimulate pancreatic secretions, allow colonocytes to absorb water and electrolytes, and stimulate growth of healthy bacteria such as bifidobacteria and lactobacillus.[1,56-61] Small RCTs showed reduced diarrhea but no difference in ventilator days, ICU length of stay, or multiorgan failure.[1,62-65] Probiotics inhibit pathogenic bacteria and help eliminate pathogenic toxins, enhance the intestinal barrier, and can modulate immune responses, but consistent outcome benefit has not been shown.[1] This may be because of the heterogeneous ICU population and probiotics. However, some studies suggest that *Lactobacillus* GG decreases the incidence of ventilator-associated pneumonia (VAP). Synbiotic Forte with *Pediococcus pentoseceus, Leuconostoc mesenteroides, Leuconostoc paracasei subsp paracasei,* and *Leuconostoc plantarum* showed reduced infectious complications when begun 1 hour after surgery (40% vs 12.5%; P < 0.05), and probiotics decrease VAP, colitis, and diarrhea in patients with liver transplants, trauma, and pancreatectomy.[1,66-77] Antioxidant vitamins and trace minerals are believed to improve patient outcomes with a significant reduction in overall mortality but do not affect infectious complications, length of stay, or duration of mechanical ventilation.[1]

Parenteral Nutrition

Parenteral nutrition is not recommend for patients with low nutritional risk in the first 7 days even if volitional intake or early EN is not possible because of infectious morbidity and minimal benefit over standard therapy in which no nutrition is provided.[1,78-80] Heyland and coworkers' aggregate analysis of four studies showed an increased mortality rate with PN (RR = 0.178l; 95% CI 1.11–2.85; P < 0.05) and trend toward greater complications (RR = 2.40; 95% CI 0.88–6.58) compared with no nutrition.[81] Regardless of nutritional risk, PN should be considered for more than 7 to 10 days if unable to

TABLE 32-1 Disease and Specific Recommendations

Disease	Recommendations
Pulmonary failure	• Use fluid-restricted energy-dense EN while monitoring phosphate closely.
Renal failure	• Use standard EN and specialty formula if the patient has electrolyte abnormalities. • Increased protein intake, 2.5 g/kg/d if on renal replacement therapy
Hepatic failure	• Use dry weight to determine energy requirements in cirrhosis or hepatic failure and avoid protein restriction. • Avoid PN because it can worsen existing liver dysfunction. • Avoid branch-chain amino acid formulations in patients with encephalopathy who are already receiving antibiotics and lactulose.
Acute pancreatitis	• Mild acute pancreatitis can be advance to an oral diet as tolerated but if the patient has a complication or is unable to advance within 7 d, specialized nutrition therapy can be considered. • Patients with moderate to severe pancreatitis should have EN even at trophic rate and advance to goal within 24–48 h of admission. • Severity may change quickly, and feeding tolerance requires frequent reassessment and need for specialized therapy. • Measures to improve tolerance should be initiated and probiotics can also be considered. • PN should only be considered after 7 d and when EN is not possible.
Trauma	• EN with high polymeric protein diet (1.2–2 g/kg/d) should be initiated within 24–48 h when the patient is hemodynamically stable. • Immunomodulation with arginine and FO is recommended in severe trauma.
Traumatic brain injury	• EN should be initiated with protein requirements 1.5–2.5 g/kg/d within 24–48 h. • Immunomodulation via arginine or EPA or DHA is recommended.
Open abdomen	• In the absence of bowel injury, EN at 24–48 h is recommended with 15–30 g/L protein loss from exudates.
Burns	• IC is used to gauge energy needs repeatedly because predictive equations have poor accuracy in burn patients. • EN is given within 4–6 h of injury, and protein should be in the range of 1.5–2 g/kg/d.
Sepsis	• EN should be initiated within 24–48 h when the patient is hemodynamically stable with trophic feeds (10–20 kcal/h or 500 kcal/d) and advanced as tolerated after 24–48 h with > 80% goal over the first week and 1.2–2 g protein/kg/d. • Supplementation with immune-modulating formulas, selenium, zinc, and antioxidants is not recommended.
Postoperative	• EN should be initiated within 24 h of surgery. • Immunomodulating formulas containing arginine and fish oils are recommended. • Although it should be judged individually, EN is recommended for patients with prolonged ileus, intestinal anastomosis, open abdomen without bowel injury, and the need for pressors. • Clear liquids are not required as the first meal.
Obesity	• Comorbidities and biomarkers of metabolic syndrome (glucose, triglycerides, and cholesterol) should be evaluated. • High protein hypocaloric feeding and low nonprotein calorie to nitrogen ratio. • EN goal should not exceed 65–70% of target energy requirements as measured by IC. • If IC not available and BMI is 30–50, use 11–14 kcal/kg/actual body weight. If BMI is > 50, use 22–25 kcal/kg IBW/d. • For a BMI 30–40, use protein 2 g/kg IBW/d. • For BMI ≥ 40 protein 2.5 g/kg IBW/d. • Additional monitoring should be done for hyperglycemia, hyperlipidemia, hypercapnia, fluid overload, and hepatic fat accumulation. • Evaluation of micronutrient deficiencies such as calcium, thiamine, vitamin B_{12}, fat-soluble vitamins, folate, iron, selenium, zinc, and copper.

BMI = body mass index; DHA = docosahexaenoic acid; EN = enteral nutrition; EPA = eicosapentaenoic acid; FO = Fish oil; IBW = ideal body weight; IC = indirect calorimetry; PN = parenteral nutrition.

Data from Taylor BE, McClave SA, Martindale RG, et al. Guidelines for the Provision and Assessment of Nutrition Support Therapy in the Adult Critically Ill Patient: Society of Critical Care Medicine (SCCM) and American Society for Parenteral and Enteral Nutrition (ASPEN). *Crit Care Med.* 2016;44:2:390-439.

meet more than 60% of energy and protein by EN.[1] When more than 60% of target energy has been delivered with EN, PN can be discontinued. Hypocaloric PN (≤ 20 kcal/kg/d or 80% estimated energy needs) with adequate protein ≥ 1.2 g/kg/d) should be considered in high-risk or severely malnourished patients in the first 7 days of the ICU stay; it has not been shown to reduce infectious complications or morbidity but is associated with a decreased incidence of hyperglycemia.[1,82-84] Table 32-1 provides a list of recommendations per disease.[1]

COMPLICATIONS WITH FEEDING

A direct association with underfeeding and mortality prompted the initiative for early feeding, but this has been recently challenged.[85]

Inadequate autophagy refers to inadequate removal of the denatured proteins and mitochondria, leading to prolonged recovery of certain organs. It has been hypothesized that early initiation of protein or lipid-rich PN or glutamine can help decrease this complication.[86]

TABLE 32-2 Feeding Regimen for Patients at Risk for Refeeding Syndrome

Day	Calorie Intake (All Feeding Routes)	Supplements
1	10 kcal/kg/d For extreme cases (BMI < 14 kg/m^2 or no food > 15 d) 5 kcal/kg/d Carbohydrate: 50–60% Fat: 30–40% Protein: 15–20%	Prophylactic supplement PO$_4^{2-}$: 0.5–0.8 mmol/kg/d K$^+$: 1–3 mmol/kg/d Mg^{2+}: 0.3–0.4 mmol/kg/d Na$^+$: <1 mmol/kg/d (restricted) IV fluids: restricted; maintain "zero" balance IV thiamine + vitamin B complex 30 min before feeding
2–4	Increase by 5 kcal/kg/d If low or no tolerance, stop or keep minimal feeding regimen	Check all biochemistry and correct any abnormality Thiamine + vitamin B complex PO or IV until day 3 Monitoring as required
5–7	20–30 kcal/kg/d	Check all electrolytes, renal and liver functions, and minerals Fluid: maintain zero balance Consider iron supplement from day 7
8–10	30 kcal/kg/d or increase to full requirement	Monitor as required

BMI = body mass index; IV = intravenous; PO = oral.

Reprinted with permission from Mehanna HM, Moledina J, Travis J. Refeeding syndrome: what it is, and how to prevent and treat it. *BMJ*. 2008;336:1495-1499.

Overfeeding can lead to hypercapnia, refeeding syndrome, azotemia, hyperglycemia, hypertriglyceridemia, and hepatic steatosis.[86] Therefore, careful monitoring of energy expenditure via use of indirect calorimetry is often advocated.

Refeeding syndrome is a potentially fatal complication of the reintroduction of feeding in a previously malnourished patient that leads to an increase in insulin secretion, which leads to increased intracellular shifts of phosphate, magnesium, and potassium and an increase in carbohydrate-dependent mechanisms and depletion of thiamine.[87,88] Patients at risk have one or more of the following: body mass index (BMI) less than 15; unintentional weight loss greater than 15% in the past 3 to 6 months; little or no nutrition in more than 10 days; low potassium, phosphate, or magnesium before initiation of feeding; or two or more of the following: BMI less than 18.5, unintentional weight loss greater than 10% in the past 3 to 6 months, little or no nutrition intake for more than 5 days, or history of alcohol abuse, drugs such as insulin, chemotherapy, antacids, or diuretics.[89] Early monitoring and administration of macronutrients, electrolytes, minerals, and vitamins, may help prevent refeeding syndrome. Table 32-2 is an example of a feeding regimen for patients at risk for refeeding syndrome.[88]

QUESTIONS

1. A 50-year-old woman with no significant past medical history has had total abdominal hysterectomy for fibroids yesterday. Her weight is 80 kg. On physical examination, the patient is noted to have clear breath sounds with a regular rate and rhythm, and her abdomen appears soft and distended. She has hypoactive bowel sounds. What is her ideal caloric intake?

A. 2400 kcal
B. 1600 kcal
C. 4800 kcal
D. 5000 kcal

2. For the patient in question 1, what is the next step?

A. Provide no enteral nutrition and start parenteral nutrition.
B. Defer on any type of nutrition.
C. Start enteral nutrition within 24 hours.
D. Start enteral nutrition and parenteral nutrition until enteral nutrition meets more than 60% of daily requirements.

3. A 67-year-old man is complaining of nausea, vomiting, diffuse abdominal pain, and diarrhea for the past 2 days. The patient is initiated on normal saline at 250 mL/h, Zofran, and morphine. His CT abdomen is seen in Figure 32-1.

Past medical history: hypertension and coronary artery disease
Social history: 43 pack-years (quit in 2008); social alcohol drinker
Allergies: no known allergies
Home medications: aspirin 81 mg orally (PO) daily, atorvastatin 40 mg PO daily, lisinopril 40 mg PO daily, prasugrel 10 mg PO daily, saw palmetto
Vital signs: 140/80, RR 18 HR 80, O$_2$ sat 99% room air
Anicteric
Clear to auscultation
Regular rate and rhythm; no murmurs

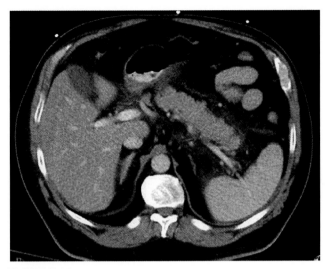

FIGURE 32-1 CT abdomen.

Soft, diffuse tenderness to palpation, hypoactive bowel sounds
Awake and alert × 4 and no neurologic deficit

Labs:

WBC	$25 \times 10^3/\mu L$	ALT	33 U/L
Hgb	14 g/dL	Alk phos	78 U/L
Plt	$197 \times 10^3/\mu L$	D. bilirubin	0.17 mg/dL
Sodium	147 mEq/L	T. bilirubin	0.9 mg/dL
Potassium	4 mEq/L	Albumin	2 g/dL
Chloride	107 mEq/L		
CO_2	24 mEq/L		
BUN	22 mg/dL		
Creatinine	1.3 mg/dL (baseline creatinine, 0.8 mg/dL)		
Lipase	1194 U/L		
Amylase	633 U/L		
Lactic acid	3.2 mmol/L		

What should be the next step?

A. The patient can be discharged home.
B. The patient should be admitted to the ICU.
C. The patient should be started on antibiotics.
D. The patient should be admitted under observation.

4. For the patient in question 3, the patient's symptoms have subsided. Lipase has been trending down. Her abdomen is slightly tender. What is the next step?

A. NPO for 7 days
B. Initiate enteral feeding
C. Start parenteral nutrition
D. NPO for now and start feeding after 24 hours

5. A 40-year-old man with no past medical history has open abdominal surgery for an abdominal aortic aneurysm.
Social history: nonsmoker, non-ETOH, vegan
Allergies: no known allergies
Family history: unknown
ROS: negative

Labs:

WBC	$14 \times 10^3/\mu L$	AST	31 U/L
Hgb	13 g/dL	ALT	33 U/L
Plt	$300 \times 10^3/\mu L$	Alk phos	78 U/L
Sodium	145 mEq/L	D. bilirubin	0.17 mg/dL
Potassium	4 mEq/L	T. bilirubin	0.9 mg/dL
Chloride	100 mEq/L	Albumin	2 g/dL
CO_2	26 mEq/L		
BUN	22 mg/dL		
Creatinine	0.87 mg/dL		
Lipase	30 U/L		
Amylase	5 U/L		
Lactic acid	0.9 mmol/L		
Ammonia	0 µmol/L		

What is the appropriate nutritional approach?

A. NPO and start parenteral nutrition
B. Enteral nutrition with 15 to 30 g of protein
C. No nutrition
D. Glutamine

6. The patient in question 5 was noted to have wheezes and hypoxia postoperatively. He does not have a history of obstructive lung disease. Chest radiographs were unremarkable. He was started on nebulizers and solumedrol 60 mg intravenously every 6 hours. A couple of days later, he becomes obtunded. Computed tomography of the head shows cerebral edema. Ammonia level is 280 µmol/L. X-ray of his abdomen shows ileus. What is the next step?

A. Lactulose
B. Initiate hemodialysis
C. Valproic acid
D. Lactulose and rifaximin

7. A 30-year-old man was found unresponsive on the street and arrived in the ED via ambulance. Past medical history consists of glycogen storage disease. His vital signs include blood pressure of 100/70 mmHg, heart rate 90 beats/min, respiratory rate 20 breaths/min, 95% on room air, and temperature of 97.8°F. Physical examination is unremarkable except for doll-like facies and a protruding abdomen. He was noted to have a glucose level of 50 mg/dL and lactic acid 7 mmol/L. He was given an amp of D50 and started on

broad-spectrum antibiotics and fluid resuscitation. He becomes more arousable.

Labs:

WBC	$10 \times 10^3/\mu L$	**AST**	31 U/L
Hgb	13 g/dL	**ALT**	33 U/L
Plt	$300 \times 10^3/\mu L$	**Alk phos**	78 U/L
Sodium	145 mEq/L	**D. bilirubin**	0.17 mg/dL
Potassium	4 mEq/L	**T. bilirubin**	0.9 mg/dL
Chloride	100 mEq/L	**Albumin**	2 g/dL
CO$_2$	26 mEq/L		
BUN	22 mg/dL		
Creatinine	0.87 mg/dL		
Lipase	30 U/L		
Amylase	5 U/L		

Bedside ultrasound after the fluid resuscitation showed the inferior vena cava was 2 cm with no respiratory variation. Repeat laboratory shows lactic acid is 7 mmol/L and glucose is 50 mg/dL. Another amp of D50 was given. What is the next best step?

A. Cornstarch with thiamine
B. Liver ultrasound
C. 1 Liter of normal saline bolus
D. D5W continuous maintenance fluid

8. A 70-year-old man with a history of dementia was admitted to the ICU for aspiration pneumonia complicated by acute respiratory distress syndrome. Today is day 4 of mechanical ventilation. He has been on tube feeds, and the nurse tells you that the patient has been having diarrhea. What would be the next step?

A. Increase tube feed rate.
B. Give a crystalloid fluid bolus.
C. Start PN in addition to EN.
D. Continue the current tube feed rate.

ANSWERS

1. **A. 2400 kcal**

   Indirect calorimetry is the ideal way to determine energy needs, but when this is not available, 25 to 30 kcal/kg/d is used. This equation has an accuracy of 40% to 75%. Choices B to D do not adhere to this equation.

2. **C. Start enteral nutrition within 24 hours.**

   It is advocated that EN should be started within 24 hours in postoperative patients. EN maybe deferred for up to 7 days in patients who are not postoperative (choice B) if they are classified as low nutritional risk via NRS-2002 (Table 32-3)[90] or NUTRIC Risk Score (Table 32-4A-C).[91]

TABLE 32-3A Nutritional Risk Screening (NRS-2002): Initial Screening

1	Is BMI < 20.5?	Yes	No
2	Has the patient lost weight within the past 3 mon?		
3	Has the patient lad a reduced dietary intake in the past week?		
4	Is the patient severely ill? (eg, in intensive therapy)		

Yes: If the answer is "yes" to any question, the screening in Table 32-3B is performed.

No: If the answer is "no" to all questions, the patient is rescreened at weekly intervals. For example, if the patient is scheduled for a major operation, a preventive nutritional care plan is considered to avoid the associated risk status.

BMI = body mass index.

PN (choice A) is not considered within the first 7 days regardless of nutritional risk because of minimal benefit and a high risk of infections. Combination nutrition via enteral and parenteral routes (choice D) is not recommended if the patient can have enteral nutrition at full capacity.

3. **B. The patient should be admitted to the ICU.**

   Acute pancreatitis is defined as two of the three features: (1) abdominal pain, (2) amylase or lipase three times greater than normal, and (3) radiologic imaging.[92,93] The severity is seen in Table 32-5.

   A severe course of acute pancreatitis is characterized by (1) patient characteristics such as age older than 55 years, obesity (BMI > 30 kg/m^2), altered mental status, or comorbidity; (2) evidence of systemic inflammatory response syndrome; (3) laboratory findings of blood urea nitrogen (BUN) > 20 mg/dL, rising BUN, hematocrit (Hct) greater than 44%, rising Hct, or elevated creatinine; and (4) pleural effusions, pulmonary infiltrates, or multiple extrapancreatic collections.[93] The patient has moderate to severe acute pancreatitis with several characteristics that suggest a severe course. With this in mind, it is best to admit the patient to the ICU. The patient should not be discharged home (choice A) or admitted under observation (choice D) because of end-organ damage.

   Complications from acute pancreatitis are listed in Table 32-6. Infection is suggested when there is extraluminal gas or if fine-needle aspiration of collections is positive for pathogens.[92] Infected necrotizing pancreatitis would warrant antimicrobials. Antibiotics are not warranted because the patient has no evidence of necrotizing pancreatitis, and there is no fluid collection to be sampled (choice C).

   There are two phases of death: the first phase is secondary to cytokine surge and lasts from 1 to 2 weeks, and the second phase is defined by persistent inflammatory response with local complications.[92] The patient may have transient

TABLE 32-3B Nutritional Risk Screening (NRS-2002): Final Screening

	Impaired Nutritional Status		Severity of Disease (≈ increase in requirements)
Absent score: 0	Normal nutritional status	Absent score: 0	Normal nutritional requirements
Mild score: 1	Weight loss > 5% in 3 mo or food intake <50–75% of normal requirement Requirement in preceding week	Mild score: I	Hip fracture;* patients with chronic disease, particularly with acute complications: cirrhosis,* COPD,* *chronic hemodialysis, diabetes, cancer*
Moderate score: 2	Weight loss > 5% in 2 mo or BMI 18.5–20.5 + impaired general condition or Food intake 25–60% of normal requirement in preceding week	Moderate score: 2	Major abdominal surgery,* stroke, * *severe pneumonia, hematologic malignancy*
Severe score: 3	Weight loss > 5% in 1 mo (> I5% in 3 mo) or BMI < 18.5 + impaired General condition or food intake 0–25% of normal requirement in preceding week.	Severe score: 3	Head injury,* bone marrow transplantation,* *intensive care patents (APACHE score>10)*
Score:	+	**Score:**	= Total score
Age if ≥ 70 years: add 1 to total score above = age-adjusted total score.			

Score ≥ 3: The patient is nutritionally at risk, and a nutritional care plan is initiated.

Score < 3: Weekly rescreening of the patient. For example, if the patient is scheduled for a major operation, a preventive nutritional care plan is considered to avoid the associated risk status.

NRS-2002 is based on an interpretation of available randomized clinical trials.
*Indicates that a trial directly supports the categorization of patients with that diagnosis. Diagnoses shown in *italics* are based on the prototypes mentioned further in Table.
Nutritional risk is defined by the present nutritional status and risk of impairment of present status due to increased requirements caused by stress metabolism of the clinical condition.

A nutritional care plan is indicated in all patients who are:
(1) severely undernourished (score = 3), (2) severely ill (score = 3), (3) moderately undernourished + mildly ill (score 2 + 1), or (4) mildly undernourished + moderately ill (score 1 + 2).
Prototypes for severity of disease score = 1: a patient with chronic disease admitted to the hospital because of complications. The patient is weak but out of bed regularly. Protein requirement is increased but can be covered by an oral diet or supplements in most cases.

Score = 2: a patient confined to bed because of illness (eg, after major abdominal surgery). Protein requirement is substantially increased but can be covered, although artificial feeding is required in many cases.
Score = 3: a patient in intensive care with assisted ventilation and so on. Protein requirement is increased and cannot be covered even by artificial feeding. Protein breakdown and nitrogen loss can be significantly attenuated.

APACHE = Acute Physiologic Assessment and Chronic Health Evaluation; BMI = body mass index; COPD = chronic obstructive pulmonary disease.

Reprinted with permission from Kondrup J, Allison SP, Elia M, Vellas B, Plauth M. ESPEN Guidelines for nutrition screening 2002. *Clin N.* 2003;22(4):415-421.

TABLE 32-4A NUTRIC Score Variables

Age	< 50	0
	50–< 75	1
	≥ 75	2
APACHE II score	< 15	0
	15–< 20	1
	20–28	2
	≥ 28	3
SOFA	6	0
	6–< 10	1
	≥ 10	2
Number of comorbidities	0–1	0
	≥ 2	1
Days from hospital to ICU admission	0–< 1	0
	≥ 1	1
IL-6	0–< 400	0
	≥ 400	1

APACHE = Acute Physiologic Assessment and Chronic Health Evaluation; ICU = intensive care unit; IL-6 = interleukin-6; NUTRIC = Nutrition Risk in the Critically Ill; SOFA = Sequential Organ Failure Assessment.

TABLE 32-4B NUTRIC Score Scoring System*

Sum of Points	Category	Explanation
6–10	High score	• Associated with worse clinical outcomes (mortality, ventilation) • These patients are the most likely to benefit from aggressive nutrition therapy
0–5	Low score	• These patients have a low malnutrition risk.

*If interleukin-6 is available.

NUTRIC = Nutrition Risk in the Critically Ill.

TABLE 32-4C NUTRIC Score Scoring System*

Sum of Points	Category	Explanation
5–9	High score	• Associated with worse clinical outcomes (mortality, ventilation) • These patients are the most likely to benefit from aggressive nutrition therapy.
0–4	Low score	• These patients have a low malnutrition risk.

*If interleukin-6 (IL-6) is not available. It is acceptable to not include IL-6 data when not routinely available; it was shown to contribute very little to the overall prediction of the Nutrition Risk in the Critically Ill (NUTRIC) score.

Data from Heyland DK, Dhaliwal R, Jiang X, Day AG. Identifying critically ill patients who benefit the most from nutrition therapy: the development and initial validation of a novel risk assessment tool. *Crit Care.* 2011;15(6):R268.

organ failure if it resolves within 48 hours or persistent if it lasts longer than 48 hours.[92] The severity and local complications are listed in Tables 32-5 and 32-6.[92,93]

4. B. Initiate enteral feeding.

The current guidelines from the American College of Gastroenterology suggest initiating EN for severe pancreatitis to prevent infectious complications.[93] PN is avoided in all types of pancreatitis because of the risk of infectious complications, organ failure, and death compared with EN (choice C). NPO status is not appropriate because early nutrition prevents disruption of gut mucosa and bacterial translocation (choices A and D).

5. B. Enteral nutrition with 15 to 30 g of protein

EN with 15 to 30 g of protein is advocated for open abdominal surgery with no colonic disruption because of the protein loss from exudates. PN (choice A) is not advocated unless the patient has been NPO for longer than 7 days or enteral nutrition is contraindicated. Glutamine and staying NPO (choices D and C) are generally avoided.

TABLE 32-5 Acute Pancreatitis Severity and Associated Mortality Rates

Acute mild pancreatitis	• Absence of organ failure and local or systemic complications	• Death rare
Moderately severe acute pancreatitis	• Transient organ failure or local or systemic complications	• Mortality rate less than severe
Severe acute pancreatitis	• Persistent organ failure with ≥ 1 local complications	• Mortality rate of 36–50% with necrosis associated with highest mortality rate

TABLE 32-6 Local Complications of Acute Pancreatitis

Acute peripancreatic fluid collection	• Associated with edematous pancreatitis with no necrosis seen within first 4 wk • Homogenous collection confined by normal pancreatic fascia; no wall encapsulation • Adjacent to pancreas
Pancreatic pseudocyst	• > 4 wk after acute interstitial edematous pancreatitis • Well-circumscribed, well-defined wall; all homogenous liquid
Acute necrotic collection	• Associated with necrotizing pancreatitis • Variable amounts of fluid and necrosis (heterogeneous) and no definite wall • Intra- or extrapancreatic
Walled-off necrosis	• > 4 wk after necrotizing pancreatitis • Heterogeneous with liquid and nonliquid components • Completely encapsulated

6. B. Initiate hemodialysis

Because ammonia is a byproduct of protein digestion, protein restriction should be the next step to help decrease ammonia production. However, there is substantial evidence to support protein restriction in cirrhosis, and it does not appear to improve hepatic encephalopathy. Because the patient has symptomatic hepatic encephalopathy, ammonia levels must be decreased rapidly. Hemodialysis can remove ammonia faster than lactulose or rifaximin (choices A and D). Even though ammonia is initially cleared by the liver, the liver enzymes do not suggest any hepatic insult (choice C).

Ammonia is a byproduct of protein digestion and bacterial metabolism in the gut and acid management in the kidneys and a consequence of seizures or exercise in skeletal muscle; it is hepatically degraded into urea via the urea cycle. Rate-limiting enzymes include carbamyl phosphatase synthetase (CPS), argininosuccinate synthetase (ASS), argininosuccinic acid lyase, and arginase.[94] If the ammonia levels exceed the capacity for hepatic degradation, it is eliminated via the kidneys by decreasing ammonia production and increasing urinary elimination and in the muscles and brain via conversion to glutamine.[94] Astrocytes supply glutamine to neurons, which convert it to glutamate, a neurotransmitter, and activate N-methyl-D-aspartate receptors.[94] Glutamate becomes glutamine in the synapse. In acute elevations of ammonia, astrocytes rapidly metabolize it to glutamine, causing swelling from increasing intracellular osmolarity, releasing inflammatory cytokines, subsequent astrocyte apoptosis, and increasing lactic acid production from metabolism of pyruvate to lactic acid because of depletion of adenosine 5 triphosphate and nicotinamide adenine dinucleotide and paralysis of the Krebs cycle.[94] Seizures, increased cerebral blood flow, cerebral edema, and herniation can result, particularly when arterial ammonia is greater than 200 μmol/L.[94] The rise in intracellular osmolarity is less acute in chronic hyperammonia and less neuroexcitation from glutamate.[94] In fulminant hepatic failure, arterial ammonia level correlates with glutamate level, which correlates with herniation.[94]

Hyperammonia can be caused by (1) increased nitrogen production from catabolism or increased protein processing such as in rapid weight loss and poor nutritional intake, internal bleeding, viral illness or stress, postpartum, changes in protein intake such as high protein strategies or malabsorption, and medications that effect catabolism such as glucocorticoids or chemotherapy; (2) diminished hepatic processing such as in vascular shunts or decreased hepatocytes such as cirrhosis or acute liver injury; or (3) urea cycle disorders from genetic defects such as cycle enzyme defects, organic academia, or fatty acid oxidation defects or from drugs such as 5-pentanoic acid, valproic acid, or cyclophosphamide.[95] Urea cycle disorders include ornithine transcarbamylase carnithine (OTC) deficiency, Argininosuccinate Synthetase deficiency, and carbamyl phosphate deficiency. Although most cases of hyperammonia secondary to urea cycle disorders are relevant in newborns, mild or partial deficiencies are asymptomatic through adulthood until specific stressors.[95-97]

This patient probably has an undiagnosed urea cycle disorder (UCD). Although family history is important, patients might not know their family history; therefore, important clues that could suggest a genetic disorder include a dietary history of veganism, psychiatric illness and prolonged flu-like illness, and exacerbation of ammonia levels greater than 100 μmol/L in the setting of stressors such as stressors, change in diet, and recent corticosteroid use.[95] Laboratory studies should include arterial blood gas analysis that shows respiratory alkalosis, serum amino acid tests, urinary orotic acid tests, urinary ketone tests, plasma and urinary organic acids, enzyme assays, DNA mutation analysis for UCD, and allopurinol testing for heterozygote carriers in OTC deficient pedigree. If the glycine and glutamine levels are elevated, the citrulline level is checked. If there is low citrulline, orotic acid is checked. Increased orotic acid suggests OTC deficiency, and normal orotic acid suggests CPS deficiency. If there is elevated citrulline, arginine is checked. If arginine is increased, there is arginase deficiency. If arginine is normal, urine arginosuccinate is evaluated. If there is no arginosuccinate, then it is citrullinemia. If there is arginosuccinate, then it is acetylsalicylic deficiency.

Treatment includes removal of ammonia, dietary protein withdrawal, reversal of catabolism from calorie supplementation and enzyme supplementation, and excess nitrogen scavenging methods.[95] Dialysis is the most effective way to remove ammonia. To reverse the catabolic state, dextrose, fluids, and intralipids should be administered. Priming dose on nitrogen scavengers include sodium phenylacetate and sodium benzoate 5.5 g/m^2 over 90 minutes with arginine HCl (10%) 200 mg/kg mixed in D10.

For carbamoyl phosphate synthetase I deficiency (CPS1), ornithine transcarbamylase (OTC), N-acetylglutamate synthetase deficiency (NAGS), or unknown deficiency, this is also the maintenance dose. For argininosuccinate synthetase (ASS) or argininosuccinate lyase (ASL) deficiency, 10% arginine HCl at 600 mg/kg/24 h is mixed with the sodium phenylacetate and sodium benzoate 5.5 g/m^2/24 h.[95] Sodium benzoate and sodium phenylacetate trap nitrogen in excretable forms (hippurate and phenylacetylglutamine, respectively), and arginine replenishes the low levels and uses part of urea cycle not affected by genetic defects to incorporate nitrogen.[95] Lactulose and rifaximin (choices A and D) do not improve ammonia levels as rapidly and are relatively contraindicated in patients with an ileus. Valproic acid increases ammonia levels (choice C).

7. B. Cornstarch with thiamine

Lactate is involved in oxidation, glucose metabolism, and cell signaling.[98,99] A total of 1.5 mol of lactate is produced daily in the skin, brain, skeletal muscle, and erthryocytes.[98] Lactate can act as fuel for mitochondrial respiration and hepatic gluconeogenesis. Mechanisms of lactate production include (1) tissue hypoxia, (2) indirectly related to tissue hypoxia, (3) increased reducing environment nictoniamide adenine dinucleotide + hydrogen/nicotinamide adenine dinucleotide NADH/NAD$^+$, (4) increased glycolytic flux, or (E) decreased lactate clearance[98] (Fig. 32-2). There is a high correlation between arterial and venous

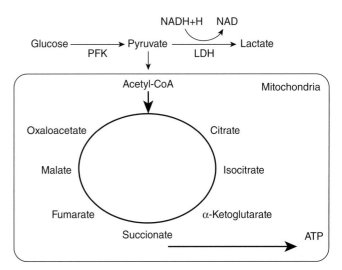

FIGURE 32-2 Glucose is metabolized to pyruvate via phosphofructokinase (PFK). In aerobic conditions, pyruvate enters the mitochondria, transforms into acetyl-coenzyme A with thiamine diphosphate, and enters the Krebs cycle to generate 38 adenosine triphosphate (ATP) molecules per 1 molecule of glucose. Pyruvate can also be converted into lactate in the cytosol. Lactate can also be produced (1) when under anaerobic conditions, the Krebs cycle cannot metabolize pyruvate; (2) there is a thiamine deficiency; (3) there is a reducing cellular environment (elevated NADH/NAD$^+$); or (4) in elevated glycolytic flux. LDH = lactate dehydrogenase.

lactate, and ice is not necessary if processed within 15 minutes.[98,99] After 15 minutes, there can be an artifactual increase secondary to the production of lactate by erythrocytes and leukocytes.[98]

The cause of elevation of lactate has been categorized into type A with evidence of inadequate tissue oxygenation and type B in which inadequate tissue oxygenation is not present. Type B is further subcategorized into type B1 in which there is an underlying disease, type B2 in which there is a drug associated, and type B3 in which there is an inborn error of metabolism.[98] Table 32-7 lists type B causes of lactic acidosis.

TABLE 32-7 Causes of Type B Lactic Acidosis

Thiamine deficiency	• Thiamine is a cofactor for cellular enzymes, and deprivation promotes anaerobic metabolism.
Malignancy	• Overexpression of glycolytic enzymes, mitochondrial dysfunction, impaired hepatic clearance +/- malnutrition
Hepatic dysfunction	• Poor clearance
Inborn errors of metabolism	• Glucose-6-phosphate deficiency • Fructose-1,6-diphosphate deficiency • Pyruvate carboxylase deficiency • Pyruvate dehydrogenase deficiency • Oxidative phosphorylation defects
Drugs • Biguanide • Acetaminophen • NRTI • Linezolid • β₂-Agonists • Propofol • Epinephrine • Theophylline • Alcohol • Cocaine • Carbon monoxide • Cyanide • Isoniazid • Sorbitol • Fructose • Inhaled nitric oxide	 • Gluconeogenesis inhibition, mitochondrial impairment, and impaired elimination • Mitochondrial impairment followed by poor hepatic clearance • Mitochondrial toxicity • Mitochondrial toxicity • Increased glycogenolysis, glycolysis, and lipolysis; free fatty acid release inhibit pyruvate dehydrogenase • Mitochondrial impairment and fatty acid oxidation impairment • B2 stimulation • Increased glycogenolysis, glycolysis, and lipolysis; free fatty acid release inhibit pyruvate dehydrogenase • Increased NADH, which inhibits pyruvate dehydrogenase • Increased glycogenolysis, glycolysis, and lipolysis; free fatty acid release inhibits pyruvate dehydrogenase and vasoconstriction • Decreased oxygen-carrying capacity of blood • Cytochrome C oxidase inhibition, causing mitochondrial dysfunction

NADH = nicotinamide adenine dicucleotide plus hydrogen; NRTI = nucleoside reverse transcriptase inhibitor. Lactate is used as an end goal for resuscitation and has prognostic implications in sepsis, asthma exacerbation, and diabetic ketoacidosis.[98-101] It usually requires intervention except in seizures, in which it is transient and resolves in 2 hours.[99] The patient appears to be well no resuscitation as per the ultrasound findings of IVC 2 cm with no respiratory variation, and giving another fluid bolus might not be helpful. However, the causes of elevated lactate are not mutually exclusive, and other etiologies should be further investigated despite having a primary diagnosis.

There are inborn errors of metabolism.[98,102-104] Most of these are apparent in neonates and infants, and some of these individuals do not survive to adulthood. In this case, the patient's physical appearance and laboratory derangement suggest glycogen storage disease type I, which is a deficiency in glucose-6-phosphatase activity or its microsomal protein transport protein.[93] It is an autosomal recessive disorder characterized by short stature, doll-like facies, hepatomegaly, and nephromegaly. The disorder also includes multiorgan dysfunction with development of liver adenomas, which can lead to hepatocellular carcinoma; bleeding diathesis secondary to platelet dysfunction with decreased adhesiveness and abnormal aggregation or von Willebrand-like defect; iron-deficiency anemia secondary to overexpression of hepcidin in adenomas and increases iron absorption; proximal renal tubular dysfunction, which can lead to renal failure; distal renal dysfunction with hypocitraturia and hypercalciuria, leading to nephrocalcinosis; polycystic ovaries with preserved fertility; neutropenia because of glucose critical for neutrophilic metabolic burst and fertility; neutropenia caused by glucose critical for neutrophilic metabolic burst; and a predisposition to gingivitis, mouth ulcers, upper respiratory infections, abscesses, and enterocolitis. The diagnosis is based on hypoglycemia, hyperuricemia, hypercholesterolemia, hypertriglyceridemia, lactic acidosis, genetic testing, and liver biopsy. Treatment consists of diet modification with avoidance of sucrose (fructose and glucose) and lactose (galactose) and use of cornstarch 1.7 to 2.5 g CS/kg every 4 to 5 hours for older children and adults sometimes with pancrelipase (lipase, protease, and amylase) to reduce side effects. Liver transplantation can improve hypoglycemia, but neutropenia and Crohn disease may still persist. Treatment includes citrate supplementation; hydration with or without thiazide to reduce hypercalciuria; low-dose angiotensin-converting enzyme inhibitors for early microalbuminuria (> 30 µg/albumin/mg creatinine); erythropoietin for glomerular filtration rate less than 50 mL/min/1.73 m² to maintain hemoglobin at 10 to 12 g/dL; granulocyte-colony stimulating factor starting at 1 µg/kg/d or every other day to maintain absolute neutrophilic count (ANC) greater than 500, up to 1×10^9/L while monitoring for splenomegaly, bone pain, and hepatomegaly and avoidance of hypoglycemic medications. Liver ultrasound will not immediately improve the lactic acid level (choice B). Continuing the D5 IV fluids might further increase the lactic acid level (choice D).

8. **D. Continue the current tube feed rate.**

Arabi et al. randomized prospective study on permissive underfeeding (40–60% of calculated calorie requirements) versus standard feeding (70–100% of calculated calorie requirements) with similar protein intake in mechanically ventilated patients showed no difference in 90-day mortality rate (121 of 445 patients [27.2%] in the permissive-underfeeding group and 127 of 440 patients [28.9] in the standard-feeding group died; RR with permissive underfeeding, 0.94; 95% CI, 0.76–1.16; *P* = 0.58).[85] Increasing the tube feeding's caloric density may increase the osmolarity and therefore diarrhea. The patient has only been on the mechanical ventilator for 4 days and therefore should not be started on PN in addition to EN. Giving fluid boluses to match the output from the diarrhea is counterproductive because conservative fluid strategies in ARDS are generally advocated.

REFERENCES

1. Taylor BE, McClave SA, Martindale RG, et al. Guidelines for the Provision and Assessment of Nutrition Support Therapy in the Adult Critically Ill Patient: Society of Critical Care Medicine (SCCM) and American Society for Parenteral and Enteral Nutrition (ASPEN). *Crit Care Med.* 2016;44:(2):390-439.
2. Heyland DK, Dhaliwal R, Jiang X, et al. Identifying critically ill patients who benefit the most from nutrition therapy: the development and initial validation of a novel risk assessment tool. *Crit Care.* 2011;15:R268.
3. Jie B, Jiang ZM, Nolan MT, et al. Impact of preoperative nutritional support on clinical outcome in abdominal surgical patients at nutritional risk. *Nutrition.* 2012;28:1022-1027.
4. Kondrup J, Allison SP, Elia M, et al. ESPEN Guidelines for nutrition screening. *Clin Nutr.* 2003;22(4):415-421.
5. Weijs PJ, Sauerwein HP, Kondrup J. Protein recommendations in the ICU: g protein/kg body weight-which body weight for underweight and obese patients? *Clin Nutr.* 2012;31:774-775.
6. Allingstrup MJ, Esmailzadeh N, Wilkens Knudsen A, et al. Provision of protein and energy in relation to measured requirements in intensive care patients. *Clin Nutr.* 2012;31:462-468.
7. Clifton GL, Robertson CS, Constant CF. Enteral hyperalimentation in head injury. *J Neurosurg.* 1985;62:186-193.
8. Scheinkestel CD, Kar L, Marschall K, et al. Prospective randomized trial to assess caloric and protein needs of critically ill, anuric, ventilated patients requiring continuous renal replacement therapy. *Nutrition.* 2003;19:909-916.
9. Plank LD. Protein for the critically ill patient—what and when? *Eur J Clin Nutr.* 2013;7:565-568.
10. Kang W, Kudsk KA. Is there evidence that the gut contributes to the mucosal immunity in humans? *JPEN J Parenter Enteral Nutr.* 2007;31:246-258.
11. Jabbar A, Chang WK, Dryden GW, et al. Gut immunology and its influence by nutrition. *Am J Surg.* 2002;183:390-398.
12. Windsor AC, Kanwar S, Li AG, et al. Compared with parenteral nutrition, enteral feeding attenuates the acute phase response and improves disease severity in acute pancreatitis. *Gut.* 1998;l42:431-435.
13. Ammori BJ. Importance of early increase in intestinal permeability in critically ill patients. *Eur J Surg.* 2002;168:660-661; author reply 662.
14. Heyland DK, Dhaliwal R, Drover JW, et al. Canadian Critical Clinical Practice Guidelines Committee: Canadian Clinical Practice Guidelines for nutrition support in mechanical ventilated critically ill adult patients. *JPEN J Parenter Enteral Nutr.* 2003;27:355-373.
15. Mark PE, Zaloga GP. Early enteral nutrition in acutely ill patients: a systemic review. *Crit Care Med.* 2001;29:2264-2270.
16. Doig GS, Heighes PT, Simpson, F et al. Early enteral nutrition provided within 24 hours of injury or intensive care unit admission; significantly reduces mortality in critically ill patients: a meta-analysis of randomized controlled trials. *Intensive Care Med.* 2008;35:2018-2027.
17. Braunschweig CL, Levy P, Seean PM, et al. Enteral compared with parenteral nutrition: a meta-analysis. *Am J Clin Nutr.* 2001;74:534-542.
18. Gramlich L, Kichian K, Pinilla J, et al. Does enteral nutritional nutrition compared to parenteral nutrition result in better outcomes in critically ill adult patients? A systemic review of the literature. *Nutrition.* 2004;20:843-848.
19. Moore FA, Feliciano DV, Andrassy RJ, et al. Early enteral feeding compared with parenteral reduces postoperative septic complications. The results of a meta-analysis . *Ann Surg.* 1992;216:172-183.
20. Simpson F, Doig GS. Parenteral vs enteral nutrition in the critically ill patient: a meta-analysis of trials using the intention to treat principle. *Intensive Care Med.* 2005;31:12-23.
21. Stechmiller JK, Treloar D, Allen N. Gut dysfunction in critically ill patients: a review of the literature. *Am J Crit Care* 1997;6:204-209.
22. Reintam A, Parm P, Kitus R, et al. Gastrointestinal symptoms in intensive care patients. *Acta Anaesthesiol Scand.* 2009;53:318-324.
23. Nguyen T, Frenette AJ, Johanson C, et al. Impaired gastrointestinal transit and its associated morbidity in the intensive care unit. *J Crit Care.* 2013;28:537e11-537e17.
24. Davies AR, Morrison SS, Bailey MJ, et al. ENTERIC Study Investigators; ANZICS Clinical Trials Group: A multicenter randomized controlled trial comparing early nasojejunal with nasogastric nutrition in critical illness. *Crit Care Med.* 2012;40:2342-2348.
25. Aosta-Escribano J, Fernandez-Vivas M, Gau Carmona T, et al. Gastric versus transpyloric feeding in severe traumatic brain injury: a prospective randomized trial. *Intensive Care Med.* 2010;36:1532-1539.
26. Hsu CW, Sun SF, Lin SL, et al. Duodenal versus gastric feeding in the medical intensive care unit patients: a prospective randomized clinical study. *Crit Care Med.* 2009;37:1866-1872.
27. Kearns PJ, Chin D, Mueller L, et al. The incidence of ventilator-associated pneumonia and success in nutrient delivery with gastric versus small intestinal feeding: a randomized clinical trial. *Crit Care Med.* 2000;28:1742-1746.
28. Montecalvo MA, Steger KA Farber HW, et al. Nutritional outcome and pneumonia in critical are patients randomized to gastric versus jejunal tube feedings. The Critical Care Research Team. *Crit Care Med.* 1992;20:1377-1387.
29. Montejo JC, Grau T, Acosta J, et al. Nutritional and Metabolic Working Group of the Spanish Society of the Intensive Care Medicine and Coronary Units: multicenter, prospective, randomized single-blind study comparing the efficacy and gastrointestinal complications of early jejunal feeding with early gastric feeding in critically ill patients. *Crit Care Med.* 2002;30:796-800.
30. Kortbeek JB, Haigh PI, Doig C. Duodenal versus gastric feeding in ventilated blunt trauma patients: a randomized controlled trial. *J Trauma.* 1999;46:992-996.
31. Taylor SJ, Fettes SB, Jewkes C, et al. Prospective randomized controlled trial to determine the effect of early enhanced enteral nutrition on clinical outcome in mechanically ventilated patients suffering head injury. *Crit Care Med.* 1999;27:2525-2531.

32. Minard G, Kudsk KA, Melton S, et al. Early versus delayed feeding with an immune-enhancing diet in patients with severe head injuries. *JPEN J Parenter Enteral Nutr.* 2000;24:145-149.

33. Day L, Stotts NA, Frankfurt A, et al. Gastric versus duodenal feeding in patients with neurological disease: a pilot Study. *J Neurosci Nurs.* 2001;33(3):148-149.

34. Davies AR, Froomes PR, Frech CJ, et al. Randomized comparison of nasojejunal and nasogastric feeding in critically ill patients. *Crit Care Med.* 2002;30:586-590.

35. White H, Sosnowski K, Tran K, et al. A randomized controlled comparison of early post-pyloric versus early gastric feeding to meet nutritional targets in ventilated intensive care patients. *Crit Care.* 2009;13:R187.

36. McClave SA, DeMeo MT, DeLegge MH, et al. North American Summit on Aspiration in the Critically Ill Patient: consensus statement. *JPEN J Parenter Enteral Nutr.* 2002;26(supp):S80-S85.

37. Elpern EH. Pulmonary aspiration in hospitalized adults. *Nutr Clin Pract.* 1997;12:5-13.

38. Mark PE. Aspiration pneumonitis and aspiration pneumonia. *N Engl J Med.* 2001;344:665-671.

39. Bonten MJ, Gaillard CA, van Tiel FH, et al. The stomach is not a source for colonization of the upper respiratory tract and pneumonia in ICU patients. *Chest.* 1994;105:878-884.

40. Heyland DK, Drover JW, MacDonald S, et al. Effect of postpyloric feeding on gastroesophageal regurgitation and pulmonary microaspiration: results of a randomized controlled trial. *Crit Care Med.* 2001;29:1495-1501.

41. Lien HC, Chang CS, Chen G. Can percutaneous endoscopic jejunostomy prevent gastroesophageal reflux in patients with preexisting esophagitis. *Am J Gastroenterol.* 2000;95:3439-3443.

42. Ibrahim EH, Mehringer L, Prentice D, et al. Early versus late enteral feeding of mechanically ventilated patients: results of a clinical trial. *JPEN J Parenter Enteral Nutr.* 2002;26:174-181.

43. MacLeod JB, Lefton J, Houghton D, et al. Prospective randomized control trial of intermittent versus continuous gastric feeds for critically ill trauma patients. *J Trauma.* 2007;63:57-61.

44. Bonten MJ, Gaillard CA, van der Hust R, et al. Intermittent enteral feeding: the influence on respiratory and digestive tract colonization in mechanically ventilated intensive care unit patients. *Am J Respir Care Med.* 1996;154:394-399.

45. Steevens EC, Lipscomb AF, Poole GV, et al. Comparison of continuous vs intermittent nasogastric enteral feeding in trauma patients: perceptions and practice. *Nutr Clin Pract.* 2002;17:118-122.

46. Hiebert JM, Brown A, Anderson RG, et al. Comparison of continuous vs intermittent tube feedings in adult burn patients. *JPEN J Parenter Enteral Nutr.* 1981;5(1):73-75.

47. Kocan MC, Hickish SM. A comparison of continuous and intermittent enteral nutrition in NICU patients. *J Neurosci Nurs.* 1986;18:333-337.

48. Ciocon JO, Galindo-Ciocon DJ, Tiessen C, et al. Continuous compared with intermitted tube feeding in the elderly. *JPEN J Parenteral Nutr.* 1992;16:525-528.

49. Berne JD, Norwood SH, McAuley CE, et al. Erythromycin reduced delayed gastric emptying in critically ill trauma patients. A randomized controlled trial. *J Trauma.* 2002;53:422-425.

50. Chapman MJ, Fraser RJ, Kluger MT, et al. Erythromycin improves gastric emptying in critically ill patients intolerant of nasogastric feeding. *Crit Care Med.* 2000;28:2334-2337.

51. Meissner W, Dohrn B, Reinhart K. Enteral Naloxone reduces gastric tube reflux and frequency of pneumonia in critical care patients during opioid analgesia. *Crit Care Med .* 2003;31:776-780.

52. Nguyen NQ, Chapman M, Frasser RJ, et al. Prokinetic therapy for feed intolerance in critical illness: one drug or two? *Crit Care Med.* 2007;35:2561-2567.

53. Nursal TZ, Erdogan B, Noyan T, et al. The effect of metoclopramide on gastric emptying in traumatic brain injury. *J Clin Neurosci.* 2007;13:344-348.

54. Yavagal DR, Karnad DR, Oak JL. Metoclopramide for preventing pneumonia in critically ill patients receiving enteral tube feeding: a randomized controlled trial. *Crit Care Med.* 2000;28:1408-1411.

55. Reignier J, Bensaid S, Perrin-Gachadoat D, et al. Erythromycin and early enteral nutrition in mechanically ventilated patients. *Crit Care Med.* 2002;30:1237-1241.

56. MacLaren R, Kiser TH, Fish DN, et al. Erythromycin vs metoclopramide for facilitating gastric emptying and tolerance to intragastric nutrition in critically ill patients. *JPEN J Parenter Enteral Nutr.* 2008;32:412-419.

57. Silk DB, Walters ER, Duncan HD, et al. The effect of a polymeric enteral formula supplemented with a mixture of six fibres on normal human bowel function and colonic motility. *Clin Nutr.* 2001;20:49-58.

58. Cummings JH, Beatty ER, Kingman SM, et al. Digestion and physiological properties of resistant starch I the human large bowel. *Br J Nutr.* 1996;75:733-747.

59. Kato Y, Nakao M, Iwasa M, et al. Soluble fiber improves management of diarrhea in elderly patients receiving enteral nutrition. *Food Nutri Sci.* 2012;3:1547-1552.

60. Shimizu K, Ogura H, Asahara T, et al. Gastrointestinal dysmotility is associated with altered gut flora and septic mortality in patients with severe systemic inflammatory response syndrome: a preliminary study. *Neurogastroenterol Motil.* 2011;23:30-35.

61. Homann HH, Jemen M, Fuessenich C, et al. Reduction in diarrhea incidence by soluble fiber in patients receiving total or supplemental enteral nutrition. *JPEN J Parenter Enteral Nutr.* 1994;18:486-490.

62. Hart GK, Dobb GJ. Effect of a fecal bulking agent on diarrhea during enteral feeding in the critically ill. *JPEN J Parenter Enteral Nutr.* 1988;12:465-468.

63. Spapen H, Diltoer M, Van Malderen C, et al. Soluble fiber reduces the incidence of diarrhea in septic patients receiving total enteral nutrition: a prospective double blind randomized and controlled trial. *Clin Nutr.* 2001;20:301-305.

64. Heather DJ, Howell L, Montana M, et al. Effect of a bulk-forming cathartic on diarrhea in tube-fed patients. *Heart Lung.* 1991;20:409-413.

65. Karakan T, Ergun M, Dogan I, et al. Comparison of early enteral nutrition in severe acute pancreatitis with prebiotic fiber supplementation versus standard enteral solution: a prospective randomized double-blind study. *World J Gastroenterol.* 2009;13:2733-2737.

66. Morrow LE, Koeef MH, Casale TB. Probiotic prophylaxis of ventilator-associated pneumonia: a blinded, randomized controlled trial. *Am J Respir Crit Care Med.* 2010;182:1058-1064.

67. Rayes N, Seehofer D, Theruvath T, et al. Effect of enteral nutrition and synbiotics on bacterial infection rates after pylorus-preserving pancreatoduodenectomy: a randomized, double blind trial. *Ann Surg.* 2007;246:36-41.

68. Bo L, Jinbao Li, Bai Y, et al. Probiotics for preventing ventilator-associated pneumonia. *Cochrane Database Syst Rev.* 2014;(10):CD009066.

69. Basselink MG, van Santvoort HC, Buskens E, et al. Dutch Acute Pancreatitis Study Group: probiotic prophylaxis in predicted severe acute pancreatitis: a randomized, double-blind placebo controlled trial. *Lancet.* 2008;37:651-659.

70. Lherm T, Monet C, Nougiere B, et al. Seven cases of fungemia with *Saccharomyces boulardii* in critically ill patients. *Intensive Care Med.* 2002;28:797-801.

71. Barraud D, Bollaert PE, Gibot S. Impact of the administration of probiotics on mortality in critically ill adult patients: a meta-analysis of randomized controlled trials. *Chest.* 2013;143:646-655.

72. Zhang Y, Chen J, Wu J, et al. Probiotic use in preventing postoperative infection in liver transplant patients. *Hepatobiliary Surg Nutr.* 2013;2:142-147.

73. Rayes N, Seehofer D, Muller AR, et al. Influence of probiotics and fibre on the incidence of bacterial infections following major abdominal surgery—results of prospective trial. *Z Gastroenterol.* 2002;40:869-876.

74. Rayes N, Seehofer D, Hansen S, et al. Early enteral supply of lactobacillus and fiber versus selective bowel decontamination: a controlled trial in liver transplant recipients. *Transplantation.* 2002;74:123-127.

75. Gu WJ, Deng T, Gong YZ, et al. The effects of probiotics in early enteral nutrition on the outcomes of trauma: a meta-analysis of randomized controlled trials. *JPEN J Parenter Enteral Nutr.* 2013;37:31-317.

76. Pattani R, Palda VA, Hwang SW, et al. Probiotics for the prevention of antibiotic-associated diarrhea and Clostridium difficile infection among hospitalized patients: systemic review and meta-analysis. *Open Med.* 2013;7(2):e56-e67.

77. Goldenberg JZ, Ma SS, Saxton JD, et al. Probiotics for the prevention of Clostridium difficile-associated diarrhea in adults and children. *Cochrane Database Syst Rev.* 2013;5:CD006095.

78. Casaser MP, Messotten D, Hermans G, et al. Early versus late parenteral nutrition in critically ill adults. *N Engl J Med.* 2011;365:506-517.

79. Kelly DG, Tappenden KA, Winkler MF. Short bowel syndrome: highlights of patient management, quality of life and survival. *JPEN J Parenter Enteral Nutr.* 2014;38:427-437.

80. Doig GS, Simpson F, Sweetman EA, et al. Early PN Investigators of the ANZICS Clinical Trials Group: early parenteral nutrition in critically ill patients with short term relative contraindications to early enteral nutrition: a randomized controlled trial. *JAMA.* 2013;309:2130-2138.

81. Heyland DK, MacDonald S, Keefe L, et al. Total parenteral nutrition in the critically ill patient: a meta-analysis. *JAMA.* 998;280:2013-2019.

82. Battistella FD, Widergren JT, Anderson JT, et al. A prospective, randomized trial of intravenous fat emulsion administration in trauma victims requiring total parenteral nutrition. *J Trauma.* 1997;43:52-8.

83. Choban PS, Burge JC, Scales D, et al. Hypoenergetic nutrition support in hospitalized obese patients: a simplified method for clinical application. *Am J Clin Nutr.* 1997;66:546-550.

84. Ahrens CL, Barletta JF, Kanji S, et al. Effect of low calorie parenteral nutrition on the incidence and severity of hyperglycemia in surgical patients: a randomized controlled trial. *Crit Care Med.* 2005;33:2507-2512.

85. Arabi YM, Aldawood AS, Haddad SH, et al. Permissive underfeeding or standard enteral feeding in critically ill adults. *N Eng J Med.* 2015;372:2398-2408.

86. Preiser JC, van Zanten AR, Berger MM, et al. Metabolic and nutritional support of critically ill patients: consensus and controversies. *Crit Care.* 2015.15;35:1-11.

87. Khan LUR, Ahmed J, Khan S, Macfie J. Refeeding syndrome: a literature review. *Gastroenterol Res Pract.* 2011;ii:410971.

88. Mehanna HM, Moledina J, Travis J. Refeeding syndrome: what it is, and how to prevent and treat it. *BMJ.* 2008; 336:1495-1499.

89. National Institute for Health and Clinical Excellence. Nutrition support in adults. Clinical Guideline CG32. 2006. http://www.nice.org.uk/page.aspx?o=cg032.

90. Kondrup J, Allison SP, Elia M, et al. ESPEN Guidelines for Nutrition Screening 2002. *Clin Nutr.* 2003;4:415-421.

91. Heyland DK, Dhaliwal R, Jiang X, Day AG. Identifying critically ill patients who benefit the most from nutrition therapy: the development and initial validation of a novel risk assessment tool. *Crit Care.* 2011;15(6):R268.

92. Banks PA, Bollen TL, Devenis C, et al. Classification of acute pancreatitis 2012: revision of the Atlanta Classification and definitions by international consensus. *Gut.* 2013;62:102-111.

93. Tenner S, Baillie J, DeWitt J, Vege SS. American College of Gastroenterology guideline: management of acute pancreatitis. *Am J Gastroenterol.* 2013;108(9):1400-1415; 1416.

94. Clay AS, Hainline BE. Hyperammonia in the ICU. *Chest.* 2007;132:1368-1378.

95. Summar ML, Barr F, Dawling S, et al. Unmasked adult-onset urea cycle disorders in the critical care setting. *Crit Care Clin.* 2005;21(Suppl):S1-S8.

96. Haberle J, Boddaert N, Burlina A, et al. Suggested guidelines for the diagnosis and management of urea cycle disorders. *Orphanet J Rare Dis.* 2012;7;32.

97. Van Vliet D, Derks TG, van Rijn M, et al. Single amino acid supplementation in aminoacidopathies: a systemic review. *Orphanet J Rare Dis.* 2014;9:7.

98. Suetrong B, Walley KR. Lactic acidosis in sepsis: it's not all anaerobic. *Chest.* 2016;149(1):252-261.

99. Andersen LW, Mackenhauer J, Roberts JC, et al. Etiology and therapeutic approach to elevated lactate levels. *Mayo Clin Proc.* 2013;88(10):1127-1140.

100. Jones AE, Shapiro NI, Trzeciak S, et al. Lactate clearance vs central venous oxygen saturation as goals of early sepsis therapy: a randomized clinical trial. *JAMA.* 2010; 303(8):252-258.

101. Puskarich MA, Trzeciak S, Shapiro NI, et al. Prognostic value and agreement of achieving lactate clearance or central venous oxygen saturation goals during early sepsis resuscitation. *Acad Emerg Med.* 2012;19(3):252-258.

102. Kishnani PS, Austin SL, Abdenur JE, et al. Diagnosis and management of glycogen storage disease type I: a practice guideline of the American College of Medical Genetics and Genomics. *Genet Med.* 2014;16(11):e1.

103. Habarou F, Brasier A, Rio M, et al. Pyruvate carboxylase deficiency: an underestimated cause of lactic acidosis. *Mol Genet Metab Rep.* 2015;2:25-31.

104. Ahmad A, Kahler SG, Kishnani P, et al. Treatment of pyruvate carboxylase deficiency with high dose of citrate and aspartate. *Am J Med Genet.* 1999;87:331-338.

Extracorporeal Life Support

Raghad Hussein, MD, Arvind Sundaram, MD, and Jason A. Stamm, MD

DEFINITION OF EXTRACORPOREAL LIFE SUPPORT

Extracorporeal life support (ECLS), also known as extracorporeal membrane oxygenation (ECMO), is an artificial form of cardiopulmonary support that allows the heart, the lungs, or both to recover from severe, but potentially reversible, pathologies. ECLS can also function in some cases as a bridge to therapies such as a ventricular assist device or heart or lung transplantation.

BACKGROUND OF EXTRACORPOREAL LIFE SUPPORT

Early work in extracorporeal support dates to 1930 when Dr. John Gibbons built a roller pump device. In 1953, Dr. Gibbons created and successfully used the first heart–lung machine during an atrial septal defect repair. Four years later, silicone rubber membranes replaced the bubbler oxygenator, allowing the prolonged use of extracorporeal machines. These membranes serve as a gas–oxygen interface and thereby prevent severe hemolysis and plasma leakage.[1,2]

In 1972, Dr. JD Hill announced the first extended use of the extracorporeal circuit outside the operating theater. Dr. Hill's patient survived posttraumatic respiratory failure after 75 hours of ECLS support. At the same time, Dr. Robert Bartlett and his colleagues at the University of Michigan took the lead in developing and implementing ECLS care, the results of which influenced ECLS care throughout the world.[3]

After the initial successful attempts, ECLS continued to make progress, albeit slowly. The medical community developed skepticism about the utility of ECLS in adults in the late 1970s when the first randomized controlled trial (RCT) reported poor survival rates.[4] Another RCT published in 1994 likewise revealed no survival benefit with ECLS.[5] ECLS regained interest in adult patients in 2009 after the publication of several landmark studies, specifically the efficacy and economic assessment of conventional ventilatory support versus extracorporeal membrane oxygenation for severe adult respiratory failure (CESAR) trial in the United Kingdom of patients with acute respiratory distress syndrome (ARDS) and observational studies from several different countries of the use of ECLS in respiratory failure caused by H1N1 influenza.[6-8] Although both the CESAR trial and the observation influenza pandemic studies had design limitations, these reports stimulated the growth of adult ECLS based on an apparent mortality benefit compared with contemporary conventional mechanical ventilation support.

In an effort to foster and organize ECLS, in 1989, the Extracorporeal Life Support Organization (ELSO) was established to support healthcare professionals and scientists who are involved in ECMO. Among its many activities, ELSO maintains a registry of both facilities trained to provide ECLS care and of patients placed on ECLS. The ELSO patient registry information is used to support clinical research, quality improvement, and regulatory action. ELSO also provides educational programs for ECLS centers and facilities that may be involved in the transfer of patients to higher levels of care.

MODES OF EXTRACORPOREAL LIFE SUPPORT

There are traditionally two modes of ECLS, venovenous (VV ECLS) and venoarterial (VA ECLS). In both modes, blood is drained from a large vein into the ECLS circuit, where gas exchange occurs, and then blood is returned to the venous side (in VV ECLS) or the arterial side (in VA ECLS).

Because ECLS is not a disease-targeted therapy, the selection criteria of the right patient and mode are fundamental to the best outcome. VV ECLS acts as an artificial lung and is connected in series with the cardiopulmonary circulation, allowing complete or partial replacement of the native lung function. It maintains pulmonary blood flow and uses the patient's own cardiac output (CO). Thus, VV ECLS does not provide hemodynamic support. Conversely, VA ECLS is connected in parallel with the heart and lungs, bypasses the pulmonary circulation, and provides nearly complete hemodynamic support (Fig. 33-1).

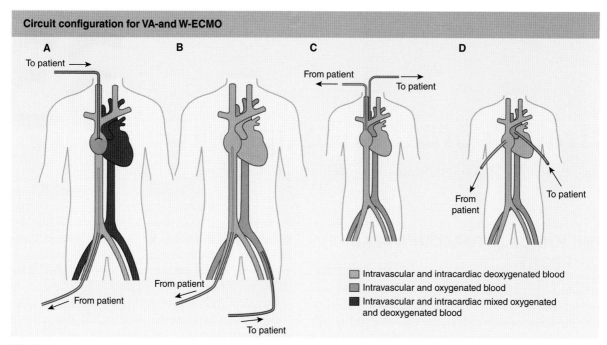

FIGURE 33-1 Different ECLS configurations with (A) VV-ECLS. Oxygenated blood is returned to the right internal jugular vein while de-oxygenated blood is right femoral vein, with catheter tip ideally near right perihepatic inferior vena cava (IVC). (B) Femoral VA-ECLS. Deoxygenated blood is drained from right femoral vein with catheter tip ideally near right perihepatic inferior vena cava and oxygenated blood returned to right femoral artery. (C) Carotid VA-ECLS. (D) Thoracic VA-ECLS. (Reprinted from Gaffney AM, Wildhirst SM, Griffin MJ, et al. Extracorporeal life support. *BMJ.* November 2, 2010;341:c5317 with permission from BMJ Publishing Group Ltd.)

INITIATION OF EXTRACORPOREAL LIFE SUPPORT

Circuit Component

The ECLS circuit is composed of three essential parts: a gas exchange device, a blood pump, and a heat exchanger device. All parts are connected by tubing along with the intravascular cannula(s) on both ends.

The Gas Exchange Device

The traditional ECLS oxygenator consists of silicone rubber membranes. They are composed of long spirals that separate the gas phase from the blood phase. The membranes inherently create high resistance to blood flow. Newer hollow, nonporous polymethylpentene (PMP) membranes were developed to mitigate the complications of the high-pressure gradient between the inlet and output circuits. The PMP-based oxygenator device comes in different sizes and shapes and is currently the most widely used oxygenator design.[9]

The Pump

Pumps drive blood into the ECLS circuit by one of two means:

• Classic roller pumps, in which blood flows passively using gravity siphon

• Centrifugal pumps, which are more commonly used and in which blood flows actively through centrifugal force

The Heat Exchanger

The heat exchanger consists of hollow, silicone-coated stainless steel tubes that are surrounded by warm water and that function to maintain body temperature as blood flows within the circuit. Heat exchangers are usually located within or after the oxygenator.[10]

The Circuit

The standard ECLS circuit tubing is made from polyvinylchloride (PVC), a commonly used synthetic polymer. This design tolerates the high pressure generated by the pump and thus prevents circuit rupture. Although there is no ideal biocompatible tubing material, the PVC circuit coated with heparin helps attenuate plasma protein adsorption and reduces the risk of thrombosis.[11]

Cannula Types

There are several kinds of ECLS cannulas. They differ in size, length, lumen(s), and fenestration. Selection of proper cannula depends on the ECLS support mode and size. As a consensus, the cannula size is reported based on the outer diameter.

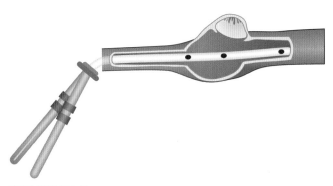

FIGURE 33-2 Catheter outflow is the upper (darker blood) port while catheter inflow is the lower port (lighter blood).

To achieve adequate blood drainage and infusion, it is important to understand the determinants of volume flow, namely the cannula's length and diameter. Short and wide cannulas are ideal for venous drainage because of reduced resistance.[12,13]

Insertion Sites

Insertion sites vary according to the cannula type and designated mode of ECLS. Cannula(s) are usually placed under vascular ultrasound, transesophageal echocardiogram (TEE), or fluoroscopy guidance.

In VV ECLS, if two cannulas are used, a typical arrangement is a single-lumen drainage catheter in the common femoral vein with blood return via an infusion cannula in the right internal jugular (RIJ) or femoral vein. Alternatively, if a double-lumen single cannula is used, the RIJ vein can be cannulated (Figs. 33-2 and 33-3). In this configuration, blood is drained

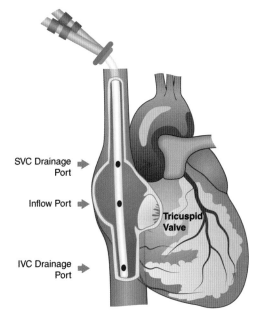

SVC Drainage Port

Inflow Port

Tricuspid Valve

IVC Drainage Port

FIGURE 33-3 For the venovenous double lumen cannula, the distal drainage is at inferior vena cava and the proximal drainage at superior vena cava. The inflow port with oxygenation blood is directed at tricuspid valve.

from the superior vena cava (SVC) and inferior vena cava (IVC) and returned through the same cannula into the right atrium.

In VA ECLS, venous blood is typically drained from the IVC and infused back into a large artery, commonly the femoral artery. In postcardiotomy operations, the drainage cannula is occasionally placed into the right atrium or SVC, and the infusing cannula is placed in the aorta.

Extracorporeal Life Support Indications and Contraindications

Extracorporeal life support is considered for cardiogenic shock or respiratory failure cases that are severe; refractory to conventional management; and most important, potentially reversible (Table 33-1).[14]

CIRCUIT MANAGEMENT

Native Oxygen Delivery and Consumption

The cardiopulmonary system is designed to deliver oxygenated blood to the tissues and eliminate carbon dioxide. Therefore, effective management of ECLS requires a robust understanding of this physiology. Oxygen delivery (DO_2) can be measured by multiplying the arterial oxygen content (Cao_2) by the CO:

$$Cao_2 \text{ (mL/dL)} = 1.39 \text{ (mL/dL)} \times \text{[Hemoglobin] (g)} \times \% \text{ } O_2 \text{ saturation} + 0.003 \text{ (mL/dL/mmHg)} \times Pao_2 \text{ (mmHg)}$$
$$Do_2 \text{ (mL/min)} = Cao_2 \times CO \times 10$$

Cao_2 represents the sum of O_2 bound to hemoglobin (Hgb) and is dissolved in plasma. The normal Cao_2 is 20 mL/dL. As seen in the formula, CO plays a major role in determining Do_2.

Oxygen consumption (Vo_2) is the difference between arterial and venous oxygen content, which can be calculated by Fick's principle:

$$Vo_2 = CO \times (Cao_2 - Cvo_2)$$

where Cvo_2 (mL/dL) = 1.39 (mL/dL) × Hgb (g) × % Svo_2 + 0.003 (mL/dL/mmHg) × Pvo_2

Svo_2 is the mixed venous oxygen saturation, and Pvo_2 is the venous partial pressure of O_2, and Hgb is hemoglobin.

Oxygen Delivery With Extracorporeal Life Support

Oxygen delivery in ECLS depends on the multiple factors, including flow through the ECLS circuit, the oxygenator membrane surface area, the contact time of the gas–blood interface and O_2 gradient, oxygenation by the native lung, and native CO. Of these, flow is the most crucial determinant of blood oxygenation during ECLS. In particular, oxygenation

TABLE 33-1 Indications and Contraindications for Extracorporeal Life Support

ECLS Mode	Indications	Contraindications
VV ECLS	• ARDS • Extracorporeal lung rest for refractory obstructive airway disease, traumatic lung contusions, and severe inhalational injuries • A bridge to lung transplant, eg, in cases of cystic fibrosis or graft dysfunction after lung transplant	There are no clearly established absolute contraindications, but the following preexisting conditions are contraindicated by most protocols: • Metastatic malignancy • Severe CNS injury • ARDS with > 7 d of mechanical ventilation • Risk of bleeding with anticoagulation • Poor candidacy for organ transplant Other relative contraindications: • Advanced age • Obesity (> 125 kg)

VA ECLS	• Cardiogenic shock
	• Myocardial ischemia
	• Myocardial depression (eg, myocarditis, drug toxicity)
	• Refractory life-threatening arrhythmia
	• Postcardiotomy
	• Inability to wean from CPB machine
	  • Heart transplant
	  • As bridge to heart transplant or VAD
	  • Postcardiac graft dysfunction	

ARDS = acute respiratory distress syndrome; CNS = central nervous system; CPB = cardiopulmonary bypass; ECLS = extracorporeal life support; VA = venoarterial; VAD = ventricular assist device; VV = venovenous

For appropriate survival prediction of ECLS candidates, ELSO and the Department of Intensive Care Medicine at the Alfred Hospital, Melbourne, developed two clinical scores, the Respiratory Extracorporeal Membrane Oxygenation Survival Prediction (RESP) (http://www.respscore.com) and Survival After Veno-Arterial ECMO (SAVE) (http://www.save-score.com) scores for respiratory and cardiac failure, respectively.[15,16]

is directly proportional to the circuit blood flow, measured in milliliters per kilogram per minute. In the adult population, a flow of 50 to 80 mL/kg/min is usually sufficient to achieve adequate tissue oxygenation. A typical ECLS circuit can achieve flows of up to 7 to 8 L/min, depending on cannula size. In general, larger flows are not necessary unless the patient has a very high CO (as seen in septic shock) or increased oxygen consumption (eg, fever). Oxygen delivery is also dependent on hemoglobin concentration, and most ECLS centers aim to keep Hgb at 7 to 8 g/dL or greater.

Extracorporeal life support flow is titrated to maintain an arterial oxyhemoglobin saturation of greater than 90% for VA ECLS or greater than 80% to 85% for VV ECLS.

Physiology of Venovenous Extracorporeal Life Support

In VV ECLS, the infused blood travels via the right atrium and right ventricle (RV) into the pulmonary circulation. The infused highly oxygenated blood from the ECLS circuit is diluted by the deoxygenated blood returning to the right side of the heart; the ratio of circuit flow to native CO is therefore an important determinant of systemic oxygenation. Because of this ever-present mixing of oxygenated and deoxygenated blood in the RV (shunt physiology), oxygen saturations are typically low in VV ECLS (goal > 80%). Assuming a lack of gas exchange across the native lung, systemic Pao_2 is equal to mixed venous Pao_2 in the pulmonary artery (PA). A return of native lung gas exchange is indicated by widened gradient between the arterial and central venous saturations. Because blood is both drained and infused on the right side of the heart, there is no hemodynamic effect of VV ECLS.

Physiology of Venoarterial Extracorporeal Life Support

The circuit augments both cardiac and pulmonary function in VA ECLS. The highly oxygenated infused blood returns to the systemic circulation, bypassing the pulmonary circulation. Depending on the nature of the disease process requiring VA ECLS, there may remain some native left ventricle (LV) CO. If lung function is normal, the oxygen content of blood leaving the LV is sufficient. However, if there is lung disease, blood leaving the LV will be relatively deoxygenated compared with blood infusing via the ECLS circuit. The location in the aorta where these two circulations meet (ie, the mixing point or watershed) varies among patients, depending on LV function and ECLS circuit flow. For this reason, measuring oxygenation in the right hand is typically performed (when the return cannula is in the femoral artery) as a surrogate to the oxygenation of the heart, coronary arteries, and brain given that the brachiocephalic and right subclavian arteries are closest to the heart. If the right hand displays insufficient oxygenation in the setting of lung disease, then the mixing point is distal to the brachiocephalic artery, and these vital organs (heart and brain) may be receiving insufficient oxygenation. The location of the mixing point will differ if the return cannula is not in the femoral artery; the concept of the mixing point should be considered in every patient receiving VA ECLS, depending on cannula location, lung function, and native CO. The adequacy of VA ECLS flow can be measured via markers of systemic oxygenation (lactic acid) or mixed venous saturation.[17]

Ventilation During Extracorporeal Life Support

Carbon dioxide removal depends on the blood flow rate and sweep gas (ventilating gas) entering the oxygenator. Typically, the sweep gas consists of 100% O_2 that flows at an equal rate to circuit blood flow rate (1:1). Alternatively, a carbogen (a mixture of 95% O_2 and 5% CO_2) can be used. CO_2 has a much higher diffusion capacity than O_2, and thus CO_2 removal is always more efficient than oxygenation during ECLS. Increasing the sweep gas rate enhances CO_2 removal without affecting oxygenation.[18]

Anticoagulation in Extracorporeal Life Support

Anticoagulation is an essential aspect of ECLS management because the circuit is a foreign substance and, despite improvements in polymer technology, continues to promote clot formation when fibrinogen and platelets adhere to its surface. The ideal anticoagulant would prevent clot formation in the circuit yet have minimal bleeding risk in native blood vessels. Also, the ideal anticoagulant should be easily titrated, monitored, and reversed. The ideal anticoagulant in ECLS does not yet exist and, consequently, there is much variability among ECLS centers in anticoagulation practices.

Unfractionated heparin (UFH) is the most widely used systemic anticoagulant in ECLS. There is no consensus on the best coagulation assay to monitor UFH activity, and possible options include activated partial thromboplastin time, activated clotting time, or anti-Xa activity (Table 33-2).

Clot-bound thrombin is relatively immune from the effects of heparin because the antithrombin site is occupied. Unlike heparin, bivalirudin, a direct thrombin inhibitor, binds directly to thrombin without a cofactor and therefore can inhibit both soluble and fibrin-bound thrombin. Bivalirudin has a short half-life of approximately 25 minutes and predictable pharmacokinetics and is not associated with heparin-induced thrombocytopenia (HIT). For these reasons, some ECLS centers use bivalirudin as the first-line anticoagulant agent.[19-22]

HEMODYNAMIC AND VENTILATOR IMPLICATIONS OF EXTRACORPOREAL LIFE SUPPORT

Hemodynamic Considerations in Extracorporeal Life Support

The hemodynamics are distinct for VV ECLS and VA ECLS. Specifically, in VV ECLS, there is no systemic hemodynamic contribution as blood is drained from and returned to the venous circulation. In contradistinction, in VA ECLS, blood is drained from the venous circulation but returned to the systemic circulation, bypassing the heart; the ECLS flow substitutes for native CO.

Several factors impact the blood flow in an ECLS circuit, including the cannulas, the pump, and native cardiac function. Most important, blood flow through a circuit is dependent on the size of the draining cannula. Based on Poiseuille law, blood flow through an ECLS circuit is highest when the drainage cannula has a short length and a large internal diameter. Furthermore, blood flow through the ECLS circuit is accomplished via a pump (most commonly a centrifugal pump) that provides the pressure needed to drain the venous blood and return blood back into the patient. The circuit pressure is always negative before the pump and positive after the pump. The centrifugal pump is preload dependent and afterload sensitive. Therefore, preload factors, such as hypovolemia, increased intrathoracic pressure (eg, tension pneumothorax), or cardiac tamponade, and afterload factors, such as kinks in the circuit or cannula or elevated systemic vascular resistance, cause reductions in the circuit blood flow for a

TABLE 33-2 Summary of Common Anticoagulation Assays in Extracorporeal Life Support

Assay	Pros	Cons
ACT (target of 180–220 sec)	Decades of experience Inexpensive Available in most centers	Sensitivity is affected by: • Hypofibrinogenemia • Anemia • Thrombocytopenia • Other coagulation factor deficiency • Hypothermia • Hemodilution
Anti-Xa level (0.3-0.7 IU/mL)	Superior correlation with UFH dose Not affected by coagulopathy, thrombocytopenia, or dilution	Interlaboratory variability False low levels with: • Dyslipidemia • Hyperbilirubinemia • Hemolysis
APTT (target of 40–50 sec)	Widely available as a laboratory test as well as POC	Unreliable with high heparin levels Sensitive to hemodilution

ACT = activated clotting time; APTT = activated partial thromboplastin time; POC = point of care; UFH = unfractionated heparin.

given pump speed (measured in rotations per minute [RPM]). The RPM of the pump can be adjusted, within certain limitations, to control circuit flow.[23]

One of the nonphysiologic factors of centrifugal pump function in severe LV failure is the generation of a continuous, nonpulsatile flow pattern. This differs from the pulsatile flow associated with the native CO or in cases of RV failure with preserved LV contractility. Physiologically, there is thought to be no difference between pulsatile and nonpulsatile flow, although with the nonpulsatile flow in VA ECLS, the usual arterial waveforms, with distinct systolic and diastolic blood pressures, are absent and are replaced by a continuous flow with minimal variation. In VA ECLS, the presence of pulsatile flow in the arterial waveform can be used to monitor the extent or recovery of native CO.

Left ventricular contractility plays an essential role in VA ECLS hemodynamics. When the native LV function is impaired, the LV may become overdistended in VA ECLS and impair LV recovery. Overdistension of the LV occurs from residual blood return to the LA and LV combined with an inability to empty against the afterload generated by VA ECLS. The lack of LV afterload reduction is an important physiologic principle of VA ELCS, one that distinguishes VA ECLS from other mechanical cardiac support modalities such as intraaortic balloon pumps or Impella devices, which augment CO while reducing LV afterload. Overdistension of the LV in VA ECLS results in both subendocardial ischemia from increasing myocardial oxygen demand and pulmonary edema. To avoid this potential negative consequence of VA ECLS, circuit flow can be reduced, or arterial vasodilators can be used to reduce LV afterload. Alternatively, the LV can be vented by invasive procedures such as thoracotomy with placement of a cannula to the left ventricle or using an Impella device in combination with VA ECLS.[24]

In a VV ECLS, blood is drained and returned at the same rate with minimal hemodynamic effect. However, with the reduction of ventilator settings and positive intrathoracic pressures with the initiation of the VV ECLS, there are an increase in the RV preload and a decrease in RV afterload, both of which can improve RV function.

Ventilator Management in Extracorporeal Life Support

In patients on VV ECLS, ventilator settings should be reduced to minimal levels to provide rest to the lungs. In distinction, patients on VA ECLS require traditional ventilator settings to ensure adequate oxygenation of blood leaving the LV (see the earlier discussion of mixing point discussion). Although there is no preferred ventilator mode in ECLS, a pressure-breath, assist-control mode is the most common (and is based on the CESAR trial). Common ventilator settings in VV ECLS include a positive end-expiratory pressure (PEEP) of 10 to 15 cm H_2O and a driving pressure of 10 cm H_2O to maintain a plateau inspiratory pressure of 25 cm H_2O or less. This may result in very low tidal volumes, sometimes lower than 4 mL/kg predicted body weight (PBW). The low tidal volume

with high PEEP combination is to minimize lung injury yet avoid alveolar collapse. The fraction of inspired oxygenation is kept low, usually at 30%. The respiratory rate is set at 5 to 10 breaths/min with prolonged inspiratory times, commonly using an inverse inspiratory:expiratory (I:E) ratio.[18,25]

SEDATION AND ANALGESIA

Analgesia and sedation are integral parts of the management of any critically ill patient, including ECLS patients. However, it is necessary to understand that the dosing and distribution of medications are altered in ECLS. In particular, the changes in the volume of distribution and the potential binding to the circuit impact the effect various medications in ECLS.

Understanding Altered Pharmacology in Extracorporeal Life Support

Although critical illness itself can impact drug pharmacokinetics, ECLS adds additional complexity to drug selection and dosing. The ECLS system increases circulating blood volume and volume of distribution, affecting pharmacokinetics.[26] Other factors contributing to the alteration in pharmacokinetics in ECLS include properties inherent to the drug, including lipophilicity and protein binding, and properties of the circuit. Drug adsorption to the circuit is increased for lipophilic drugs, such as midazolam and fentanyl. Because of altered pharmacokinetics, such medications require larger doses to achieve effects like those before induction of ECLS (Fig. 33-4).[27-29]

Analgesia and Sedation in Extracorporeal Life Support Patients

Pain is common in intensive care unit (ICU) patients and is often associated with an increase in metabolic demand, agitation, and delirium. ECLS patients, like all ICU patients, can have

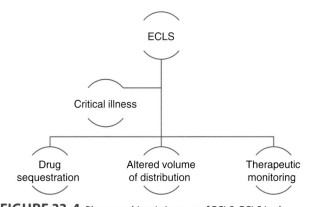

FIGURE 33-4 Pharmacokinetic impact of ECLS. ECLS in the context of critical illness (and associated organ dysfunction) has multiple impacts on drug pharmacokinetics, including sequestration in the ECLS circuit and increased volumes of distribution. Therapeutic monitoring of drug concentrations is only available for certain medications (eg, vancomycin). For many drugs, measuring levels is not practically available.

pain from prolonged bed rest and immobilization, devices, or procedures. A vital part of pain management includes assessment of pain using validated pain scales and scoring systems. After analgesia is addressed, some patients require sedatives to promote ventilator synchrony and treatment of agitation. Apart from the traditional uses of sedatives, sedation in ECLS patients helps to prevent accidental catheter decannulation.

Drugs commonly used for analgesia and sedation in the ICU include opiates, benzodiazepines, propofol, and dexmedetomidine.

Opiates are the preferred analgesics in ECLS. Among the opioids, fentanyl, morphine, and hydromorphone are commonly used drugs. Fentanyl is highly lipophilic and protein bound, and hence the levels are remarkably reduced in ECLS, requiring higher doses than typical. In contrast, morphine is hydrophilic and is less absorbed by the circuit and produces analgesia at lower doses.[28-30] However, many patients receiving ECLS commonly have associated renal dysfunction. Morphine's effect is exerted through its active metabolite, morphine-6-glucuronide, which is renally excreted and which may accumulate in ECLS patients who have kidney dysfunction. Hydromorphone is a semisynthetic opiate that has not been as well studied in ECLS. Hydromorphone has intermediate lipophilicity and has been increasingly used for analgesia and sedation in ECLS patients. In addition, ketamine, an N-methyl-D-aspartate (NMDA) antagonist with both analgesic and sedative properties, has also been used in ECLS patients.[31-33]

Among sedative medications, benzodiazepines, including lorazepam and midazolam, are commonly used in ECLS. Both lorazepam and midazolam are highly lipophilic and hence are sequestered by the circuit, leading to higher dosage requirements for sedation. The clearance of midazolam increases rapidly, and only 25% of the initial concentration has been noticed in the circuit 24 hours after the patient was placed on ECLS.

Propofol is an anesthetic and sedative agent that is highly lipophilic and hence rapidly bound by the ECLS circuit. Studies have shown that 70% of the baseline concentration of propofol is lost within the first 30 minutes of introduction into the circuit, 90% is lost by 5 hours, and only a negligible fraction is present at the end of 24 hours (Fig. 33-5). In addition, because of its lipophilicity, propofol has the potential to occlude the oxygenator. For these reasons, propofol is generally avoided in ECLS patients.[34]

Dexmedetomidine is an α_2-agonist similar in activity to clonidine, which has been used as an anxiolytic medication in ICU patients as an alternative to benzodiazepines and propofol. Small studies suggest that dexmedetomidine is effective in ECLS and facilitates sedation and weaning from ECLS.[35]

EXTRACORPOREAL LIFE SUPPORT PROBLEM SOLVING AND COMPLICATIONS

Extracorporeal life support involves several complex machines that interface with human physiology; understanding how to troubleshoot is essential knowledge for those who manage ECLS patients. Some of the common problems that arise in ECLS are described next.

Chattering

"Chattering" is a commonly seen complication with ECLS circuits and can happen any time the pump is running. Pump "chatter" or "rattling" is a low-frequency swaying movement of the drainage cannula caused by hypovolemia or other causes of reduced preload (eg, decreased venous return from tension pneumothorax) and is rarely caused by malposition of the cannula. In the setting of hypovolemia or cannula malposition, there is an imbalance between the circuit volume and negative pressure generated by the centrifugal pump, leading to the "chatter." If these excessive negative pressures are maintained, chattering can be associated with cavitation and hemolysis. Chattering can be managed either by turning down the pump RPMs or by giving back volume. More serious causes of chattering, such as pneumothorax, tamponade, or circuit occlusion by a clot, should always be considered.[36]

Recirculation

Recirculation is one of the factors that determines systemic oxygenation, along with pump flow and CO, in VV ECLS. Recirculation (R) is defined as the fraction of the oxygenated blood that exits the infusion cannula that is subsequently and immediately returned to the ECLS circuit via the drainage cannula, bypassing the patient's circulation. Effective flow (EF) in liters per minute is the actual flow of oxygenated blood that gets delivered into the patient's circulation. Effective flow is calculated from the formula:

$$EF = (1 - R)\,PF$$

where R is fraction of pump flow that is recirculated and PF is the pump flow.

Therefore, as recirculation increases, EF decreases. Systemic oxygen saturation is directly proportional to the EF and inversely proportional to the recirculation. Although increasing pump flow can improve EF in the presence of recirculation, at some level of PF, recirculation tends to increase, mitigating any impact on oxygenation of increasing pump flow. Recirculation can be diagnosed by measuring the oxygen saturation of the arterial blood (Sao$_2$) and the drainage cannula blood (Sdo$_2$). The cardinal sign of recirculation is the presence of low Sao$_2$ in the setting of high Sdo$_2$. Another means by which to assess for recirculation is to measure preoxygenator blood oxygen saturation (PreoxSO$_2$); if this is greater than 80%, there is likely recirculation. TEE can be done to confirm and reposition catheter position if recirculation is present.[37]

North–South Syndrome

The north–south (or Harlequin) syndrome can be seen in VA ECLS patients when LV contractility is present but lung function is poor. In such conditions, the blood ejected from the

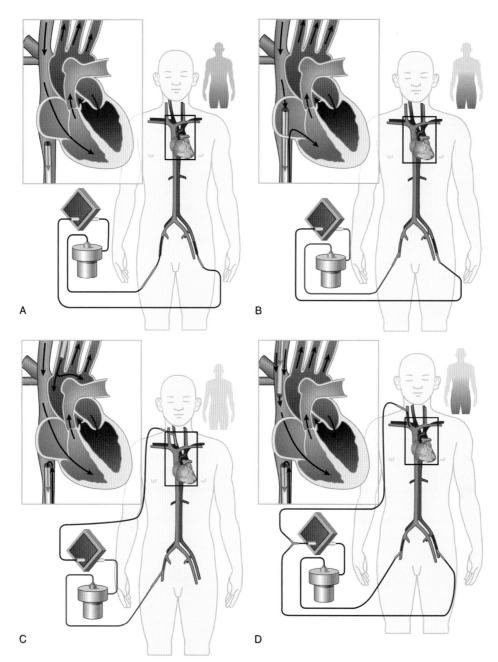

FIGURE 33-5 (A) Deoxygenated blood from a diseased lung returns to the left ventricle and preferentially supplies the upper part of the body (north) after it pushes the mixing point distally, leading to cyanosis. On the other hand, the lower part of the body (south) receives a highly oxygenated blood via the femoral artery return cannula. Deoxygenated blood returning to the SVC will not pass through the oxygenator if the drainage cannula ends in the IVC, perpetuating the differential cyanosis. In (B), the drainage cannula is pushed toward the SVC which allows the poorly oxygenated blood to pass through the oxygenator while allowing more oxygenated blood from the lower half of the body to enter the right ventricle; this mitigates the differential cyanosis (north–south syndrome). (C) and (D) depict different cannulation arrangement which eliminate the North–South syndrome by placing the return cannula(s) in the carotid artery and the RIJ vein, respectively. (Source: Hou X, Yang X, Du Z, et al. Superior vena cava drainage improves upper body oxygenation during veno-arterial extracorporeal membrane oxygenation in sheep. *Crit Care.* 2015;19:68.)

LV is deoxygenated and pushes the mixing point, the point at which the native CO pressure equals the pressure of VA ECLS infusion, distal to the great vessels of the aortic arch. Under these circumstances, the brain, heart, and upper extremities will be perfused with deoxygenated blood and appear blue.

At the same time, the trunk and lower extremities, perfused by VA ECLS, will appear pink (Fig. 33-5). A two-circulation scenario can exacerbate this situation if blood is drained only from the IVC. Blood from the lower half of the body, well oxygenated, returns via the IVC drainage cannula and ECLS circuit to be reoxygenated. Conversely, blood entering the SVC from the upper half of the body, already severely deoxygenated from the aforementioned distal mixing point, now preferentially enters the pulmonary circulation and returns to the LV and again bypasses the ECLS circuit (see Fig. 33-5). As discussed previously, the best way to measure cerebral and coronary oxygenation in VA ECLS with femoral arterial return cannula is by measurement of arterial blood gas (ABG) from the right radial artery. Management of north–south syndrome includes improving lung function or increasing VA ECLS flow, although the latter approach will increase LV afterload. Alternative solutions include changing the placement of the arterial return cannula (right subclavian artery) or by diverting some of the oxygenated blood from the ECLS circuit into a second return cannula placed in the RIJ vein (VAV ECLS configuration). This will result in some oxygenated blood traversing the pulmonary circulation and leaving the LV.[23,38]

Bleeding

Bleeding is one of the more common complications in ECLS, affecting 6% to 33% of patients and associated with a high rate of morbidity and mortality. Major bleeding, defined by a decrement of 2 g/dL or greater in a 24-hour period, can be caused by hemorrhage in the retroperitoneal space or lungs. Central nervous system hemorrhage is another potentially fatal complication associated with ECLS.[20] Minor bleeding is typically associated with cannula sites.[39] The causes of bleeding in ECLS patients are multifactorial and include the use of anticoagulation, coagulation factor consumption caused by both severe illness and the ECLS circuit, increased fibrinolysis, and thrombocytopenia.[40] Although there are no strict transfusion thresholds in ECLS and the risks of blood product transfusion must always be balanced against the benefits, most centers maintain platelets at 100,000/mm³ or greater and fibrinogen levels at 150 mg/dL or greater. Likewise, although Hgb is essential for systemic oxygenation delivery, most centers are tending toward more restrictive Hgb thresholds of 7 to 8 g/dL, absent signals of ischemia.

Thrombosis

Thrombosis, like bleeding, is another serious complication seen in ECLS patients. The incidence of thromboembolic complications is often underestimated because of the subclinical or occult presentation and by the lack of autopsy results. However, a recent ELSO report suggests that the rate of clot identification within the circuits is about 20%.[38] Risk factors for thrombus formation include activation of coagulation pathway and complement-mediated inflammatory response, stasis of blood within the circuit, and HIT. The incidence of deep vein thrombosis (DVT) has been estimated to be 8 per 1000 catheter days, and some centers routinely screen for DVT using ultrasound. Other systemic thrombotic events include cerebral infarction and bowel ischemia.[39,41] The main strategy to manage or prevent thrombosis is systemic anticoagulation (see earlier section on anticoagulation).

Hemolysis

Hemolysis occurs in ECLS from the mechanical factors associated with ECLS, including the type of pump used, pressure gradients, and the presence of turbulent flow or clots. ELSO defines hemolysis complicating ECLS as a plasma-free hemoglobin level greater than 0.5 g/L. Centrifugal pumps produce lesser hemolysis than the classic roller pumps, but hemolysis can still occur happen if the negative pressure across the centrifugal pump is very high. Similarly, high pump speed also contributes to hemolysis. If extensive clot burden is present in the circuit, hemolysis can be prevented by changing the circuit.

Accidental Decannulation

Unexpected decannulation can be a catastrophic and usually results from inadvertent tension on, or inadequate protection of, the cannula. Accidental decannulation can result in massive blood loss or air embolism, both potentially fatal events.

WEANING OFF EXTRACORPOREAL LIFE SUPPORT

Weaning or discontinuing a patient from an ECLS differs between VV and VA ECLS. The first step is determining if the patient is ready to begin weaning from ECLS:

A patient can be a considered for a VV ECLS weaning trial if the respiratory condition improves, which can be assessed by the following metrics:

- The respiratory mechanics are improving. Specifically, static compliance increases, and airway resistance decreases. This is usually associated with an improving chest radiograph.
- Gas exchange is improving. This is indicated by improving systemic oxygenation and ventilation as the lung injury resolves.

The weaning process of VV ECLS happens in parallel with the improvement of the native lung parameters. Depending on the cause of the respiratory failure, ECLS blood flow and sweep gas are adjusted as the lung function recovers. During the lung recovery process, sedative medications are reduced, and spontaneous respiration is encouraged to reduce lung atelectasis.

Weaning trials from VV ECLS are performed by simply turning down the sweep gas flow rate and placing the patient on acceptable ventilator settings, typically fraction of inspired oxygen (Fio_2) of 60% or less and PEEP of 10 to 12 cm H_2O. There is no oxygenation or ventilation via ECLS when the sweep gas is turned down. ECLS flow is typically maintained during the weaning trial to reduce the risk of clot formation (although gas exchange is not occurring). The duration of VV ECLS weaning trials differs among centers but generally lasts from 6 to 24 hours. If the patient continues to be stable and maintains gas exchange with ventilator support, she or he can be decannulated and ECLS stopped.[42]

Weaning VA ECLS must consider the following parameters:

- The LV is recovering as evidence by echocardiography and the presence of a pulsatile waveform.
- The shock state is resolving with adequate mean arterial pressure and perfusion absent significant vasopressor support.

If these conditions are met, the VA ECLS blood flow is gradually reduced by 0.5 to 1 L/min to a level of approximately 1 to 1.5 L/min. During this low-flow state, hemodynamics must remain stable, including adequate LV and RV function and minimal increases in central venous pressure and pulmonary capillary wedge pressure (if a right heart catheter is present). Alternatively, measures of systemic perfusion can be assessed, such as lactate or $Scvo_2$. If these measures show adequate perfusion, the patient can be decannulated and ECLS stopped.[43]

CLINICAL EVIDENCE FOR EXTRACORPOREAL LIFE SUPPORT

The evolution of early adult ECLS was described earlier. Adult ECLS has seen a resurgence since the publication of the CESAR trial in 2009. In the CESAR trial, patients with ARDS were randomized to conventional therapy or transfer to an ARDS center capable of ECLS support. This study demonstrated significant survival benefit at 6 months (63% vs 47%).[6] During the same period, an observational study conducted in Australia and New Zealand during the H1N1 pandemic of 2009 reported a mortality rate of 21% in patients undergoing ECMO, much lower than expected in patients with severe ARDS.[7]

More recently, a study of the ELSO patient registry of patients with ARDS treated with ECLS between 1986 and 2006 reported a mortality rate of 50%, similar to other ECMO studies.[44] These survival outcomes correlate with the ELSO registry outcome for adult respiratory failure requiring ECLS in which 66% survive ECLS and 57% survive to discharge. Although these studies suggest that ECLS improves outcomes, there has not been a robust study comparing ECLS with best ARDS care, including prone ventilation. The EOLIA (ECMO to rescue Lung Injury in severe ARDS) trial compares the role of early ECLS with protocolized mechanical ventilation setting, including low tidal volume ventilation with prone positioning. The EOLIA study, which is ongoing, will hopefully answer the question of whether VV ECLS improves outcomes in ARDS compared with best current care.

ETHICAL ISSUES ASSOCIATED WITH EXTRACORPOREAL LIFE SUPPORT

Extracorporeal life support has been successfully used in the management of severe cardiopulmonary failure until the patient shows signs of recovery or ECLS can be used as a bridge to destination therapy in appropriate candidates, either transplant or a ventricular assist device. However, ECLS is not a treatment per se for any condition but is only a supportive measure. Therefore, it is incumbent on ECLS physicians to assess the potential for recovery or destination therapy in all potential ECLS patients and to communicate clearly with patients and families before initiating ECLS that, absent recovery or destination therapy, ECLS may need to be eventually withdrawn. Informed consent in ECLS situations is essential, and the patient and family members should be provided with detailed risks associated with the ECLS procedure and potential complications and outcomes.

Extracorporeal life support therapy should generally be offered as a "time-limited trial" because the longer the duration of ECLS, the lower the survival rate. The patient and family must be made aware that the likelihood of ECLS success will be periodically evaluated and that the management can turn futile. This can help families prepare themselves emotionally if their loved one's survival chances are low. A palliative medicine team, if available, can help guide the patient and family through these difficult scenarios.

QUESTIONS

1. A 35-year-old man with ARDS and severe refractory hypoxia was placed on VV ECLS 1 hour ago. While on conventional mechanical ventilation, his Pao_2 was 59 mmHg, with an Sao_2 of 70% despite protective ventilation strategy and a 100% Fio_2.

   The patient weighs 95 kg, his blood pressure is 110/83 mmHg, and his Hgb is 11 g/dL. He now has a right common femoral drainage cannula and an RIJ infusion cannula. The ECLS flow rate is 60 mL/kg/min with a corresponding centrifugal pump speed of 3200 RPM. The inlet (drainage) Sao_2 is 80%, and the outlet (return) Sao_2 is 84%. The flow rate is increased to 70 mL/kg/min, corresponding to a pump speed of 3500 RPM, with no change in oxygenation. What is the best next step?

   A. Increase the flow rate to 80 mL/kg/min.
   B. Transfuse 1 unit of packed red blood cells.
   C. Obtain TEE to assess the infusion cannula flow pattern.
   D. Continue the current ELCS settings.

2. You are called to evaluate a 34-year-old woman for ECLS initiation. She was admitted to the ICU 7 days ago after a high-speed motor vehicle accident. She was intubated in the field for a Glasgow Coma Scale score of 4. The computed tomography (CT) scan of the head showed frontal lobe edema and subarachnoid hemorrhage. She was diagnosed with aspiration pneumonia on day 2 and was started on broad-spectrum antibiotics. Over the course of the next 5 days, she had persistent and worsening hypoxia despite

multiple ventilator adjustments, paralysis, and prone positioning. She is receiving 8 μg/kg/min of norepinephrine and broad-spectrum antibiotics and has been off sedation and paralytic medications for multiple hours. Her complete blood count, basic metabolic profile, and liver function tests are unremarkable except for a white blood cell count of 18×10^3 K/μL. On physical examination, her heart rate is 110 beats/min, blood pressure is 97/55 mmHg, and Spo_2 is 85% on 6 mL/kg predicted body weight tidal volume, 80% Fio_2, and 10 cm H_2O of PEEP. She has coarse breaths sounds with diffuse rhonchi. She does not open her eyes and extends all extremities to pain. What is the best next step?

A. Initiate VA ECLS now.
B. Initiate VV ECLS now.
C. Continue the protective ventilation strategy.
D. Continue antibiotics for another day, repeat the CT scan of the head, and initiate ECLS in the next 48 hours.

3. A 45-year-old active smoker is brought to emergency department (ED) after several days of flulike symptoms. He is in respiratory distress and requires urgent intubation and mechanical ventilation. He is diagnosed with influenza A. An early arterial blood gas analysis shows returns with the following values on PEEP 10 and FiO 100% 7.26/58/70. A chest radiograph shows diffuse airspace disease without pleural effusions. A bedside transthoracic echocardiogram shows preserved LV function, and the patient is not requiring vasopressor support. Despite optimization of his ventilator settings and paralysis, his oxygenation continues to worsen. He is placed on VV ECLS for severe ARDS with a dual-lumen 31-Fr catheter in his RIJ vein. After he is placed on VV ECLS, what are the preferred ventilator settings?

A. Pressure breath, AC mode, Vt 6 mL/kg PBW, PEEP 5, Fio_2 80%, RR 24, PPlat goal less than 35 cm H_2O
B. Pressure breath, AC mode, Vt 8 mL/kg PBW, PEEP 10, Fio_2 60%, RR 10, PPlat goal less than 30 cm H_2O
C. Pressure breath, AC mode, Vt 4 mL/kg PBW, PEEP 10, Fio_2 40%, RR 10, PPlat goal less than 25 cm H_2O
D. Pressure breath, AC mode, Vt 4 mL/kg PBW, PEEP 20, FiO_2 60%, RR 24, PPlat goal less than 30 cm H_2O

4. A 60-year-old man with type 1 diabetes is brought to the ED after a witnessed cardiac arrest requiring defibrillations and cardiopulmonary resuscitation for 45 minutes. After the return of circulation, he is diagnosed with anterior wall ST-segment elevation myocardial infarction, and an emergent left anterior descending coronary artery stent is placed. He is found to have an ejection fraction of 10% and is in cardiogenic shock. A chest radiograph shows diffuse pulmonary edema. An intravascular microaxial blood pump placement (Impella) fails, and the patient is placed on VA ECLS support with a 21-Fr venous drainage cannula in the left internal jugular vein and 17-Fr arterial cannula in the left femoral artery. Over the next several hours, the patient has increased

cyanosis of his upper extremities and head despite adjustments to the ventilator and ECLS pump. An ABG obtained from the right radial arterial line reveals a Pao_2 of 50 mmHg. What is the most likely diagnosis?

A. North–south syndrome
B. Acute limb ischemia
C. HIT syndrome
D. Compartment syndrome

5. A 25-year old man is on day 5 of VV ECLS for severe ARDS secondary to adenovirus-induced pneumonia. He is hemodynamically stable and is maintaining systemic oxygen saturation consistently above 92%. He is being diuresed to maintain euvolemia, and in the past 48 hours, and he is net negative 2 Liters. Over the past few hours, there was "chattering" in the drainage limb, and his ECLS circuit flow has dropped to 3 L/min despite increasing the pump speed to 4000 RPM. In addition, his blood gas oxygen has been between 85% to 88%. What is the most likely cause for the fall in pump flow in the above scenario?

A. Fever
B. Recirculation
C. Hypovolemia
D. Membrane oxygenator obstruction

ANSWERS

1. C. Obtain TEE to assess the infusion cannula flow pattern.

   The high-inlet (drainage) Sao_2 indicates the presence of recirculation. Increasing the flow to 80 mL/kg/min will increase recirculation and reduce effective flow and hence systemic oxygenation (choice A). Although increasing the Hgb can increase the oxygen content and Do_2, the patient's current Hgb is satisfactory (choice B). Continuing the same ECLS settings will not resolve recirculation (choice D). Recirculation is a phenomenon that occurs in VV ECMO, especially with two-site cannulation in which the returning jet is close to the inlet (drainage) cannula. Thus, obtaining TEE to assess the infusion cannula flow pattern (choice C) will confirm the diagnosis and allows cannula(s) repositioning. The use of a double-lumen cannula can reduce the risk of recirculation.

2. C. Continue the protective ventilation strategy.

   Although this patient is young, she is not a good candidate for ECLS (choices A, B, and D). She has evidence of traumatic brain injury with no signs of neurologic recovery, and she is at risk of worsening subarachnoid hemorrhage after systemic anticoagulation initiation. In this case, continuing protective lung ventilation is appropriate (choice C). Initiating ECLS 7 days after the onset of ARDS and mechanical ventilation is a relative contraindication.

3. C. Pressure breath, AC mode, Vt 4 mL/kg PBW, PEEP 10, Fio$_2$ 40%, RR 10, PPlat goal less than 25 cm H$_2$O

   During the initiation of VV ECLS, it is preferred to keep the ventilator in rest mode to give time for the lungs to recover. Although some debate exists about the ideal settings, most ECLS centers use low tidal volumes of approximately 4 mL/kg PBW, PEEP of 10 to 15 cm H$_2$O, a lower respiratory rate with prolonged inspiratory time, and a goal PPlat of 20 to 25 cm H$_2$O. Oxygen is likewise kept to a minimum concentration. Hence, choice C is the best choice. To prevent complete lung atelectasis, a moderate amount of PEEP is maintained, typically 10 to 15 cm H$_2$O, and thus choice A is incorrect. The tidal volume set is as per the ARDSnet protocol, and in patients on VV ECLS, lower tidal volumes (less than 6 mL/Kg PBW) are preferred to reduce volutrauma, so choice B is incorrect. The goal PPlat is less than 25 cm H$_2$O, so choice D is incorrect.

4. A. North–south syndrome

   North–south syndrome (or Harlequin syndrome) is a two-circulation consequence of VA ECLS, particularly in the setting of lung injury and some degree of residual LV function. As described in the text, the result is a mixing point between deoxygenated blood via native CO and highly oxygenated blood from the ECLS circuit. As the mixing point between these two circulations moves farther away from the aortic valve (because of improving LV function or decreased ECLS flow), deoxygenated blood will reach the great vessels of the aortic arch, including the brachiocephalic artery and carotid arteries, leading to cardiac and cerebral hypoxia and upper extremity cyanosis. The right radial artery is the most easily accessed proximal point at which to detect a mixing point. Acute limb ischemia is a documented complication arising from the cannulations, but the timing and relation to the ABG from the right radial arterial line are more consistent with the north–south syndrome (choice B). HIT syndrome is less likely because there is no documentation of thrombocytopenia or necrotic skin changes, the onset over several hours is not typical, and the differential cyanosis is not expected (choice C). Compartment syndrome usually arises secondary to acute limb ischemia in VA ECLS patients, but there is no mention of the signs or symptoms in the case scenario (choice D).

5. C. Hypovolemia

   The most common cause of a fall in pump flow is hypovolemia. Other possible causes are kinking of the drainage cannula or obstruction of the circuit or oxygenator by thrombus. A fall in the circuit flow secondary to hypovolemia can cause a phenomenon called chattering in which the ECLS cannulas produce vibratory swaying motion because of the development of higher negative pressure within the drainage cannula. Additional causes of relative hypovolemia that may contribute to decreasing ECLS flows and chattering include hemorrhage, tension pneumothorax or pericardial effusion (decreased venous return), or the development of distributive shock, as associated with sepsis. Because this patient is hemodynamically stable and is being diuresed, hypovolemia is the most likely explanation (choice C), although the other more serious causes described should be considered as well. His systemic oxygenation will decrease as the ratio of ECLS pump flow to native CO is reduced. Fever will increase metabolic demand and native CO, both of which will decrease systemic oxygenation. However, fever is not typically associated with decreased pump flows (choice A). Recirculation can cause increase arterial hypoxemia, although it is not usually associated with decreasing flows and chattering (choice B). Membrane oxygenator obstruction can cause oxygen desaturation, but chattering is not typical (choice D).

REFERENCES

1. Bartlett RH. John H Gibbon Jr Lecture. Extracorporeal life support: Gibbon fulfilled. *J Am Coll Surg.* 2014;218:317-327.

2. Kammermeyer K. Silicone rubber as a selective barrier. *Ind Eng Chem.* 1957;49(10):1685-1686.

3. Hill JD, O'Brien TG, Murray JJ, et al. Prolonged extracorporeal oxygenation for acute post-traumatic respiratory failure (shock-lung syndrome). Use of the Bramson membrane lung. *N Engl J Med.* 1972;286:629-634.

4. Zapol WM, Snider MT, Hill JD, et al. Extracorporeal membrane oxygenation in severe acute respiratory failure. A randomized prospective study. *JAMA.* 1979;242:2193-2196.

5. Morris AH, Wallace CJ, Menlove RL, et al. Randomized clinical trial of pressure-controlled inverse ratio ventilation and extracorporeal CO$_2$ removal for adult respiratory distress syndrome. *Am J Respir Crit Care Med.* 1994;149:295-305.

6. Peek GJ, Mugford M, Tiruvoipati R, et al. Efficacy and economic assessment of conventional ventilatory support versus extracorporeal membrane oxygenation for severe adult respiratory failure (CESAR): a multicentre randomised controlled trial. *Lancet.* 2009;374:1351-1363.

7. Australia and New Zealand Extracorporeal Membrane Oxygenation (ANZ ECMO) Influenza Investigators, Davies A, Jones D, et al. Extracorporeal Membrane Oxygenation for 2009 Influenza A(H1N1) Acute Respiratory Distress Syndrome. *JAMA.* 2009;302:1888-1895.

8. In: Farcy DA, Chiu WC, Marshall JP, Osborn TM, eds. *Critical Care Emergency Medicine.* 2nd ed. New York: McGraw Hill Professional; 2016.

9. Motomura T, Maeda T, Kawahito S, et al. Development of silicone rubber hollow fiber membrane oxygenator for ECMO. *Artif Organs.* 2003;27:1050-1053.

10. Peter Papadakos BL. Extracorporeal membrane oxygenator (ECMO) in pediatric and neonatal patients, heat exchanger. In: Houmes R-J, Gischler S, Tibboel E, eds. *Mechanical Ventilation: Clinical Applications and Pathophysiology.* 1st ed. St. Louis: Saunders Elsevier; 2008: 563.

11. In: Hess DR, Kacmarek RM, eds. *Essentials of Mechanical Ventilation.* 3rd ed. New York: McGraw Hill Education; 2014.

12. Lequier L, Horton SB, McMullan DM, Bartlett RH. Extracorporeal membrane oxygenation circuitry. *Pediatr Crit Care Med.* 2013;5(Suppl 1):S7-S12.

13. Montoya JP, Merz SI, Bartlett RH. A standardized system for describing flow/pressure relationships in vascular access devices. *ASAIO Trans.* 1991;37:4-8.

14. Guillermo Martinez, Alain Vuylsteke. Extracorporeal membrane oxygenation in adults. *Contin Education Anaesthes Critical Care Pain.* 2012;12(2):57-61.

15. Schmidt M, Bailey M, Sheldrake J, et al. Predicting survival after extracorporeal membrane oxygenation for severe acute respiratory failure. The Respiratory Extracorporeal Membrane Oxygenation Survival Prediction (RESP) score. *Am J Respir Crit Care Med.* 2014;189:1374-1382.

16. Schmidt M, Burrell A, Roberts L, et al. Predicting survival after ECMO for refractory cardiogenic shock: the survival after veno-arterial-ECMO (SAVE)-score. *Eur Heart J.* 2015;36:2246-2256.

17. Bartlett RH. Physiology of extracorporeal life support. In: Zwischenberger JB, Toomasian JM, Drake K, et al, eds. *ECMO: Extracorporeal Cardiopulmonary Support in Critical Care.* 2nd ed. Extracorporeal Life Support Organization; 2000: 41-66.

18. Annich GM, Lynch WR, MacLAren G, Wilson JM, Bartlett RH. *ECMO Extracorporeal Cardiopulmonary Support in Critical Care (The Red Book).* 4th ed. University of Washington Press.

19. Extracorporeal Life Support Organization. ELSO Anticoagulation Guideline. https://www.elso.org/resources/guidelines.aspx.

20. Koster A, Weng Y, Böttcher W, et al. Successful use of bivalirudin as anticoagulant for ECMO in a patient with acute HIT. *Ann Thorac Surg.* 2007;83:1865-1867.

21. Pieri M, Agracheva N, Bonaveglio E, et al. Bivalirudin versus heparin as an anticoagulant during extracorporeal membrane oxygenation: a case-control study. *J Cardiothorac Vasc Anesth.* 2013;27:30-34.

22. Xiao Z, Theroux P. Platelet activation with unfractionated heparin at therapeutic concentrations and comparisons with a low-molecular-weight heparin and with a direct thrombin inhibitor. *Circulation.* 1998;97:251-256.

23. Chung M, Shiloh AL, Carlese A. Monitoring of the adult patient on venoarterial extracorporeal membrane oxygenation. *Sci World J.* 2014;2014:10.

24. Doufle G, Roscoe A, Billia F, Fan E. Echocardiography for adult patients supported with extracorporeal membrane oxygenation. *Crit Care.* 2015;19:326.

25. Schmidt M, Stewart C, Bailey M, et al. Mechanical ventilation management during extracorporeal membrane oxygenation for acute respiratory distress syndrome: a retrospective international multicenter study. *Crit Care Med.* 2015;43(3):654-664.

26. Buck ML. Pharmacokinetic changes during extracorporeal membrane oxygenation: implications for drug therapy of neonates. *Clin Pharmacokinet.* 2003;42(5):403-417.

27. Bhatt-Mehta V, Annich G. Sedative clearance during extracorporeal membrane oxygenation. *Perfusion.* 2005;20(6):309-315.

28. Wildschut ED, Ahsman MJ, Allegaert K, et al. Determinants of drug absorption in different ECMO circuits. *Intensive Care Med.* 2010;36(12):2109-2116.

29. Shekar K, Fraser JF, Smith MT, Roberts JA. Pharmacokinetic changes in patients receiving extracorporeal membrane oxygenation. *J Crit Care.* 2012;27(6):741.e9-e18.

30. Shekar K, Roberts JA, McDonald CI, et al. Sequestration of drugs in the circuit may lead to therapeutic failure during extracorporeal membrane oxygenation. *Crit Care.* 2012;16(5):R194.

31. Kielstein JT, Heiden AM, Beutel G, et al. Renal function and survival in 200 patients undergoing ECMO therapy. *Nephrol Dial Transplant.* 2013;28:86-90.

32. Franck LS, Vilardi J, Durand D, Powers R. Opioid withdrawal in neonates after continuous infusions of morphine or fentanyl during extracorporeal membrane oxygenation. *Am J Crit Care.* 1998;7(5):364-369.

33. Tellor B, Shin N, Graetz TJ, Avidan MS. Ketamine infusion for patients receiving extracorporeal membrane oxygenation support: a case series. *F1000Res.* 2015;4:16.

34. Lemaitre F, Hasni N, Leprince P, et al. Propofol, midazolam, vancomycin and cyclosporine therapeutic drug monitoring in extracorporeal membrane oxygenation circuits primed with whole human blood. *Crit Care.* 2015;19:40.

35. Cozzolino M, Franci A, Peris A, et al. Weaning from extracorporeal membrane oxygenation: experience with dexmedetomidine in seven adult ARDS patients. *Crit Care.* 2015;19(Suppl 1): P485.

36. Sidebotham D. Troubleshooting adult ECMO. *J Extra Corpor Technol.* 2011;43(1):P27-P32.

37. Messai E, Bouguerra A, Harmelin G, et al. A numerical model of blood oxygenation during veno-venous ECMO: analysis of the interplay between blood oxygenation and its delivery parameters. *J Clin Monit Comput.* 2016;30(3):327-332.

38. Hou X, Yang X, Du Z, et al. Superior vena cava drainage improves upper body oxygenation during veno-arterial extracorporeal membrane oxygenation in sheep. *Crit Care.* 2015;19:68.

39. Aubron C, DePuydt J, Belon F, et al. Predictive factors of bleeding events in adults undergoing extracorporeal membrane oxygenation. *Ann Intensive Care.* 2016;6(1):97.

40. Murphy DA, Hockings LE, Andrews RK, et al. Extracorporeal membrane oxygenation-hemostatic complications. *Transfus Med Rev.* 2015;29(2):90-101.

41. Cooper E, Burns J, Retter A, et al. Prevalence of venous thrombosis following venovenous extracorporeal membrane oxygenation in patients with severe respiratory failure. *Crit Care Med.* 2015;43(12):e581-e584.

42. Sangalli F, Patroniti N, Pesenti A. *ECMO—Extracorporeal Life Support in Adults.* Milan: Springer; 2014.

43. Aissaoui N, El-Banayosy A, Combes A. How to wean a patient from veno-arterial extracorporeal membrane oxygenation. *Intensive Care Med.* 2015;41(5):902-905.

44. Brogan TV, Thiagarajan RR, Rycus PT, et al. Extracorporeal membrane oxygenation in adults with severe respiratory failure: a multi-center database. *Intensive Care Med.* 2009;35(12):2105-2114.

Hypothermia and Hyperthermia

Ronaldo Collo Go, MD

INTRODUCTION

Normal body temperature changes during the course of the day and is regulated by the thermoregulatory center in the anterior hypothalamus. The normal temperature at 6 AM is 37.2°C and at 4 PM is 37.7°C. Rectal temperatures are normally higher than oral temperatures because of mouth breathing. To obtain core temperature, readings should be obtained in the esophagus or tympanic membrane. During a fever, the setpoint in the hypothalamus is shifted upward. During hyperthermia, the setpoint is unchanged, but the rest of the body overcompensates to remove heat. At the other end of the spectrum, hypothermia is defined as core temperature less than 35°C. This chapter discusses the therapeutic and pathologic implications of hypothermia and hyperthermia.

THERAPEUTIC AND PATHOLOGIC HYPOTHERMIA

Therapeutic hypothermia (TH) is part of targeted temperature management (TTM). It is currently advocated as part of the postresuscitation care that includes optimization of oxygen supplementation and blood pressure and treatment of acute coronary syndromes. The consequences of anoxia are secondary to loss of adenosine triphosphate (ATP) and glucose, loss of cellular integrity, mitochondrial damage, and loss of calcium homeostasis.[1] Increased calcium and glutamate perpetuates necrosis or apoptosis. In addition, restoration of perfusion leads to reperfusion injury caused by reactive oxygen species that further exacerbates endothelial dysfunction, vasomotor dysregulation, and edema.[2] Hypothermia reduces release of excitatory amino acids and free radicals and improves oxygen supply and demand mismatch with reduction of cerebral metabolic rate of oxygen, blood volume, and pressure.[2]

Therapeutic hypothermia is indicated for patients who received return of spontaneous circulation (ROSC) after cardiac arrest from ventricular tachycardia or ventricular fibrillation (Class I) or ROSC after cardiac arrest from nonshockable rhythm (Class IIb).[2] These patients must be comatose, which was initially defined by the Glasgow Coma Scale but has been broadened to include patients who are not answering verbal commands.[2] Contraindications include sepsis, surgery within 14 days, and bleeding diathesis.

The temperature goals have evolved but every hour of delay of initiation increases the mortality rate by 20%.[3] Therefore, it is advocated that TH is initiated within 6 hours. Initially, the temperature goal is 32°C to 34°C for 24 hours as per the 2010 guidelines.[3-5] By 2015, the guidelines suggest 32° to 36°C because one randomized control trial suggested no survival or neurologic benefit between 32° and 36°C. (Class I; Level of Evidence: B).[3-5] In 2017, The American Academy of Neurology (AAN) further stratified the recommendations. AAN recommendations are based on the following levels of evidence. Level A Recommendation is established effectiveness, ineffectiveness, or harmful and requires two Class I studies.[6] Level B Recommendation is probably effective, ineffective, or harmful and requires one or more than one Class I study or two Class II studies.[6] Level C Recommendation is possibly effective, ineffective, or harmful with at ≥ 1 Class II study or more than two Class III studies.[6] Class I study is a prospective randomized controlled clinical trial (RCT) with (a) cleared defined outcomes, (b) exclusion/inclusion criteria, (c) adequate accounts for dropouts and crossovers, and (d) relevant baseline characteristics.[6] Class II is a prospective matched group cohort study or RCT which lacks one of a-d criteria.[6] Class III are other controlled trials in a representative population.[6] Class IV are case studies, case reports, or expert opinion.[6] For comatose patients with initial rhythm of pulseless ventricular tachycardia or ventricular fibrillation, AAN favors a TH goal of 32-34°C for 24 hours (Level A) over of 36°C for 24 hours (Level B) due to better evidence.[6] 36°C is considered in high risk of bleeding, and is followed by 8 hours of rewarming to 37°C and maintenance below 37.5°C until 72 hours.[6] TH is weakly recommended for comatose patients with initial rhythm of PEA or asystole since it possibly improves neurologic outcomes and survival[6] (Level C).

Cooling is achieved via ice bags, cooling blankets, and temperature-regulated surface devices. Shivering occurs between 35° and 37°C, increases the metabolic rate, and delays achieving the temperature goal.[2] Nonpharmacologic approaches to prevent shivering include warm blankets on the face, hands, or feet. Magnesium sulfate is sometimes given to increase the shivering threshold.[7] Patients often are placed on analgesics or sedation with or without a neuromuscular blocking agent.

After ROSC is achieved, hypotension may result from vasodilation from inflammation and cardiac dysfunction. During the initiation of TH, tachycardia and hypertension are expected because of cutaneous vasoconstriction. However, after cooling is initiated, bradycardia with a prolonged PR interval is noted. Further cooling can lead to junctional rhythm, sinus bradycardia, or ventricular escape rhythms. Despite prolonged QTc, there is no higher risk of torsade de pointes.[2] If significant hemodynamic instability is the result of TH, temperature can be increased up to 35°C at a rate of 0.25°C per hour.[2] Mean arterial pressure (MAP) should be maintained at greater than 80 mmHg.

Increased insulin resistance and decreased insulin secretion can cause hyperglycemia, but administration of insulin can cause a precipitous drop in glucose level. Therefore, the glucose goal is greater than 200 mg/mL.

Hypokalemia can result inward potassium influx and diuretic effect of TH. Potassium should be kept at above 3.5 mEq/L but repletion held 4 hours before rewarming because it causes reversal of influx.

Rewarming occurs 12 to 24 hours after cooling at a rate of 0.25°C every hour until the patient is normothermic (37°C). The patient is maintained normothermic for 48 hours. Neurologic prognostication is performed at least 72 hours after ROSC in patients who have not used TH and 4.5 to 5 days after TH.[3,8]

The Hypothermia after Cardiac Arrest Study Group conducted a multicenter trial with blinded assessment of the outcome of patients with cardiac arrest after ventricular fibrillation who were randomly assigned to undergo TH (32–34°C for 24 hours) compared with normothermia showed that 55% of the hypothermia group had favorable neurologic outcome compared with 39% in the normothermic group. The mortality rate at 6 months was 41% in the hypothermic group compared with 55% in the normothermic group.[9] A randomized controlled trial by Bernard and coworkers had similar results: 49% of patients in hypothermia had a good outcome (ie, discharged home or to a rehabilitation facility) compared with 26% of patients in normothermia.[10] After adjustment for age and time from collapse to ROSC, the odds ratio of a good outcome with hypothermia compared with normothermia was 5.25 (5% confidence interval [CI], 1.47–18.76; $P = 0.011$).[10] TH is used for both out-of-hospital and in-hospital cardiac arrest. Another study by Chan and colleagues showed that in-hospital cardiac arrest in patients who had TH had lower in-hospital survival rates (27.4% vs 29.2%; relative risk [RR], 0.88; 95% CI, 0.80–0.97; risk difference, −3.6%; 95% CI, 6.3–0.9%; $P = 0.01$).[11]

PATHOLOGIC HYPOTHERMIA

Heat is lost because of radiation (55–65%), conduction and convection (15%), and respiration and evaporation, although conduction and convection are the most common causes of accidental hypothermia.[12,13] The stages of accidental hypothermia, clinical symptoms, core temperature, and treatment are shown in Table 34-1.[14]

THERAPEUTIC AND PATHOLOGIC HYPERTHERMIA

Therapeutic hyperthermia is proposed as an adjunct to radiation therapy or chemotherapy to treat malignancies such as breast and cervical cancer. The mechanisms of action of therapeutic hyperthermia are heat-induced necrosis and protein inactivation with alterations in tumor cytoskeletal and

TABLE 34-1 Hypothermia Staging and Management*

Hypothermia Stage	Core Temperature (°C)†	Management
I	32–35	Warm environment, warm sweet drinks and movement
II	28–32	Monitoring for arrhythmias, immobilization, full boy insulation, external and minimally invasive warming techniques like warm environment, chemical, electrical or forced air heating packs, warm parenteral fluids
III	24–28	Stage II management and consider Extracorporeal Membrane Oxygenation (ECMO) or Cardiopulmonary Bypass (CPB)
IV	< 24	Vital signs maybe absent there if in cardiac arrest, proceed to cardiopulmonary resuscitation and Stage III management

*Hypothermia maybe determined clinically on the basis of vital signs with the use of the Swiss staging system.

†Measurement of body core temperature is helpful but not mandatory.

CPB = cardiopulmonary bypass; ECMO = extracorporeal membrane oxygenation.

Data from Brown DJA, Brugger H, Boyd J, Paal P. Accidental hypothermia. *N Engl J Med.* 2012;15;367(20):1930-1938.

membrane structures.[15] Therapeutic hyperthermia has limited relevance in the critical care setting, so the focus will be shifted toward pathologic hyperthermia.

Malignant Hyperthermia

This is an autosomal dominant disorder secondary to a gene mutation affecting the RYR-1 channel that helps release calcium in skeletal muscle during excitation and contraction and serves a binding site for ATP, magnesium, inhaled anesthetics, and dantrolene. Disease is triggered with exposure to halothane, sevoflurane, desflurane, succinylcholine, and stress. The mutation causes excessive elevation of calcium within myocytes, leading to increased cell metabolism, heat production, lactic acidosis, and rhabdomyolysis.[16,17] Clinically, patients present with the triad of muscle rigidity, usually affecting the masseter muscles first; hyperthermia; and metabolic acidosis. This can progress to multiorgan failure. Treatment begins with external cooling devices with control of shivering. Dantrolene which reduces release of calcium is administered at 1 to 2.5 mg/kg until symptoms subside or 10 mg/kg intravenously has been given.[16] Symptoms subside within 30 minutes. To prevent recurrence, dantrolene 1 mg/kg every 4 hours for 24 hours followed by dantrolene 4 to 8 mg/d orally (PO) is given for 1 to 3 days.[16,17]

Anticholinergic Syndrome

Hyperthermia is a consequence of increased muscle activity and an inability to remove heat through sweat by the blockade of central and peripheral muscarinic acetylcholine receptors.[18,19] Medications include antispasmodics, antihistamines, tricyclic antidepressants (TCAs), antiparkinsonian medications, neuroleptics, atropine, and belladonna.[18] Central muscarinic symptoms include altered mental status, tremor, and myoclonus, and peripheral muscarinic symptoms include a lack of sweat, mydriasis, blurred vision, flushing, urinary retention, and decreased bowel sounds.[18] Treatment includes external cooling measures; benzodiazepine; and physostigmine, an acetylcholinesterase inhibitor, at a dose 1 to 2 mg intravenously.[20]

Sympathomimetics

Amphetamines, including MDMA (3,4-methylenedioxymethamphetamine), cocaine, and monamine oxidase inhibitors, cause hyperthermia because of central and peripheral thermoregulatory disturbances via changes in levels of norepinephrine, dopamine, and serotonin (5-HT).[14] MDMA causes increased dopamine and 5-HT release; cocaine increases release of catecholamines and blocks reuptake; and amphetamines release norepinephrine, dopamine, and 5-HT from presynaptic terminals and inhibit reuptake.[15-21] Symptoms include altered mental status, adrenergic state, seizures, and coma. MDMA can cause hyperkalemia, hypo- or hypercalcemia, hyponatremia, hypoglycemia, and coagulopathy.

Treatment includes external cooling measures, benzodiazepines, barbiturates, and sometimes paralytics. Beta-blockers are avoided in cocaine because of vasospasm from unopposed α stimulation.[22]

Neuroleptic Malignant Syndrome

Hyperthermia is caused by dopamine depletion or blockade in the hypothalamus secondary to antipsychotics, dopamine antagonists, prochlorperazine, metoclopramide, droperidol, and promethazine. Although neuroleptic malignant syndrome is a diagnosis if exclusion, diagnostic criteria have been used. Diagnosis via the Diagnostic Statistic Manual of Mental Disorders (DSMMD) criteria includes neuroleptic medications with severe muscle rigidity; an elevated temperature; and two or more of the following: diaphoresis, dysphagia, tremor, incontinence, altered mental status, mutism, tachycardia, labile blood pressure, leukocytosis, and elevated creatine kinase.[23] Levenson and colleagues' criteria include three of the following major manifestations: hyperthermia, rigidity, and elevated creatine kinase, or four minor criteria such as tachycardia, abnormal blood pressure, tachypnea, altered mental status, diaphoresis, or leukocytosis.[24] Symptoms may manifest from 24 hours to 30 days.[17] They may take up to 2 weeks to resolve after the offending medication is removed. Treatment includes discontinuation of medication, external cooling devices, benzodiazepines, bromocriptine, and dantrolene. Bromocriptine increases dopamine activity in the hypothalamus and is given at 2.5 mg every 8 hours with a total dose of 45 mg/d. Complications include hypotension and vomiting. Dantrolene can be used as monotherapy or adjunct therapy and is given as 1 to 2.5 mg intravenously with a cumulative dose of 10 mg/kg. Complications include muscle weakness and phlebitis.

Serotonin Syndrome

Hyperthermia is the result of excessive 5-HT concentration in the synapse, leading to stimulation of serotonergic neurons in midline raphe nuclei that has thermoregulation processes. Norepinephrine, NMDA, and γ-aminobutyric acid are also associated with serotonin syndrome.[25-27] Medications implicated include serotonin reuptake inhibitors, serotonin–norepinephrine reuptake inhibitors, monoamine oxidase inhibitors, TCAs, tramadol, amphetamines, dextromethorphan, linezolid, sumatriptan, lithium, fentanyl, meperidine, MDMA, St. John's wort, and tryptophan.[25-27] There are two diagnostic criteria. Sternbach criteria requires exposure to medication and three or more of the following: mental status changes, agitation, myoclonus, shivering, diaphoresis, hyperreflexia, tremor, diarrhea, incoordination, and fever.[28] Dunkley and coworkers' criteria are based on Hunter's criteria, which include spontaneous, inducible ocular clonus; agitation; diaphoresis; hyperreflexia; hypertonicity; tremor; and body temperature greater than 38°C.[29] Symptoms can manifest within minutes. Treatment includes removal of the offending medication, external cooling measures, benzodiazepines, and cyproheptadine (an antihistamine with 5-HT$_{1a}$ and 5-HT$_{2a}$ antagonistic properties). The dosage is 12 mg PO followed by 2 mg every 2 hours until symptoms resolved with maintenance of 8 mg every 6 hours.[30]

Heat Stroke

Heat stroke is defined as hyperthermia greater than 40°C (>104°F) with signs of organ system failure, usually of the central nervous system. There is a disproportionate heat production relative to heat loss, leading to hyperkalemia, rhabdomyolysis, acute renal failure, disseminated intravascular coagulation, multiorgan failure, and death.[31,32] There are two forms: exertional and classical (the latter is seen in heat waves). Treatment is a prompt reduction of core temperature, with improved survival rates if it is lowered to 38.9°C within 60 minutes.[31,32] The technique includes immersion in cold water with a temperature cutoff 101–102°F (38.3–38.9°C) to prevent hypothermia.

QUESTIONS

1. A 48-year-old man suddenly collapsed at the mall. An automated external defibrillator was applied, and he was found to have ventricular fibrillation. Advanced Cardiac Life Support was initiated, and ROSC was achieved. He was transferred to the emergency department (ED), and TH was initiated. He was noted to have shivering on his neck, torso, and upper extremities. Which is not an intervention to control shivering?

   A. Warm blanket on the face
   B. Acetaminophen
   C. Buspirone
   D. None of the above

2. A 45-year-old woman with a history of diabetes mellitus, obesity, and hypotension was admitted after cardiac arrest for ventricular tachycardia. ROSC was achieved, but the patient was not responsive and was subsequently placed on hypothermic protocol. What would be the next step?

   A. Initiate tube feeds during the cooling phase.
   B. Initiate tube feeds during the warming phase.
   C. Glucose goal less than 200 mg/dL
   D. Start dopamine for sinus bradycardia 40 with MAP above 80.

3. A 56-year-old man with cerebral palsy and depression was noted to have altered mental status. His home medications include lisinopril, Celexa, and a baclofen pump. He was recently started on a selective serotonin reuptake inhibitor, and his baclofen pump was recently manipulated. He was seen in the ED, and vital signs on admission showed a blood pressure of 90/60 mmHg, heart rate of 140 beats/min, respiratory rate of 18 breaths/min, temperature of 104.5°F, and O$_2$ saturation of 95% on room air. Physical examination noted rigid movements of his extremities.

WBC	$10 \times 10^3/\mu L$
Hgb	12.4 g/dL
Plt	$245 \times 10^3/\mu L$
Na	134 mEq/L
K	5.4 mEq/L
Creatinine	3.4 mg/dL
CPK	5000 IU/L

What is the next step?

   A. Baclofen PO
   B. Increase baclofen dose in the pump
   C. Dantrolene
   D. Cyproheptadine

4. A 30-year-old woman at 30 weeks of gestation is complaining of shortness of breath, fever, and diaphoresis. She has a history of depression, and her citalopram dosage was recently increased. Her vital signs are blood pressure of 90/60 mmHg, heart rate of 120 beats/min, respiratory rate of 24 breaths/min, O$_2$ sat of 98% on room air, and temperature of 103°C. She is agitated and diaphoretic. Her pupils are dilated and noted to have slow, continuous horizontal movements. Her lungs are clear to auscultation. Her heart sounds were tachycardic. Her abdomen was distended with fetal heart sounds and bowel sounds. Her extremities showed muscle rigidity, tremors, and deep tendon hyperreflexia. Home medications were discontinued, and external cooling measures were started.

WBC	$10 \times 10^3/\mu L$
Hgb	10 g/dL
Plt	$300 \times 10^3/\mu L$
Na	145 mEq/L
K	4 mEq/L
CO$_2$	24 mg/dL
Crea	1 mg/DL
Ca	8 mg/dL
CPK	100
AST	25
ALT	25

Chest radiographs are unremarkable.

The patient is given cyproheptadine 12 mg PO followed by 2 mg PO every 2 hours for two more doses. There was no improvement with her symptoms. What is the next step?

   A. Cyproheptadine
   B. Bromocriptine
   C. Dantrolene
   D. Flumazenil

TABLE 34-2 **Columbia Antishivering Protocol**

Step		Intervention	Dose
0	Baseline	Acetaminophen Buspirone Magnesium sulfate Skin counterwarming	650–1000 mg every 4–6 h 30 mg every 8 h 0.5–1 mg/h IV goal (3–4 mg/dL) 43°C, maximum temperature
1	Mild sedation	Dexmedetomidine or Opioid	0.2–1.5 mcg/kg/h Fentanyl starting dose: 25 mcg/h Meperidine 50–100 mg IM or IV
2	Moderate sedation	Dexmedetomidine and opioid	Doses as above
3	Deep sedation	Propofol	50–75 mcg/kg/min
4	Neuromuscular blockade	Vecuronium	0.1 mg/kg IV

IM = intramuscular; IV = intravenous.

Reprinted with permission from Choi HA, Sang-Bae K, Presciutti M, et al. Prevention of shivering during therapeutic temperature modulation: the Columbia anti-shivering protocol. *Neurocrit Care*. 2011;1-6.

ANSWERS

1. A. None of the above

   Control of shivering is necessary for affective TH. The Bedside Shivering Assessment Scale (BSAS) is used to gauge the appropriate medication. Scores are 0 = none; 1 = mild with shivering in the neck or thorax; 2 = moderate with shivering in upper extremities, including the neck and thorax; and 3 = gross movements of the truck and upper and lower extremities.[33,34] An example of the shivering stepwise protocol is derived from Columbia University.[34] Step 1 is for a BSAS score of 2 or 3 despite baseline interventions. Step 2 is used if step 1 is ineffective and so forth. The goal is BSAS of 1 or less.[34] See Table 34-2.

   Skin counterwarming decreases shivering because it provides 20% of hypothalamic input regarding temperature[34,35] (choice A). Acetaminophen lowers the hypothalamic setpoint because of prostaglandin synthesis[36-39] (choice B). Buspirone act of 5-HT_{1a} and lowers the shivering threshold (choice C).

2. C. Glucose goal less than 200 mg/dL

   Nutrition is avoided during initiation, maintenance, and rewarming (choices A and B). Bradycardia, as low as less than 40 beats/min is common and should not be treated unless associated with hypotension (choice D). Tight glucose control is advocated.

3. B. Increase baclofen dose in the pump

   Baclofen is used for spasticity, and intrathecal pumps are preferred because they can reach higher levels in the cerebrospinal fluid (CSF) compared with oral baclofen. Baclofen withdrawal is considered when there is recent manipulation of the intrathecal pump. It is characterized by hyperthermia, rhabdomyolysis, seizures, and renal failure. Treatment consists of hydration, benzodiazepines, and increasing intrathecal administration of baclofen. Oral baclofen does not increase the CSF levels of baclofen adequately[40,41] (choice A). Increasing the baclofen dose should be considered. Dantrolene (choice C) and cyproheptadine (choice D) have been postulated to have some effect with baclofen withdrawal but are not the first choice in this case.

4. A. Cyproheptadine

   The patient has serotonin syndrome via the Hunter criteria. Cyproheptadine is safe to use during pregnancy (Category B) and can be continued every 2 hours until there is a clinical response. Patients might become sedated or might have hypotension. Therefore, intubation and fluid boluses or pressors might be necessary. Bromocriptine exacerbates symptoms (choice B). Dantrolene has no proven effect (choice C). Flumazenil is used to treat patients with benzodiazepine poisoning (choice D).

REFERENCES

1. Polderman KH. Mechanisms of action, physiological effects, and complications of hypothermia. *Crit Care Med*. 2009;37(Suppl):S186-S202.

2. Scirica BM. Therapeutic hypothermia after cardiac arrest. *Circulation*. 2013;127:244-250.

3. Callaway CW, Donnino MW, Fink EL, et al. Part 8: Post-Cardiac Arrest Care 2015 American Heart Association Guidelines Update for Cardiopulmonary Resuscitation and Emergency Cardiovascular Care. *Circulation*. 2015;132(Suppl): S465-S482.

4. Nielsen N, Wetterslev J, Cronberg T, et al; TTM Trial Investigators. Targeted temperature management at 33°C versus 36°C after cardiac arrest. *N Engl J Med*. 2013;369:2197-2206.

5. Musselman ME, Saely S. Diagnosis and treatment of drug-induced hyperthermia. *Am J Health-Syst Pharm*. 2013;70:34-42.

6. Geocadin RG, Wijdicks E, Armstrong MN, et al. Practice Guideline Summary: Reducing brain injury following cardiopulmonary resuscitation: Report of the Guideline Development, Dissemination, and Implementation Subcommittee of the American Academy of Neurology. *Neurology*. 2017;88(22):2141-2149.

7. Wadha A, Sengupta P, Durrani J, et al. Magnesium sulphate only slightly reduces the shivering threshold in humans. *Br J Anaesth.* 2005;94:756-762.

8. Sandroni C, Cavallaro F, Callaway CW, et al. Predictors of poor neurological outcome in adult comatose survivors of cardiac arrest: a systematic review and meta-analysis. Part 2: patients treated with therapeutic hypothermia. *Resuscitation.* 2013;84:1324-1338.

9. The Hypothermia after Cardiac Arrest Study Group. Mild therapeutic hypothermia to improve neurologic outcome after cardiac arrest. *N Engl J Med.* 2002;346:549-556.

10. Bernard SA, Gray TW, Buist MD, et al. Treatment of comatose survivors of out-of-hospital cardiac arrest with induced hypothermia. *N Engl J Med.* 2002;346:557-563.

11. Chan PS, Berg RA, Tang Y, et al. Association between therapeutic hypothermia and survival after in-hospital cardiac arrest. *JAMA.* 2016;316(13):1375-1382.

12. Hanania NA, Zimmerman JL. Accidental hypothermia. *Crit Care Clin.* 1999;15(2):235-249.

13. Jolly BT, Ghezzi KT. Accidental hypothermia. *Emerg Med Clin North Am.* 1992;10(2):311-327.

14. Brown DJA, Brugger H, Boyd J, Paal P. Accidental hypothermia. *N Engl J Med.* 2012;367:1930-1938.

15. Mallory M, Gorgineni E, Jones GC, et al. Therapeutic hyperthermia: the old, the new and the upcoming. *Crit Rev Oncol Hematol.* 2016;97:56-64.

16. Musselman ME, Saely S. Diagnosis and treatment of drug-induced hyperthermia. *Am J Health Syst Pharm.* 2013;70:34-42.

17. Rosenberg H, Davis M, James D, et al. Malignant hyperthermia. *Orphanet J Rare Dis.* 2007;2:21.

18. Chan TC, Evans SD, Clark RF. Drug induced hyperthermia. *Crit Care Clin.* 1997;13:785-808.

19. Eyer F, Zilker T. Bench-to-bedside review: mechanisms and management of hyperthermia due to toxicity. *Crit Care.* 2007;11:236.

20. Howland MA. Physostigmine salicylate: antidote in depth (A12): In: Nelson L, Goldfrank LR, eds. *Goldfrank's Toxicologic Emergencies.* 9th ed. New York: McGraw-Hill Medical; 2010: 759-762.

21. Hadad E, Weinbroum AA, Ben-Abraham R. Drug-induced hyperthermia and muscle rigidity: a practical approach. *Eur J Emerg Med.* 2003;10:149-154.

22. Ramoska E, Sacchetti AD. Propranolol-induced hypertension in treatment of cocaine intoxication. *Ann Emerg Med.* 1985;14:1112-1113.

23. American Psychiatric Association. *Diagnostic and Statistical Manual of Mental Disorders.* 4th ed. Washington, DC: American Psychiatric Association; 2000.

24. Levenson JL. Neuroleptic malignant syndrome. *Am J Psychiatry.* 1985;142:1137-1145.

25. Boyer EW, Shannon M. The serotonin syndrome. *N Engl J Med.* 2005;352:1112-20. [Errata, *N Engl J Med.* 2009;361:1714, and *N Engl J Med.* 2007;356:2437.]

26. Nisijima K, Shioda K, Yoshino T, et al. Memantine, an NMDA antagonist, prevents the development of hyperthermia in an animal model for serotonin syndrome. *Pharmacopsychiatry.* 2004;37:57-62.

27. Done CJ, Sharp T. Biochemical evidence for the regulation of central noradrenergic activity by 5-HT1A and 5-HT2 receptors: microdialysis studies in the awake and anaesthetized rat. *Neuropharmacology.* 1994;33:411-421.

28. Sternbach H. The serotonin syndrome. *Am J Psychiatry.* 1991;148:705-713.

29. Dunkley EJ, Isbister GK, Sibbritt D, et al. The Hunter Serotonin Toxicity Criteria: simple and accurate diagnostic decision rules for serotonin toxicity. *QJM.* 2003;96:635-642.

30. Boyer EW, Shannon M. The serotonin syndrome. *N Engl J Med.* 2005;352:1112-1120. [Errata, *N Engl J Med.* 2009;361:1714, and *N Engl J Med.* 2007;356:2437.]

31. Water E, Venn R, Stevenson T. Exertional heat stroke—the athlete's nemesis. *JICS.* 2012;13(4):304-308.

32. Binkley HM, Beckett J, Casa DJ, et al. National Athletic Trainers' Association Position Statement: exertional heat illnesses. *J Athl Train.* 2002;37(3):329-343.

33. Badjatia N, Strongilis E, Gordon E, et al. Metabolic impact of shivering during therapeutic temperature modulation: the bedside shivering assessment scale. *Stroke.* 2008;39(12):3242-3247.

34. Choi HA, Presciutti M, Fernandez L, et al. Prevention of shivering during therapeutic temperature modulation: the Columbia anti-shivering protocol. *Neurocrit Care.* 2011;1-6.

35. Kimberger O, Ali SZ, Markstaller M, et al. Meperidine and skin surface warming additively reduce the shivering threshold: a volunteer study. *Crit Care.* 2007;11:R29.

36. Lennon RL, Hosking MP, Conover MA, Perkins WJ. Evaluation of a forced-air system for warming hypothermic postoperative patients. *Anesth Analg.* 1990;70:424-427.

37. Kasner SE, Wein T, Piriyawat P, et al. Acetaminophen for altering body temperature in acute stroke: a randomized clinical trial. *Stroke.* 2002;33:130-134.

38. Dippel DW, van Breda EJ, van Gemert HM, et al. Effect of paracetamol (acetaminophen) on body temperature in acute ischemic stroke: a double-blind, randomized phase II clinical trial. *Stroke.* 2001;32:1607-1612.

39. Dippel DW, van Breda EJ, van der Worp HB, et al. Effect of paracetamol (acetaminophen) and ibuprofen on body temperature in acute ischemic stroke PISA, a phase II double-blind, randomized, placebo-controlled trial [ISRCTN98608690]. *BMC Cardiovasc Disord.* 2003;3:2.

40. Ross JC, Cook AM, Stewart GL, Fahy BG. Acute intrathecal baclofen withdrawal: a brief review of treatment options. *Neurocrit Care.* 2011;14(1):103-108.

41. Imran M, Hussain A. Intrathecal baclofen withdrawal syndrome—a life threatening complication of baclofen pump: a case report. *BMC Clin Pharmacol.* 2005;4:1-5.

35

Biostatistics

Kartik Ramakrishna, MD

INTRODUCTION

We are in an era of evidence-based medicine, with an exponentially increasing information base arising from descriptive and interventional studies. Clinicians are required to use this evidence to guide their clinical strategies for diagnosis and management of patients. This chapter discusses the basic principles of epidemiology and medical biostatistics.

TYPES OF EPIDEMIOLOGIC STUDIES

Epidemiologic studies are broadly divided into observational studies and experimental studies.[1-6]

Observational studies are based on naturally occurring phenomena and do not involve an intervention by the study team. There are several types:

1. Case reports and case series: These are descriptive studies that report the characteristics of the disease and frequency of events. They tend to report sentinel events that are useful in generating a hypothesis but cannot test them. They are useful for describing very rare diseases. In the hierarchy of the evidence pyramid, laboratory research and animal studies are at the very bottom followed by editorials, case reports, and case series.

2. Cross-sectional studies: These are analytic studies that evaluate a specified population for a given time. They may be used to determine the number of cases of a disease in the population at a particular point in time (ie, prevalence of a disease) and hence are also called prevalence studies. They are not suitable to evaluate incidence rates or to evaluate rare diseases or exposures. These are the weakest form of evidence among analytical observational studies, falling just above case series in the evidence pyramid.

3. Case-control studies: These are a form of analytic observational studies in which patients with a disease are selected for the case arm, and appropriate matched participants are selected for the control arm. These studies start with the disease and attempt to retrospectively identify causal associations. The advantages include that they are fast and inexpensive to conduct. They are well suited to study uncommon diseases and allow evaluation for multiple causal exposures. They are, however, subject to significant bias such as recall bias. Appropriate matching of control participants may be difficult. Case-control studies rank above cross-sectional studies but below cohort studies in the hierarchy of evidence.

4. Cohort studies: These are observational studies that follow a group of participants or a cohort with a known exposure as well as a cohort without the exposure, until development of the disease, to look for a difference in the incidence of the disease in the two groups. These studies may be prospective, retrospective, or mixed. They are suitable to estimate incidence, evaluate rare exposures, and evaluate for multiple outcomes. They can, however, be expensive and require long periods of follow-up.

Experimental studies involve an active controlled intervention such as an exposure or treatment.

1. Randomized controlled trials (RCTs): These are the most well-known experimental design. These are the best design to prove the relationship between exposure and event. Randomization and blinding are usually performed to minimize bias. They may be expensive and time consuming and are of limited value in evaluating exposures that are known to have harmful outcomes. When reviewing these studies, one must question the internal validity as well as external validity of the study. RCTs rank higher than observational studies in the evidence pyramid, with systematic reviews and meta-analyses at the top.

BIAS IN EPIDEMIOLOGIC STUDIES

Bias in a study is an error in the design or execution of a study that consistently encourages one outcome or answer over others.[1] The sources and types of bias vary depending on the study design (eg, observational studies such as case-control studies or experimental studies such as RCTs).

Common types of bias include:

1. Bias due to confounders: A confounding factor or covariate is a factor that is associated with the exposure or

risk factor and disease being studied and is distributed unequally between the study groups. Bias due to confounders can be minimized in observational studies by matching cases and control participants to ensure equal distribution of known confounding variables. The effect of confounders can also be minimized by analytical strategies such as multivariable analysis.

2. Selection bias: This occurs when the method of selecting participants in the study results in a difference between the study population and the target population. There is a distortion in the magnitude of the association between the exposure and disease in the study versus the target population.

3. Exclusion bias: This can occur when the study is designed to exclude people with certain conditions to prevent confounding. This occurs more often when the exclusion criteria are different for cases versus control participants. An example is if a study were designed to evaluate the association between chronic obstructive pulmonary disease (COPD) and lung cancer and smokers were excluded from the control arm to prevent undiagnosed cases of COPD but smokers were included in the cases arm. A significant association would be noted between COPD and lung cancer; however, the differential exclusion of smokers would be a source of bias.

4. Nonresponse bias: This occurs because people who volunteer to enroll in studies or respond to calls to enroll in studies tend to behave differently from those who do not and hence may not fully represent the target population.

5. Berkson bias: This is a form of selection bias or hospital admission bias that occurs in hospital-based case-control studies. This can occur if the exposure increases the chance of admission, leading to a higher number of participants with that exposure.

6. Recall bias: This occurs predominantly because of one of two reasons. One tends to recall more recent events compared with distant events, as well as more severe or traumatic events compared with less severe events.

7. Reporting bias: Participants tend to report and emphasize events or exposures that they believe to be more important or relevant.

8. Hawthorne effect: The behavior or response of a participant can change if he knows he is being observed.

9. Placebo effect: This can occur when patients subjected to the exposure or intervention report feeling better as a result of knowing that they are receiving treatment.

10. Observer bias and ascertainment bias: These can occur when knowing the arm of the study that the participant is in subconsciously influences the person determining the outcome.

The design of RCTs may incorporate a number of methods to reduce bias:

1. Randomization: Randomization helps prevent selection bias, preventing the allotting of a certain cohort of patients to one arm of the trial versus the other.

Although matching allows for equitable distribution of known confounding factors, it has little effect of unknown confounders. Randomization aids in the equitable distribution of unknown confounders.

2. Stratification: Stratification during randomization assists with equal distribution of known confounding factors such as stratification by age or by center in multicenter trials.

3. Single blinding or blinding of patients: This involves use of a placebo or sham procedure to minimize the placebo effect.

4. Double blinding: This involves blinding of the patient and the physician as well as outcomes assessor. This minimizes observer or ascertainment bias, as well as deviations in care based on the treating physicians bias toward the intervention.

5. Triple blinding: In addition to double blinding, the person analyzing the data and the monitoring committee is also blinded. This can minimize bias in analysis and evaluation. Triple-blinded studies are rarely done because of the need to monitor safety of the intervention.

SAMPLE SIZE, POWER, ACCURACY, AND PRECISION

A study with inadequate sample size would be underpowered to reject the null hypothesis and hence would be a waste of time and resources. Similarly, a study with too many participants would also be a waste of time and resources.

Null hypothesis: This is the default position that there is no statistically significant association between the variables in the hypothesis.

Type I error: This is the incorrect rejection of a true null hypothesis, also known as a false-positive or alpha error. The alpha level (or level of significance) is the probability of making a type I error, and the acceptable level is typically considered to be 0.05.

Type II error: This is the incorrect acceptance of a false null hypothesis, also known as a false-negative or beta error. Beta level is the probability of making a type II error, and the acceptable level is typically considered to be 10% to 20%.

Power: This is the probability of detecting a statistically significant difference if one really exists. Power is related to beta (power = 1 – beta level), and hence the acceptable level is typically considered to be 80% to 90%.

Sample size: Multiple variables are required for sample size calculation, such as prevalence rate, incidence rate, odds ratio (OR), and means, as well as exposure or treatment effect size, the alpha level, and the power. The smaller the effect size or the higher the power, the larger the sample size that will result.

Precision: This is the reproducibility of the results if the study were repeated under the same conditions. Improved precision translates to reduced sampling or random error.

Standard error of measurement is an estimate of precision. A narrower standard error indicates increased precision. Increasing the sample size reduces the standard error and increases the precision.

Accuracy: This is degree to which a measured value represents the true population value. Accuracy is an estimate of error in measurement due to systematic error or error due to bias. Good precision does not necessarily mean good accuracy. Larger sample sizes do not ensure absence of bias and hence do not necessarily improve accuracy.

PREVALENCE AND INCIDENCE RATES

Incidence and prevalence are measures used to describe the frequency of an event. Incidence is the number of new cases of a disease as a percentage of the population at risk, which is the people who do not already have the disease. Incidence is useful to evaluate the effectiveness of preventive measures.

Prevalence is the number of people with the disease divided by the total population and measures the magnitude of disease burden in a community and to help identify high-risk populations. It is influenced by the incidence of the disease, as well as the average duration of the illness. It is directly proportional to the incidence of a disease as well as the average duration of illness. Lifetime prevalence is the proportion of persons in a given population that will develop the disease in their lifetime.

ODDS RATIO AND CONFIDENCE INTERVALS

The OR is used in case-control studies to measure the association between a causal factor and a disease by comparing the frequency of occurrence of a causal factor in those with and without the outcome of interest.[2,3]

Risk is the probability of occurrence of the event or disease of interest. It is calculated as the number of people with the outcome of interest divided by the number of people with all possible outcomes. For example, if three in four people who smoke develop lung cancer, the risk is 3 divided by 4, which is 0.75.

Odds is the probability of developing the outcome divided by the probability of not developing that outcome. In the above scenario, the odds of developing lung cancer with

TABLE 35-1 Odd's Ratio Table

	Disease Present (Case)	Disease Absent (Control)
Exposure present	A	B
Exposure absent	C	D

smoking would be 3 divided by 1, which is 3. The OR is more appropriate for case-control studies than relative risk (RR) because the total number of people with the exposure is not known, and hence the denominator would be unknown for calculating the RR.

The OR is best calculated by drawing a 2 × 2 table as shown in Table 35-1.

The OR of developing the disease with exposure is calculated by dividing the odds of presence of exposure in the case arm (A/C) with the odds of presence of exposure in the control arm (B/D). Therefore,

$$OR = (A/C) \div (B/D) = (A/C) \times (D/B) = AD/CB$$

Interpreting the OR:

OR of 1 indicates no difference in the odds in each group.

OR more than 1 indicates increased odds of occurrence of disease in those with the exposure.

OR less than 1 indicates decreased odds of occurrence of disease in those with the exposure.

The OR is often expressed with the 95% confidence interval (95% CI). The 95% CI is the range around the result within which the populations true value is likely to be 95% of the time.

The narrower the CI, the smaller the P value. The size of the CI may also be related to the sample size of the study. However, an OR with a 95% CI that crosses the value 1 is not significant.

SENSITIVITY, SPECIFICITY, PREDICTIVE VALUES, AND LIKELIHOOD RATIOS

These statistics are used to evaluate the diagnostic value of clinical tests or screening tools and help assess the probability of whether the patient does or does not have the disease in question. These are best determined using a 2 × 2 table as illustrated in Table 35-2.

TABLE 35-2 Table for Sensitivity, Specificity, Positive Predictive Value, and Negative Predictive Value

	Disease Present	Disease Absent	
Test positive	True positive (TP)	False positive (FP)	PPV = TP/(TP + FP)
Test negative	False negative (FN)	True negative (TN)	NPV = TN/(TN+FN)
	Sensitivity = TP/(TP + FN)	Specificity = TN/(TN+FP)	

NPV = negative predictive value; PPV = positive predictive value.

Sensitivity is the ability of a test to correctly identify those with the disease. It is the proportion of those with the disease who test positive for the disease.

$$Sensitivity = TP/(TP + FN)$$

where TP is true positive and FN is false negative.

Specificity is the ability of the test to accurately exclude disease in healthy individuals. It is the proportion of those without the disease who test negative for the disease.

$$Specificity = TN/(TN + FP)$$

where TN is true negative and FP is false positive.

Positive predictive value (PPV) is the likelihood that the patient will have the disease if the test result is positive. It is the proportion of patients who test positive who have the disease.

$$PPV = TP/(TP + FP)$$

Negative predictive value (NPV) is the likelihood that the patient is healthy if the test result is negative. It is the proportion of patients who test negative who do not have the disease.

$$NPV = TN/(TN + FN)$$

Sensitivity and specificity are measures of test characteristics and are independent of the prevalence in the population.

However, PPV and NPV can be influenced significantly by the prevalence of the disease. For example, if the test were used in a population with a low prevalence of the disease, the FP would increase, resulting in a decrease in PPV. The TN would also increase, resulting in an increase in the NPV.

The likelihood ratio (LR) is another measure used in clinical practice. The positive LR is the probability that those with the disease test positive compared with the probability that those without the disease test positive.

$$LR+ = Sensitivity/(1 - Specificity)$$

Similarly, the negative LR can be calculated as:

$$LR- = (1 - Sensitivity)/Specificity$$

RELATIVE RISK REDUCTION AND NUMBER NEEDED TO TREAT

These are statistics used to evaluate the magnitude of effect of a risk factor or a treatment.

Relative risk is the ratio of the probability of developing a disease or an outcome event with the experimental intervention to the probability of developing a disease or outcome event without the experimental intervention (ie, in the control arm). The RR may exaggerate the treatment effect, especially if the outcome is uncommon.

The absolute risk reduction (ARR), also called the risk difference (RD), is the difference in the rate of events between the control arm (CER) and experimental arm (EER). The relative risk reduction (RRR) is the ratio of the ARR to the CER.

The number needed to treat (NNT) is defined as the number of patients needing to receive an intervention for one additional patient to benefit. It provides a better estimate of the effect size than the RR. The NNT is calculated as the inverse of the ARR, as demonstrated below.

1. CER % = Number of Events/Number of Patients in the Control Arm × 100
2. EER % = Number of Events/Number of Patients in the Intervention Arm × 100
3. RR = EER/CER
4. ARR = CER – EER
5. RRR = (CER – EER)/CER
6. NNT = 1/(CER – EER) = 1/ARR

QUESTIONS

1. Intensive care unit (ICU) delirium is an increasingly recognized problem in ICUs, with multiple risk factors identified. You want to know the prevalence of preexisting cognitive impairment among patients admitted to your ICU. Which of the following types of study designs would be most appropriate to answer this question?

   A. Case series
   B. Cross-sectional study
   C. Cohort study
   D. Case-control study

2. You review different studies regarding ICU delirium to discuss in journal club. All of the following statements regarding studies of different designs are true except

   A. Bias is more common in observational studies than in RCTs.
   B. Cohort studies are well suited to evaluate rare diseases.
   C. Incidence rate can be calculated from cohort studies.
   D. Case-control studies fall below cohort studies in the hierarchy of evidence.

3. Match the study objective with the most appropriate study design.
   1. To study the effect of an uncommon exposure
   2. To study the prevalence of a disease
   3. To study the cause of a rare disease
   4. To study the effectiveness of a new drug

   A. Case-control study
   B. Randomized controlled trial
   C. Cohort study
   D. Cross-sectional study

4. A large academic center has designed a new protocol for severe sepsis and septic shock. They plan to perform an RCT to compare this new protocol with the current standard therapy. In a study to establish current practices, questionnaires are sent to all the ICU providers. Half the providers return the completed questionnaire. Which of the following types of bias is likely to result in this scenario?

   A. Nonresponse bias
   B. Berkson bias
   C. Selection bias
   D. Reporting bias

5. The Rivers trial was a randomized controlled trial published in the *New England Journal of Medicine* (*NEJM*) in 2001, which showed that early goal-directed therapy reduced mortality rates in severe sepsis and septic shock. Patients were randomized to standard care versus protocolized early goal-directed therapy in computer-generated blocks of two to eight. Randomization is done to prevent which of the following?

   A. Recall bias
   B. Hawthorne effect
   C. Selection bias
   D. Placebo effect

6. Match the type of bias to the appropriate method used to minimize the bias.
   1. Bias due to known confounders and covariates
   2. Ascertainment bias
   3. Bias due to unknown confounders
   4. Placebo effect

   A. Blinding data collectors and outcome adjudicators
   B. Blinding patients
   C. Stratification during randomization
   D. Randomization

7. You review a recently published RCT assessing for mortality benefit with catheter-directed thrombolysis versus current standard of care (anticoagulation with heparin). The results show the mortality rate to be no different with the new intervention compared with the current standard of care. On careful review of the paper, however, you note that to detect a 20% decrease in mortality rate, with a power of 80% and an alpha level of 0.05, a sample size of 500 patients in each arm is required. However, only 300 patients could be recruited to each arm of the study. Other adequately powered studies published since then have shown a significant mortality benefit with this new intervention. Which of the following statements regarding the initial study is correct?

   A. This is an example of a type I error.
   B. To detect a smaller mortality benefit, a smaller sample size would be required.

C. This is an example of a type II error.
D. If the power were increased to 90% when designing the study, a smaller sample size would be required.

8. Regarding sample size calculation, which of the following statements is incorrect?

   A. Increasing the power would increase the sample size.
   B. Increasing the sample size would decrease the standard error of measurement.
   C. Increasing the sample size will increase the precision.
   D. Increasing the sample size will increase accuracy.

9. Staphylococcal drug resistance is becoming an increasing problem in your ICU. You are monitoring methicillin-resistant *Staphylococcus aureus* (MRSA) in the community. You are following 5000 people, of whom 1000 people have tested positive as MRSA carriers. You continue to follow these patients for 1 year, and now an additional 200 patients test positive as MRSA carriers. What is the point prevalence of MRSA per 1000 people at the start of the study, and what is the yearly incidence?

   A. Prevalence: 200; incidence: 5%
   B. Prevalence: 400; incidence: 2%
   C. Prevalence: 100; incidence: 4%
   D. Prevalence: 500; incidence: 20%

10. Assuming the prevalence of the disease has been fairly constant for the past 10 years, all of the following would decrease the prevalence of the disease except

    A. Measures are introduced that decrease the incidence of disease.
    B. A large number of healthy people immigrate to the area.
    C. Because of improved therapy, people with the disease live longer with the disease.
    D. A disproportionately large number of people with the disease die in an influenza pandemic.

11. You have multiple patients who develop *Clostridium difficile*–associated diarrhea (CDAD) in your ICU. You decide to do a study to see if this could be related to the use of proton pump inhibitors (PPIs). You review the charts of 100 patients with CDAD and 100 control participants matched for antibiotic use. You note that 80 patients in the CDAD arm had been taking PPIs, and 40 patients in the control arm had been taking PPIs. What is the OR for development of CDAD with use of PPIs in this study?

    A. 5
    B. 6
    C. 4
    D. 8

12. The 95% CI is 3.18 to 11.29. Which of the following statements is true?

    A. The *P* value is 0.07.
    B. 95% of the data fall between these two values.
    C. The chance that the true value falls in this range is 95%.
    D. The result would be significant if the 95% CI crossed 1.

13. A patient is admitted to the ICU with hypoxemic respiratory failure and a clear chest radiograph. Computed tomographic pulmonary artery angiography (CTPA) is negative for pulmonary embolism (PE). You decide to review the literature regarding this test.

    You review the Prospective Investigation of Pulmonary Embolism (PIOPED) II trial published in the *NEJM* in 2006. This was a prospective multicenter trial evaluating the accuracy of CTPA compared with a composite gold standard. A total of 7284 patients with clinical suspicion for PE were screened, and 1090 patients were enrolled. Of these, 773 were included in the final analysis because the remainder had incomplete evaluations, missing data, or suboptimal imaging. A total of 181 of the 773 included patients who were confirmed to have PE based on the composite gold standard test. A total of 175 patients had a CTPA study positive for PE, of whom only 150 patients were confirmed to have PE on the composite gold standard. Based on the above data, what is the sensitivity and specificity of CTPA in the above cohort?

    A. Sensitivity = 85.7%; specificity = 94.8%
    B. Sensitivity = 94.8%; specificity = 85.7%
    C. Sensitivity = 82.8%; specificity = 95.7%
    D. Sensitivity = 95.7%; specificity = 82.8%

14. If the study in question 13 was repeated in all patients with any respiratory complaint, irrespective of the presence of suspicion for PE, which of the following will one expect to see?

    A. Sensitivity: decreased; specificity: similar; PPV: decreased; NPV: similar
    B. Sensitivity: decreased; specificity: decreased; PPV: decreased; NPV: decreased
    C. Sensitivity: similar; specificity: similar; PPV: decreased; NPV: increased
    D. Sensitivity: similar; specificity: increased; PPV: similar; NPV: increased

15. The ARDSnet trial published in *NEJM* in 2000 compared ventilation with lower tidal volumes (6 mL/kg) with traditional tidal volumes (12 mL/kg) in acute lung injury (ALI) and acute respiratory distress syndrome (ARDS). The primary outcome was breathing without assistance before discharge to home. The trial was stopped after the fourth interim analysis, having enrolled 861 patients.

The mortality rate was found to be significantly lower in the low tidal volume group compared with the traditional tidal volume group (31% vs 39.8%, respectively; $P = 0.007$). What is the RRR for mortality with low tidal volume ventilation compared with traditional tidal volume ventilation?

    A. 8.8%
    B. 22%
    C. 78%
    D. 28%

16. In reference to the ARDsnet trial in question 15, how many patients must receive low tidal volume ventilation to prevent one death?

    A. 11.3% patients
    B. 8.8% patients
    C. 7.8% patients
    D. 22% patients

17. Which of the following is not associated with the Choosing Wisely Campaign?

    A. Transfuse to hemoglobin greater than 7 in hemodynamically unstable patients.
    B. Daily blood draws
    C. Discussion regarding comfort measures only in a patient who has anoxic encephalopathy after cardiac arrest
    D. Deep sedation in a patient with ARDS on continuous neuromuscular blockade with a positive end-expiratory pressure of 15 and a fraction of inspired oxygen (FiO_2) of 100 %

ANSWERS

1. B. Cross-sectional study

    Case series describe the characteristics of a disease and are particularly useful to describe rare diseases. They cannot determine the incidence or prevalence of the disease (choice A).

    A cross-sectional study determines the number of cases of a disease in a population in a particular point in time and hence can determine the prevalence (choice B).

    A cohort study follows a group of participants with a known exposure and a group without the exposure to compare the incidence in both groups (choice C).

    A case-control study compares those who already have the disease with matched control participants to retrospectively identify the cause of the disease and hence cannot be used to estimate prevalence of the disease (choice D).

2. B. Cohort studies are well suited to evaluate rare diseases.

Case-control studies are better suited to study rare diseases (choice B). Cohort studies compare the incidence of an event or disease in those with an exposure compared with those without an exposure (choice C). They are useful to evaluate the effect of rare exposures. They, however, are of limited value in evaluating rare diseases because very few participants are likely to develop the disease.

RCTs use methods such as randomization, stratification, and blinding to reduce bias and are higher on the hierarchy of evidence that observational studies (choice A). At the bottom of the evidence pyramid are animal and in vitro studies followed by case reports and series, cross-sectional studies, case-control studies, cohort studies, RCTs, and finally meta-analysis and reviews (choice D).

3. 1 C, 2 D, 3 A, and 4 B

A cohort study is the appropriate study design to evaluate the effect of an uncommon exposure. Cross-sectional studies are designed to study the prevalence of a disease. Case-control studies are well suited to study the cause of an uncommon or rare disease. RCTs are the best study design to evaluate the effectiveness of a new therapy.

4. A. Nonresponse bias

In this scenario of a survey trying to establish current practice, only half of the providers responded. In such a scenario, the people who respond are likely to behave different than those who do not and may have different clinical practice from those who do not respond. This is known as nonresponse bias (choice A).

Berkson bias is a form of a selection bias that occurs in hospital based case-control studies (choice B).

Selection bias occurs when the method of selecting participants in the study results in a difference between the study population and the target population. In this scenario, questionnaires were sent to all ICU providers (choice C).

Reporting bias occurs as enrolled participants tend to report or emphasize exposures that they believe to be more important (choice D).

5. C. Selection bias

Randomization prevents the allotting of a certain subset of patients to one arm of the trial versus the other. It ensures that investigators cannot select the arm of the study that the patient is allotted to, thereby minimizing selection bias (choice C).

Recall bias occurs as participants interviewed tend to recall more recent and more severe events. Randomization is not targeted at minimizing this (choice A).

The Hawthorne effect is the change in the behavior of a participant when she knows she is being observed. This is unaffected by randomization (choice B).

The placebo effect is the subjective improvement felt because of knowledge that one is receiving treatment and is unaffected by randomization (choice D).

6. 1 C, 2 A, 3 D, and 4 B

Bias due to known confounders can be minimized by stratification during randomization so as to ensure equitable distribution of the confounders in both arms of the trial.

Ascertainment bias occurs when the person determining the outcome is influenced by knowing which are the study the participant is in. This can be minimized by blinding data collectors and outcome adjudicators.

Randomization helps minimize selection bias; it also aides in the equitable distribution of known as well as unknown confounders.

The placebo effect occurs when patients report improvement as a result of knowing that they are receiving treatment. This can be minimized by blinding the patients to the arms of the study that they are in, with the use of placebos or sham treatments.

7. C. This is an example of a type II error.

In this hypothetical scenario, the above negative study falsely accepts the null hypothesis, which is that there is no benefit with the new intervention. This is an example of a type II error, which is the acceptance of a false null hypothesis (choice C).

A type I error is the false rejection of a true null hypothesis, or a false positive finding (choice A).

A larger sample size would be required (choice B) to detect a smaller treatment benefit or effect.

Increasing the power to 90% when designing the study would result in a larger sample size (choice D).

8. D. Increasing the sample size will increase accuracy.

Accuracy is the degree to which an obtained result represents the true population result and is an estimate of error due to bias. Larger sample sizes do not necessarily minimize reduce bias and hence would not improve accuracy (choice D).

Increasing the power of the study to detect a difference would increase the sample size (choice A).

Precision is the reproducibility of the result if the study were to be repeated under similar circumstances. Increasing the sample size would increase the precision (choice C) and decrease the standard error of measurement, which is an estimate of precision (choice B). A narrower standard error indicates increased precision.

9. A. Prevalence: 200; incidence: 5%

Prevalence is the number of people with the disease divided by the total population. Here, the number with the disease at the start of the study is 1000, and the total population is 5000. Thus, the point prevalence at the start of the study is 1000/5000 = 20% or 200 per 1000 people (choice A).

The incidence is the number of new cases of a disease as a percentage of the population at risk, which is the people who do not already have the disease. In this scenario, of the 5000 people, 1000 have the disease to begin with; hence, the at-risk population is 4000, of which 200 develop the condition. Hence the incidence is 200/4000 = 0.05 or 5% (choice A).

10. C. Because of improved therapy, people with the disease live longer with the disease.

The prevalence of a disease is influenced by the incidence of the disease, as well as the average duration of the illness. A decrease in the incidence of disease would decrease the number of cases being added to the population and hence decrease the prevalence (choice A). An increased average duration of the disease would increase the number of people in the population who have the disease and hence increase the prevalence rather than reduce it (choice C). Large-scale immigration of healthy people to the region would increase the total population (the denominator) and hence decrease the prevalence (choice B). The death of a large number of those with the disease would decrease the total number in the population with the disease (the numerator) and hence decrease the prevalence (choice D).

11. B. 6

The OR is best calculated by drawing a 2 × 2 table as shown in Table 35-3.

The OR of developing CDAD with PPI use is calculated by dividing the odds of PPI use in the CDAD arm (A/C) with the odds of PPI use in the non-CDAD or control arm (B/D). Therefore,

$$OR = AD/CB = (80 \times 60)/(20 \times 40) = 6$$

TABLE 35-3 Table of CDAD

	CDAD Present (Case)	CDAD Absent (Control)
PPI use present	80 (A)	40 (B)
PPI use absent	20 (C)	60 (D)

CDAD = *Clostridium difficile*–associated diarrhea; PPI = proton pump inhibitor.

12. C. The chance that the true value falls in this range is 95%.

The 95% CI is the range around the result within which the populations true value is likely to be 95% of the time

(choice C). It does not mean that 95% of the data falls between these values (choice B). An OR with a 95% CI that crosses 1 is not significant (choice D). In this case, the 95% CI does not cross 1, and a corresponding P value would be less than 0.05 (choice A).

13. C. Sensitivity = 82.8%; specificity = 96%

In this scenario, we are provided the total number included in the final analysis (773), the number in whom PE is present (181), and hence those without PE (592), total test positive (TTP = 175), and the true positive (TP = 150). With this, we can calculate the false positive (FP = TTP – TP = 175 – 150 = 25), true negative (TN = PE absent – FP = 592 – 25 = 567), and false negative (FN = PE present – TP = 181 – 150 = 31) and populate the 2 × 2 table as shown in Table 35-4.

Sensitivity = TP/(TP + FN) = 150/(150 + 31) = 0.827 or 82.7%

Specificity = TN/(TN + FP) = 567/(567 + 25) = 0.957 or 95.7%

PPV = TP/(TP + FP) = 150/(150 + 25) = 0.857 or 85.7%

NPV = TN/(TN + FN) = 567/(567 + 31) = 0.948 or 94.8%

Hence choice C is the correct answer to question 13.

TABLE 35-4 Table for Pulmonary Embolism

	PE Present (181)	PE Absent (592)
Test positive (TP)	TP = 150	FP = 25
Test negative (TN)	FN = 31	TN = 567

FN = false negative; FP = false positive; PE = pulmonary embolism; TN = true negative; TP = true positive.
Predictive Value NPV = negative predictive value; PPV = positive predictive value.

14. C. Sensitivity: similar; specificity: similar; PPV: decreased; NPV: increased

If this study were to be repeated in all patients with respiratory symptoms, irrespective of the presence of clinical suspicion for PE, the prevalence of the disease would be significantly lower. And as discussed previously, the sensitivity and specificity of a test are unaffected by the prevalence of a disease in the population being tested. However, the PPV would decrease in a population with a low prevalence because the number of false positives would increase relative to the number of true positives. Similarly, the NPV would increase, and the number of true negatives would increase relative to the number of false negatives.

15. B. 22%

The CER and EER are provided in the scenario and are 39.8% and 31%, respectively.

The RR of mortality with low tidal volume ventilation compared with the traditional strategy is EER/CER = 31%/39.8% = 0.78 (choice C).

The ARR is the CER – EER = 39.8% – 31% = 8.8%.

The RRR is the ratio of the ARR to the CER and is calculated as (CER – EER)/CER = 8.8/39.8 = 0.22 or 22%.

16. A. 11.3 patients

The number of patients that must receive low tidal volume ventilation to prevent one death is the NNT, which is the inverse of the ARR.

NNT = 1/ARR = 1/(CER – EER) = 1/8.8% = 11.3 patients

17. B. Daily blood draws

To combat the rising costs of health care without compromising the quality of care, the Choosing Wisely Campaign was developed.[7] Recommendations from this campaign include: (1) diagnostic tests should be ordered as a response to a specific clinical question and not at regular intervals, (2) blood transfusions should not be performed on hemodynamically stable, nonbleeding patients with hemoglobin greater than 7 g/dL, (3) parenteral nutrition should not be used during the first 7 days of ICU stay in an adequately nourished patient, (4) deep sedation should not be used in mechanically ventilation without a specific indication and without daily attempts to lighten sedation, and (5) life support should not be continued for patients at high risk for death or severely impaired functional recovery without offering patients and their families alternative care focused on comfort.[7]

REFERENCES

1. Pannucci CJ, Wilkins EG. Identifying and avoiding bias in research. *Plast Reconstr Surg.* 2010;126:619-625.
2. Szumilas M. Explaining odds ratios. *J Can Acad Child Adolesc Psychiatry.* 2010;19:227-229.
3. Ranganathan P, Aggarwal R, Pramesh CS. Common pitfalls in statistical analysis: odds versus risk. *Perspect Clin Res.* 2015;6:222-224.
4. Park K. *Park's Textbook of Preventive and Social Medicine.* 23rd edition. Jabalpur; Banarsidas Bhanot; 2015.
5. Harris M, Taylor G. *Medical Statistics Made Easy.* New York: Springer-Verlag; 2003.
6. Indrayan A. *Basic Methods of Medical Research.* 3rd ed. Delhi, India: AITBS Publishers; 2012.
7. Halpern SD, Becker D, Curtis JR, et al; Choosing Wisely Taskforce. An official American Thoracic Society/American Association of Critical-Care Nurses/American College of Chest Physicians/Society of Critical Care Medicine policy statement: the Choosing Wisely Top 5 list in Critical Care Medicine. *Am J Respir Crit Care Med.* 2014;190(7):818-826.
8. Centers for Medicare & Medicaid Services. Hospital Value-Based Purchasing. http://www.cms.gov/Medicare/Quality-Initiatives-Patient-Assessment-Instruments/hospital-value-based-purchasing.

Ethics, Death, and Organ Donation

Chika Nwulu, MD, and Ronaldo Collo Go, MD

INTRODUCTION

Ethics is a moral code of what we believe to be universally accepted principles of rightness and wrongness that influences our medical decisions. Ever-advancing technology and therapies constantly challenge and call into question previously established ethical norms. The most accessible approach is committing to the following principles: respect for autonomy, beneficence, nonmaleficence, and justice.[1] These principles are dependent on a thorough understanding of the patient's illness and how medical interventions, or the lack of will, impact his quality of life. What to advise may not be so easy and often the progress of the clinical course and morbidity and predictive scores are used to give the physician, patient, and family the global perspective into his illness.

MORBIDITY AND MORTALITY PREDICTIVE SCORES

These scores help benchmark the quality of care and aide with triage of patients who would benefit from care in the intensive care unit. They are also helpful with prognostication and guide the physician's goals of care discussion with the patient or family members, particularly when the clinical course is equivocal.

APACHE

In 1985, The Acute Physiology and Chronic Health Evaluation (APACHE) II is a scoring classification of disease severity using acute physiologic score (APS) based on 12 physiologic measurements, age, and chronic health points.[2,3] APACHE II score of less than 25 points has less than or equal to 50% mortality with more than or equal to 35 points had 80% mortality.[3] Criticism to APACHE II is that it provided information regarding severity of illness of patient groups but not individual patients.[2,4] In 1991, the APACHE III revision provided risk stratification of individual patients within defined patient groups and the APACHE III Score and reference data on disease categories and treatment location allowed risk estimate for hospital mortality.[5] There was a greater emphasis on the impact of the APS and the APACHE III Score range from 0-299.

Along with Simplified Acute Physiology Score (SAPS) II and Mortality Probability Model (MPM) II, APACHE III was believed to have significantly different predicted mortality from observed.[6-8] In 2006, APACHE IV (Score 0-252) remodeled the physiologic variables and weights and included 4 new predictor variables: (1) presence of mechanical ventilation; (2) use to thrombolytic therapy for acute myocardial infarction; (3) adjustments for prognostic implications of Glasgow Coma Scale (GCS) and Pao_2 and Fio_2; and (4) inability to assess GCS due to sedation or paralysis.[8] APACHE IV has excellent discrimination with an area under a receive operating characteristic curve (AU-ROC) of 0.88. AU-ROC more than 0.80 indications good discrimination.[8] Observed and mean predicted mortality were 13.5% and 13.55% (p = 0.76)[8] (Table 36-1).

SAPS

Another scoring system to predict mortality is the Simplified Acute Physiology Score (SAPS) II created in 1993.[9] It used physiologic variables, age, type of admission, and three disease variables (acquired immunodeficiency syndrome, metastatic disease, and hematologic malignancy) and found to have Goodness of fit test P = 0.883 and P = .103 in developmental and validated samples.[9] The ROC is 0.88 developmental and 0.86 in validated sample.[9]

It has been hypothesized that SAPS II needs to be updated because: (1) there is a major change in prevalence of disease and therapeutic interventions; (2) SAPS II is based on data from Europe and North America only; (3) the development of computers; and (4) need for country-representative database.[10,11] In 2005, SAPS III was developed to assess disease severity and predict status on hospital discharge based on data upon ICU admission.[10,11] SAPS III admission score is based on three "boxes." Box I involves patient characteristics such as age, previous health status, comorbidities, location before ICU admission, length of stay in hospital before ICU, and use of major therapeutic options such as vasoactive drugs before ICU admission.[10,11] Box II involves circumstances of ICU admission like reason for admission, anatomic site of surgery, planned or unplanned ICU admission, surgical status and infection.[10,11] Box III is degree of physiologic derangement at ICU admission or within 1 hour before or after admission.[10,11] The physiologic

TABLE 36-1 APACHE IV Variables: Data Items Collected and Used for Predicting Hospital Mortality Among Patients Admitted to Intensive Care Unit (ICU) Who Did Not Have Coronary Artery Bypass Graft (CABG) Surgery

Age	Continuous Measure Plus Five Spline Terms
APS variables	Weight determined by most abnormal value within first APACHE day; sum of weights equals the APS, which ranges from 0 to 252. Five spline terms added. Variables include pulse rate, mean blood pressure, temperature, respiratory rate. Pao_2/Fio_2 ratio (or $P(A-a)o_2$ for intubated patients with $Fio_2 \geq 0.5$), hematocrit, white blood cell count, creatinine, urine output, blood urea nitrogen, sodium, albumin, bilirubin, glucose, acid base abnormalities, and neurological abnormalities based on Glasgow Coma Score
Chronic health variables	AIDS, cirrhosis, hepatic failure, immunosupression, lymphoma, leukemia or myeloma, metastatic tumor. Not used for elective surgery patients.
ICU admission diagnosis	116 categories
ICU admission source	Floor, emergency room, operating/recovery room, stepdown unit, direct admission, other ICU, other hospital, other admission source
Length of stay before ICU admission	Square root plus four spline terms
Emergency surgery	Y/N
Unable to assess Glasgow	Y/N
Coma Scale score	
Thrombolytic therapy	For patients with acute myocardial infarction (Y/N)
Glasgow Coma Scale score rescaled	15 minus measured Glasgow Coma Scale score
Pao_2/Fio_2 ratio	
Mechanical ventilation	Y/N

APS, acute physiology score; APACHE, Acute Physiology and Chronic Health Evaluation. All predictor variables use ICU day 1 data.

Reprinted with permission from Zimmerman JE, Kramer AA, McNair DS, et al. Acute physiology and chronic health evaluation (APACHE) IV: hospital mortality assessment for today's critically ill patients. *Crit Care Med.* 2006;34(5):1297-1310.

variables include lowest GCS, highest heart rate, lowest systolic blood pressure, highest bilirubin, highest temperature, highest creatinine, highest leukocytes, lowest platelets, lowest pH, and ventilator support and oxygenation.[10,11] ROC was 0.848 and the Hosmer-Lemeshow goodness-of-fit test H of 10.56 (p = 0.39) and Hosmer-Lemeshow goodness of fits test C of 14.29 (p = 0.16)[10,11] (Table 36-2).

MPP₀

MPM₀

Mortality Probability Model (MPM_0) II, another severity scoring system that predicts mortality from 15 variables within 1 hour of ICU admission was thought to overpredict mortality.[12,13] The updated Mortality Probability Model (MPM_0) III had new variables: "zero factor" for low risk mortality risk in elective surgery patients with no other mortality risk, "full code" variable, and 7 age related interaction terms.[13] MPM_0 III was found to have area under the ROC 0.826 (95% confidence interval 0.822-0.831) and Hosmer-Lemeshow statistic of 11.52 (p = 0.1740).[13]

SOFA

A prospective multicenter study where the median length of ICU stay was 5 days and the ICU mortality was 22% multiple organ dysfunction and high Sequential Organ Failure Assessment (SOFA) score were associated with increased

mortality.[14-16] A subgroup of patients who had an ICU stay of more than or equal to 1 week had higher respiratory, cardiovascular, and neurologic scores. SOFA score increased to 44% in nonsurvivors but only 20% in survivors (P < 0.001) and decreased by 33% in survivors compared to 21% in nonsurvivors (P < 0.001).[16] With a SOFA score >15, mortality was 90% (Sensitivity 31%, Specificity 99%, correct classification 84%).[16] Primarily used in sepsis, modified versions of SOFA have been used in critical care triage of patients in mass disasters and cardiac patients.[17,18] In the modified version for critical care triage of patients from mass disasters, platelet count is removed, arterial oxygen saturation replaces partial pressure of arterial oxygen, and clinical assessment of jaundice replaces serum bilirubin. Area under the receiver operating characteristic curve (ROC) decreased from day 1 (ROC = 0.83) to Day 5 (ROC = 0.74).[17] Another study on post cardiac surgical patients showed good correlation with mortality with ROC 0.841 on admission to area under ROC 0.82 on postoperative day 4, and area under ROC 0.77 on postoperative day 7.[18] A recent retrospective cohort suggested that SOFA's score prediction of mortality from sepsis diminishes after fifth ICU day[19] (Table 36-3).

MODS

In 1995, Marshall et al created the multiple organ dysfunction score (MODS).[20] The score correlated to ICU mortality when

TABLE 36-2 SAPS III Box I, II, and III: SAPS 3 Admission Scoresheet—Part 1

Box I	0	3	5	6	7	8	9	11	13	15	18
Age, years	<40		≥40 <60				≥60 <70		≥70 <75	≥75 <80	≥80
Co-morbidities		Cancer therapy[2]		Chron, HF (NYHA IV), Haematological cancer[3,4]		Cirrhosis, AIDS[3]		Cancer[5]			
Length of stay before ICU admission, days[1]	<14			≥14 <28	≥28						
Intra-hospital location before ICU admission			Emergency room		Other ICU	Other[6]					
Use of major therapeutic options before ICU admission		Vasoactive drugs									

Moreno RP, Metnitz PG, Almeida E, et al. SAPS 3 – from evaluation of the patient to evaluation of the intensive care unit. Part 2: development of a prognostic model for hospital mortality at ICU admission. *Intensive Care Med.* 2005;31(10):1345-1355.

Box II	0	3	4	5	6
ICU admission: Planned or Unplanned		Unplanned			
Reason(s) for ICU admission	please see Part 2 of the scoresheet				
Surgical status at ICU admission	Scheduled surgery			No surgery[7]	Emergency surgery
Anatomical site of surgery	please see Part 2 of the scoresheet				
Acute infection at ICU admission			Nosocomial[8]	Respiratory[9]	

(Continued)

TABLE 36-2 SAPS III Box I, II, and III: SAPS 3 Admission Scoresheet—Part 1 (Continued)

Box III	15	13	11	10	8	7	5	3	2	0	2	4	5	7	8
Estimated Glasgow Coma Scale (lowest), points	3–4			5		6			7–12	≥13					
Total bilirubin (highest), mg/dL										<2		≥2 <6	≥6		
Total bilirubin (highest), µmol/L										<34.2		≥34.2 <102.6	≥102.6		
Body temperature (highest), Degrees Celsius						<35				≥35					
Creatinine (highest), mg/dL										<1.2	≥1.2 <2			≥2 <3.5	≥3.5
Creatinine (highest), µmol/L										<106.1	≥106.1 <176.8			≥176.8 <309.4	≥309.4
Heart rate (highest), beats/min										<120			≥120 <160	≥160	
Leukocytes (highest), G/L										<15	≥15				
Hydrogen ion concentration (lowest), pH								≤7.25		>7.25					
Plateletes (lowest), G/L		<20			≥20 <50		≥50 <100			≥100					
Systolic blood pressure (lowest), mm Hg			<40		≥40 <70			≥70 <120		≥120					
Oxygenation [10), 11]			Pao₂/Fio₂ <100 and MV			Pao₂/Fio₂ ≥100 and MV	Pao₂ <60 and no MV			Pao₂ ≥60 and no MV					

The definition for all variables can be found in detail in Appendix C of the ESM. For names and abbreviations which are differing from those in the ESM, explanations are given below. Generally, it should be noted that no mutually exclusive conditions exist for the following fields: Comorbidities, Reasons for ICU admission, and Acute infection at ICU admission. Thus, if a patient has more than one condition listed for a specific variable, points are assigned for all applicable combinations.

[1] This variable is calculated from the two data fields: ICU Admission date and time—Hospital admission date and time (see Appendix C of the ESM)

[2] Cancer Therapy refers to the data definitions in Appendix C of the ESM: Co-Morbidities: Chemotherapy, Immunosupression other, Radiotherapy, Steroid treatment

[3] If a patient has both conditions he/she gets double points.

[4] Chronic HF (NYHA IV)/Haematological cancer refer both to the data definitions in Appendix C of the ESM: Co-Morbidities: Chronic heart failure class IV NYHA, Haematological cancer.

[5] Cancer refers to the data definitions in Appendix C of the ESM: Co-Morbidities: Metastatic cancer.

[6] Other refers to the data definitions in Appendix C of the ESM: Intra-hospital location before ICU admission: Ward, Other.

[7] No surgery refers to the data definitions in Appendix C of the ESM: Surgical Status at ICU Admission: Patient not submitted to surgery.

[8] Nosocomial refers to the data definitions in Appendix C of the ESM: Acute infection at ICU admission—Acquisition: Hospital-acquired.

[9] Respiratory refers to the data definition in Appendix C of the ESM: Acute infection at ICU admission—Site: Lower respiratory tract: Pneumonia, Lung asbcess, other.

[10] Pao₂, Fio₂ refer to the data definitions in Appendix C of the ESM: Arterial oxygen partial pressure (lowest), Inspiratory oxygen concentration.

[11] MV refers to the data definition in Appendix C of the ESM: Ventilatory support and mechanical ventilation.

740

TABLE 36-2 SAPS III Admission Scoresheet—Part 2

Box II – (Continued)	
ICU admission [12]	16
Reason(s) for ICU admission	
Cardiovascular: Rhythm disturbances [13]	–5
Neurologic: Seizures [13]	–4
Cardiovascular: Hypovolemic hemorrhagic shock, hypovolemic non-hemorrhagic shock/Digestive: Acute abdomen, other [3]	3
Neurologic: coma, stupor, obtuned patient, vigilance disturbances, confusion, agitation, delirium	4
Cardiovascular: Septic shock/Cardiovascular: anaphylactic shock, mixed and undefined shock	5
Hepatic: Liver failure	6
Neurologic: Focal neurologic deficit	7
Digestive: Severe pancreatitis	9
Neurologic: Intracranial mass effect	10
All others	0
Anatomical site of surgery	
Transplantation surgery: Liver, kidney, pancreas, kidney and pancreas, Transplantation other	–11
Trauma—other, isolated: (includes thorax, abdomen, limb); trauma—multiple	–8
Cardiac surgery: CABG without valvular repair	–6
Neurosurgery: Cerebrovascular accident	5
All others	0

[12]Every patient gets an offset of 16 points for being admitted (to avoid negative SAPS 3 Scores).

[13]If both reasons for admission are present, only the worse valve (–4) is scored.

applied during first ICU day and over course of ICU stay. At 9-12 points, mortality was 25%; at 13-16 points, mortality was 50%; at 17-20 points, mortality was 75%; and more than 20 points mortality was 100%. ROC was 0.928-0.936.[20] (See Table 36-4).

AUTONOMY, BENEFICENCE, AND NONMALEFICENCE

Autonomy is the right to self-governance. A patient has the right to accept or refuse the care that is offered provided that the patient has a well-rounded perspective regarding the present clinical condition and any proposed treatment or procedure and has decision-making capacity. The benefits and complications of an intervention must carefully be explained.

Beneficence and nonmaleficence are considered together because the first refers to the principle of treating patients in a way that will benefit them, and the latter demands we act in such a way that will not harm our patients.

Because what one patient would consider beneficial, another may consider harm, combining respect for autonomy with commitment to beneficence and nonmaleficence is essential. Take, for example, leg amputation for gangrene. It may represent lifesaving benefit for one patient with a mostly sedentary lifestyle, but the same surgery could represent unacceptable harm (absence of mobility) to another patient whose quality of life hinges on being mobile.

GOALS OF CARE

Healthcare workers desire to cure and eradicate disease wherever present. For patients with chronic disease, those who are critically ill, and those who present at end of life, achieving goals such as "relief of suffering," "self-sufficiency," and "a good death" may be of higher priority than sustaining life through cardiopulmonary resuscitation (CPR) and mechanical ventilation, which may, to the patient, be deemed an unacceptable harm.[21] Too often we discover, far into a treatment regimen, that either our treatment goals do not align with those of the patient or that the patient has expectations of treatment that were never a possible outcome.[22] Therefore, it is good practice to establish goals of care with patients preferably at the initiation of every encounter because not only do patients want to discuss such things,[23] but these goals also positively impact the quality of end-of-life care.[24] Goals of care are dynamic and frequently need to be reassessed based on clinical course. Most often this also implies the healthcare professional's understanding of the disease and clinical condition.

Decisions are often dependent on the patient's wishes, the severity and reversibility of the patient's acute disease, chronic diseases such as cancer, functional status, age, social support, and compliance. Therefore, healthcare providers must be aware of the current trends and developments for that particular disease. For example, it is true that patients with cancer have lower survival rates than patients without cancer, but their in-hospital mortality rate is not higher compared with other patients with chronic disease.[25-30] In fact, a substantial high survival rate can be achieved even in critically ill cancer patients.[28-30] This has been attributed to improved survival in cancer patients, development of more potent and targeted therapies, improved intensive care unit (ICU) management, and improved diagnostics skills.[25] Therefore, a 72-hour trial of critical care is sometimes recommended before end-of-care discussion.[25]

PALLIATIVE CARE

Discussion of goals of care frequently leads to discussions about palliative care and hospice care. Palliative care is a multidisciplinary specialty that treats patients with the primary goals of relieving suffering. A patient does not have to be dying to be appropriate for palliative care. With the prerequisite of a chronic or life-limiting illness, patients with frequent

TABLE 36-3 SOFA Score

	SOFA Score				
	0	1	2	3	4
Respiration					
Pao_2/Fio_2 (torr)	> 400	≤ 400	≤300	≤ 200 With respiratory support	≤ 100 With respiratory support
Coagulation					
Platelets (x $10^3/mm^3$)	> 150	≤ 150	≤100	≤ 50	≤ 20
Liver					
Bilirubin (mg/dL)	< 1.2	1.2-1.9	2.0-5.9	6.0-11.9	> 12.0
(μmol/L)	< 20	20-32	33-101	102-204	> 204
Cardiovascular					
Hypotension	No hypotension	MAP < 70 mm Hg	Dopamine ≤ 5 or dobutamine (any dose)[a]	Dopamine > 5 or epi ≤ 0.1 or norepi ≤ 0.1[a]	Dopamine > 15 or epi > 0.1 or norepi > 0.1[a]
Central Nervous System					
Glasgow Coma Score	15	13-14	10-12	6-9	< 6
Renal					
Creatinine (mg/dL)	< 1.2	1.2-1.9	2.0-3.4	3.5-4.9	> 5.0
(μmol/L) or urine output	< 110	110-170	171-299	300-440 or < 500 mL/d	> 440 or < 200 mL/d

epi, epinephrine; norepi, norepinephrine.

[a]Adrenergic agents administered for at least 1 hour (doses given are in μg/kg/min).

To convert torr to kPa, multiply the value by 0.1333.

Reprinted with permission from Vincent JL, deMendonca A, Cantraine F, et al. Use of the SOFA score to assess the incidence of organ dysfunction/failure in intensive care units: results of a multicenter, prospective study. Working group on "sepsis-related problems" of the European Society of Intensive Care Medicine. *Crit Care Med.* 1998;26(11):1793-1800.

admissions for the same condition, patients with admissions for uncontrolled symptoms, patients with failure to thrive, or patients whose daily cares are excessively complex are all candidates for palliative care. Patients receiving palliative care need not forgo curative or life-prolonging treatments.

HOSPICE CARE

Hospice care is reserved for patients with a life expectancy of less than 6 months. Hospice care also focuses on symptom management for the patient and emotional and spiritual

TABLE 36-4 MODS

Organ system	Score				
	0	1	2	3	4
Respiratory Pao_2/Fio_2	> 300	226-300	151-225	76-150	≤ 75
Renal creatinine (μmol/L)	≤ 100	101-200	201-350	251-500	> 500
Hepatic bilirubin (μmol/L)	≤ 20	21-60	61-120	121-240	> 240
Cardiovascular PAR[1]	< 10.0	10.1-15	15.1-20	20.1-30	> 30.0
Cardiovascular HR (beats/min)	< 120	120-140	> 140	Dopamine > 3 mg/g per min	Lactate > 5 mmoL/L
Hematologic platelet count (/L)	> 120	81-120	51-80	21-50	≤ 20
Neurologic Glasgow coma score	15	13-14	10-12	7-9	≤ 6

PAR = Heart Rate × Central Venous Pressure/Mean Arterial Blood Pressure.

Reprinted with permission from Marshall J, Cook DJ, Christou NV, et al. Multiple organ dysfunction score: a reliable descriptor of a complex clinical outcome. *Crit Care Med.* 1995;23(10):1638-1652.

support for the patient and family and provides bereavement services to family after the patient has passed. All hospice care is palliative care but not vice versa. Hospice care is palliative treatment for a dying patient with the goal of accepting the imminence of death and achieving a comfortable death with dignity. To this end, although inpatient and facility hospice care is available, the patient's home is the preferred location for hospice care—a familiar, comfortable, and dignified setting. At home, the burden of the care of the patient (bathing, medicating, feeding) falls primarily on family members with hospice providing weekly or biweekly visiting nurses and 24-hour on call hospice assistance via phone.

When addressing goals of care, the healthcare provider should be aware of the patient and their families' views regarding death and dying with consideration for religion and culture. If a pregnant patient's religion dictates that she does not receive blood products, for example, even if transfusion is the patient's and her unborn child's only chance at survival, this needs to be respected. Certain cultures believe that only a higher power dictates one's time to die. Under this belief, they insist that extraordinary measures be taken to keep nonviable patients alive. Simply discussing quality of life with family members in these situations may not make much headway because these beliefs are frequently woven into fabric of their belief system and identity. Ethics consult can be helpful in these cases.

SURROGATE, POWER OF ATTORNEY, AND WARD OF THE STATE

In certain instances, patients are unable to make their own decisions. In these situations, we turn to surrogate decision makers. Ideally, every patient would have a durable power of attorney for health care (also known as a healthcare proxy) drawn up before hospitalization, effectively providing an individual (surrogate) to make decisions regarding the patient's health (consenting to or refusing to consent to procedures, medications, and so on) if they become unable to. If a healthcare proxy is not in place, the surrogate decision maker is the patient's next of kin, which is determined by state law.

The most important concept of surrogate decision making is that of substituted judgment. This is striving to make decisions based on what the patient, if she or he were able, would have decided. If this is not known, then making decisions that are in the patient's best interests is the next priority.

If a patient is incompetent or incapable of making independent decisions, has no relatives, and has no designated surrogate, a state-appointed legal guardianship would need to be pursued, and the patient becomes a ward of the state.

WITHDRAWAL OF CARE AND DOUBLE EFFECT

There is no standard set of criteria that dictates when withdrawal of care should be discussed. However, when there are no more available medical interventions to accomplish a patient's goals of care, when further measures would violate patient's known wishes, and when continuation of medical care is futile, withdrawal of care can be discussed. Although withdrawal of care is not uncommon,[31] it remains an understandably challenging issue to navigate,[32] fraught with many misconceptions.[33]

First, when the physician withdraws ventilator support, this is not synonymous with cessation of care. The physician will still be actively caring for the patient until death occurs. Second, withdrawing ventilator support does not necessarily mean the physician is violating his or her obligation to act in a way to benefit the patient because frequently patients consider death preferable to "being kept alive on machines." Finally, withdrawing ventilator support frequently results in a dyspneic patient's need for the administration of analgesics and sedatives for palliation, which can be misconstrued as administering medications to hasten or cause death. In this example, the more correct way to view administration of analgesia and sedation can be explained by the principle of double effect.

The principle of double effect is actualized when an intervention benefits a patient but simultaneously has a harmful side ("double") effect. The harmful side effect is acceptable because the intention was for good. This principle is frequently called into effect when dying patients are given palliative analgesia and sedation to ease pain and dyspnea, and death follows, which is acceptable. On the contrary, giving analgesia and sedation to cause death as a means to end a patient's suffering would not be acceptable.[34]

ETHICS OF ORGAN DONATION

The gap between the supply and demand of solid organs is increasing,[35] and there is an argument for physicians to advocate for organ donation based on ethical principles of beneficence and justice. It would be impossible to predict if current healthy patients or future patients would need solid organ transplants; however, if and when that need occurs, it would benefit them to have a larger pool of available organs. Hence, adhering to the principle of beneficence does demand physicians to at least not be neutral in the discussion to donate organs. Justice, the fair allocation of scarce resources, demands that we do what we can to make available the resources, in this case organs, to our patients who are in need. Respect for patient autonomy can conflict with the prior two responsibilities based on patients' culture, personal preference, or religion. In these cases, a deliberative approach can be taken[36] to physician–patient decision making. In this approach, the physician plays the role of clarifying health-related values associated with available treatments and suggesting why certain values are worthier. In this way, respect for patient autonomy is always maintained, but physicians can also fulfill obligations to being just and beneficent.

DEATH

Death occurs when there is either irreversible cessation of brain or respiratory-circulatory function.[37] Part of the assessment is subjective and not evidence based; thus, a standard approach has been formulated in declaring a patient dead.[38]

Determination of brain death is based on neurologic clinical examination, apnea test, and ancillary testing. The process of declaring a patient brain dead begins with radiographic evidence of a catastrophic neurologic event and exclusion of confounding conditions such as shock, acid–base disorders, electrolyte disorders, high cervical neck injury, Guillain-Barré syndrome (GBS), locked-in syndrome, hypothermia, and drug toxicity.[37-41] Therefore, the patient's temperature must be at least 36°C. Pupillary reflexes are lost when the temperature is 32°C or less, and brainstem functions cease at 28°C or less. Drug clearance must be calculated by multiplying 5 times its half-life or drug levels below therapeutic levels.[37] Clinical evaluation includes (1) evidence that the patient is comatose with no response to any stimuli or environment, (2) absence of brainstem function (Table 36-5), and (3) the apnea test.[37-39] A patient is considered comatose if there is no eye opening or movement or motor response to noxious stimuli. Absence of brainstem reflexes is defined as (1) absence of pupillary reflex to bring light in both eyes with the eyes and usually fixed and dilated, (2) absence of ocular movements via oculocephalic testing (no movement of eyes relative to head movement) or oculovestibular testing (no movement of eyes for 1 minute after irrigation of external auditory canal with 50 mL of ice saline), (3) absence of corneal reflex with no eyelid movement noted after touching the cornea, (4) absence of facial muscle movement after deep pressure on the condyles at the temporomandibular joints and supraorbital ridge, and (5) absence of gag reflex after stimulation of posterior pharynx with tongue blade or suction device.[42] "Spontaneous movements" can still be seen and are derived from peripheral or spinal cord reflexes and are not derived from the brainstem. These can be spontaneous or induced and include facial nerve innervation muscles; finger flexor movements; tonic neck reflex; triple flexion with flexion at the hip, knee, and ankle with foot stimulation; opisthotonic trunk posturing; abdominal reflexes; alternating flexion–extension of the toes with passive foot displacement; upper limb protonation extension reflex; and fasciculations.

Apnea test assesses respiratory drive when subjected to CO_2 challenge. Prerequisites include (1) normotensive (systolic blood pressure ≥ 100 mmHg), (2) normothermic, (3) PCO_2 of 35 to 45 mmHg, (4) not hypoxic, (5) euvolemic, and (6) no prior CO_2 retention. The patient is then administered 100% oxygen to eliminate nitrogen stores for 10 minutes to a maximum Pao_2 of 200 mmHg. The patient is disconnected from the ventilator, and 6 to 8 L/min of oxygen is administered with nasal cannula prongs attached to endotracheal tube. Respiratory movements, defined as chest or abdominal movements, is observed for 5 to 10 minutes. This process is aborted if the systolic blood pressure drops less than 90 mmHg, arrhythmia develops, or the patient has hypoxia to less than 85% for 30 seconds. If the patient has hypoxia, she or who should be placed on T-piece, continuous positive airway pressure 10 mmH_2O, or oxygen supplementation with 12 L/min.[37] The apnea test result is considered positive if there is no visible signs of respirations and a PCO_2 greater than 60 mmHg or a 20-mmHg increase over baseline arterial PCO_2.[37] If the test results are inconclusive, it can be repeated again after a longer preoxygenation time or obtain ancillary tests. The apnea test may not apply in patients with high cervical neck injuries or neuromuscular disease.

Indications for ancillary testing include conditions that can alter consciousness such as medications or severe metabolic derangements; conditions that prevent assessment of cranial nerves (CNs) such as facial trauma, neuromuscular diseases, or neuropathies; contraindications to apnea tests; posterior fossa mass effect; brainstem pathology 24 hours after cardiac arrest and return of spontaneous circulation; abnormal movements; uncertainty of brain death diagnosis; and family's request.[41] (Table 36-5).

TABLE 36-5 Ancillary Tests for Brain Death

Ancillary Tests	Positive Test Result If:	Specificity/Sensitivity	Considerations
EEG	No reactivity to somatosensory or audiovisual stimuli or absence of EEG activity > 2 uV amp when recorded from scalp electrode pairs ≥ 10 cm apart with impedance < 10,000 ohms	90%/90%	
Cerebral angiography	No intracranial filling at entry of the carotid or vertebral artery to the skull or circle of Willis; external carotid patent	100%/75%	False negative with lowered intracranial pressure from surgery, trauma, or shunts
Transcranial Doppler	Reverberating flow or small systolic peaks in early systole	91–99%/100%	Temporal bone thickening
Cerebral scintigraphy	Hollow skull phenomenon—no radionuclide localization in MCA, ACA, or basilar artery		
Magnetic resonance angiography	Absence of blood flow		

ACA = anterior cerebral artery; EEG = electroencephalography; MCA = middle cerebral artery.

TABLE 36-6 Requesting Team, Clinical Studies, and Timing for Organ Donation

Team Requesting or Performing Studies	Clinical Studies	Timing
Organ donor network	Serum: HIV1 and -2 antibody, HTLV1 and -2 antibody, hepatitis B surface antigen, hepatitis B core antibody, hepatitis B core IgM, hepatitis C antibody, hepatitis B/C and HIV RNA testing, CMV IgM and IgG, EBV IgM and IgG, RPR, toxoplasmosis IgG, Chagas disease antibody (for patients with travel to Texas or South America)	Once
Primary care team	Serum: CBC; ABG; LFTs, including GGT, coagulation studies, fibrinogen, troponin/CK; chemistry panel, including calcium, phosphorous, and magnesium; LDH; amylase; lipase	Every 6 h
Primary care team	CXR, ECG, blood culture, urine culture, urinalysis, sputum culture and Gram stain, Hgb_{A1c} (once), type and screen (once)	Daily and as needed
Primary care team	Two-dimensional transthoracic echocardiography	At least once; may repeat depending on hemodynamic status
Organ donor network, primary care team, cardiology team, cardiology	Coronary catheterization	May be required for potential heart donors
Organ donor network, primary care team, pulmonology	Bronchoscopy	Required for potential lung donors

ABG, arterial blood gas; CBC = complete blood count; CK = creatine kinase; CMV = cytomegalovirus; CXR = chest radiography; EBV = Epstein-Barr virus; ECG = electrocardiography; EEG = electroencephalography; GGT = γ-glutamyl transferase; Hgb_{A1c}, hemoglobin A1c; HTLV = human T lymphotrophic virus; IgG = immunoglobulin G; IgM = immunoglobulin M; LDH = lactate dehydrogenase; LFT, liver function test; RPR = rapid plasma reagin.

Reprinted with permission from Frontera JA, Kalb T. How I manage the adult potential organ donor: donation after neurological death. Part 1. *Neurocrit Care.* 2010;12:103-110.

ORGAN DONATION

All potential organ donors, such as those with impending brain death, withdrawal of care or circulatory death, or death within 1 hour, should have the local organ donor network contacted.[43] Contraindications can vary but generally include a history of cancer except for certain skin cancers such as melanoma, primary brain tumors, remote prostate cancer, viral infections, bacterial infections, fungal infections, parasitic infections, and prions.[43] The routine studies are seen in Table 36-6.[43]

Donation After Brain Death

The care of a potential donor from brain death includes maintaining hemodynamic instability and ventilator management.

The hemodynamic instability secondary to brain death usually is a three-phase course with (1) sympathetic surge leading to hypertension, cardiac stunning and left ventricular dysfunction, pulmonary edema, and arrythmias; (2) herniation leading to loss of sympathetic tone and therefore hypotension; and (3) decreased pituitary hormone secretion leading to low triiodothyronine (T_3), thyroxine (T_4), cortisol, insulin, and antidiuretic hormone.[43-47] Therefore, conventional management of hypotension in these patients might be inadequate. In addition to fluid resuscitation and pressors, hormonal therapy is advocated. See Table 36-7.[43]

Because improved oxygenation has not been shown to improve outcomes, ventilator management is focused on decreasing incident of ventilator-induced lung injury.[37]

TABLE 36-7 Hormonal Therapy

Drug	Dosage	Comments
Thyroxine (T_4)	Administer 10 U of regular insulin with 1 ampule of D50 (unless glucose > 300 mg/dL); then	Inotropic effect; can be used as a pressor
	20 mcg T_4 IV bolus (mixed 200 mcg in 500 mL NS followed by	Causes hyperkalemia with bolus; must administer insulin and D50 before initiation
	10 mcg/h of T_4 IV; maximum dose, 20 mcg	T_4 shown to be more beneficial than triiodothyronine (T_3)[4,18,20,24]
Vasopressin	0.5 units/h IV (25 u in 250 mL NS or D5W); maximum dose, 6 U/h	Check for DI: UOP ≥ 5 cc/kg/h for ≥ 2 h, urine-specific gravity < 1.005, serum Na > 145 mEq/L, *or* serum osmolality > 300 mOsm/kg and urine osmolarity < 200 mOsm/kg
Insulin	1 unit/h IV (25 u in 250 mL of NS)	Adjust to maintain glucose at 100–140 mg/dL
Methylprednisolone	15 mg/kg IV bolus; repeat daily	Improves potential for lung donation

D50 = 50% dextrose solution; DI = diabetes insipidus; IV = intravenous; NS = normal saline; UOP = urine output.

Reprinted with permission from Frontera JA, Kalb T. How I manage the adult potential organ donor: donation after neurological death. Part 1. *Neurocrit Care.* 2010;12:103-110.

TABLE 36-8 Organs Available for Donation After Cardiac Death

Organ	WIT Threshold
Kidneys	WIT < 120 min; GFR > 30 ml/min/1.732 m²; not on HD; no ATN via biopsy
Liver	WIT < 30 min; noncirrhotic or no history of portal vein thrombosis
Pancreas	WIT < 30 min; no DM; BMI < 35; age < 65 y
Lung	WIT < 60 min

ATN = acute tubular necrosis; BMI = body mass index; DM = diabetes mellitus; GFR = glomerular filtration rate; HD = hemodialysis; WIT = warm ischemia time.

The current approach is to use pressure cycle modes because they can reduce preload, cardiac arrhythmias, and hyperoxic lung injury.

Donation After Cardiac Death

Patients who do not meet the criteria for brain death or who have an irreversible disease in which death is imminent can be considered for donation after cardiac death (DCD).[48-50] A major difference between donation after brain death (DBD) and DCD is the duration of warm ischemia time (WIT) and cold ischemia time (CIT). WIT is defined as the time to inadequate perfusion, oxygenation, or both as defined by systolic arterial pressure less than 50 mmHg, O_2 saturation less than 70%, or both.[48] This can lead to accumulation of ischemic metabolites. CIT is initiation of cold preservation to warming after transplantation.[48] In DBD, CIT is initiated before organ removal, and WIT is minimized.[48,49] In DCD, there is some degree of WIT before organ removal.[47,49] This makes DCD less ideal than DBD for organ donation. DCD donors can be further be subclassified as either controlled, in which donation is planned before death, or uncontrolled, in which death has occurred before planned donation or via modified Maastricht classificication.[48] In addition to skin, bone, cornea, and heart valves, Table 36-8 lists the organs available for DCD.[48-51]

Death occurs with irreversible cessation of brain or respiratory-circulatory function, with the former requiring both clinical assessment and at times radiographic and other ancillary testing. Organ donation should be pursued when possible, and the local organ donor network should be called early in the process. DBD is preferable to DCD.

QUESTIONS

1. What is a contraindication to apnea test?

    A. The use of pressors
    B. Chronic carbon dioxide retainers
    C. Locked-in syndrome
    D. Temperature of 36.5°C

2. A 52-year-old man with past medical history of cerebrovascular accident (CVA) causing trochlear nerve palsy, was brought in by emergency medical services after sustaining ventricular fibrillation arrest outside of the hospital. Family members report that patient was likely down for 10 minutes before initiation of CPR. The patient had return of circulation (ROSC) after 12 minutes of CPR and was intubated in the field. A cooling protocol was initiated, and the patient is now 24 hours after rewarming. He shows no response to external stimuli. A neurologist is present and is performing a neurologic examination to initiate certification of brain death. In this patient, which element of the neurologic examination may not be accurate given patient's past medical history?

    A. Oculocephalic reflex
    B. Vestibulocephalic reflex
    C. Corneal reflex
    D. All of the above

3. For the patient in question 2, the neurologic examination shows absent corneal reflex, gag, and oculocephalic and vestibulocephalic reflexes. The patient does at times have spontaneous raising of arms. An apnea test cannot be performed at this time because of acute respiratory distress syndrome. Computed tomography (CT) of the head shows cerebral edema. Organ donation has already been contacted, and the patient's liver and kidneys in addition to others are to be harvested for donation. Given the patient's arm movement, the family refuses to believe that patient is brain dead. What is the next best step?

    A. Declare the patient brain dead because brain death is a clinical determination
    B. Perform electroencephalography (EEG)
    C. B and D
    D. Obtain four-vessel angiography

4. An 84-year-old woman with a past medical history of diabetes mellitus, hepatitis C, and CVA presented with altered mental status, shortness of breath, and abdominal pain. Her ammonia level was elevated at 80 mcg/dL. Abdominal ultrasound showed large ascites. The patient is now feeling better after large-volume paracentesis. Alfa-feto protein (AFP) is noted to be above 500 ng/mL, and subsequent CT of the abdomen and pelvis has shown likely hepatocellular carcinoma with abdominal lymphadenopathy and multiple spinal lesions concerning for metastases. The patient's daughter has asked that you not to share the diagnosis with patient. What is the next step?

    A. Discuss the diagnosis with the daughter only.
    B. Discuss the diagnosis with the patient.
    C. Assess the patient's mental status.
    D. Ask other family members to weigh in on the daughter's request.

5. Initiation of morphine drip for palliation presents what type of ethical issue?

   A. Double effect
   B. Beneficence
   C. Maleficence
   D. Autonomy

ANSWERS

1. C. Locked-in syndrome

High cervical cord lesions; GBS; toxicities such as organophosphate, baclofen, lidocaine, and vecuronium; and locked-in syndrome can be mimics of brain death with temporary or permanent absence of brainstem reflexes and even unresponsive pupils.[39] Although eucapnia is a prerequisite for the apnea test, some authors suggest it can be used in CO_2 retainers. First, the CO_2 baseline is reached. During the test, a PCO_2 greater than 20 mmHg from baseline with a pH less than 7.28 suggest a positive apnea test.[37,39] (choice B). Despite hypotension being the main complication of the apnea test, the use of pressors before the apnea test does not exclude them from the test. Pressors are titrated to maintain a mean arterial pressure above 100 mmHg[37,38] (choice A). The cutoff temperature to perform the apnea test is 36°C.[37] (choice D).

2. A. Oculocephalic reflex

To test this reflex, the patient's eyelids are held open, and the head is flexed and extended; if the reflex is intact, the eyes will move in the contralateral direction to head movement. This reflex, along with the oculocephalic (doll's eyes) is usually specifically the vertical portion of oculocephalic testing. Vestibular cephalic reflexes (choice B) test CNs III, VI, and VIII. Because the doll's eyes reflex involves vertical movement of the eyes and this patient has some unspecified problem with one of the CNs that is involved in vertical eye movement (CN IV, trochlear), this may confound the test. The corneal reflex tests CNs V and VII (choice C).

3. B. Perform electroencephalography (EEG).

The American Academy of Neurology has EEG, transcranial Doppler, cerebral angiography, and hexamethylpropyleneamine oxime (HMPAO) singe-photon emission computed tomography as approved ancillary tests to help confirm or otherwise add more evidence to the diagnosis of brain death; therefore, evoked potentials is incorrect. Declaring the patient brain dead without further testing would be remiss and would likely be unacceptable to the family. Angiography could potentially harm the patient's organs for donation (choice D); therefore, EEG is probably the best and most readily available of the listed answer choices. Brain death is not solely a clinical determination (choice A).

4. C. Assess the patient's mental status.

Assess the patient's mental status. If she still has altered mental status or encephalopathy and you have no indication that the patient would be able to comprehend the information or diagnosis, then you can defer providing patient with this information (choice A). If the patient is alert and with capacity, discuss further with daughter to find out why she doesn't want the patient to know the diagnosis (choice A). The patient may come from a culture in which the family make decisions for a sick member, or the daughter herself may be fearful, anxious, or overwhelmed. Knowing this can help facilitate the discussion. Notwithstanding, invoking the principle of autonomy, patient should be told her diagnosis unless she has specifically stated she does not want to know. If the patient is awake, alert, and able to comprehend the diagnosis, then the discussion with the patient can take place (choice B).

5. A. Double effect

Morphine drip can be an ethical dilemma. It has a beneficence component that it will benefit the patient to relieve pain (choice B). It also has a nonmaleficence component because it will alleviate harm since pain is harmful emotionally and physiologically (choice C). The initiation of morphine drip in end-of-life care is more an example of double effect. Treatment is provided to meet the end desired, which is the cessation of pain. The intention to achieve this effect must outweigh an unintended bad effect, which might be to hasten death, although this is not always the case. Patients cannot exercise their right to self-governing if they are not coherent or are in intractable pain (choice D).

REFERENCES

1. Beauchamp TL, Childress JF. *Principles of Biomedical Ethics.* 5th ed. New York, NY: Oxford University Press; 2001.
2. Moemen ME. Prognostic categorization of intensive care septic patients. *World J Crit Care Med.* 2012;1(3):67-79.
3. Knaus WA, Draper EA, Wagner DP, Zimmerman JE. APACHE II: A severity of disease classification system. *Crit Care Med.* 1985;13(10):818-829.
4. Chang RW. Individual outcome prediction models for intensive care units. Lancet. 1989;2(8655):143-146.
5. Knaus WA, Wagner DP, Draper EA, et al. The APACHE III Prognostic System risk prediction of hospital mortality for critically ill hospitalized adults. *Chest.* 1991;100(6):1619-1636.
6. Zimmerman JE, Draper EA, Wagner DP. Comparing ICU populations: Background and current methods. In: Sibbald WJ, Bion JF, eds. *Evaluating Critical Care.* New York: Springer Verlag; 2001: 121-139.

7. Glance LG, Osler TM, Dick AW. Identifying quality outliers in a large, multiple-institution database by using customized versions of the Simplified Acute Physiology Score II and the Mortality Probability Model IIo. *Crit Care Med.* 2002;30(9):1995-2002.

8. Zimmerman JE, Kramer AA, McNair DS, Malila FM. Acute Physiology and Chronic Health Evaluation (APACHE) IV: Hospital mortality assessment for today's critically ill patients. *Crit Care Med.* 2006;34(5):1297-1310.

9. Le Gall JR, Lemeshow S, Saulnier F. A New Simplified Acute Physiology Score (SAPS II) based on a European/North American Multicenter Study. JAMA. 1993;270(24):2957-2963.

10. Metnitz PG, Moreno RP, Almeida E, et al. SAPS 3 – From evaluation of the patient to evaluation of the intensive care unit. Part 1: Objectives, methods, and cohort design. *Intensive Care Med.* 2005;31(10):1336-1344.

11. Moreno RP, Metnitz PG, Almeida E, et al. SAPS 3–From Evaluation of the patient to evaluation of the intensive care unit. Part 2: Development of a prognostic model for hospital mortality at ICU admission. *Intensive Care Med.* 2005;31(10):1345-1355.

12. Lemeshow S, Teres D, Klar J, Avrunin JS, Gehlbach SH, Rapoport J. Mortality Probability Models (MPM II) based on an international cohort of intensive care unit patients. *JAMA.* 1993;270(20):2478-2486.

13. Higgins TL, Teres D, Copes WS, Nathanson BH, Stark M, Kramer AA. Assessing contemporary intensive care unit outcome: An Updated Mortality probability Admission Model (MPM$_0$-III). *Crit Care Med.* 2007;35(3):827-835.

14. Vincent JL, Moreno R. Clinical Review: Scoring systems in the critically ill. *Crit Care.* 2010;14(2):207.

15. Vincent JL, Moreno R, Takala J, et al. The SOFA (Sepsis-related Organ Failure Assessment) score to describe organ dysfunction/failure. On behalf of the Working Group on Sepsis-Related Problems of the European Society of Intensive Care Medicine. *Intensive Care Med.* 1996;22(7):707-710.

16. Vincent JL, deMendonca A, Cantraine F, et al. Use of the SOFA Score to assess the incidence of organ dysfunction/failure in intensive care units: results of a multicenter, prospective study. Working group on "sepsis-related problems" of the European Society of Intensive Care Medicine. *Crit Care Med.* 1998;26(11):1793-1800.

17. Grissom CK, Brown SM, Kuttler KG, et al. A modified sequential organ failure assessmen score for critical care triage. *Disaster Med Public Health Prep.* 2010;4(4):277-284.

18. Wilson B, Tran D, Dupuis JY, McDonald B. Validation of a modified SOFA score as a mortality risk prediction model in cardiac surgical ICU. *Crit Care Med.* 2016;44(12):109.

19. Holder AL, Overton E, Lyu P, et al. Serial daily organ failure assessment beyond ICU Day 5 does not independently add precision to ICU risk of death prediction. *Crit Care Med.* 2017;45(12):2014-2022.

20. Marshall J, Cook DJ, Christou NV, Bernard GR, Sprung CL, Sibbald WJ. Multiple Organ Dysfunction Score: A reliable descriptor of a complex clinical outcome. *Crit Care Med.* 1995;23(10):1638-1652.

21. Naik AD, Martin LA, Moye J, Karel MJ. Health values and treatment goals of older, multimorbid adults facing life-threatening illness. *J Am Geriatr Soc.* 2016;64:625.

22. Weeks JC, Catalano PJ, Cronin A, et al. Patients' expectations about effects of chemotherapy for advanced cancer. *N Engl J Med.* 2012;367(17):1616-1625.

23. Kaldjian LC, Erekson ZD, Haberle TH, et al. Code status discussions and goals of care among hospitalized adults. *J Med Ethics.* 2009;35(6):338-334.

24. Detering KM, Hancock AD, Reade MC, Silvester W. The impact of advance care planning on end of life care in elderly patients: randomised controlled trial. *BMJ.* 2010;340:c1345.

25. Azoulay E, Soars M, Darmon M, et al. Intensive care of the cancer patient: recent achievements and remaining challenges. *Ann Intensive Care.* 2011;1(1):5.

26. Tanvetyanon T, Leighton JC. Life-sustaining treatments in patients who died of chronic congestive heart failure compared with metastatic cancer. *Crit Care Med.* 2003;31:60-64.

27. Benoit DD, Vandewoude KH, Decruyenaere JM, et al. Outcome and early prognostic indicators in patients with a hematologic malignancy admitted to the intensive care unit for a life-threatening complication. *Crit Care Med.* 2003;31:104-112.

28. Lecuyer L, Chevret S, Thiery G, et al. The ICU trial: a new admission policy for cancer patients requiring mechanical ventilation. *Crit Care Med.* 2007;35:808-814.

29. Soares M, Azoulay E. Critical care management of lung cancer patients to prolong life without prolonging dying. *Intensive Care Med.* 2009;35:2012-2014.

30. Azoulay E, Afessa B. The intensive care support of patients with malignancy: do everything that can be done. *Intensive Care Med.* 2006;32:3-5.

31. Smedira NG, Evans BH, Grais LS, et al. Withholding and withdrawal of life support from the critically ill. *N Engl J Med.* 1990;322:309-315.

32. Helft PR, Siegler M, Lantos J. The rise and fall of the futility movement. *N Engl J Med.* 2000;343:293-296.

33. Truog RD, Campbell ML, Curtis JR, et al. Recommendations for end-of-life care in the intensive care unit. American Academy of Critical Care Medicine. *Crit Care Med.* 2008;36(3):953.

34. Wilson WC, Smedira NG, Fink C, et al. Ordering and administration of sedatives and analgesics during the withholding and withdrawal of life support from critically ill patients. *JAMA.* 1992;267(7):949-953.

35. 2013 Annual Data Report: introduction. *Am J Transplant.* 2015;15(Suppl 2):8-10.

36. Emanuel EJ, Emanuel LL. Four models of the physician-patient relationship. *JAMA.* 1992;267(16):2221-2226.

37. Wijdicks E, Varelas PN, Gronseth GS, Greer D. Determining brain death in adults. *Neurology.* 20120;74:1911-1918.

38. Wijdicks EFM. Brain death guidelines explained. *Semin Neurol.* 2015;35:105-115.

39. Busl KM, Greer DM. Pitfalls in the diagnosis of brain death. *Neurocrit Care.* 2009;11:276-287.

40. Spinello IM. Brain death determination. *J Intensive Care Med.* 2015;30(6):326-337.

41. Kramer AH. Ancillary tests for brain death. *Semin Neurol.* 2015;35:125-138.

42. Wijdicks EFM, Varelas P, Gronseth GS, Greer DM. Evidence-based guideline update: determining brain death in adults. *Neurology.* 2010;74:1911-1918.

43. Frontera JA, Kalb T. How I manage the adult potential organ donor: donation after neurological death. Part 1. *Neurocrit Care.* 2010;12:103-110.

44. Novitzky D, Horak A, Cooper DK, Rose AG. Electrocardiographic and histopathologic changes developing during experimental brain death in the baboon. *Transplant Proc.* 1989;21(1 Pt 3):2567-2569.

45. Cooper DK, Novitzky D, Wicomb WN. The pathophysiological effects of brain death on potential donor organs, with particular reference to the heart. *Ann R Coll Surg Engl.* 1989;71(4):261-266.

46. Shivalkar B, Van Loon J, Wieland W, et al. Variable effects of explosive or gradual increase of intracranial pressure on myocardial structure and function. *Circulation.* 1993;87(1):230-239.

47. Novitzky D, Cooper DK, Rosendale JD, Kauffman HM. Hormonal therapy of the brain-dead organ donor: experimental and clinical studies. *Transplantation.* 2006;82(11):1396-1401.

48. Dunne K, Doherty P. Donation after circulatory death. *Contin Educ Anesthes Crit Care Pain.* 2011;11:82-86.

49. Reich DJ, Mulligan DC, Abt PL, et al. ASTS recommended practice guidelines for controlled donation after cardiac death organ procurement and transplantation. *Am J Transplant.* 2009;9:2004-2011.

50. Frontera JA. How I manage the adult potential organ donor: donation after cardiac arrest (part 2). *Neurocrit Care.* 2010;12:111-116.

51. Organ Donation after Circulatory Death. Report of a consensus meeting. Intensive Care Society, NHS Blood and Transplant, and British Transplantation Society, 2010. http://www.ics.ac.uk/intensive_care_professional/standards_and_guidelines/dcd.

Appendix

Normal Laboratory Values

Hemoglobin	13.3–17 g/dL	AST	15–41 μ/L
Hematocrit	40.3–50.3%	ALT	17–63 μ/L
White blood cells	4.3–10.6 × 10^3 μL	Lactic acid	0.5–2.2 mmol/L
Platelets	132–337 × 10^3 μ/L	Total CK	49–397 μL
Protime	9.8–12.8 seconds	CK-MB	0.6–6.3 ng/mL
APTT	25.1–36.5 seconds	Troponin I	< 0.03 ng/mL
International		TSH	0.450–5.330 μ/mL
normalized ratio	0.86–1.14	T3 uptake ratio	32–48.4%
Sodium	136–144 mEq/L	Free T4	0.61–1.12 g/dL
Chloride	101–111 mEq/L	Total T4	6.1–12.2 ug/dL
Potassium	3.5–5.1 mEq/L	Cortisol	10–20 ug/dL (morning)
Creatinine	0.55–1.02 mg/dL		3–10 ug/dL (4 pm)
Blood urea nitrogen	8–20 mg/dL		< 5 ug/dL (nighttime)
GFR	> 60.0 mL/min/1.732 m^2	Serum osmolality	275–295 mOsm/kg
Calcium	8.5–10.1 mg/dL	Urine osmolality	500–800 mOsm/kg
Phosphorus	2.5–4.9 mg/dL	Fibrinogen	200–393 mg/dL
Magnesium	1.8–2.5 mg/dL	Fibrin degradation	
Total bilirubin	0.3–1.2 mg/dL	products	< 5 ug/mL
Albumin	3.5–4.8 g/dL	LDH	84–246 μ/L
Total protein	6.4–8.3 g/dL	Ammonia	11–35 umol/L
Alkaline phosphate	45–117 μ/L		

Urinalysis

Color	clear, straw
Specific gravity	1.001–1.035
pH	5–8
Protein	negative
Glucose	negative
Ketone	negative
Bilirubin	negative
Blood	negative
Leukocytes	negative
Nitrite	negative
Urobilinogen	< 2 mg/dL

Index

Note: Page numbers followed by *f* indicate figures; those followed by *t* indicate tables.